Contents

Part IV Maternal-neonatal care

Part V Care of the child

Part VI Issues in nursing

Appendices

Contributors and consultants

Melody C. Antoon, RN, MSN
Lamar University
Beaumont, Tex.

Laura Aromando, MSN, ARNP
Department Chair, Nursing Programs
Seminole Community College
Sanford, Fla.

Adrianne E. Avillion, RN, DEd
President
AEA Consulting
York, Pa.

Peggy D. Baikie, RN, MS, CNNP, CPNP
Senior Instructor and Nurse Practitioner
University of Colorado School of Nursing
Denver

Pennie Sessler Branden, CNM, BSN, MS
Consultant
Maternal Instinct Corp.
Woodbridge, Conn.

Barbara S. Broome, RN, PhD, CNS
Chair Community/Mental Health
University of South Alabama
Mobile

Garry Brydges, RN, MSN, ACNP
Medical Consultant
Houston

Michelle Byrne, RN, PhD, CNOR
Instructor of Nursing and Independent Nurse Consultant
North Georgia College & State University
Dahlonega

Nan S. Carey, RN, MSN
Assistant Professor
Baptist College of Health Sciences
Memphis

Rebecca Sue Chamberlain, RN, MSN, CRNP
CV Surgery Advanced Practice Nurse
Children's National Medical Center
Washington, D.C.

Linda Carman Copel, RN, PhD, CS, DAPA
Associate Professor
Villanova (Pa.) University College of Nursing

Arlene Coughlin, RN, MSN
Nursing Faculty
Holy Name Hospital School of Nursing
Teaneck, N.J.

Sheryl L. Currie, RN, MN
Lead Instructor
Butler County Community College
El Dorado, Kans.

Louise Diehl-Oplinger, RN, MSN, APRN, BC, CCRN, CLNC
Staff Development Instructor
Warren Hospital
Philipsburg, N.J.

Jennifer Elizabeth DiMedio, RN, MSN, CRNP
Family Nurse Practitioner
University of Pennsylvania: West Chester Family Practice

Shelba Durston, RN, MSN, CCRN
Adjunct Faculty
San Joaquin Delta College
Stockton, Calif.

Emilie M. Fedorov, RN, MSN, CS
Clinical Nurse Manager – Department of Neurology
The Cleveland Clinic Foundation

Karla Jones, RN, MS
Nursing Faculty
Treasure Valley Community College
Ontario, Ore.

Gwendolyn L. Jordan, RN, MSN
Faculty
Carolinas College of Health Sciences
Charlotte, N.C.

Jacqueline M. Lamb, RN, PhD
Instructor
University of Pittsburgh School of Nursing

Jennifer McWha, RN, MSN
Nursing Instructor
Del Mar College
Corpus Christi, Tex.

Karin K. Roberts, RN, PhD
Associate Professor
Research College of Nursing
Kansas City, Mo.

Judith A. Robertson, RN, MN
Instructor
Seminole Community College
Sanford, Fla.

Debra Siela, RN, DNSc, CCNS, CCRN, CNS, CS, RRT
Assistant Professor of Nursing
Ball State University School of Nursing
Muncie, Ind.

Linda Wood, RN, MSN
Director of Practical Nursing
Massanutten Technical Center
Harrisonburg, Va.

Foreword

For more than 20 years, I've been helping students prepare for the NCLEX, and I've learned that the keys to success lie in thinking positively about the ability to pass (yes, I *can* do it! I *can* pass!) and in studying seriously. *NCLEX-RN Questions & Answers Made Incredibly Easy,* Second Edition, has been written and designed expressly to help you do both. This edition, which includes new chapters covering management and leadership topics as well as ethical and legal issues, provides more than 3,500 practice questions and answers with rationales plus six 75-question comprehensive tests that simulate the NCLEX experience. You'll also find helpful hints in many questions that lead you to the correct answer.

To get the most from this enormously helpful book, follow these strategies:

Start studying early and study often. About 6 weeks before your scheduled test, set aside daily review time. Begin by reading Part I, which deals with the NCLEX-RN. It discusses studying and test-taking strategies, describes the test format in detail, and gives helpful information on computer adaptive testing to help you fully prepare. Next, complete review questions in at least one chapter from parts II through V daily. Each part is subdivided into chapters covering specific disorders. For instance, Part IV (Maternal-neonatal care) is subdivided into four chapters: Antepartum, Intrapartum, Postpartum, and Neonatal care. Conclude your studies by taking one comprehensive test each day during the week preceding the NCLEX.

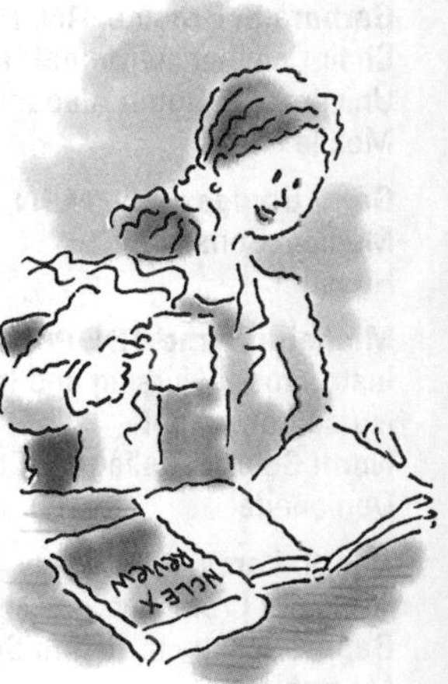

Follow a specific pattern for answering questions. After reading the question and before looking at the four answer options, form an answer in your mind. Then read the choices provided. At this point, key words or ideas should be easy to identify, and this approach also helps avoid information overload. As you take the practice tests, use the tear-off insert to cover the four options; cover the rationales as well.

Note the test-taking hints. The NCLEX is a test of nursing knowledge, so look for nursing actions and remember the steps of the nursing process: Assess before you intervene. Consider Maslow's hierarchy of needs, for example, a client can't learn if he's in pain or hypoxic. Think "client safety" when setting priorities, for example, position the client for effective breathing before checking the equipment. Select answers that use the principles of therapeutic communication, for example, open-ended questioning or reflective techniques.

When you finally sit down at the computer testing station, take a moment and imagine Joy once again offering words of encouragement and support. As you reach for the mouse, relax, feel confident that you've prepared well, and be positive about your ability to pass. You're the future of nursing — welcome!

Robyn M. Nelson DNSc, RN
Chair and Professor
California State University – Sacramento
Division of Nursing

Part I Surviving the NCLEX

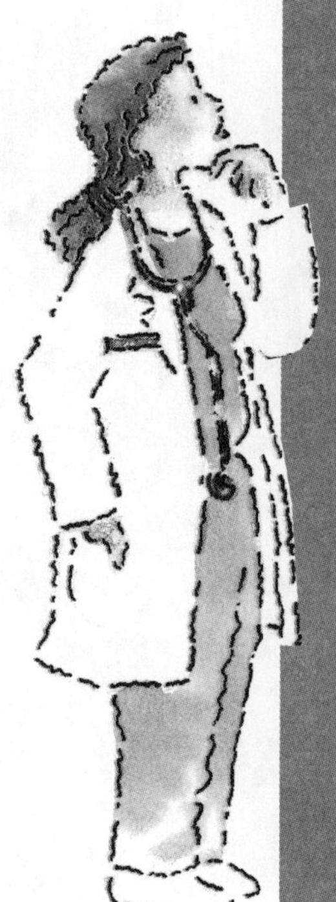

Understanding the NCLEX goals and structure is an important first step in proper preparation for the test. This chapter explains how best to prepare for this important examination.

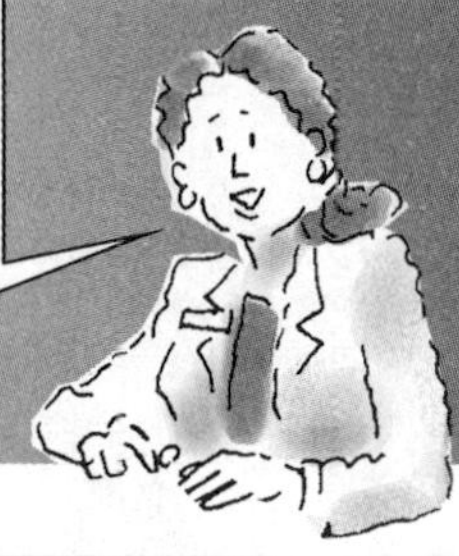

Chapter 1 Preparing for the NCLEX

Just the facts

In this chapter, you'll learn:

- about the NCLEX examination and why you must take it
- what you need to know about taking the NCLEX by computer
- strategies to use when answering NCLEX questions
- how to avoid common mistakes when taking an NCLEX examination.

All about the NCLEX

Passing the National Council Licensure Examination (NCLEX) is a vital step in your career as a nurse. The first step on your way to passing the NCLEX is to understand what the NCLEX is and how it's administered.

NCLEX structure

The NCLEX is a multiple-choice test written by nurses who, like most of your nursing instructors, have master's degrees and clinical expertise in particular areas. Only one small difference distinguishes nurses who write NCLEX questions: They're trained to write questions in a style particular to the NCLEX.

If you've completed an accredited nursing program, you've already taken numerous tests written by nurses with backgrounds and experiences similar to those of the nurses who write for the NCLEX. The test-taking experience you've gained will help you pass the NCLEX. So your NCLEX review should be *just* that — a review.

The point of it all

The NCLEX is designed for one purpose: To determine whether it's appropriate for you to receive a license to practice as a nurse. By passing the NCLEX, you demonstrate that you possess the minimum level of knowledge necessary to practice nursing safely.

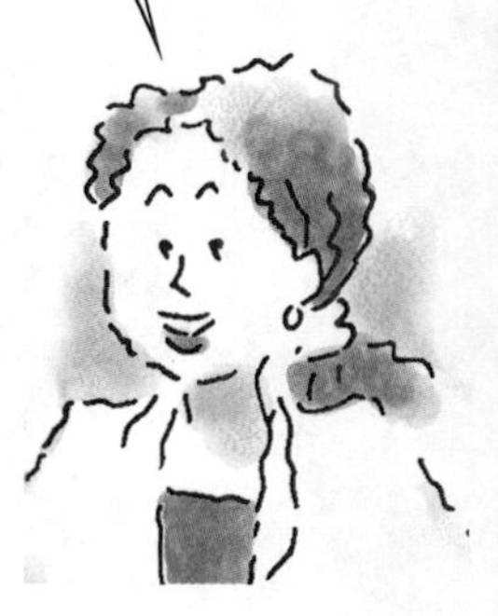

Believe me, you're more ready for the NCLEX than you probably know.

An integrated exam

In nursing school, you probably took courses organized by the medical model. Courses were separated into such subjects as medical-surgical, pediatrics, and psychiatric nursing. By contrast, the NCLEX is integrated, meaning that different subjects are mixed together.

As you answer NCLEX questions, you may encounter patients in any stage in life, from neonatal to geriatric. These patients — clients, in NCLEX lingo — may be of any background and may be completely well or extremely ill and have any of a variety of disorders.

What you need to know about client needs

The NCLEX draws questions from four categories of client needs that were developed by the National Council of State Boards of Nursing, the organization that sponsors and manages the NCLEX. Client needs categories ensure that a wide variety of topics appear on every NCLEX examination.

The National Council of State Boards of Nursing developed client needs categories after conducting a work-study analysis of new nurses. All aspects of nursing care observed in the study were broken down into categories. Categories were broken down further into subcategories. (See *Client needs categories.*)

The categories and subcategories are used to develop the NCLEX test plan, the content guidelines for the distribution of test questions. Question-writers and the people who put the NCLEX examination together use the test plan and client needs categories to make sure that a full spectrum of nursing activities are covered in the NCLEX. Client needs categories appear in most NCLEX review and question-and-answer books, including this one. The truth is, however, that as a test-taker you don't have to concern yourself with client needs categories. You'll see those categories for each question and answer in this book but they'll be invisible on the actual NCLEX.

Testing by computer

The NCLEX, like many standardized tests today, is administered by computer. That means you won't be filling in empty circles, sharpening pencils, or erasing frantically. It also means that you must become familiar with computer tests, if you're not already. Fortunately, the skills required to take the NCLEX on a comput-

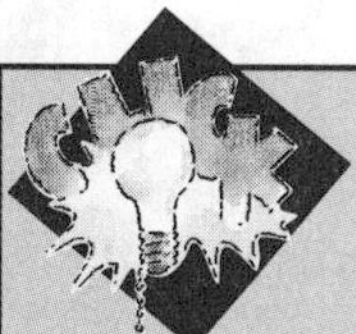

Now I get it!

Client needs categories

The NCLEX assigns each question a certain category based on client needs. This chart lists client needs categories and subcategories and the percentages of each type of question that appear on an NCLEX examination.

Category	Subcategories	Percentage of NCLEX questions
Safe, effective care environment	Management of care	7% to 13%
	Safety and infection control	5% to 11%
Health promotion and maintenance	Growth and development through the life span	7% to 13%
	Prevention and early detection of disease	5% to 11%
Psychosocial integrity	Coping and adaptation	5% to 11%
	Psychosocial adaptation	5% to 11%
Physiological integrity	Basic care and comfort	7% to 13%
	Pharmacological and parenteral therapies	5% to 11%
	Reduction of risk potential	12% to 18%
	Physiological adaptation	12% to 18%

er are simple enough to allow you to focus on the questions, not the keyboard.

Eek! A mouse

You'll use a mouse to select your answer to each question. A tutorial will tell you how to choose and register your answer. You'll have a chance to practice using the mouse on three sample questions before you begin the test. (See *A sample NCLEX question,* page 6.)

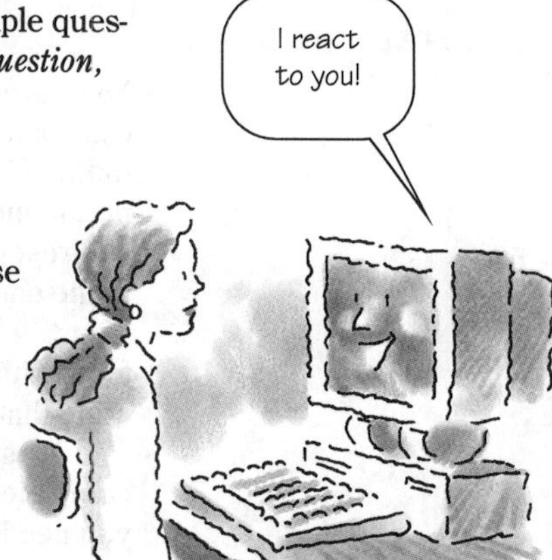

Onscreen calculations

During the test you may use an on-screen calculator to calculate medication dosages. You'll be shown how to use the calculator during the tutorial before the test begins.

There's no going back

When you take the NCLEX, the computer will show you only one question at a time on the screen. Take a reasonable amount of time to answer each question. Once your answer is recorded you can't go back to re-

A sample NCLEX question

NCLEX examinations, given on a computer, present a question and four options. Many questions present a clinical scenario. Here's an example of a typical NCLEX question.

42. After a stroke, a client develops aphasia. Which assessment finding *most* typifies aphasia?

1. Arm and leg weakness
2. Absence of gag reflex
3. Difficulty swallowing
4. Inability to speak clearly

(Correct answer: 4. Inability to speak clearly.)

view the question or change your answer. And, you can't skip a question — they must all be answered.

Computer-adaptive testing

The NCLEX is a computer-adaptive test, meaning that the computer reacts to the answers you give, supplying more difficult questions if you answer correctly and slightly easier questions if you answer incorrectly. Each test is thus uniquely adapted to the individual test taker.

The goal of computer-adaptive testing is to find the point at which each student answers 50% of the questions correctly. Imagine the questions all lined up, from easiest to most difficult. At some point you would be answering more questions incorrectly than correctly. This is where you reach your 50% mark or competency level. Once you've answered the minimum number of questions, the computer compares your competency level to the standard required for passing. If your level is above the passing standard, you pass the test.

A matter of time

You have a great deal of flexibility with the amount of time you can spend on individual questions. The examination lasts a maximum of 5 hours, however, so don't waste time. The 5-hour time period includes the mouse tutorial, three sample test questions, and rest periods. There's a mandatory 10-minute rest period at the end of 2 hours and an optional 10-minute rest period after 3½ hours. If you fail to answer a set number of questions within 5 hours, the computer may determine that you lack minimum competency.

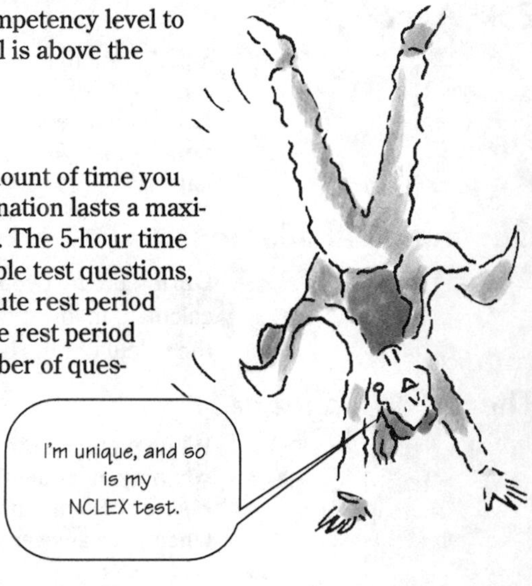

Most students have plenty of time to complete the test, so take as much time as you need to get the question right without wasting time. Keep moving at a decent pace to help you maintain concentration. A good rule-of-thumb is to answer one question per minute.

Difficult items = *Good news*

If you find as you progress through the test that the questions seem to be increasingly more difficult, it's a good sign. The more questions you answer correctly, the more difficult the questions become.

Some students, though, knowing that questions get progressively harder, focus on the degree of difficulty of subsequent questions to try to figure out if they're answering questions correctly. Avoid the temptation to do this. Stay focused on selecting the best answer for each question put before you.

Finished

The computer test finishes when one of the following events occurs:

- You demonstrate minimum competency, according to the computer program.
- You demonstrate a lack of minimum competency, according to the computer program.
- You've answered the maximum number of questions (265 total questions).
- You've used the maximum time allowed (5 hours).

Answering NCLEX questions

NCLEX questions are often fairly long. As a result, it's easy to become overloaded with information. (See *Anatomy of an NCLEX question,* page 8.) To focus on the question and avoid becoming overwhelmed, apply proven strategies for answering NCLEX questions, including:

- determining what the question asks
- determining relevant facts about the client
- rephrasing the question
- choosing the best option.

What is the question asking?

Read the question twice. If the answer isn't apparent, rephrase the question in simpler, more personal terms. Breaking down the question into easier, less intimidating terms may help you to focus more accurately on the correct answer.

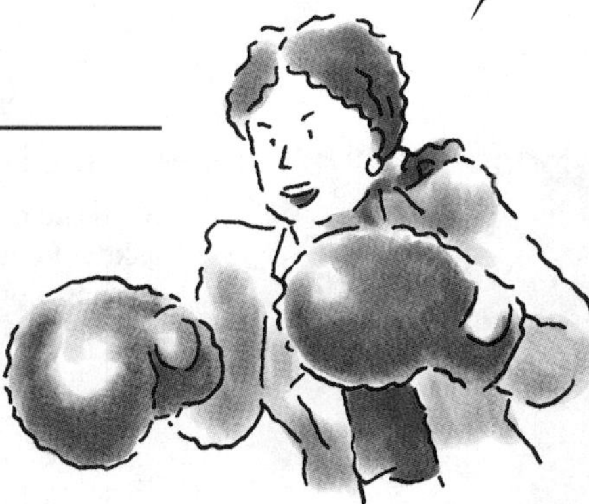

Can't figure out what the question is asking? Knock it down into smaller pieces.

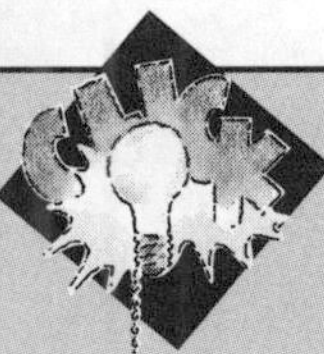

Now I get it!

Anatomy of an NCLEX question

When taking the NCLEX, you may note that the structure and tone of questions is repetitive. That is no accident. NCLEX questions are constructed according to strict standards. As shown below, each question has a stem and four options: a key (correct answer) and three distractors (incorrect answers). A brief case study may precede the question.

Case study

A 36-year-old client is admitted with a gunshot wound to the abdomen. After an exploratory laparotomy, the client is transferred to the surgical intensive care unit.

Stem	Options
Which assessment finding suggests that the client is now developing acute renal failure?	**1.** Urine output of 400 ml in 24 hours (key) **2.** Blood urea nitrogen level of 22 mg/dl (distractor) **3.** Serum creatinine level of 1.2 mg/dl (distractor) **4.** Temperature of 100.2° F (37.9° C) (distractor)

Sample question

For example, a question might be, "A 74-year-old client with a history of heart failure is admitted to the coronary care unit with pulmonary edema. He is intubated and placed on a mechanical ventilator. Which of the following parameters should the nurse monitor closely to assess the client's response to a bolus dose of furosemide (Lasix) I.V.?"

The options for this question — numbered from 1 to 4 — might include:

1. Daily weight
2. 24-hour intake and output
3. Serum sodium levels
4. Hourly urine output

Hocus, focus on the question

Read the question again, ignoring all details except what is being asked. Focus on the last line of the question. It asks you to select the appropriate assessment for monitoring a client who received a bolus of furosemide I.V.

What facts about the client are relevant?

Next, sort out the relevant client information. Start by asking whether any of the information provided about the client is *not* relevant? For instance, do you need to know that the client has been admitted to the coronary care unit? Probably not; his reaction to I.V. furosemide won't be affected by his location in the hospital.

Determine what you *do* know about the client. In the example, you know that:

- he just received an I.V. bolus of furosemide, a crucial fact
- he has pulmonary edema, the most fundamental aspect of the client's underlying condition
- he's intubated and placed on a mechanical ventilator, suggesting that his pulmonary edema is serious
- he's 74 years old and has a history of heart failure, a fact that may or may not be relevant.

Rephrase the question

After you've determined relevant information about the client and the question being asked, consider rephrasing the question to make it more clear. Eliminate jargon and put the question in simpler, more personal terms. Here's how you might rephrase the question in the example: "My client has pulmonary edema. He requires intubation and mechanical ventilation. He's 74 years old and has a history of heart failure. He received an I.V. bolus of furosemide. What assessment parameter should I monitor?"

Choose the best option

Armed with all the information you now have, it's time to select an option. You know that the client received an I.V. bolus of furosemide, a diuretic. You know that monitoring fluid intake and output is a key nursing intervention for a client taking a diuretic, a fact that eliminates options 1 and 3 (daily weight and serum sodium levels), narrowing the answer down to options 2 or 4 (24-hour intake and output or hourly urine output).

You also know that the drug was administered by I.V. bolus, suggesting a rapid effect. (In fact, furosemide administered by I.V. bolus takes effect almost immediately.) Monitoring the client's 24-hour intake and output would be appropriate for assessing the effects of repeated doses of furosemide. Hourly urine output, however, is most appropriate in this situation because it monitors the immediate effect of this rapid-acting drug.

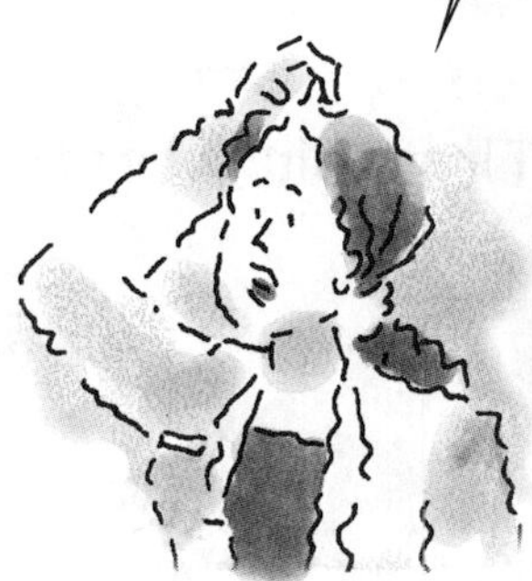
Hmmm, what happens when two options seem correct?

When more than one option seems correct

What if you encounter a question for which two or more options appear correct? You're most likely facing a common NCLEX question, one for which there may be two or more appropriate options. NCLEX questions commonly include phrases such as:
- most appropriate
- best
- first
- last
- next
- most helpful
- most suitable.

Such questions ask you to determine priority. Determining priority means deciding which answer is best, most appropriate, or should be implemented first.

Key strategies

Regardless of the type of question or the number of seemingly correct options, four key strategies will help you determine the correct answer for each question. (See *Strategies for success.*) These strategies are:
- considering the nursing process
- referring to Maslow's hierarchy of needs
- reviewing patient safety
- reflecting on principles of therapeutic communication.

Nursing process

One of the ways to determine which answer takes priority is to apply the nursing process. Steps in the nursing process include:
- assessment
- analysis
- planning
- implementation
- evaluation.

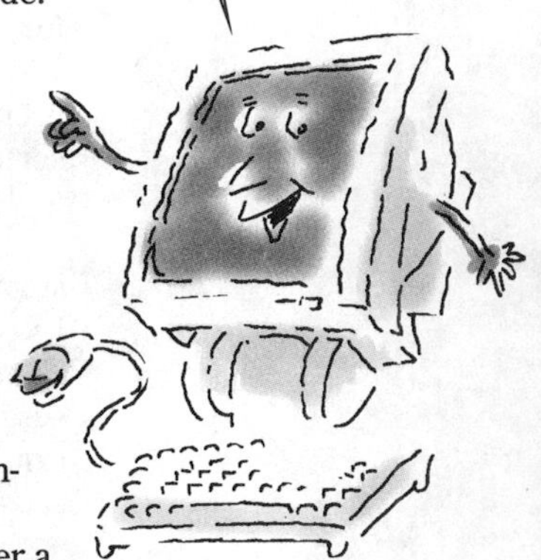

Put that ol' nursing process to work for you to answer my questions.

First things first

The nursing process may provide insights to help you analyze a question and eliminate incorrect options. According to the nursing process, assessment comes before analysis, which comes before planning, which comes before implementation, which comes before evaluation.

You're halfway to the correct answer when you encounter a question that asks you to assess the situation and then provides two assessment options and two implementation options. You

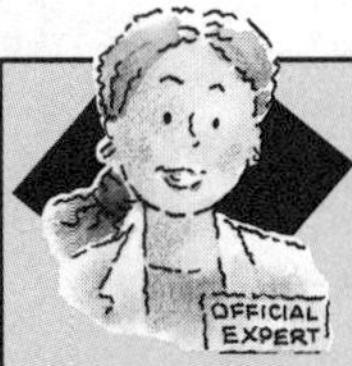

Advice from the experts

Strategies for success

Keeping a few main strategies in mind as you answer each NCLEX question can help ensure greater success. These four strategies are critical for answering NCLEX questions correctly:

- If the question asks what you should do in a situation, use the nursing process to determine which step in the process would be next.
- If the question asks what the client needs, use Maslow's hierarchy to determine which need to address first.
- If the question indicates that the client doesn't have an urgent physiologic need, focus on the client's safety.
- If the question involves communicating with a patient, use the principles of therapeutic communication.

can immediately eliminate the implementation options, which then gives you, at worst, a 50-50 chance of selecting the correct answer. Use the following sample question to apply the nursing process.

A client returns from an endoscopic procedure during which he was sedated. Before offering the client food, which of the following actions should the nurse take?

1. Assess the client's respiratory status.
2. Check the client's gag reflex.
3. Place the client in a side-lying position.
4. Have the client drink a few sips of water.

Assess before intervening

According to the nursing process, the nurse must assess a client before performing an intervention. Does the question indicate that the client has been properly assessed? No, it doesn't. Therefore, you can eliminate options 3 and 4 because they're both interventions.

That leaves options 1 and 2, both of which are assessments. Your nursing knowledge should tell you the correct answer — in this case, option 2. The sedation required for an endoscopic procedure may impair the client's gag reflex, so you would assess the gag reflex before giving food to the client to reduce the risk of aspiration and airway obstruction.

Final elimination

Why not select option 1, assessing the client's respiratory status? You might select this option but the question is specifically asking about offering the client food, an action that wouldn't be taken if the client's respiratory status was at all compromised. In this case, you're making a judgment based on the phrase, "Before offering the client food." If the question was trying to test your knowledge of respiratory depression following an endoscopic procedure, it probably wouldn't mention a function — such as giving food to a client — that so clearly occurs only after the client's respiratory status has been stabilized.

Maslow's hierarchy

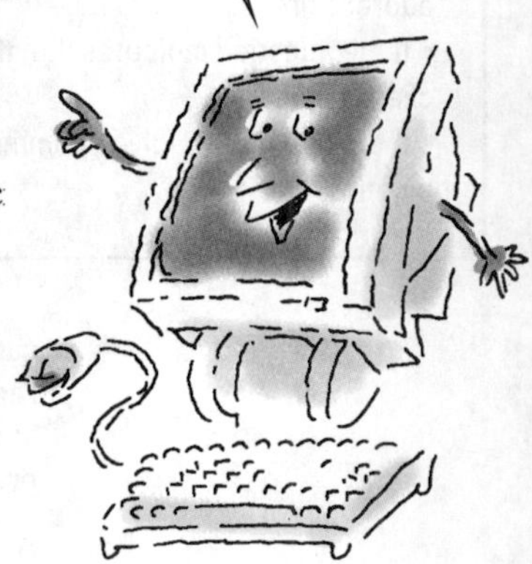

Maslow? Who is this Maslow? Oh, you mean *that* Maslow.

Knowledge of Maslow's hierarchy of needs can be a vital tool for establishing priorities on the NCLEX examination. Maslow's theory states that physiologic needs are the most basic human needs of all. Only after physiologic needs have been met can safety concerns be addressed. Only after safety concerns are met can concerns involving love and belonging be addressed, and so forth. (See *Maslow's hierarchy of needs.*) Apply the princ ples of Maslow's hierarchy of needs to the following sample question:

A client complains of severe pain 2 days after surgery. Which of the following actions should the nurse perform first?

1. Offer reassurance to the client that he will feel less pain tomorrow.
2. Allow the client time to verbalize his feelings.
3. Check the client's vital signs.
4. Administer an analgesic.

Phys before psyche

In this example, two of the options — 3 and 4 — address physiological needs. The other two answer choices — 1 and 2 — address psychosocial concerns. According to Maslow, physiological needs must be met before psychosocial needs, so you can eliminate options 1 and 2.

Final elimination

Now use your nursing knowledge to choose the best answer from the two remaining options. In this case, 3 is correct because the client's vital signs should be checked before administering an analgesic (assessment before intervention). When prioritizing according to Maslow's hierarchy, remember your ABCs — airway, breathing, circulation — to help you further prioritize. Check for a patent airway before addressing breathing. Check breathing before checking the health of the cardiovascular system.

One caveat...

Just because an option appears on an NCLEX examination doesn't mean it's a viable choice for the client referred to in the question. Always examine your choice in light of your knowledge and experience. Ask yourself, "Does this choice make sense for

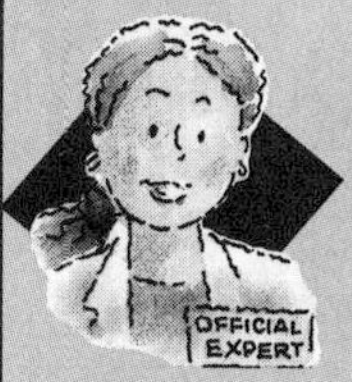

Advice from the experts

Maslow's hierarchy of needs

Maslow's hierarchy of needs is a vital tool for establishing priorities on the NCLEX examination. These illustrations show Maslow's hierarchy of needs and a definition for each stage in the hierarchy. The stages, from most basic to most complex, are physiologic needs, safety and security, love and belonging, self-esteem, and self-actualization.

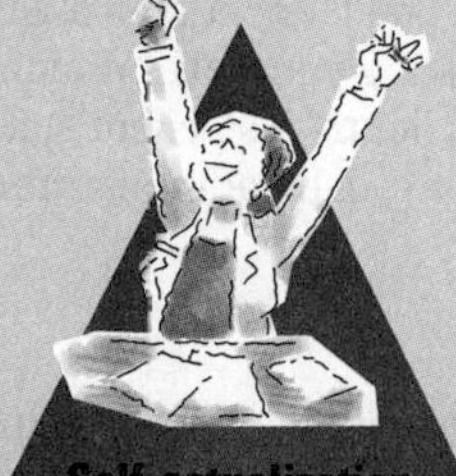

Self-actualization
Recognition and realization of one's potential growth, health, and autonomy

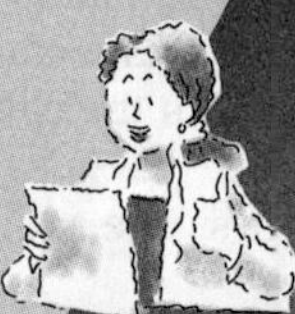

Self-esteem
Sense of self-worth, self-respect, independence, dignity, privacy, and self-reliance

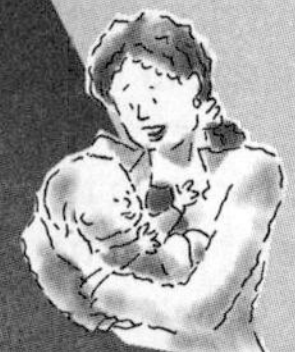

Love and belonging
Affiliation, affection, intimacy, support, and reassurance

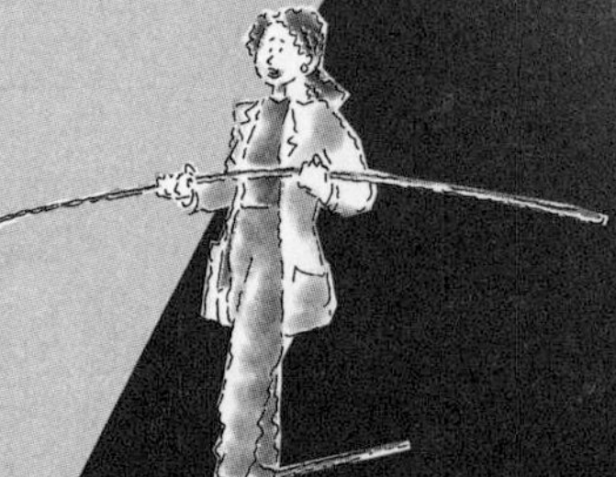

Safety and security
Safety from physiologic and psychological threat, protection, continuity, stability, and lack of danger

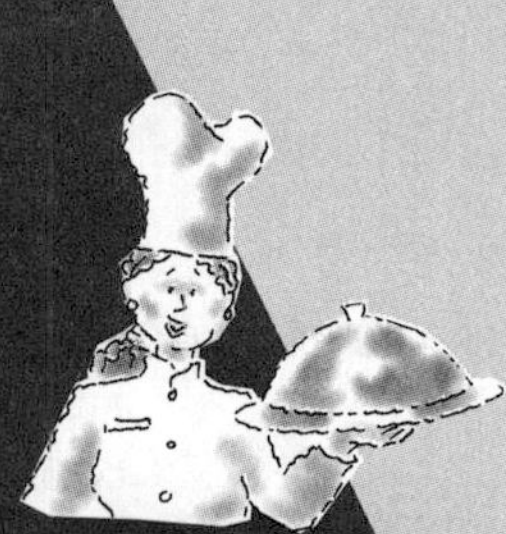

Physiologic needs
Oxygen, food, elimination, temperature control, sex, movement, rest, and comfort

this client?" Allow yourself to eliminate choices — even ones that might normally take priority — if they don't make sense for a particular client's situation.

Remember, client safety takes high priority on the NCLEX.

Client safety

As you might expect, client safety takes high priority on NCLEX examinations. You'll encounter many questions that can be answered by asking yourself, "Which answer will best ensure the safety of this client?" Use client safety criteria for situations involving lab values, drug administration, or nursing care procedures.

Client 1st, equipment 2nd

You may encounter a question in which some options address the client and others address the equipment. When in doubt, select an option relating to the client; never place equipment before a client.

For instance, suppose a question asks what the nurse should do first when entering a client's room where an infusion pump alarm is sounding. If two options deal with the infusion pump, one with the infusion tubing, and another with the client's catheter insertion site, select the one relating to the client's catheter insertion site. Always check the client first; the equipment can wait.

The best therapeutic communication responds to the client's feelings and provides accurate information.

Therapeutic communication

Some NCLEX questions focus on the nurse's ability to communicate effectively with the client. Therapeutic communication incorporates verbal or non-verbal responses and involves:

- listening to the client
- understanding the client's needs
- promoting clarification and insight about the client's condition.

Poor therapeutic communication

Like other NCLEX questions, questions dealing with therapeutic communication commonly require choosing the best response from among the four options. First, eliminate options that indicate the use of poor therapeutic communication techniques, such as those in which the nurse:

- tells the client what to do without regard to the client's feelings or desires (the "do this" response)

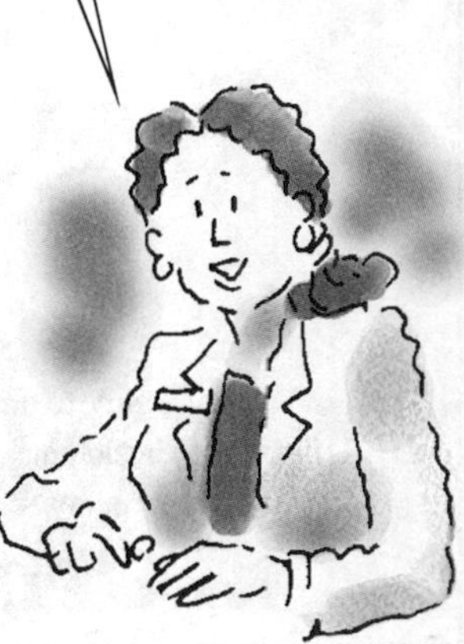

• asks a question that can be answered "yes" or "no" or with another one-syllable response
• seeks reasons for the client's behavior
• implies disapproval of the client's behavior
• offers false reassurances
• attempts to interpret the client's behavior rather than allowing the client to verbalize his own feelings
• offers a response that focuses on the nurse, not the client.

Good therapeutic communication

When answering NCLEX questions, look for responses that:
• allow the client time to think and reflect
• encourage the client to talk
• encourage the client to describe a particular experience
• reflect that the nurse has listened to the client such as through paraphrasing the client response.

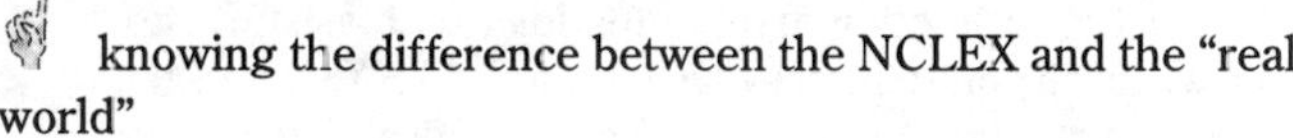

Avoiding pitfalls

Even the most knowledgeable students can get tripped up on certain NCLEX questions. (See *Handling further teaching questions,* page 16.) Students commonly cite three areas that can be difficult for unwary test takers:

 knowing the difference between the NCLEX and the "real world"

 delegating care

knowing laboratory values.

NCLEX versus the real world

Some students who take the NCLEX have extensive practical experience in health care. For example, many test takers have worked as licensed practical nurses or nurse's assistants. In one of those capacities, test takers might have been exposed to less than optimum clinical practice and may carry those experiences over to the NCLEX.

However, the NCLEX is a textbook examination — not a test of clinical skills. Take the NCLEX with the understanding that what happens in the real world may differ from what the NCLEX and your nursing school say *should* happen.

Remember, this is the real world. The NCLEX may not always reflect what happens in it.

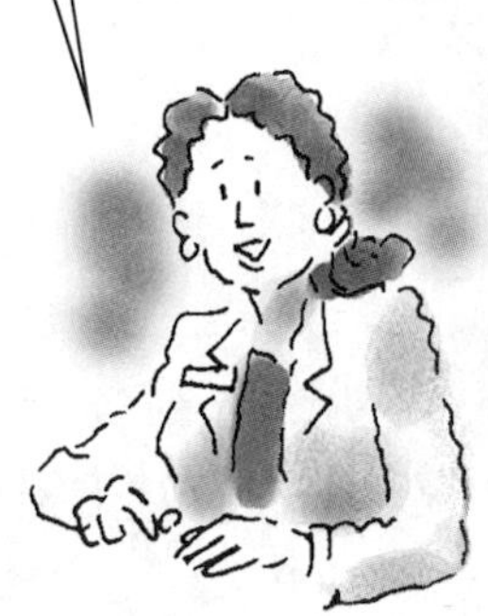

Don't take shortcuts

If you've had practical experience in health care, you may know a quicker way to perform a procedure or tricks to get by when you

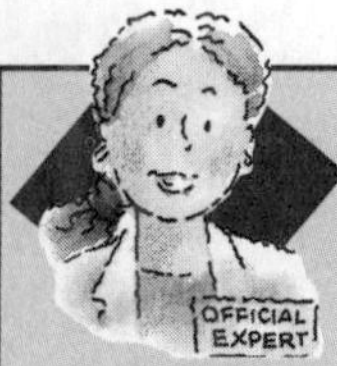

Advice from the experts

Handling further teaching questions

The NCLEX occasionally asks a particular kind of question called the "further teaching" question, which involves client-teaching situations. These questions can be tricky. You'll have to choose the response that suggests that the client has *not* learned the correct information. Here's an example:

37. Which statement by a client who takes nitroglycerin (Nitrostat) as needed for anginal pain indicates that further teaching is necessary?

1. "I store the tablets in a dark bottle."
2. "I take the tablet with a full glass of water."
3. "I check for my tongue to tingle when I take a tablet."
4. "I'll go to the hospital if three tablets, 5 minutes apart, don't relieve the pain."

The answer you should choose is 2 because it indicates the client has a poor understanding of how nitroglycerin should be taken and needs further teaching. *Remember:* If you see the phrase *further teaching* or *further instruction,* you're looking for a wrong answer by the client.

don't have the right equipment. Situations such as staff shortages may force you to improvise. On the NCLEX, such scenarios can lead to trouble. Always check your practical experiences against textbook nursing care, taking care to select the response that follows the textbook.

Delegating care

On the NCLEX, you may encounter questions that assess your ability to delegate care. Delegating care involves coordinating the efforts of other health care workers to provide effective care for your client. On the NCLEX, you may be asked to assign duties to:

- licensed practical nurses or licensed vocational nurses
- nursing assistants
- other support staff.

In addition, you'll be asked to decide when to notify a physician, social worker, or other hospital staff member. In each case, you'll have to decide when, where, and how to delegate.

Shoulds and shouldn'ts

As a general rule, it's OK to delegate actions that involve stable clients or standard, unchanging procedures. Bathing, feeding, dressing, and transferring clients are examples of procedures that can be delegated.

Be careful not to delegate complicated or complex activities. In addition, don't delegate activities that involve assessment, evaluation, or your own nursing judgment. On the NCLEX and in the real world, these duties fall squarely on your shoulders. Make sure that you take primary responsibility for assessing and evaluating the client and for making decisions about the client's care. Never hand off those responsibilities to someone with less training.

Calling in reinforcements

Deciding when to notify a physician, social worker, or other hospital staff comprises an important element of nursing care. On the NCLEX, however, choices that involve notifying the physician are usually incorrect. Remember that the NCLEX wants to see you, the nurse, at work.

If you're sure the correct answer is to notify the physician, however, make sure the client's safety has been addressed before notifying a physician or other staff member. On the NCLEX, the client's safety has a higher priority than notifying other health care providers.

Knowing lab values

Some NCLEX questions supply laboratory results without indicating normal levels. As a result, answering questions involving laboratory values requires you to have the normal range of the most common laboratory values memorized to make an informed decision.

Normal lab values

- Blood urea nitrogen 8 to 25 mg/dl
- Creatinine 0.6 to 1.5 mg/dl
- Sodium 135 to 145 mmol/L
- Potassium 3.5 to 5.5 mEq/L
- Chloride 97 to 110 mmol/L
- Glucose (fasting plasma) 65 to 115 mg/dl
- Hemoglobin
  - –Male: 13.8 to 17.2 g/dl
  - –Female: 12.1 to 15.1 g/dl
- Hematocrit
  - –Male: 40.7 to 50.3%
  - –Female: 36.1 to 44.3%

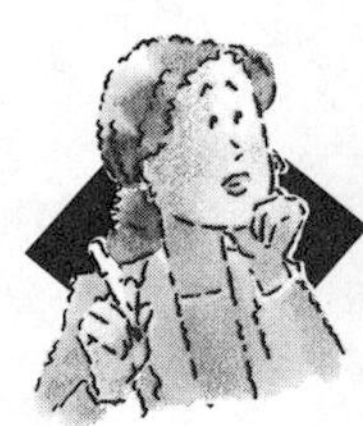

Quick quiz

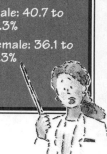

1. To register your answer for an NCLEX question, you'll:

A. press the ENTER key.

B. touch the appropriate answer on the screen.

C. click the mouse.

Answer: C. After deciding the option you want and double-checking to make sure that option is the one you want, click the mouse to register the answer.

2. Because the NCLEX is a computer-adaptive test, the computer provides questions according to:

A. the number of questions you answer correctly.

B. a random selection of questions in specific client needs categories.

C. a strict pattern established after studying the responses of new nurses.

Answer: A. The NCLEX is a computer-adaptive test, meaning that the computer reacts to the answers you give, supplying more difficult questions if you answer correctly and slightly easier questions if you answer incorrectly.

3. When delegating responsibilities, keep in mind that you should *not* delegate:

A. basic tasks to a nursing assistant.
B. tasks that require evaluation skills to a licensed practical nurse or licensed vocational nurse.
C. tasks that require advanced assessment to a physician.

Answer: B. Be careful not to delegate complicated or complex activities. In addition, don't delegate activities that involve assessment, evaluation, or your own nursing judgment. On the NCLEX and in the real world, these duties fall squarely on your shoulders.

Scoring

☆☆☆ If you answered all three questions correctly, wowsa, wowsa, *wowsa!* You're not only ready for the NCLEX, you could probably write questions for it!

☆☆ If you answered two questions correctly, super! You can delegate for us *anytime!*

☆ If you answered fewer than two questions correctly, shake it easy, kiddo! By the time you finish working with this book, you'll be so ready for the NCLEX that you won't be able to *stand* it. *That's* how ready you'll be. Promise.

As you count down the weeks, days, and finally hours to the NCLEX, refer back to the information in this chapter. It's a recipe for NCLEX success!

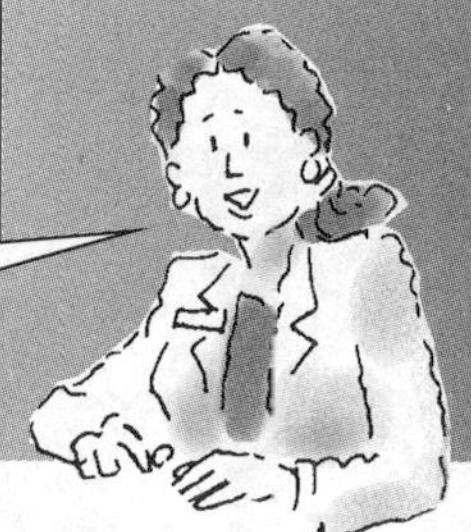

Chapter 2 Passing the NCLEX

Just the facts

In this chapter, you'll learn:

- how to properly prepare for the NCLEX
- how to concentrate during difficult study times
- ways to make more effective use of your time
- why creative studying strategies can enhance learning
- how to get the most out of NCLEX practice tests.

Study preparations

Most students pass the NCLEX on the first try. I know you can pass it too!

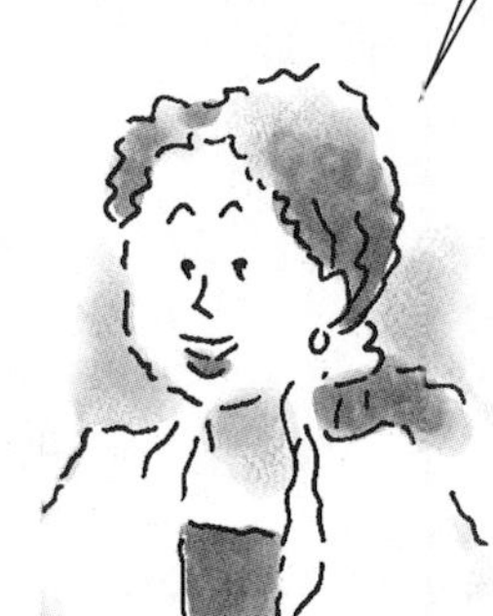

If you're like most people preparing to take the test, you're probably feeling nervous, anxious, or concerned. Keep in mind that most test-takers pass the NCLEX the first time around.

Passing the test won't happen by accident, though; you'll need to prepare carefully and efficiently. To help jump-start your preparations:

- determine your strengths and weaknesses
- create a study schedule
- set realistic goals
- find an effective study space
- think positively
- start studying sooner rather than later.

Strengths and weaknesses

Most students recognize that, even at the end of their nursing studies, they know more about some topics than others. Because the NCLEX covers a broad range of material, you should make some decisions about how intensively you'll review each topic.

Make a list

Base those decisions on a list. Divide a sheet of paper in half vertically. On one side, list topics you think you know well. On the other side, list topics you feel less secure about. Pay no attention if one side is longer than the other. When you're done studying, you'll feel strong in every area.

Where the list comes from

To make sure your list reflects a comprehensive view of all the areas you studied in school, look at the contents page in the front of this book. For each topic listed, place it in the "know well" column or "needs review" column. Separating content areas this way shows immediately which topics need less study time and which need more time.

Because I'm strong in certain areas, I'll spend less time studying them.

Scheduling study time

Study when you're most alert. Most people can identify a period of the day when they feel most alert. If you feel most alert and energized in the morning, for example, set aside sections of time in the morning for topics that need a lot of review. Then you can use the evening, a time of lesser alertness, for topics that need some refreshing. The opposite is true as well; if you're more alert in the evening, study difficult topics at that time.

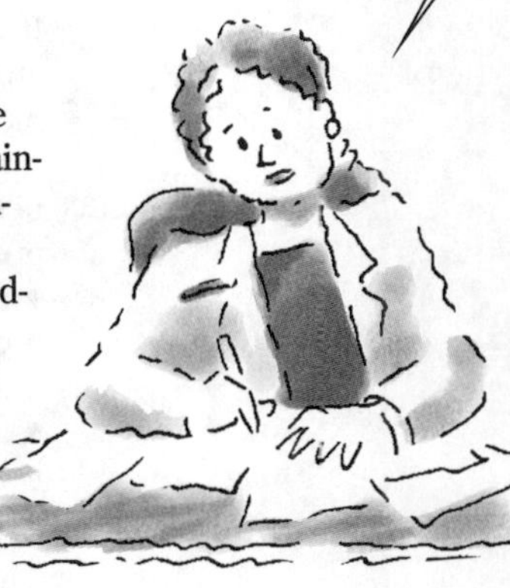

Because I'm most alert in the morning, that is when I'll cover difficult topics.

What you'll do, when

Set up a basic schedule for studying. Using a calendar or organizer, determine how much time remains before you'll take the NCLEX. (See *2 to 3 months before the NCLEX.*) Fill in the remaining days with specific times and topics to be studied. For example, you might schedule the respiratory system on a Tuesday morning and the GI system that afternoon. Remember to schedule difficult topics during your most alert times.

Keep in mind that you shouldn't fill each day with studying. Be realistic and set aside time for normal activities. Try to create ample study time before the NCLEX and then stick to the schedule.

Set goals you can meet

Part of creating a schedule means setting goals you can accomplish. You no doubt studied a great deal in nursing school, and by now you have a sense of your own capabilities. Ask yourself, "How much can I cover in a day?" Set that amount of time aside and then stay on task. You'll feel better about yourself — and your chances of passing the NCLEX — when you meet your goals regularly.

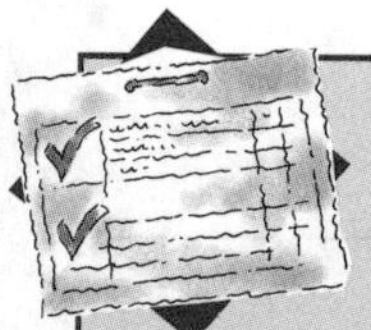

To-do list

2 to 3 months before the NCLEX

With 2 to 3 months remaining before you plan to take the examination, take these steps:

- Establish a study schedule. Set aside ample time to study but also leave time for social activities, exercise, family or personal responsibilities, and other matters.
- Become knowledgeable about the NCLEX-RN examination, its content, the types of questions it asks, and the testing format.
- Begin studying your notes, texts, other study materials.
- Take some NCLEX practice questions to help you diagnose strengths and weaknesses as well as to become familiar with NCLEX-style questions.

Study space

Find a space conducive to effective learning and then study there. Whatever you do, don't study with a television on in the room. Instead, find a quiet, inviting study space that:

- is located in a quiet, convenient place, away from normal traffic patterns
- contains a solid chair that encourages good posture (Avoid studying in bed; you'll be more likely to fall asleep and not accomplish your goals.)
- uses comfortable, soft lighting with which you can see clearly without eye strain
- has a temperature between 65° and 70° F
- contains flowers or green plants, familiar photos or paintings, and easy access to soft, instrumental background music.

Accentuate the positive

Consider taping positive messages around your study space. Make signs with words of encouragement, such as, "You can do it!" "Keep studying!" and "Remember the goal!" These upbeat messages can help keep you going when your attention begins to waver.

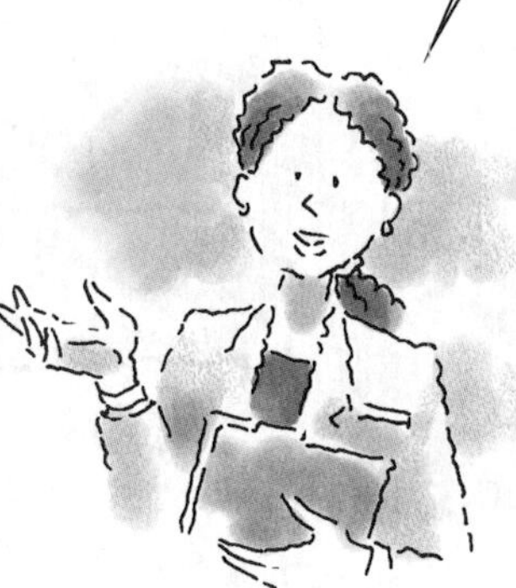

I know how much I can study in one day, so I've made up my schedule taking that into account.

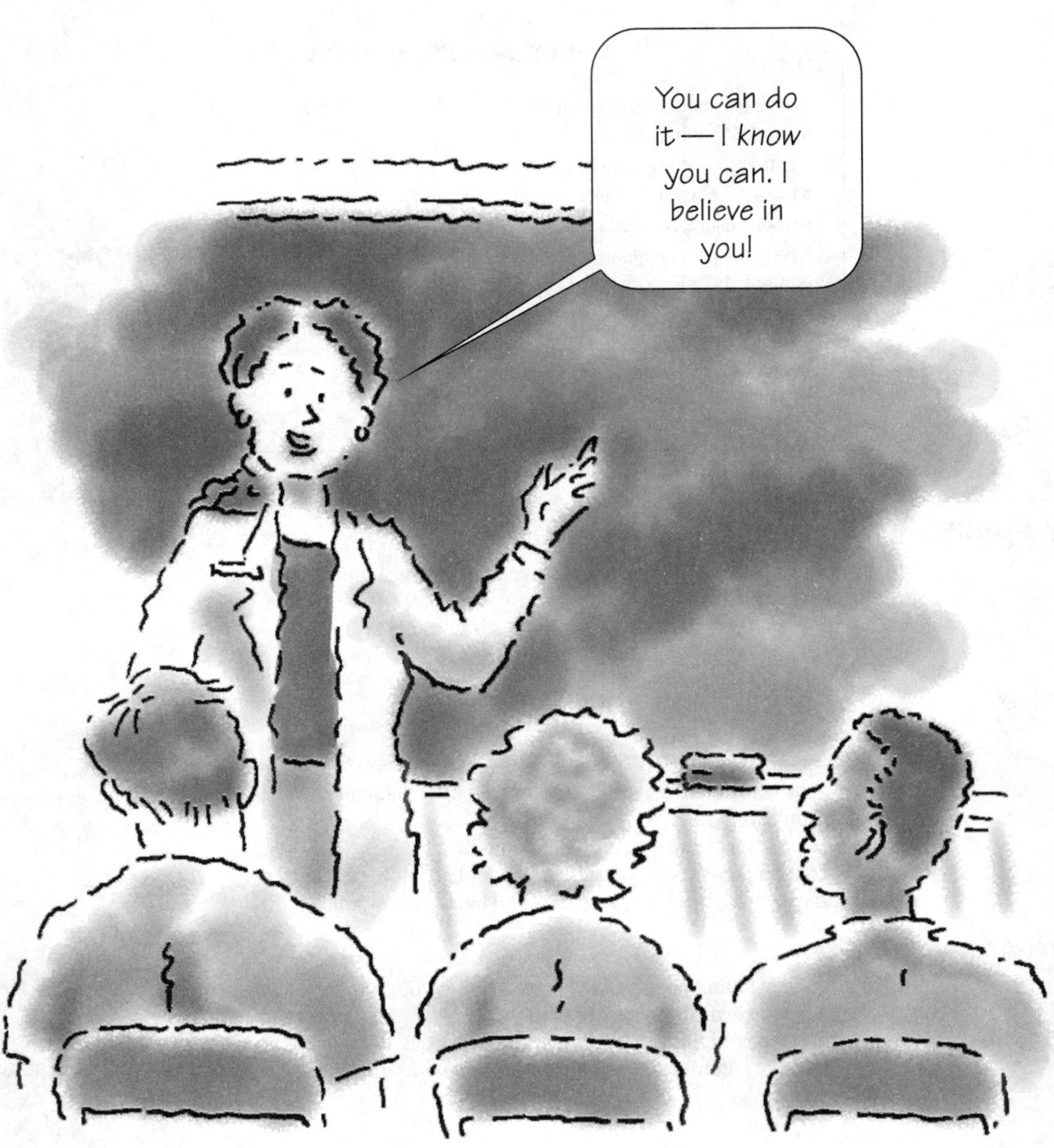
You can do it — I *know* you can. I believe in you!

Feel free to hang this upbeat message in your study area.

Maintaining concentration

When you're faced with reviewing the amount of information covered by the NCLEX, it's easy to become distracted and lose your concentration. When you lose concentration, you make less effective use of valuable study time. To help stay focused, keep these tips in mind:

- Alternate the order of the subjects you study during the day to add variety to your study. Try alternating between topics you find most interesting and those you find least interesting.
- Approach your studying with enthusiasm, sincerity, and determination.
- Once you've decided to study, begin immediately. Don't let anything interfere with your thought processes once you've begun.
- Concentrate on accomplishing one task at a time, to the exclusion of everything else.
- Don't try to do two things at once, such as studying and watching television or conversing with friends.
- Work continuously without interruption for a while, but don't study for such a long period that the whole experience becomes grueling or boring.
- Allow time for periodic breaks to give yourself a change of pace. Use these breaks to ease your transition into studying a new topic.
- When studying in the evening, wind down from your studies slowly. Don't progress directly from studying to sleeping.

Taking care of yourself

Never neglect your physical and mental well-being in favor of longer study hours. Maintaining physical and mental health are critical for success in taking the NCLEX. (See *4 to 6 weeks before the NCLEX,* page 24.)

A few simple rules

You can increase your likelihood of passing the test by following these simple health rules:

- Get plenty of rest. You can't think deeply or concentrate for long periods when you're tired.
- Eat nutritious meals. Maintaining your energy level is impossible when you're undernourished.
- Exercise regularly. Regular exercise helps you work harder and think more clearly. As a result, you'll study more efficiently and increase the likelihood of success on the all-important NCLEX.

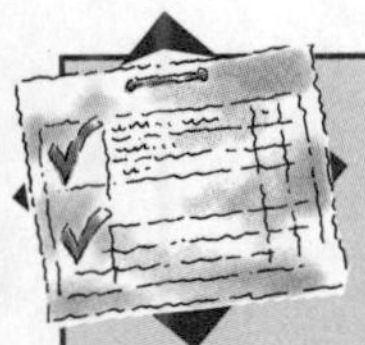

To-do list

4 to 6 weeks before the NCLEX

With 4 to 6 weeks remaining before you plan to take the examination, take these steps:

- Focus on your areas of weakness. That way, you'll have time to review these areas again before the test date.
- Find a study partner or form a study group.
- Take a practice test to gauge your skill level early.
- Take time to eat, sleep, exercise, and socialize to avoid burnout.

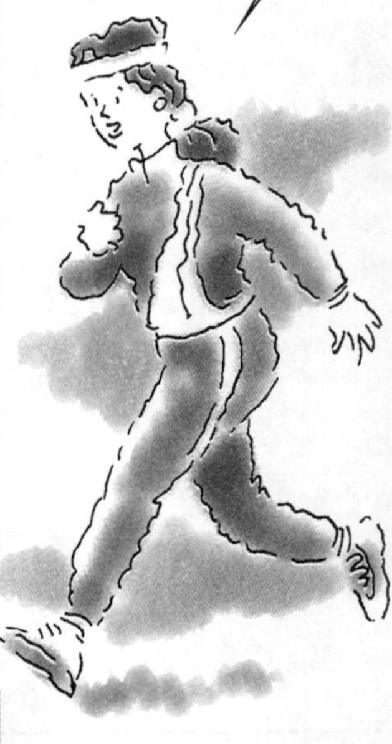

A short jog now wi l help me to concentrate later.

Memory powers, activate!

If you're having trouble concentrating but would rather push through than take a break, try making your studying more active by reading out loud. Active studying can renew your powers of concentration. By reading review material out loud to yourself, you're engaging your ears as well as your eyes — and making your studying a more active process. Hearing the material out loud also fosters memory and subsequent recall.

You can also rewrite in your own words a few of the more difficult concepts you're reviewing. Explaining these concepts in writing forces you to think through the material and can jump-start your memory.

Study schedule

When you were creating your schedule, you might have asked yourself, "How long should I study? One hour at a stretch? Two hours? Three?" To make the best use of your study time, you'll need to answer those questions.

Optimum study time

Experts are divided about the optimum length of study time. Some say you should study no more than an hour at a time several times a day. Their reasoning: You remember the material you study at the beginning and end of a session best and tend to remember less material studied in the middle of the session.

Other experts say you should hold longer study sessions because you lose time in the beginning, when you're just getting warmed up, and again at the end, when you're cooling down.

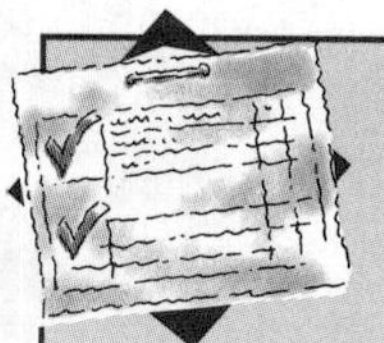

To-do list

1 week before the NCLEX

With 1 week remaining before the NCLEX examination, take these steps:
- Take a review test to measure your progress.
- Record key ideas and principles on note cards or audiotapes.
- Rest, eat well, and avoid thinking about the examination during nonstudy times.
- Treat yourself to one special event. You've been working hard, and you deserve it!

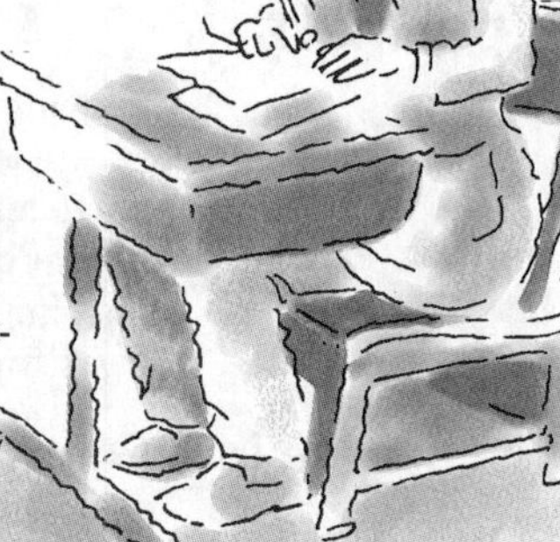

I've found that hour-and-a-half sessions work best for me.

Therefore, say those experts, a long, concentrated study period will allow you to cover more material.

To thine own self be true

So what's the answer? It doesn't matter as long as you determine what's best for *you*. At the beginning of your NCLEX study schedule, try study periods of varying lengths. Pay close attention to those that seem more successful.

Remember that you're a trained nurse who is competent at assessment. Think of yourself as a patient, and assess your own progress. Then implement the strategy that works best for you.

Finding time to study

So does that mean that short sections of time are useless? Not at all. We all have spaces in our day that might otherwise be dead time. (See *1 week before the NCLEX.*) These are perfect times to review for the NCLEX but not to cover new material because by the time you get deep into new material, your time will be over. Always keep some flashcards or a small notebook handy for situations when you have a few extra minutes.

You'll be amazed how many short sessions you can find in a day and how much reviewing you can do in five minutes. The following places offer short stretches of time you can use:
- eating breakfast
- waiting for, or riding on, a train or bus
- waiting in line at the bank, post office, bookstore, or other places.

Creative studying

Even when you study in a perfect study space and concentrate better than ever, studying for the NCLEX can get a little, well, dull. Even people with terrific study habits occasionally feel bored or sluggish. That is why it's important to have some creative tricks in your study bag to liven up your studying during those down times.

Creative studying doesn't have to be hard work. It involves making efforts to alter your study habits a bit. Some techniques that might help include studying with a partner or group and creating flash cards or other audiovisual study tools.

Study partners

Studying with a partner or group of students can be an excellent way to energize your studying. Working with a partner allows you to test each other on the material you've reviewed. Your partner can give you encouragement and motivation. Perhaps most important, working with a partner can provide a welcome break from solitary studying.

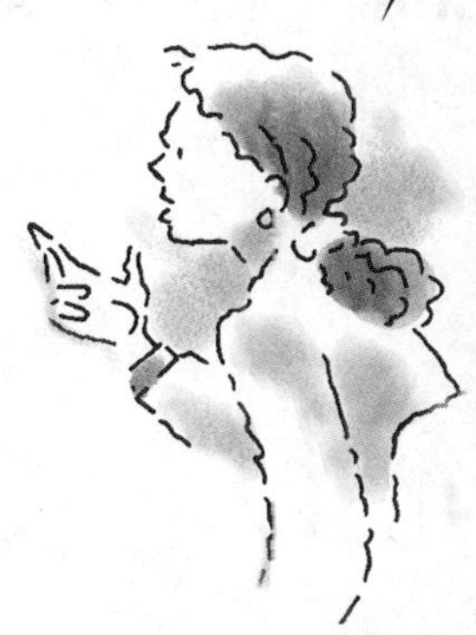

Find a partner with similar goals and strengths. But remember to stay focused!

I'll take the one in the red hat

Exercise some care when choosing a study partner or assembling a study group. A partner who doesn't fit your needs won't help you make the most of your study time. Look for a partner who:

- possesses similar goals to yours. For example, someone taking the NCLEX at approximately the same date who feels the same sense of urgency as you do might make an excellent partner.
- possesses about the same level of knowledge as you. Tutoring someone can sometimes help you learn, but partnering should be give-and-take so both partners can gain knowledge.
- can study without excess chatting or interruptions. Socializing is an important part of creative study, but remember, you've still got to pass the NCLEX — so stay serious!

Audiovisual tools

Flash cards and other audiovisual tools foster retention and make learning and reviewing fun.

Flash Gordon? No, it's Flash Card!

Flash cards can provide you with an excellent study tool. The process of writing material on a flash card will help you remember it. In addition, flash cards are small and easily portable, per-

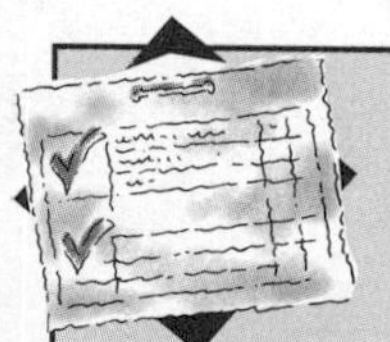

To-do list

The day before the NCLEX

With one day before the NCLEX examination, take these steps:

- Drive to the test site, review traffic patterns, and find out where to park. If your route to the test site occurs during heavy traffic or if you're expecting bad weather, set aside extra time to ensure prompt arrival.
- Do something relaxing during the day.
- Avoid concentrating on the test.
- Rest, eat well, and avoid dwelling on the NCLEX during nonstudy periods.
- Call a supportive friend or relative for some last-minute words of encouragement.

fect for those 5-minute slivers of time that show up during the day.

Creating a flash card should be fun. Use magic markers, highlighters, and other colorful tools to make them visually stimulating. The more effort you put into creating your flash cards, the better you'll remember the material contained on the cards.

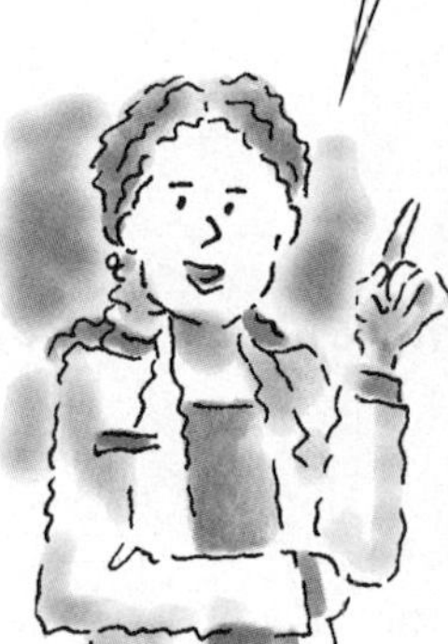

Charts, drawings, and diagrams help me learn more efficiently.

Other visual tools

Flowcharts, drawings, diagrams, and other image-oriented study aids can also help you learn material more effectively. Substituting images for text can be a great way to give your eyes a break and recharge your brain. Remember to use vivid colors to make your creations visually engaging.

Hear's the thing

If you learn more effectively when you hear information rather than see it, consider recording key ideas using a handheld tape recorder. Recording information helps promote memory because you say the information aloud when taping and then listen to it when playing it back. Like flash cards, tapes are portable and perfect for those short study periods during the day. (See *The day before the NCLEX.*)

Practice tests

Practice questions should comprise an important part of your NCLEX study strategy. Practice questions can improve your studying by helping you review material and familiarizing yourself with the exact style of questions you'll encounter on the NCLEX.

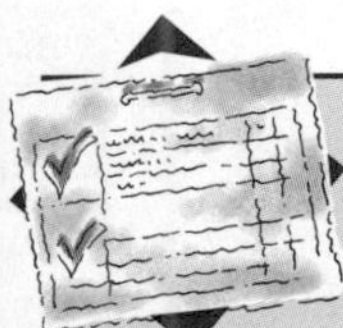

To-do list

The day of the NCLEX

On the day of the NCLEX examination, take these steps:

- Get up early.
- Wear comfortable clothes, preferably with layers you can adjust to fit the room temperature.
- Leave your house early.
- Arrive at the test site early.
- Avoid looking at your notes as you wait for your test computer.
- Listen carefully to the instructions given before entering the test room.
- Succeed, succeed, *succeed!*

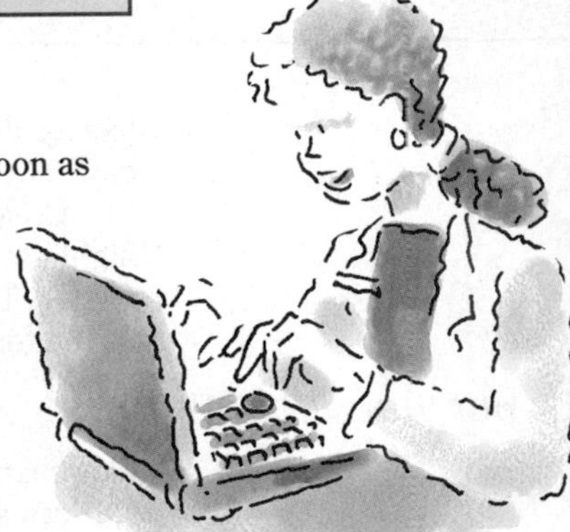

Because I've taken lots of practice tests, I understand how the questions work.

Practice at the beginning

Consider working through some practice questions as soon as you begin studying for the NCLEX. For example, you might try a half-dozen questions from each chapter in this book.

If you score well, you probably know the material contained in that chapter fairly well and can spend less time reviewing that particular topic. If you have trouble with the questions, spend extra study time on that topic.

I'm getting there

Practice questions can also provide an excellent means of marking your progress. Don't worry if you have trouble answering the first few practice questions you take; you'll need time to adjust to the way the questions are asked. Eventually you'll become accustomed to the question format and begin to focus more on the questions themselves.

If you make practice questions a regular part of your study regimen, you'll be able to notice areas in which you're improving. You can then adjust your study time accordingly.

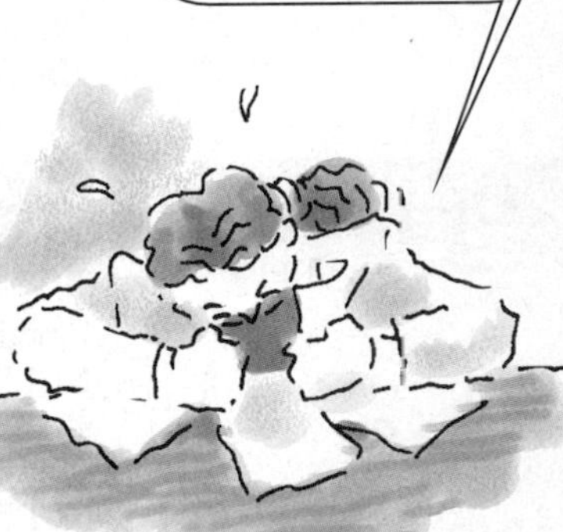

The test is getting awfully close. I'm not nervous. Do I look nervous? I'm NOT!

Practice makes perfect

As you near the examination date, continue to answer practice questions, but also set aside time to take an entire NCLEX practice test. (We've included six at the back of this book.) That way, you'll know exactly what to expect. (See *The day of the NCLEX.*) The more you know ahead of time, the better you're likely to do on the NCLEX.

Taking an entire practice test is also a way to gauge your progress. When you find yourself answering questions correctly, it will give you the confidence you need to conquer the NCLEX for real.

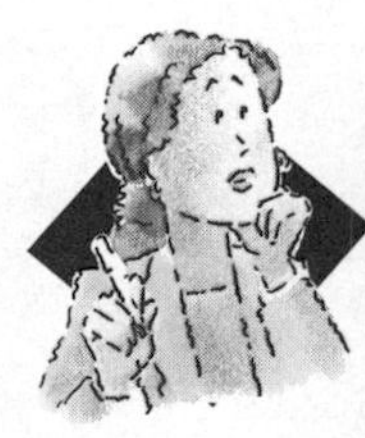

Quick quiz

1. The best time to study is:
- A. in the morning.
- B. early in the evening.
- C. when you feel most alert.

Answer: C. Study when you're most alert. If you feel most alert and energized in the morning, for example, set aside sections of time in the morning for topics that need a lot of review.

2. The temperature of the ideal study area should be between:
- A. 60° and 65° F.
- B. 65° and 70° F.
- C. 70° and 75° F.

Answer: B. The ideal study area has a temperature between 65° and 70° F.

3. To help you maintain concentration during long study periods, recommended study strategies include:
- A. Study the topics you find most interesting first, followed by the topics you find least interesting.
- B. Study the topics you find least interesting first, followed by the topics you find most interesting.
- C. Alternate the order of the subjects you study during the day.

Answer: C. Alternating the order of the subjects you study during the day adds variety to your study and helps you remain focused and make the most of your study time.

4. When selecting a study partner, choose one who:
- A. possesses similar goals as you.
- B. is highly social and will keep you entertained.
- C. isn't as knowledgeable as you so you can tutor him.

Answer: A. A partner who doesn't fit your needs won't help you make the most of your study time. Look for a partner who possesses similar goals to yours, possesses about the same level of knowledge as you, and won't spend too much time socializing.

Scoring

☆☆☆ If you answered all four questions correctly, that's *it!* We're calling the NCLEX testing center right now. You're *ready!*

☆☆ If you answered three questions correctly, outstanding! All you need now is a snack before the test, and you'll be rarin' to go!

☆ If you answered fewer than three questions correctly, fear not. You've got *NCLEX success* written all over your future!

Part II Care of the adult

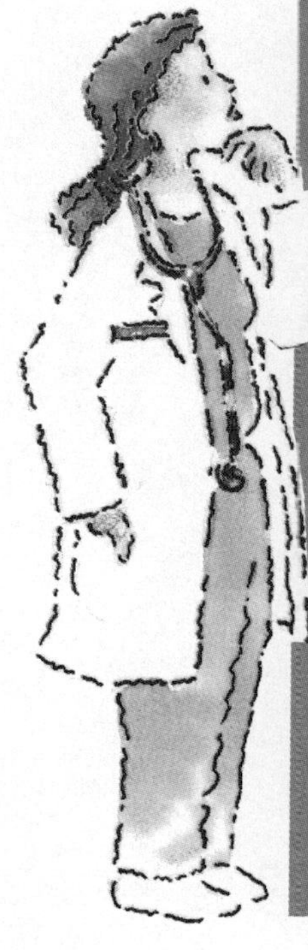

Chapter 3 Cardiovascular disorders

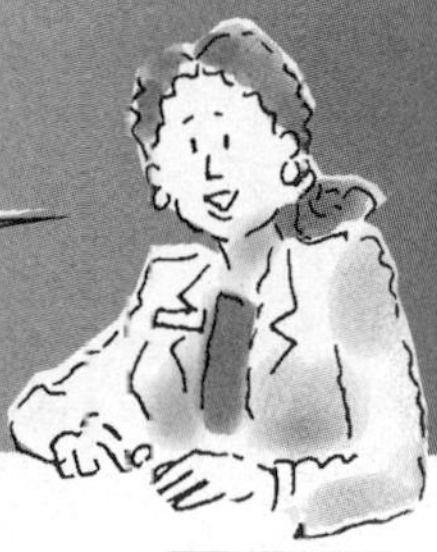

If you'd like to rummage through a Web site dedicated to cardiovascular disorders, check out the American Heart Association's **www.americanheart.org/.** Go for it!

1. Which of the following arteries primarily feeds the anterior wall of the heart?

1. Circumflex artery
2. Internal mammary artery
3. Left anterior descending artery
4. Right coronary artery

2. When do coronary arteries primarily receive blood flow?

1. During inspiration
2. During diastole
3. During expiration
4. During systole

3. Which of the following illnesses is the leading cause of death in the United States?

1. Cancer
2. Coronary artery disease
3. Liver failure
4. Renal failure

4. Which of the following conditions most commonly results in coronary artery disease (CAD)?

1. Atherosclerosis
2. Diabetes mellitus
3. Myocardial infarction
4. Renal failure

5. Atherosclerosis impedes coronary blood flow by which of the following mechanisms?

1. Plaques obstruct the vein
2. Plaques obstruct the artery
3. Blood clots form outside the vessel wall
4. Hardened vessels dilate to allow blood to flow through

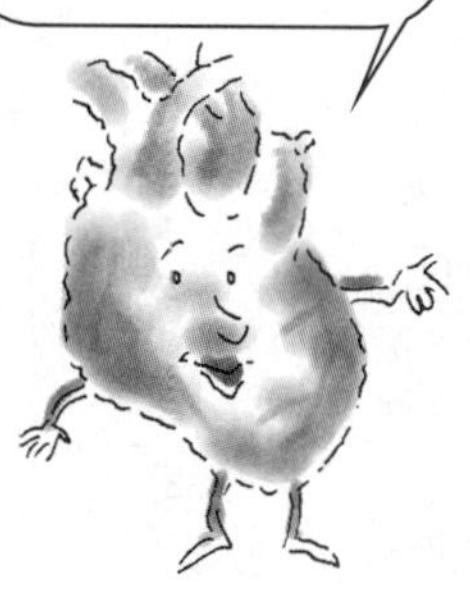

Different arteries supply my different sections with the blood I need to stay healthy.

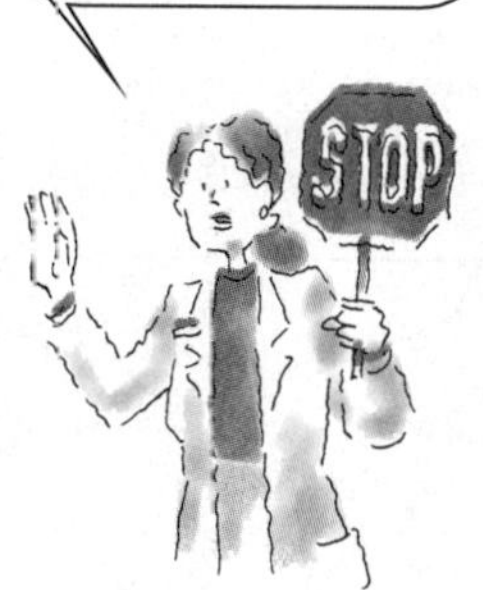

Stop and think! Although all of the answers relate to CAD, only one answer is correct.
STOP

1. 3. The left anterior descending artery is the primary source of blood for the anterior wall of the heart. The circumflex artery supplies the lateral wall, the internal mammary artery supplies the mammary, and the right coronary artery supplies the inferior wall of the heart.
NP: Evaluation; CN: Physiological integrity; CNS: Physiological adaptation; CL: Knowledge

2. 2. Although the coronary arteries may receive a minute portion of blood during systole, most of the blood flow to coronary arteries is supplied during diastole. Breathing patterns are irrelevant to blood flow.
NP: Analysis; CN: Physiological integrity; CNS: Physiological adaptation; CL: Knowledge

3. 2. Coronary artery disease accounts for over 50% of all deaths in the United States. Cancer accounts for approximately 20%. Liver failure and renal failure account for less than 10% of all deaths in the United States.
NP: Analysis; CN: Health promotion and maintenance; CNS: Prevention and early detection of disease; CL: Knowledge

4. 1. Atherosclerosis, or plaque formation, is the leading cause of CAD. Diabetes mellitus is a risk factor for CAD but it isn't the most common cause. Renal failure doesn't cause CAD, but the two conditions are related. Myocardial infarction is commonly a result of CAD.
NP: Analysis; CN: Physiological integrity; CNS: Physiological adaptation; CL: Analysis

5. 2. Arteries, not veins, supply the coronary arteries with oxygen and other nutrients. Atherosclerosis is a direct result of plaque formation in the artery. Hardened vessels can't dilate properly and, therefore, constrict blood flow.
NP: Analysis; CN: Physiological integrity; CNS: Physiological adaptation; CL: Knowledge

NP: Nursing process CN: Client needs category CNS: Client needs subcategory CL: Cognitive level

6. Which of the following risk factors for coronary artery disease cannot be corrected?
1. Cigarette smoking
2. Diabetes mellitus
3. Heredity
4. Hypertension

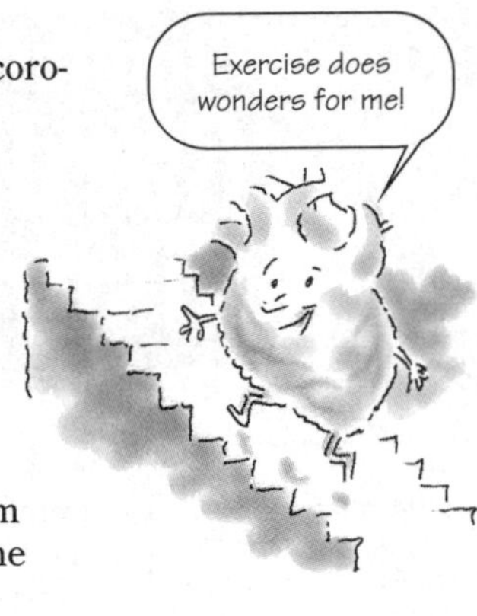
Exercise does
wonders for me!

6. 3. Because "heredity" refers to our genetic makeup, it can't be changed. Cigarette smoking cessation is a lifestyle change that involves behavior modification. Diabetes mellitus is a risk factor that can be controlled with diet, exercise, and medication. Altering one's diet, exercise, and medication can correct hypertension.
NP: Evaluation; CN: Physiological integrity; CNS: Reduction of risk potential; CL: Analysis

7. Exceeding which of the following serum cholesterol levels significantly increases the risk of coronary artery disease?
1. 100 mg/dl
2. 150 mg/dl
3. 175 mg/dl
4. 200 mg/dl

7. 4. Cholesterol levels above 200 mg/dl are considered excessive. They require dietary restriction and perhaps medication. Exercise also helps reduce cholesterol levels. The other levels listed are all below the nationally accepted levels for cholesterol and carry a lesser risk for coronary artery disease.
NP: Analysis; CN: Physiological integrity; CNS: Reduction of risk potential; CL: Comprehension

8. Which of the following actions is the first priority of care for a client exhibiting signs and symptoms of coronary artery disease?
1. Decrease anxiety.
2. Enhance myocardial oxygenation.
3. Administer sublingual nitroglycerin.
4. Educate the client about his symptoms.

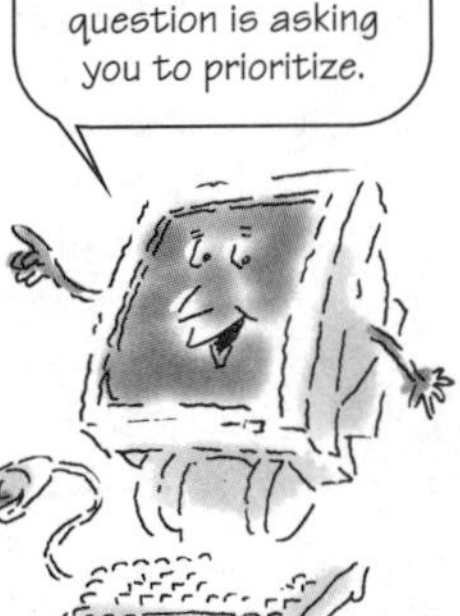
Careful! This
question is asking
you to prioritize.

8. 2. Enhancing myocardial oxygenation is always the first priority when a client exhibits signs or symptoms of cardiac compromise. Without adequate oxygen, the myocardium suffers damage. Sublingual nitroglycerin is administered to treat acute angina, but its administration isn't the first priority. Although educating the client and decreasing anxiety are important in care delivery, neither are priorities when a client is compromised.
NP: Implementation; CN: Physiological integrity; CNS: Physiological adaptation; CL: Application

9. Medical treatment of coronary artery disease includes which of the following procedures?
1. Cardiac catheterization
2. Coronary artery bypass surgery
3. Oral medication administration
4. Percutaneous transluminal coronary angioplasty

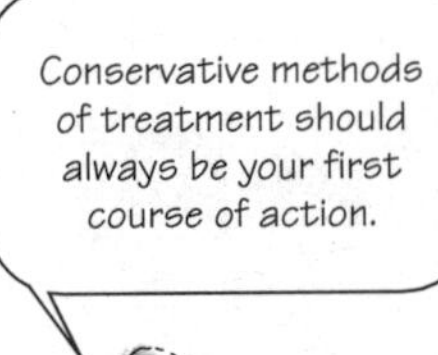
Conservative methods
of treatment should
always be your first
course of action.

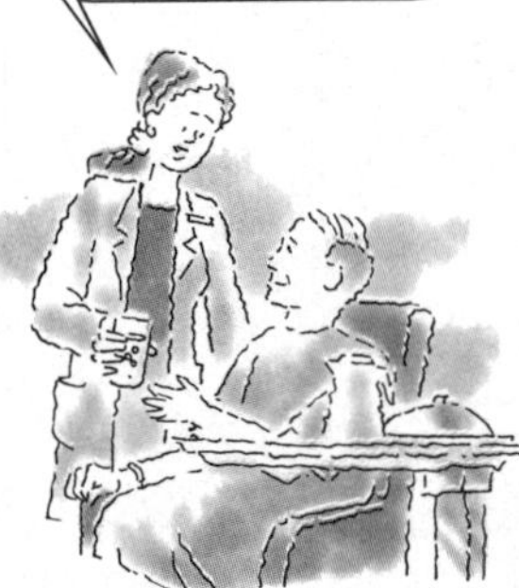

9. 3. Oral medication administration is a noninvasive, medical treatment for coronary artery disease. Cardiac catheterization isn't a treatment but a diagnostic tool. Coronary artery bypass surgery and percutaneous transluminal coronary angioplasty are invasive, surgical treatments.
NP: Evaluation; CN: Physiological integrity; CNS: Physiological adaptation; CL: Analysis

10. Prolonged occlusion of the right coronary artery produces an infarction in which of the following areas of the heart?
1. Anterior
2. Apical
3. Inferior
4. Lateral

10. 3. The right coronary artery supplies the right ventricle, or the inferior portion of the heart. Therefore, prolonged occlusion could produce an infarction in that area. The right coronary artery doesn't supply the anterior portion (left ventricle), lateral portion (some of the left ventricle and the left atrium), or the apical portion (left ventricle) of the heart.
NP: Analysis; CN: Physiological integrity; CNS: Physiological adaptation; CL: Knowledge

11. Which of the following is the most common symptom of myocardial infarction (MI)?

1. Chest pain
2. Dyspnea
3. Edema
4. Palpitations

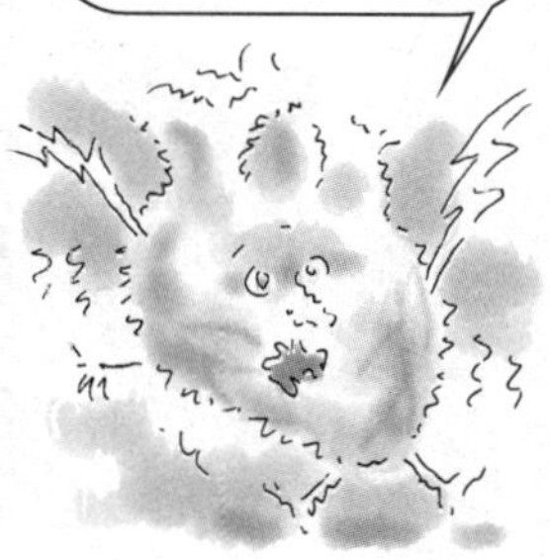

I may experience many symptoms during a heart attack, but which one are you most likely to see?

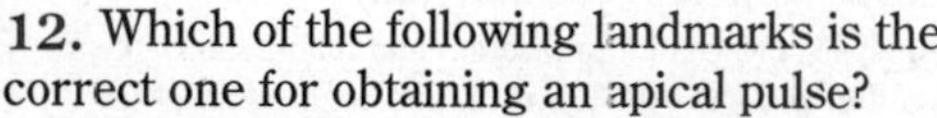

12. Which of the following landmarks is the correct one for obtaining an apical pulse?

1. Left fifth intercostal space, midaxillary line
2. Left fifth intercostal space, midclavicular line
3. Left second intercostal space, midclavicular line
4. Left seventh intercostal space, midclavicular line

13. Which of the following systems is the most likely origin of pain the client describes as knifelike chest pain that increases in intensity with inspiration?

1. Cardiac
2. Gastrointestinal
3. Musculoskeletal
4. Pulmonary

14. A murmur is heard at the second left intercostal space along the left sternal border. Which valve area is this?

1. Aortic
2. Mitral
3. Pulmonic
4. Tricuspid

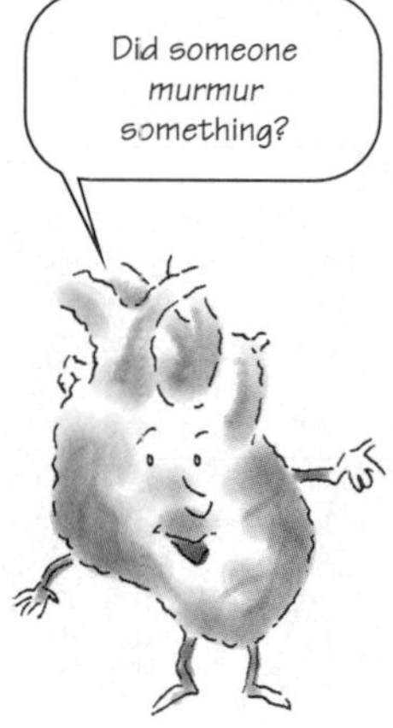

Did someone murmur something?

11. 1. The most common symptom of an MI is chest pain, resulting from deprivation of oxygen to the heart. Dyspnea is the second most common symptom, related to an increase in the metabolic needs of the body during an MI. Edema is a later sign of heart failure, often seen after an MI. Palpitations may result from reduced cardiac output, producing arrhythmias.

NP: Analysis; CN: Safe, effective care environment; CNS: Management of care; CL: Analysis

12. 2. The correct landmark for obtaining an apical pulse is the left fifth intercostal space in the midclavicular line. This is the point of maximum impulse and the location of the left ventricular apex. The left second intercostal space in the midclavicular line is where pulmonic sounds are auscultated. Normally, heart sounds aren't heard in the midaxillary line or the seventh intercostal space in the midclavicular line.

NP: Analysis; CN: Physiological integrity; CNS: Basic care and comfort; CL: Application

13. 4. Pulmonary pain is generally described by these symptoms. Musculoskeletal pain only increases with movement. Cardiac and GI pains don't change with respiration.

NP: Evaluation; CN: Physiological integrity; CNS: Physiological adaptation; CL: Analysis

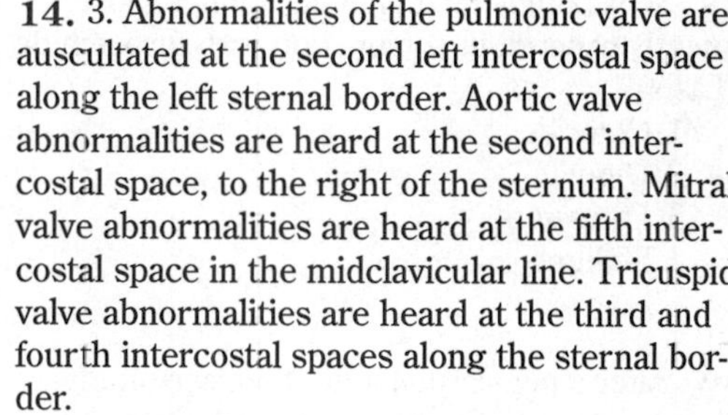

14. 3. Abnormalities of the pulmonic valve are auscultated at the second left intercostal space along the left sternal border. Aortic valve abnormalities are heard at the second intercostal space, to the right of the sternum. Mitral valve abnormalities are heard at the fifth intercostal space in the midclavicular line. Tricuspid valve abnormalities are heard at the third and fourth intercostal spaces along the sternal border.

NP: Evaluation; CN: Physiological integrity; CNS: Physiological adaptation; CL: Knowledge

15. Which of the following blood tests is most indicative of cardiac damage?

1. Lactate dehydrogenase
2. Complete blood count (CBC)
3. Troponin I
4. Creatine kinase (CK)

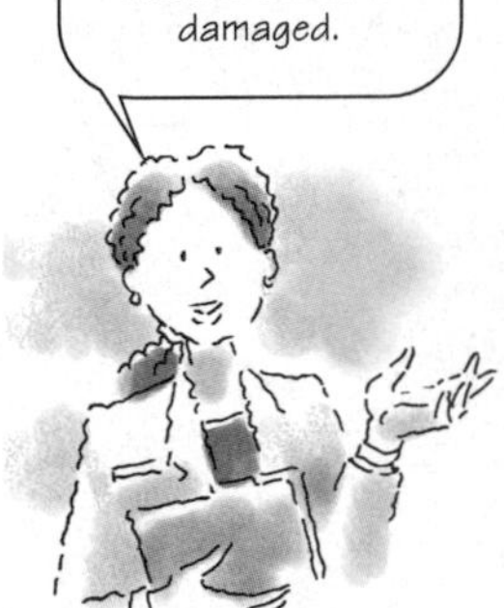

Think of what happens when cardiac tissue is damaged.

15. 3. Troponin I levels rise rapidly and are detectable within 1 hour of myocardial injury. Troponin I levels aren't detectable in people without cardiac injury. Lactate dehydrogenase (LDH) is present in almost all body tissues and not specific to heart muscle. LDH isoenzymes are useful in diagnosing cardiac injury. CBC is obtained to review blood counts, and a complete chemistry is obtained to review electrolytes. Because CK levels may rise with skeletal muscle injury, CK isoenzymes are required to detect cardiac injury.

NP: Analysis; CN: Health promotion and maintenance; CNS: Prevention and early detection of disease; CL: Analysis

16. What is the primary reason for administering morphine to a client with a myocardial infarction?

1. To sedate the client
2. To decrease the client's pain
3. To decrease the client's anxiety
4. To decrease oxygen demand on the client's heart

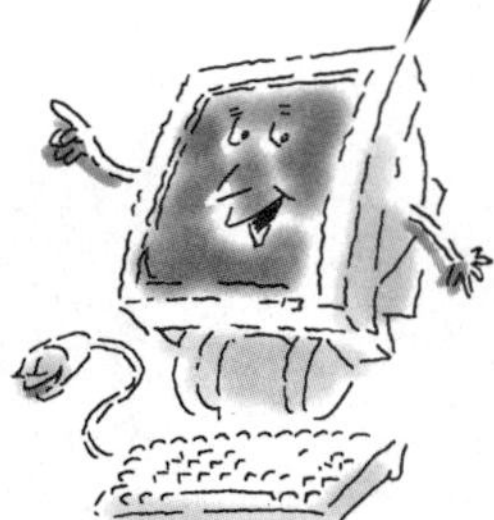

This question is looking for the most common cause of myocardial infarction.

16. 4. Morphine is administered because it decreases myocardial oxygen demand. Morphine will also decrease pain and anxiety while causing sedation, but it isn't primarily given for those reasons.

NP: Implementation; CN: Physiological integrity; CNS: Pharmacological and parenteral therapies; CL: Application

17. Which of the following conditions is most commonly responsible for myocardial infarction (MI)?

1. Aneurysm
2. Heart failure
3. Coronary artery thrombosis
4. Renal failure

17. 3. Coronary artery thrombosis causes an occlusion of the artery, leading to myocardial death. An aneurysm is an outpouching of a vessel and doesn't cause an MI. Renal failure can be associated with MI but isn't a direct cause. Heart failure is usually the result of an MI.

NP: Analysis; CN: Physiological integrity; CNS: Physiological adaptation; CL: Knowledge

18. What supplemental medication is most frequently ordered in conjunction with furosemide (Lasix)?

1. Chloride
2. Digoxin
3. Potassium
4. Sodium

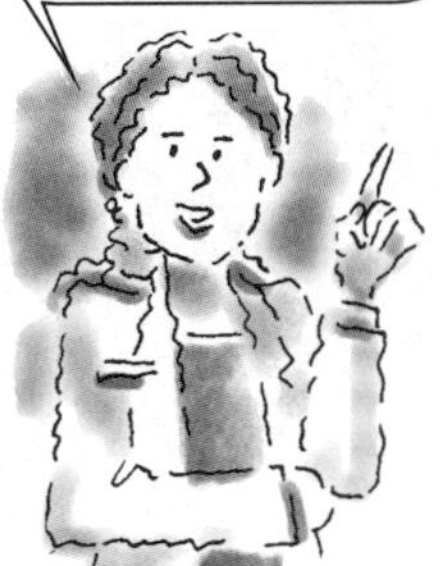

It's important to know what physiologic changes occur in your client after a heart attack.

18. 3. Supplemental potassium is given with furosemide because of the potassium loss that occurs as a result of this diuretic. Chloride and sodium aren't lost during diuresis. Digoxin acts to increase contractility but isn't given routinely with furosemide.

NP: Analysis; CN: Physiological integrity; CNS: Pharmacological and parenteral therapies; CL: Knowledge

19. After a myocardial infarction, serum glucose levels and free fatty acid production both increase. What type of physiologic changes are these?

1. Electrophysiologic
2. Hematologic
3. Mechanical
4. Metabolic

19. 4. Both glucose and fatty acids are metabolites whose levels increase after a myocardial infarction. Mechanical changes are those that affect the pumping action of the heart, and electrophysiologic changes affect conduction. Hematologic changes would affect the blood.

NP: Analysis; CN: Physiological integrity; CNS: Physiological adaptation; CL: Knowledge

20. Which of the following complications is indicated by a third heart sound (S_3)?
1. Ventricular dilation
2. Systemic hypertension
3. Aortic valve malfunction
4. Increased atrial contractions

21. After an anterior wall myocardial infarction (MI), which of the following problems is indicated by auscultation of crackles in the lungs?
1. Left-sided heart failure
2. Pulmonic valve malfunction
3. Right-sided heart failure
4. Tricuspid valve malfunction

22. Which of the following diagnostic tools is most commonly used to determine the location of myocardial damage?
1. Cardiac catheterization
2. Cardiac enzymes
3. Echocardiogram
4. Electrocardiogram (ECG)

23. What is the first intervention for a client experiencing myocardial infarction (MI)?
1. Administer morphine.
2. Administer oxygen.
3. Administer sublingual nitroglycerin.
4. Obtain an electrocardiogram (ECG).

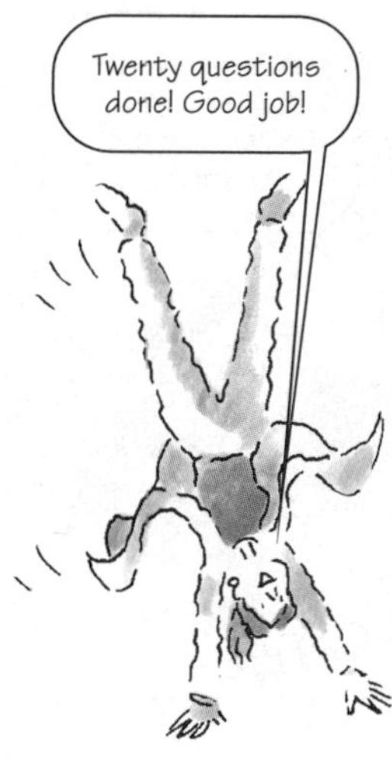

Twenty questions done! Good job!

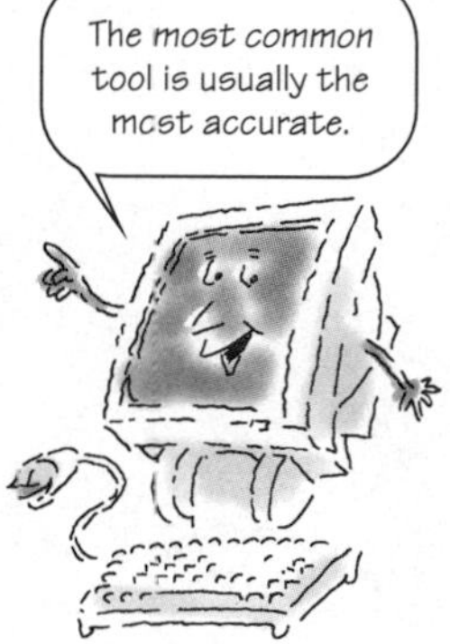

The most common tool is usually the most accurate.

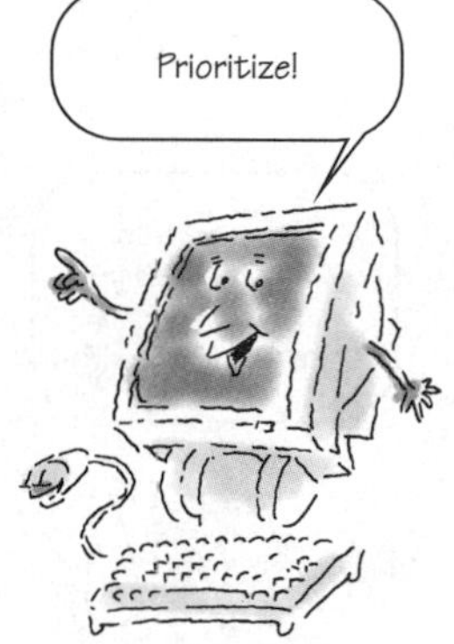

Prioritize!

20. 1. Rapid filling of the ventricle causes vasodilation that is auscultated as S_3. Increased atrial contraction or systemic hypertension can result in a fourth heart sound. Aortic valve malfunction is heard as a murmur.

NP: Analysis; CN: Health promotion and maintenance; CNS: Prevention and early detection of disease; CL: Analysis

21. 1. The left ventricle is responsible for most of the cardiac output. An anterior wall MI may result in a decrease in left ventricular function. When the left ventricle doesn't function properly, resulting in left-sided heart failure, fluid accumulates in the interstitial and alveolar spaces in the lungs and causes crackles. Pulmonic and tricuspid valve malfunction causes right-sided heart failure.

NP: Analysis; CN: Physiological integrity; CNS: Physiological adaptation; CL: Analysis

22. 4. The ECG is the quickest, most accurate, and most widely used tool to determine the location of myocardial infarction (MI). Cardiac enzymes are used to diagnose MI but can't determine the location. An echocardiogram is used most widely to view myocardial wall function after an MI has been diagnosed. Cardiac catheterization is an invasive study for determining coronary artery disease and may also indicate the location of myocardial damage, but the study may not be performed immediately.

NP: Analysis; CN: Safe, effective care environment; CNS: Management of care; CL: Knowledge

23. 2. Administering supplemental oxygen to the client is the first priority of care. The myocardium is deprived of oxygen during an infarction, so additional oxygen is administered to assist in oxygenation and prevent further damage. Morphine and sublingual nitroglycerin are also used to treat MI, but they're more commonly administered after the oxygen. An ECG is the most common diagnostic tool used to evaluate MI.

NP: Implementation; CN: Physiological integrity; CNS: Pharmacological and parenteral therapies; CL: Application

24. What is the most appropriate nursing response to a myocardial infarction client who is fearful of dying?
1. "Tell me about your feelings right now."
2. "When the doctor arrives, everything will be fine."
3. "This is a bad situation, but you'll feel better soon."
4. "Please be assured we're doing everything we can to make you feel better."

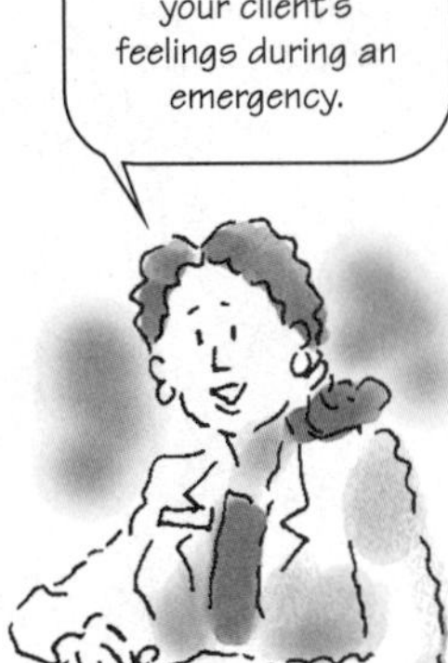

Be sensitive to your client's feelings during an emergency.

24. 1. Validation of a client's feelings is the most appropriate response. It gives the client a feeling of comfort and safety. The other three responses give the client false hope. No one can determine if a client experiencing a myocardial infarction will feel or get better and, therefore, these responses are inappropriate.
NP: Analysis; CN: Psychosocial integrity; CNS: Coping and adaptation; CL: Comprehension

25. Which of the following classes of medications protects the ischemic myocardium by blocking catecholamines and sympathetic nerve stimulation?
1. Beta-adrenergic blockers
2. Calcium channel blockers
3. Narcotics
4. Nitrates

25. 1. Beta-adrenergic blockers work by blocking beta receptors in the myocardium, reducing the response to catecholamines and sympathetic nerve stimulation. They protect the myocardium, helping to reduce the risk of another infarction by decreasing the workload of the heart and decreasing myocardial oxygen demand. Calcium channel blockers reduce the workload of the heart by decreasing the heart rate. Narcotics reduce myocardial oxygen demand, promote vasodilation, and decrease anxiety. Nitrates reduce myocardial oxygen consumption by decreasing left ventricular end-diastolic pressure (preload) and systemic vascular resistance (afterload).
NP: Analysis; CN: Physiological integrity; CNS: Pharmacological and parenteral therapies; CL: Application

26. What is the most common complication of a myocardial infarction (MI)?
1. Cardiogenic shock
2. Heart failure
3. Arrhythmias
4. Pericarditis

26. 3. Arrhythmias, caused by oxygen deprivation to the myocardium, are the most common complication of an MI. Cardiogenic shock, another complication of MI, is defined as the end stage of left ventricular dysfunction. The condition occurs in approximately 15% of clients with MI. Because the pumping function of the heart is compromised by an MI, heart failure is the second most common complication. Pericarditis most commonly results from a bacterial or viral infection but may occur after MI.
NP: Analysis; CN: Physiological integrity; CNS: Physiological adaptation; CL: Knowledge

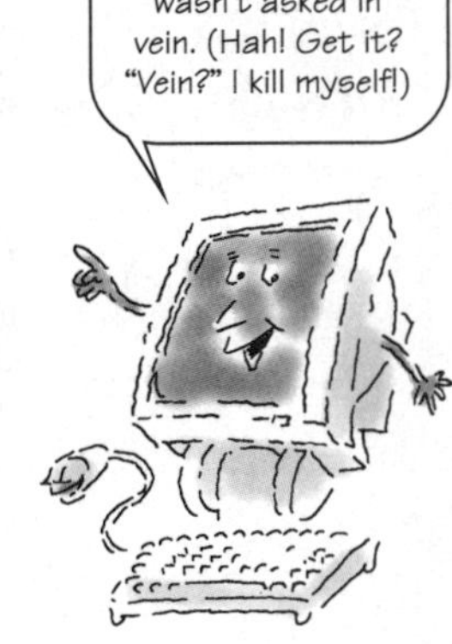

This question wasn't asked in vein. (Hah! Get it? "Vein?" I kill myself!)

27. With which of the following disorders is jugular vein distention most prominent?
1. Abdominal aortic aneurysm
2. Heart failure
3. Myocardial infarction (MI)
4. Pneumothorax

27. 2. Elevated venous pressure, exhibited as jugular vein distention, indicates a failure of the heart to pump. Jugular vein distention isn't a symptom of abdominal aortic aneurysm or pneumothorax. An MI, if severe enough, can progress to heart failure; however, in and of itself, an MI doesn't cause jugular vein distention.
NP: Analysis; CN: Physiological integrity; CNS: Physiological adaptation; CL: Analysis

28. What position should the nurse place the head of the bed in to obtain the most accurate reading of jugular vein distention?
1. High Fowler's
2. Raised 10 degrees
3. Raised 30 degrees
4. Supine position

28. 3. Jugular venous pressure is measured with a centimeter ruler to obtain the vertical distance between the sternal angle and the point of highest pulsation with the head of the bed inclined between 15 and 30 degrees. Increased pressure can't be seen when the client is supine or when the head of the bed is raised 10 degrees because the point that marks the pressure level is above the jaw (therefore, not visible). In high Fowler's position, the veins would be barely discernible above the clavicle.
NP: Evaluation; CN: Physiological integrity; CNS: Reduction of risk potential; CL: Analysis

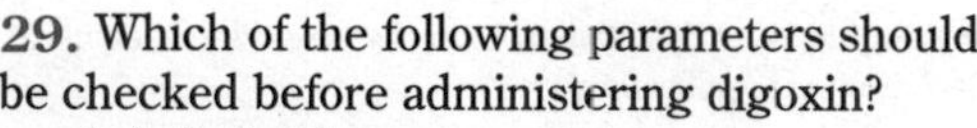

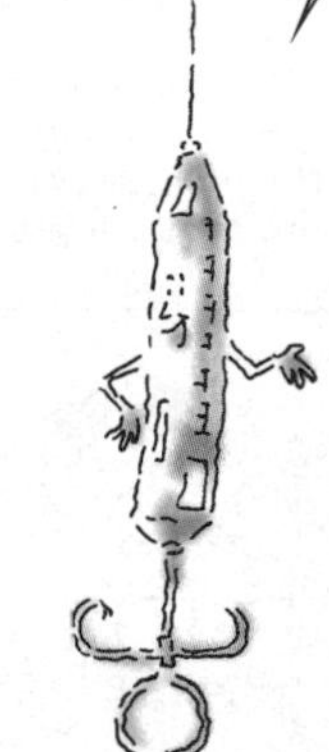

Keep in mind that digoxin strengthens myocardial contraction.

29. Which of the following parameters should be checked before administering digoxin?
1. Apical pulse
2. Blood pressure
3. Radial pulse
4. Respiratory rate

29. 1. An apical pulse is essential for accurately assessing the client's heart rate before administering digoxin. The apical pulse is the most accurate pulse point in the body. Blood pressure is usually only affected if the heart rate is too low, in which case the nurse would withhold digoxin. The radial pulse can be affected by cardiac and vascular disease and, therefore, won't always accurately depict the heart rate. Digoxin has no effect on respiratory function.
NP: Analysis; CN: Physiological integrity; CNS: Pharmacological and parenteral therapies; CL: Knowledge

30. Toxicity from which of the following medications may cause a client to see a green halo around lights?
1. Digoxin
2. Furosemide (Lasix)
3. Metoprolol (Lopressor)
4. Enalapril (Vasotec)

30. 1. One of the most common signs of digoxin toxicity is the visual disturbance known as the green halo sign. The other medications aren't associated with such an effect.
NP: Evaluation; CN: Physiological integrity; CNS: Pharmacological and parenteral therapies; CL: Knowledge

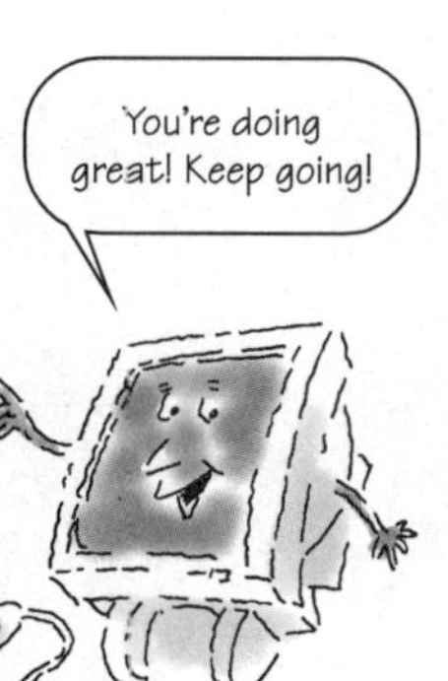

31. Which of the following symptoms is most commonly associated with left-sided heart failure?
1. Crackles
2. Arrhythmias
3. Hepatic engorgement
4. Hypotension

31. 1. Crackles in the lungs are a classic sign of left-sided heart failure. These sounds are caused by fluid backing up into the pulmonary system. Arrhythmias can be associated with both right- and left-sided heart failure. Hepatic engorgement is associated with right-sided heart failure. Left-sided heart failure causes hypertension secondary to an increased workload on the system.
NP: Analysis; CN: Physiological integrity; CNS: Physiological adaptation; CL: Knowledge

32. In which of the following disorders would the nurse expect to assess sacral edema in a bedridden client?

1. Diabetes mellitus
2. Pulmonary emboli
3. Renal failure
4. Right-sided heart failure

33. Which of the following symptoms might a client with right-sided heart failure exhibit?

1. Adequate urine output
2. Polyuria
3. Oliguria
4. Polydipsia

34. Which of the following classes of medications maximizes cardiac performance in clients with heart failure by increasing ventricular contractility?

1. Beta-adrenergic blockers
2. Calcium channel blockers
3. Diuretics
4. Inotropic agents

35. Stimulation of the sympathetic nervous system produces which of the following responses?

1. Bradycardia
2. Tachycardia
3. Hypotension
4. Decreased myocardial contractility

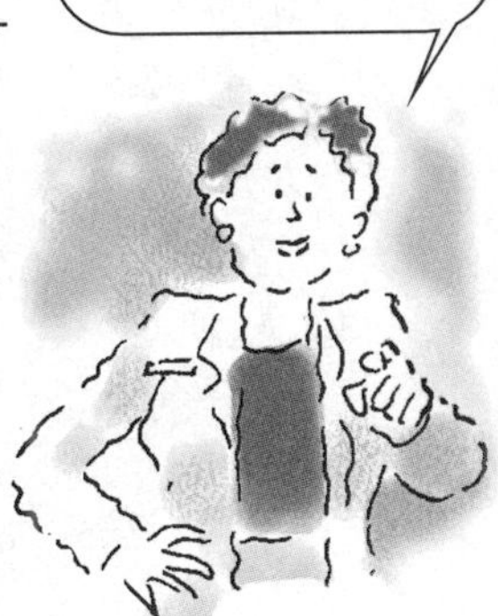

Make sure you understand how these different drugs work to benefit the heart.

32. 4. The most accurate area on the body to assess dependent edema in a bedridden client is the sacral area. Sacral, or dependent, edema is secondary to right-sided heart failure. Diabetes mellitus, pulmonary emboli, and renal disease aren't directly linked to sacral edema.
NP: Analysis; CN: Physiological integrity; CNS: Physiological adaptation; CL: Analysis

33. 3. Inadequate deactivation of aldosterone by the liver after right-sided heart failure leads to fluid retention, which causes oliguria. Adequate urine output, polyuria, and polydipsia aren't associated with right-sided heart failure.
NP: Analysis; CN: Physiological integrity; CNS: Physiological adaptation; CL: Application

34. 4. Inotropic agents are administered to increase the force of the heart's contractions, thereby increasing ventricular contractility and ultimately increasing cardiac output. Beta-adrenergic blockers and calcium channel blockers decrease the heart rate and ultimately decrease the workload of the heart. Diuretics are administered to decrease the overall vascular volume, also decreasing the workload of the heart.
NP: Analysis; CN: Physiological integrity; CNS: Pharmacological and parenteral therapies; CL: Comprehension

35. 2. Stimulation of the sympathetic nervous system causes tachycardia and increased contractility. The other symptoms listed are related to the parasympathetic nervous system, which is responsible for slowing the heart rate.
NP: Analysis; CN: Physiological integrity; CNS: Physiological adaptation; CL: Knowledge

36. Which of the following conditions is most closely associated with weight gain, nausea, and a decrease in urine output?
1. Angina pectoris
2. Cardiomyopathy (left sided heart failure)
3. Left-sided heart failure
4. Right-sided heart failure

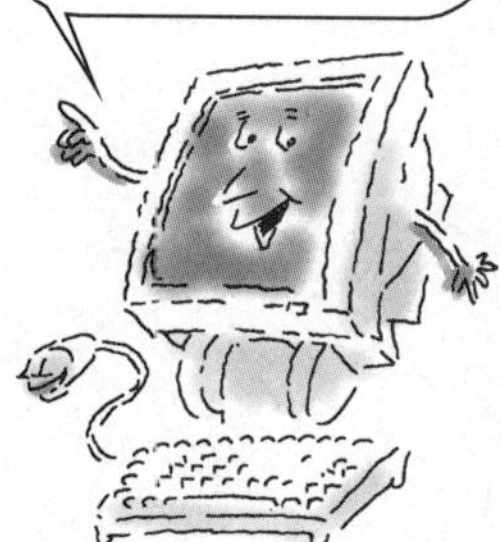
This question asks you to distinguish between symptoms of left- and right-sided heart failure.

36. 4. Weight gain, nausea, and a decrease in urine output are secondary effects of right-sided heart failure. Cardiomyopathy is usually identified as a symptom of left-sided heart failure. Left-sided heart failure causes primarily pulmonary symptoms rather than systemic ones. Angina pectoris doesn't cause weight gain, nausea, or a decrease in urine output.
NP: Evaluation; CN: Physiological integrity; CNS: Physiological adaptation; CL: Application

37. What is the most common cause of an abdominal aortic aneurysm?
1. Atherosclerosis
2. Diabetes mellitus
3. Hypertension
4. Syphilis

37. 1. Atherosclerosis accounts for 75% of all abdominal aortic aneurysms. Plaques build up on the wall of the vessel and weaken it, causing an aneurysm. Although the other conditions are related to the development of an aneurysm, none is a direct cause.
NP: Analysis; CN: Health promotion and maintenance; CNS: Prevention and early detection of disease; CL: Knowledge

38. In which of the following areas is an abdominal aortic aneurysm most commonly located?
1. Distal to the iliac arteries
2. Distal to the renal arteries
3. Adjacent to the aortic arch
4. Proximal to the renal arteries

38. 2. The portion of the aorta distal to the renal arteries is more prone to an aneurysm because the vessel isn't surrounded by stable structures, unlike the proximal portion of the aorta. Distal to the iliac arteries, the vessel is again surrounded by stable vasculature, making this an uncommon site for an aneurysm. There is no area adjacent to the aortic arch, which bends into the thoracic (descending) aorta.
NP: Analysis; CN: Physiological integrity; CNS: Physiological adaptation; CL: Knowledge

39. A pulsating abdominal mass usually indicates which of the following conditions?
1. Abdominal aortic aneurysm
2. Enlarged spleen
3. Gastric distention
4. Gastritis

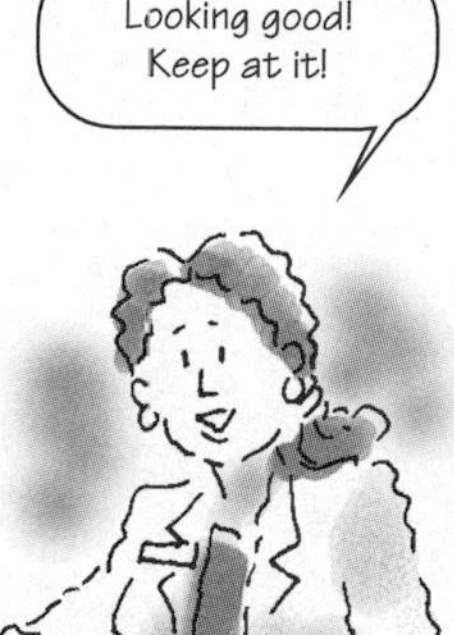

39. 1. The presence of a pulsating mass in the abdomen is an abnormal finding, usually indicating an outpouching in a weakened vessel, as in abdominal aortic aneurysm. The finding, however, can be normal on a thin person. Neither an enlarged spleen, gastritis, nor gastric distention cause pulsation.
NP: Evaluation; CN: Health promotion and maintenance; CNS: Prevention and early detection of disease; CL: Application

40. What is the most common symptom in a client with abdominal aortic aneurysm?
1. Abdominal pain
2. Diaphoresis
3. Headache
4. Upper back pain

40. 1. Abdominal pain in a client with an abdominal aortic aneurysm results from the disruption of normal circulation in the abdominal region. Lower back pain, not upper, is a common symptom, usually signifying expansion and impending rupture of the aneurysm. Headache and diaphoresis aren't associated with abdominal aortic aneurysm.
NP: Analysis; CN: Physiological integrity; CNS: Basic care and comfort; CL: Comprehension

41. Which of the following symptoms usually signifies rapid expansion and impending rupture of an abdominal aortic aneurysm?

1. Abdominal pain
2. Absent pedal pulses
3. Angina
4. Lower back pain

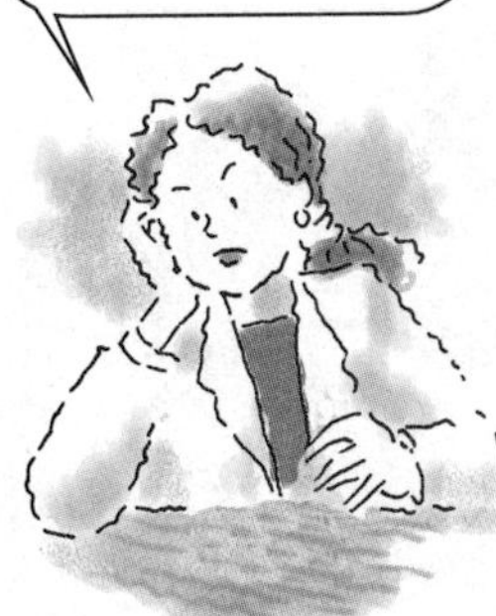

Knowing which symptom relates to which complication will help you to make a more accurate diagnosis.

41. 4. Lower back pain results from expansion of the aneurysm. The expansion applies pressure in the abdominal cavity, and the pain is referred to the lower back. Abdominal pain is the most common symptom resulting from impaired circulation. Absent pedal pulses are a sign of no circulation and would occur after a ruptured aneurysm or in peripheral vascular disease. Angina is associated with atherosclerosis of the coronary arteries.

NP: Analysis; CN: Physiological integrity; CNS: Basic care and comfort; CL: Comprehension

42. What is the definitive test used to diagnose an abdominal aortic aneurysm?

1. Abdominal X-ray
2. Arteriogram
3. Computed tomography (CT) scan
4. Ultrasound

42. 2. An arteriogram accurately and directly depicts the vasculature; therefore, it clearly delineates the vessels and any abnormalities. An abdominal aneurysm would only be visible on an X-ray if it were calcified. CT scan and ultrasound don't give a direct view of the vessels and don't yield as accurate a diagnosis as the arteriogram.

NP: Analysis; CN: Health promotion and maintenance; CNS: Prevention and early detection of disease; CL: Knowledge

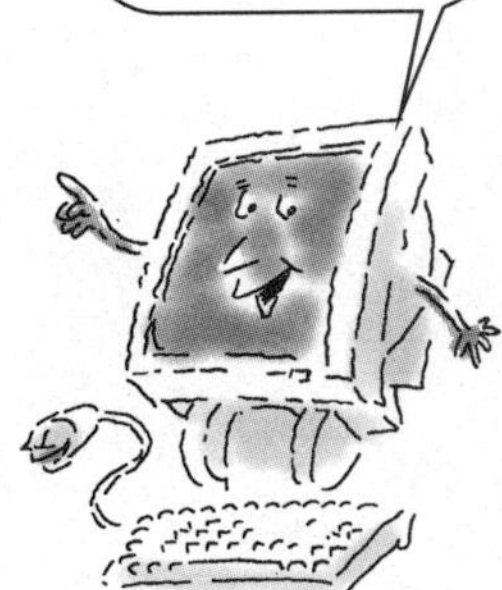

This question is asking you to prioritize, once again.

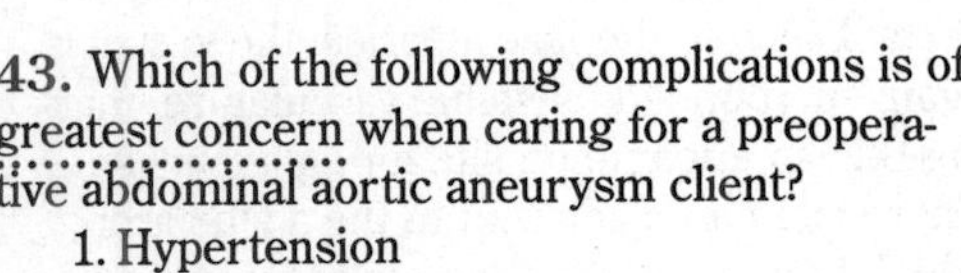

43. Which of the following complications is of greatest concern when caring for a preoperative abdominal aortic aneurysm client?

1. Hypertension
2. Aneurysm rupture
3. Cardiac arrhythmias
4. Diminished pedal pulses

43. 2. Rupture of the aneurysm is a life-threatening emergency and is of the greatest concern for the nurse caring for this type of client. Hypertension should be avoided and controlled because it can cause the weakened vessel to rupture. Diminished pedal pulses, a sign of poor circulation to the lower extremities, are associated with an aneurysm but aren't life-threatening. Cardiac arrhythmias aren't directly linked to an aneurysm.

NP: Evaluation; CN: Physiological integrity; CNS: Basic care and comfort; CL: Analysis

44. Which of the following blood vessel layers may be damaged in a client with an aneurysm?

1. Externa
2. Interna
3. Media
4. Interna and media

44. 3. The factor common to all types of aneurysms is a damaged media. The media has more smooth muscle and less elastic fibers, so it's more capable of vasoconstriction and vasodilation. The interna and externa are generally not damaged in an aneurysm.

NP: Analysis; CN: Physiological integrity; CNS: Physiological adaptation; CL: Knowledge

45. When assessing a client for an abdominal aortic aneurysm, which area of the abdomen is most commonly palpated?
1. Right upper quadrant
2. Directly over the umbilicus
3. Middle lower abdomen to the left of the midline
4. Middle lower abdomen to the right of the midline

45. 3. The aorta lies directly left of the umbilicus; therefore, any other region is inappropriate for palpation.
NP: Evaluation; CN: Physiological integrity; CNS: Basic care and comfort; CL: Application

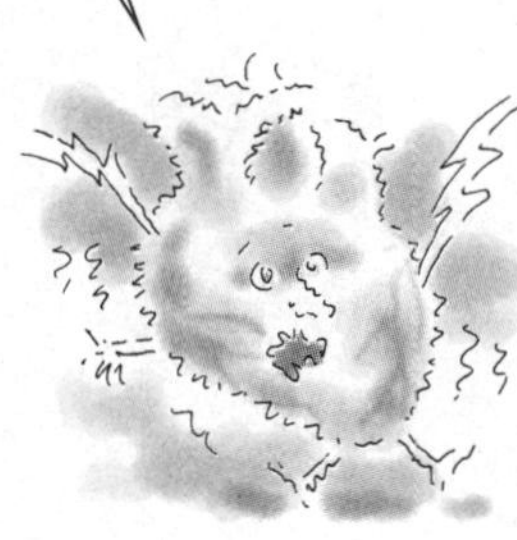

I'm suddenly feeling a little tense, a little hyper. (Get it?)

46. Which of the following conditions is linked to more than 50% of clients with abdominal aortic aneurysms?
1. Diabetes mellitus
2. Hypertension
3. Peripheral vascular disease
4. Syphilis

46. 2. Continuous pressure on the vessel walls from hypertension causes the walls to weaken and an aneurysm to occur. Atherosclerotic changes can occur with peripheral vascular diseases and are linked to aneurysms, but the link isn't as strong as it is with hypertension. Only 1% of clients with syphilis experience an aneurysm. Diabetes mellitus doesn't have a direct link to aneurysm.
NP: Analysis; CN: Health promotion and maintenance; CNS: Prevention and early detection of disease; CL: Comprehension

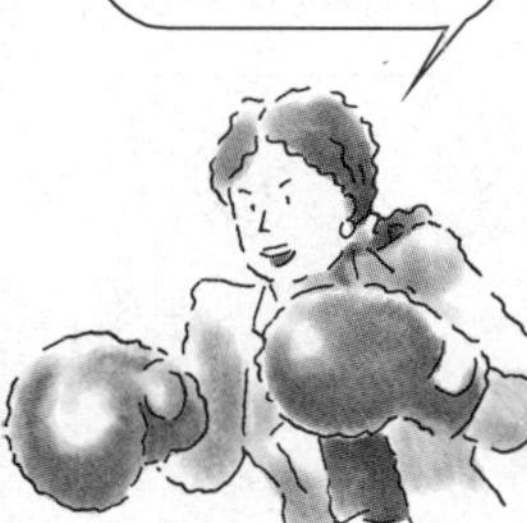

This is a real bruit of a question.

47. Which of the following sounds is distinctly heard on auscultation over the abdominal region of an abdominal aortic aneurysm client?
1. Bruit
2. Crackles
3. Dullness
4. Friction rubs

47. 1. A bruit, a vascular sound resembling heart murmur, suggests partial arterial occlusion. Crackles are indicative of fluid in the lungs. Dullness is heard over solid organs, such as the liver. Friction rubs indicate inflammation of the peritoneal surface.
NP: Evaluation; CN: Physiological integrity; CNS: Basic care and comfort; CL: Comprehension

48. Which of the following groups of symptoms indicates a ruptured abdominal aortic aneurysm?
1. Lower back pain, increased blood pressure, decreased red blood cell (RBC) count, increased white blood cell (WBC) count
2. Severe lower back pain, decreased blood pressure, decreased RBC count, increased WBC count
3. Severe lower back pain, decreased blood pressure, decreased RBC count, decreased WBC count
4. Intermittent lower back pain, decreased blood pressure, decreased RBC count, increased WBC count

48. 2. Severe lower back pain indicates an aneurysm rupture, secondary to pressure being applied within the abdominal cavity. When rupture occurs, the pain is constant because it can't be alleviated until the aneurysm is repaired. Blood pressure decreases due to the loss of blood. After the aneurysm ruptures, the vasculature is interrupted and blood volume is lost, so blood pressure wouldn't increase. For the same reason, the RBC count is decreased — not increased. The WBC count increases as cells migrate to the site of injury.
NP: Analysis; CN: Physiological integrity; CNS: Physiological adaptation; CL: Knowledge

49. Which of the following complications of an abdominal aortic repair is indicated by detection of a hematoma in the perineal area?
1. Hernia
2. Stage 1 pressure ulcer
3. Retroperitoneal rupture at the repair site
4. Rapid expansion of the aneurysm

49. 3. Blood collects in the retroperitoneal space and is exhibited as a hematoma in the perineal area. This rupture is most commonly caused by leakage at the repair site. A hernia doesn't cause vascular disturbances, nor does a pressure ulcer. Because no bleeding occurs with rapid expansion of the aneurysm, a hematoma won't form.
NP: Evaluation; CN: Physiological integrity; CNS: Physiological adaptation; CL: Comprehension

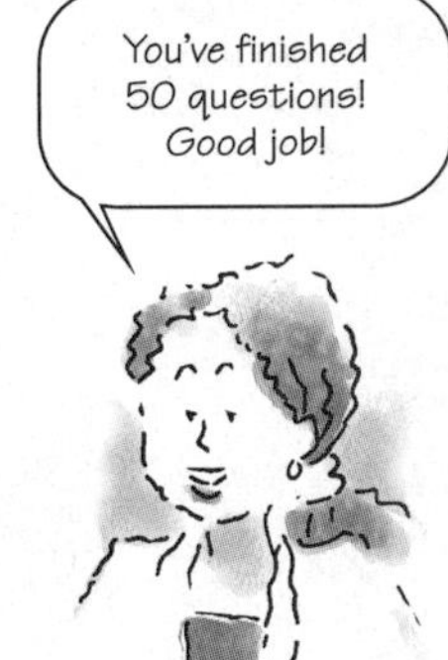

You've finished 50 questions! Good job!

50. Which hereditary disease is most closely linked to aneurysm?
1. Cystic fibrosis
2. Lupus erythematosus
3. Marfan's syndrome
4. Myocardial infarction

50. 3. Marfan's syndrome results in the degeneration of the elastic fibers of the aortic media. Therefore, clients with the syndrome are more likely to develop an aneurysm. Although cystic fibrosis is hereditary, it hasn't been linked to aneurysms. Lupus erythematosus isn't hereditary. Myocardial infarction is neither hereditary nor a disease.
NP: Analysis; CN: Health promotion and maintenance; CNS: Prevention and early detection of disease; CL: Knowledge

51. Which of the following treatments is the definitive one for a ruptured aneurysm?
1. Antihypertensive medication administration
2. Aortogram
3. Beta-adrenergic blocker administration
4. Surgical intervention

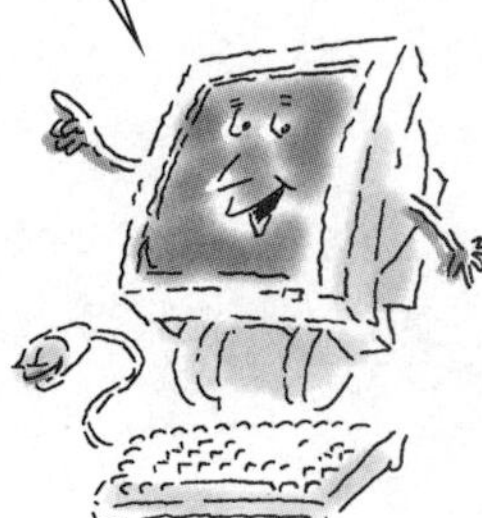

This question is asking for a treatment, not a preventive measure.

51. 4. When the vessel ruptures, surgery is the only intervention that can repair it. Administration of antihypertensive medications and beta-adrenergic blockers can help control hypertension, reducing the risk of rupture. An aortogram is a diagnostic tool used to detect an aneurysm.
NP: Intervention; CN: Physiological integrity; CNS: Basic care and comfort; CL: Application

52. Which of the following heart muscle diseases is unrelated to other cardiovascular disease?
1. Cardiomyopathy
2. Coronary artery disease
3. Myocardial infarction
4. Pericardial effusion

52. 1. Cardiomyopathy isn't usually related to an underlying heart disease such as atherosclerosis. The etiology in most cases is unknown. Coronary artery disease and myocardial infarction are directly related to atherosclerosis. Pericardial effusion is the escape of fluid into the pericardial sac, a condition associated with pericarditis and advanced heart failure.
NP: Analysis; CN: Physiological integrity; CNS: Physiological adaptation; CL: Knowledge

53. Which of the following types of cardiomyopathy can be associated with childbirth?
1. Dilated
2. Hypertrophic
3. Myocarditis
4. Restrictive

53. 1. Although the cause isn't entirely known, cardiac dilation and heart failure may develop during the last month of pregnancy or the first few months after birth. The condition may result from a preexisting cardiomyopathy not apparent prior to pregnancy. Hypertrophic cardiomyopathy is an abnormal symmetry of the ventricles that has an unknown etiology but a strong familial tendency. Myocarditis isn't specifically associated with childbirth. Restrictive cardiomyopathy indicates constrictive pericarditis; the underlying cause is usually myocardial.

NP: Analysis; CN: Physiological integrity; CNS: Physiological adaptation; CL: Knowledge

54. Septal involvement occurs in which type of cardiomyopathy?
1. Congestive
2. Dilated
3. Hypertrophic
4. Restrictive

54. 3. In hypertrophic cardiomyopathy, hypertrophy of the ventricular septum — not the ventricle chambers — is apparent. This abnormality isn't seen in other types of cardiomyopathy.

NP: Analysis; CN: Physiological integrity; CNS: Physiological adaptation; CL: Knowledge

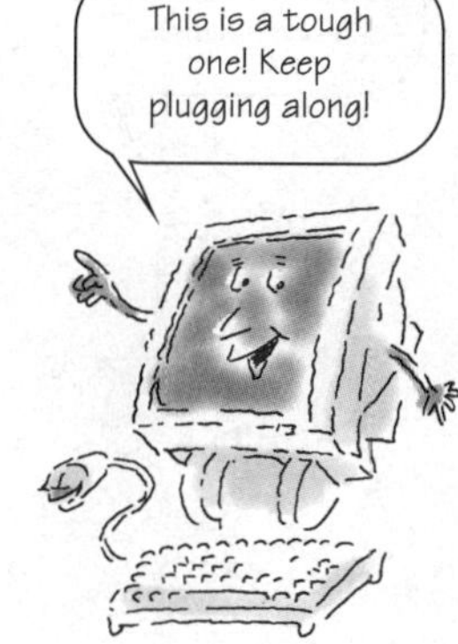

This is a tough one! Keep plugging along!

55. Which of the following recurring conditions most commonly occurs in clients with cardiomyopathy?
1. Heart failure
2. Diabetes mellitus
3. Myocardial infarction
4. Pericardial effusion

55. 1. Because the structure and function of the heart muscle is affected, heart failure most commonly occurs in clients with cardiomyopathy. Myocardial infarction results from prolonged myocardial ischemia due to reduced blood flow through one of the coronary arteries. Pericardial effusion is most predominant in clients with pericarditis. Diabetes mellitus is unrelated to cardiomyopathy.

NP: Analysis; CN: Physiological integrity; CNS: Physiological adaptation; CL: Comprehension

56. What is the term used to describe an enlargement of the heart muscle?
1. Cardiomegaly
2. Cardiomyopathy
3. Myocarditis
4. Pericarditis

56. 1. Cardiomegaly denotes an enlarged heart muscle. Cardiomyopathy is a heart muscle disease of unknown origin. Myocarditis refers to inflammation of heart muscle. Pericarditis is an inflammation of the pericardium, the sac surrounding the heart.

NP: Analysis; CN: Physiological integrity; CNS: Physiological adaptation; CL: Knowledge

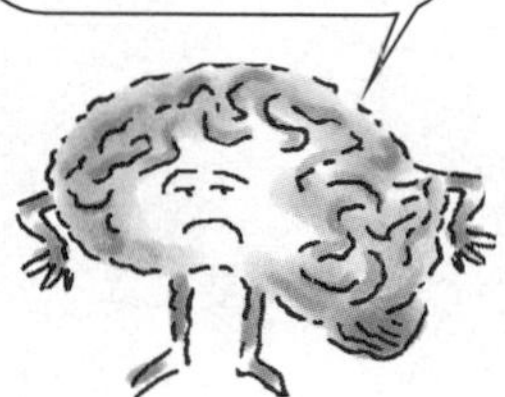

I don't know about you, but along about now, I'm getting kinda fried.

57. Dyspnea, cough, expectoration, weakness, and edema are classic signs and symptoms of which of the following conditions?
1. Pericarditis
2. Hypertension
3. Myocardial infarction
4. Heart failure

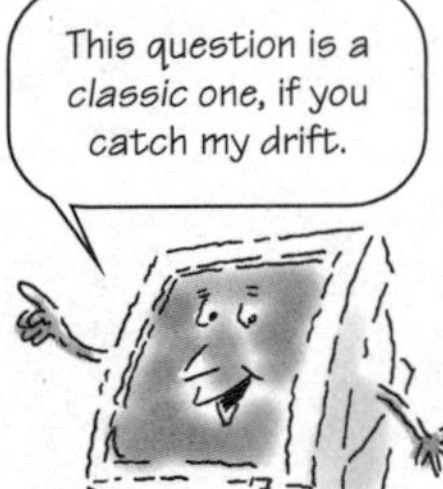

This question is a classic one, if you catch my drift.

57. 4. These are the classic symptoms of heart failure. Pericarditis is exhibited by a feeling of fullness in the chest and auscultation of a pericardial friction rub. Hypertension is usually exhibited by headaches, visual disturbances, and a flushed face. Myocardial infarction causes heart failure but isn't related to these symptoms.
NP: Evaluation; CN: Physiological integrity; CNS: Reduction of risk potential; CL: Knowledge

58. In which of the following types of cardiomyopathy does cardiac output remain normal?
1. Dilated
2. Hypertrophic
3. Obliterative
4. Restrictive

58. 2. Cardiac output isn't affected by hypertrophic cardiomyopathy because the size of the ventricle remains relatively unchanged. Dilated cardiomyopathy, obliterative cardiomyopathy, and restrictive cardiomyopathy all decrease cardiac output.
NP: Analysis; CN: Physiological integrity; CNS: Physiological adaptation; CL: Comprehension

59. Which of the following cardiac conditions does a fourth heart sound (S_4) indicate?
1. Dilated aorta
2. Normally functioning heart
3. Decreased myocardial contractility
4. Failure of the ventricle to eject all the blood during systole

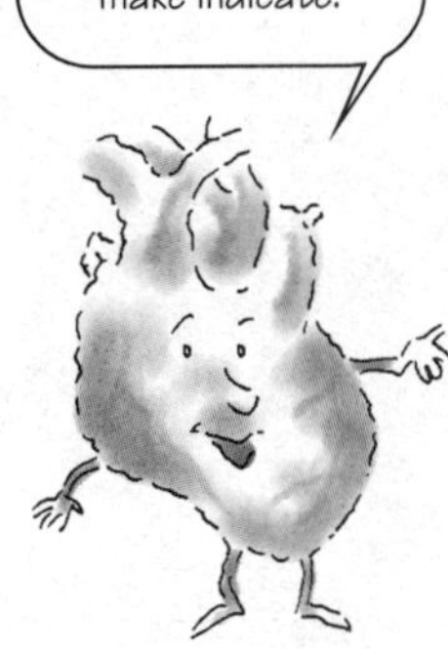

It's important to know what the different sounds I make indicate.

59. 4. An S_4 occurs as a result of increased resistance to ventricular filling after atrial contraction. This increased resistance is related to decreased compliance of the ventricle. A dilated aorta doesn't cause an extra heart sound, though it does cause a murmur. Decreased myocardial contractility is heard as a third heart sound. An S_4 isn't heard in a normally functioning heart.
NP: Evaluation; CN: Health promotion and maintenance; CNS: Prevention and early detection of disease; CL: Application

60. Which of the following classes of drugs is most widely used in the treatment of cardiomyopathy?
1. Antihypertensives
2. Beta-adrenergic blockers
3. Calcium channel blockers
4. Nitrates

60. 2. By decreasing the heart rate and contractility, beta-adrenergic blockers improve myocardial filling and cardiac output, which are primary goals in the treatment of cardiomyopathy. Antihypertensives aren't usually indicated because they would decrease cardiac output in clients who are often already hypotensive. Calcium channel blockers are sometimes used for the same reasons as beta-adrenergic blockers; however, they aren't as effective as beta-adrenergic blockers and cause increased hypotension. Nitrates aren't used because of their dilating effects, which would further compromise the myocardium.
NP: Analysis; CN: Physiological integrity; CNS: Pharmacological and parenteral therapies; CL: Comprehension

61. If medical treatments fail, which of the following invasive procedures is necessary for treating cardiomyopathy?

1. Cardiac catheterization
2. Coronary artery bypass graft (CABG)
3. Heart transplantation
4. Intra-aortic balloon pump (IABP)

61. 3. The only definitive treatment for cardiomyopathy that can't be controlled medically is a heart transplant because the damage to the heart muscle is irreversible. Cardiac catheterization is an invasive diagnostic procedure for coronary artery disease. CABG is a surgical intervention used for atherosclerotic vessels. An IABP is an invasive treatment that assists the failing heart; however, it can't be used for an extended time because it's only a temporary solution.

NP: Analysis; CN: Physiological integrity; CNS: Physiological adaptation; CL: Comprehension

Stress can be a real pain in the heart.

62. Which of the following conditions is associated with a predictable level of pain that occurs as a result of physical or emotional stress?

1. Anxiety
2. Stable angina
3. Unstable angina
4. Variant angina

62. 2. The pain of stable angina is predictable in nature, builds gradually, and quickly reaches maximum intensity. Anxiety generally isn't described as painful. Unstable angina doesn't always need a trigger, is more intense, and lasts longer than stable angina. Variant angina usually occurs at rest — not as a result of exertion or stress.

NP: Evaluation; CN: Physiological integrity; CNS: Physiological adaptation; CL: Analysis

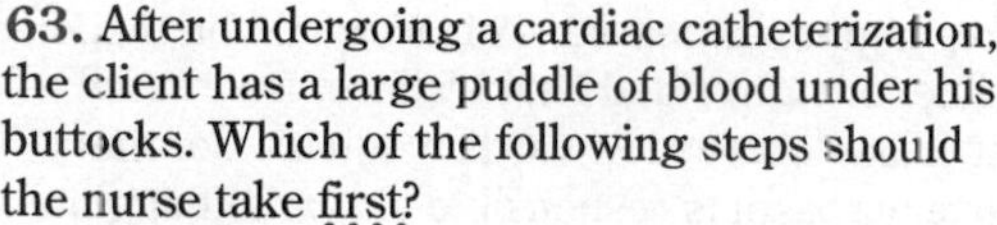

63. After undergoing a cardiac catheterization, the client has a large puddle of blood under his buttocks. Which of the following steps should the nurse take *first*?

1. Call for help.
2. Obtain vital signs.
3. Ask the client to "lift up."
4. Apply gloves and assess the groin site.

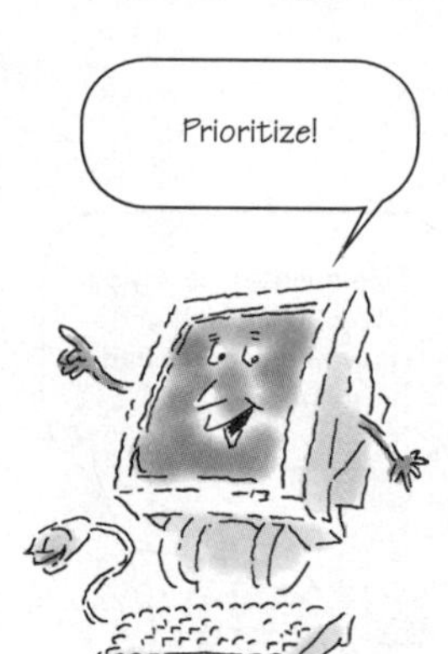

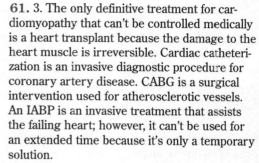

63. 4. Observing standard precautions is the first priority when dealing with any body fluid. Assessment of the groin site is the second priority. This establishes where the blood is coming from and determines how much blood has been lost. The goal in this situation is to stop the bleeding. The nurse would call for help if it were warranted after the assessment of the situation. After determining the extent of the bleeding, vital signs assessment is important. The nurse should never move the client, in case a clot has formed. Moving can disturb the clot and cause rebleeding.

NP: Evaluation; CN: Safe, effective care environment; CNS: Management of care; CL: Comprehension

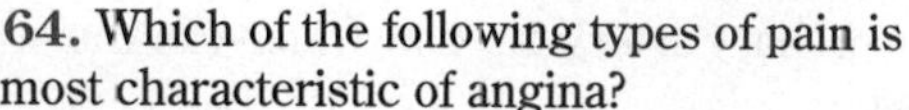

64. Which of the following types of pain is most characteristic of angina?

1. Knifelike
2. Sharp
3. Shooting
4. Tightness

64. 4. The pain of angina usually ranges from a vague feeling of tightness to heavy, intense pain. Pain impulses originate in the most visceral muscles and may move to such areas as the chest, neck, and arms. Pain described as knifelike, sharp, or shooting is more characteristic of pulmonary or pleuritic pain.

NP: Analysis; CN: Physiological integrity; CNS: Basic care and comfort; CL: Knowledge

65. Which of the following types of angina is most closely associated with an impending myocardial infarction (MI)?
1. Angina decubitus
2. Chronic stable angina
3. Nocturnal angina
4. Unstable angina

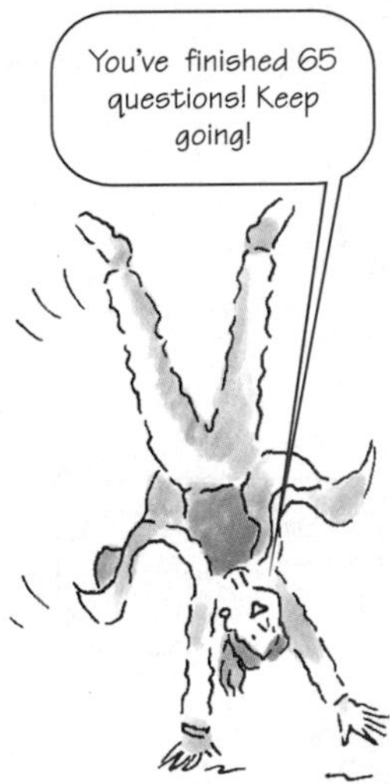

You've finished 65 questions! Keep going!

65. 4. Unstable angina progressively increases in frequency, intensity, and duration and is related to an increased risk of MI within 3 to 18 months. Angina decubitus, chronic stable angina, and nocturnal angina aren't associated with an increased risk of MI.
NP: Analysis; CN: Physiological integrity; CNS: Physiological adaptation; CL: Knowledge

66. Which of the following medications is the drug of choice for angina pectoris?
1. Aspirin
2. Furosemide (Lasix)
3. Nitroglycerin
4. Nifedipine (Procardia)

66. 3. Nitroglycerin is administered to reduce the myocardial demand, which decreases ischemia and relieves pain. In addition, nitroglycerin dilates the vasculature, thereby reducing preload. Aspirin is administered to reduce the risk of myocardial infarction in patients with unstable angina. Furosemide is a loop diuretic that won't directly reduce pain or prevent angina. Nifedipine is a calcium channel blocker primarily used to decrease coronary artery spasm, as in variant angina.
NP: Analysis; CN: Physiological integrity; CNS: Pharmacological and parenteral therapies; CL: Knowledge

67. Which of the following conditions is the predominant cause of angina?
1. Increased preload
2. Decreased afterload
3. Coronary artery spasm
4. Inadequate oxygen supply to the myocardium

67. 4. Inadequate oxygen supply to the myocardium is responsible for the pain accompanying angina. Increased preload would be responsible for right-sided heart failure. Decreased afterload causes low cardiac output. Coronary artery spasm is responsible for variant angina.
NP: Analysis; CN: Physiological integrity; CNS: Physiological adaptation; CL: Knowledge

68. Which of the following tests is used most often to diagnose angina?
1. Chest X-ray
2. Echocardiogram
3. Cardiac catheterization
4. 12-lead electrocardiogram (ECG)

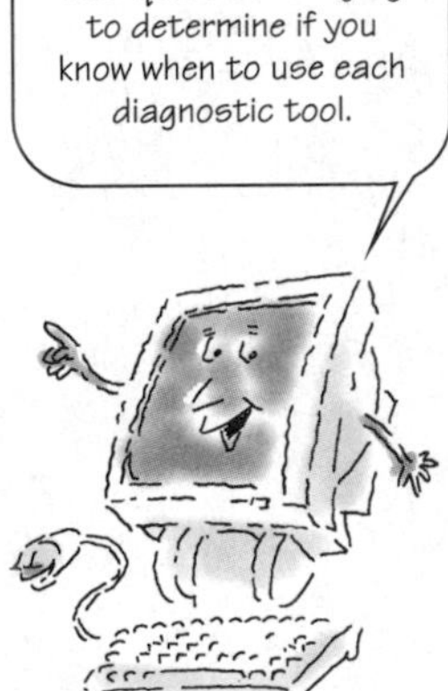

This question is trying to determine if you know when to use each diagnostic tool.

68. 4. The 12-lead ECG will indicate ischemia, showing T-wave inversion. In addition, with variant angina, the ECG shows ST-segment elevation. A chest X-ray will show heart enlargement or signs of heart failure but isn't used to diagnose angina. An echocardiogram is used to detect wall function and valvular function and is most accurate in diagnosing myocardial infarction. Cardiac catheterization is used to diagnose coronary artery disease, which can cause angina.
NP: Analysis; CN: Health promotion and maintenance; CNS: Prevention and early detection of disease; CL: Knowledge

69. Which of the following results is the primary treatment goal for angina?

1. Reversal of ischemia
2. Reversal of infarction
3. Reduction of stress and anxiety
4. Reduction of associated risk factors

69. 1. Reversal of the ischemia is the primary goal, achieved by reducing oxygen consumption and increasing oxygen supply. An infarction is permanent and can't be reversed. Reduction of associated risk factors, such as stress and anxiety, is a progressive, long-term treatment goal that has cumulative effects. Reduction of these factors will decrease the risk for angina but this usually isn't an immediate goal.

NP: Analysis; CN: Physiological integrity; CNS: Physiological adaptation; CL: Comprehension

70. Which of the following treatments is a suitable surgical intervention for unstable angina?

1. Cardiac catheterization
2. Echocardiogram
3. Nitroglycerin
4. Percutaneous transluminal coronary angioplasty (PTCA)

70. 4. PTCA can alleviate the blockage and restore blood flow and oxygenation. An echocardiogram is a noninvasive diagnostic test. Nitroglycerin is an oral or sublingual medication. Cardiac catheterization is a diagnostic tool — not a treatment.

NP: Analysis; CN: Physiological integrity; CNS: Physiological adaptation; CL: Knowledge

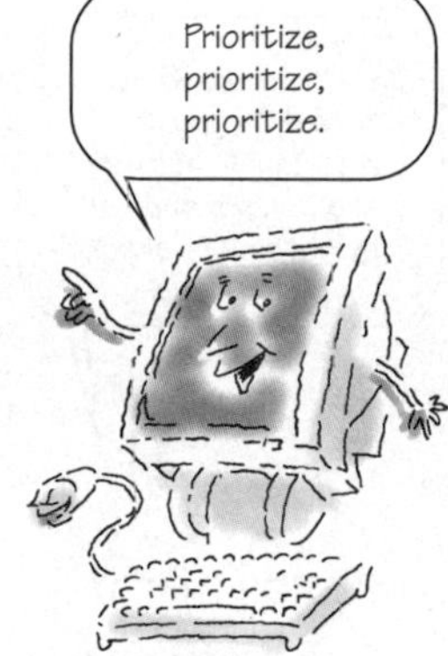

Prioritize, prioritize, prioritize.

71. Which of the following interventions should be the first priority when treating a client experiencing chest pain while walking?

1. Sit the client down.
2. Get the client back to bed.
3. Obtain an electrocardiogram (ECG).
4. Administer sublingual nitroglycerin.

71. 1. The initial priority is to decrease the oxygen consumption; this would be achieved by sitting the client down. An ECG can be obtained after the client is sitting down. After the ECG, sublingual nitroglycerin would be administered. When the client's condition is stabilized, he can be returned to bed.

NP: Implementation; CN: Physiological integrity; CNS: Basic care and comfort; CL: Application

72. Which of the following terms is used to describe reduced cardiac output and perfusion impairment due to ineffective pumping of the heart?

1. Anaphylactic shock
2. Cardiogenic shock
3. Distributive shock
4. Myocardial infarction (MI)

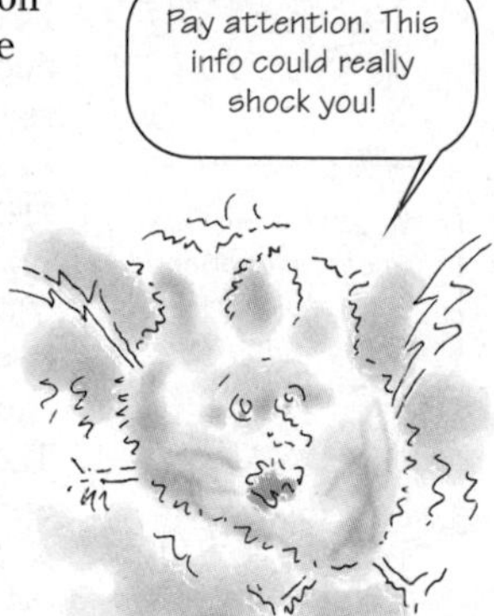

Pay attention. This info could really shock you!

72. 2. Cardiogenic shock is shock related to ineffective pumping of the heart. Anaphylactic shock results from an allergic reaction. Distributive shock results from changes in the intravascular volume distribution and is usually associated with increased cardiac output. MI isn't a shock state, though a severe MI can lead to shock.

NP: Analysis; CN: Physiological integrity; CNS: Physiological adaptation; CL: Knowledge

73. Which of the following conditions most commonly causes cardiogenic shock?
1. Acute myocardial infarction (MI)
2. Coronary artery disease
3. Decreased hemoglobin level
4. Hypotension

73. 1. Of all clients with an acute MI, 15% suffer cardiogenic shock secondary to the myocardial damage and decreased function. Coronary artery disease causes MI. Hypotension is the result of a reduced cardiac output produced by the shock state. A decreased hemoglobin level is a result of bleeding.
NP: Analysis; CN: Physiological integrity; CNS: Reduction of risk potential; CL: Knowledge

74. Which of the following percentages represents the amount of damage the myocardium must sustain before signs and symptoms of cardiogenic shock develop?
1. 10%
2. 25%
3. 40%
4. 90%

74. 3. At least 40% of the heart muscle must be involved for cardiogenic shock to develop. In most circumstances, the heart can compensate for up to 25% damage. An infarction involving 90% of the heart would result in death.
NP: Analysis; CN: Physiological integrity; CNS: Physiological adaptation; CL: Comprehension

75. Myocardial oxygen consumption increases as which of the following parameters increase?
1. Preload, afterload, and cerebral blood flow
2. Preload, afterload, and renal blood flow
3. Preload, afterload, contractility, and heart rate
4. Preload, afterload, cerebral blood flow, and heart rate

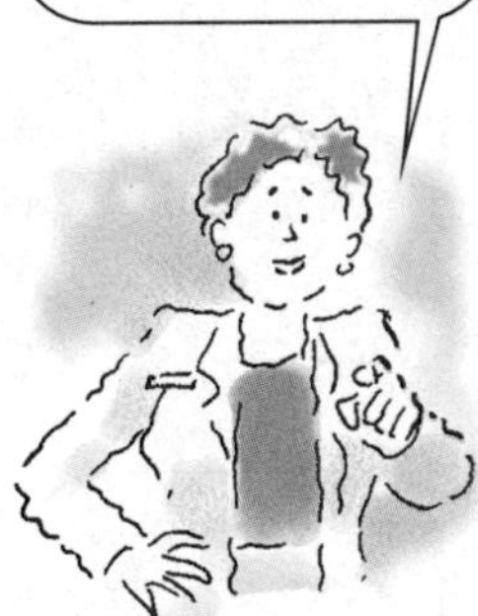

Question 76 is asking you to distinguish between the causes and the symptoms of shock.

75. 3. Myocardial oxygen consumption increases as preload, afterload, renal contractility, and heart rate increase. Cerebral blood flow doesn't directly affect myocardial oxygen consumption.
NP: Analysis; CN: Physiological integrity; CNS: Physiological adaptation; CL: Comprehension

76. Which of the following factors would be most useful in detecting a client's risk of developing cardiogenic shock?
1. Decreased heart rate
2. Decreased cardiac index
3. Decreased blood pressure
4. Decreased cerebral blood flow

76. 2. The cardiac index, a figure derived by dividing the cardiac output by the client's body surface area, is used for identifying whether the cardiac output is meeting a client's needs. Decreased cerebral blood flow, blood pressure, and heart rate are less useful in detecting the risk of cardiogenic shock.
NP: Analysis; CN: Physiological integrity; CNS: Physiological adaptation; CL: Analysis

77. Which of the following symptoms is one of the earliest signs of cardiogenic shock?
1. Tachycardia
2. Decreased urine output
3. Presence of fourth heart sound (S_4)
4. Altered level of consciousness

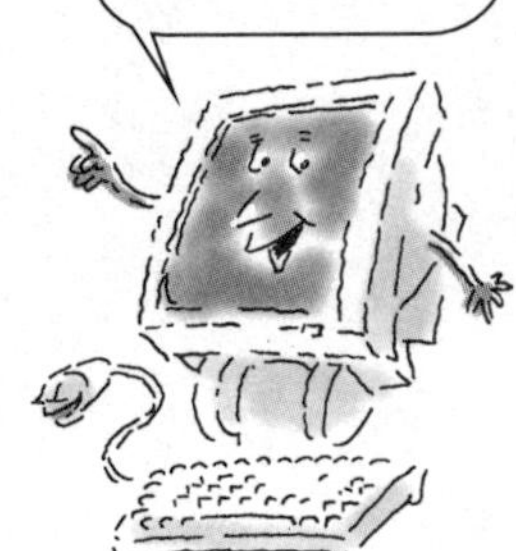

Pay attention. This question involves assessing the order of symptoms.

77. 4. Initially, the decrease in cardiac output results in a decrease in cerebral blood flow that causes restlessness, agitation, or confusion. Tachycardia, decreased urine output, and presence of an S_4 are all later signs of shock.
NP: Evaluation; CN: Physiological integrity; CNS: Basic care and comfort; CL: Application

78. Which of the following diagnostic studies can determine when cellular metabolism becomes anaerobic and when pH decreases?

1. Arterial blood gas (ABG) levels
2. Complete blood count (CBC)
3. Electrocardiogram (ECG)
4. Lung scan

78. 1. ABG levels reflect cellular metabolism and indicate hypoxia. A CBC is performed to determine various constituents of venous blood. An ECG shows the electrical activity of the heart. A lung scan is performed to view functionality of the lungs.

NP: Analysis; CN: Health promotion and maintenance; CNS: Prevention and early detection of disease; CL: Analysis

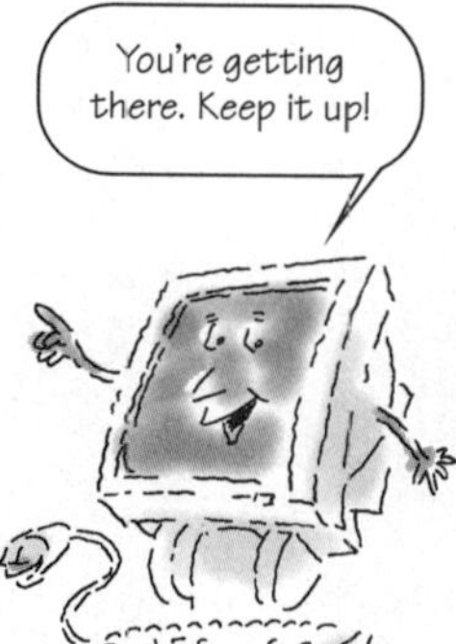

You're getting there. Keep it up!

79. Which of the following is the initial treatment goal for cardiogenic shock?

1. Correct hypoxia
2. Prevent infarction
3. Correct metabolic acidosis
4. Increase myocardial oxygen supply

79. 4. A balance must be maintained between oxygen supply and demand. In a shock state, the myocardium requires more oxygen. If it can't get more oxygen, the shock worsens. Increasing the oxygen will also play a large role in correcting metabolic acidosis and hypoxia. Infarction typically causes the shock state, so prevention isn't an appropriate goal for this condition.

NP: Implementation; CN: Physiological integrity; CN: Physiological adaptation; CL: Comprehension

80. Which of the following drugs is most commonly used to treat cardiogenic shock?

1. Dopamine (Intropin)
2. Enalapril (Vasotec)
3. Furosemide (Lasix)
4. Metoprolol (Lopressor)

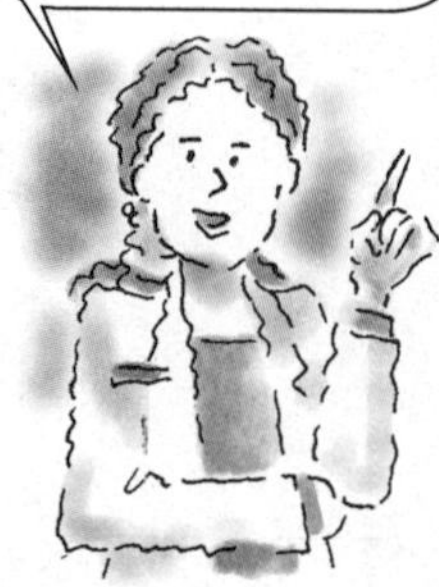

When answering questions, look for phrases such as most commonly. These are often hints.

80. 1. Dopamine, a sympathomimetic drug, improves myocardial contractility and blood flow through vital organs by increasing perfusion pressure. Enalapril is an angiotensin-converting enzyme inhibitor that directly lowers blood pressure. Furosemide is a diuretic and doesn't have a direct effect on contractility or tissue perfusion. Metoprolol is a beta-adrenergic blocker that slows heart rate and lowers blood pressure, neither a desired effect in the treatment of cardiogenic shock.

NP: Analysis; CN: Physiological integrity; CNS: Pharmacological and parenteral therapies; CL: Application

81. Which of the following instruments is used as a diagnostic and monitoring tool for determining the severity of a shock state?

1. Arterial line
2. Indwelling urinary catheter
3. Intra-aortic balloon pump (IABP)
4. Pulmonary artery catheter

81. 4. A pulmonary artery catheter is used to give accurate pressure measurements within the heart, which aids in determining the course of treatment. An arterial line is used to directly assess blood pressure continuously. An indwelling urinary catheter is used to drain the bladder. An IABP is an assistive device used to rest the damaged heart.

NP: Analysis; CN: Physiological integrity; CNS: Pharmacological and parenteral therapies; CL: Knowledge

82. Which of the following parameters represents stage 1 hypertension according to the Sixth Joint National Committee (JNC VI) on the prevention, detection, evaluation, and treatment of high blood pressure?

1. Systolic blood pressure of 160 to 179 mm Hg, or diastolic blood pressure of 100 to109 mm Hg
2. Systolic blood pressure of 180 mm Hg or higher, or diastolic blood pressure of 110 mm Hg or higher
3. Systolic blood pressure of 140 to 159 mm Hg, or diastolic blood pressure of 90 to 99 mm Hg
4. Systolic blood pressure of 130 to 139 mm Hg, or diastolic blood pressure of 85 to 89 mm Hg

82. 3. According to the JNC VI, a systolic blood pressure of 140 to 159 mm Hg or a diastolic pressure of 90 to 99 mm Hg represents stage 1 hypertension. A systolic pressure of 160 to 179 mm Hg or diastolic pressure of 100 to 109 mm Hg represents stage 2 hypertension. A systolic pressure of 180 mm Hg or higher or a diastolic pressure of 110 mm Hg or higher represents stage 3 hypertension. A systolic pressure of 130 to 139 mm Hg or diastolic pressure of 85 to 89 mm Hg is in the high-normal range.

NP: Evaluation; CN: Health promotion and maintenance; CNS: Prevention and early detection of disease; CL: Knowledge

83. Which of the following sounds will be heard during the first phase of Korotkoff's sounds?

1. Disappearance of sounds
2. Faint, clear tapping sounds
3. A murmur or swishing sounds
4. Soft, muffling sounds

83. 2. In phase I, auscultation produces a faint, clear tapping sound that gradually increases in intensity. Phase II produces a murmur sound, and precedes Phase III, the phase marked by an increased intensity of sound. Phase IV produces a muffling sound that gives a soft blowing noise. Phase V, the final phase, is marked by the disappearance of sounds.

NP: Evaluation; CN: Physiological integrity; CNS: Basic care and comfort; CL: Application

84. Which of the following parameters is the major determinant of diastolic blood pressure?

1. Baroreceptors
2. Cardiac output
3. Renal function
4. Vascular resistance

84. 4. Vascular resistance is the impedance of blood flow by the arterioles that most predominantly affects the diastolic pressure. Baroreceptors are nerve endings that are embedded in the blood vessels and respond to the stretching of vessel walls. They don't directly affect diastolic blood pressure. Cardiac output determines systolic blood pressure. Renal function helps control blood volume and indirectly affects diastolic blood pressure.

NP: Analysis; CN: Physiological integrity; CNS: Physiological adaptation; CL: Knowledge

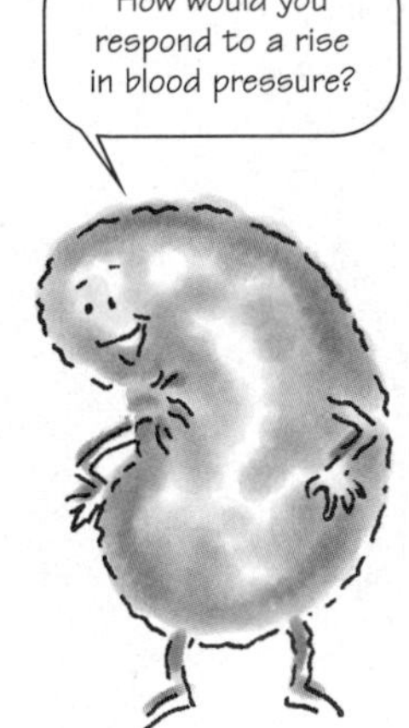
How would you respond to a rise in blood pressure?

85. Which of the following factors can cause blood pressure to drop to normal levels?

1. Kidneys' excretion of sodium only
2. Kidneys' retention of sodium and water
3. Kidneys' excretion of sodium and water
4. Kidneys' retention of sodium and excretion of water

85. 3. The kidneys respond to a rise in blood pressure by excreting sodium and excess water. This response ultimately affects systolic blood pressure by regulating blood volume. Sodium or water retention would only further increase blood pressure. Sodium and water travel together across the membrane in the kidneys; one can't travel without the other.

NP: Analysis; CN: Physiological integrity; CNS: Physiological adaptation; CL: Comprehension

86. Baroreceptors in the carotid artery walls and aorta respond to which of the following conditions?

1. Changes in blood pressure
2. Changes in arterial oxygen tension
3. Changes in arterial carbon dioxide tension
4. Changes in heart rate

86. 1. Baroreceptors located in the carotid arteries and aorta sense pulsatile pressure. Decreases in pulsatile pressure cause a reflex increase in heart rate. Chemoreceptors in the medulla are primarily stimulated by carbon dioxide. Peripheral chemoreceptors in the aorta and carotid arteries are primarily stimulated by oxygen.

NP: Analysis; CN: Physiological integrity; CNS: Physiological adaptation; CL: Knowledge

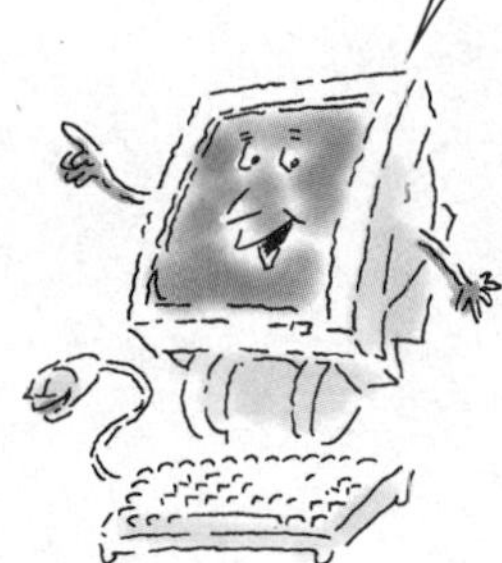

Don't get two tense to answer this question. (Oh, I am just two, er, too clever for words.)

87. Which of the following hormones is responsible for raising arterial pressure and promoting venous return?

1. Angiotensin I
2. Angiotensin II
3. Thyroid hormone
4. Insulin

87. 2. Angiotensin II is a potent vasoconstrictor, thereby promoting venous return. Angiotensin I is a precursor that is converted in the pulmonary vasculature to angiotensin II. Neither thyroid hormone nor insulin have vasoconstrictive properties.

NP: Analysis; CN: Physiological integrity; CNS: Physiological adaptation; CL: Knowledge

88. Which of the following terms is used to describe persistently elevated blood pressure with an unknown cause that accounts for approximately 90% of hypertension cases?

1. Accelerated hypertension
2. Malignant hypertension
3. Primary hypertension
4. Secondary hypertension

88. 3. Characterized by a progressive, usually asymptomatic blood pressure increase over several years, primary hypertension is the most common type. Malignant hypertension, also known as accelerated hypertension, is rapidly progressive, uncontrollable, and causes a rapid onset of complications. Secondary hypertension occurs secondary to a known, correctable cause.

NP: Evaluation; CN: Physiological integrity; CNS: Reduction of risk potential; CL: Analysis

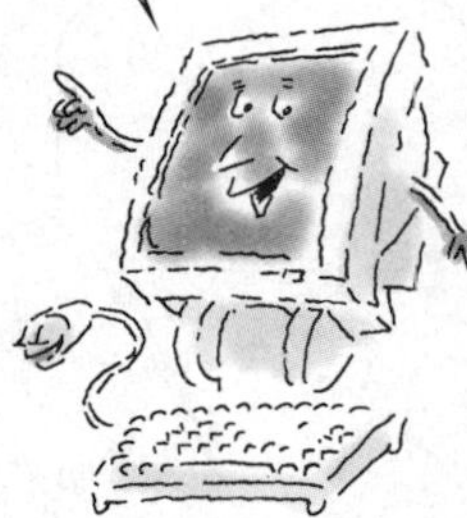

89. Which of the following symptoms of hypertension is most common?

1. Blurred vision
2. Epistaxis
3. Headache
4. Peripheral edema

89. 3. An occipital headache is typical of hypertension secondary to continued increased pressure on the cerebral vasculature. Epistaxis (nosebleed) occurs far less frequently than a headache but can also be a diagnostic sign of hypertension. Blurred vision can result from hypertension due to the arteriolar changes in the eye. Peripheral edema can also occur from an increase in sodium and water retention but is usually a latent sign.

NP: Evaluation; CN: Health promotion and maintenance; CNS: Prevention and early detection of disease; CL: Comprehension

90. The bell of the stethoscope is most commonly placed over which of the following arteries to obtain a blood pressure measurement?

1. Brachial
2. Brachiocephalic
3. Radial
4. Ulnar

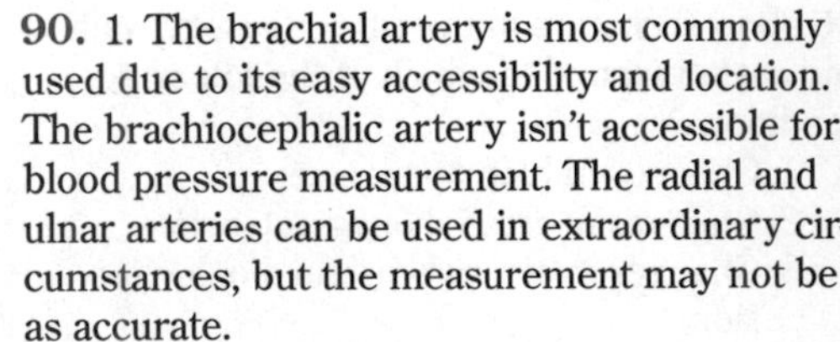

90. 1. The brachial artery is most commonly used due to its easy accessibility and location. The brachiocephalic artery isn't accessible for blood pressure measurement. The radial and ulnar arteries can be used in extraordinary circumstances, but the measurement may not be as accurate.

NP: Analysis; CN: Physiological integrity; CNS: Basic care and comfort; CL: Application

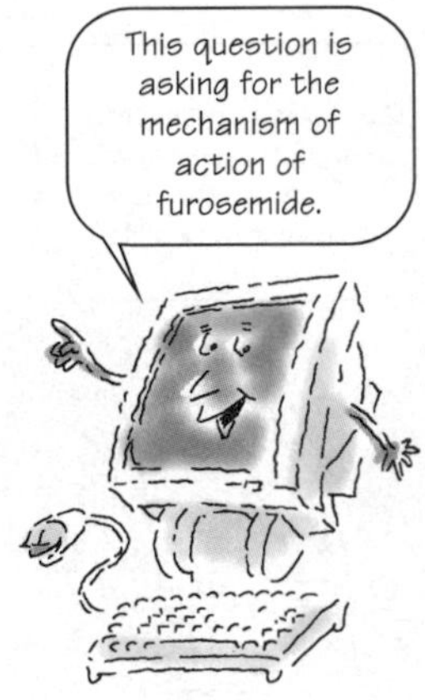

This question is asking for the mechanism of action of furosemide.

91. Which of the following statements explains why furosemide (Lasix) is administered to treat hypertension?

1. It dilates peripheral blood vessels.
2. It decreases sympathetic cardioacceleration.
3. It inhibits the angiotensin-converting enzyme.
4. It inhibits reabsorption of sodium and water in the loop of Henle.

91. 4. Furosemide is a loop diuretic that inhibits sodium and water reabsorption in the loop of Henle, thereby causing a decrease in blood pressure. Vasodilators cause dilation of peripheral blood vessels, directly relaxing vascular smooth muscle and decreasing blood pressure. Adrenergic blockers decrease sympathetic cardioacceleration and decrease blood pressure. Angiotensin-converting enzyme inhibitors decrease blood pressure due to their action on angiotensin.

NP: Analysis; CN: Physiological integrity; CNS: Pharmacological and parenteral therapies; CL: Comprehension

92. The hypothalamus responds to a decrease in blood pressure by secreting which of the following substances?

1. Angiotensin
2. Antidiuretic hormone (ADH)
3. Epinephrine
4. Renin

92. 2. ADH acts on the renal tubules to promote water retention, which increases blood pressure. Angiotensin, epinephrine, and renin aren't stored in the hypothalamus but they all help to increase blood pressure.

NP: Analysis; CN: Physiological integrity; CNS: Physiological adaptation; CL: Knowledge

93. Which of the following parts of the eye is examined to see arterial changes caused by hypertension?

1. Cornea
2. Fovea
3. Retina
4. Sclera

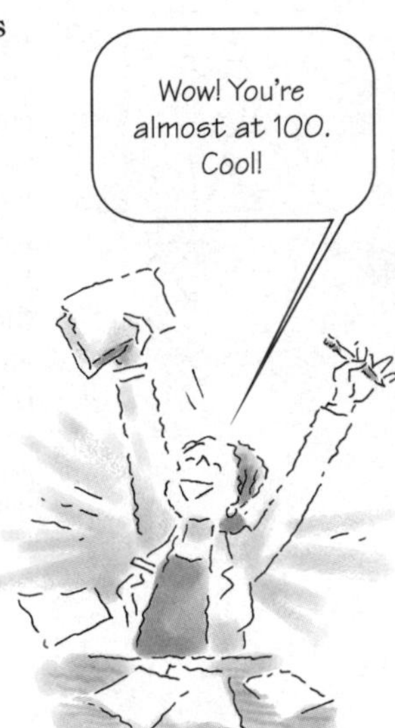

Wow! You're almost at 100. Cool!

93. 3. The retina is the only site in the body where arteries can be seen without invasive techniques. Changes in the retinal arteries signal similar damage to vessels elsewhere. The cornea is the nonvascular, transparent fibrous coat where the iris can be seen. The fovea is the point of central vision. The sclera is the fibrous tissue that forms the outer protective covering over the eyeball.

NP: Analysis; CN: Health promotion and maintenance; CNS: Prevention and early detection of disease; CL: Knowledge

94. Which of the following conditions causes varicose veins?
1. Tunica media tear
2. Intraluminal occlusion
3. Intraluminal valvular compression
4. Intraluminal valvular incompetence

94. 4. Varicose veins, dilated tortuous surface veins engorged with blood, result from intraluminal valvular incompetence. An intraluminal occlusion would result from plaque or thrombosis. The valves aren't outside the lumen (intraluminal) and a tear would result in a hematoma.

NP: Analysis; CN: Physiological integrity; CNS: Physiological adaptation; CL: Knowledge

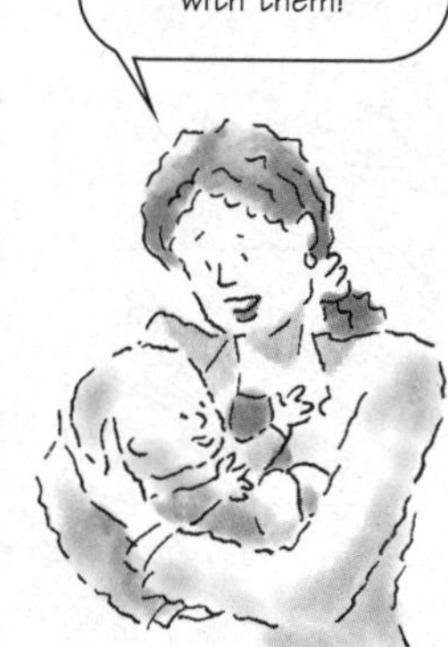

Oooh, I love babies. But not the varicose veins that go with them!

95. Which of the following factors causes primary varicose veins?
1. Hypertension
2. Pregnancy
3. Thrombosis
4. Trauma

95. 2. Primary varicose veins have a gradual onset and progressively worsen. In pregnancy, the expanding uterus and increased vascular volume impede blood return to the heart. The pressure places increased stress on the veins. Hypertension has no role in varicose vein formation. Thrombosis and trauma cause valvular incompetence and so are secondary causes of varicosities — not primary.

NP: Analysis; CN: Health promotion and maintenance; CNS: Prevention and early detection of disease; CL: Comprehension

96. Which of the following symptoms commonly occur in a client with varicose veins?
1. Fatigue and pressure
2. Fatigue and cool feet
3. Sharp pain and fatigue
4. Sharp pain and cool feet

96. 1. Fatigue and pressure are classic signs of varicose veins, secondary to increased blood volume and edema. Sharp pain and cool feet are symptoms of alteration in arterial blood flow.

NP: Evaluation; CN: Physiological integrity; CNS: Physiological adaptation; CL: Comprehension

97. In which of the following veins do varicose veins most commonly occur?
1. Brachial
2. Femoral
3. Renal
4. Saphenous

97. 4. Varicose veins occur most frequently in the saphenous veins of the lower extremities. They don't develop in the brachial, femoral, or renal veins.

NP: Analysis; CN: Physiological integrity; CNS: Physiological adaptation; CL: Knowledge

98. Which of the following conditions is caused by increased hydrostatic pressure and chronic venous stasis?
1. Venous occlusion
2. Cool extremities
3. Nocturnal calf muscle cramps
4. Diminished blood supply to the feet

98. 3. Calf muscle cramps result from increased pressure and venous stasis secondary to varicose veins. An occlusion is a blockage of blood flow. Cool extremities and diminished blood supply to the feet are symptoms of arterial blood flow changes.

NP: Analysis; CN: Health promotion and maintenance; CNS: Prevention and early detection of disease; CL: Analysis

99. Which of the following activities should a client with varicose veins avoid?
1. Exercise
2. Leg elevations
3. Prolonged lying
4. Wearing tight clothing

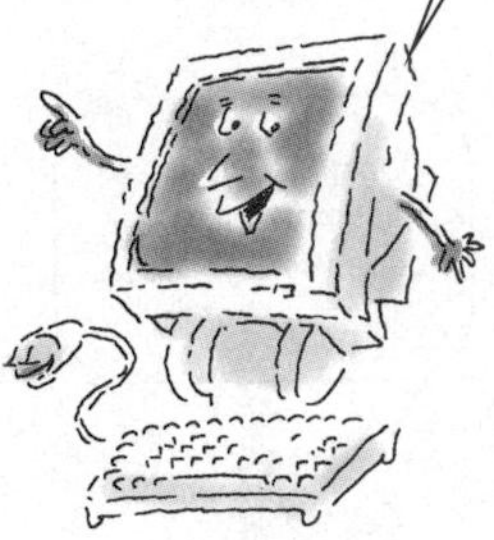

Be careful. Using the word *avoid* makes this almost a negative question.

99. 4. Tight clothing, especially below the waist, increases vascular volume and impedes blood return to the heart. Exercise, leg elevations, and lying down usually relieve symptoms of varicose veins.
NP: Analysis; CN: Health promotion and maintenance; CNS: Prevention and early detection of disease; CL: Comprehension

100. Which of the following tests demonstrates the backward flow of blood through incompetent valves of superficial veins?
1. Trendelenburg's test
2. Manual compression test
3. Perthes' test
4. Plethysmography

100. 1. Trendelenburg's test is the most accurate tool used to determine retrograde venous filling. The manual compression test is a quick, easy test done by palpation and usually isn't diagnostic of the backward flow of blood. Perthes' test easily indicates whether the deeper venous system and communicating veins are competent. Plethysmography allows measurement of changes in venous blood volume.
NP: Analysis; CN: Health promotion and maintenance; CNS: Prevention and early detection of disease; CL: Application

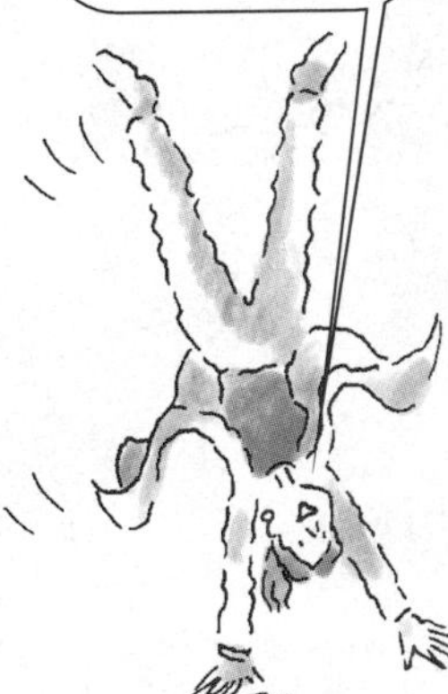

Congratulations! You've finished 100 questions! You're almost there!

101. Which of the following signs and symptoms are produced by secondary varicose veins?
1. Pallor and severe pain
2. Severe pain and edema
3. Edema and pigmentation
4. Absent hair growth and pigmentation

101. 3. Secondary varicose veins result from an obstruction of the deep veins. Incompetent valves lead to impaired blood flow, and edema and pigmentation result from venous stasis. Severe pain, pallor, and absent hair growth are symptoms of an altered arterial blood flow.
NP: Analysis; CN: Physiological integrity; CNS: Physiological adaptation; CL: Comprehension

102. Which of the following treatments can be used to eliminate varicose veins?
1. Ablation therapy
2. Cold therapy
3. Ligation and stripping
4. Radiation

102. 3. Ligation and stripping of the vein can rid the vein of varicosity. This invasive procedure will take care of current varicose veins only; it won't prevent others from forming. The other procedures aren't used for varicose veins.
NP: Analysis; CN: Physiological integrity; CNS: Pharmacological and parenteral therapies; CL: Knowledge

103. Which of the following treatments is recommended for postoperative management of a client who has undergone ligation and stripping?
1. Sitting
2. Bed rest
3. Ice packs
4. Elastic leg compression

103. 4. Elastic leg compression helps venous return to the heart, thereby decreasing venous stasis. Sitting and bed rest are contraindicated because both promote decreased blood return to the heart and venous stasis. Although ice packs would help reduce edema, they would also cause vasoconstriction and impede blood flow.
NP: Implementation; CN: Physiological integrity; CNS: Basic care and comfort; CL: Application

104. Which of the following factors usually causes deep vein thrombosis (DVT)?
1. Aerobic exercise
2. Inactivity
3. Pregnancy
4. Tight clothing

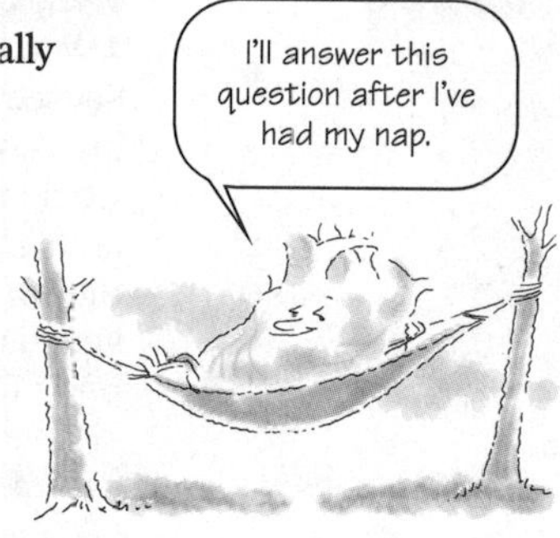

I'll answer this question after I've had my nap.

104. 2. A thrombus lodged in a vein can cause venous occlusion as a result of venous stasis. Inactivity can cause venous stasis, leading to DVT. Aerobic exercise helps to prevent venous stasis. Pregnancy and tight clothing can cause varicose veins, which can lead to venous stasis and eventually DVT, but these aren't primary causes.

NP: Analysis; CN: Health promotion and maintenance; CNS: Prevention and early detection of disease; CL: Knowledge

105. Which of the following terms is used to describe a thrombus lodged in the lungs?
1. Hemothorax
2. Pneumothorax
3. Pulmonary embolism
4. Pulmonary hypertension

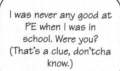

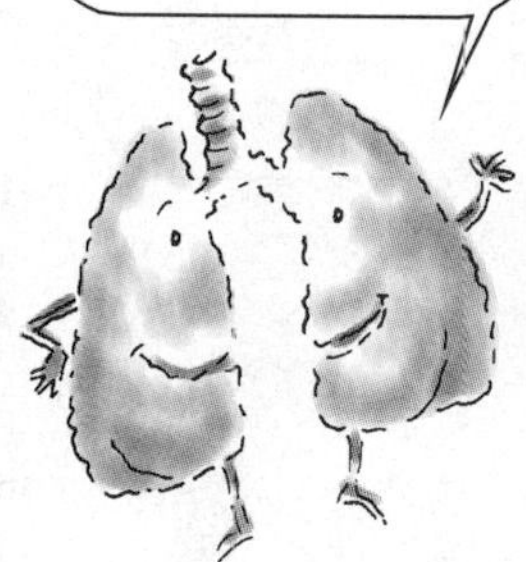

I was never any good at PE when I was in school. Were you? (That's a clue, don'tcha know.)

105. 3. A pulmonary embolism is a blood clot lodged in the pulmonary vasculature. A hemothorax refers to blood in the pleural space. A pneumothorax is caused by an opening in the pleura. Pulmonary hypertension is an increase in pulmonary artery pressure, which increases the workload of the right ventricle.

NP: Analysis; CN: Physiological integrity; CNS: Physiological adaptation; CL: Knowledge

106. Which of the following terms refers to the condition of blood coagulating faster than normal, causing thrombin and other clotting factors to multiply?
1. Embolus
2. Hypercoagulability
3. Venous stasis
4. Venous wall injury

106. 2. Hypercoagulability is the condition of blood coagulating faster than normal, causing thrombin and other clotting factors to multiply. This condition, along with venous stasis and venous wall injury, accounts for the formation of deep vein thrombosis. An embolus is a blood clot or fatty globule that formed in one area and is carried through the bloodstream to another area.

NP: Analysis; CN: Physiological integrity; CNS: Physiological adaptation; CL: Comprehension

107. Which of the following characteristics is typical of the pain associated with deep vein thrombosis (DVT)?
1. Dull ache
2. No pain
3. Sudden onset
4. Tingling

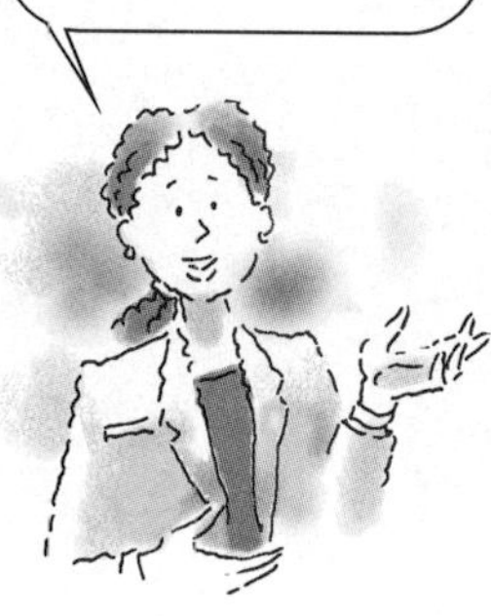

This question is asking you to characterize the type of pain experienced during deep vein thrombosis.

107. 3. DVT is associated with deep leg pain of sudden onset, which occurs secondary to the occlusion. A dull ache is more commonly associated with varicose veins. A tingling sensation is associated with an alteration in arterial blood flow. If the thrombus is large enough, it will cause pain.

NP: Analysis; CN: Physiological integrity; CNS: Basic care and comfort; CL: Analysis

108. Which of the following treatments can relieve pain from deep vein thrombosis (DVT)?
1. Application of heat
2. Bed rest
3. Exercise
4. Leg elevation

108. 4. Leg elevation alleviates the pressure caused by thrombosis and occlusion by assisting venous return. The application of heat would dilate the vessels and pool blood in the area of the thrombus, increasing the risk of further thrombus formation. Bed rest adds to venous stasis by increasing the risk of thrombosis formation. When DVT is diagnosed, exercise isn't recommended until the clot has dissolved.

NP: Analysis; CN: Physiological integrity; CNS: Basic care and comfort; CL: Comprehension

109. Which of the following terms best describes the findings on cautious palpation of the vein in typical superficial thrombophlebitis?
1. Dilated
2. Knotty
3. Smooth
4. Tortuous

109. 2. The knotty feeling is secondary to the emboli adhering to the vein wall. Varicose veins may be described as dilated and tortuous. Normal veins feel smooth.

NP: Evaluation; CN: Physiological integrity; CNS: Physiological adaptation; CL: Application

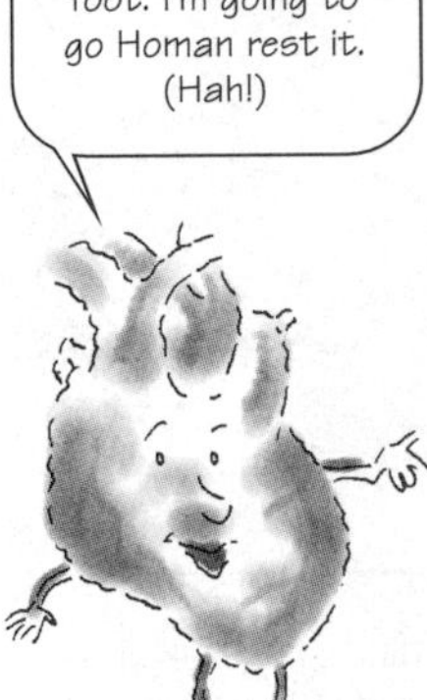

I have a pain in my foot. I'm going to go Homan rest it. (Hah!)

110. Which of the following terms is used to describe pain in the calf due to sharp dorsiflexion of the foot?
1. Dyskinesia
2. Eversion
3. Positive Babinski's reflex
4. Positive Homans' sign

110. 4. A positive Homans' sign (elicited by quickly dorsiflexing the foot), when accompanied by other findings, is diagnostic of deep vein thrombosis (DVT). Alone, however, Homans' sign can't be used to diagnose DVT because other conditions of the calf can produce a positive Homans' sign. Dyskinesia is the inability to perform voluntary movement. Eversion is the outward movement of the transverse tarsal joint. A positive Babinski's reflex is an extensor plantar response.

NP: Evaluation; CN: Health promotion and maintenance; CNS: Prevention and early detection of disease; CL: Comprehension

111. Which of the following conditions causes intermittent claudication (cramplike pains in the calves)?
1. Inadequate blood supply
2. Elevated leg position
3. Dependent leg position
4. Inadequate muscle oxygenation

111. 4. When a muscle is starved of oxygen, it produces pain much like that of angina. Inadequate blood supply would cause necrosis. Leg position either alleviates or aggravates the condition.

NP: Analysis; CN: Physiological integrity; CNS: Physiological adaptation; CL: Knowledge

112. Which of the following medical treatments should be administered to treat intermittent claudication?
1. Analgesics
2. Warfarin (Coumadin)
3. Heparin
4. Pentoxifylline (Trental)

112. 4. Pentoxifylline decreases blood viscosity, increases red blood cell flexibility, and improves flow through small vessels. Analgesics are administered for pain relief. Warfarin and heparin are anticoagulants.

NP: Analysis; CN: Physiological integrity; CNS: Pharmacological and parenteral therapies; CL: Knowledge

113. Which of the following oral medications is administered to prevent further thrombus formation?
1. Warfarin (Coumadin)
2. Heparin
3. Furosemide (Lasix)
4. Metoprolol (Lopressor)

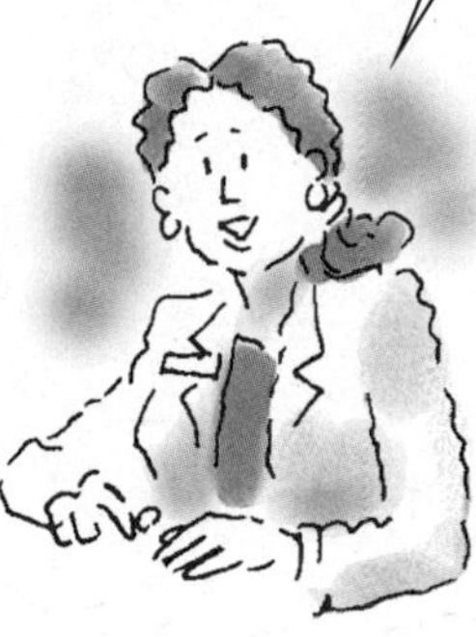

This question requires you to know how certain drugs are administered.

113. 1. Warfarin prevents vitamin K from synthesizing certain clotting factors. This oral anticoagulant can be given long-term. Heparin is a parenteral anticoagulant that interferes with coagulation by readily combining with antithrombin; it can't be given by mouth. Neither furosemide nor metoprolol affect anticoagulation.

NP: Analysis; CN: Physiological integrity; CNS: Pharmacological and parenteral therapies; CL: Application

114. Which of the following positions would best aid breathing for a client with acute pulmonary edema?
1. Lying flat in bed
2. Left side-lying
3. In high Fowler's position
4. In semi-Fowler's position

114. 3. A high Fowler's position promotes ventilation and facilitates breathing by reducing venous return. Lying flat and side-lying positions worsen the breathing and increase workload of the heart. Semi-Fowler's position won't reduce the workload of the heart as well as Fowler's position will.

NP: Implementation; CN: Physiological integrity; CNS: Basic care and comfort; CL: Comprehension

115. Which of the following blood gas abnormalities is initially most suggestive of pulmonary edema?
1. Anoxia
2. Hypercapnia
3. Hyperoxygenation
4. Hypocapnia

115. 4. In an attempt to compensate for increased work of breathing due to hyperventilation, carbon dioxide (CO_2) decreases, causing hypocapnia. If the condition persists, CO_2 retention occurs and hypercapnia results. Although oxygenation is relatively low, the client isn't anoxic. Hyperoxygenation would result if the client was given oxygen in excess. However, secondary to fluid build-up, the client would have a low oxygenation level.

NP: Analysis; CN: Physiological integrity; CNS: Physiological adaptation; CL: Analysis

116. Which of the following is a compensatory response to decreased cardiac output?
1. Decreased blood pressure
2. Alteration in level of consciousness (LOC)
3. Decreased blood pressure and diuresis
4. Increased blood pressure and fluid volume

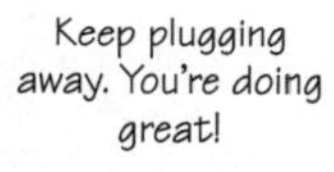

Keep plugging away. You're doing great!

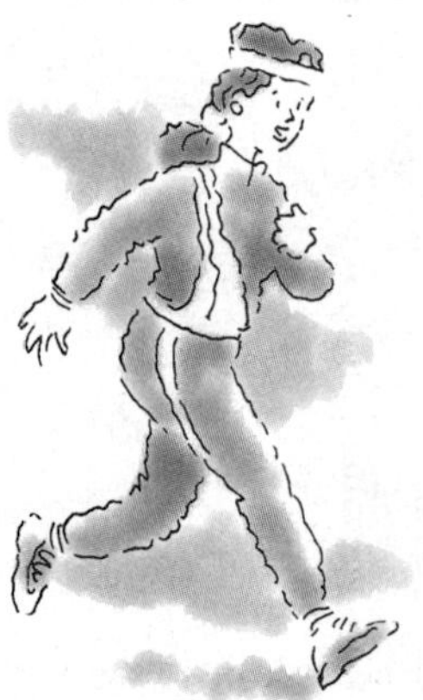

116. 4. The body compensates for a decrease in cardiac output with a rise in blood pressure, due to the stimulation of the sympathetic nervous system and an increase in blood volume as the kidneys retain sodium and water. Blood pressure doesn't initially drop in response to the compensatory mechanism of the body. Alteration in LOC will occur only if the decreased cardiac output persists.

NP: Analysis; CN: Physiological integrity; CNS: Physiological adaptation; CL: Knowledge

117. Which of the following actions is the appropriate initial response to a client coughing up pink, frothy sputum?

1. Call for help.
2. Call the physician.
3. Start an I.V. line.
4. Suction the client.

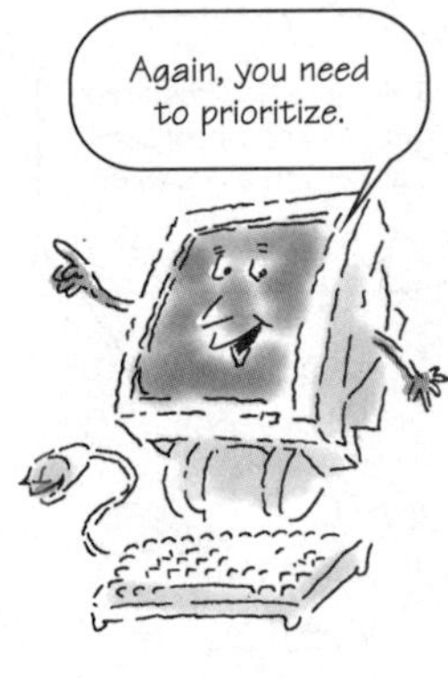

Again, you need to prioritize.

117. 1. Production of pink, frothy sputum is a classic sign of acute pulmonary edema. Because the client is at high risk for decompensation, the nurse should call for help but not leave the room. The other three interventions would immediately follow.
NP: Evaluation; CN: Physiological integrity; CNS: Physiological adaptation; CL: Comprehension

118. Which of the following precautions should a client be instructed to take after an episode of acute pulmonary edema?

1. Limit caloric intake.
2. Restrict carbohydrates.
3. Measure weight twice per day.
4. Call the physician if there is weight gain of more than 3 lb (1.5 kg) in 1 day.

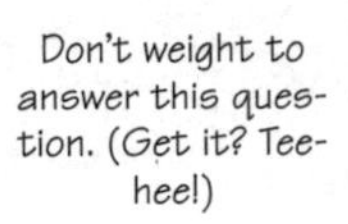

Don't weight to answer this question. (Get it? Tee-hee!)

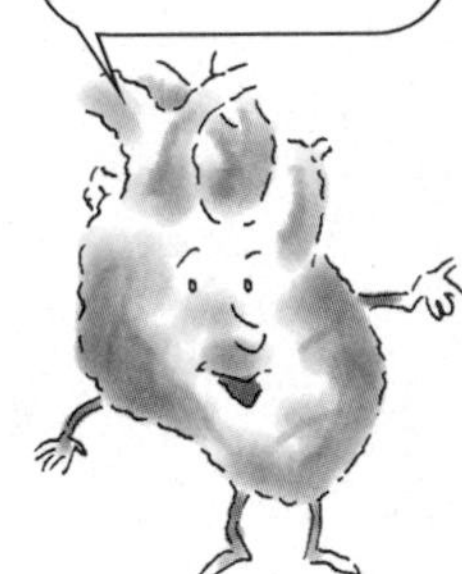

118. 4. Gaining 3 lb in 1 day is indicative of fluid retention that would increase the workload of the heart, thereby putting the client at risk for acute pulmonary edema. Restricting carbohydrates wouldn't affect fluid status. Limiting caloric intake doesn't influence fluid status. The body needs carbohydrates for energy and healing. The client must be weighed in the morning after the first urination. If the client is weighed later in the day, the finding wouldn't be accurate because of fluid intake during the day.
NP: Analysis; CN: Physiological integrity; CNS: Reduction of risk potential; CL: Knowledge

119. Which of the following terms describes the force against which the ventricle must expel blood?

1. Afterload
2. Cardiac output
3. Overload
4. Preload

119. 1. Afterload refers to the resistance normally maintained by the aortic and pulmonic valves, the condition and tone of the aorta, and the resistance offered by the systemic and pulmonary arterioles. Cardiac output is the amount of blood expelled from the heart per minute. Overload refers to an abundance of circulating volume. Preload is the volume of blood in the ventricle at the end of diastole.
NP: Analysis; CN: Physiological integrity; CNS: Physiological adaptation; CL: Knowledge

120. After recovery from an episode of acute pulmonary edema, why would an angiotensin-converting enzyme (ACE) inhibitor be administered?

1. To promote diuresis
2. To increase contractility
3. To decrease contractility
4. To reduce blood pressure

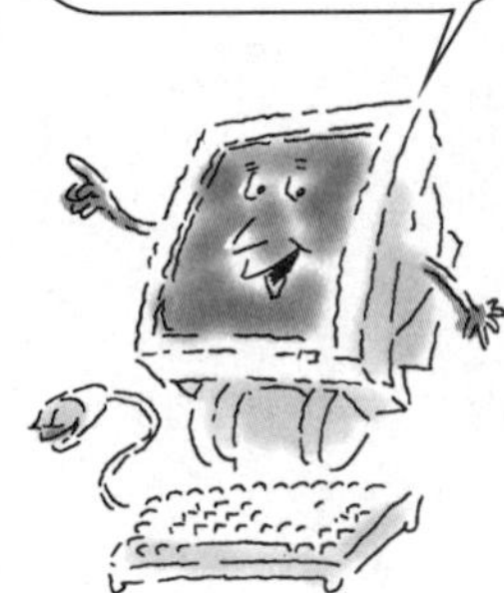

This is another question that tests your knowledge of what certain drugs do.

120. 4. ACE inhibitors are given to reduce blood pressure by inhibiting aldosterone production, which in turn decreases sodium and water reabsorption. ACE inhibitors also reduce production of angiotensin II, a potent vasoconstrictor. Diuretics are given to promote diuresis. Inotropic agents increase contractility. Negative inotropic agents decrease contractility.
NP: Analysis; CN: Physiological integrity; CNS: Pharmacological and parenteral therapies; CL: Knowledge

NP: Nursing process CN: Client needs category CNS: Client needs subcategory CL: Cognitive level

121. Acute pulmonary edema caused by heart failure is usually a result of damage to which of the following areas of the heart?
1. Left atrium
2. Right atrium
3. Left ventricle
4. Right ventricle

121. 3. The left ventricle is responsible for the majority of force for the cardiac output. If the left ventricle is damaged, the output decreases and fluid accumulates in the interstitial and alveolar spaces, causing pulmonary edema. Damage to the left atrium would contribute to heart failure but wouldn't affect cardiac output or, therefore, the onset of pulmonary edema. If the right atrium and right ventricle were damaged, right-sided heart failure would result.
NP: Analysis; CN: Physiological integrity; CNS: Physiological adaptation; CL: Comprehension

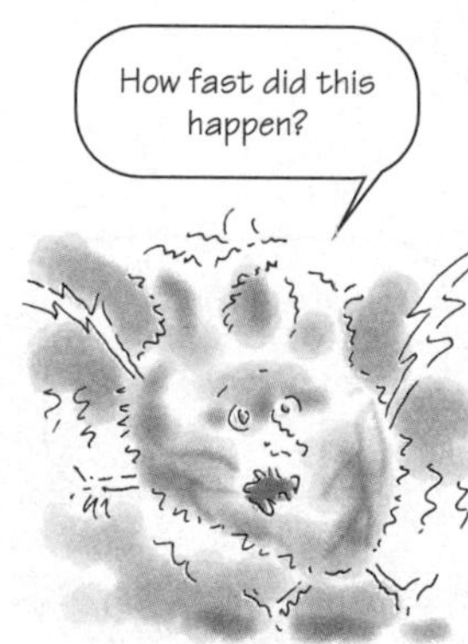

How fast did this happen?

122. How quickly can an episode of acute pulmonary edema develop?
1. In minutes
2. In ½ hour
3. In 1 hour
4. In 3 hours

122. 1. Pulmonary edema can develop in minutes, secondary to a sudden fluid shift from the pulmonary vasculature to the lung interstitial alveoli.
NP: Evaluation; CN: Physiological Integrity; CNS: Physiological adaptation; CL: Comprehension

123. Which of the following terms is used to describe the amount of stretch on the myocardium at the end of diastole?
1. Afterload
2. Cardiac index
3. Cardiac output
4. Preload

123. 4. Preload is the amount of stretch of the cardiac muscle fibers at the end of diastole. The volume of blood in the ventricle at the end of diastole determines preload. Afterload is the force against which the ventricle must expel blood. Cardiac index is the individualized measurement of cardiac output, based on the client's body surface area. Cardiac output is the amount of blood the heart is expelling per minute.
NP: Analysis; CN: Physiological integrity; CNS: Physiological adaptation; CL: Knowledge

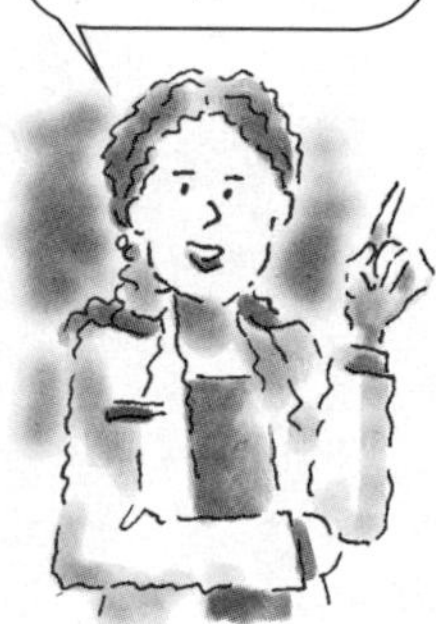

Which answer best promotes compliance?

124. Which of the following actions should a nurse take when administering a new blood pressure medication to a client?
1. Administer the medication to the client without explanation.
2. Inform the client of the new drug only if he asks about it.
3. Inform the client of the new medication, its name, use, and the reason for the change in medication.
4. Administer the medication, and inform the client that the physician will later explain the medication.

124. 3. Informing the client of the medication, its use, and the reason for the medication change is important to the care of the client. Teaching the client about his treatment regimen promotes compliance. The other responses are inappropriate.
NP: Implementation; CN: Safe, effective care environment; CNS: Management of care; CL: Application

125. Antihypertensives should be used cautiously in clients taking which of the following drugs?

1. Ibuprofen (Advil)
2. Diphenhydramine (Benadryl)
3. Thioridazine (Mellaril)
4. Vitamins

125. 3. Thioridazine affects the neurotransmitter norepinephrine, which causes hypotension and other cardiovascular effects. Administering an antihypertensive to a client who already has hypotension could have serious adverse effects. Ibuprofen is an anti-inflammatory that doesn't interfere with the cardiovascular system. Although diphenhydramine does have histaminic effects, such as sedation, it isn't known to decrease blood pressure. Vitamins aren't drugs and don't interfere with cardiovascular function.

NP: Analysis; CN: Physiological integrity; CNS: Pharmacological and parenteral therapies; CL: Knowledge

126. A 57-year-old client with a history of bronchial asthma is prescribed propranolol (Inderal) to control hypertension. Before administering propranolol, which of the following actions should the nurse take first?

1. Monitor the apical pulse rate.
2. Instruct the client to take the medication with food.
3. Question the physician about the order.
4. Caution the client to rise slowly when standing.

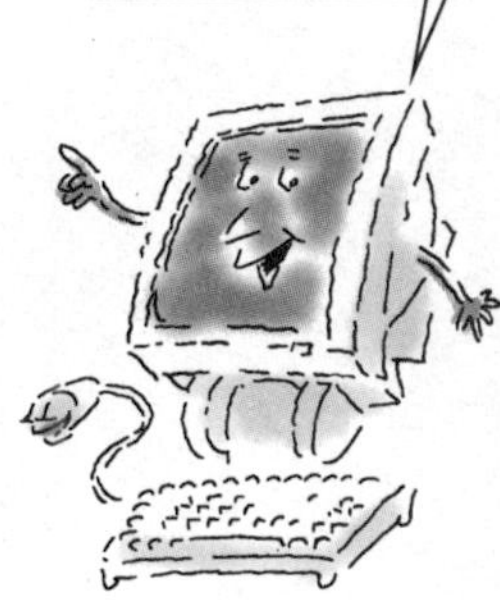
Note the first in question 126. It's the key to the right answer.

126. 3. Propranolol and other beta-adrenergic blockers are contraindicated in a client with bronchial asthma, so the nurse should question the physician before giving the dose. The other responses are appropriate actions for a client receiving propranolol, but questioning the physician takes priority. The client's apical pulse should always be checked before giving propranolol; if the pulse rate is extremely low, the nurse should withhold the drug and notify the physician. Taking propranolol with food enhances its absorption. Because propranolol can cause light-headedness, the client should be told to rise slowly when standing.

NP: Implementation; CN: Physiological integrity; CNS: Pharmacological and parenteral therapies; CL: Application

127. One hour after administering I.V. furosemide (Lasix) to a client with heart failure, a short burst of ventricular tachycardia appears on the cardiac monitor. Which of the following electrolyte imbalances should the nurse suspect?

1. Hypocalcemia
2. Hypermagnesemia
3. Hypokalemia
4. Hypernatremia

127. 3. Furosemide is a potassium-depleting diuretic that can cause hypokalemia. In turn, hypokalemia increases myocardial excitability, leading to ventricular tachycardia. Hypocalcemia, which slows conduction through the atrioventricular junction, can cause such bradyarrhythmias as atrioventricular block. Hypermagnesemia may lead to bradycardia, not tachycardia. Hypernatremia may cause sinus tachycardia as a result of water loss.

NP: Assessment; CN: Physiological integrity; CNS: Physiological adaptation; CL: Analysis

128. A client has a reduced serum high-density lipoprotein (HDL) level and an elevated low-density lipoprotein (LDL) level. Which of the following dietary modifications is not appropriate for this client?

1. Fiber intake of 25 to 30 g daily
2. Less than 30% of calories from fat
3. Cholesterol intake of less than 300 mg daily
4. Less than 10% of calories from saturated fat

128. 2. A client with low serum HDL and high serum LDL levels should get less than 30% of daily calories from fat. The other modifications are appropriate for this client.

NP: Planning; CN: Physiological integrity; CNS: Reduction of risk potential; CL: Application

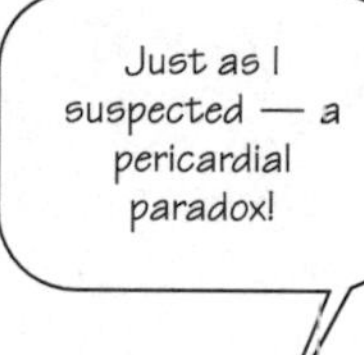
Just as I
suspected — a
pericardial
paradox!

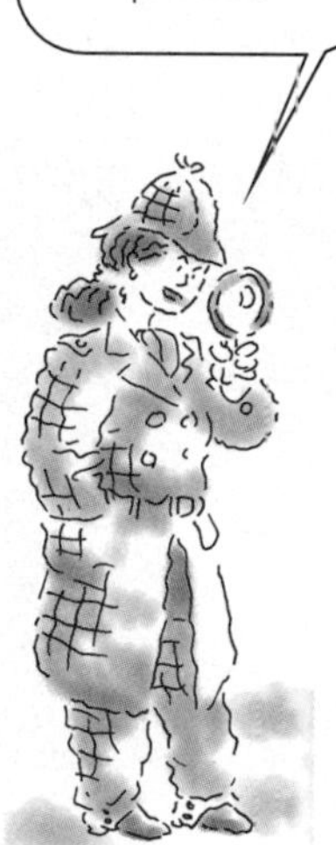

129. A paradoxical pulse occurs in a client who had coronary artery bypass graft (CABG) surgery 2 days ago. Which of the following surgical complications should the nurse suspect?

1. Left-sided heart failure
2. Aortic regurgitation
3. Complete heart block
4. Pericardial tamponade

129. 4. A paradoxical pulse (a palpable decrease in pulse amplitude on quiet inspiration) signals pericardial tamponade, a complication of CABG surgery. Left-sided heart failure can cause pulsus alternans (pulse amplitude alternation from beat to beat, with a regular rhythm). Aortic regurgitation may cause bisferious pulse (an increased arterial pulse with a double systolic peak). Complete heart block may cause a bounding pulse (a strong pulse with increased pulse pressure).

NP: Assessment; CN: Physiological integrity; CNS: Physiological adaptation; CL: Application

130. A 35-year-old client was admitted to the coronary care unit (CCU) 2 days ago with an acute myocardial infarction. Which of the following actions would breach client confidentiality?

1. The CCU nurse gives a verbal report to the nurse on the telemetry unit before transferring the client to that unit.
2. The CCU nurse notifies the on-call physician about a change in the client's condition.
3. The emergency department nurse calls up the latest electrocardiogram results to check the client's progress.
4. At the client's request, the CCU nurse updates the client's wife on his condition.

130. 3. The emergency department nurse is no longer directly involved with the client's care and thus has no legal right to information about his present condition. Anyone directly involved in his care (such as the telemetry nurse and the on-call physician) has the right to information about his condition. Because the client requested that the nurse update his wife on his condition, doing so doesn't breach confidentiality.

NP: Evaluation; CN: Safe, effective care environment; CNS: Management of care; CL: Application

131. A client arriving in the emergency department is receiving cardiopulmonary resuscitation from paramedics, who are giving ventilations through an endotracheal (ET) tube that they placed in the client's home. During a pause in compressions, the cardiac monitor shows narrow QRS complexes and a heart rate of 55 beats/minute with a palpable pulse. Which of the following actions should the nurse take first?

1. Start an I.V. line and administer amiodarone (Cordarone), 300 mg I.V. over 10 minutes.
2. Check endotracheal tube placement.
3. Obtain an arterial blood gas (ABG) sample.
4. Administer atropine, 1 mg I.V.

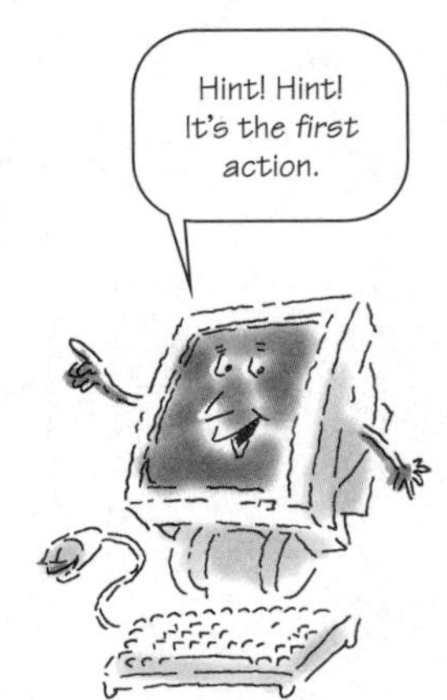
Hint! Hint!
It's the first action.

131. 2. ET tube placement should be confirmed as soon as the client arrives in the emergency department. Once the airway is secured, oxygenation and ventilation should be confirmed using an end-tidal carbon dioxide monitor and pulse oximetry. Next, the nurse should make sure I.V. access is established. If the client experiences symptomatic bradycardia, atropine is administered as ordered, 0.5 to 1 mg every 3 to 5 minutes to a total of 3 mg. Then the nurse should try to find the cause of the client's arrest by obtaining an ABG sample. Amiodarone is indicated for ventricular tachycardia, ventricular fibrillation, and atrial flutter—not symptomatic bradycardia.

NP: Implementation; CN: Physiological integrity; CNS: Physiological adaptation; CL: Application

132. After unsuccessful cardiopulmonary resuscitation efforts, the nurse must prepare an Islamic client for the morgue. Which nursing action is appropriate when caring for a client of the Islamic faith?

1. Allowing the client's family to perform the ritualistic washing
2. Doing nothing; the Burial Society will perform a ritual cleansing
3. Doing nothing; only the family and close friends may touch the body
4. Providing routine postmortem care

132. 1. Physical care at death for a person of the Islamic faith consists of ritualistic washing by the family, with the client's body positioned toward Mecca. The Burial Society may perform ritual cleansing for clients of the Jewish faith. Hindu clients believe that only family and close friends should touch the body. Routine postmortem care is appropriate for Christian clients.

NP: Implementation; CN: Psychosocial integrity; CNS: Coping and adaptation; CL: Comprehension

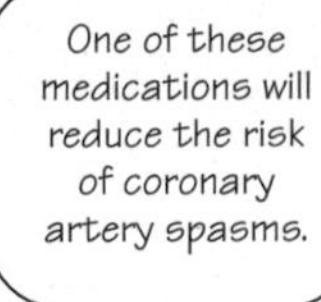
One of these medications will reduce the risk of coronary artery spasms.

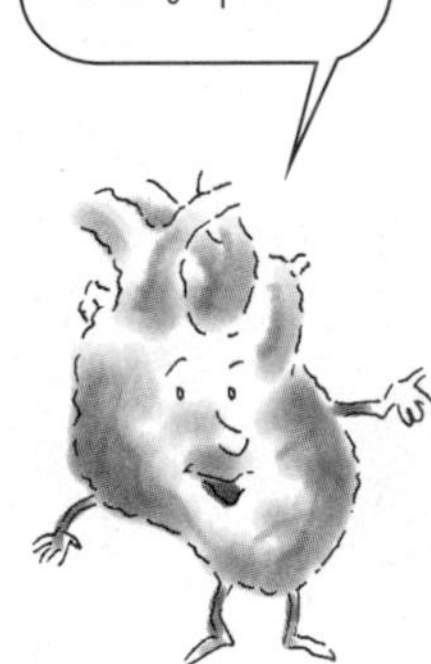

133. A 63-year-old client has Prinzmetal's angina. To reduce the risk of coronary artery spasms, which type of medication is the physician most likely to prescribe?

1. Beta-adrenergic blocker
2. Angiotensin-converting enzyme (ACE) inhibitor
3. Inotropic vasodilator
4. Calcium channel blocker

133. 4. A calcium channel blocker, such as diltiazem (Cardizem), is indicated in managing Prinzmetal's angina because it reduces the incidence of coronary artery spasm. A beta-adrenergic blocker, such as metoprolol (Lopressor), treats angina by decreasing myocardial oxygen needs and has no effect on coronary artery spasms. An ACE inhibitor, such as enalapril (Vasotec), is used to manage hypertension. An inotropic vasodilator, such as milrinone (Primacor), is indicated for short-term I.V. therapy in heart failure.

NP: Planning; CN: Physiological integrity; CNS: Pharmacological and parenteral therapies; CL: Application

134. An 86-year-old client with heart failure is receiving furosemide (Lasix), 40 mg I.V. The physician orders 40 mEq of potassium chloride in 100 ml of dextrose 5% in water, to infuse over 4 hours. The client's most recent serum potassium level is 3.0 mEq/L. At which infusion rate should the nurse set the I.V. pump?

1. 25 ml/hour
2. 10 ml/hour
3. 100 ml/hour
4. 50 ml/hour

134. 1. Use the following formula to determine the infusion rate:

$$\text{ml/hour} = \frac{\text{total volume (in ml) to be infused}}{\text{total time of infusion in hours}}$$

$$\text{ml/hour} = \frac{100 \text{ ml}}{4 \text{ hours}}$$

$$\text{ml/hour} = 25$$

NP: Implementation; CN: Physiological integrity; CNS: Pharmacological and parenteral therapies; CL: Application

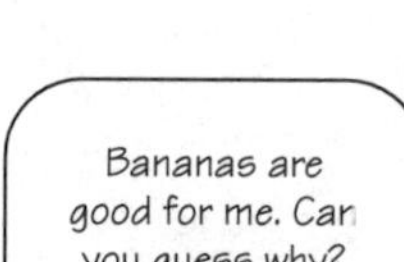
Bananas are
good for me. Can
you guess why?

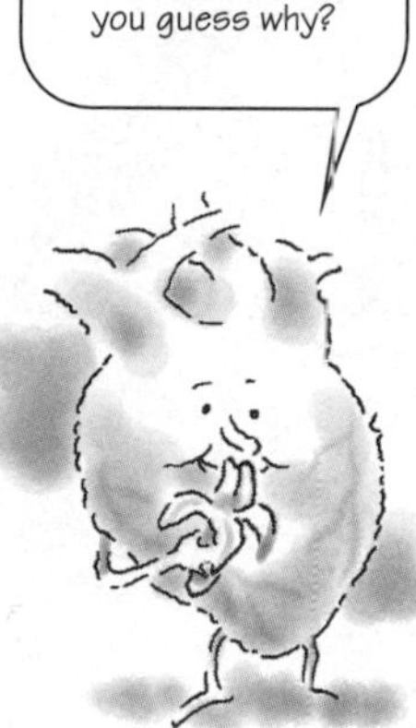

135. For a client who is being treated for ventricular tachycardia, why should the teaching plan include an instruction to eat foods such as bananas?

1. Because bananas are high in carbohydrate
2. Because bananas are high in potassium
3. Because bananas are low in sodium
4. Because bananas are high in fiber

135. 2. A low serum potassium level increases the risk of ventricular tachycardia. Therefore, the client should be instructed to eat potassium-rich foods such as bananas.

NP: Planning; CN: Health promotion and maintenance; CNS: Prevention and early detection of disease; CL: Comprehension

136. After cardiac surgery, a client's blood pressure measures 126/80 mm Hg. The nurse determines that mean arterial pressure (MAP) is which of the following?

1. 46 mm Hg
2. 80 mm Hg
3. 95 mm Hg
4. 90 mm Hg

136. 3. Use the following formula to calculate MAP:

$$\text{MAP} = \frac{\text{systolic} + 2\ (\text{diastolic})}{3}$$

$$\text{MAP} = \frac{126 \text{ mm Hg} + 2\ (80 \text{ mm Hg})}{3}$$

$$\text{MAP} = \frac{286 \text{ mm Hg}}{3}$$

$$\text{MAP} = 95 \text{ mm Hg}$$

NP: Assessment; CN: Physiological integrity; CNS: Reduction of risk potential; CL: Analysis

137. The charge nurse is preparing client care assignments for the next shift. A client who underwent femoral-popliteal bypass surgery is scheduled to return from the postanesthesia care unit. Which of the following staff members should receive this client?

1. Registered nurse with 1 year of experience
2. Licensed practical nurse (LPN) with 5 years of experience
3. Client care attendant with 15 years of experience
4. Charge nurse with 10 years of experience

137. 1. Because this client requires frequent neurovascular assessments, a registered nurse should receive him. An LPN, although she's experienced and can collect data, doesn't have the education to perform the physical assessment required by this client. The client care attendant lacks the necessary assessment skills. The charge nurse needs to be available to direct the care of other clients.

NP: Assessment; CN: Safe, effective care environment; CNS: Management of care; CL: Analysis

138. An 18-year-old client who recently had an upper respiratory infection is admitted with suspected rheumatic fever. Which assessment findings confirm this diagnosis?

1. Erythema marginatum, subcutaneous nodules, and fever
2. Tachycardia, finger clubbing, and a loud second heart sound (S_2)
3. Dyspnea, cough, and palpitations
4. Dyspnea, fatigue, and syncope

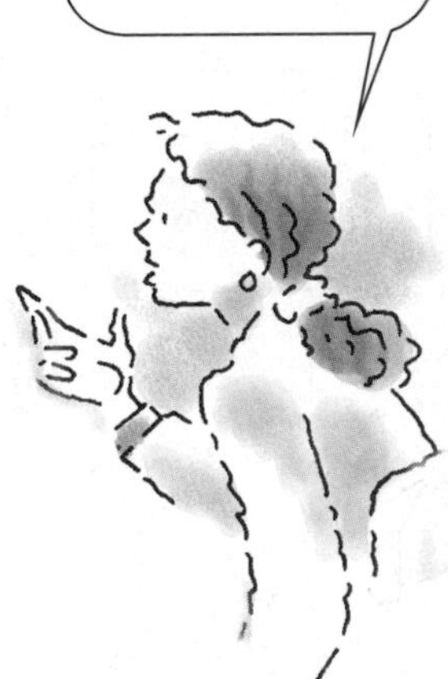

There are several findings here. Which answer confirms the diagnosis?

138. 1. Diagnosis of rheumatic fever requires that the client have either two major Jones criteria or one minor criterion plus evidence of a previous streptococcal infection. Major criteria include carditis, polyarthritis, Sydenham's chorea, subcutaneous nodules, and erythema marginatum (transient, nonpruritic macules on the trunk or inner aspects of the upper arms or thighs). Minor criteria include fever, arthralgia, elevated levels of acute phase reactants, and a prolonged PR interval on electrocardiography. Tachycardia, finger clubbing, and a loud S_2 suggest transposition of the great arteries (a cyanotic congenital heart defect). Dyspnea, cough, and palpitations occur with mitral insufficiency. Dyspnea, fatigue, and syncope indicate aortic insufficiency.

NP: Assessment; CN: Physiological integrity; CNS: Physiological adaptation; CL: Application

139. A client with new onset of atrial fibrillation is receiving warfarin (Coumadin) to help prevent thromboemboli. The warfarin dosage will reach therapeutic levels when the International Normalized Ratio (INR) falls within which range?

1. 1 to 2
2. 1.5 to 2.5
3. 2 to 3
4. 2.5 to 3.5

139. 3. In a client with atrial fibrillation, warfarin reaches therapeutic levels when the INR is 2 to 3. Lower ratios are below the therapeutic range. A range of 2.5 to 3.5 is too high for a client on warfarin and increases the hemorrhage risk.

NP: Evaluation; CN: Physiological integrity; CNS: Reduction of risk potential; CL: Application

140. A 38-year-old client comes to the emergency department complaining that her heart "suddenly began to race." After attaching her to the cardiac monitor, the nurse observes atrial tachycardia. Which of the following rhythm strip characteristics indicate this arrhythmia?

1. Atrial rate greater than the ventricular rate, sawtooth P waves
2. Irregular rhythm, indiscernible atrial rate, absent P waves
3. Regular atrial and ventricular rhythms, rate of 123 beats/minute
4. Regular atrial and ventricular rhythms, P wave hidden in the T wave, rate of 210 beats/minute

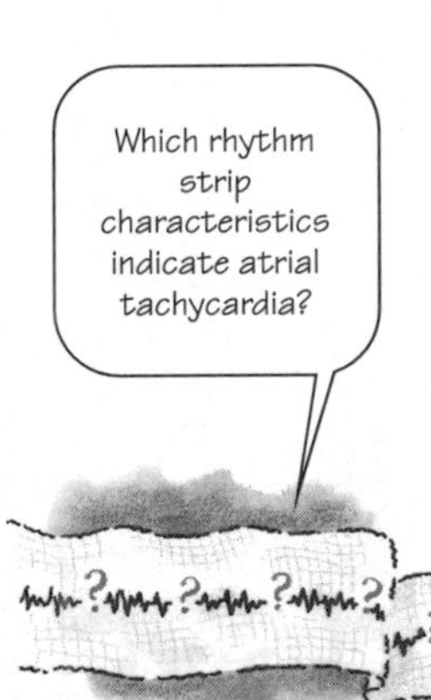

140. 4. With atrial tachycardia, the rhythm is regular, the P wave is hidden in the preceding T wave, and the rate ranges from 140 to 250 beats/minute. A ventricular rate that varies with the degree of atrioventricular block, along with sawtooth P waves, characterizes atrial flutter. Irregular ventricular response and absent P waves characterize atrial fibrillation. Regular and equal atrial and ventricular rhythms and a rate of 100 to 160 beats/minute characterize sinus tachycardia.

NP: Assessment; CN: Physiological integrity; CNS: Physiological adaptation; CL: Application

141. A client is receiving spironolactone to treat hypertension. Which of the following instructions should the nurse provide?

1. "Eat foods high in potassium."
2. "Take daily potassium supplements."
3. "Discontinue sodium restrictions."
4. "Avoid salt substitutes."

141. 4. Because spironolactone is a potassium-sparing diuretic, the client should avoid salt substitutes because of their high potassium content. The client should also avoid potassium-rich foods and potassium supplements. To reduce fluid volume overload, sodium restrictions should continue.

NP: Implementation; CN: Physiological integrity; CNS: Pharmacological and parenteral therapies; CL: Application

142. A 23-year-old client develops cardiac tamponade when the car he was driving hits a telephone pole; he wasn't wearing a seat belt. The nurse helps the physician perform pericardiocentesis. Which of the following outcomes would indicate that pericardiocentesis has been effective?

1. Neck vein distention
2. Pulsus paradoxus
3. Increased blood pressure
4. Muffled heart sounds

142. 3. Cardiac tamponade is associated with decreased cardiac output, which in turn reduces blood pressure. By removing a small amount of blood, pericardiocentesis increases blood pressure. Neck vein distention, pulsus paradoxus, and muffled heart sounds indicate persistent cardiac tamponade, meaning that pericardiocentesis hasn't been effective.

NP: Evaluation; CN: Physiological integrity; CNS: Physiological adaptation; CL: Application

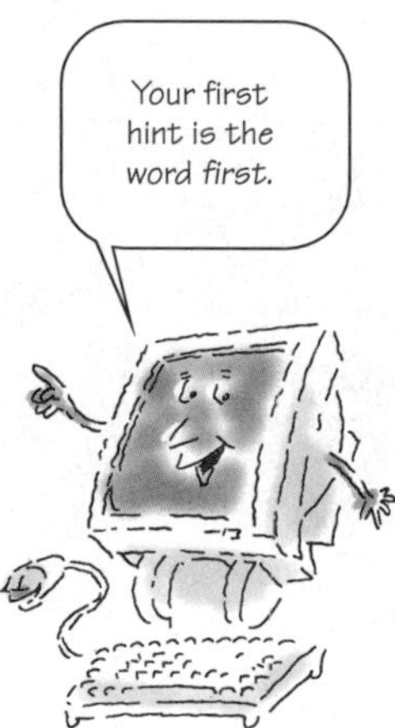
Your first hint is the word first.

143. A client admitted with angina complains of severe chest pain and suddenly becomes unresponsive. After establishing unresponsiveness, which of the following actions should the nurse take first?

1. Activate the resuscitation team.
2. Open the client's airway.
3. Check for breathing.
4. Check for signs of circulation.

143. 1. Immediately after establishing unresponsiveness, the nurse should activate the resuscitation team. The next step is to open the airway using the head-tilt, chin-lift maneuver and check for breathing (looking, listening, and feeling for no more than 10 seconds). If the client isn't breathing, give two slow breaths using a bag mask or pocket mask. Next, check for signs of circulation by palpating the carotid pulse.

NP: Implementation; CN: Physiological integrity; CNS: Physiological adaptation; CL: Application

144. A 54-year-old client is admitted with an acute inferior-wall myocardial infarction (MI). During the admission interview, he says he stopped taking his metoprolol (Lopressor) 5 days ago because he was feeling better. Which of the following nursing diagnoses takes priority for this client?

1. Anxiety
2. Ineffective tissue perfusion (cardiopulmonary)
3. Acute pain
4. Ineffective therapeutic regimen management

144. 2. MI results from prolonged myocardial ischemia caused by reduced blood flow through the coronary arteries. Therefore, the priority nursing diagnosis for this client is *Ineffective tissue perfusion (cardiopulmonary)*. Anxiety, acute pain, and ineffective therapeutic regimen management are appropriate but don't take priority.

NP: Analysis; CN: Safe, effective care environment; CNS: Management of care; CL: Analysis

145. A client comes to the emergency department with acute shortness of breath and a cough that produces pink, frothy sputum. Admission assessment reveals crackles and wheezes, a blood pressure of 82/45 mm Hg, a heart rate of 120 beats/minute, and a respiratory rate of 38 breaths/minute. The client's medical history includes diabetes mellitus, hypertension, and heart failure. Which of the following disorders should the nurse suspect?

1. Pulmonary edema
2. Pneumothorax
3. Cardiac tamponade
4. Pulmonary embolus

145. 1. Shortness of breath, tachypnea, low blood pressure, tachycardia, diffuse crackles, and a cough producing pink, frothy sputum are late signs of pulmonary edema. Pneumothorax causes sudden, sharp pleuritic pain exacerbated by chest movement, breathing, and coughing; shortness of breath; and absent breath sounds on the affected side. Cardiac tamponade produces muffled heart sounds, pulsus paradoxus, and jugular vein distention. Pulmonary embolus may cause fever, cough, hemoptysis, and a pleural friction rub.

NP: Assessment; CN: Physiological integrity; CNS: Physiological adaptation; CL: Application

146. A 57-year-old client with acute arterial occlusion of the left leg undergoes an emergency embolectomy. Six hours later, the nurse isn't able to obtain pulses in his left foot using Doppler ultrasound. She immediately notifies the physician, who asks her to prepare the client for surgery. As the nurse enters the client's room to prepare him, he states that he won't have any more surgery. Which of the following is the best initial response by the nurse?

1. Explaining the risks of not having the surgery
2. Notifying the physician immediately
3. Notifying the nursing supervisor
4. Recording the client's refusal in the nurses' notes

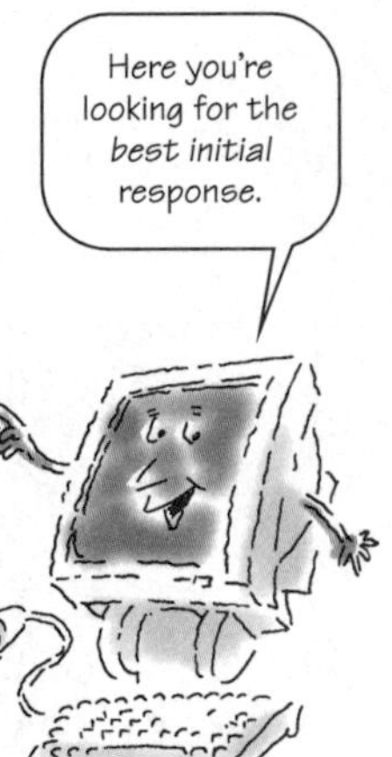
Here you're looking for the best initial response.

146. 1. The best initial response is to explain the risks of not having the surgery. If the client understands the risks but still refuses, the nurse should notify the physician and the nursing supervisor and then record the client's refusal in the nurses' notes.

NP: Implementation; CN: Safe, effective care environment; CNS: Management of care; CL: Application

147. The nurse coming on duty receives the report from the nurse going off duty. Which of the following clients should the on-duty nurse assess first?

1. The 58-year-old client who was admitted 2 days ago with heart failure, blood pressure of 126/76 mm Hg, and a respiratory rate of 22 breaths/minute
2. The 89-year-old client with end-stage right-sided heart failure, blood pressure of 78/50 mm Hg, and a "Do not resuscitate" order
3. The 62-year-old client who was admitted 1 day ago with thrombophlebitis and is receiving I.V. heparin
4. The 75-year-old client who was admitted 1 hour ago with new-onset atrial fibrillation and is receiving I.V. diltiazem (Cardizem)

147. 4. The client with atrial fibrillation has the greatest potential to become unstable and is on I.V. medication that requires close monitoring. After assessing this client, the nurse should assess the client with thrombophlebitis who is receiving a heparin infusion, and then the 58-year-old client admitted 2 days ago with heart failure (his signs and symptoms are resolving and don't require immediate attention). The lowest priority is the 89-year-old with end-stage right-sided heart failure, who requires time-consuming supportive measures.

NP: Assessment; CN: Safe, effective care environment; CNS: Management of care; CL: Analysis

148. When developing a teaching plan for a client with endocarditis, which of the following points is most essential for the nurse to include?

1. "Report fever, anorexia, and night sweats to the physician."
2. "Take prophylactic antibiotics after dental work and invasive procedures."
3. "Include potassium-rich foods in your diet."
4. "Monitor your pulse rate daily."

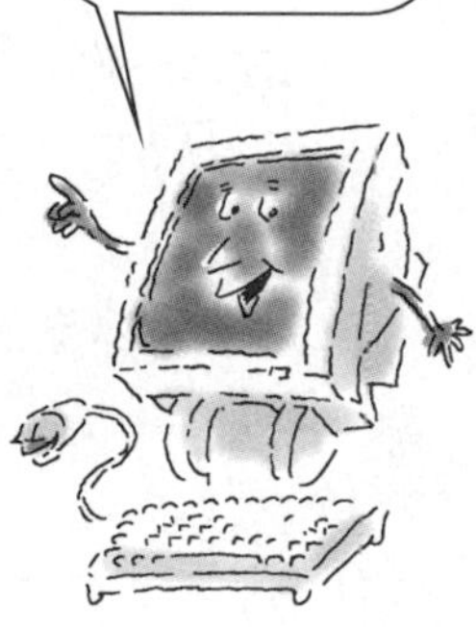
It's essential
with this
question that
you choose the
most essential
answer.

148. 1. The most essential teaching point is to report signs of relapse, such as fever, anorexia, and night sweats, to the physician. To prevent further endocarditis episodes, prophylactic antibiotics are taken before and sometimes after dental work, childbirth, or genitourinary, GI, or gynecologic procedures. A potassium-rich diet and daily pulse monitoring aren't necessary for a client with endocarditis.

NP: Planning; CN: Health promotion and maintenance; CNS: Prevention and early detection of disease; CL: Application

149. Which finding suggests that fluid resuscitation has been effective for a 23-year-old client admitted in hypovolemic shock?

1. Urine output of 15 ml/hour
2. Urine output of 20 ml/hour
3. Urine output of 25 ml/hour
4. Urine output of 30 ml/hour

149. 4. In an adult, urine output below 30 ml/hour indicates inadequate blood flow to the kidneys. Therefore, urine output of 30 ml/hour or greater reflects adequate fluid resuscitation.

NP: Evaluation; CN: Physiological integrity; CNS: Physiological adaptation; CL: Analysis

150. A 22-year-old client complains of substernal chest pain and states that her heart feels like "it's racing out of my chest." She reports no history of cardiac disorders. The nurse attaches her to a cardiac monitor and notes sinus tachycardia with a rate of 136 beats/minute. Breath sounds are clear and the respiratory rate is 26 breaths/minute. Which of the following drugs should the nurse question the client about using?

1. Barbiturates
2. Opioids
3. Cocaine
4. Benzodiazepines

150. 3. Because of the client's age and negative medical history, the nurse should question her about cocaine use. Cocaine increases myocardial oxygen consumption and can cause coronary artery spasm, leading to tachycardia, ventricular fibrillation, myocardial ischemia, and myocardial infarction. Barbiturate overdose may trigger respiratory depression and a slow pulse. Opioids can cause marked respiratory depression, while benzodiazepines can cause drowsiness and confusion.

NP: Assessment; CN: Physiological integrity; CNS: Physiological adaptation; CL: Analysis

151. A client seems anxious immediately after the physician tells him that he has suffered an acute myocardial infarction. Which of the following actions should the nurse take?

1. Leave the room to give the client privacy.
2. Walk over to the client and say, "You seem anxious."
3. Offer the client a sedative.
4. Ask the chaplain to spend time with the client.

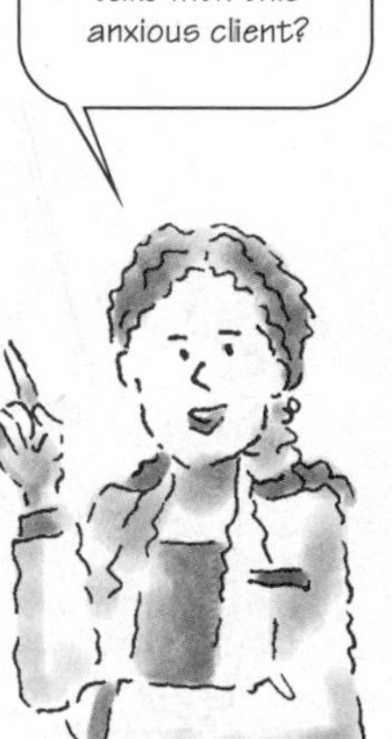
What action
should the nurse
take with this
anxious client?

151. 2. Walking over to the client and making an observation that he seems anxious gives him a chance to verbalize his concerns while receiving support and assistance from the nurse. If he remains anxious after the nurse speaks with him, the nurse can offer a sedative, if ordered. Leaving the room to give the client privacy doesn't address his problem and most likely would increase his anxiety. Calling the chaplain is appropriate only when done at the client's request.

NP: Implementation; CN: Psychosocial integrity; CNS: Coping and adaptation; CL: Application

152. The physician orders total serum calcium measurement in a client who experiences an arrhythmia. To ensure an accurate calcium level, which other laboratory value should be measured?

1. Serum albumin
2. Serum potassium
3. Serum magnesium
4. Serum vitamin D

I measure up — when it comes to lab values.

152. 1. The serum albumin level should be measured along with total serum calcium because serum calcium decreases 0.8 mg/dl for every 1-g decrease in serum albumin. The serum calcium measurement is adjusted upward by the amount of the serum albumin decrease. Ionized calcium is estimated to be approximately half the adjusted calcium value. Although serum potassium and magnesium levels should be measured when a client experiences an arrhythmia, they don't affect the accuracy of serum calcium measurement. Vitamin D helps regulate calcium balance; however, measuring the serum vitamin D level won't ensure an accurate calcium level.

NP: Implementation; CN: Physiological integrity; CNS: Reduction of risk potential; CL: Analysis

153. After a client undergoes abdominal aortic aneurysm repair, the nurse should monitor for which of the following complications?

1. Arrhythmias
2. Hypertension
3. Acute renal failure
4. Bounding peripheral pulses

153. 3. Surgical repair of the aorta commonly interrupts blood flow to the kidneys, so the nurse should monitor urine output closely for signs of acute renal failure. Arrhythmias rarely follow abdominal aortic aneurysm repair. Hypotension — not hypertension — commonly accompanies increased blood loss. Weak or absent pulses may occur if emboli occlude peripheral arteries.

NP: Assessment; CN: Physiological integrity; CNS: Reduction of risk potential; CL: Application

154. A 45-year-old client admitted with an acute inferior myocardial infarction (MI) undergoes emergency cardiac catheterization. The nurse should expect an occlusion in which coronary artery?

1. Right coronary artery
2. Circumflex artery
3. Left anterior descending artery, diagonal branch
4. Left anterior descending artery, septal branch

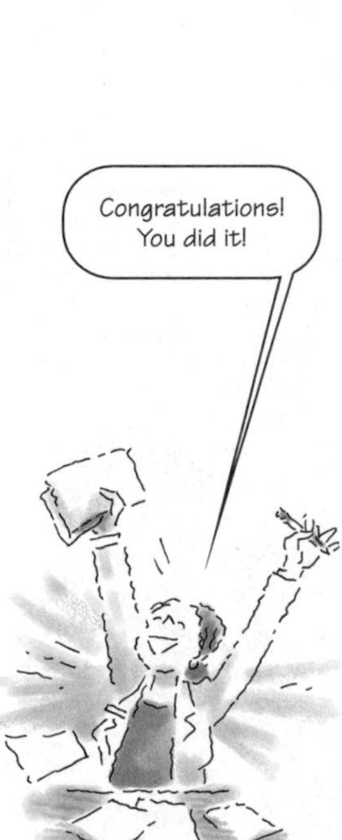
Congratulations! You did it!

154. 1. An inferior MI typically results from occlusion of the right coronary artery. A lateral wall results from occlusion of the circumflex artery; an anterior wall MI, from occlusion of the diagonal branch of the left anterior descending artery; and a septal MI, from occlusion of the septal branch of the left anterior descending artery.

NP: Assessment; CN: Physiological integrity; CNS: Reduction of risk potential; CL: Analysis

155. When auscultating the heart of a client with heart failure, the nurse hears an extra heart sound immediately after an S_2. How should the nurse document this sound?

1. As a first heart sound (S_1)
2. As a third heart sound (S_3)
3. As a fourth heart sound (S_4)
4. As a murmur

155. 2. An S_3 follows an S_2, which commonly occurs in heart failure because of increased filling pressures. An S_1 is a normal heart sound caused by closure of the mitral and tricuspid valves. An S_4 occurs just before an S_1 and results from resistance to ventricular filling. A murmur reflects turbulent blood flow across the valves.

NP: Assessment; CN: Physiological integrity; CNS: Physiological adaptation; CL: Analysis

NP: Nursing process CN: Client needs category CNS: Client needs subcategory CL: Cognitive level

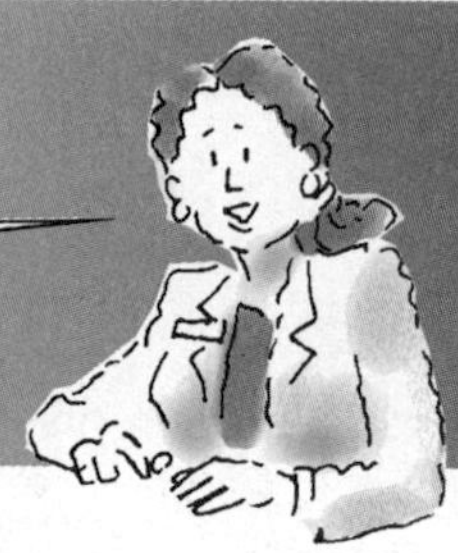

This challenging chapter covers HIV infection, AIDS, rheumatoid arthritis, ITP, and lots of other complex disorders. You can handle it, though, I know you can. Go for it!

Chapter 4
Hematologic & immune disorders

1. For a client to be diagnosed with acquired immunodeficiency syndrome (AIDS), which of the following conditions must be present?

1. Infection with human immunodeficiency virus (HIV), tuberculosis, and cytomegalovirus infection
2. Infection with HIV, an alternative lifestyle, and a T-cell count above 200 cells/µl
3. Infection with HIV, $CD4^+$ count below 200 cells/µl, and a T-cell count above 400 cells/µl
4. Infection with HIV, a history of acute HIV infection, and a $CD4^+$ T-cell count below 200 cells/µl

1. 4. Three criteria must be met for a client to be diagnosed with AIDS. He must be HIV-positive, have a $CD4^+$ T-cell count below 200 cells/µl, and have one or more specific conditions that include acute infection with HIV. Because HIV attaches to the $CD4^+$ receptor sites of the T cell, a T-cell value alone is incorrect.

NP: Assessment; CN: Safe, effective care environment; CNS: Management of care; CL: Knowledge

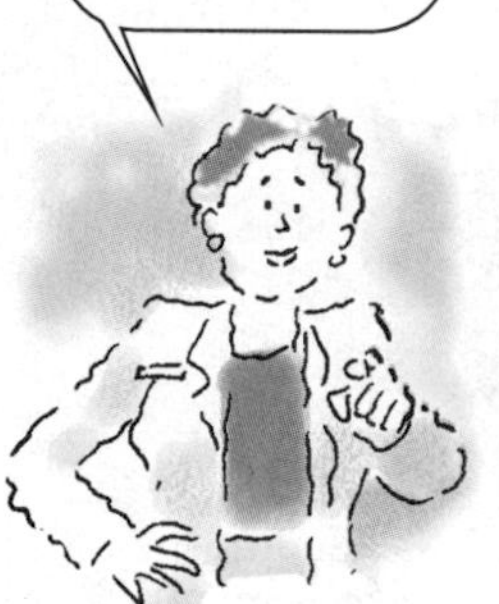

More than one answer may seem correct. Be careful to choose the best answer.

2. Which of the following body substances most easily transmits human immunodeficiency virus (HIV)?

1. Feces and saliva
2. Blood and semen
3. Breast milk and tears
4. Vaginal secretions and urine

2. 2. HIV is most easily transmitted in blood, semen, and vaginal secretions. However, it has also been found in urine, feces, saliva, tears, and breast milk.

NP: Assessment; CN: Health promotion and maintenance; CNS: Prevention and early detection of disease; CL: Knowledge

3. Immediately after giving an injection, a nurse is accidentally stuck with the needle when a client becomes agitated. When is the best time for the employer to test the nurse for human immunodeficiency virus (HIV) antibodies to determine if she became infected as a result of the needle stick?

1. Immediately and then again in 6 weeks
2. Immediately and then again in 3 months
3. In 2 weeks and then again in 6 months
4. In 2 weeks and then again in 1 year

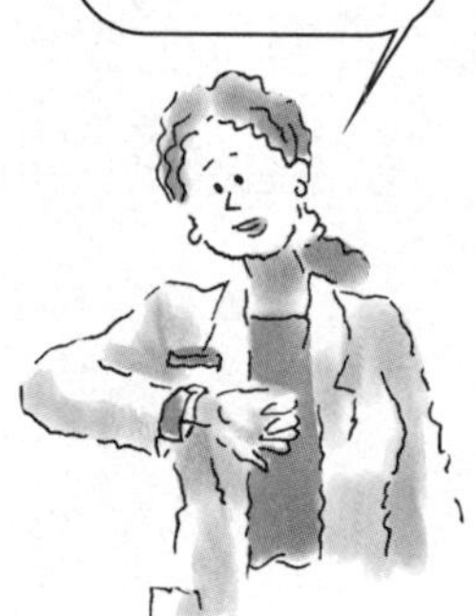

Time is often a crucial element in testing for HIV.

3. 2. The employer will want to test the nurse immediately to determine whether a preexisting infection is present, and then again in 3 months to detect seroconversion as a result of the needle stick. Waiting 2 weeks to perform the first test is too late to detect preexisting infection. Testing sooner than 3 months may yield false-negative results.

NP: Implementation; CN: Health promotion and maintenance; CNS: Prevention and early detection of disease; CL: Application

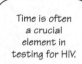

4. Which of the following blood tests is used first to identify a response to human immunodeficiency virus (HIV) infection?

1. Western blot
2. $CD4^+$ T-cell count
3. Erythrocyte sedimentation rate
4. Enzyme-linked immunosorbent assay (ELISA)

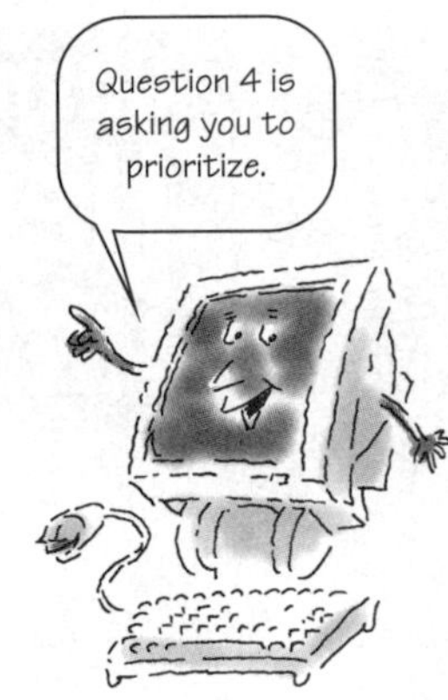

Question 4 is asking you to prioritize.

4. 4. The ELISA is the first screening test for HIV. A Western blot test confirms a positive ELISA test. Other blood tests that support the diagnosis of HIV include $CD4^+$ and $CD8^+$ counts, complete blood counts, immunoglobulin levels, p24 antigen assay, and quantitative ribonucleic acid assays.

NP: Assessment; CN: Health promotion and maintenance; CNS: Prevention and early detection of disease; CL: Knowledge

5. Which of the following factors makes it difficult to develop a vaccine for human immunodeficiency virus (HIV)?

1. HIV is a virus.
2. HIV matures early.
3. HIV mutates easily.
4. HIV spreads through body secretions.

5. 3. HIV was first identified in 1983. By 1986, two strains existed, HIV-1 and HIV-2. The fact that HIV is a virus, matures early, and spreads through body secretions doesn't affect the potential for vaccine development against the virus.

NP: Implementation; CN: Physiological integrity; CNS: Pharmacological and parenteral therapies; CL: Knowledge

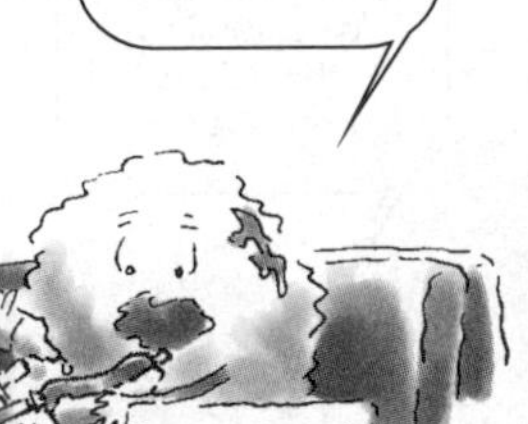

6. Which of the following dietary recommendations may help the client with rheumatoid arthritis reduce inflammation?

1. Fish oil
2. Vitamin D
3. Iron-rich foods
4. Calcium carbonate

6. 1. The therapeutic effect of fish oil suppresses inflammatory mediator production (such as prostaglandins); how it works is unknown. Iron-rich foods are recommended to decrease the anemia associated with rheumatoid arthritis. Calcium and vitamin D supplements may help reduce bone resorption.

NP: Planning; CN: Physiological integrity; CNS: Physiological adaptation; CL: Knowledge

7. Which of the following is a nonsteroidal anti-inflammatory drug (NSAID) used most often to treat rheumatoid arthritis?

1. Furosemide
2. Haloperidol
3. Ibuprofen
4. Methotrexate

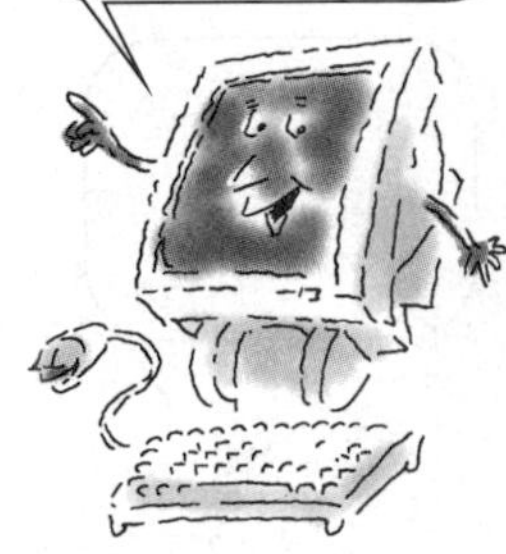

More than one answer may seem right. Read the key words carefully.

7. 3. Ibuprofen, fenoprofen, naproxen, piroxicam, and indomethacin are NSAIDs used for clients with rheumatoid arthritis. Furosemide is a loop diuretic and haloperidol is an antipsychotic agent, neither of which is used to treat rheumatoid arthritis. Methotrexate is an immunosuppressant used in the *early* treatment of rheumatoid arthritis.

NP: Implementation; CN: Physiological integrity; CNS: Pharmacological and parenteral therapies; CL: Knowledge

8. Which of the following methods of transmission has the most risk for exposure to human immunodeficiency virus (HIV)?

1. Routine teeth cleaning at the dentist's office
2. Intercourse with your spouse
3. Unprotected, noninsertive relations
4. Intercourse with a new partner without a condom

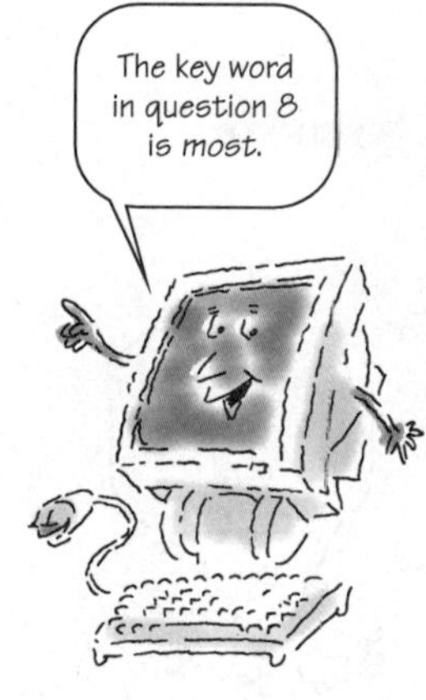
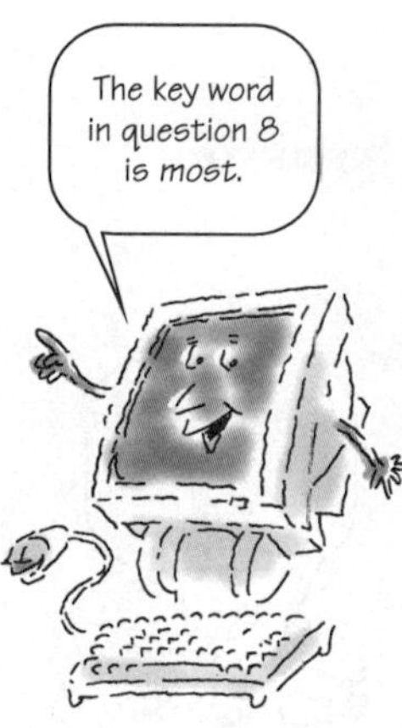

The key word in question 8 is most.

8. 4. Having intercourse with a new partner is risky because of the unknown I.V. drug use and sexual history. Use of a condom may increase the protection against HIV exposure. Absolutely safe sex practices include autosexual activities, abstinence, and relations in a monogamous uninfected couple. Very safe practices include noninsertive relations. Having your teeth cleaned is not a risk factor if the dental office properly sterilizes the equipment.

NP: Planning; CN: Health promotion and maintenance; CNS: Prevention and early detection of disease; CL: Comprehension

9. Which of the following clients is most at risk for developing rheumatoid arthritis?

1. A 25-year-old woman
2. A 40-year-old man
3. A 65-year-old woman
4. A 70-year-old man

9. 3. Rheumatoid arthritis affects women three times more often than men. The average age of onset is age 55.

NP: Assessment; CN: Health promotion and maintenance; CNS: Prevention and early detection of disease; CL: Analysis

10. To which of the following classifications does human immunodeficiency virus (HIV) belong?

1. *Hantavirus*
2. Retrovirus
3. Rhinovirus
4. Rotavirus

10. 2. HIV is a retrovirus that has ribonucleic acid–dependent reverse transcriptase. HIV doesn't belong to the other viruses.

NP: Assessment; CN: Safe, effective care environment; CNS: Safety and infection control; CL: Knowledge

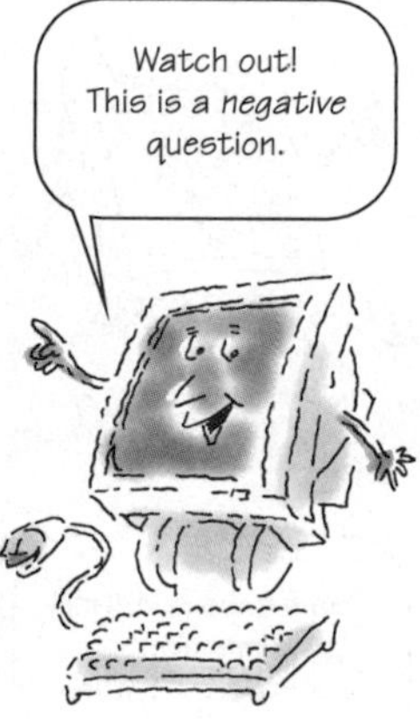

Watch out! This is a negative question.

11. A pregnant woman has just been diagnosed with human immunodeficiency virus (HIV). Which of the following methods or actions does not put the baby at risk for infection by the virus?

1. Vaginal birth
2. Substance abuse
3. Breast-feeding after birth
4. Changing diapers after birth

11. 4. A vaginal birth, breast-feeding after birth, and I.V. substance abuse are all associated with higher rates of mother-to-child transmission of HIV. Changing diapers doesn't put the baby at risk for HIV.

NP: Implementation; CN: Safe, effective care environment; CNS: Safety and infection control; CL: Application

12. Which of the following groups or factors is linked to higher morbidity and mortality in human immunodeficiency virus (HIV)–infected clients?

1. Homosexual men
2. Lower socioeconomic levels
3. Treatment in a large teaching hospital
4. Treatment by a physician who specializes in HIV infection

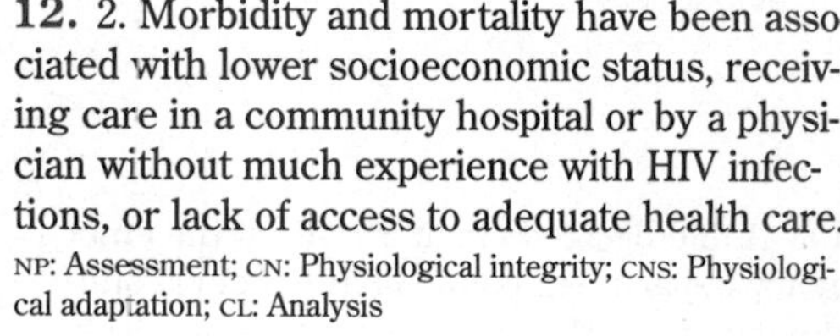

12. 2. Morbidity and mortality have been associated with lower socioeconomic status, receiving care in a community hospital or by a physician without much experience with HIV infections, or lack of access to adequate health care.

NP: Assessment; CN: Physiological integrity; CNS: Physiological adaptation; CL: Analysis

13. After teaching a client about rheumatoid arthritis, which of the following statements indicates the client understands the disease process?
1. "It will get better and worse again."
2. "Once it clears up, it will never come back."
3. "I will definitely have to have surgery for this."
4. "It will never get any better than it is right now."

13. 1. The client with rheumatoid arthritis needs to understand it is a somewhat unpredictable disease characterized by periods of exacerbation and remission. There's no cure, but symptoms can be managed at times. Surgery may be indicated in some cases but not always.

NP: Evaluation; CN: Psychosocial integrity; CNS: Coping and adaptation; CL: Application

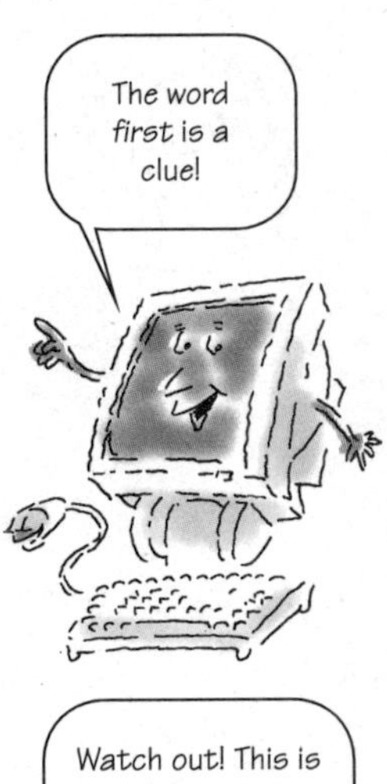

The word *first* is a clue!

14. Which of the following medications would be prescribed first for a client with rheumatoid arthritis?
1. Aspirin
2. Cytoxan
3. Ferrous sulfate
4. Prednisone

14. 1. Nonsteroidal anti-inflammatory drugs (NSAIDs) such as aspirin are considered first-line therapy by some physicians. Cytoxan may be used in cases of severe synovitis, rather than as first-line therapy. Ferrous sulfate isn't used to treat rheumatoid arthritis. Prednisone may be used to control inflammation when NSAIDs aren't tolerated.

NP: Implementation; CN: Physiological integrity; CNS: Pharmacological and parenteral therapies; CL: Application

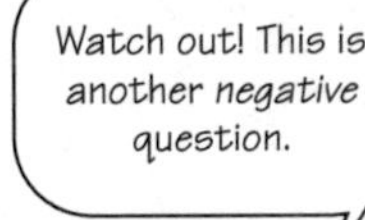

Watch out! This is another *negative* question.

15. Human immunodeficiency virus (HIV) primarily attacks the immune system. HIV does not cause which of the following illnesses?
1. Anemia
2. Arthritis
3. Cardiomyopathy
4. Glaucoma

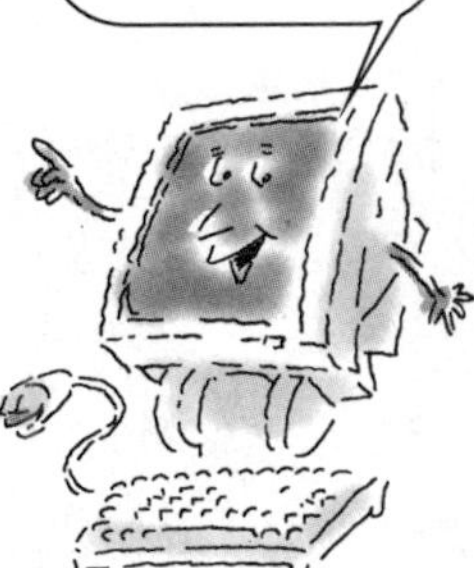

15. 4. HIV has been shown to cause neuropathy, cardiomyopathy, psoriasis, arthritis, cervicitis, uveitis, pneumonia, malabsorption of the small bowel, nephritis, gonad dysfunction, anemia, thrombocytopenia, granulocytopenia, and adrenalitis. Glaucoma hasn't been associated with HIV infection.

NP: Evaluation; CN: Physiological integrity; CNS: Reduction of risk potential; CL: Knowledge

16. Which of the following blood components is decreased in anemia?
1. Erythrocytes
2. Granulocytes
3. Leukocytes
4. Platelets

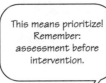

16. 1. Anemia is defined as a decreased number of erythrocytes (red blood cells). Leukopenia is a decreased number of leukocytes (white blood cells). Thrombocytopenia is a decreased number of platelets. Lastly, granulocytopenia is a decreased number of granulocytes (a type of white blood cell).

NP: Assessment; CN: Health promotion and maintenance; CNS: Prevention and early detection of disease; CL: Knowledge

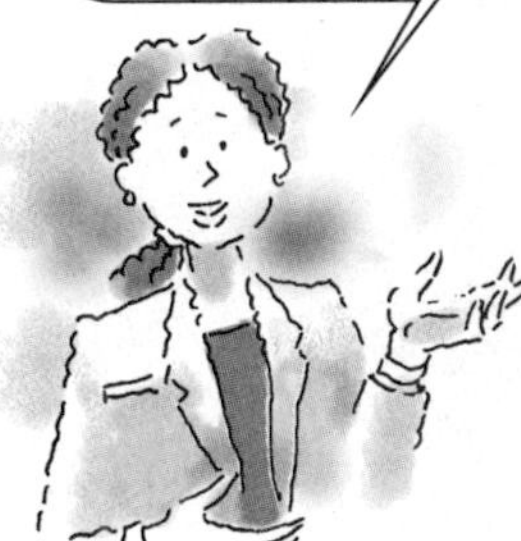

This means prioritize! Remember: assessment before intervention.

17. A middle-aged client arrives at the emergency department complaining of chest and stomach pain. He also reports passing black stools for a month. Which of the following interventions is done first?
1. Give nasal oxygen.
2. Take his vital signs.
3. Begin cardiac monitoring.
4. Draw blood for laboratory analysis.

17. 2. His vital signs will show hemodynamic stability, and monitoring his heart rhythm may be indicated based on your findings. Giving nasal oxygen and drawing blood require a physician's order and wouldn't be part of a screening evaluation.

NP: Assessment; CN: Physiological integrity; CNS: Physiological adaptation; CL: Application

18. A client arrives at the emergency department with chest and stomach pain and a report of black, tarry stools for several months. Which of the following orders should the nurse anticipate?

1. Cardiac monitor, oxygen, creatine kinase and lactate dehydrogenase levels
2. Prothrombin time, partial thromboplastin time, fibrinogen and fibrin split product values
3. Electrocardiogram, complete blood count, testing for occult blood, comprehensive serum metabolic panel
4. Electroencephalogram, alkaline phosphatase and aspartate aminotransferase levels, basic serum metabolic panel

18. 3. An electrocardiogram evaluates the complaint of chest pain, laboratory tests determine anemia, and the stool test for occult blood determines blood in the stool. Cardiac monitoring, oxygen, and creatine kinase and lactate dehydrogenase levels are appropriate for a cardiac primary problem. A basic metabolic panel and alkaline phosphatase and aspartate aminotransferase levels assess liver function. Prothrombin time, partial thromboplastin time, fibrinogen and fibrin split products are measured to verify bleeding dyscrasias. An electroencephalogram evaluates brain electrical activity.

NP: Evaluation; CN: Physiological integrity; CNS: Reduction of risk potential; CL: Analysis

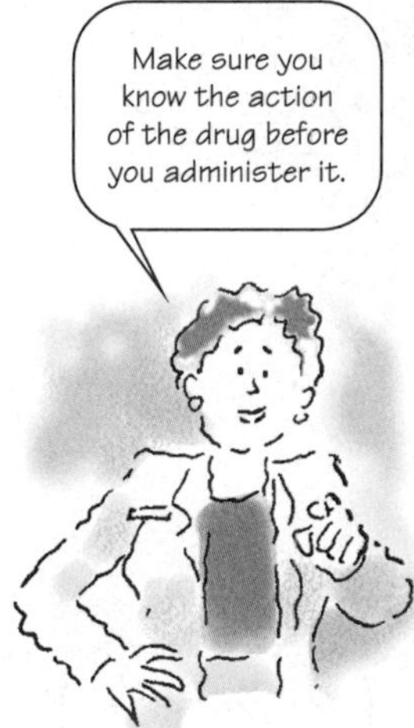

Make sure you know the action of the drug before you administer it.

19. Which of the following goals for medications prescribed to treat rheumatoid arthritis is accurate?

1. To cure the disease
2. To prevent osteoporosis
3. To control inflammation
4. To encourage bone regeneration

19. 3. The goal of medications in the treatment of rheumatoid arthritis is to control inflammation. There is no cure for rheumatoid arthritis. Rheumatoid arthritis causes bone erosion at the joints, not osteoporosis. Medications aren't available to replace bone lost through erosion.

NP: Implementation; CN: Physiological integrity; CNS: Pharmacological and parenteral therapies; CL: Comprehension

20. A client with anemia may be tired due to a tissue deficiency of which of the following substances?

1. Carbon dioxide
2. Factor VIII
3. Oxygen
4. T-cell antibodies

20. 3. Anemia stems from a decreased number of red blood cells and the resulting deficiency in oxygen in body tissues. Clotting factors, such as factor VIII, relate to the body's ability to form blood clots and aren't related to anemia, nor is carbon dioxide or T antibodies.

NP: Assessment; CN: Physiological integrity; CNS: Physiological adaptation; CL: Application

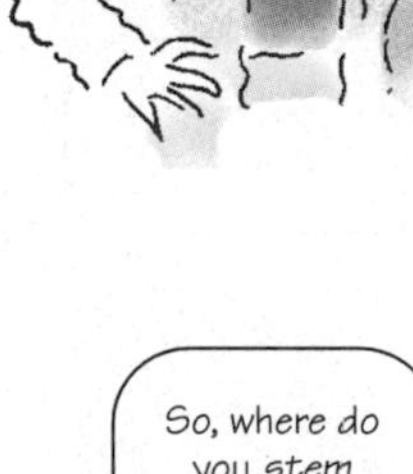

So, where do you stem from?

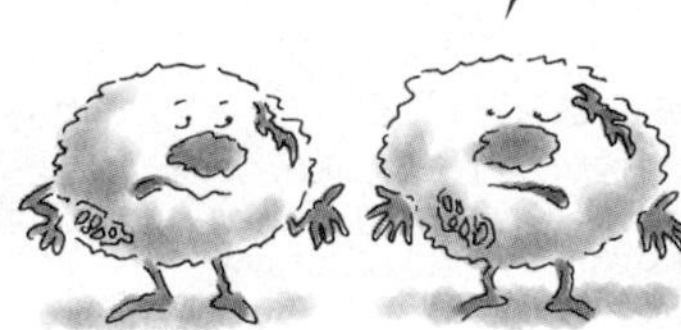

21. Which of the following cells is the precursor to the red blood cell (RBC)?

1. B cell
2. Macrophage
3. Stem cell
4. T cell

21. 3. The precursor to the RBC is the stem cell. B cells, macrophages, and T cells are lymphocytes, not RBC precursors.

NP: Assessment; CN: Physiological integrity; CNS: Physiological adaptation; CL: Knowledge

22. Which of the following conditions is not a cause of blood disorders such as anemia?

1. Chronic disease
2. Malnutrition
3. Medications
4. Rhinovirus infection

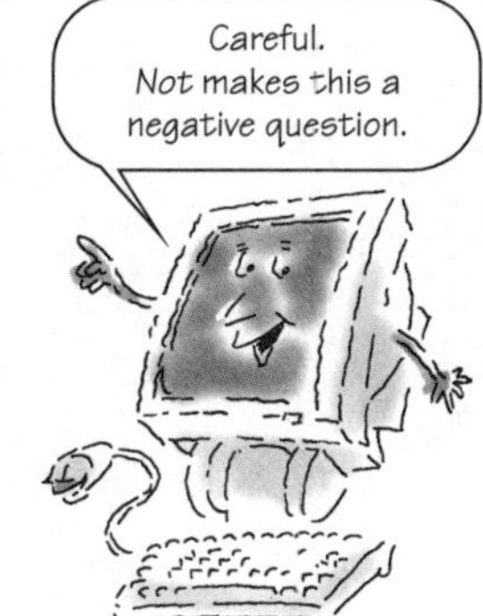

Careful.
Not makes this a negative question.

22. 4. Trauma, chronic illness, surgery, malnutrition, medication, toxins, radiation, genetic and congenital disorders, and sepsis can cause anemia. It isn't caused by a rhinovirus infection, which causes the common cold.

NP: Evaluation; CN: Health promotion and maintenance; CNS: Prevention and early detection of disease; CL: Comprehension

23. Which of the following diagnostic tests does not confirm a diagnosis of rheumatoid arthritis (RA)?
1. Antinuclear antibody (ANA) titer
2. Complete blood count (CBC)
3. Erythrocyte sedimentation rate (ESR)
4. Immunoglobulin G (IgG)

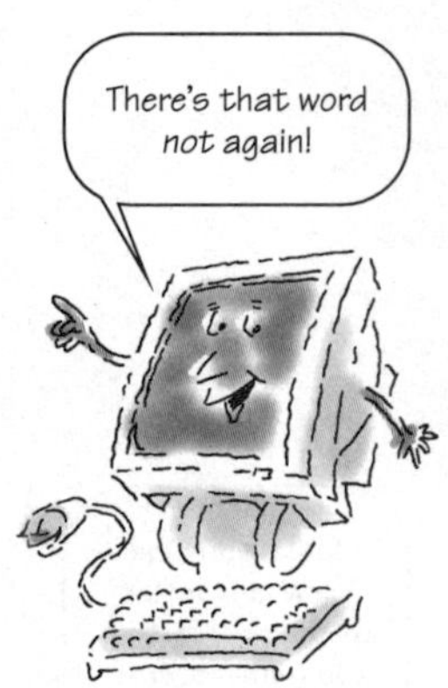
There's that word not again!

23. 4. Although RA is believed to be an autoimmune disorder involving the interaction of IgG with rheumatoid factor, measuring IgG levels isn't commonly used to assess for RA. The CBC (anemia and leukocytosis), ANA titer (elevated), and ESR (elevated) are all measured when evaluating a client for RA.
NP: Assessment; CN: Health promotion and maintenance; CNS: Prevention and early detection of disease; CL: Application

24. Which of the following symptoms is expected with a hemoglobin level of 10 g/dl?
1. None
2. Pallor
3. Palpitations
4. Shortness of breath

24. 1. Mild anemia usually has no clinical signs. Palpitations, shortness of breath, and pallor are associated with *severe* anemia.
NP: Assessment; CN: Physiological adaptation; CNS: Reduction of risk potential; CL: Application

25. Which of the following is not a common cause of anemia?
1. Lack of dietary iron
2. Vitamin C deficiency
3. GI bleeding
4. Hereditary disorders of the red blood cells

25. 2. Anemia can be caused by a lack of vitamin B_{12}, iron, and folic acid, not by a lack of vitamin C. It can also be caused by bleeding from any organ or system, hereditary disorders, and hematopoietic disorders.
NP: Assessment; CN: Physiological integrity; CNS: Physiological adaptation; CL: Comprehension

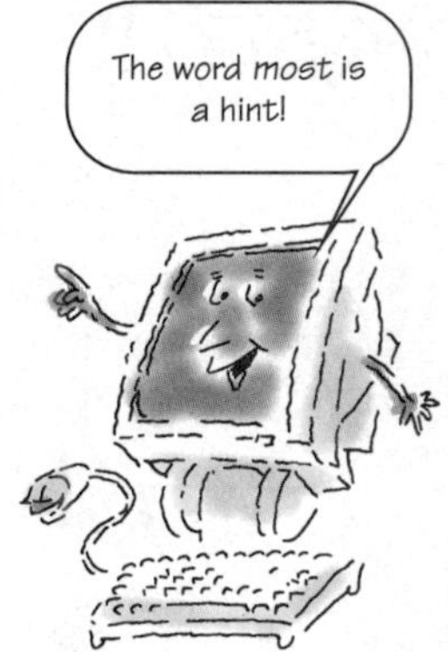
The word most is a hint!

26. Which of the following age-groups is most at risk for developing anemia?
1. Younger than 24 months
2. 18 to 30 years
3. 30 to 65 years
4. 65 years and older

26. 4. The elderly are most at risk for anemia, often due to financial concerns affecting protein intake or poor dentition that interferes with chewing meat.
NP: Assessment; CN: Health promotion and maintenance; CNS: Prevention and early detection of disease; CL: Comprehension

27. Which of the following countries has the highest rate of anemia?
1. Brazil
2. Canada
3. Russia
4. Zimbabwe

27. 4. Anemia is more prevalent in third-world countries such as Zimbabwe, where malnutrition and parasitic infestations are common.
NP: Assessment; CN: Health promotion and maintenance; CNS: Prevention and early detection of disease; CL: Knowledge

28. For which of the following conditions is a client who has just had an appendectomy most at risk?
1. Anemia
2. Polycythemia
3. Purpura
4. Thrombocytopenia

28. 1. Surgery is a risk factor for anemia. Polycythemia can occur from severe hypoxia due to congenital heart and pulmonary disease. Purpura and thrombocytopenia may result from decreased bone marrow production of platelets and doesn't result from surgery.
NP: Assessment; CN: Physiological integrity; CNS: Reduction of risk potential; CL: Application

29. Which of the following terms describes a decreased number of platelets?
1. Thrombectomy
2. Thrombocytopenia
3. Thrombocytopathy
4. Thrombocytosis

29. 2. Thrombocytopenia is a decreased number of platelets. Thrombocytosis is an excess number of platelets, and thrombocytopathy is platelet dysfunction. Thrombectomy is the surgical removal of a thrombus.
NP: Assessment; CN: Physiological integrity; CNS: Physiological adaptation; CL: Knowledge

30. Which of the following symptoms are classic for thrombocytopenia?
1. Weakness and fatigue
2. Dizziness and vomiting
3. Bruising and petechiae
4. Light-headedness and nausea

30. 3. Platelets are necessary for clot formation, so petechiae and bruising are signs of a decreased number of platelets. Weakness and fatigue are signs of anemia. Light-headedness, nausea, dizziness, and vomiting are *not* usual signs of thrombocytopenia.
NP: Assessment; CN: Health promotion and maintenance; CNS: Prevention and early detection of disease; CL: Analysis

31. Which of the following substances are involved in clot lysis?
1. Factors X and XII
2. Fibrin and fibrinogen
3. Plasmin and plasminogen
4. Thrombin and prothrombin

31. 3. Plasmin and plasminogen are necessary for the clot to be dissolved. All other substances are needed only for clot formation.
NP: Assessment; CN: Physiological integrity; CNS: Physiological adaptation; CL: Knowledge

32. A client had coronary artery bypass graft (CABG) surgery 3 days ago. Which of the following conditions is suspected when a decrease in platelet count from 230,000 μl to 5,000 μl is noted?
1. Pancytopenia
2. Idiopathic thrombocytopenic purpura (ITP)
3. Disseminated intravascular coagulation (DIC)
4. Heparin-associated thrombosis and thrombocytopenia (HATT)

32. 4. HATT may occur after CABG surgery due to heparin use during surgery. Although DIC and ITP cause platelet aggregation and bleeding, neither is common in a client after revascularization surgery. Pancytopenia is a reduction in all blood cells.
NP: Implementation; CN: Physiological integrity; CNS: Physiological adaptation; CL: Application

33. Disseminated intravascular coagulation (DIC) often results in complications initially associated with which of the following organs?
1. Brain
2. Kidney
3. Lung
4. Stomach

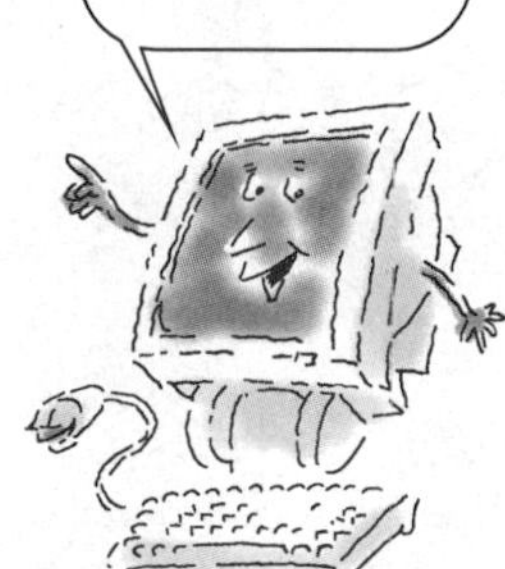

Pay close attention to the word *initially* before choosing an answer.

33. 2. DIC usually affects the kidneys and extremities, but if it isn't treated, it will affect the lungs, brain, stomach, and adrenal and pituitary glands.
NP: Assessment; CN: Physiological integrity; CNS: Reduction of risk potential; CL: Comprehension

34. A pregnant woman arrives at the emergency department with abruptio placentae at 34 weeks' gestation. She is at risk for which of the following blood dyscrasias?

1. Thrombocytopenia
2. Idiopathic thrombocytopenic purpura (ITP)
3. Disseminated intravascular coagulation (DIC)
4. Heparin-associated thrombosis and thrombocytopenia (HATT)

34. 3. Abruptio placentae is a cause of DIC because of activation of the clotting cascade after hemorrhage. Thrombocytopenia results from decreased bone marrow production. ITP can result in DIC but isn't associated with abruptio placentae. A client with abruptio placentae wouldn't receive heparin and, as a result, wouldn't be at risk for HATT.

NP: Assessment; CN: Physiological integrity; CNS: Reduction of risk potential; CL: Application

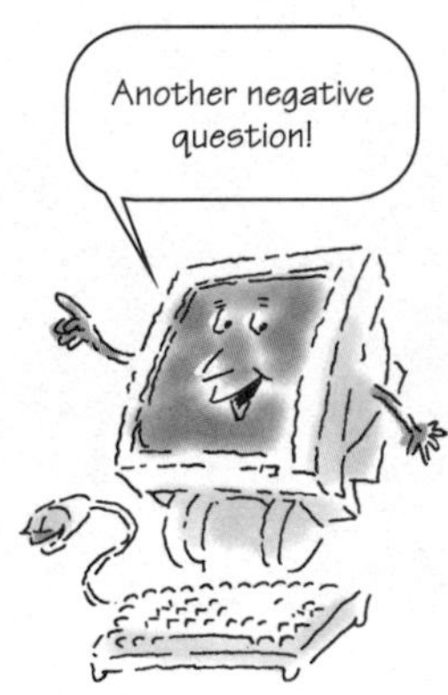
Another negative question!

35. Which of the following conditions is not caused by disseminated intravascular coagulation (DIC)?

1. Organ tissue damage
2. Depletion of circulating clotting factors
3. Thrombus formation in the large vessels
4. Activation of the clotting-dissolving process

35. 3. DIC occurs in response to a primary problem that initiates the clotting cascade, resulting in hypercoagulability. This hypercoagulable state produces clots that can block the microcirculation. As the clotting factors are depleted and fibrinolysis occurs, a hypocoagulable state results. Clotting and bleeding in the microcirculation can cause tissue damage.

NP: Assessment; CN: Physiological integrity; CNS: Physiological adaptation; CL: Comprehension

36. A 36-year-old client complains of fatigue, weight loss, and a low-grade fever. He also has pain in his fingers, elbows, and ankles. Which of the following conditions is suspected?

1. Anemia
2. Leukemia
3. Rheumatic arthritis
4. Systemic lupus erythematosus (SLE)

36. 3. Fatigue, weight loss, and a low-grade fever are all early signs of many immune system diseases, including anemia, leukemia, and SLE. However, only rheumatic arthritis is associated with pain in the fingers, elbows, wrists, ankles, and knees.

NP: Assessment; CN: Health promotion and maintenance; CNS: Prevention and early detection of disease; CL: Application

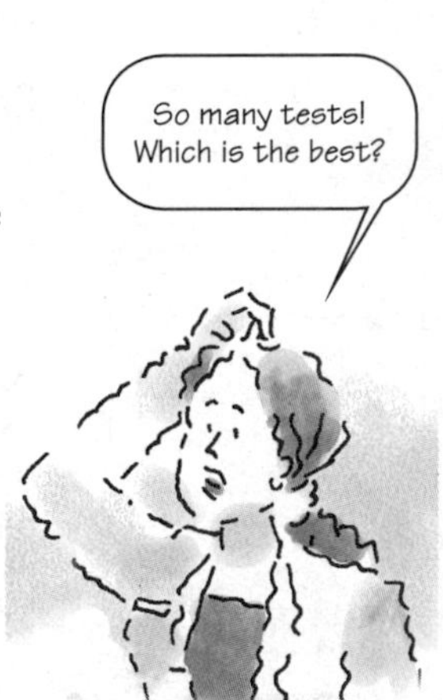
So many tests! Which is the best?

37. Which of the following laboratory tests, besides a platelet count, is best to confirm the diagnosis of essential thrombocytopenia?

1. Bleeding time
2. Complete blood count
3. Immunoglobulin (Ig) G level
4. Prothrombin time and international normalized ratio (INR)

37. 1. After a platelet count, the best test to determine thrombocytopenia is a bleeding time. The platelet count is decreased and bleeding time is prolonged. IgG assays are nonspecific but may help determine the diagnosis. A complete blood count shows the hemoglobin levels, hematocrit levels, and white blood cell values, and the prothrombin time and INR evaluate the effect of warfarin therapy.

NP: Assessment; CN: Physiological integrity; CNS: Physiological adaptation; CL: Application

38. Which of the following drugs would be ordered to improve the platelet count in a client with idiopathic thrombocytopenic purpura (ITP)?
1. Acetylsalicylic acid (ASA)
2. Corticosteroids
3. Methotrexate
4. Vitamin K

38. 2. Corticosteroid therapy can decrease antibody production and phagocytosis of the antibody-coated platelets, retaining more functioning platelets. Methotrexate can cause thrombocytopenia. Vitamin K is used to treat an excessive anticoagulable state from warfarin overload, and ASA decreases platelet aggregation.
NP: Assessment; CN: Physiological integrity; CNS: Pharmacological and parenteral therapies; CL: Application

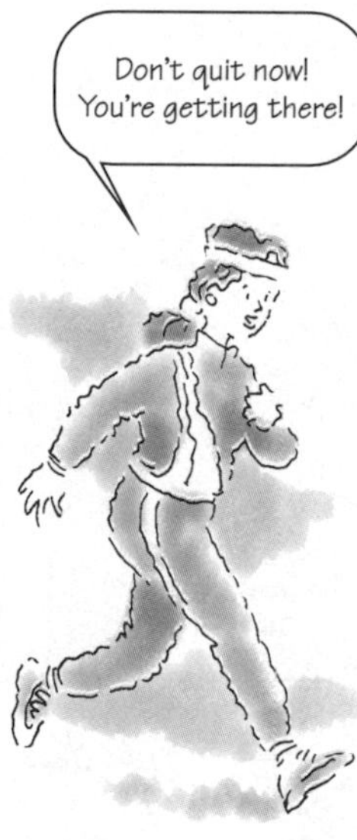

Don't quit now!
You're getting there!

39. Which of the following organs are part of the immune system?
1. Adenoids and tonsils
2. Adrenals and kidneys
3. Lymph nodes and thymus
4. Pancreas and liver

39. 3. The immune system includes the lymph nodes, thymus, spleen, and tonsils. Adenoids and tonsils are part of the respiratory system. The adrenals are endocrine organs. Kidneys belong to the genitourinary system. The liver and pancreas are part of the GI system.
NP: Assessment; CN: Physiological integrity; CNS: Physiological adaptation; CL: Knowledge

40. Which of the following definitions best explains the function of the thymus gland in the immune system?
1. The thymus gland is a reservoir for blood.
2. The thymus gland stores blood cells until they mature.
3. The thymus gland protects the body against ingested pathogens.
4. The thymus gland removes bacteria and toxins from the circulatory system.

40. 2. Bone marrow produces immature blood cells (stem cells). Those that become lymphocytes migrate to the bone marrow for maturation (to B lymphocytes) or to the thymus for maturation (to T lymphocytes). These lymphocytes are responsible for cell-mediated immunity. The spleen is a reservoir for blood cells. The tonsils shield against airborne and ingested pathogens, and the lymph nodes remove bacteria and toxins from the bloodstream.
NP: Evaluation; CN: Physiological integrity; CNS: Physiological adaptation; CL: Knowledge

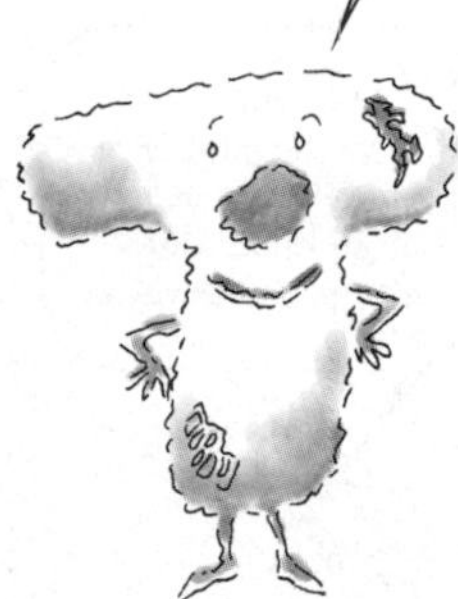

Let's see, what kind of immunity do I have a hankering for today?

41. T cells are involved in which of the following types of immunity?
1. Humoral immunity
2. Cell-mediated immunity
3. Antigen-mediated immunity
4. Immunoglobulin-mediated immunity

41. 2. T cells are responsible for cell-mediated immunity, in which the T cells respond directly to the antigen. B cells are responsible for humoral or immunoglobulin-mediated immunity. There is *no* antigen-mediated immunity.
NP: Assessment; CN: Physiological integrity; CNS: Physiological adaptation; CL: Knowledge

42. A client is scheduled to receive a heart valve replacement with a porcine valve. Which of the following types of transplant is this?
1. Allogeneic
2. Autologous
3. Syngeneic
4. Xenogeneic

42. 4. An xenogeneic transplant is between humans and another species. A syngeneic transplant is between identical twins, allogeneic transplant is between two humans, and autologous is a transplant from the same individual.
NP: Assessment; CN: Physiological integrity; CNS: Physiological adaptation; CL: Comprehension

43. Which of the following clients is most at risk for developing malignant lymphoma?

1. A 22-year-old man with a history of mononucleosis
2. A 25-year-old man who smokes a pack of cigarettes a day
3. A 33-year-old man with a sister with Hodgkin's lymphoma
4. A 40-year-old woman with a history of human immunodeficiency virus (HIV) infection

43. 1. Malignant lymphoma has a peak incidence between ages 20 and 30 and after age 50. It's more common in men than women and is associated with a history of Epstein-Barr virus (which causes mononucleosis). There is also an increased incidence of the disease among siblings. There is no reported association between malignant lymphoma and smoking, I.V. drug use, or HIV infection.

NP: Assessment; CN: Health promotion and maintenance; CNS: Prevention and early detection of disease; CL: Comprehension

44. What is the life span for normal platelets?

1. 1 to 3 days
2. 3 to 5 days
3. 7 to 10 days
4. 3 to 4 months

44. 3. The life span of a normal platelet is 7 to 10 days. However, in idiopathic thrombocytopenia, the platelet life span is reduced to 1 to 3 days.

NP: Planning; CN: Physiological integrity; CNS: Physiological adaptation; CL: Knowledge

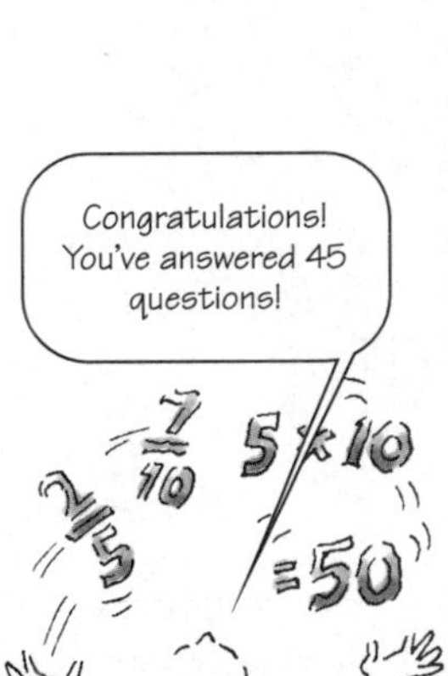

45. What is the normal life span for healthy red blood cells?

1. 60 days
2. 90 days
3. 120 days
4. 240 days

45. 3. A healthy red blood cell lives for about 120 days.

NP: Assessment; CN: Physiological integrity; CNS: Physiological adaptation; CL: Knowledge

46. Which of the following statements indicates that a client with thrombocytopenia understands the function of platelets in her body?

1. "Platelets regulate acid-base balance."
2. "Platelets regulate the immune response."
3. "Platelets protect the body from infection."
4. "Platelets stop the bleeding when arteries and veins are injured."

46. 4. Platelets clump together to plug small breaks in blood vessels. They also initiate the clotting cascade by releasing thromboplastin, which (in the presence of calcium) converts prothrombin into thrombin. Platelets don't perform the other functions.

NP: Evaluation; CN: Physiological integrity; CNS: Reduction of risk potential; CL: Application

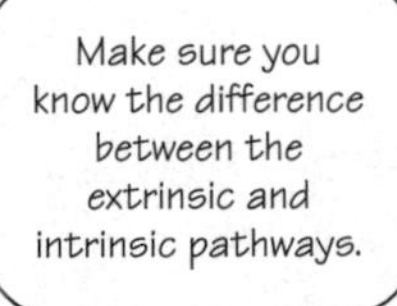

Make sure you know the difference between the extrinsic and intrinsic pathways.

47. A client falls off his bicycle and injures his ankle. Which of the following actions shows the initial response to the injury in the extrinsic pathway?

1. Release of calcium
2. Release of tissue thromboplastin
3. Conversion of factor XII to factor XIIa
4. Conversion of factor VIII to factor VIIIa

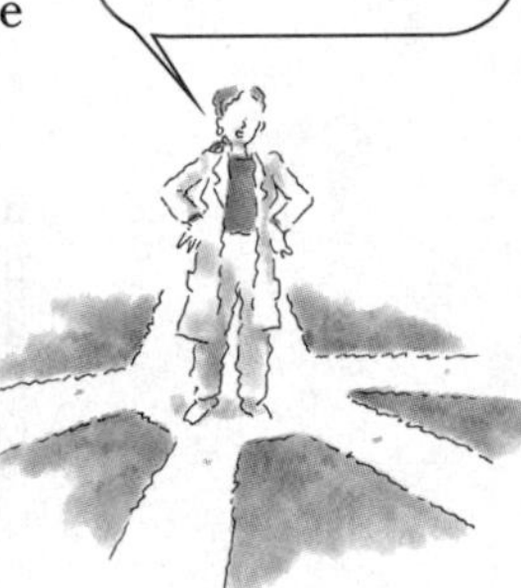

47. 2. Tissue thromboplastin is released when damaged tissue comes in contact with clotting factors. Calcium is released to assist the conversion of factor X to Xa. Conversion of factors XII to XIIa and VIII to VIIIa are part of the *intrinsic* pathway.

NP: Assessment; CN: Physiological integrity; CNS: Physiological adaptation; CL: Knowledge

48. A 16-year-old client involved in a motor vehicle accident arrives in the emergency department unconscious and severely hypotensive. He is suspected to have several fractures (pelvis and legs). Which of the following parenteral fluids is the best choice for his current condition?

1. Whole blood
2. Normal saline solution
3. Lactated Ringer's solution
4. Packed red blood cells

48. 4. In a trauma situation, the first blood product given is unmatched (O negative) packed red blood cells. Fresh frozen plasma is often used to replace clotting factors. Normal saline or lactated Ringer's solution is used to increase volume and blood pressure, but too much colloid will hemodilute the blood and won't improve oxygen-carrying capacity, as red blood cells would.

NP: Planning; CN: Physiological integrity; CNS: Physiological adaptation; CL: Application

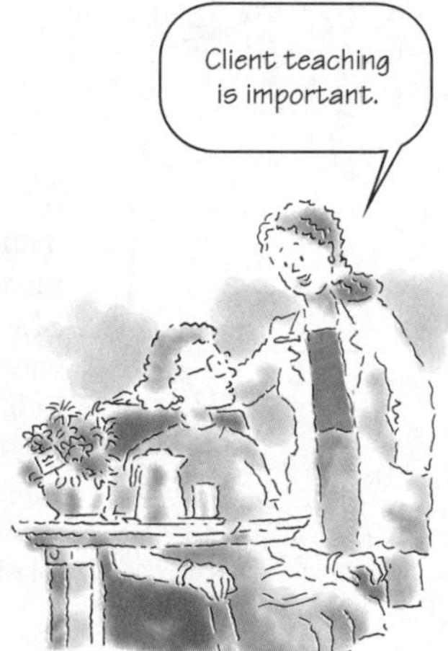
Client teaching
is important.

49. Instructions for a client with systemic lupus erythematosus (SLE) would include information about which of the following blood dyscrasias?

1. Dressler's syndrome
2. Polycythemia
3. Essential thrombocytopenia
4. von Willebrand's disease

49. 3. Essential thrombocytopenia is linked to immunologic disorders, such as SLE and human immunodeficiency virus. The disorder known as von Willebrand's disease is a type of hemophilia and isn't linked to SLE. Moderate to severe anemia is associated with SLE, not polycythemia. Dressler's syndrome is pericarditis that occurs after a myocardial infarction and isn't linked to SLE.

NP: Planning; CN: Health promotion and maintenance; CNS: Prevention and early detection of disease; CL: Knowledge

50. Which of the following clients is most at risk for systemic lupus erythematosus (SLE)?

1. A 20-year-old White man
2. A 25-year-old Black woman
3. A 45-year-old Hispanic man
4. A 65-year-old Black woman

50. 2. SLE affects women eight times more often than men and usually strikes during childbearing age. It's three times more common in Black women than in White women.

NP: Assessment; CN: Health promotion and maintenance; CNS: Prevention and early detection of disease; CL: Comprehension

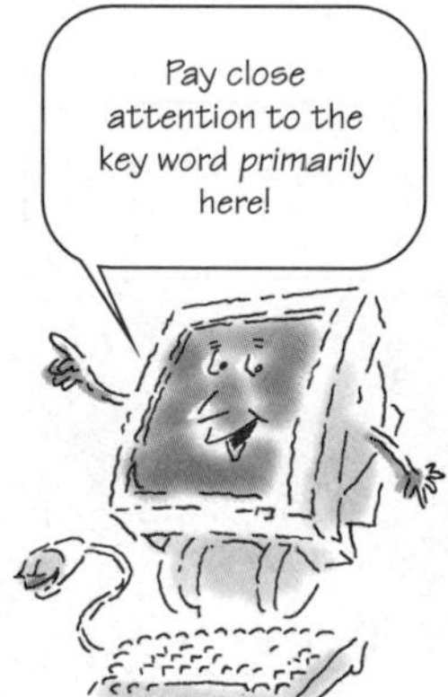
Pay close
attention to the
key word primarily
here!

51. Systemic lupus erythematosus (SLE) primarily attacks which of the following tissues?

1. Connective
2. Heart
3. Lung
4. Nerve

51. 1. SLE is a chronic, inflammatory, autoimmune disorder that primarily affects connective tissue. It also affects the skin and kidneys and may affect the pulmonary, cardiac, neural, and renal systems.

NP: Assessment; CN: Physiological integrity; CNS: Physiological adaptation; CL: Knowledge

52. Which of the following symptoms is most commonly an early indication of stage I Hodgkin's disease?

1. Pericarditis
2. Night sweats
3. Splenomegaly
4. Persistent hypothermia

52. 2. In stage I, symptoms include a single enlarged lymph node (usually), unexplained fever, night sweats, malaise, and generalized pruritis. Although splenomegaly may be present in some clients, night sweats are generally more prevalent. Pericarditis isn't associated with Hodgkin's disease, nor is hypothermia. Moreover, splenomegaly and pericarditis aren't symptoms. Persistent hypothermia is associated with Hodgkin's but isn't an early sign of the disease.

NP: Assessment; CN: Health promotion and maintenance; CNS: Prevention and early detection of disease; CL: Knowledge

53. Which of the following statements shows that a client does not understand the cause of an exacerbation of systemic lupus erythematosus (SLE)?

1. "I need to stay away from sunlight."
2. "I don't have to worry if I get a strep throat."
3. "I need to work on managing stress in my life."
4. "I don't have to worry about changing my diet."

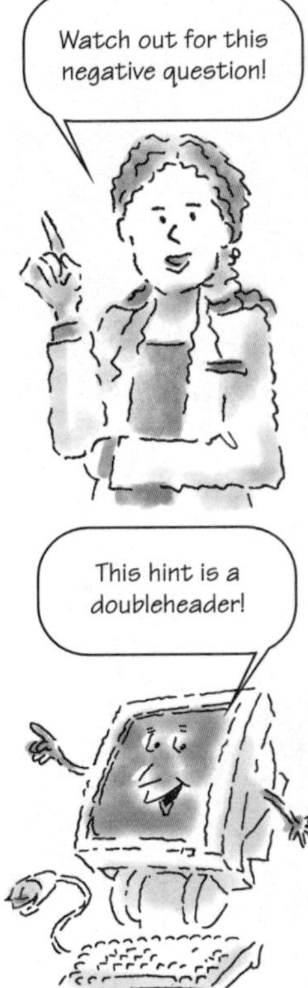

Watch out for this negative question!
This hint is a doubleheader!

53. 2. Infection may cause an exacerbation of SLE. Other factors that can precipitate an exacerbation are immunizations, sunlight exposure, and stress.

NP: Evaluation; CN: Health promotion and maintenance; CNS: Prevention and early detection of disease; CL: Application

54. Which of the following complications of systemic lupus erythematosus (SLE) is most common and most serious?

1. Arthritis
2. Nephritis
3. Pericarditis
4. Pleural effusion

54. 2. About 50% of the clients with SLE have some type of nephritis, and kidney failure is the most common cause of death for clients with SLE. Pericarditis is the most common cardiovascular manifestation of SLE, but it isn't usually life-threatening. Arthritis is very common (95%), as are pleural effusions (50%), but neither is life-threatening.

NP: Assessment; CN: Physiological integrity; CNS: Physiological adaptation; CL: Analysis

55. Which of the following conditions is a sign of neurologic involvement in systemic lupus erythematosus (SLE)?

1. Facial tic
2. Psychosis
3. Extremity weakness
4. Cerebrovascular accidents

55. 2. Neurologic involvement may be shown by psychosis, seizures, and headaches. Tics and cerebrovascular accidents aren't related to SLE. Weakness may be present, but it's usually related to muscle atrophy, not neurologic involvement.

NP: Assessment; CN: Physiological integrity; CNS: Physiological adaptation; CL: Knowledge

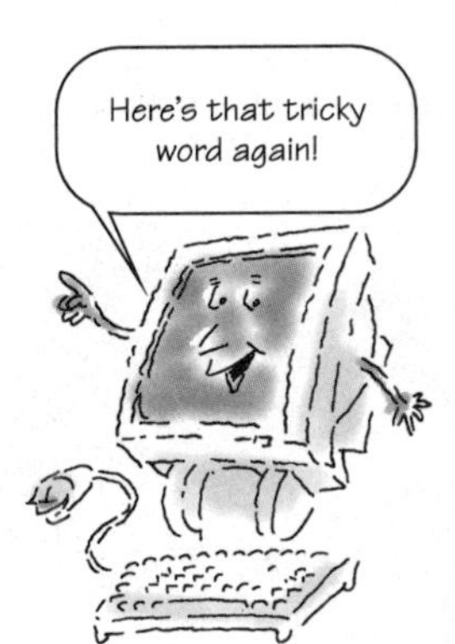

Here's that tricky word again!

56. Which of the following conditions is not a complication of Hodgkin's disease?

1. Anemia
2. Infection
3. Myocardial infarction
4. Nausea

56. 3. Complications of Hodgkin's disease are pancytopenia, nausea, and infection. Cardiac involvement usually doesn't occur.

NP: Assessment; CN: Physiological integrity; CNS: Physiological adaptation; CL: Knowledge

57. Which of the following symptoms is a classic sign of systemic lupus erythematosus (SLE)?

1. Vomiting
2. Weight loss
3. Difficulty urinating
4. Superficial lesions over the cheeks and nose

57. 4. Although all these symptoms can be signs of SLE, the classic sign is the butterfly rash over the cheeks and nose.

NP: Assessment; CN: Physiological integrity; CNS: Physiological adaptation; CL: Knowledge

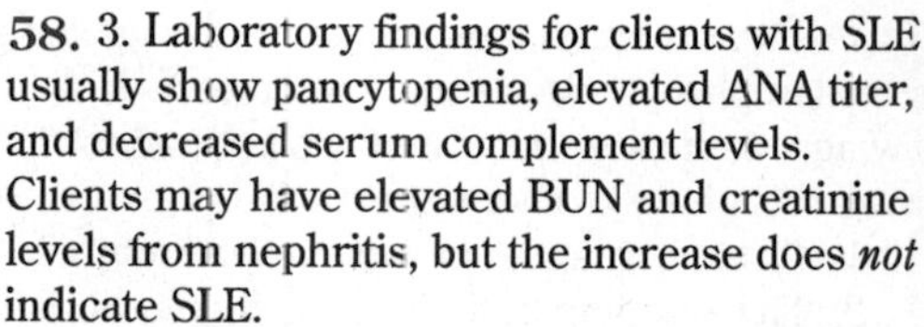

58. Which of the following laboratory test results supports the diagnosis of systemic lupus erythematosus (SLE)?

1. Elevated serum complement level
2. Thrombocytosis, elevated sedimentation rate
3. Pancytopenia, elevated antinuclear antibody (ANA) titer
4. Leukocytosis, elevated blood urea nitrogen (BUN) and creatinine levels

58. 3. Laboratory findings for clients with SLE usually show pancytopenia, elevated ANA titer, and decreased serum complement levels. Clients may have elevated BUN and creatinine levels from nephritis, but the increase does *not* indicate SLE.

NP: Assessment; CN: Physiological integrity; CNS: Physiological adaptation; CL: Application

59. Which of the following laboratory values is expected for a client just diagnosed with chronic lymphocytic leukemia?

1. Elevated sedimentation rate
2. Uncontrolled proliferation of granulocytes
3. Thrombocytopenia and increased lymphocytes
4. Elevated aspartate aminotransferase and alanine aminotransferase levels

59. 3. Chronic lymphocytic leukemia shows a proliferation of small abnormal mature B lymphocytes and decreased antibody response. Thrombocytopenia also is often present. Uncontrolled proliferation of granulocytes occurs in myelogenous leukemia. Aspartate aminotransferase, alanine aminotransferase, and erythrocyte sedimentation rate values are *not* affected.

NP: Assessment; CN: Physiological integrity; CNS: Physiological adaptation; CL: Knowledge

60. At the time of diagnosis of Hodgkin's lymphoma, which of the following areas is often involved?

1. Back
2. Chest
3. Groin
4. Neck

60. 4. At the time of diagnosis, a painless cervical lesion is often present. The back, chest, and groin areas aren't involved.

NP: Assessment; CN: Physiological integrity; CNS: Physiological adaptation; CL: Knowledge

61. According to a standard staging classification of Hodgkin's disease, which of the following criteria reflects stage II?

1. Involvement of extralymphatic organs or tissues
2. Involvement of a single lymph node region or structure
3. Involvement of two or more lymph node regions or structures
4. Involvement of lymph node regions or structures on both sides of the diaphragm

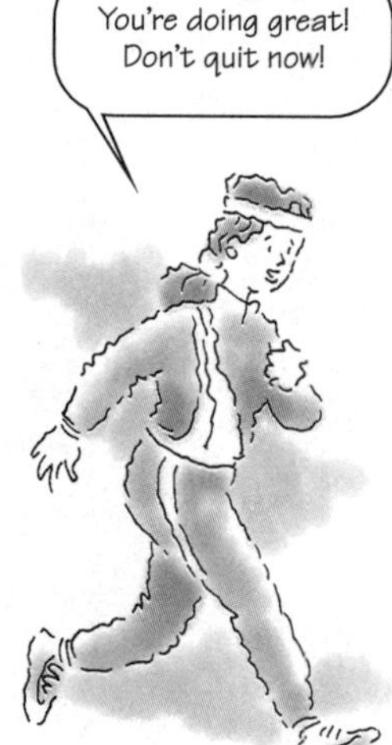
You're doing great!
Don't quit now!

61. 3. Stage II involves two or more lymph node regions. Stage I involves only one lymph node region; stage III involves nodes on both sides of the diaphragm; and stage IV involves extralymphatic organs or tissues.

NP: Assessment; CN: Physiological integrity; CNS: Physiological adaptation; CL: Knowledge

62. A client is about to start chemotherapy for acute lymphocytic leukemia. Which of the following statements shows he does not understand this phase of chemotherapy?
1. "I'll have treatments only once a month."
2. "I'll be getting high doses of chemotherapy."
3. "I won't get sick at this stage of the treatment."
4. "The purpose of these treatments is to induce a remission."

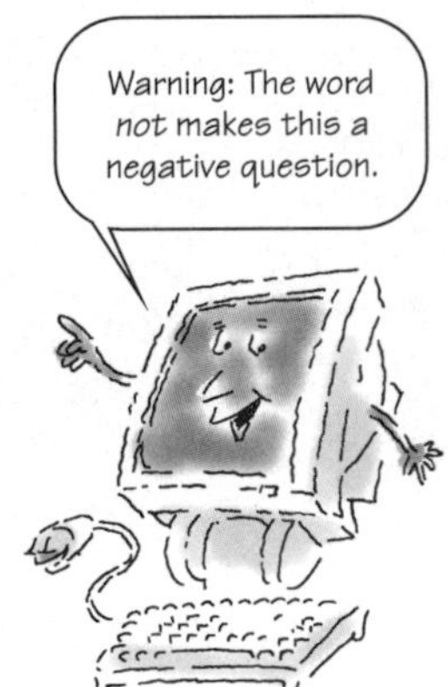

Warning: The word not makes this a negative question.

62. 1. The initial phase of chemotherapy is called the induction phase and is designed to put the client into remission by giving high doses of the drugs. Treatments will be closer together than once each month. Monthly treatments usually occur during the maintenance phase of chemotherapy. The other options indicate that the client understands chemotherapy.
NP: Evaluation; CN: Physiological integrity; CNS: Basic care and comfort; CL: Knowledge

63. Which of the following statements is correct about the rate of cell growth in relation to chemotherapy?
1. Faster growing cells are less susceptible to chemotherapy.
2. Nondividing cells are more susceptible to chemotherapy.
3. Faster growing cells are more susceptible to chemotherapy.
4. Slower growing cells are more susceptible to chemotherapy.

63. 3. The faster the cell grows, the more susceptible it is to chemotherapy and radiation therapy. Slow-growing and nondividing cells are less susceptible to chemotherapy. Repeated cycles of chemotherapy are used to destroy nondividing cells as they begin active cell division.
NP: Assessment; CN: Physiological integrity; CNS: Physiological adaptation; CL: Application

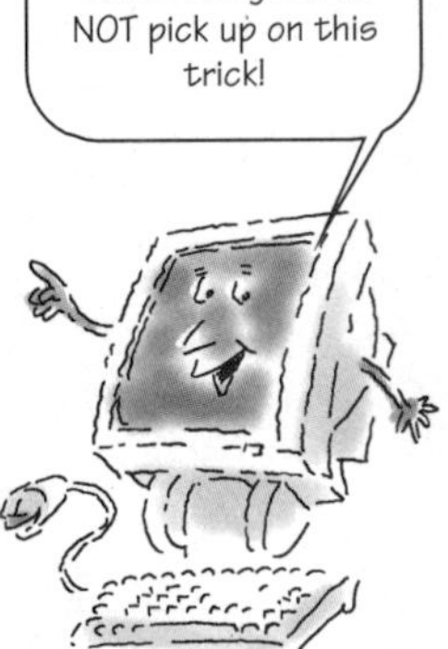

You're too good to NOT pick up on this trick!

64. Which of the following tests will not be used to diagnose tumor lysis syndrome?
1. Complete blood count (CBC)
2. Chest X-ray
3. Electrocardiogram (ECG)
4. Electrolytes

64. 2. A chest X-ray wouldn't be indicated. CBC, electrolytes, and ECG would all confirm the diagnosis of tumor lysis syndrome. The client is at risk for infection and anemia because of the cell destruction.
NP: Assessment; CN: Physiological integrity; CNS: Physiological adaptation; CL: Application

65. Which of the following treatments is most appropriate for the client with tumor lysis syndrome?
1. Give antibiotics.
2. Give I.V. hydration.
3. Give packed red blood cells.
4. Give potassium chloride I.V.

65. 2. The treatment for tumor lysis syndrome is I.V. hydration, allopurinol, and alkalizing the urine. Transfusions of red blood cells aren't given until the body is able to produce mature cells. Antibiotics are given when infection is first detected. The potassium level is often elevated in tumor lysis syndrome, so potassium chloride wouldn't be indicated.
NP: Implementation; CN: Physiological integrity; CNS: Pharmacological and parenteral therapies; CL: Knowledge

66. Which of the following foods should a client with leukemia avoid?
1. White bread
2. Carrot sticks
3. Stewed apples
4. Medium rare steak

66. 2. A low-bacteria diet would be indicated which excludes raw fruits and vegetables.
NP: Planning; CN: Health promotion and maintenance; CNS: Prevention and early detection of disease; CL: Application

67. A client with leukemia has neutropenia. Which of the following functions must be frequently assessed?

1. Blood pressure
2. Bowel sounds
3. Heart sounds
4. Breath sounds

67. 4. Pneumonia, both viral and fungal, is a common cause of death in clients with neutropenia, so frequent assessment of respiratory rate and breath sounds is required. Although assessing blood pressure, bowel sounds, and heart sounds is important, it won't help detect pneumonia.

NP: Assessment; CN: Physiological integrity; CNS: Physiological adaptation; CL: Application

68. Which of the following processes removes excess white blood cells from the body?

1. Erythrapheresis
2. Granulapheresis
3. Leukapheresis
4. Plasmapheresis

68. 3. Leukapheresis is the removal of excess white blood cells. Plasmapheresis is the filtering of the plasma. There are no processes called granulapheresis or erythrapheresis.

NP: Assessment; CN: Physiological integrity; CNS: Basic care and comfort; CL: Knowledge

69. Which of the following clients is most at risk for developing multiple myeloma?

1. A 20-year-old Asian woman
2. A 30-year-old White man
3. A 50-year-old Hispanic woman
4. A 60-year-old Black man

69. 4. Multiple myeloma is more common in middle-aged and older clients (the median age at diagnosis is 60 years) and is twice as common in Blacks as Whites. It occurs most often in Black men.

NP: Assessment; CN: Health promotion and maintenance; CNS: Prevention and early detection of disease; CL: Comprehension

Forget the weights. Keep an eye on those "abs."

70. Which of the following substances has abnormal values early in the course of multiple myeloma (MM)?

1. Immunoglobulins
2. Platelets
3. Red blood cells (RBCs)
4. White blood cells (WBCs)

70. 1. MM is characterized by malignant plasma cells that produce an increased amount of immunoglobulin that isn't functional. As more malignant plasma cells are produced, there's less space in the bone marrow for RBC production. In late stages, platelets and WBCs are reduced as the bone marrow is infiltrated by malignant plasma cells.

NP: Assessment; CN: Health promotion and maintenance; CNS: Prevention and early detection of disease; CL: Knowledge

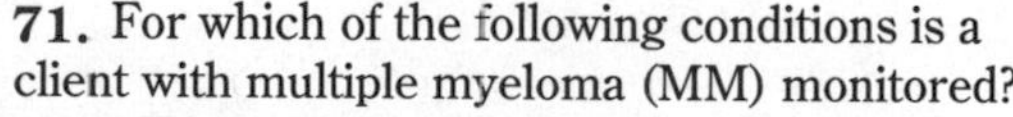

71. For which of the following conditions is a client with multiple myeloma (MM) monitored?

1. Hypercalcemia
2. Hyperkalemia
3. Hypernatremia
4. Hypermagnesemia

71. 1. Calcium is released when bone is destroyed. This causes an increase in serum calcium levels. MM doesn't affect potassium, sodium, or magnesium levels.

NP: Planning; CN: Physiological integrity; CNS: Physiological adaptation; CL: Application

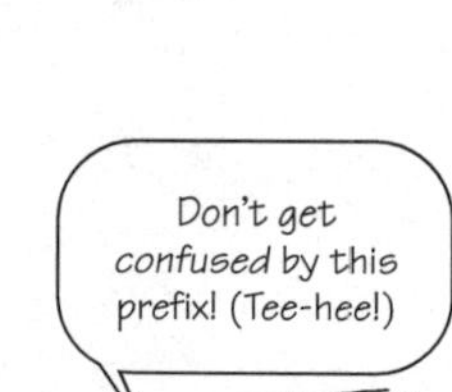

Don't get confused by this prefix! (Tee-hee!)

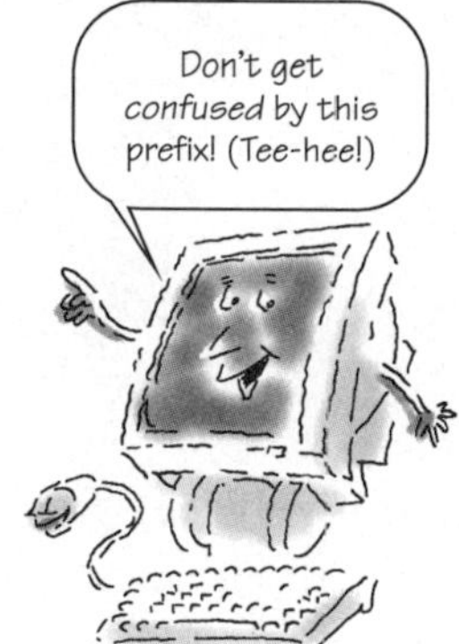

72. Which of the following symptoms commonly occurs with hypercalcemia?

1. Tremors
2. Headache
3. Confusion
4. Muscle weakness

72. 3. Signs of hypercalcemia include confusion, anorexia, nausea, vomiting, abdominal pain, ileus, constipation, and eventually impaired renal function. Tremors, headache, and muscle weakness are not common symptoms of hypercalcemia.

NP: Assessment; CN: Physiological integrity; CNS: Physiological adaptation; CL: Application

73. Which of the following conditions or symptoms is often a secondary complication of hypercalcemia in a client with multiple myeloma (MM)?

1. Pneumonia
2. Muscle spasms
3. Renal dysfunction
4. Myocardial irritability

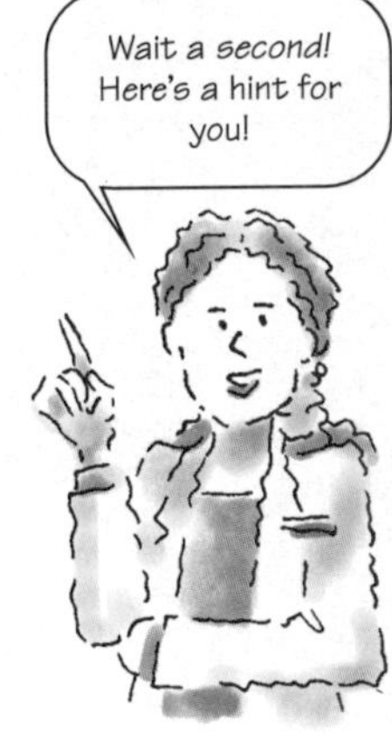

Wait a second! Here's a hint for you!

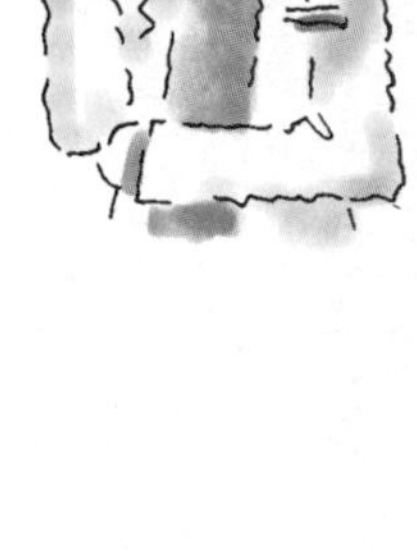

74. The neurologic complications of multiple myeloma (MM) usually involve which of the following body systems?

1. Brain
2. Spinal column
3. Autonomic nervous system
4. Parasympathetic nervous system

75. Which of the following interventions is stressed in teaching about multiple myeloma (MM)?

1. Maintain bed rest.
2. Enforce fluid restriction.
3. Drink 3 L of fluid daily.
4. Keep the lower extremities elevated.

76. Although a client's physiologic response to a health crisis is important to the health outcome, which of the following nursing interventions also must be addressed?

1. Teach the family how to care for the client.
2. Help the client effectively cope with the crisis.
3. Maintain I.V. access, medications, and diet.
4. Teach the client basic information about the illness.

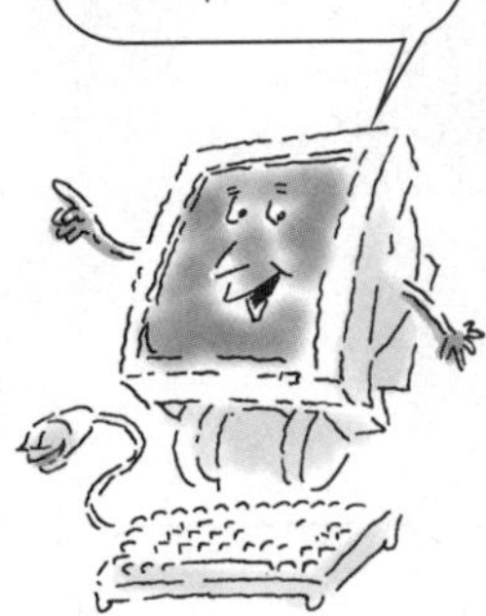

Here's a question that uses a clever little technique — *must* — to get you to prioritize.

73. 3. Twenty percent of MM clients with hypercalcemia and hyperuricemia develop renal insufficiency. Hypocalcemia causes muscle spasms and hypokalemia causes myocardial irritability. Pneumonia doesn't result from hypercalcemia.

NP: Planning; CN: Health promotion and maintenance; CNS: Prevention and early detection of disease; CL: Comprehension

74. 2. Back pain or paresthesia in the lower extremities may indicate impending spinal cord compression from a spinal tumor. This should be recognized and treated promptly as progression of the tumor may result in paraplegia. The other options, which reflect parts of the nervous system, aren't usually affected by MM.

NP: Assessment; CN: Physiological integrity; CNS: Physiological adaptation; CL: Application

75. 3. The client needs to drink 3 to 5 L of fluid each day to dilute calcium and uric acid to try to reduce the risk of renal dysfunction. Walking is encouraged to prevent further bone demineralization. The lower extremities don't need to be elevated.

NP: Planning; CN: Physiological integrity; CNS: Basic care and comfort; CL: Application

76. 2. Although all of the answers are important in the care of the client, if the individual isn't able to cope with the emotional, spiritual, and psychological aspects of his crisis, the other components of care may be ineffective as well.

NP: Implementation; CN: Psychosocial integrity; CNS: Coping and adaptation; CL: Application

77. To promote healing of a laceration, which of the following interventions is correct?
1. Elevate the body part.
2. Monitor the blood pressure.
3. Apply a pressure dressing and heat.
4. Apply a pressure dressing and ice pack.

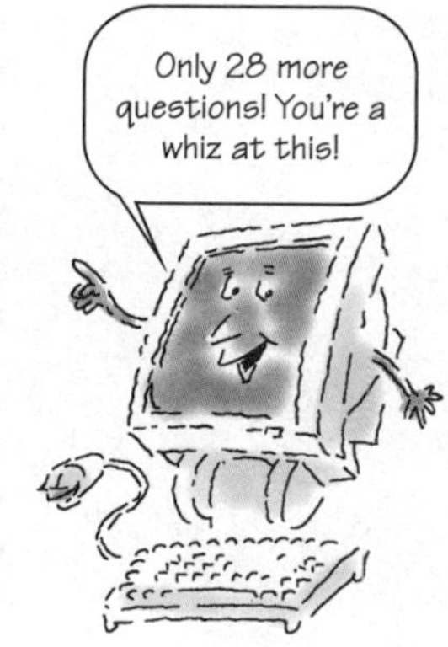

Only 28 more questions! You're a whiz at this!

77. 4. Pressure dressings help clotting by promoting the localization of microorganisms and the development of meshwork for repair and healing. Ice decreases blood flow to the site, slowing the bleeding. Heat increases blood flow to the site, increasing the bleeding. Monitoring blood pressure is important when the individual is bleeding but does nothing to promote clotting. Elevating the body part helps reduce edema but doesn't directly promote healing.

NP: Implementation; CN: Physiological integrity; CNS: Physiological adaptation; CL: Application

78. An elderly client has a wound that isn't healing normally. Interventions should be based on which of the following principles or test results?
1. Laboratory test results
2. Kidney function test results
3. Poor wound healing expected as part of the aging process
4. Diminished immune function interfering with ability to fight infection

78. 4. Immune function is important in the healing process and diminished response may slow or prevent the healing process from taking place. Although immune function declines with age, there are healthy behaviors that will enhance the elderly individual's response to tissue trauma (nutrition, exercise). Kidney function and laboratory results are important but are *not* solely responsible for health outcomes.

NP: Analysis; CN: Physiological integrity; CNS: Physiological adaptation; CL: Analysis

79. Which of the following conditions or symptoms is an appropriate immune response?
1. Allergies
2. Autoimmune disorder
3. Inflammation and increased temperature
4. Insufficient protection (immune deficiency)

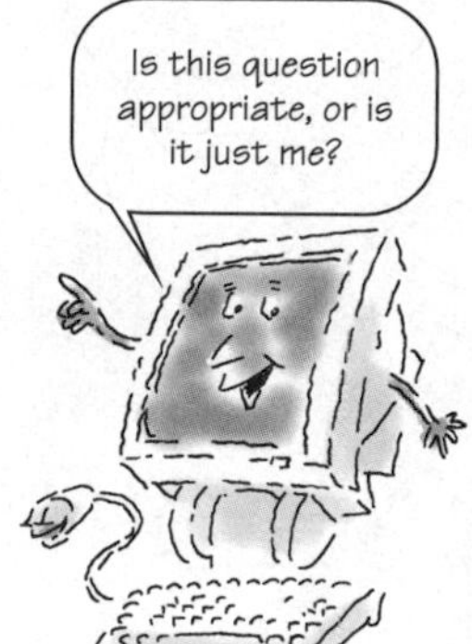

Is this question appropriate, or is it just me?

79. 3. Inflammation and increased temperature are a normal immune response to antigens. Allergies are heightened responses to antigens to which the body was previously exposed. Autoimmune disorders result when immune cells attack self cells and result in long-term diseases. Insufficient protection results in immune deficiency disorders that compromise the individual's ability to ward off infections.

NP: Analysis; CN: Physiological integrity; CNS: Reduction of risk potential; CL: Analysis

80. What is the average length of time from human immunodeficiency virus (HIV) infection to the development of acquired immunodeficiency syndrome (AIDS)?
1. Less than 5 years
2. 5 to 7 years
3. 10 years
4. More than 10 years

80. 3. Epidemiologic studies show the average time from initial contact with HIV to the development of AIDS is 10 years.

NP: Planning; CN: Health promotion and maintenance; CNS: Prevention and early detection of disease; CL: Knowledge

81. Which of the following conditions or factors may cause an acquired immune deficiency?

1. Age
2. Genetics
3. Environment
4. Medical treatments

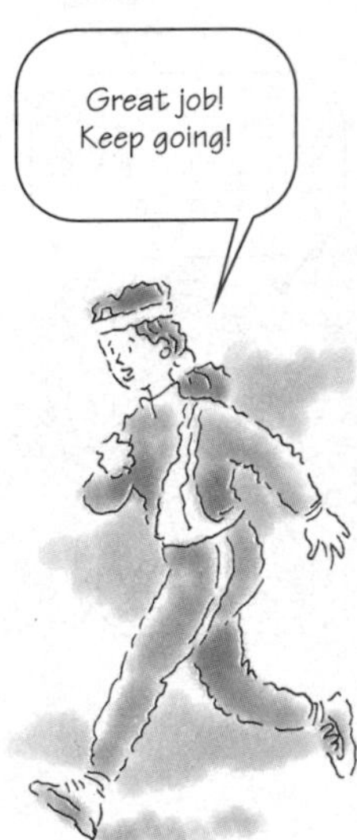
Great job!
Keep going!

81. 4. Immune deficiencies may result from medical treatments, such as medications, radiation, or transplants. Immune function may decline with age, but it isn't considered the cause of acquired immune deficiency. Genetics and environment haven't been shown to be factors in acquired immune deficiency.

NP: Evaluation; CN: Physiological integrity; CNS: Physiological adaptation; CL: Analysis

82. Which of the following statements best explains the reason for using stress management with clients?

1. Everyone is stressed.
2. It has become an accepted practice.
3. Eastern health practices have shown its effectiveness.
4. Prolonged psychological stress may contribute to the development of physical illness.

82. 4. Psychological and emotional stress stimulate the central nervous system, increasing the levels of corticotropin and cortisol, which result in harmful effects on immune, cardiac, neural, and endocrine function. Although stress management may be a common therapy for stressed individuals, and Eastern countries may promote its use, nursing interventions must have research-based rationales. Many people report high levels of stress, but not everyone would claim to be stressed.

NP: Planning; CN: Psychosocial integrity; CNS: Coping and adaptation; CL: Knowledge

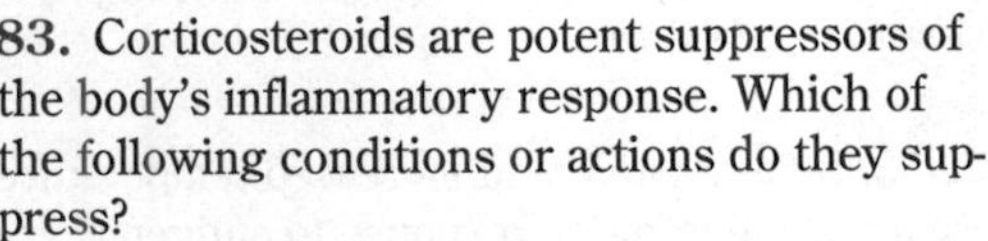

83. Corticosteroids are potent suppressors of the body's inflammatory response. Which of the following conditions or actions do they suppress?

1. Sympathetic response
2. Pain receptors
3. Immune response
4. Neural transmission

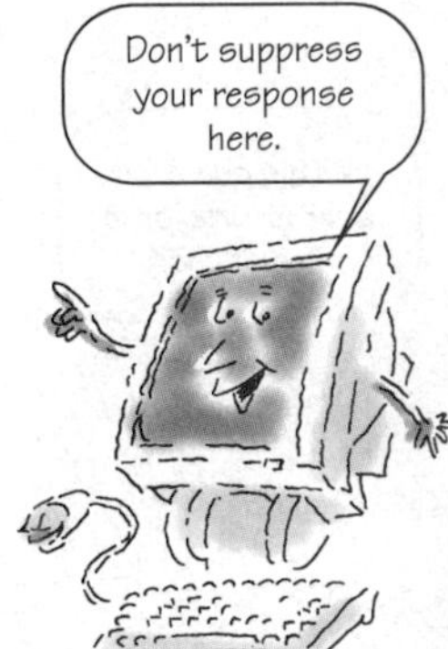
Don't suppress
your response
here.

83. 3. Corticosteroids suppress eosinophils, lymphocytes, natural-killer cells, and other microorganisms, inhibiting the natural inflammatory process in an infected or injured part of the body. This promotes resolution of inflammation, stabilizes lysosomal membranes, decreases capillary permeability, and depresses phagocytosis of tissues by white blood cells, thus blocking the release of more inflammatory materials. Corticosteroids don't affect neural transmission, pain receptors, or the sympathetic response.

NP: Assessment; CN: Physiological integrity; CNS: Pharmacological and parenteral therapies; CL: Comprehension

84. Which statement made by a client indicates that he understands the results of a negative human immunodeficiency virus (HIV) test?

1. "I'm not infected with HIV."
2. "I haven't produced antibodies to HIV."
3. "I'm immune to HIV."
4. "I have antibodies to HIV."

84. 2. A negative HIV test means that HIV antibodies weren't in the client's blood at the time the test was performed. Antibodies may take 3 weeks to 6 months or longer to develop. A negative test result doesn't indicate immunity. If antibodies to HIV are present, the test result is positive.

NP: Assessment; CN: Psychosocial integrity; CNS: Psychosocial adaptation; CL: Application

85. In community health and epidemiologic studies, which of the following definitions of disease prevalence is correct?

1. The number of individuals affected by a particular disease at a specific time
2. The rate at which individuals without a specific disease develop that disease
3. The proportion of individuals affected by the disease who live for a particular period of time
4. The proportion of individuals without the disease who eventually develop the disease within a specific period of time

85. 1. Prevalence is the number of individuals affected by the disease at a specific time. Risk is the proportion of individuals without the disease who develop the disease within a particular time period. Incidence rate is the rapidity with which individuals without the disease contract it. Survival is the proportion of individuals affected by the disease who live for a particular length of time.

NP: Assessment; CN: Health promotion and maintenance; CNS: Prevention and early detection of disease; CL: Analysis

86. Hepatitis B immunizations shouldn't be given to which of the following groups?

1. Immunosuppressed clients
2. Immigrants
3. Health care professionals
4. Individuals older than age 65

86. 1. The immune system of immunosuppressed clients can't handle the hepatitis B vaccine. Elderly clients, health care professionals, and immigrants are all candidates for the vaccine and may need the protection.

NP: Assessment; CN: Physiological integrity; CNS: Pharmacological and parenteral therapies; CL: Analysis

87. Epidemiologic research has contributed to our knowledge of acquired immunodeficiency syndrome (AIDS) by which of the following actions?

1. Finding a cure
2. Developing vaccines for future use
3. Requiring the reporting of all diagnosed clients and their partners
4. Identifying risk factors that compare between affected and unaffected individuals

87. 4. Epidemiologic research has been pivotal in identifying the behaviors that place individuals at risk for AIDS. No vaccine has been shown to be effective to date, but work is ongoing. Not all states require the reporting of sexual partners for AIDS clients. No cure has been found.

NP: Assessment; CN: Health promotion and maintenance; CNS: Prevention and early detection of disease; CL: Knowledge

88. A 32-year-old client is admitted with a tentative diagnosis of acquired immunodeficiency syndrome (AIDS). The preliminary report of biopsies done on her facial lesions indicates Kaposi's sarcoma. Which of the following approaches would be most appropriate?

1. Tell the client that Kaposi's sarcoma is common in people with AIDS.
2. Pretend not to notice the lesions on the client's face.
3. Inform the client of the biopsy results and support her emotionally.
4. Explore the client's feelings about her facial disfigurement.

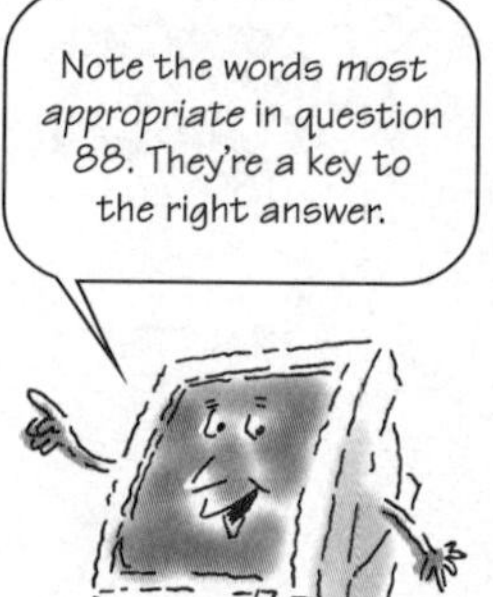
Note the words *most appropriate* in question 88. They're a key to the right answer.

88. 4. Facial lesions can contribute to decreased self-esteem and an altered body image. Discussing AIDS with a client whose diagnosis isn't final may be inappropriate and doesn't provide emotional support. Pretending not to notice visible lesions ignores the client's concerns. The primary care provider — not the nurse — should inform the client of the biopsy results.

NP: Implementation; CN: Psychosocial integrity; CNS: Psychosocial adaptation; CL: Application

89. A client infected with human immunodeficiency virus (HIV) begins zidovudine (AZT) therapy. Which of the following statements best describes the action of this drug?

1. It destroys the outer wall of the virus and kills it.
2. It interferes with viral replication.
3. It stimulates the immune system.
4. It promotes excretion of viral antibodies.

89. 2. Zidovudine inhibits deoxyribonucleic acid synthesis in HIV, thus interfering with viral replication. The drug doesn't destroy the viral wall, stimulate the immune system, or promote HIV antibody excretion.

NP: Analysis; CN: Physiological integrity; CNS: Pharmacological and parenteral therapies; CL: Knowledge

90. For a client with acquired immunodeficiency syndrome (AIDS), the nurse should follow standard precautions and take which of the following actions to protect herself when performing mouth care on the client?

1. Use reverse isolation.
2. Place the client in a private room.
3. Put on a mask, gloves, and a gown.
4. Wear gloves.

90. 4. Standard precautions stipulate that a health care worker who anticipates coming into contact with a client's blood or body fluids must wear gloves. Reverse isolation is used to protect the client from the health care worker, not the other way around. A private room doesn't provide barrier protection, an essential step in standard precautions. A mask and gloves are needed only for anticipated contact with airborne droplets of blood or body fluids; a gown is needed only for anticipated contact with splashes of blood or body fluids. Neither is the case when performing oral hygiene.

NP: Planning; CN: Psychosocial integrity; CNS: Psychosocial adaptation; CL: Application

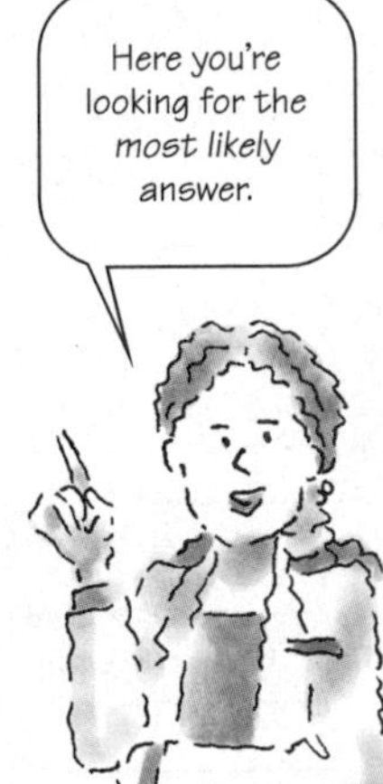

Here you're looking for the most likely answer.

91. Which of the following diagnostic findings are most likely for a client with aplastic anemia?

1. Decreased production of T-helper cells
2. Decreased levels of white blood cells (WBCs), red blood cells (RBCs), and platelets
3. Increased levels of WBCs, RBCs, and platelets
4. Reed-Sternberg cells and lymph node enlargement

91. 2. In aplastic anemia, the most likely diagnostic findings are decreased levels of all the cellular elements of the blood (pancytopenia). T-helper cell production doesn't decrease in aplastic anemia. Reed-Sternberg cells and lymph node enlargement occur with Hodgkin's disease.

NP: Assessment; CN: Health promotion and maintenance; CNS: Prevention and early detection of disease; CL: Comprehension

92. A client with iron deficiency anemia is scheduled for discharge. Which instruction about prescribed ferrous gluconate therapy should the nurse include in the teaching plan?

1. "Take the medication with an antacid."
2. "Take the medication with a glass of milk."
3. "Take the medication with cereal."
4. "Take the medication on an empty stomach."

92. 4. Preferably, ferrous gluconate should be taken on an empty stomach. Ferrous gluconate should not be taken with antacids, milk, or whole-grain cereals because these foods reduce iron absorption.

NP: Planning; CN: Physiological integrity; CNS: Pharmacological and parenteral therapies; CL: Application

93. A client with ankylosing spondylitis is most likely to report which of the following initial symptoms?

1. Red, painful, swollen joints
2. Fatigue and night sweats
3. Low back pain
4. Neck pain and stiffness

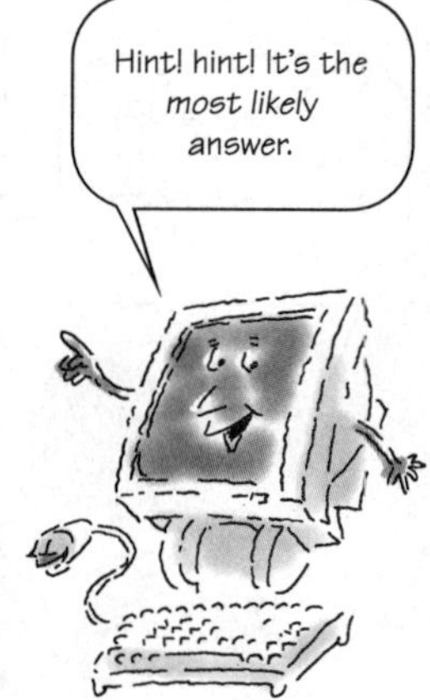

Hint! hint! It's the most likely answer.

93. 3. Typically, intermittent low back pain is the first indication of ankylosing spondylitis. Red, painful, swollen joints occur with rheumatoid arthritis. Although ankylosing spondylitis may cause fatigue, it rarely produces night sweats. Neck pain and stiffness from involvement of the cervical spine are relatively late manifestations.

NP: Assessment; CN: Physiological integrity; CNS: Physiological adaptation; CL: Comprehension

94. A female client with the beta-thalassemia trait plans to marry a man of Italian ancestry who also has the trait. Which client statement would indicate that she understands the teaching provided by the nurse?

1. "Thalassemia is treated with iron supplements."
2. "I need to learn how to give myself vitamin B_{12} injections."
3. "I'll see a genetic counselor before starting a family."
4. "If my fiancé were of Middle Eastern descent, I wouldn't be worried about having children."

94. 3. Two people with the beta-thalassemia trait have a 25% chance of having a child with thalassemia major, a potentially life-threatening disease. Iron supplements aren't used to treat thalassemia; in fact, they could contribute to iron overload. Vitamin B_{12} injections are used to treat pernicious anemia, not thalassemia. Thalassemia occurs primarily in people of Italian, Greek, African, Asian, Middle Eastern, East Indian, and Caribbean descent.

NP: Evaluation; CN: Health promotion and maintenance; CNS: Prevention and early detection of disease; CL: Application

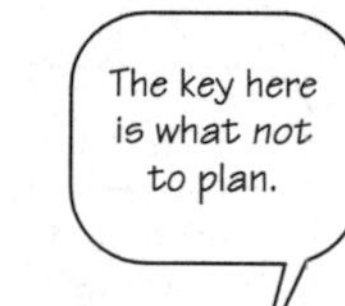

The key here is what not to plan.

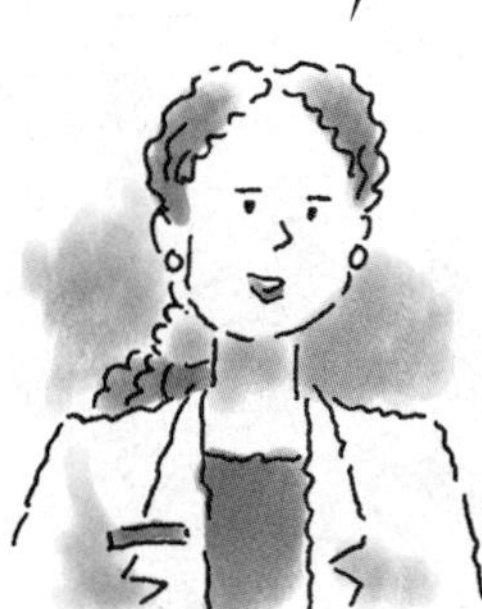

95. A young African-American woman with a history of sickle cell disease is complaining of severe abdominal pain. Which of the following nursing interventions should the nurse not plan for this client?

1. Forcing oral fluid intake
2. Keeping the client nothing by mouth (NPO)
3. Administering oxygen therapy
4. Preparing the client for a CT scan of the abdomen

95. 1. Although the client may be in a sickle cell crisis and experiencing acute abdominal pain caused by sickling in the mesenteric circulation, it's important to remember that clients with sickle cell disease aren't spared appendicitis or other intra-abdominal events. Important nursing interventions would include preparing the client for possible surgery by keeping her NPO and for diagnostic studies such as computer tomography scanning. Administering oxygen will help most clients in a sickle cell crisis.

NP: Planning; CN: Physiological integrity; CNS: Reduction of risk potential; CL: Application

96. Which of the following precautions should the nurse include in the care plan for a neutropenic client with leukemia?

1. Have the client use a soft toothbrush and electric razor, avoid using enemas, and watch for signs of bleeding.
2. Put on a mask, gown, and gloves when entering the client's room.
3. Provide a clear liquid, low-sodium diet.
4. Eliminate fresh fruits and vegetables, avoid using enemas, and practice frequent handwashing.

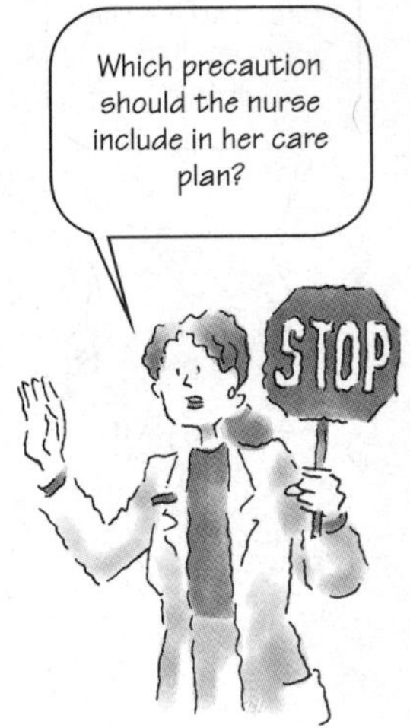

96. 4. Neutropenia occurs when the absolute neutrophil count falls below 1,000/mm³, reflecting a severe risk for infection. The nurse should provide a low-bacterial diet, which means eliminating fresh fruits and vegetables; avoid invasive procedures, such as enemas, because they increase the infection risk; and practice frequent handwashing to lower the infection risk. Using a soft toothbrush, avoiding straight-edged razors and enemas, and monitoring for bleeding are thrombocytopenia precautions. Putting on a mask, gown, and gloves when entering the client's room are reverse isolation measures. A neutropenic patient doesn't need a clear liquid diet or sodium restrictions.

NP: Planning; CN: Safe, effective care environment; CNS: Safety and infection control; CL: Application

97. Which of the following disorders results from a deficiency of factor VIII?

1. Sickle cell disease
2. Christmas disease
3. Hemophilia A
4. Hemophilia B

97. 3. Hemophilia A results from a deficiency of factor VIII. Sickle cell disease is caused by a defective hemoglobin molecule. Christmas disease, also called hemophilia B, results from a factor IX deficiency.

NP: Assessment; CN: Physiological integrity; CNS: Physiological adaptation; CL: Knowledge

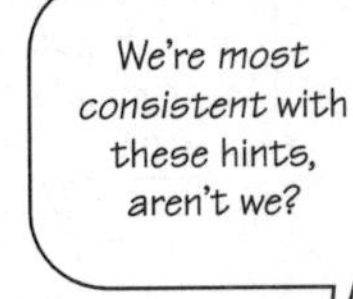

We're most consistent with these hints, aren't we?

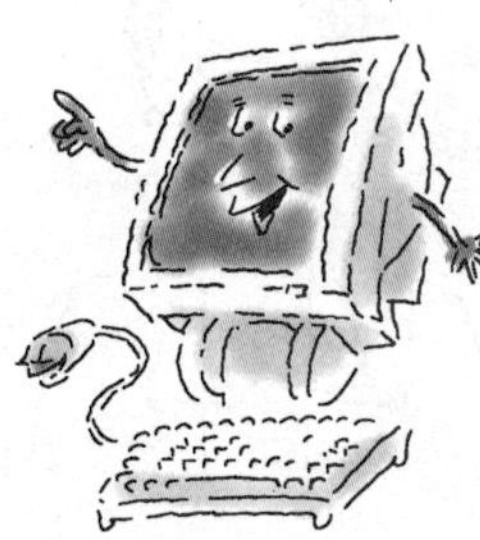

98. A 19-year-old client admitted with heat stroke begins to show signs of disseminated intravascular coagulation (DIC). Which of the following laboratory findings is most consistent with DIC?

1. Low platelet count
2. Elevated fibrinogen levels
3. Low levels of fibrin degradation products
4. Reduced prothrombin time

98. 1. In DIC, platelets and clotting factors are consumed, resulting in microthrombi and excessive bleeding. As clots form, fibrinogen levels decrease and the prothrombin time increases. Fibrin degradation products increase as fibrinolysis takes place.

NP: Assessment; CN: Physiological integrity; CNS: Physiological adaptation; CL: Knowledge

99. A client comes to the clinic complaining of fever, drenching night sweats, and unexplained weight loss over the past 3 months. Physical examination reveals a single enlarged supraclavicular lymph node. Which of the following is the most probable diagnosis?

1. Influenza
2. Sickle cell anemia
3. Leukemia
4. Hodgkin's disease

99. 4. Hodgkin's disease typically causes fever, night sweats, weight loss, and lymph node enlargement. Influenza doesn't last for months. Clients with sickle cell anemia manifest signs and symptoms of chronic anemia with pallor of the mucous membranes, fatigue, and decreased tolerance for exercise; they don't show fever, night sweats, weight loss or lymph node enlargement. Leukemia doesn't cause lymph node enlargement.

NP: Assessment; CN: Health promotion and maintenance; CNS: Prevention and early detection of disease; CL: Application

100. A client learns from the physician that he has Hodgkin's disease. After the physician leaves the room, the client tells the nurse he's afraid of dying. Which response by the nurse is appropriate?

1. "Don't worry, many people survive this disease."
2. "Hodgkin's disease is very treatable."
3. "You're afraid of dying?"
4. "You should speak with your minister."

100. 3. Repeating what the client has said (or describing his feelings) encourages the client to elaborate on his thoughts and feelings. Telling him not to worry and saying that Hodgkin's disease is very treatable ignores his feelings and offers false reassurance. Telling a client what to do, such as calling his minister, also ignores his feelings.

NP: Analysis; CN: Psychosocial integrity; CNS: Coping and adaptation; CL: Application

101. Before starting treatment for leukemia, a client receives I.V. fluids and allopurinol (Zyloprim). The goal of these interventions is to reduce the risk of which complication of chemotherapy?

1. Disseminated intravascular coagulation (DIC)
2. Pancytopenia
3. Tumor lysis syndrome
4. Mucositis

101. 3. During chemotherapy for leukemia, tumor lysis syndrome may occur as cell destruction releases intracellular components, resulting in hyperuricemia. Large fluid quantities and allopurinol therapy help prevent urine crystallization. Although DIC, pancytopenia, and mucositis are possible chemotherapy complications, they're not treated with I.V. fluids and allopurinol.

NP: Planning; CN: Physiological integrity; CNS: Pharmacological and parenteral therapies; CL: Application

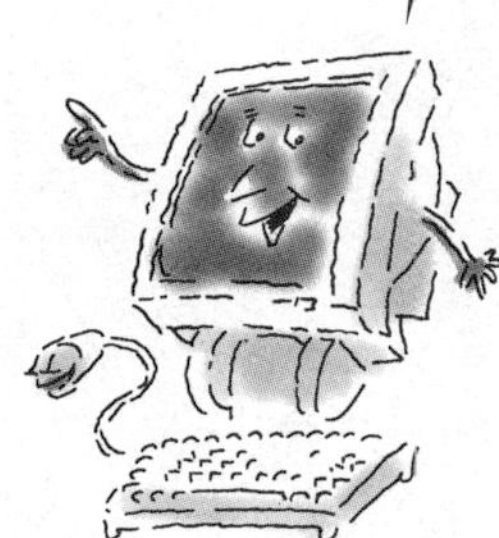

Be on the safe side and choose the safest type.

102. A client with a gunshot wound requires an emergency blood transfusion. His blood type is AB negative. Which blood type would be the safest for him to receive?

1. AB Rh-positive
2. A Rh-positive
3. A Rh-negative
4. O Rh-positive

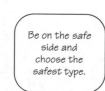

102. 3. Human blood can sometimes contain an inherited D antigen. Persons with the D antigen have Rh-positive blood type; those lacking the antigen have Rh-negative blood. It's important that a person with Rh-negative blood receives Rh-negative blood. If Rh-positive blood is administered to an Rh-negative person, the recipient develops anti-Rh agglutinins, and subsequent transfusions with Rh-positive blood may cause serious reactions with clumping and hemolysis of red blood cells.

NP: Implementation; CN: Physiological integrity; CNS: Pharmacological and parenteral therapies; CL: Application

103. In North America, the incidence of multiple myeloma is significantly higher in which of the following groups?

1. Whites
2. Children
3. Blacks
4. Asians

103. 3. In North America, the incidence of multiple myeloma is 8 to 10 per 100,000 for Blacks, 4 to 5 per 100,000 for Whites, and 1 to 2 per 100,000 for people of Chinese or Japanese origin. The median age at diagnosis is 72, and less than 3% of cases occur in people under age 40.

NP: Assessment; CN: Health promotion and maintenance; CNS: Prevention and early detection of disease; CL: Knowledge

104. A client with polycythemia vera is at risk for thrombosis from which of the following conditions?

1. Thrombocytopenia
2. Increased blood viscosity
3. Increased blood velocity
4. Chemotherapy treatment

104. 2. In polycythemia vera, increased red blood cell mass leads to hyperviscosity and inhibited blood flow through the microcirculation. Increased viscosity, thrombocytosis (not thrombocytopenia), and decreased blood velocity promote intravascular thrombosis. Chemotherapy may be used to treat polycythemia vera, but it doesn't increase the thrombosis risk.

NP: Assessment; CN: Health promotion and maintenance; CNS: Prevention and early detection of disease; CL: Application

105. A client with severe anemia needs a transfusion of packed red blood cells (RBCs). To prepare for the transfusion, the nurse should hang which of the following I.V. solutions?

1. Normal saline (0.9% NaCl)
2. Dextrose 5% in water (D_5W)
3. Lactated Ringer's
4. Dextrose 5% in normal saline (D_5 in 0.9% NaCl)

105. 1. Normal saline solution should be given during a packed RBC transfusion. Solutions containing dextrose or lactated Ringer's shouldn't be used because they can cause RBC hemolysis.

NP: Planning; CN: Physiological integrity; CNS: Pharmacological and parenteral therapies; CL: Comprehension

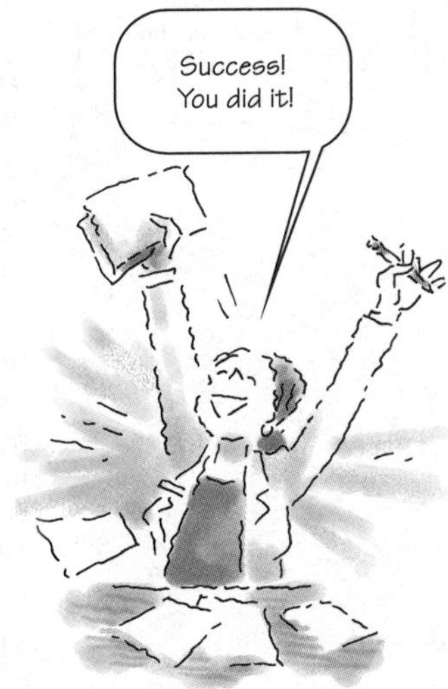

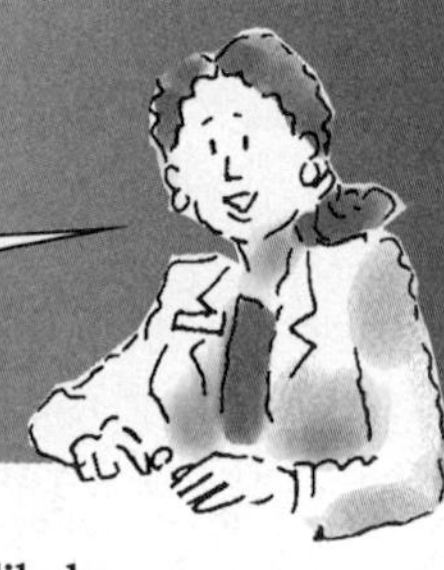

Chapter 5 Respiratory disorders

1. Clients with chronic illnesses are more likely to get pneumonia when which of the following situations is present?

1. Dehydration
2. Group living
3. Malnutrition
4. Severe periodontal disease

1. 2. Clients with chronic illnesses generally have poor immune systems. Often, residing in group living situations increases the chance of disease transmission. Adequate fluid intake, adequate nutrition, and proper oral hygiene help maintain normal defenses and can reduce the incidence of getting such diseases as pneumonia.

NP: Analysis; CN: Physiological integrity; CNS: Physiological adaptation; CL: Comprehension

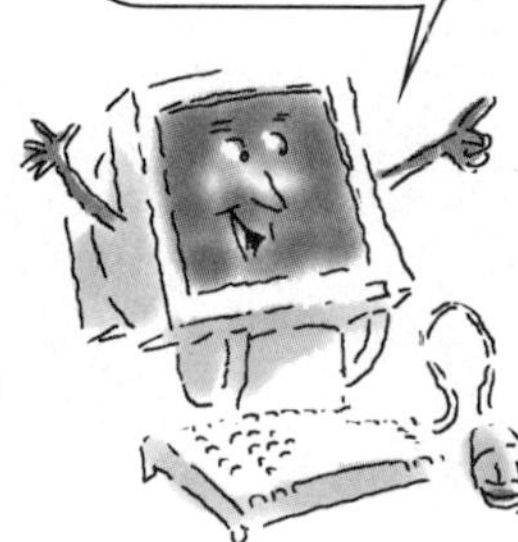

In question 1, the term *more likely* is a hint for finding the correct answer.

2. Which of the following pathophysiological mechanisms that occur in the lung parenchyma allows pneumonia to develop?

1. Atelectasis
2. Bronchiectasis
3. Effusion
4. Inflammation

2. 4. The common feature of all types of pneumonia is an inflammatory pulmonary response to the offending organism or agent. Atelectasis and bronchiectasis indicate a collapse of a portion of the airway that doesn't occur in pneumonia. An effusion is an accumulation of excess pleural fluid in the pleural space, which may be a secondary response to pneumonia.

NP: Analysis; CN: Physiological integrity; CNS: Physiological adaptation; CL: Knowledge

3. Which of the following organisms most commonly causes community-acquired pneumonia in adults?

1. *Haemophilus influenzae*
2. *Klebsiella pneumoniae*
3. *Streptococcus pneumoniae*
4. *Staphylococcus aureus*

3. 3. Pneumococcal or streptococcal pneumonia, caused by *Streptococcus pneumoniae,* is the most common cause of community-acquired pneumonia. *Haemophilus influenzae* is the most common cause of infection in children. *Klebsiella* species is the most common gram-negative organism found in the hospital setting. *Staphylococcus aureus* is the most common cause of hospital-acquired pneumonia.

NP: Evaluation; CN: Physiological integrity; CNS: Physiological adaptation; CL: Knowledge

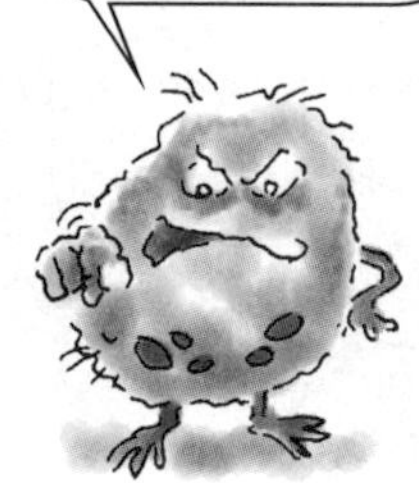

Pssst. Yeah, I'm talking to you. You'd better strep lively — er, I mean, step lively. Got it?

4. An elderly client with pneumonia may appear with which of the following symptoms first?

1. Altered mental status and dehydration
2. Fever and chills
3. Hemoptysis and dyspnea
4. Pleuritic chest pain and cough

4. 1. Fever, chills, hemoptysis, dyspnea, cough, and pleuritic chest pain are the common symptoms of pneumonia, but elderly clients may first appear with only an altered mental status and dehydration due to a blunted immune response.

NP: Assessment; CN: Physiological integrity; CNS: Physiological adaptation; CL: Application

5. When auscultating the chest of a client with pneumonia, the nurse would expect to hear which of the following sounds over areas of consolidation?

1. Bronchial
2. Bronchovesicular
3. Tubular
4. Vesicular

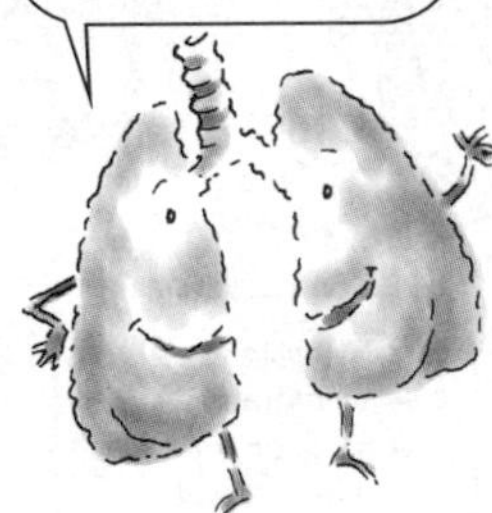

For question 5, think of where you normally hear each type of breath sound.

5. 1. Chest auscultation reveals bronchial breath sounds over areas of consolidation. Bronchovesicular breath sounds are normal over midlobe lung regions, tubular sounds are commonly heard over large airways, and vesicular breath sounds are commonly heard in the bases of the lung fields.

NP: Assessment; CN: Physiological integrity; CNS: Physiological adaptation; CL: Application

6. A diagnosis of pneumonia is typically achieved by which of the following diagnostic tests?

1. Arterial blood gas (ABG) analysis
2. Chest X-ray
3. Blood cultures
4. Sputum culture and sensitivity

6. 4. Sputum culture and sensitivity is the best way to identify the organism causing the pneumonia. Chest X-ray will show the area of lung consolidation. ABG analysis will determine the extent of hypoxia present due to the pneumonia, and blood cultures will help determine if the infection is systemic.

NP: Implementation; CN: Physiological integrity; CNS: Physiological adaptation; CL: Application

7. A 78-year-old client is admitted with a diagnosis of dehydration and change in mental status. He's being hydrated with I.V. fluids. When the nurse takes his vital signs, she notes he has a fever of 103° F (39.4° C), a cough producing yellow sputum, and pleuritic chest pain. The nurse suspects this client may have which of the following conditions?

1. Adult respiratory distress syndrome (ARDS)
2. Myocardial infarction (MI)
3. Pneumonia
4. Tuberculosis (TB)

7. 3. Fever, productive cough, and pleuritic chest pain are common signs and symptoms of pneumonia. The client with ARDS has dyspnea and hypoxia, with worsening hypoxia over time, if not treated aggressively. Pleuritic chest pain varies with respiration, unlike the constant chest pain during an MI, so this client most likely isn't having an MI. The client with TB typically has a cough producing blood-tinged sputum. A sputum culture should be obtained to confirm the nurse's suspicions.

NP: Assessment; CN: Physiological integrity; CNS: Physiological adaptation; CL: Application

8. A client with pneumonia develops dyspnea with a respiratory rate of 32 breaths/minute and difficulty expelling his secretions. The nurse auscultates his lung fields and hears bronchial sounds in the left lower lobe. The nurse determines that the client requires which of the following treatments *first*?

1. Antibiotics
2. Bed rest
3. Oxygen
4. Nutritional intake

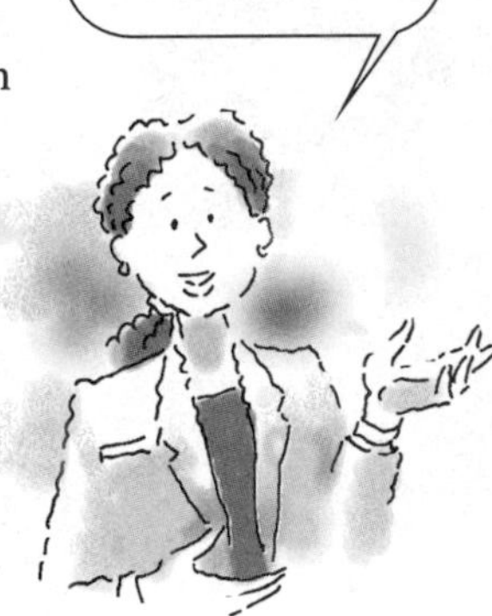

The nurse can give oxygen without a physician's order to help her client breathe easier.

8. 3. The client is having difficulty breathing and is probably becoming hypoxic. As an emergency measure, the nurse can provide oxygen without waiting for a physician's order. Antibiotics may be warranted, but this isn't a nursing decision. The client should be maintained on bed rest if he's dyspneic to minimize his oxygen demands, but providing additional oxygen will deal more immediately with his problem. The client will need nutritional support, but while dyspneic, he may be unable to spare the energy needed to eat and at the same time maintain adequate oxygenation.

NP: Assessment; CN: Physiological integrity; CNS: Physiological adaptation; CL: Application

9. A client has been treated with antibiotic therapy for right lower-lobe pneumonia for 10 days and will be discharged today. Which of the following physical findings would lead the nurse to believe it is appropriate to discharge this client?

1. Continued dyspnea
2. Fever of 102° F (38.9° C)
3. Respiratory rate of 32 breaths/minute
4. Vesicular breath sounds in right base

9. 4. If the client still has pneumonia, the breath sounds in the right base will be bronchial, not the normal vesicular breath sounds. If the client still has dyspnea, fever, and increased respiratory rate, he should be examined by the physician before discharge because he may have another source of infection or still have pneumonia.

NP: Evaluation; CN: Physiological integrity; CNS: Physiological adaptation; CL: Analysis

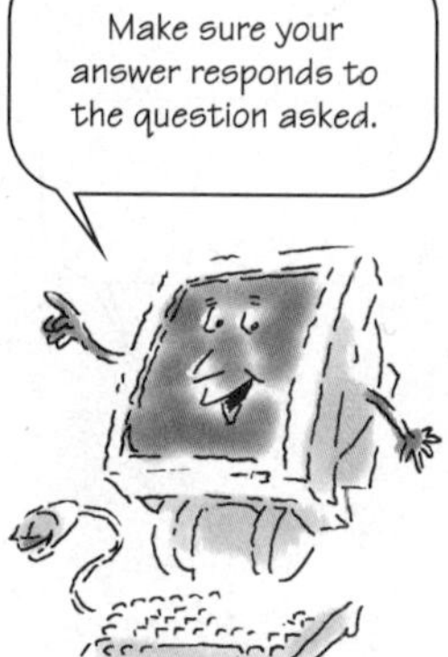

10. A 20-year-old client is being treated for pneumonia. He has a persistent cough and complains of severe pain on coughing. What type of instruction could be given to help the client reduce the discomfort he is having?

1. "Hold in your cough as much as possible."
2. "Place the head of your bed flat to help with coughing."
3. "Restrict fluids to help decrease the amount of sputum."
4. "Splint your chest wall with a pillow for comfort."

10. 4. Showing this client how to splint his chest wall will help decrease discomfort when coughing. Holding in his coughs will only increase the amount of pain he has. Placing the head of the bed flat may increase the frequency of his cough and require more work; a 45-degree angle may help his cough more efficiently and with less pain. Increasing fluid intake will help thin his secretions, making it easier for him to clear them. Promoting fluid intake is appropriate in this situation.

NP: Implementation; CN: Physiological integrity; CNS: Physiological adaptation; CL: Application

11. A client in a long-term care facility has been receiving tube feedings around the clock. The nurse notices he has a cough producing tan sputum, much like the content of his tube feedings, and is now febrile to 102° F. The nurse auscultates his lung fields and hears bronchial breath sounds in his right middle lobe. The nurse suspects he may have developed which of the following conditions?

1. Atelectasis
2. Bronchitis
3. Pneumonia
4. Pulmonary embolism

11. 3. The client probably has aspirated the contents of his tube feedings and developed aspiration pneumonia. This is the most common cause of pneumonia in clients with tube feedings. Atelectasis wouldn't be associated with a productive cough, and breath sounds would be decreased in the areas of atelectasis. The client most likely hasn't developed bronchitis because in that condition, he may have a nonproductive or productive cough but secretions are usually clear. A client with a pulmonary embolism wouldn't have a cough producing tan sputum, and pulmonary embolisms aren't typically associated with high fever.

NP: Assessment; CN: Physiological integrity; CNS: Physiological adaptation; CL: Analysis

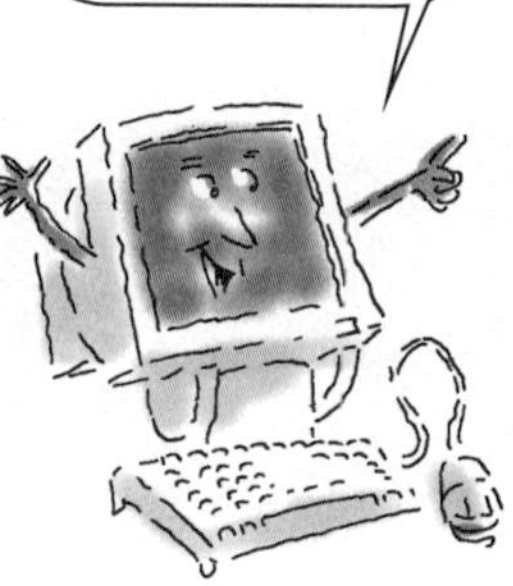

Another test-taking hint! Choose the most likely response about today's population.

12. A nurse is working in a walk-in clinic. She has been alerted that there is an outbreak of tuberculosis (TB). Which of the following clients entering the clinic today is most likely to have TB?

1. A 16-year-old female high school student
2. A 33-year-old day-care worker
3. A 43-year-old homeless man with a history of alcoholism
4. A 54-year-old businessman

12. 3. Clients who are economically disadvantaged, malnourished, and have reduced immunity, such as a client with a history of alcoholism, are at extremely high risk for developing TB. A high school student, day-care worker, and businessman probably have a much lower risk of contracting TB.

NP: Planning; CN: Physiological integrity; CNS: Physiological adaptation; CL: Comprehension

13. Tuberculosis (TB) is a communicable disease transmitted by which of the following methods?

1. Sexual contact
2. Using dirty needles
3. Using an infected person's eating utensils
4. Inhaling droplets exhaled from an infected person

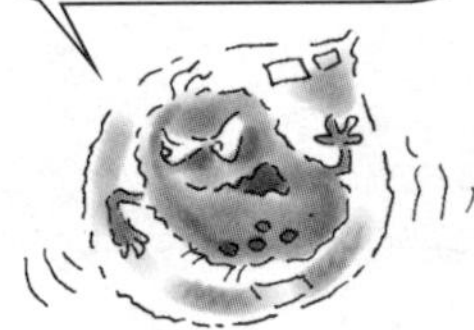

This droplet transmission stuff sure beats the subway! Wheeee!

13. 4. The TB bacillus is airborne and carried in droplets exhaled by an infected person who is coughing, sneezing, laughing, or singing. Sexual contact and dirty needles don't spread the TB bacillus, but may spread other communicable diseases. It's never advisable to use dirty utensils, but if they're cleaned normally, it isn't necessary to dispose of eating utensils used by someone infected with TB.

NP: Analysis; CN: Physiological integrity; CNS: Physiological adaptation; CL: Knowledge

14. An adult client is being screened in the clinic today for tuberculosis. He reports having negative purified protein derivative (PPD) test results in the past. The nurse performs a PPD test on his right forearm today. When should he return to have the test read?

1. Right after performing the test
2. 24 hours after performing the test
3. 48 hours after performing the test
4. 1 week after performing the test

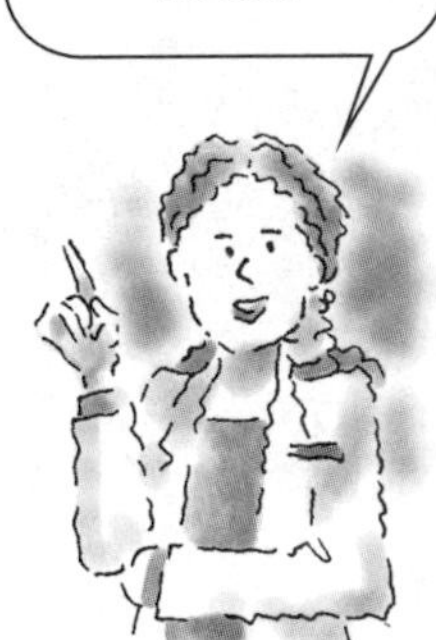

The timing is the clue!

14. 3. PPD tests should be read in 48 to 72 hours. If read too early or too late, the results won't be accurate.

NP: Assessment; CN: Physiological integrity; CNS: Physiological adaptation; CL: Knowledge

15. The right forearm of a client who had a purified protein derivative (PPD) test for tuberculosis (TB) is reddened and raised about 3 mm where the test was given. This PPD would be read as having which of the following results?

1. Indeterminate
2. Needs to be redone
3. Negative
4. Positive

15. 3. This test would be classed as negative. A 3-mm raised area would be a positive result if a client had recent close contact with someone diagnosed with or suspected of having infectious TB. Follow-up should be done with this client, and a chest X-ray should be ordered. *Indeterminate* isn't a term used to describe results of a PPD test. The test can be redone in 6 months to see if the client's test results change. If the PPD test is reddened and raised 10 mm or more, it's considered positive according to the Centers for Disease Control and Prevention.

NP: Evaluation; CN: Physiological integrity; CNS: Physiological adaptation; CL: Knowledge

16. A client with a primary tuberculosis (TB) infection can expect to develop which of the following conditions?

1. Active TB within 2 weeks
2. Active TB within 1 month
3. A fever that requires hospitalization
4. A positive skin test

16. 4. A primary TB infection occurs when the bacillus has successfully invaded the entire body after entering through the lungs. At this point, the bacilli are walled off and skin tests read positive. However, all but infants and immunosuppressed people will remain asymptomatic. The general population has a 10% risk of developing active TB over their lifetime, in many cases because of a break in the body's immune defenses. The active stage shows the classic symptoms of TB: fever, hemoptysis, and night sweats.

NP: Analysis; CN: Physiological integrity; CNS: Physiological adaptation; CL: Application

17. A client was infected with tuberculosis (TB) bacillus 10 years ago but never developed the disease. He's now being treated for cancer. The client begins to develop signs of TB. This is known as which of the following types of infection?

1. Active infection
2. Primary infection
3. Superinfection
4. Tertiary infection

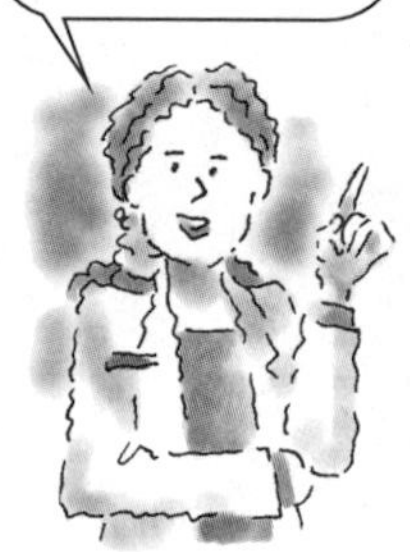

Think: How does cancer affect the immune system?

17. 1. Some people carry dormant TB infections that may develop into active disease. In addition, primary sites of infection containing TB bacilli may remain latent for years and then activate when the client's resistance is lowered, as when a client is being treated for cancer. There's no such thing as tertiary infection, and superinfection doesn't apply in this case.
NP: Analysis; CN: Physiological integrity; CNS: Physiological adaptation; CL: Application

18. A client has active tuberculosis (TB). Which of the following symptoms will he exhibit?

1. Chest and lower back pain
2. Chills, fever, night sweats, and hemoptysis
3. Fever of more than 104° F (40° C) and nausea
4. Headache and photophobia

18. 2. Typical signs and symptoms are chills, fever, night sweats, and hemoptysis. Chest pain may be present from coughing, but isn't usual. Clients with TB typically have low-grade fevers, not higher than 102° F (38.9° C). Nausea, headache, and photophobia aren't usual TB symptoms.
NP: Assessment; CN: Physiological integrity; CNS: Physiological adaptation; CL: Application

19. Which of the following diagnostic tests is definitive for tuberculosis?

1. Chest X-ray
2. Mantoux test
3. Sputum culture
4. Tuberculin test

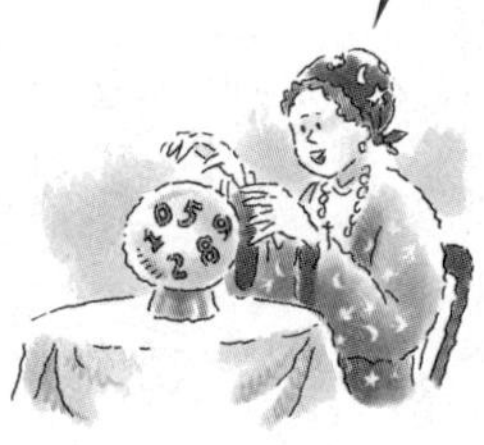

You don't need to be a fortune teller! The right diagnostic test can give you the answer!

19. 3. The sputum culture for *Mycobacterium tuberculosis* is the only method of confirming the diagnosis. Lesions in the lung may not be big enough to be seen on X-ray. Skin tests may be falsely positive or falsely negative.
NP: Assessment; CN: Physiological integrity; CNS: Physiological adaptation; CL: Knowledge

20. A client with a positive Mantoux test result will be sent for a chest X-ray. For which of the following reasons is this done?

1. To confirm the diagnosis
2. To determine if a repeat skin test is needed
3. To determine the extent of lesions
4. To determine if this is a primary or secondary infection

20. 3. If the lesions are large enough, the chest X-ray will show their presence in the lungs. Sputum culture confirms the diagnosis. There can be false-positive and false-negative skin test results. A chest X-ray can't determine if this is a primary or secondary infection.
NP: Analysis; CN: Physiological integrity; CNS: Physiological adaptation; CL: Application

21. A chest X-ray shows a client's lungs to be clear. His Mantoux test is positive, with 10 mm of induration. His previous test was negative. These test results are possible because:

1. he had tuberculosis (TB) in the past and no longer has it.
2. he was successfully treated for TB, but skin tests always stay positive.
3. he's a "seroconverter," meaning the TB has gotten to his bloodstream.
4. he's a "tuberculin converter," which means he has been infected with TB since his last skin test.

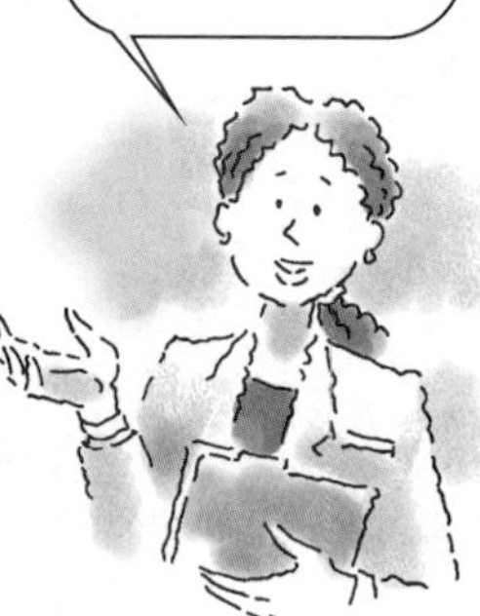

21. 4. A tuberculin converter's skin test will be positive, meaning he has been exposed to and infected with TB and now has a cell-mediated immune response to the skin test. The client's blood and X-ray results may stay negative. It doesn't mean the infection has advanced to the active stage. Because his X-ray is negative, he should be monitored every 6 months to see if he develops changes in his chest X-ray or pulmonary examination. Being a seroconverter doesn't mean the TB has gotten into his bloodstream; it means it can be detected by a blood test.
NP: Analysis; CN: Physiological integrity; CNS: Physiological adaptation; CL: Application

22. A client with a positive skin test for tuberculosis (TB) isn't showing signs of active disease. To help prevent the development of active TB, the client should be treated with isoniazid, 300 mg daily, for how long?
1. 10 to 14 days
2. 2 to 4 weeks
3. 3 to 6 months
4. 9 to 12 months

22. 4. Because of the increasing incidence of resistant strains of TB, the disease must be treated for up to 24 months in some cases, but treatment typically lasts from 9 to 12 months. Isoniazid is the most common medication used for the treatment of TB, but other antibiotics are added to the regimen to obtain the best results.
NP: Analysis; CN: Physiological integrity; CNS: Physiological adaptation; CL: Application

23. A client with a productive cough, chills, and night sweats is suspected of having active tuberculosis (TB). The physician should take which of the following actions?
1. Admit him to the hospital in respiratory isolation.
2. Prescribe isoniazid and tell him to go home and rest.
3. Give a tuberculin test and tell him to come back in 48 hours to have it read.
4. Give a prescription for isoniazid, 300 mg daily for 2 weeks, and send him home.

23. 1. This client is showing signs and symptoms of active TB and, because of the productive cough, is highly contagious. He should be admitted to the hospital, placed in respiratory isolation, and three sputum cultures should be obtained to confirm the diagnosis. He would most likely be given isoniazid and two or three other antitubercular antibiotics until the diagnosis is confirmed, and then isolation and treatment would continue if the cultures were positive for TB. After 7 to 10 days, three more consecutive sputum cultures will be obtained. If they're negative, he would be considered noncontagious and may be sent home, although he'll continue to take the antitubercular drugs for 9 to 12 months.
NP: Implementation; CN: Physiological integrity; CNS: Physiological adaptation; CL: Application

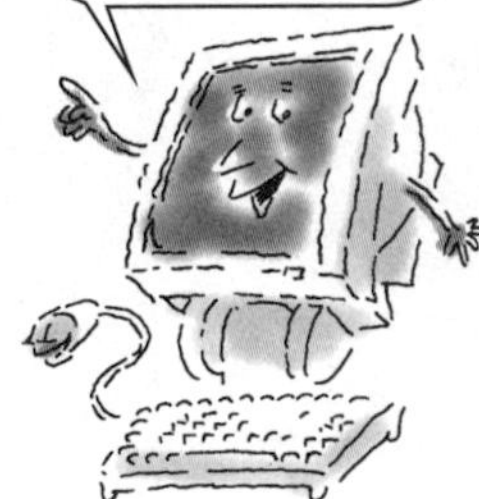

Read question 24 carefully! It's easy to miss the two little letters in front of "adequate."

24. A client is diagnosed with active tuberculosis and started on triple antibiotic therapy. What signs and symptoms would the client show if therapy is inadequate?
1. Decreased shortness of breath
2. Improved chest X-ray
3. Nonproductive cough
4. Positive acid-fast bacilli in a sputum sample after 2 months of treatment

24. 4. Continuing to have acid-fast bacilli in the sputum after 2 months indicates continued infection. The other choices would all indicate improvement with therapy.
NP: Evaluation; CN: Physiological integrity; CNS: Physiological adaptation; CL: Application

25. Which of the following instructions should the nurse give a client about his active tuberculosis (TB)?
1. "It's OK to miss a dose every day or two."
2. "If side effects occur, stop taking the medication."
3. "Only take the medication until you feel better."
4. "You must comply with the medication regimen to treat TB."

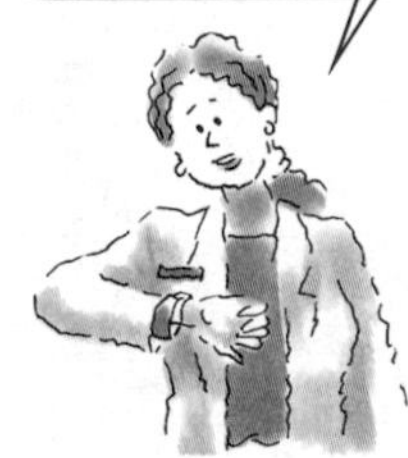

25. 4. The regimen may last up to 24 months. It's essential that the client comply with therapy during that time or resistance will develop. At no time should he stop taking the medications before his physician tells him to.
NP: Evaluation; CN: Physiological integrity; CNS: Physiological adaptation; CL: Analysis

26. A client diagnosed with active tuberculosis (TB) would be hospitalized primarily for which of the following reasons?

1. To evaluate his condition
2. To determine his compliance
3. To prevent spread of the disease
4. To determine the need for antibiotic therapy

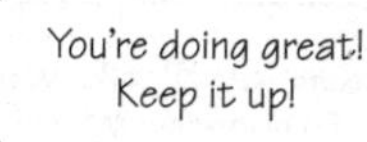

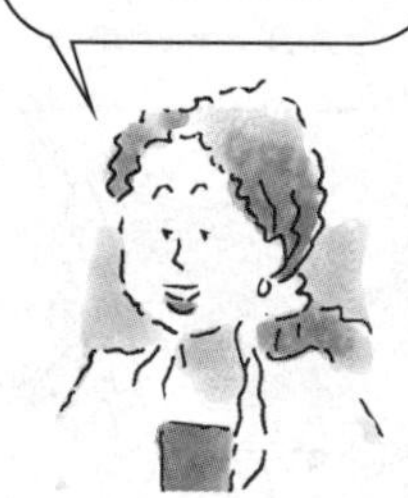

26. 3. The client with active TB is highly contagious until three consecutive sputum cultures are negative, so he's put in respiratory isolation in the hospital. Neither assessment of physical condition, determinations of compliance, nor antibiotic therapy are primary reasons for hospitalization in this case.

NP: Implementation; CN: Physiological integrity; CNS: Physiological adaptation; CL: Application

27. A 7-year-old client is brought to the emergency department. He's tachypneic and afebrile and has a respiratory rate of 36 breaths/minute and a nonproductive cough. He recently had a cold. From this history, the client may have which of the following conditions?

1. Acute asthma
2. Bronchial pneumonia
3. Chronic obstructive pulmonary disease (COPD)
4. Emphysema

27. 1. Based on the client's history and symptoms, acute asthma is the most likely diagnosis. He's unlikely to have bronchial pneumonia without a productive cough and fever and he's too young to have developed COPD and emphysema.

NP: Assessment; CN: Physiological integrity; CNS: Physiological adaptation; CL: Analysis

28. Which of the following assessment findings would help confirm a diagnosis of asthma in a client suspected of having the disorder?

1. Circumoral cyanosis
2. Increased forced expiratory volume
3. Inspiratory and expiratory wheezing
4. Normal breath sounds

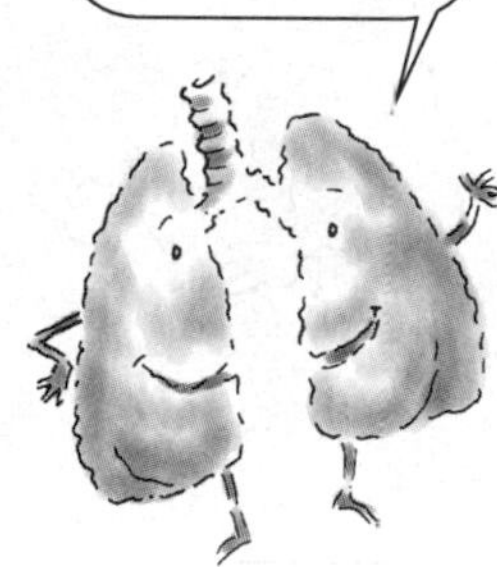

Listen to how we sound — any changes from normal are clues.

28. 3. Inspiratory and expiratory wheezes are typical findings in asthma. Circumoral cyanosis may be present in extreme cases of respiratory distress. The nurse would expect the client to have a decreased forced expiratory volume because asthma is an obstructive pulmonary disease. Breath sounds will be "tight" sounding or markedly decreased; they won't be normal.

NP: Assessment; CN: Physiological integrity; CNS: Physiological adaptation; CL: Analysis

29. Which of the following types of asthma involves an acute asthma attack brought on by an upper respiratory infection?

1. Emotional
2. Extrinsic
3. Intrinsic
4. Mediated

29. 3. Intrinsic asthma doesn't have an easily identifiable allergen and can be triggered by the common cold. Asthma caused by emotional reasons is considered to be in the extrinsic category. Extrinsic asthma is caused by dust, molds, and pets; easily identifiable allergens. Mediated asthma doesn't exist.

NP: Assessment; CN: Physiological integrity; CNS: Physiological adaptation; CL: Knowledge

30. A client with acute asthma showing inspiratory and expiratory wheezes and a decreased forced expiratory volume should be treated with which of the following classes of medication right away?

1. Beta-adrenergic blockers
2. Bronchodilators
3. Inhaled steroids
4. Oral steroids

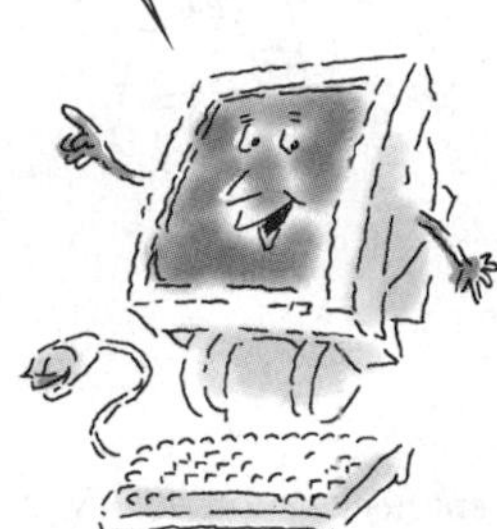

Another hint! Question 30 asks you to set priorities.

30. 2. Bronchodilators are the first line of treatment for asthma because bronchoconstriction is the cause of reduced airflow. Beta-adrenergic blockers aren't used to treat asthma and can cause bronchoconstriction. Inhaled or oral steroids may be given to reduce the inflammation but aren't used for emergency relief.

NP: Implementation; CN: Physiological integrity; CNS: Physiological adaptation; CL: Application

31. A 19-year-old client comes to the emergency department with acute asthma. His respiratory rate is 44 breaths/minute, and he appears in acute respiratory distress. Which of the following actions should be taken first?

1. Take a full medical history.
2. Give a bronchodilator by nebulizer.
3. Apply a cardiac monitor to the client.
4. Provide emotional support to the client.

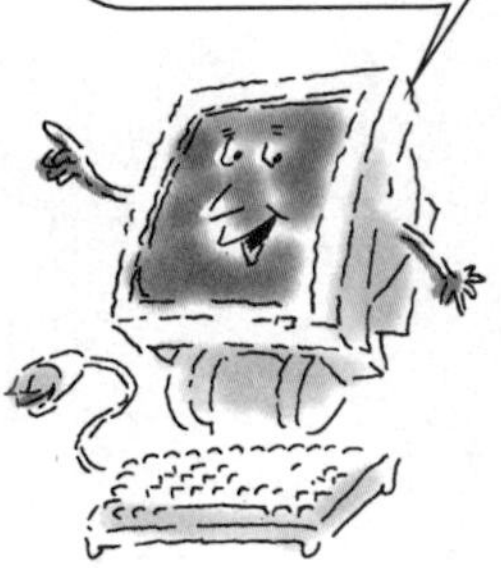

Question 31 asks you to prioritize. Which action comes first?

31. 2. The client having an acute asthma attack needs to increase oxygen delivery to the lung and body. Nebulized bronchodilators open airways and increase the amount of oxygen delivered. First resolve the acute phase of the attack, then obtain a full medical history to determine the cause of the attack and how to prevent attacks in the future. It may not be necessary to place the client on a cardiac monitor because he's only 19 years old, unless he has a past medical history of cardiac problems.

NP: Implementation; CN: Physiological integrity; CNS: Physiological adaptation; CL: Application

32. A client is found to be allergic to Chinese food, which causes acute asthma. Which of the following instructions should the nurse give the client?

1. "Only eat Chinese food once per month."
2. "Use your inhalers before eating Chinese food."
3. "Avoid Chinese food because this is a trigger for you."
4. "Determine other causes because Chinese food wouldn't cause such a violent reaction."

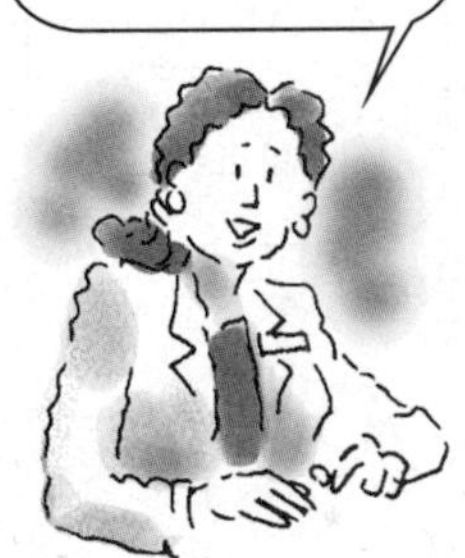

32. 3. If the trigger of an acute asthma attack is known, this trigger should be avoided at all times. Using an inhaler before eating wouldn't prevent the attack, and food frequently is a trigger for an acute asthma attack.

NP: Implementation; CN: Physiological integrity; CNS: Physiological adaptation; CL: Application

33. A 58-year-old client with a 40-year history of smoking one to two packs of cigarettes per day has a chronic cough producing thick sputum, peripheral edema, and cyanotic nail beds. Based on this information, he most likely has which of the following conditions?

1. Adult respiratory distress syndrome (ARDS)
2. Asthma
3. Chronic obstructive bronchitis
4. Emphysema

33. 3. Because of his extensive smoking history and symptoms, the client most likely has chronic obstructive bronchitis. Clients with ARDS have acute symptoms of hypoxia and typically need large amounts of oxygen. Clients with asthma and emphysema tend not to have a chronic cough or peripheral edema.

NP: Implementation; CN: Physiological integrity; CNS: Physiological adaptation; CL: Application

34. The term "blue bloater" refers to which of the following conditions?

1. Adult respiratory distress syndrome (ARDS)
2. Asthma
3. Chronic obstructive bronchitis
4. Emphysema

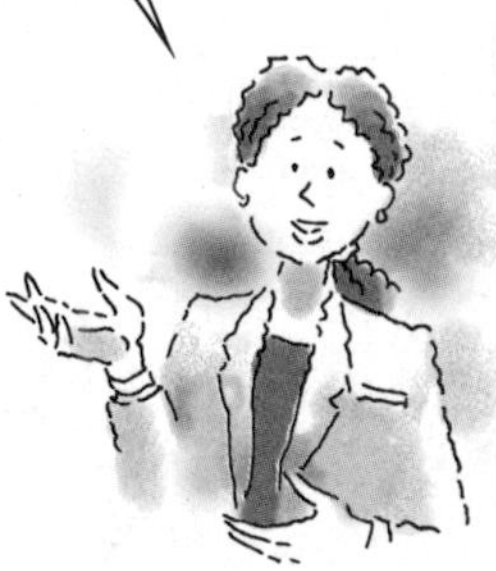

Terms such as *blue bloater* can help you remember the symptoms of some diseases.

34. 3. Clients with chronic obstructive bronchitis appear bloated; they have large barrel chests and peripheral edema, cyanotic nail beds and, at times, circumoral cyanosis. Clients with ARDS are acutely short of breath and frequently need intubation for mechanical ventilation and large amounts of oxygen. Clients with asthma don't exhibit characteristics of chronic disease, and clients with emphysema appear pink and cachectic.

NP: Assessment; CN: Physiological integrity; CNS: Physiological adaptation; CL: Application

35. The term "pink puffer" refers to the client with which of the following conditions?
1. Adult respiratory distress syndrome (ARDS)
2. Asthma
3. Chronic obstructive bronchitis
4. Emphysema

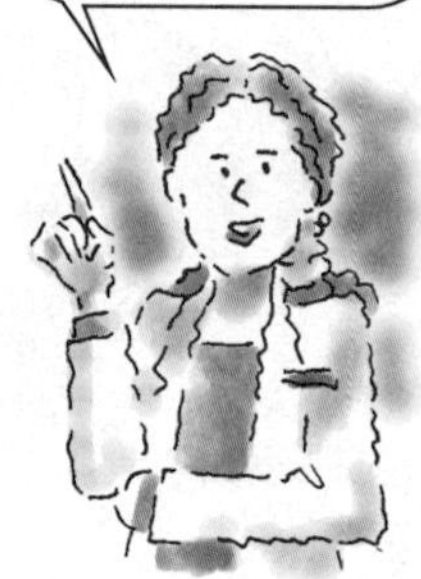

Here's another term to help remember symptoms.

35. 4. Because of the large amount of energy it takes to breathe, clients with emphysema are usually cachectic. They're pink and usually breathe through pursed lips, hence the term "puffer." Clients with ARDS are usually acutely short of breath. Clients with asthma don't have any particular characteristics, and clients with chronic obstructive bronchitis are bloated and cyanotic in appearance.

NP: Assessment; CN: Physiological integrity; CNS: Physiological adaptation; CL: Application

36. A 66-year-old client has marked dyspnea at rest, is thin, and uses accessory muscles to breathe. He's tachypneic, with a prolonged expiratory phase. He has no cough. He leans forward with his arms braced on his knees to support his chest and shoulders for breathing. This client has symptoms of which of the following respiratory disorders?
1. Adult respiratory distress syndrome (ARDS)
2. Asthma
3. Chronic obstructive bronchitis
4. Emphysema

36. 4. These are classic signs and symptoms of a client with emphysema. Clients with ARDS are acutely short of breath and require emergency care; those with asthma are also acutely short of breath during an attack and appear very frightened. Clients with chronic obstructive bronchitis are bloated and cyanotic in appearance.

NP: Assessment; CN: Physiological integrity; CNS: Physiological adaptation; CL: Application

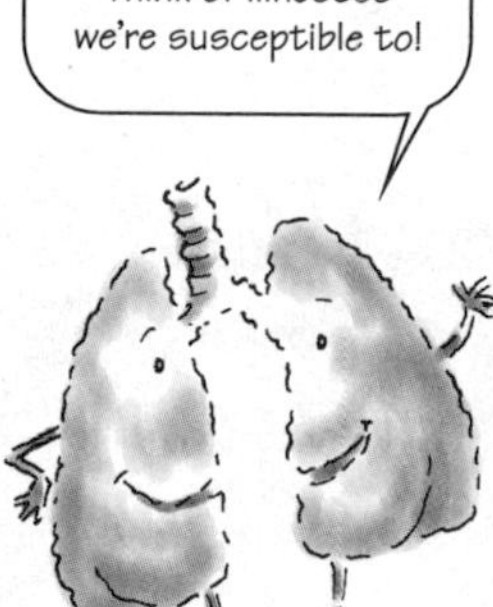

Think of illnesses we're susceptible to!

37. It's highly recommended that clients with asthma, chronic bronchitis, and emphysema have Pneumovax and flu vaccinations for which of the following reasons?
1. All clients are recommended to have these vaccines.
2. These vaccines produce bronchodilation and improve oxygenation.
3. These vaccines help reduce the tachypnea these clients experience.
4. Respiratory infections can cause severe hypoxia and possibly death in these clients.

37. 4. It's highly recommended that clients with respiratory disorders be given vaccines to protect against respiratory infection. Infections can cause these clients to need intubation and mechanical ventilation, and it may be difficult to wean these clients from the ventilator. The vaccines have no effect on bronchodilation or respiratory rate.

NP: Implementation; CN: Physiological integrity; CNS: Physiological adaptation; CL: Application

38. Exercise has which of the following effects on clients with asthma, chronic bronchitis, and emphysema?
1. It enhances cardiovascular fitness.
2. It improves respiratory muscle strength.
3. It reduces the number of acute attacks.
4. It worsens respiratory function and is discouraged.

38. 1. Exercise can improve cardiovascular fitness and help the client tolerate periods of hypoxia better, perhaps reducing the risk of heart attack. Most exercise has little effect on respiratory muscle strength, and these clients can't tolerate the type of exercise necessary to do this. Exercise won't reduce the number of acute attacks. In some instances, exercise may be contraindicated, and the client should check with his physician before starting any exercise program.

NP: Implementation; CN: Physiological integrity; CNS: Physiological adaptation; CL: Application

39. Clients with chronic obstructive bronchitis are given diuretic therapy. Which of the following reasons *best* explains why?

1. Reducing fluid volume reduces oxygen demand.
2. Reducing fluid volume improves clients' mobility.
3. Reducing fluid volume reduces sputum production.
4. Reducing fluid volume improves respiratory function.

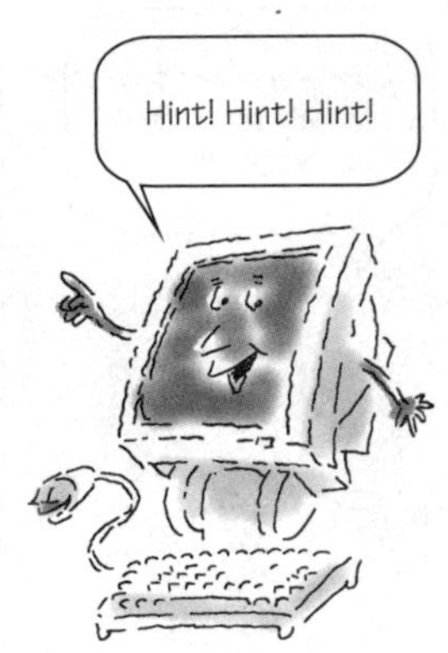

39. 1. Reducing fluid volume reduces the workload of the heart, which reduces oxygen demand and, in turn, reduces the respiratory rate. It also may reduce edema and improve mobility a little, but exercise tolerance will still be poor. Sputum may get thicker and make it harder to clear airways. Reducing fluid volume won't improve respiratory function, but may improve oxygenation.

NP: Implementation; CN: Physiological integrity; CNS: Physiological adaptation; CL: Application

40. A 69-year-old client appears thin and cachectic. He's short of breath at rest and his dyspnea increases with the slightest exertion. His breath sounds are diminished even with deep inspiration. These signs and symptoms fit which of the following conditions?

1. Adult respiratory distress syndrome (ARDS)
2. Asthma
3. Chronic obstructive bronchitis
4. Emphysema

40. 4. In emphysema, the wall integrity of the individual air sacs is damaged, reducing the surface area available for gas exchange. Very little air movement occurs in the lungs because of bronchiole collapse, as well. In ARDS, the client's condition is more acute and typically requires mechanical ventilation. In asthma and bronchitis, wheezing is prevalent.

NP: Implementation; CN: Physiological integrity; CNS: Physiological adaptation; CL: Application

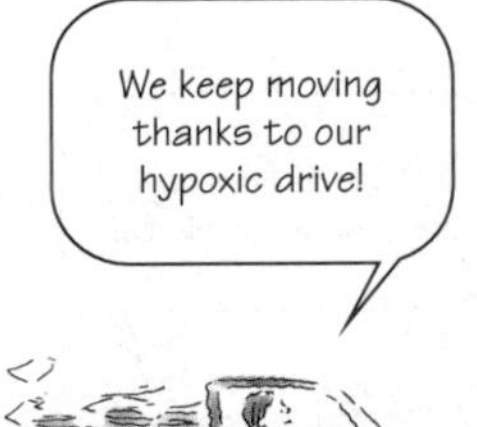

We keep moving thanks to our hypoxic drive!

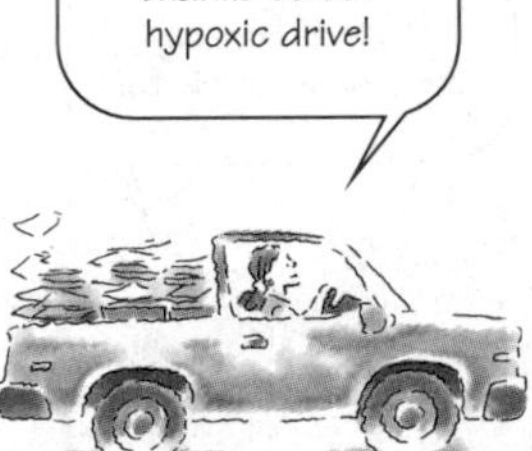

41. A client with emphysema should receive only 1 to 3 L/minute of oxygen, if needed, or he may lose his hypoxic drive. Which of the following statements is correct about hypoxic drive?

1. The client doesn't notice he needs to breathe.
2. The client breathes only when his oxygen levels climb above a certain point.
3. The client breathes only when his oxygen levels dip below a certain point.
4. The client breathes only when his carbon dioxide level dips below a certain point.

41. 3. Clients with emphysema breathe when their oxygen levels drop to a certain level; this is known as the hypoxic drive. They don't take a breath when their levels of carbon dioxide are higher than normal, as do those with healthy respiratory physiology. If too much oxygen is given, the client has little stimulus to take another breath. In the meantime, his carbon dioxide levels continue to climb, and the client will pass out, leading to a respiratory arrest.

NP: Implementation; CN: Physiological integrity; CNS: Physiological adaptation; CL: Application

42. Teaching for a client with chronic obstructive pulmonary disease should include which of the following topics?

1. How to listen to his own lungs
2. How to increase his oxygen therapy
3. How to treat respiratory infections without going to the physician
4. How to recognize the signs of an impending respiratory infection

42. 4. Respiratory infection in clients with a respiratory disorder can be fatal. It's important that the client understands how to recognize the signs and symptoms of an impending respiratory infection. It isn't appropriate to teach a client how to listen to his own lungs or change his oxygen therapy regimen. If the client has signs and symptoms of an infection, he should contact his physician at once.

NP: Implementation; CN: Physiological integrity; CNS: Physiological adaptation; CL: Application

43. Which of the following respiratory disorders is most common in the first 24 to 48 hours after surgery?
1. Atelectasis
2. Bronchitis
3. Pneumonia
4. Pneumothorax

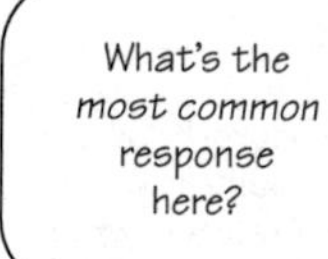

What's the most common response here?

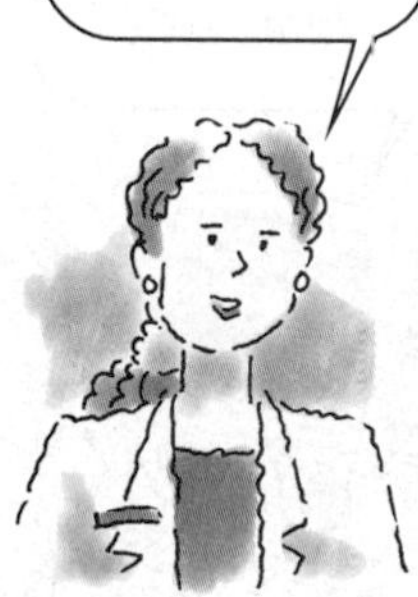

43. 1. Atelectasis develops when there's interference with the normal negative pressure that promotes lung expansion. Clients in the postoperative phase often splint their breathing because of pain and positioning, which causes hypoxia. It's uncommon for any of the other respiratory disorders to develop.
NP: Implementation; CN: Physiological integrity; CNS: Physiological adaptation; CL: Application

44. Which of the following measures can reduce or prevent the incidence of atelectasis in a postoperative client?
1. Chest physiotherapy
2. Mechanical ventilation
3. Reducing oxygen requirements
4. Use of an incentive spirometer

44. 4. Using an incentive spirometer requires the client to take deep breaths and promotes lung expansion. Chest physiotherapy helps mobilize secretions but won't prevent atelectasis. Reducing oxygen requirements or placing someone on mechanical ventilation doesn't affect the development of atelectasis.
NP: Implementation; CN: Physiological integrity; CNS: Physiological adaptation; CL: Application

45. Emergency treatment of a client in status asthmaticus includes which of the following medications?
1. Inhaled beta-adrenergic agents
2. Inhaled corticosteroids
3. I.V. beta-adrenergic agents
4. Oral corticosteroids

45. 1. Inhaled beta-adrenergic agents help promote bronchodilation, which improves oxygenation. I.V. beta-adrenergic agents can be used but have to be monitored because of their greater systemic effects. They're typically used when the inhaled beta-adrenergic agents don't work. Corticosteroids are slow acting, so their use won't reduce hypoxia in the acute phase.
NP: Implementation; CN: Physiological integrity; CNS: Physiological adaptation; CL: Application

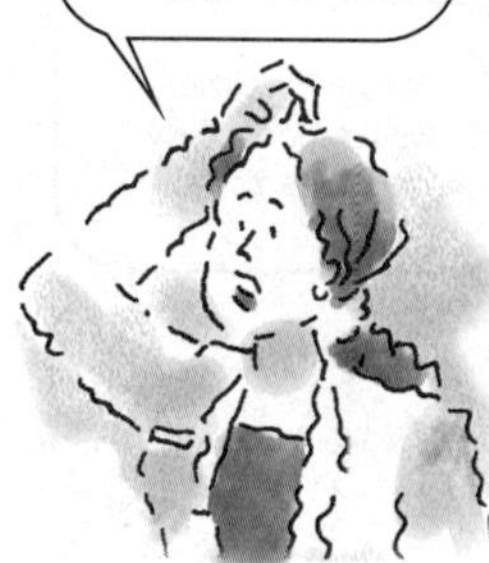

For question 46, you need to choose the best out of several possible goals.

46. Which of the following treatment goals is best for the client with status asthmaticus?
1. Avoiding intubation
2. Determining the cause of the attack
3. Improving exercise tolerance
4. Reducing secretions

46. 1. Inhaled beta-adrenergic agents, I.V. corticosteroids, and supplemental oxygen are used to reduce bronchospasm, improve oxygenation, and avoid intubation. Determining the trigger for the client's attack and improving exercise tolerance are later goals. Typically, secretions aren't a problem in status asthmaticus.
NP: Implementation; CN: Physiological integrity; CNS: Physiological adaptation; CL: Application

47. A client was given morphine sulfate for pain. He's sleeping and his respiratory rate is 4 breaths/minute. If action isn't taken quickly, he might have which of the following reactions?
1. Asthma attack
2. Respiratory arrest
3. Seizure
4. Wake up on his own

47. 2. Narcotics can cause respiratory arrest if given in large quantities. It's unlikely the client will have an asthma attack or a seizure or wake up on his own.
NP: Implementation; CN: Physiological integrity; CNS: Physiological adaptation; CL: Application

48. Which of the following additional assessment data should immediately be gathered to determine the status of a client with a respiratory rate of 4 breaths/minute?

1. Arterial blood gas (ABG) and breath sounds
2. Level of consciousness and a pulse oximetry value
3. Breath sounds and reflexes
4. Pulse oximetry value and heart sounds

Ask yourself, "Which assessment would help first, and which could wait?"

49. A client is in danger of respiratory arrest following the administration of a narcotic analgesic. An arterial blood gas value is obtained. The nurse would expect the $Paco_2$ to be which of the following values?

1. 15 mm Hg
2. 30 mm Hg
3. 40 mm Hg
4. 80 mm Hg

50. A client's arterial blood gas (ABG) results are as follows: pH, 7.16; $Paco_2$, 80 mm Hg; Pao_2, 46 mm Hg; HCO_3^-, 24 mEq/L; Sao_2, 81%. This ABG result represents which of the following conditions?

1. Metabolic acidosis
2. Metabolic alkalosis
3. Respiratory acidosis
4. Respiratory alkalosis

51. Clients at high risk for respiratory failure include those with which of the following diagnoses?

1. Breast cancer
2. Cervical sprains
3. Fractured hip
4. Guillain-Barré syndrome

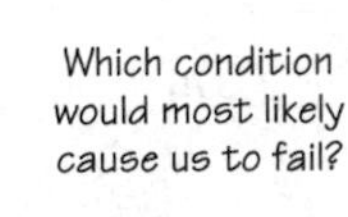

Which condition would most likely cause us to fail?

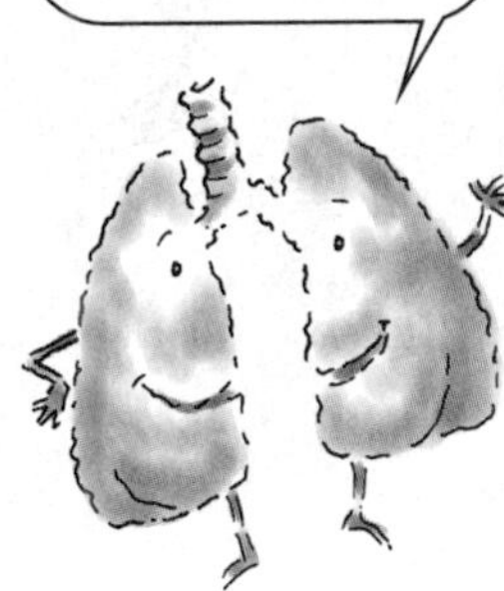

48. 2. First, the nurse should attempt to rouse the client because this should increase the client's respiratory rate. If available, a spot pulse oximetry check should be done and breath sounds should be checked. The physician should be notified immediately of the findings. He'll probably order ABG analysis to determine specific carbon dioxide and oxygen levels, which will indicate the effectiveness of ventilation. Reflexes and heart sounds will be part of the more extensive examination done after these initial actions are completed.

NP: Assessment; CN: Physiological integrity; CNS: Physiological adaptation; CL: Application

49. 4. A client about to go into respiratory arrest will have inefficient ventilation and will be retaining carbon dioxide. The value expected would be around 80 mm Hg. All other values are lower than expected.

NP: Implementation; CN: Physiological integrity; CNS: Physiological adaptation; CL: Application

50. 3. Because the $Paco_2$ is high at 80 mm Hg and the metabolic measure, HCO_3^-, is normal, the client has respiratory acidosis. The pH is less than 7.35, acidemic, which eliminates metabolic and respiratory alkalosis as possibilities. If the HCO_3^- was below 22 mEq/L the client would have metabolic acidosis.

NP: Implementation; CN: Physiological integrity; CNS: Physiological adaptation; CL: Application

51. 4. Guillain-Barré syndrome is a progressive neuromuscular disorder that can affect the respiratory muscles and cause respiratory failure. The other conditions typically don't affect the respiratory system.

NP: Implementation; CN: Physiological integrity; CNS: Physiological adaptation; CL: Application

52. A client has started a new drug for hypertension. Thirty minutes after he takes the drug, he develops chest tightness and becomes short of breath and tachypneic. He has a decreased level of consciousness. These signs indicate which of the following conditions?

1. Asthma attack
2. Pulmonary embolism
3. Respiratory failure
4. Rheumatoid arthritis

52. 3. The client was reacting to the drug with respiratory signs of impending anaphylaxis, which could lead to eventual respiratory failure. Although the signs are also related to an asthma attack or a pulmonary embolism, consider the new drug first. Rheumatoid arthritis doesn't manifest these signs.

NP: Implementation; CN: Physiological integrity; CNS: Physiological adaptation; CL: Application

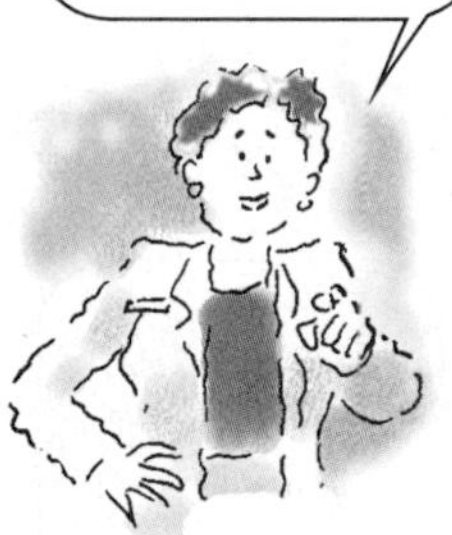

Set your priorities properly. What should be done first?

53. Emergency treatment for a client with impending anaphylaxis secondary to hypersensitivity to a drug should include which of the following actions first?

1. Administering oxygen
2. Inserting an I.V. catheter
3. Obtaining a complete blood count (CBC)
4. Taking vital signs

53. 1. Giving oxygen would be the best first action in this case. Vital signs then should be checked and the physician immediately notified. If the client doesn't already have an I.V. catheter, one may be inserted now if anaphylactic shock is developing. Obtaining a CBC wouldn't help the emergency situation.

NP: Implementation; CN: Physiological integrity; CNS: Physiological adaptation; CL: Application

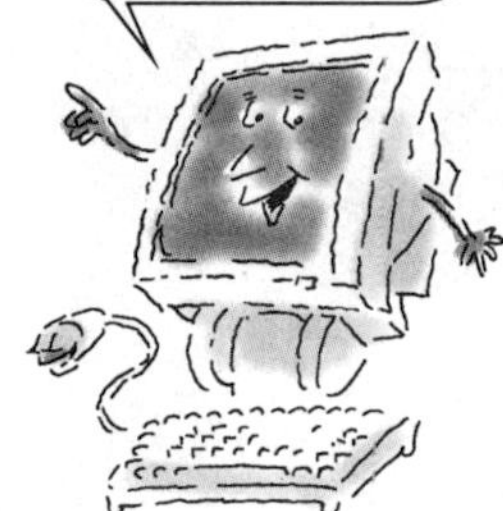

Next is another hint that means to prioritize.

54. Following the initial care of a client with asthma and impending anaphylaxis from hypersensitivity to a drug, the nurse should take which of the following steps next?

1. Administer beta-adrenergic blockers.
2. Administer bronchodilators.
3. Obtain serum electrolyte levels.
4. Have the client lie flat in the bed.

54. 2. Bronchodilators would help open the client's airway and improve his oxygenation status. Beta-adrenergic blockers aren't indicated in the management of asthma because they may cause bronchospasm. Obtaining laboratory values wouldn't be done on an emergency basis, and having the client lie flat in bed could worsen his ability to breathe.

NP: Implementation; CN: Physiological integrity; CNS: Physiological adaptation; CL: Application

55. A 19-year-old client went to a party, took "some pills," and drank beer. He's brought to the emergency department because he won't wake up. When assessing him, the nurse would expect to find which of the following reactions?

1. Hyperreflexive reflexes
2. Muscle spasms
3. Shallow respirations
4. Tachypnea

55. 3. The client probably can't be roused from the combination of pills and alcohol he's taken. This has probably caused him to breathe shallowly, which, if not monitored closely, could lead to respiratory arrest. The nurse wouldn't expect to find tachypnea and doesn't have enough information about which drugs he took to expect muscle spasms or hyperreflexia.

NP: Assessment; CN: Physiological integrity; CNS: Physiological adaptation; CL: Application

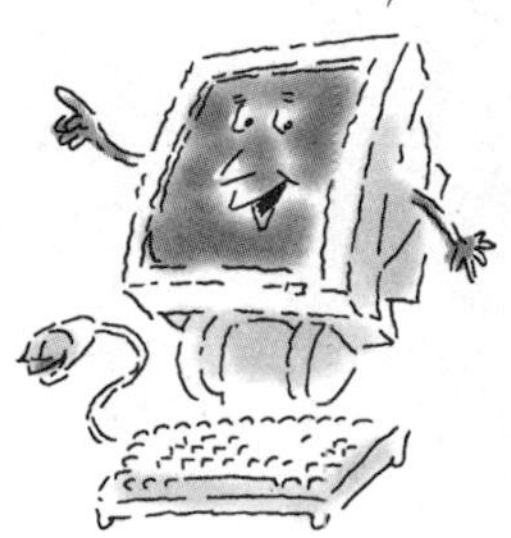

In a drug overdose, you'll want to do only one of these first. Which one?

56. Which of the following actions should be taken first in response to an initial assessment of probable drug overdose complicated with alcohol ingestion?

1. Administer I.V. fluids.
2. Administer I.V. naloxone (Narcan).
3. Continue close monitoring of vital signs.
4. Draw blood for a drug screen.

56. 2. If the client took narcotics, giving naloxone could reverse the effects and awaken the client. I.V. fluids will most likely be administered, and he'll be closely monitored over a period of several hours to several days. A drug screen should be drawn but results may not come back for several hours.

NP: Implementation; CN: Physiological integrity; CNS: Physiological adaptation; CL: Application

57. An unconscious client who overdosed on a narcotic receives naloxone (Narcan) to reverse the overdose. After he awakens, which of the following actions by the nurse would be the best?

1. Feed the client.
2. Teach the client about the effects of taking pills and alcohol together.
3. Discharge the client from the hospital.
4. Admit the client to a psychiatric facility.

57. 2. This client needs information about the dangers of taking pills and alcohol together. It may not be advisable to feed the client at first, in case his level of consciousness decreases again, increasing the possibility of aspiration Discharge at this point is inappropriate. Unless the client was trying to commit suicide, admission to a psychiatric facility isn't necessary.
NP: Implementation; CN: Physiological integrity; CNS: Physiological adaptation; CL: Application

58. A firefighter was involved in extinguishing a house fire and is being treated for smoke inhalation. He develops severe hypoxia 48 hours after the incident, requiring intubation and mechanical ventilation. He most likely has developed which of the following conditions?

1. Adult respiratory distress syndrome (ARDS)
2. Atelectasis
3. Bronchitis
4. Pneumonia

58. 1. Severe hypoxia after smoke inhalation is typically related to ARDS. The other conditions listed aren't typically associated with smoke inhalation and severe hypoxia.
NP: Implementation; CN: Physiological integrity; CNS: Physiological adaptation; CL: Application

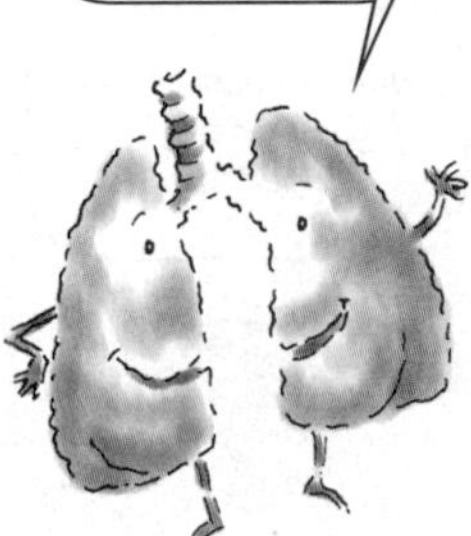

Crackle, wheeze, or rattle? Each sound is another clue.

59. In a client with smoke inhalation, the nurse would expect to hear which of the following breath sounds?

1. Crackles
2. Decreased breath sounds
3. Inspiratory and expiratory wheezing
4. Upper airway rhonchi

59. 1. In adult respiratory distress syndrome, the most frequently heard sounds are crackles throughout the lung fields. Decreased breath sounds or inspiratory and expiratory wheezing are associated with asthma, and rhonchi are heard when there's sputum in the airways.
NP: Assessment; CN: Physiological integrity; CNS: Physiological adaptation; CL: Application

60. Which of the following areas would differentiate between adult respiratory distress syndrome (ARDS) and heart failure?

1. Cardiac function, because heart failure has a cardiac cause and ARDS doesn't
2. Chest X-ray results, which appear differently in the two diagnoses
3. Prognosis, which is worse with ARDS
4. Sputum production, because copious amounts of thin clear sputum are produced in ARDS

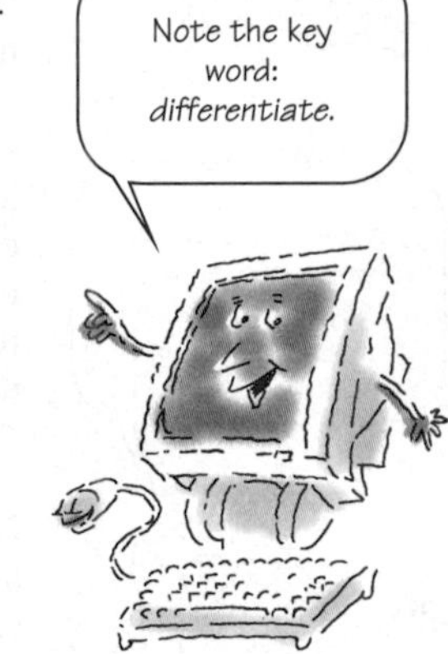

60. 1. ARDS is referred to as noncardiogenic pulmonary edema because heart failure and pulmonary edema have cardiac causes whereas ARDS doesn't. Chest X-rays appear the same for heart failure and ARDS, and the prognosis for ARDS is typically worse than it is for heart failure. Clear sputum production is a symptom associated with ARDS.
NP: Implementation; CN: Physiological integrity; CNS: Physiological adaptation; CL: Application

61. Which of the following statements best describes what happens to the alveoli in adult respiratory distress syndrome (ARDS)?

1. Alveoli are overexpanded.
2. Alveoli increase perfusion.
3. Alveolar spaces are filled with fluid.
4. Alveoli improve gaseous exchange.

61. 3. In ARDS, the alveolar membranes are more permeable and the spaces are fluid-filled. Alveoli collapse, impairing gas exchange. The fluid interferes with gas exchange and reduces perfusion.
NP: Implementation; CN: Physiological integrity; CNS: Physiological adaptation; CL: Application

NP: Nursing process CN: Client needs category CNS: Client needs subcategory CL: Cognitive level

62. A 69-year-old client develops acute shortness of breath and progressive hypoxia requiring mechanical ventilation after repair of a fractured right femur. The hypoxia was probably caused by which of the following conditions?

1. Asthma attack
2. Atelectasis
3. Bronchitis
4. Fat embolism

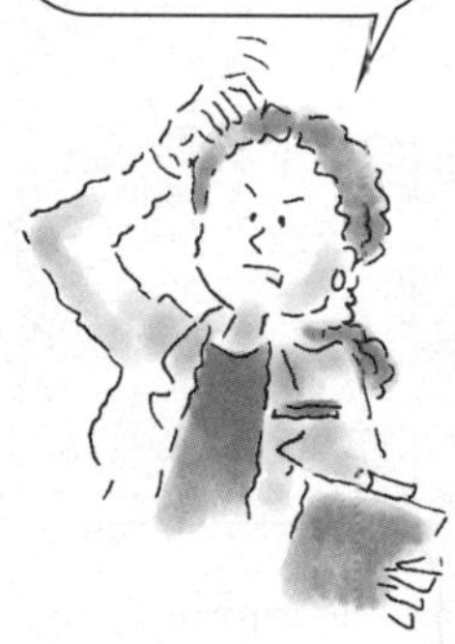

Several answers may seem correct, but *probably* points to the best one.

62. 4. Long bone fractures are correlated with fat emboli, which cause shortness of breath and hypoxia. It's unlikely the client has developed asthma or bronchitis without a previous history. He could develop atelectasis, but it typically doesn't produce progressive hypoxia.

NP: Implementation; CN: Physiological integrity; CNS: Physiological adaptation; CL: Application

63. A client with a fat embolism is receiving 100% fraction of inspired oxygen (FIO_2) on a mechanical ventilator and continues to be hypoxic. Which of the following measures can improve his oxygenation?

1. Add positive end-expiratory pressure (PEEP).
2. Give beta-adrenergic blockers.
3. Give diuretics.
4. Increase the FIO_2 on the ventilator.

63. 1. PEEP can be added to open up alveoli and keep them open. There's no reason to give the client beta-adrenergic blockers. He may benefit from diuresis, but in the meantime, PEEP should be added to improve oxygenation. The highest amount of oxygen that can be delivered is 100% FIO_2.

NP: Implementation; CN: Physiological integrity; CNS: Physiological adaptation; CL: Application

64. If a client with a fat embolism continues to be hypoxic following therapy with positive end-expiratory pressure, what can be done to reduce oxygen demand?

1. Give diuretics.
2. Give neuromuscular blockers.
3. Put the head of the bed flat.
4. Use bronchodilators.

64. 2. Neuromuscular blockers cause skeletal muscle paralysis, reducing the amount of oxygen used by the restless skeletal muscles. This should improve oxygenation. Diuretics can be administered to reduce pulmonary congestion and the head of the bed should be partially elevated to facilitate diaphragm movement. Bronchodilators may be used, but they typically don't have enough of an effect to reduce the amount of hypoxia present. However, diuretics, head elevation, and bronchodilators would improve oxygen delivery, not reduce oxygen demand.

NP: Implementation; CN: Physiological integrity; CNS: Physiological adaptation; CL: Application

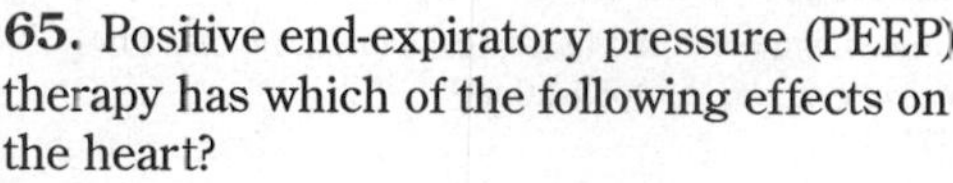

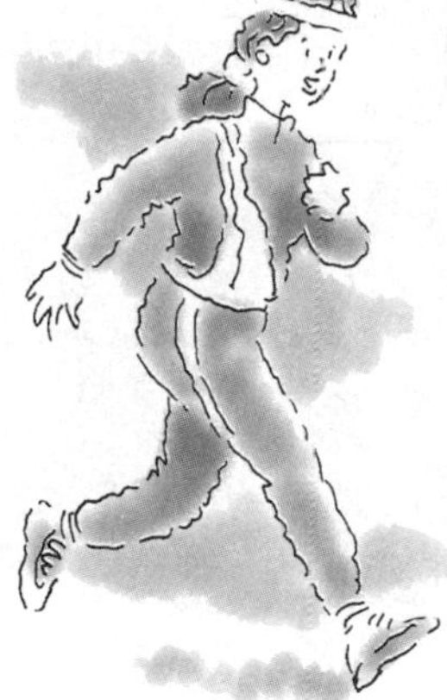

You're almost there! Keep a' going!

65. Positive end-expiratory pressure (PEEP) therapy has which of the following effects on the heart?

1. Bradycardia
2. Tachycardia
3. Increased blood pressure
4. Reduced cardiac output

65. 4. PEEP reduces cardiac output by increasing intrathoracic pressure and reducing the amount of blood delivered to the left side of the heart, thereby reducing cardiac output. It doesn't affect heart rate, but a decrease in cardiac output may reduce blood pressure, commonly causing a compensatory tachycardia.

NP: Implementation; CN: Physiological integrity; CNS: Physiological adaptation; CL: Application

66. Occasionally clients with adult respiratory distress syndrome (ARDS) are placed in the prone position. How does this position help the client?

1. It improves cardiac output.
2. It makes the client more comfortable.
3. It prevents skin breakdown.
4. It recruits more alveoli.

66. 4. A supine position may reduce the ability of posterior alveoli to open and remain open. Turning the client to the prone position may recruit new alveoli in the posterior region of the lung and improve oxygenation status. Cardiac output shouldn't be affected by the prone position. Generally, the client is obtunded when this measure is used. If not, he should be well-sedated. Skin breakdown can still occur over the new pressure points.

NP: Implementation; CN: Physiological integrity; CNS: Physiological adaptation; CL: Application

67. Which of the following conditions could lead to adult respiratory distress syndrome (ARDS)?

1. Appendicitis
2. Massive trauma
3. Receiving conscious sedation
4. Right meniscus injury

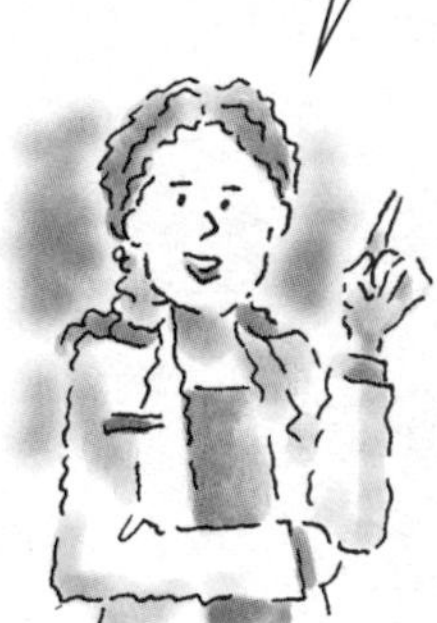

It's important to know which values to monitor.

67. 2. The client with massive trauma will require multiple transfusions. Blood products are preserved with citrate, which causes increased permeability in the lungs, the defect that allows ARDS to develop. Appendicitis, unless it causes overwhelming sepsis, won't lead to ARDS. Conscious sedation and injuries to the meniscus don't lead to ARDS.

NP: Implementation; CN: Physiological integrity; CNS: Physiological adaptation; CL: Application

68. Which of the following indicators would show if the condition of the client with adult respiratory distress syndrome (ARDS) is improving?

1. Arterial blood gas (ABG) values
2. Bronchoscopy results
3. Increased blood pressure
4. Sputum culture and sensitivity results

68. 1. Improved ABG results would indicate that the client's oxygenation status is improved. Hypoxia is the problem in ARDS, so bronchoscopy and sputum culture results may have no bearing on the improvement of ARDS. Increased blood pressure isn't relative to the client's respiratory condition.

NP: Evaluation; CN: Physiological integrity; CNS: Physiological adaptation; CL: Analysis

69. A high level of oxygen exerts which of the following effects on the lung?

1. Improves oxygen uptake
2. Increases carbon dioxide levels
3. Stabilizes carbon dioxide levels
4. Reduces amount of functional alveolar surface area

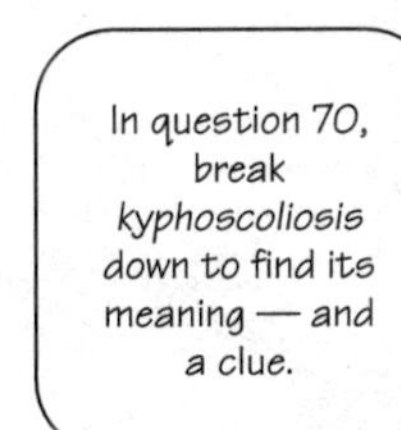

In question 70, break kyphoscoliosis down to find its meaning — and a clue.

69. 4. Oxygen toxicity causes direct pulmonary trauma, reducing the amount of alveolar surface area available for gaseous exchange, which results in increased carbon dioxide levels and decreased oxygen uptake.

NP: Implementation; CN: Physiological integrity; CNS: Physiological adaptation; CL: Application

70. Which of the following effects can thoracic kyphoscoliosis have on lung function?

1. Improves lung expansion
2. Obstructs lung deflation
3. Reduces alveolar compression during expiration
4. Restricts lung expansion

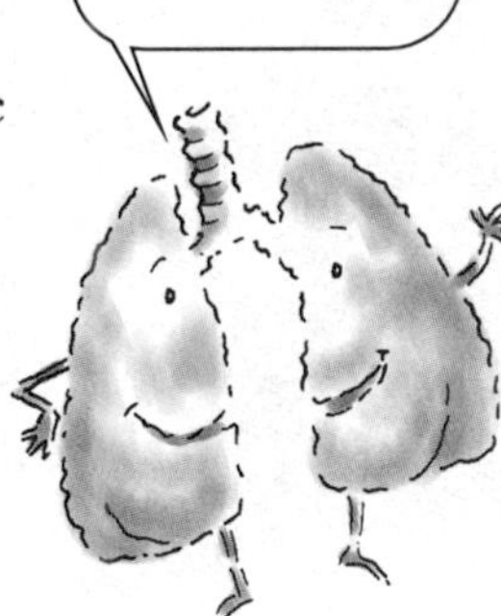

70. 4. Thoracic kyphoscoliosis causes lung compression, restricts lung expansion, and results in more rapid and shallow respiration. It doesn't improve lung expansion because of the compression. It also doesn't cause obstruction or reduce alveolar compression during expiration.

NP: Implementation; CN: Physiological integrity; CNS: Physiological adaptation; CL: Application

71. A 24-year-old client comes into the clinic complaining of right-sided chest pain and shortness of breath. He reports that it started suddenly. The assessment should include which of the following interventions?

1. Auscultation of breath sounds
2. Chest X-ray
3. Echocardiogram
4. Electrocardiogram (ECG)

71. 1. Because the client is short of breath, listening to breath sounds is a good idea. He may need a chest X-ray and an ECG, but a physician must order these tests. Unless a cardiac source for the client's pain is identified, he won't need an echocardiogram.

NP: Implementation; CN: Physiological integrity; CNS: Physiological adaptation; CL: Application

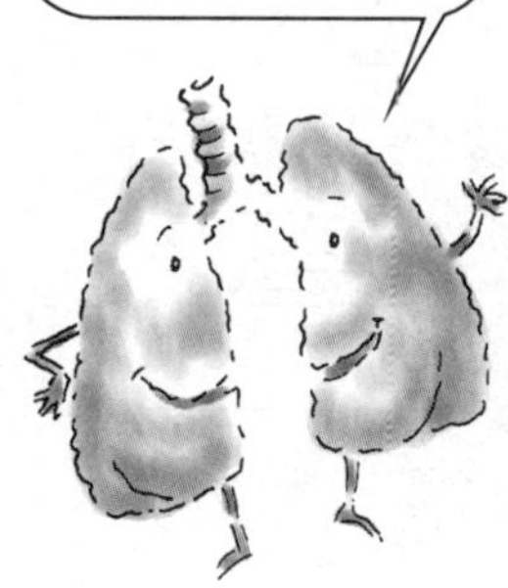
Listening to breath sounds sure helps diagnose a lot of conditions, doesn't it?

72. A client with shortness of breath has decreased to absent breath sounds on the right side, from the apex to the base. Which of the following conditions would best explain this?

1. Acute asthma
2. Chronic bronchitis
3. Pneumonia
4. Spontaneous pneumothorax

72. 4. A spontaneous pneumothorax occurs when the client's lung collapses, causing an acute decrease in the amount of functional lung used in oxygenation. The sudden collapse was the cause of his chest pain and shortness of breath. An asthma attack would show wheezing breath sounds, and bronchitis would have rhonchi. Pneumonia would have bronchial breath sounds over the area of consolidation.

NP: Implementation; CN: Physiological integrity; CNS: Physiological adaptation; CL: Application

73. Which of the following treatments would the nurse expect for a client with spontaneous pneumothorax?

1. Antibiotics
2. Bronchodilators
3. Chest tube placement
4. Hyperbaric chamber

73. 3. The only way to reexpand the lung is to place a chest tube on the right side so the air in the pleural space can be removed and the lung reexpanded. Antibiotics and bronchodilators would have no effect on lung reexpansion, nor would the hyperbaric chamber.

NP: Implementation; CN: Physiological integrity; CNS: Physiological adaptation; CL: Application

74. A 60-year-old client was in a motor vehicle accident as an unrestrained driver. He's now in the emergency department complaining of difficulty breathing and chest pain. On auscultation of his lung fields, no breath sounds are present in the left upper lobe. This client may have which of the following conditions?

1. Bronchitis
2. Pneumonia
3. Pneumothorax
4. Tuberculosis (TB)

74. 3. From the trauma the client experienced, it's unlikely he has bronchitis, pneumonia, or TB; rhonchi with bronchitis, bronchial breath sounds with pneumonia, and rhonchorous breath sounds with TB would be heard.

NP: Implementation; CN: Physiological integrity; CNS: Physiological adaptation; CL: Application

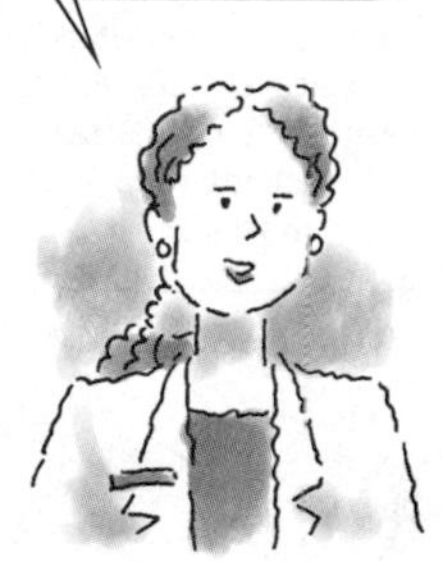
You're doing great! Keep going!

75. Which of the following methods is the best way to confirm the diagnosis of a pneumothorax?

1. Auscultate breath sounds.
2. Have the client use an incentive spirometer.
3. Take a chest X-ray.
4. Stick a needle in the area of the decreased breath sounds.

75. 3. A chest X-ray will show the area of collapsed lung if a pneumothorax is present as well as the volume of air in the pleural space. Listening to breath sounds won't confirm a diagnosis. An incentive spirometer is used to encourage deep breathing. A needle thoracostomy is done only in an emergency and only by someone trained to do it.

NP: Implementation; CN: Physiological integrity; CNS: Physiological adaptation; CL: Application

76. A client is about to have a chest tube inserted in the left upper chest. When the tube is inserted, it begins to drain a large amount of serosanguineous fluid. Which of the following explanations best describes what caused this?

1. The chest tube was inserted improperly.
2. This always happens when a chest tube is inserted.
3. An artery was nicked when the chest tube was placed.
4. The client had a hemothorax instead of a pneumothorax.

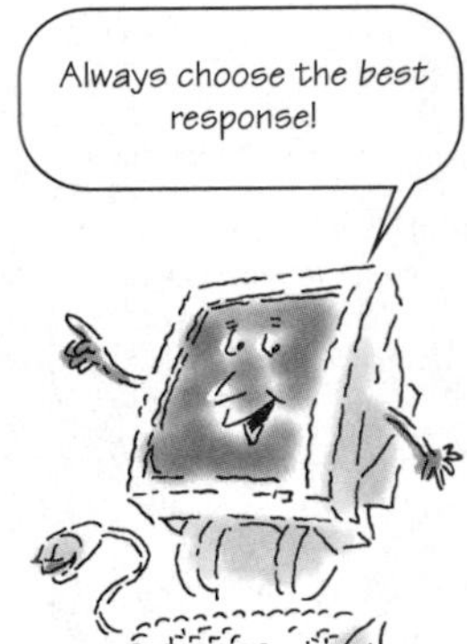

Always choose the best response!

76. 4. Because of the traumatic cause of injury, the client had a hemothorax, in which blood collection causes the collapse of the lung. The placement of the chest tube will drain the blood from the space and reexpand the lung. There's a very slight chance of nicking an intercostal artery during insertion, but it's fairly unlikely if the person placing the chest tube has been trained. The initial chest X-ray would help confirm whether there was blood in the pleural space or just air.

NP: Implementation; CN: Physiological integrity; CNS: Physiological adaptation; CL: Application

77. A hospitalized client needs a central I.V. catheter inserted. The physician places the catheter in the subclavian vein. Shortly afterward, the client develops shortness of breath and appears restless. Which of the following actions would the nurse do first?

1. Administer a sedative.
2. Advise the client to calm down.
3. Auscultate breath sounds.
4. Check to see if the client can have medication.

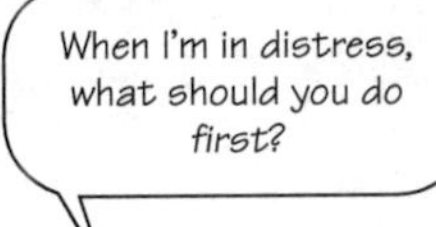

When I'm in distress, what should you do first?

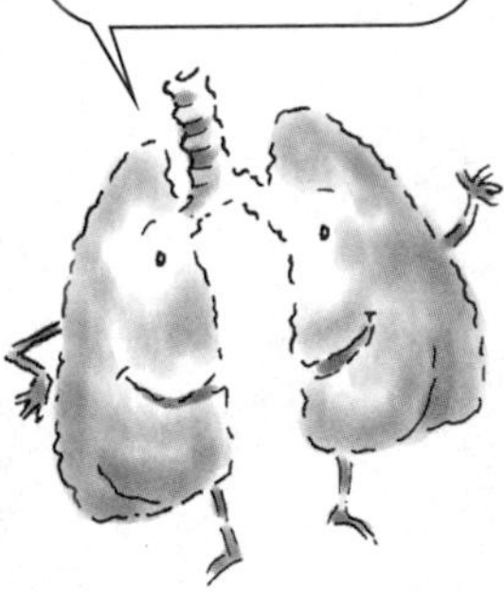

77. 3. Because this is an acute episode, listen to the client's lungs to see if anything has changed. Don't give this client medication, especially sedatives, if he's having difficulty breathing. Give the client emotional support and contact the physician who placed the central venous access.

NP: Assessment; CN: Physiological integrity; CNS: Physiological adaptation; CL: Application

78. Which of the following measures would be ordered for a client who recently had a central venous catheter inserted and who now appears short of breath and anxious?

1. Chest X-ray
2. Electrocardiogram
3. Laboratory tests
4. Sedation

78. 1. Inserting an I.V. catheter in the subclavian vein can result in a pneumothorax, so a chest X-ray should be done. If it's negative, then other tests should be done but they aren't appropriate as the first intervention. Sedation may depress respirations.

NP: Implementation; CN: Physiological integrity; CNS: Physiological adaptation; CL: Application

79. A client needs to have a chest tube inserted in the right upper chest. Which of the following actions is part of the nurse's role?

1. The nurse isn't needed.
2. Prepare the chest tube drainage system.
3. Bring the chest X-ray to the client's room.
4. Insert the chest tube.

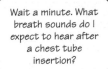

79. 2. The nurse must anticipate that a drainage system is required and set this up before insertion so the tube can be directly connected to the drainage system. The chest X-ray need not be brought to the client's room. A physician will insert the chest tube.

NP: Implementation; CN: Physiological integrity; CNS: Physiological adaptation; CL: Application

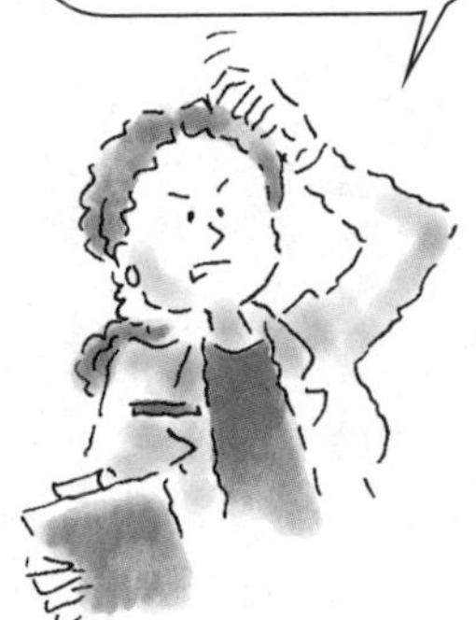

80. Which of the following results shows that a chest tube insertion was done correctly?

1. Bronchial sounds heard at both bases
2. Vesicular sounds heard over upper lung fields
3. Bronchovesicular sounds heard over both lung fields
4. Crackles heard on the affected side

80. 3. If the chest tube is inserted correctly, normal bronchovesicular breath sounds in that area will be heard and the client's oxygenation status will improve. A chest X-ray should be done to ensure reexpansion. All other sounds noted are abnormal.

NP: Evaluation; CN: Physiological integrity; CNS: Physiological adaptation; CL: Analysis

81. Which of the following measures best determines that a chest tube is no longer needed for a client who had a pneumothorax?

1. The drainage from the chest tube is minimal.
2. Arterial blood gas (ABG) levels are obtained to ensure proper oxygenation.
3. It's removed and the client is assessed to see if he's breathing adequately.
4. No fluctuation in the water seal chamber occurs when no suction is applied.

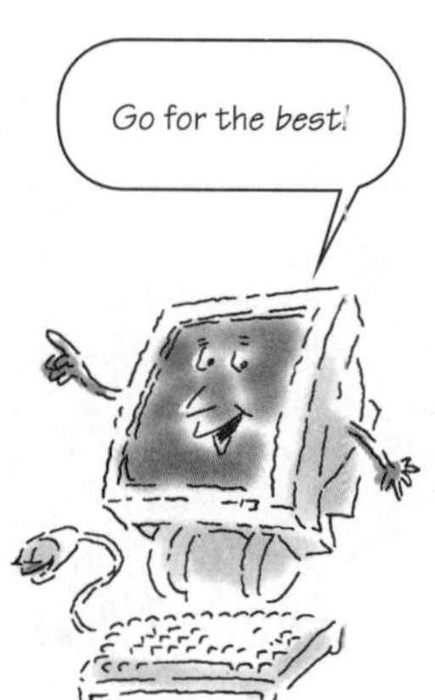

Go for the best!

81. 4. One indication of reexpansion is the cessation of fluctuation in the water seal chamber when suction isn't applied. Drainage should be minimal before the chest tube is removed. An ABG analysis may be done to ensure proper oxygenation but isn't necessary if clinical assessment criteria are met. The chest tube isn't removed until it's determined the client's lung has adequately reexpanded and will stay that way. After the lung stays expanded, the chest tube is removed.

NP: Implementation; CN: Physiological integrity; CNS: Physiological adaptation; CL: Application

82. Which of the following interventions should be done before a chest tube is removed?

1. Disconnect the drainage system from the tube.
2. Obtain a chest X-ray to document reexpansion.
3. Obtain an arterial blood gas level to document oxygen status.
4. Sedate the client, and the physician will slip the tube out without warning the client.

82. 2. A chest X-ray should be done to ensure and document the lung is reexpanded and has remained expanded since suction was discontinued. The drainage system shouldn't be disconnected from the tube while still in the client because that could cause a pneumothorax to recur. A pulse oximetry measurement is sufficient to track oxygenation before the tube is removed. Client cooperation is desirable; if the client can hold his breath while the chest tube is removed, there's less chance that air will be drawn back into the pleural space during removal.

NP: Implementation; CN: Physiological integrity; CNS: Physiological adaptation; CL: Application

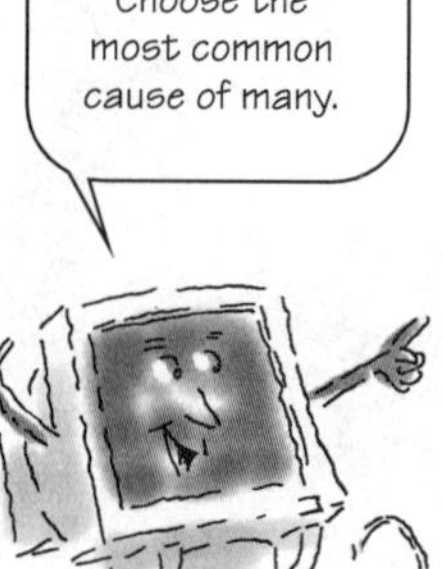

Choose the most common cause of many.

83. Which of the following actions or conditions is the number one cause of lung cancer?

1. Genetics
2. Occupational exposures
3. Smoking a pipe
4. Smoking cigarettes

83. 4. As many as 90% of clients with lung cancer smoke cigarettes. Cigarette smoke contains several organ-specific carcinogens. There may be a genetic predisposition for the development of cancer. Occupational hazards such as pollutants can cause cancer. Pipe smokers inhale less often and tend to develop cancers of the lip and mouth.

NP: Implementation; CN: Physiological integrity; CNS: Physiological adaptation; CL: Application

84. The client with which of the following types of lung cancer has the best prognosis?

1. Adenocarcinoma
2. Oat cell
3. Squamous cell
4. Small cell

84. 3. Squamous cell carcinoma is a slow-growing, rarely metastasizing type of cancer. Adenocarcinoma is the next best lung cancer to have in terms of prognosis. Oat cell and small cell carcinoma are the same. Small cell carcinoma grows rapidly and is quick to metastasize.

NP: Implementation; CN: Physiological integrity; CNS: Physiological adaptation; CL: Application

85. Warning signs and symptoms of lung cancer include persistent cough, bloody sputum, dyspnea, and which of the following other symptoms?
1. Dizziness
2. Generalized weakness
3. Hypotension
4. Recurrent pleural effusions

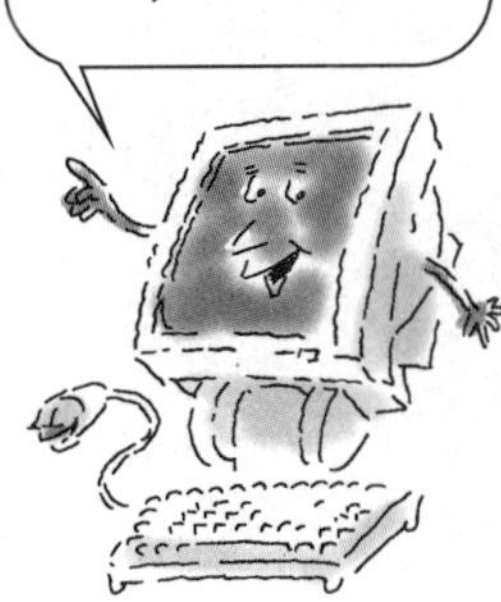

Centrally located. That's your clue for question 86.

86. A centrally located tumor would produce which of the following symptoms?
1. Coughing
2. Hemoptysis
3. Pleuritic pain
4. Shoulder pain

87. A definitive diagnosis of lung cancer is obtained by which of the following evaluations?
1. Bronchoscopy
2. Chest X-ray
3. Computerized tomography of the chest
4. Surgical biopsy

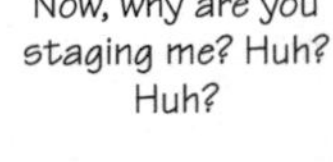

Now, why are you staging me? Huh? Huh?

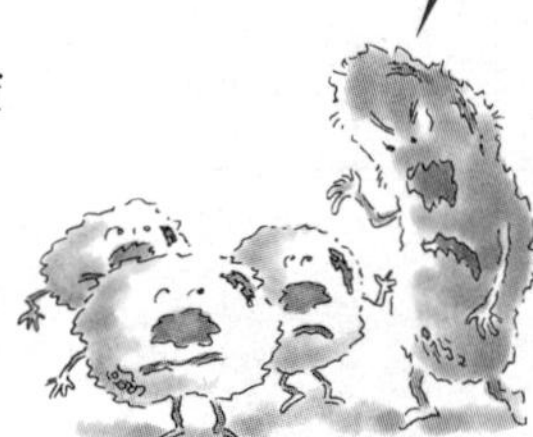

88. Staging of lung cancer is done for which of the following reasons?
1. To identify the type of cancer
2. To identify the best treatment
3. To identify if metastasis occurred
4. To identify the location of the lesion

89. Which of the following interventions is the key to increasing the survival rates of clients with lung cancer?
1. Early bronchoscopy
2. Early detection
3. High-dose chemotherapy
4. Smoking cessation

85. 4. Recurring episodes of pleural effusions can be caused by the tumor and should be investigated. Dizziness, generalized weakness, and hypotension aren't typically considered warning signals, but may occur in advanced stages of cancer.
NP: Implementation; CN: Physiological integrity; CNS: Physiological adaptation; CL: Application

86. 1. Centrally located pulmonary tumors are found in the upper airway (vocal cords) and usually obstruct airflow, producing such symptoms as coughing, wheezing, and stridor. Small cell tumors tend to be located in the lower airways and often cause hemoptysis. As the tumor invades the pleural space, it may cause pleuritic pain. Pancoast tumors that occur in the apices may cause shoulder pain.
NP: Implementation; CN: Physiological integrity; CNS: Physiological adaptation; CL: Application

87. 4. Only surgical biopsy and cytologic examination of the cells can give a definitive diagnosis of the type of cancer. Bronchoscopy gives positive results in only 30% of the cases. Chest X-ray and computerized tomography can identify location, but don't diagnose the type of cancer.
NP: Implementation; CN: Physiological integrity; CNS: Physiological adaptation; CL: Application

88. 2. Staging the cancer allows the physician to determine appropriate therapies and estimate the client's prognosis. The staging information may include whether the cancer has metastasized, but this information is obtained by a body scan, such as magnetic resonance imaging or computerized tomography. The location and type of cancer has already been identified before the staging is done.
NP: Implementation; CN: Physiological integrity; CNS: Physiological adaptation; CL: Application

89. 2. Early detection of cancer when the cells may be premalignant and potentially curable would be most beneficial. However, a tumor must be 1 cm in diameter before it's detectable on a chest X-ray, so this is difficult. A bronchoscopy may help identify cell type but may not increase survival rate. High-dose chemotherapy has minimal effect on long-term survival. Smoking cessation won't reverse the process but may prevent further decompensation.
NP: Implementation; CN: Physiological integrity; CNS: Physiological adaptation; CL: Application

90. A client with a chest tube has accidentally removed it. What should be done first?
1. Lie the client down on his left side.
2. Lie the client down on his right side.
3. Apply an occlusive dressing over the site.
4. Reinsert the chest tube that fell out.

90. 3. To prevent the client from sucking air into the pleural space and causing a pneumothorax, an occlusive dressing should be put over the hole where the tube came out. The physician should be called and the client checked for signs of respiratory distress. Positioning the client on either the left or right side won't make a difference. It isn't advisable for the physician to reinsert the old tube because it's no longer sterile.

NP: Implementation; CN: Physiological integrity; CNS: Physiological adaptation; CL: Application

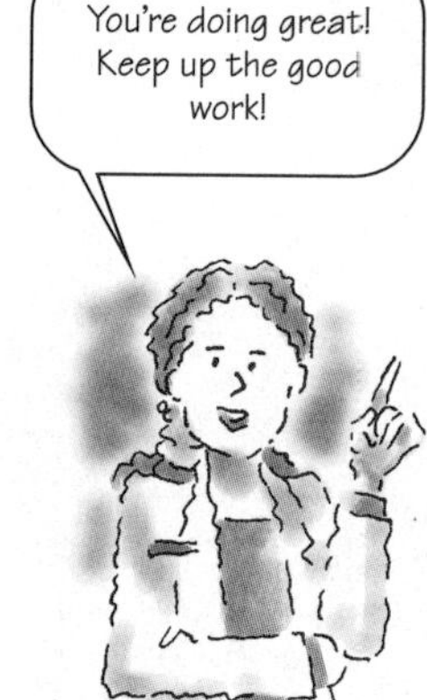

91. A client has been diagnosed with lung cancer and requires a wedge resection. How much of the lung is removed?
1. One entire lung
2. A lobe of the lung
3. A small, localized area near the surface of the lung
4. A segment of the lung, including a bronchiole and its alveoli

91. 3. A small area of tissue close to the surface of the lung is removed in a wedge resection. An entire lung is removed in a pneumonectomy. A segment of the lung is removed in a segmental resection and a lobe is removed in a lobectomy.

NP: Implementation; CN: Physiological integrity; CNS: Physiological adaptation; CL: Application

92. When a client has a lobectomy, what fills the space where the lobe was?
1. The space stays empty.
2. The surgeon fills the space with a gel.
3. The lung space fills up with serous fluid.
4. The remaining lobe or lobes overexpand to fill the space.

92. 4. The remaining lobe or lobes overexpand slightly to fill the space previously occupied by the removed tissue. The diaphragm is carried higher on the operative side to further reduce the empty space. The space can't remain "empty," because truly empty would imply a vacuum, which would interfere with the intrathoracic pressure changes that allow breathing. The surgeon doesn't use gel to fill the space. Serous fluid overproduction would compress the remaining lobes, diminish their function and, possibly, cause a mediastinal shift.

NP: Implementation; CN: Physiological integrity; CNS: Physiological adaptation; CL: Application

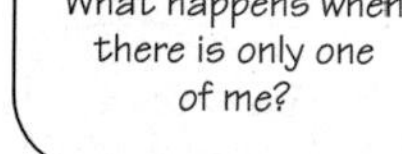

What happens when there is only one of me?

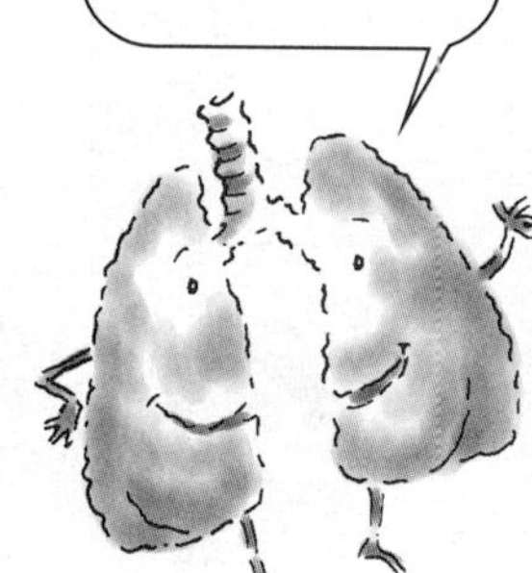

93. If a client requires a pneumonectomy, what fills the area of the thoracic cavity?
1. The space remains filled with air only.
2. The surgeon fills the space with a gel.
3. Serous fluid fills the space and consolidates the region.
4. The tissue from the other lung grows over to the other side.

93. 3. Serous fluid fills the space and eventually consolidates, preventing extensive mediastinal shift of the heart and remaining lung. Air can't be left in the space. There's no gel that can be placed in the pleural space. The tissue from the other lung can't cross the mediastinum, although a temporary mediastinal shift exists until the space is filled.

NP: Implementation; CN: Physiological integrity; CNS: Physiological adaptation; CL: Application

94. During a pneumonectomy, the phrenic nerve on the surgical side is usually cut to cause hemidiaphragm paralysis. Why is this done?

1. Paralyzing the diaphragm reduces oxygen demand.
2. Cutting the phrenic nerve is a mistake during surgery.
3. The client isn't using that lung to breathe.
4. Paralyzing the diaphragm reduces the space left by the pneumonectomy.

94. 4. Because the hemidiaphragm is a muscle that doesn't contract when paralyzed, an uncontracted hemidiaphragm remains in an "up" position, which reduces the space left by the pneumonectomy. Serous fluid has less space to fill, thus reducing the extent and duration of mediastinal shift after surgery. Paralyzing the hemidiaphragm doesn't significantly decrease total-body oxygen demand. Although it's true that the client no longer needs the hemidiaphragm on the operative side to breathe, this alone wouldn't be sufficient justification for cutting the phrenic nerve.

NP: Implementation; CN: Physiological integrity; CNS: Physiological adaptation; CL: Application

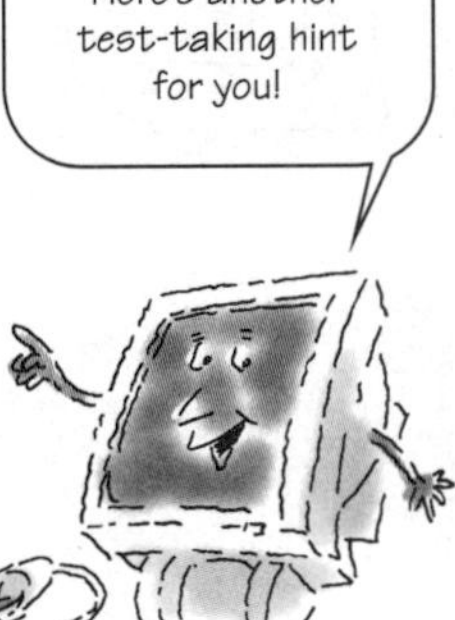

Here's another test-taking hint for you!

95. Which of the following is the primary goal of surgical resection for lung cancer?

1. To remove the tumor and all surrounding tissue
2. To remove the tumor and as little surrounding tissue as possible
3. To remove all the tumor and any collapsed alveoli in the same region
4. To remove as much of the tumor as possible, without removing any alveoli

95. 2. The goal of surgical resection is to remove the lung tissue that has a tumor in it while saving as much surrounding tissue as possible. It may be necessary to remove alveoli and bronchioles, but care is taken to make sure only what's absolutely necessary is removed.

NP: Implementation; CN: Physiological integrity; CNS: Physiological adaptation; CL: Application

96. If the client with lung cancer also has preexisting pulmonary disease, which of the following statements best describes how this affects the extent of surgery that can be performed?

1. It doesn't affect it.
2. It may require a whole lung to be removed.
3. The entire tumor may not be able to be removed.
4. It may prevent surgery if the client can't tolerate lung tissue removal.

96. 4. If the client's preexisting pulmonary disease is restrictive and advanced, it may be impossible to remove the tumor, and the client may have to be treated with only chemotherapy and radiation.

NP: Implementation; CN: Physiological integrity; CNS: Physiological adaptation; CL: Application

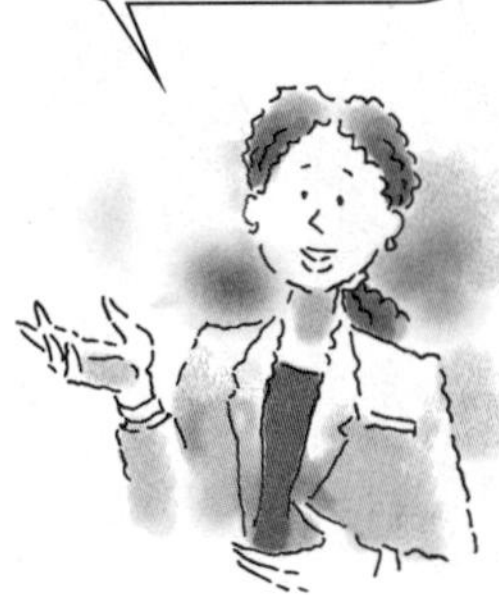

The nurse does a lot of teaching but in this case, what would be the main focus?

97. Preoperative teaching for the client having surgery should focus on which of the following areas?

1. Deciding if the client should have the surgery
2. Giving emotional support to the client and his family
3. Giving minute details of the surgery to the client and his family
4. Providing general information to reduce client and family anxiety

97. 4. The nurse's role is to provide general information about the surgery and what to expect before and after surgery, and to give emotional support during this time. The nurse's role isn't to decide if the client should have surgery or to give minute details of the surgery unless the client or family requests them, in which case the surgeon should answer the questions. Emotional support alone during this time isn't sufficient.

NP: Implementation; CN: Physiological integrity; CNS: Physiological adaptation; CL: Application

98. The client with a benign tumor is treated in which of the following ways?

1. The tumor is treated with radiation only.
2. The tumor is treated with chemotherapy only.
3. The tumor is left alone unless symptoms are present.
4. The tumor is removed, involving the least possible amount of tissue.

98. 4. The tumor is removed to prevent further compression of lung tissue as the tumor grows, which could lead to respiratory decompensation. If for some reason it can't be removed, then radiation or chemotherapy may be used to try to shrink the tumor.

NP: Implementation; CN: Physiological integrity; CNS: Physiological adaptation; CL: Application

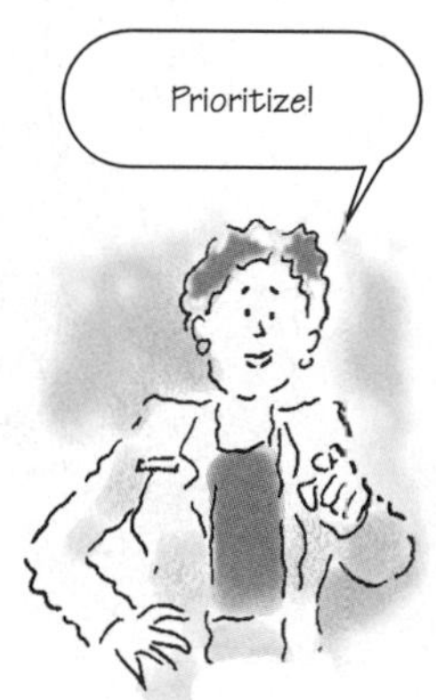

99. In the client with terminal lung cancer, the focus of nursing care is on which of the following nursing interventions?

1. Provide emotional support.
2. Provide nutritional support.
3. Provide pain control.
4. Prepare the client's will.

99. 3. The client with terminal lung cancer may have extreme pleuritic pain and should be treated to reduce his discomfort. Preparing the client and his family for the impending death and providing emotional support is also important but shouldn't be the primary focus until pain is under control. Nutritional support may be provided, but as the terminal phase advances, the client's nutritional needs greatly decrease. Nursing care doesn't focus on helping the client prepare a will.

NP: Implementation; CN: Physiological integrity; CNS: Physiological adaptation; CL: Application

100. Which of the following statements best defines a pulmonary embolism?

1. It's a blood clot that originates in the lung.
2. It's a blood clot that has occluded an alveolus.
3. It's a blood clot that has occluded a bronchiole.
4. It's a blood clot that has occluded a pulmonary blood vessel.

100. 4. A pulmonary embolism is a blood clot or some other material that, after traveling from some other place in the body through the bloodstream, becomes lodged in one of the pulmonary blood vessels. An embolism remains in the bloodstream and specifically isn't in the bronchial tree, the "air side" of the lung architecture; therefore, it isn't in the alveoli or the bronchiole.

NP: Implementation; CN: Physiological integrity; CNS: Physiological adaptation; CL: Application

101. Which of the following is the most common origin for a pulmonary embolism?

1. Amniotic fluid
2. Bone marrow
3. Septic thrombi
4. Venous thrombi

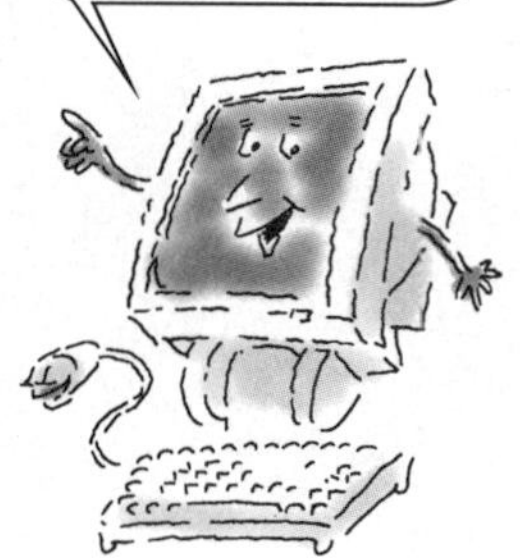

This clue asks you to select the most common, even when all answers are correct.

101. 4. Venous thrombi in the thigh and pelvis are the most common sources for pulmonary emboli. Clients who are immobile form clots from this source. When dislodged, the clots are carried through the bloodstream and lodge in the pulmonary vasculature. The other options are also sources, but not the most common.

NP: Implementation; CN: Physiological integrity; CNS: Physiological adaptation; CL: Application

102. Clients most at risk for pulmonary embolism are those with which of the following conditions?

1. Arthritis
2. Diabetes
3. Pregnancy
4. Trauma to the pelvis or lower extremities

102. 4. Trauma to the pelvis or lower extremities requires the client to be immobile for a long recovery period, which allows the blood to pool and clot in this region and ultimately become an embolus. Clients with the other conditions aren't at as much risk for pulmonary embolism.

NP: Implementation; CN: Physiological integrity; CNS: Physiological adaptation; CL: Application

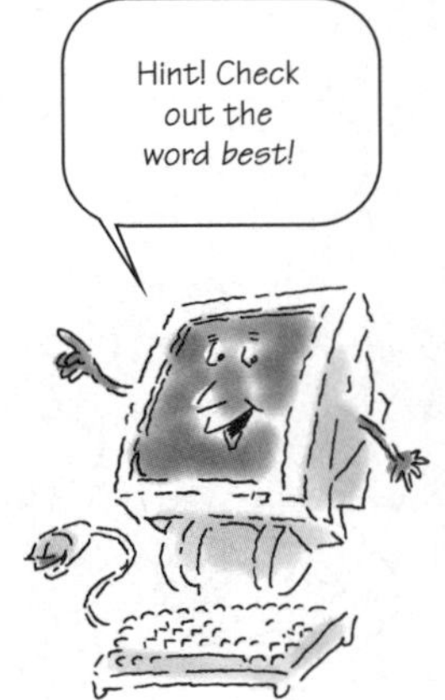
Hint! Check out the word best!

103. Which of the following measures to prevent pulmonary embolism after lower extremity surgery is the best?

1. Early ambulation
2. Frequent chest X-rays to find a pulmonary embolism
3. Frequent lower extremity scans
4. Intubation of the client

103. 1. Early ambulation helps reduce pooling of blood, which reduces the tendency of the blood to form a clot that could then dislodge. Frequent chest X-rays or lower extremity scans don't prevent pulmonary embolism. Intubation of the client won't prevent the occurrence of a pulmonary embolism.

NP: Implementation; CN: Physiological integrity; CNS: Physiological adaptation; CL: Application

104. Which of the following physiologic effects of a pulmonary embolism would initially affect oxygenation?

1. A blood clot blocks ventilation; perfusion is unaffected.
2. A blood clot blocks ventilation, producing hypoxia despite normal perfusion.
3. A blood clot blocks perfusion and ventilation, producing profound hypoxia.
4. A blood clot blocks perfusion, producing hypoxia despite normal or supernormal ventilation.

104. 4. The blood clot blocks blood flow to a region of the lung tissue. That area remains ventilated, but because blood flow is blocked, no gas exchange can occur in that region and a ventilation-perfusion mismatch is present. Ventilation isn't initially affected by a blood clot because air can still move normally through the bronchial tree.

NP: Implementation; CN: Physiological integrity; CNS: Physiological adaptation; CL: Application

105. Which of the following statements best describes the ventilation-perfusion mismatch that occurs with a pulmonary embolism?

1. The area of the lung being ventilated isn't being perfused.
2. The area of the lung being perfused isn't being ventilated.
3. The area of the lung being ventilated is also being perfused.
4. The amount of ventilation occurring doesn't equal perfusion.

105. 1. A pulmonary embolism blocks the flow of blood past a region of the lung tissue, which is still being ventilated because no disorder of the bronchial tree exists. A pulmonary embolism blocks the pulmonary vasculature, not allowing blood to flow to the distal region of the lung and interfering with gas exchange. Blood must flow around each alveolus, or perfuse, for the exchange of carbon dioxide and oxygen to occur across the alveolar-capillary membrane. When an area of lung is ventilated but not perfused, there is a ventilation-perfusion mismatch specific to pulmonary embolism. A mismatch that shows impaired ventilation but normal perfusion indicates a pathological state in the bronchial tree, such as pneumonia or atelectasis.

NP: Implementation; CN: Physiological integrity; CNS: Physiological adaptation; CL: Application

106. When a client has a pulmonary embolism, he develops chest pain caused by which of the following conditions?

1. Costochondritis
2. Myocardial infarction (MI)
3. Pleuritic pain
4. Referred pain from the pelvis to the chest

106. 3. Pleuritic pain is caused by the inflammatory reaction of the lung parenchyma. The pain isn't associated with costochondritis, MI, or referred pain from the pelvis to the chest.

NP: Implementation; CN: Physiological integrity; CNS: Physiological adaptation; CL: Application

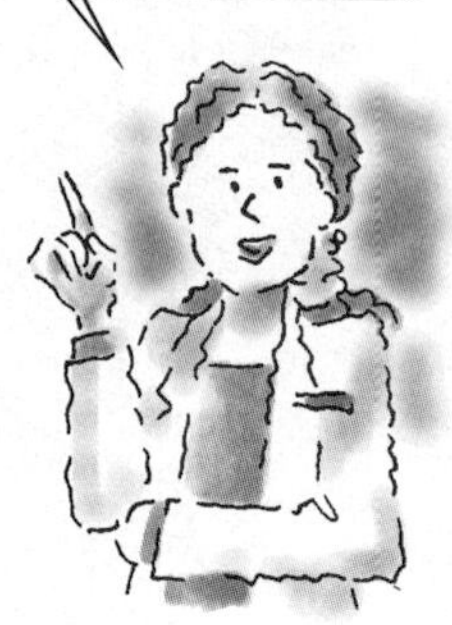

Here's a hint for question 107: Think about what causes the condition.

107. The client with a pulmonary embolism frequently feels apprehension or a sense of "impending doom" because of which of the following reasons?

1. Inflammatory reaction in the lung parenchyma
2. Loss of chest expansion
3. Loss of lung tissue
4. Sudden reduction in adequate oxygenation

107. 4. The client with a pulmonary embolism has less lung involved in oxygenation, causing the client to feel apprehensive. If the area involved is large, the apprehension can be great, giving the client the feeling of "impending doom." The inflammatory reaction in the lung causes chest pain. There's no actual loss of lung tissue, and chest expansion isn't affected.

NP: Implementation; CN: Physiological integrity; CNS: Physiological adaptation; CL: Application

108. Hemoptysis may be present in the client with a pulmonary embolism because of which of the following reasons?

1. Alveolar damage in the infarcted area
2. Involvement of major blood vessels in the occluded area
3. Loss of lung parenchyma
4. Loss of lung tissue

108. 1. The infarcted area produces alveolar damage that can lead to the production of bloody sputum, sometimes in massive amounts. Clot formation usually occurs in the legs. There's a loss of lung parenchyma and subsequent scar tissue formation.

NP: Implementation; CN: Physiological integrity; CNS: Physiological adaptation; CL: Application

109. A client with a massive pulmonary embolism will have an arterial blood gas analysis performed to determine the extent of hypoxia. The acid-base disorder that may be present is:

1. metabolic acidosis.
2. metabolic alkalosis.
3. respiratory acidosis.
4. respiratory alkalosis.

109. 4. A client with a massive pulmonary embolism will have a large region of lung tissue unavailable for perfusion. This causes the client to hyperventilate and blow off large amounts of carbon dioxide, which crosses the unaffected alveolar-capillary membrane more readily than does oxygen and results in respiratory alkalosis.

NP: Implementation; CN: Physiological integrity; CNS: Physiological adaptation; CL: Application

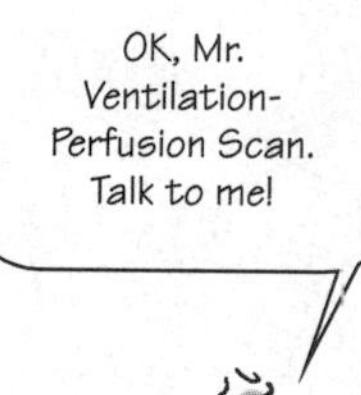

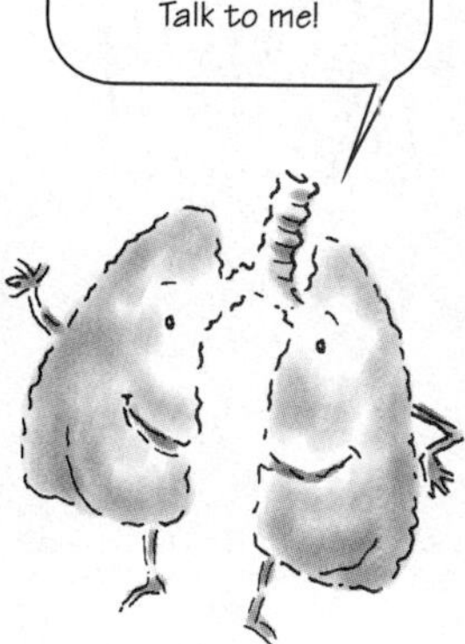

110. A ventilation-perfusion scan is frequently performed to diagnose a pulmonary embolism. This test provides what type of information?

1. Amount of perfusion present in the lung
2. Extent of the occlusion and amount of perfusion lost
3. Location of the pulmonary embolism
4. Location and size of the pulmonary embolism

110. 2. The ventilation-perfusion scan provides information on the extent of occlusion caused by the pulmonary embolism and the amount of lung tissue involved in the area not perfused.

NP: Implementation; CN: Physiological integrity; CNS: Physiological adaptation; CL: Application

111. Which of the following tests can be used to definitively diagnose a pulmonary embolism?

1. Arterial blood gas (ABG) analysis
2. Computed tomography (CT) scan
3. Pulmonary angiogram
4. Ventilation-perfusion scan

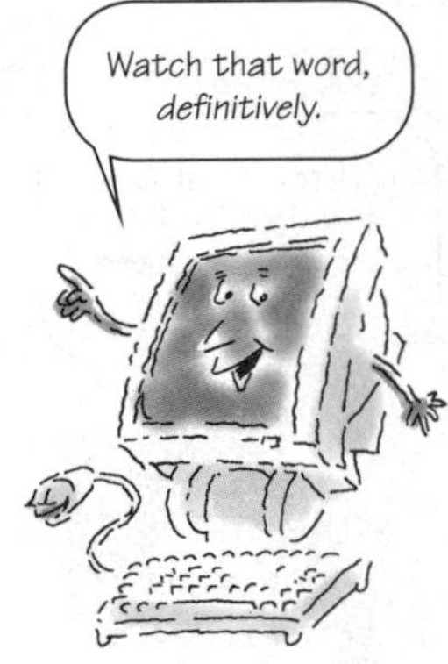

Watch that word, definitively.

111. 3. Pulmonary angiogram is used to definitively diagnose a pulmonary embolism. A catheter is passed through the circulation to the region of the occlusion; the region can be outlined with an injection of contrast medium and viewed by fluoroscopy. This shows the location of the clot, as well as the extent of the perfusion defect. ABG levels can define the amount of hypoxia present. CT scan can show the location of infarcted or ischemic tissue. The ventilation-perfusion scan can report whether there's a ventilation-perfusion mismatch present and define the amount of tissue involved.
NP: Implementation; CN: Physiological integrity; CNS: Physiological adaptation; CL: Application

112. Which of the following medications is prescribed after a pulmonary embolism is diagnosed?

1. Warfarin (Coumadin)
2. Heparin
3. Streptokinase
4. Urokinase

112. 2. Heparin is started I.V. once a pulmonary embolism is diagnosed to reduce further clot formation. When a therapeutic level of heparin is established, warfarin is started. It can take up to 3 days before a therapeutic level of warfarin is achieved. Streptokinase and urokinase are both fibrinolytics, and their usefulness in the management of pulmonary embolism is unclear.
NP: Implementation; CN: Physiological integrity; CNS: Physiological adaptation; CL: Application

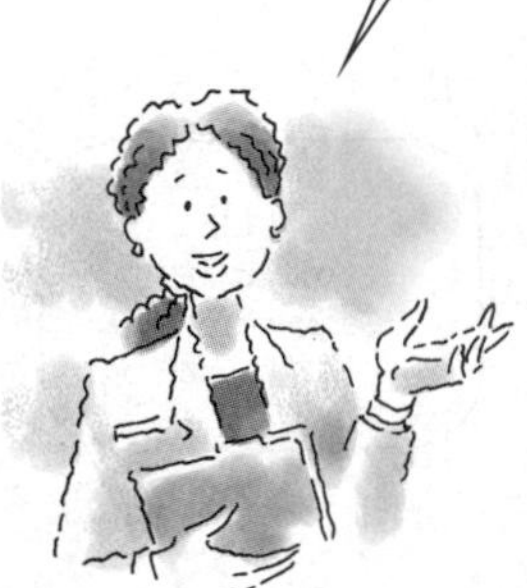

Knowing what a treatment should achieve will help you monitor the response.

113. I.V. heparin is given to clients with pulmonary embolism for which of the following reasons?

1. To dissolve the clot
2. To break up the pulmonary embolism
3. To slow the development of other clots
4. To prevent clots from breaking off and embolizing to the lung

113. 3. Heparin doesn't break up pulmonary embolisms or dissolve clots already formed, but it slows the development of other clots. Heparin doesn't stop clots from going to the lung.
NP: Implementation; CN: Physiological integrity; CNS: Physiological adaptation; CL: Application

114. A client with a pulmonary embolism is discharged but will remain on warfarin (Coumadin) therapy for up to 6 months to:

1. prevent further embolism formation.
2. minimize the growth of new or existing thrombi.
3. continue to reduce the size of the pulmonary embolism.
4. break up the existing pulmonary embolism until it's totally gone.

114. 2. Warfarin minimizes the growth of new or existing thrombi. It's impossible to tell whether a client who developed a thrombus that became a pulmonary embolism will develop more thrombi. Therefore, current therapy is to treat clients who had a pulmonary embolism with warfarin for up to 6 months, as long as it isn't contraindicated. Warfarin doesn't reduce the size of existing pulmonary emboli or break them up.
NP: Implementation; CN: Physiological integrity; CNS: Physiological adaptation; CL: Application

115. The goal of oxygen therapy for a client with a pulmonary embolism is to obtain which of the following values?

1. $Paco_2$ above 40 mm Hg
2. $Paco_2$ below 40 mm Hg
3. Pao_2 above 60 mm Hg
4. Pao_2 below 60 mm Hg

115. 3. The goal of oxygen therapy for a client with a pulmonary embolism is to have a Pao_2 greater than 60 mm Hg on an Fio_2 of 40% or less. The normal range of the $Paco_2$ is 35 to 45 mm Hg. In the absence of other pathologic states, it should reach normal levels before the Pao_2 does on room air because carbon dioxide crosses the alveolar-capillary membrane with greater ease.
NP: Implementation; CN: Physiological integrity; CNS: Physiological adaptation; CL: Application

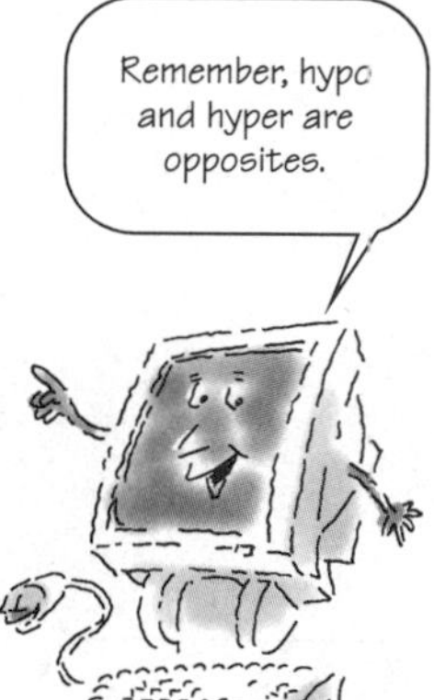

Remember, hypo and hyper are opposites.

116. A client may develop hypotension caused by a pulmonary embolism that produces which of the following results?

1. Pressure on the heart and reduced cardiac output
2. Reduced blood flow to the lung, which causes hypotension
3. Reduced blood return to the right side of the heart leading to lower blood pressure
4. Increased pulmonary vascular resistance and reduced blood delivery to the left side of the heart

116. 4. Blood meets resistance and can't perfuse the pulmonary vasculature because of the embolism. Pulmonary vascular resistance is increased, which reduces the amount of blood returned to the left side of the heart, lowers the cardiac output of the heart, and reduces blood pressure, sometimes significantly.
NP: Implementation; CN: Physiological integrity; CNS: Physiological adaptation; CL: Application

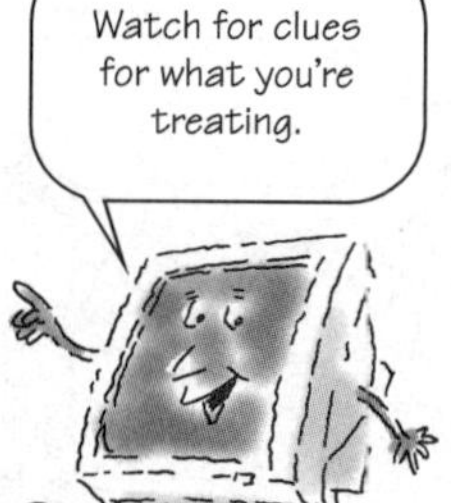

Watch for clues for what you're treating.

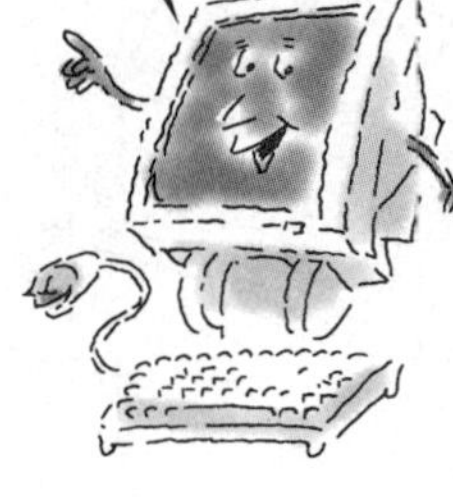

117. A client with a pulmonary embolism typically has chest pain and apprehension, which can be treated by which of the following methods?

1. Administering analgesics
2. Using guided imagery
3. Positioning the client on his left side
4. Providing emotional support

117. 1. Once the pulmonary embolism has been diagnosed and the amount of hypoxia determined, apprehension can be treated with analgesics as long as respiratory status isn't compromised by analgesics. Using guided imagery and providing emotional support can be used as alternatives. Positioning the client on his left side when a pulmonary embolism is suspected may prevent a clot that has extended through the capillaries and into the pulmonary veins from breaking off and traveling through the heart into the arterial circulation, leading to a massive stroke.
NP: Implementation; CN: Physiological integrity; CNS: Physiological adaptation; CL: Application

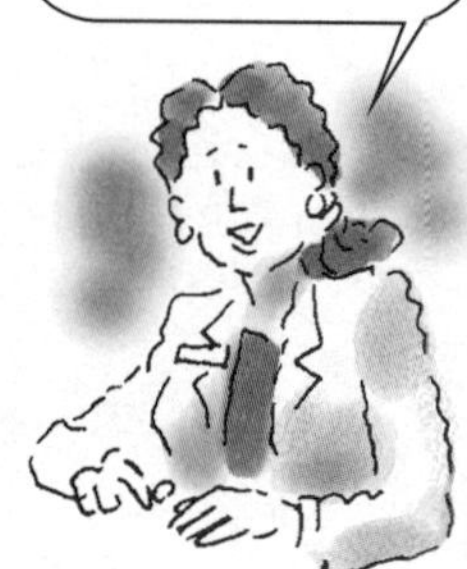

Always know the whys of a condition, especially the most common ones, like this one.

118. A client with a pulmonary embolism may have an umbrella filter placed in the vena cava for which of the following reasons?

1. The filter prevents further clot formation.
2. The filter collects clots so they don't go to the lung.
3. The filter breaks up clots into insignificantly small pieces.
4. The filter contains anticoagulants that are slowly released, dissolving any clots.

118. 3. The umbrella filter is placed in a client at high risk for the formation of more clots that could potentially become pulmonary emboli. The filter breaks the clots into small pieces that won't significantly occlude the pulmonary vasculature. The filter doesn't prevent further clot formation and doesn't release anticoagulants. The filter doesn't collect the clots, because if it did, it would have to be emptied periodically, causing the client to require surgery in the future.
NP: Implementation; CN: Physiological integrity; CNS: Physiological adaptation; CL: Application

119. A client with a pulmonary embolism may need an embolectomy, which involves which of the following actions?

1. Removing an embolism in the lower extremity
2. Sucking the embolism out of the lung by bronchoscopy
3. Surgically removing the embolism source in the pelvis
4. Surgically removing the embolism in the pulmonary vasculature

119. 4. If the pulmonary embolism is large and doesn't respond to treatment, surgical removal may be necessary to restore perfusion to the area of the lung. This is rarely done because of the associated high mortality risk. It's impossible to remove a pulmonary embolism through bronchoscopy because the defect isn't in the bronchial tree. A thrombectomy can be performed at other sources of clot, but when a pulmonary embolism has already occurred, it would have little effect on oxygenation.

NP: Implementation; CN: Physiological integrity; CNS: Physiological adaptation; CL: Application

120. Nursing management of a client with a pulmonary embolism focuses on which of the following actions?

1. Assessing oxygenation status
2. Monitoring the oxygen delivery device
3. Monitoring for other sources of clots
4. Determining whether the client requires another ventilation-perfusion scan

120. 1. Nursing management of a client with a pulmonary embolism focuses on assessing oxygenation status and ensuring that treatment is adequate. If the client's status begins to deteriorate, it's the nurse's responsibility to contact the physician and attempt to improve oxygenation. Ensuring that the oxygen delivery device is working properly and monitoring for other clot sources are other nursing responsibilities, but they aren't the focus of care.

NP: Implementation; CN: Physiological integrity; CNS: Physiological adaptation; CL: Application

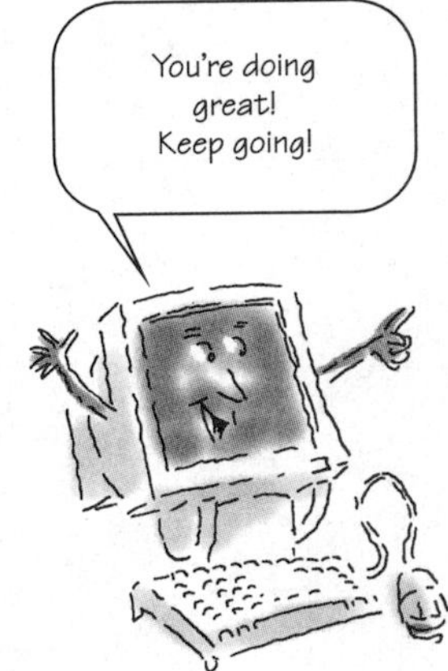
You're doing great!
Keep going!

121. A pulse oximeter gives what type of information about the client?

1. Amount of carbon dioxide in the blood
2. Amount of oxygen in the blood
3. Percentage of hemoglobin carrying oxygen
4. Respiratory rate

121. 3. The pulse oximeter determines the percentage of hemoglobin carrying oxygen. This doesn't ensure that the oxygen being carried through the bloodstream is actually being taken up by the tissue. The pulse oximeter doesn't provide information about the amount of carbon dioxide or oxygen in the blood or the client's respiratory rate.

NP: Implementation; CN: Physiological integrity; CNS: Physiological adaptation; CL: Application

122. What effect does hemoglobin amount have on oxygenation status?

1. No effect
2. More hemoglobin reduces the client's respiratory rate
3. Low hemoglobin levels cause reduced oxygen-carrying capacity
4. Low hemoglobin levels cause increased oxygen-carrying capacity

122. 3. Hemoglobin carries oxygen to all tissues in the body. If the hemoglobin level is low, the amount of oxygen-carrying capacity is also low. More hemoglobin will increase oxygen-carrying capacity and thus increase the total amount of oxygen available in the blood. If the client has been tachypneic during exertion, or even at rest, because oxygen demand is higher than the available oxygen content, then an increase in hemoglobin may decrease the respiratory rate to normal levels.

NP: Implementation; CN: Physiological integrity; CNS: Physiological adaptation; CL: Application

123. How does positive end-expiratory pressure (PEEP) improve oxygenation?

1. It provides more oxygen to the client.
2. It opens up bronchioles and allows oxygen to get in the lungs.
3. It opens up collapsed alveoli and helps keep them open.
4. It adds pressure to the lung tissue, which improves gaseous exchange.

123. 3. PEEP delivers positive pressure to the lung at the end of expiration. This helps open collapsed alveoli and helps them stay open so gas exchange can occur in these newly opened alveoli, improving oxygenation. The bronchioles don't participate in gas exchange except to act as a conduit for inspired and expired air. The walls are rigid enough they generally don't collapse. PEEP doesn't directly add pressure to the lung tissue or provide more oxygen to the client.

NP: Implementation; CN: Physiological integrity; CNS: Physiological adaptation; CL: Application

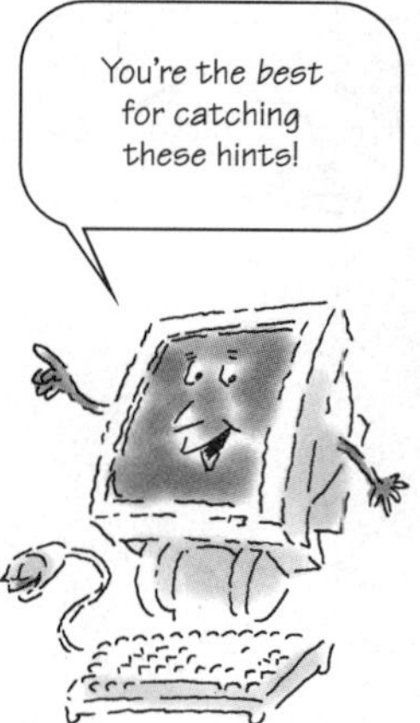

You're the best for catching these hints!

124. Which of the following statements best explains how opening up collapsed alveoli improves oxygenation?

1. Alveoli need oxygen to live.
2. Alveoli have no effect on oxygenation.
3. Collapsed alveoli increase oxygen demand.
4. Gaseous exchange occurs in the alveolar membrane.

124. 4. Gaseous exchange occurs in the alveolar membrane, so if the alveoli collapse, no exchange occurs. Collapsed alveoli receive oxygen, as well as other nutrients, from the bloodstream. Collapsed alveoli have no effect on oxygen demand, though by decreasing the surface area available for gas exchange, they decrease oxygenation of the blood.

NP: Implementation; CN: Physiological integrity; CNS: Physiological adaptation; CL: Application

125. Continuous positive airway pressure can be provided through an oxygen mask to improve oxygenation in hypoxic clients by which of the following methods?

1. The mask provides 100% oxygen to the client.
2. The mask provides continuous air that the client can breathe.
3. The mask provides pressurized oxygen so the client can breathe more easily.
4. The mask provides pressurized oxygen at the end of expiration to open collapsed alveoli.

125. 3. The mask provides pressurized oxygen continuously through both inspiration and expiration. The mask can be set to deliver any amount of oxygen needed. By providing a client with pressurized oxygen, the client has less resistance to overcome in taking in his next breath, making it easier to breathe. Pressurized oxygen delivered at the end of expiration is positive end-expiratory pressure, not continuous positive airway pressure.

NP: Implementation; CN: Physiological integrity; CNS: Physiological adaptation; CL: Application

126. Bilevel positive airway pressure (BiPAP) is delivered though a special oxygen mask that performs which of the following functions?

1. The mask provides 100% oxygen at both inspiration and expiration.
2. The mask provides pressurized oxygen so the client can breathe more easily.
3. The mask provides pressurized oxygen at the end of expiration to open collapsed alveoli.
4. The mask provides both continuous positive airway pressure (CPAP) and positive end-expiratory pressure (PEEP) to provide optimal oxygenation and ventilation.

126. 4. BiPAP delivers both CPAP and PEEP. It provides the differing pressures throughout the respiratory cycle, attempting to optimize a client's oxygenation and ventilation. It's used in an effort to avoid intubation for mechanical ventilation. Inspiratory and expiratory pressures are set separately to optimize the client's ventilatory status, and the fraction of inspired oxygen is adjusted to optimize oxygenation. The second choice describes only the CPAP component of BiPAP, and the third choice describes the PEEP component.

NP: Implementation; CN: Physiological integrity; CNS: Physiological adaptation; CL: Application

127. Which of the following states best describes pleural effusion?
1. The collapse of alveoli
2. The collapse of a bronchiole
3. The fluid in the alveolar space
4. The accumulation of fluid between the linings of the pleural space

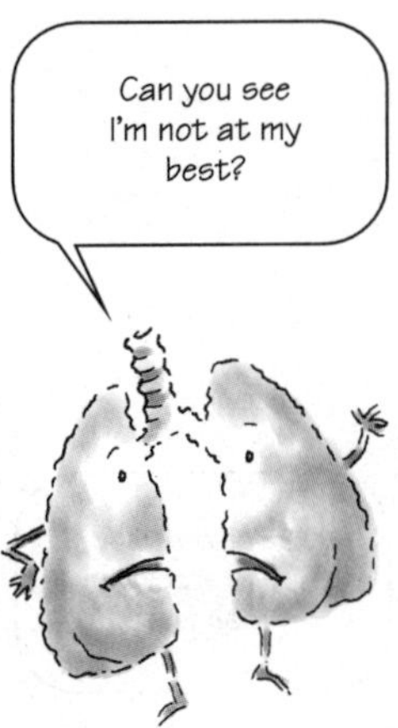

Can you see I'm not at my best?

127. 4. Pleural fluid normally seeps continually into the pleural space from the capillaries lining the parietal pleura and is reabsorbed by the visceral pleural capillaries and lymphatics. Any condition that interferes with either the secretion or drainage of this fluid will lead to a pleural effusion. The collapse of alveoli or a bronchiole has no particular name. Fluid within the alveolar space can be caused by heart failure or adult respiratory distress syndrome.
NP: Implementation; CN: Physiological integrity; CNS: Physiological adaptation; CL: Application

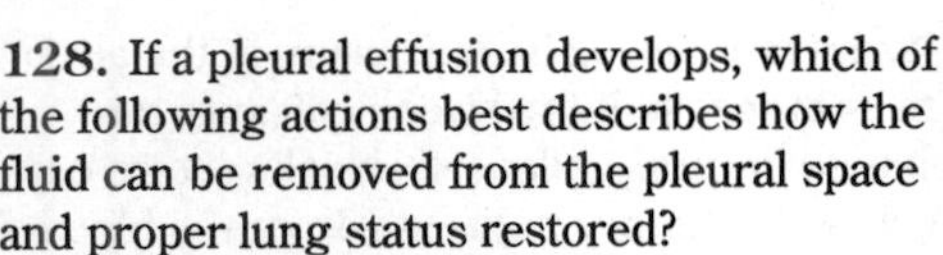

128. If a pleural effusion develops, which of the following actions best describes how the fluid can be removed from the pleural space and proper lung status restored?
1. Inserting a chest tube
2. Performing thoracentesis
3. Performing paracentesis
4. Allowing the pleural effusion to drain by itself

128. 2. Thoracentesis is used to remove excess pleural fluid. The fluid is then analyzed to determine if it's transudative or exudative. Transudates are substances that have passed through a membrane and usually occur in low protein states. Exudates are substances that have escaped from blood vessels. They contain an accumulation of cells and have a high specific gravity and a high lactate dehydrogenase level. Exudates usually occur in response to a malignancy, infection, or inflammatory process. A chest tube is rarely necessary because the amount of fluid typically isn't large enough to warrant such a measure. Paracentesis is the removal of fluid from the abdomen. Pleural effusions can't drain by themselves.
NP: Analysis; CN: Physiological integrity; CNS: Physiological adaptation; CL: Knowledge

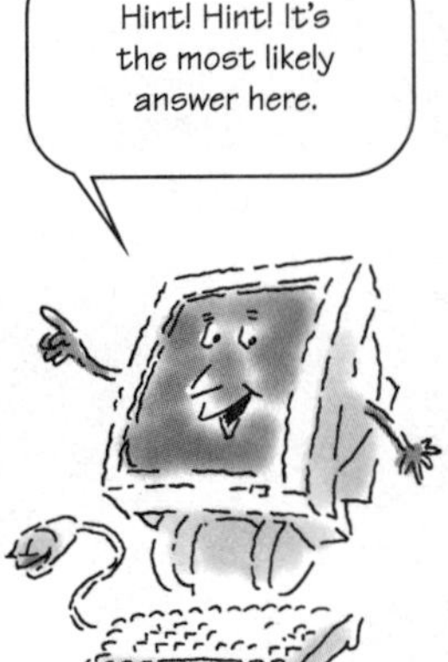

Hint! Hint! It's the most likely answer here.

129. After a motor vehicle accident, an 18-year-old client is admitted with a pneumothorax. The surgeon inserts a chest tube and attaches it to a chest drainage system. Bubbling soon appears in the water seal chamber. Which of the following is the most likely cause of the bubbling?
1. Air leak
2. Adequate suction
3. Inadequate suction
4. Kinked chest tube

129. 1. Bubbling in the water seal chamber of a chest drainage system stems from an air leak. In pneumothorax, an air leak can occur as air is pulled from the pleural space. Bubbling doesn't normally occur with either adequate or inadequate suction. A kinked chest tube can stop the suction and any preexisting bubbling in the water seal chamber.
NP: Assessment; CN: Physiological integrity; CNS: Reduction of risk potential; CL: Application

130. A comatose client needs a nasopharyngeal airway for suctioning. After the airway is inserted, he gags and coughs. Which action should the nurse take?

1. Remove the airway and insert a shorter one.
2. Reposition the airway.
3. Leave the airway in place until the client gets used to it.
4. Remove the airway and attempt suctioning without it.

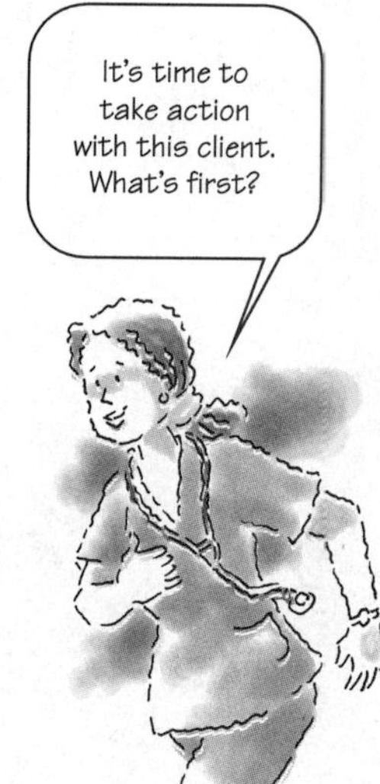

It's time to take action with this client. What's first?

130. 1. If the client gags or coughs after nasopharyngeal airway placement, the tube may be too long. The nurse should remove it and insert a shorter one. Simply repositioning the airway won't solve the problem. The client won't get used to the tube because it's the wrong size. Suctioning without a nasopharyngeal airway causes trauma to the natural airway.

NP: Implementation; CN: Physiological integrity; CNS: Reduction of risk potential; CL: Application

131. An 87-year-old client requires long-term ventilator therapy. He has a tracheostomy in place and requires frequent suctioning. Which of the following techniques is correct?

1. Using intermittent suction while advancing the catheter
2. Using continuous suction while withdrawing the catheter
3. Using intermittent suction while withdrawing the catheter
4. Using continuous suction while advancing the catheter

131. 3. Intermittent suction should be applied during catheter withdrawal. To prevent hypoxia, suctioning shouldn't last more than 10 seconds at a time. Suction shouldn't be applied while the catheter is being advanced.

NP: Implementation; CN: Physiological integrity; CNS: Reduction of risk potential; CL: Application

132. A client's arterial blood gas (ABG) analysis reveals a pH of 7.18, $Paco_2$ of 73 mm Hg, Pao_2 of 77 mm Hg, and HCO_3^- of 24 mEq/L. What do these values indicate?

1. Metabolic acidosis
2. Respiratory alkalosis
3. Metabolic alkalosis
4. Respiratory acidosis

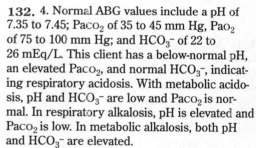

132. 4. Normal ABG values include a pH of 7.35 to 7.45; $Paco_2$ of 35 to 45 mm Hg, Pao_2 of 75 to 100 mm Hg; and HCO_3^- of 22 to 26 mEq/L. This client has a below-normal pH, an elevated $Paco_2$, and normal HCO_3^-, indicating respiratory acidosis. With metabolic acidosis, pH and HCO_3^- are low and $Paco_2$ is normal. In respiratory alkalosis, pH is elevated and $Paco_2$ is low. In metabolic alkalosis, both pH and HCO_3^- are elevated.

NP: Assessment; CN: Physiological integrity; CNS: Physiological adaptation; CL: Analysis

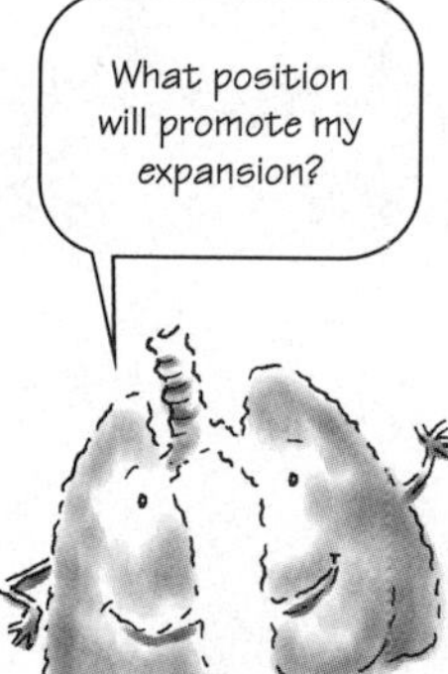

What position will promote my expansion?

133. A 67-year-old client is in distress after being admitted with an exacerbation of chronic obstructive pulmonary disease. In which position should the nurse put the client to promote optimal lung expansion?

1. Prone
2. Semi-Fowler's
3. Reverse Trendelenburg's
4. Supine

133. 2. Semi-Fowler's position (with the head of the bed elevated 30 degrees) promotes optimal lung expansion. A prone position (lying on the abdomen) improves oxygenation in a client with adult respiratory distress syndrome who is receiving mechanical ventilation. Reverse Trendelenburg's position (in which the entire bed is raised to a 45-degree angle) may improve lung expansion but is less effective than semi-Fowler's position. Supine positioning (lying flat on the back) doesn't aid lung expansion.

NP: Implementation; CN: Physiological integrity; CNS: Reduction of risk potential; CL: Application

134. A nursing home client is transferred to the hospital with dehydration and pneumonia. After receiving the client from the emergency department, the nurse notices that his I.V. infusion has infiltrated. Which of the following is the best initial response by the nurse?

1. Stop the infusion, remove the I.V. catheter, and restart the infusion in another site.
2. Remove the I.V. catheter and apply a cool compress to the site.
3. Apply moist heat to the site.
4. Gently massage the site.

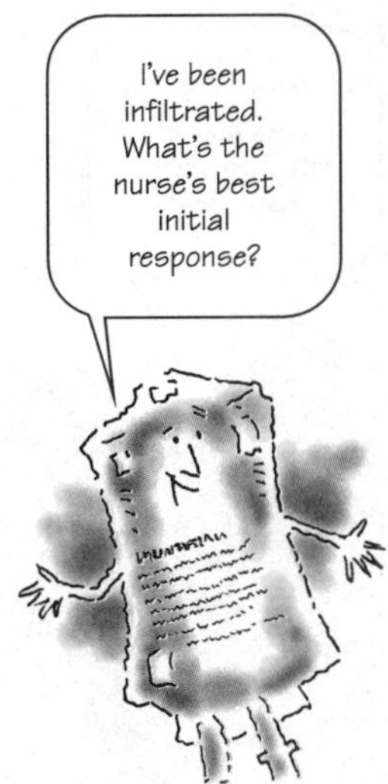

I've been infiltrated. What's the nurse's best initial response?

134. 1. Immediately after discovering an I.V. infiltration, the nurse should stop the infusion, remove the I.V. catheter, restart the infusion in another site, and apply a warm compress to the infiltrated site. A cool compress doesn't promote fluid absorption. Moist heat shouldn't be applied until the infusion is stopped, the catheter is removed, and another catheter is inserted at a different site. Massaging the site is likely to cause pain and isn't effective in treating an infiltration.

NP: Implementation; CN: Physiological integrity; CNS: Pharmacological and parenteral therapies; CL: Application

135. A police officer brings a 45-year-old homeless client to the emergency department. A chest X-ray suggests he has tuberculosis. The physician orders an intradermal injection of 5 tuberculin units/0.1 ml of tuberculin purified protein derivative. Which needle is appropriate for this injection?

1. ⅝″ to ½″ 25G to 27G needle
2. 1″ to 3″ 20G to 25G needle
3. ½″ to ⅜″ 26G or 27G needle
4. 1″ 20G needle

135. 3. Intradermal injections like those used in tuberculin skin tests are administered in small volumes (usually 0.5 ml or less) into the outer skin layers to produce a local effect. A tuberculin syringe with a ½″ to ⅜″ 26G or 27G needle should be inserted about ⅛″ below the epidermis. A ⅝″ to ½″ 25G to 27G needle is appropriate for a subcutaneous injection; a 1″ to 3″ 20G to 25G needle, for an I.M. injection; and a 1″ 20G needle, for an I.V. bolus injection.

NP: Implementation; CN: Physiological integrity; CNS: Pharmacological and parenteral therapies; CL: Application

136. After a right lower lobectomy for lung cancer, a client returns to her room with a chest tube in place. The nurse formulates a care plan with a primary nursing diagnosis of *Impaired gas exchange related to lung surgery.* Which expected outcome is appropriate for this diagnosis?

1. The client will sit upright, leaning slightly forward.
2. The client will request pain medication as needed.
3. The client will maintain a pulse oximetry level above 93%.
4. The client will be pain-free.

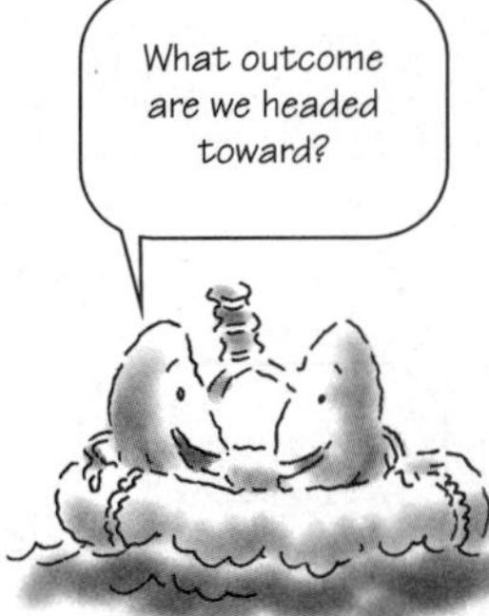

What outcome are we headed toward?

136. 3. A pulse oximetry level above 93% and a normal respiratory rate demonstrate probable lung expansion and normal chest tube functioning. Sitting upright and leaning slightly forward suggests that the client has impaired gas exchange because this position increases lung expansion. Requesting pain medication as needed and remaining pain-free are expected outcomes associated with a nursing diagnosis of *Acute pain.*

NP: Evaluation; CN: Physiological integrity; CNS: Physiological adaptation; CL: Analysis

137. An unrestrained passenger is thrown 20′ (6.1 m) from a car. On admission to the emergency department, he has a heart rate of 130 beats/minute, shallow respirations at a rate of 32 breaths/minute, and a blood pressure of 90/60 mm Hg. His skin is pale and cool, and capillary refill is delayed. Breath sounds are diminished on the right side and paradoxical chest wall movement appears on the right side. Arterial blood gas analysis shows increased pH and decreased $Paco_2$ and Pao_2 levels. A chest X-ray reveals a right pneumothorax with multiple rib fractures (4th to 7th right ribs). Which of the following diagnoses is the most probable?

1. Tension pneumothorax
2. Flail chest
3. Ruptured diaphragm
4. Massive hemothorax

138. A healthy client comes to the clinic for a routine examination. When auscultating his lower lung lobes, the nurse should expect to hear which type of breath sound?

1. Bronchial
2. Tracheal
3. Vesicular
4. Bronchovesicular

139. A 76-year-old client is admitted for elective knee surgery. Physical examination reveals shallow respirations but no signs of respiratory distress. Which of the following is a normal physiologic change related to aging?

1. Increased elastic recoil of the lungs
2. Increased number of functional capillaries in the alveoli
3. Decreased residual volume
4. Decreased vital capacity

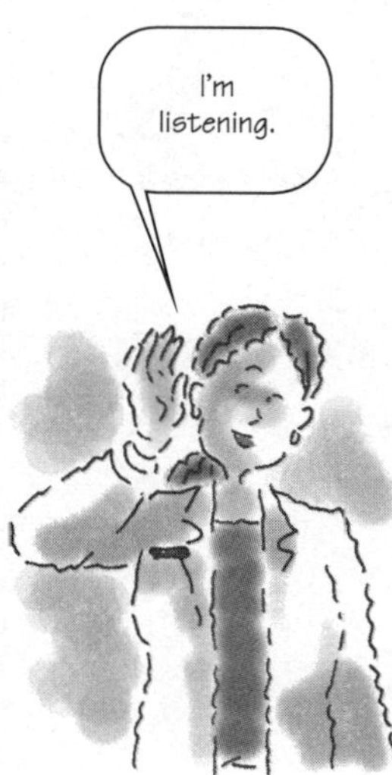

137. 2. Multiple rib fractures and paradoxical chest wall movement confirm a diagnosis of flail chest. Tension pneumothorax causes severe respiratory distress, hypotension, diminished breath sounds over the affected area, hyperresonance, distended neck veins, eventual tracheal shift and, possibly, paradoxical chest movement on the injured side. A ruptured diaphragm leads to hyperresonance on percussion, hypotension, dyspnea, dysphagia, and shifting of heart and bowel sounds in the lower to middle chest. A massive hemothorax produces signs of shock (such as tachycardia and hypotension), dullness on percussion on the injured side, decreased breath sounds on the injured side, respiratory distress and, possibly, mediastinal shift.

NP: Assessment; CN: Physiological integrity; CNS: Physiological adaptation; CL: Analysis

138. 3. Vesicular breath sounds are soft, low-pitched sounds normally heard over the lower lobes of the lung. They're prolonged on inhalation and shortened on exhalation. Bronchial breath sounds are loud, high-pitched sounds normally heard next to the trachea; discontinuous, they're loudest during exhalation. Tracheal breath sounds are harsh, discontinuous sounds heard over the trachea during inhalation or exhalation. Bronchovesicular breath sounds are medium-pitched, continuous sounds that occur during inhalation or exhalation and are best heard over the upper third of the sternum and between the scapulae.

NP: Assessment; CN: Health promotion and maintenance; CNS: Prevention and early detection of disease; CL: Application

139. 4. Reduction in vital capacity is a normal physiologic change in the older adult. Other normal physiologic changes include decreased elastic recoil of the lungs, fewer functional capillaries in the alveoli, and an increase in residual volume.

NP: Assessment; CN: Health promotion and maintenance; CNS: Growth and development through the life span; CL: Application

140. A 79-year-old client is admitted with pneumonia. Which nursing diagnosis should take priority?

1. Acute pain related to lung expansion secondary to lung infection
2. Risk for imbalanced fluid volume related to increased insensible fluid losses secondary to fever
3. Anxiety related to dyspnea and chest pain
4. Ineffective airway clearance related to retained secretions

140. 4. Pneumonia is an acute infection of the lung parenchyma. The inflammatory reaction may cause an outpouring of exudate into the alveolar spaces, leading to ineffective airway clearance related to retained secretions. Pneumonia also can cause acute pain related to lung expansion and anxiety related to dyspnea and chest pain. However, these diagnoses take lower priority than ineffective airway clearance. Fever associated with pneumonia places the client at risk for imbalanced fluid volume—but this diagnosis also doesn't take priority.

NP: Analysis; CN: Physiological integrity; CNS: Physiological adaptation; CL: Analysis

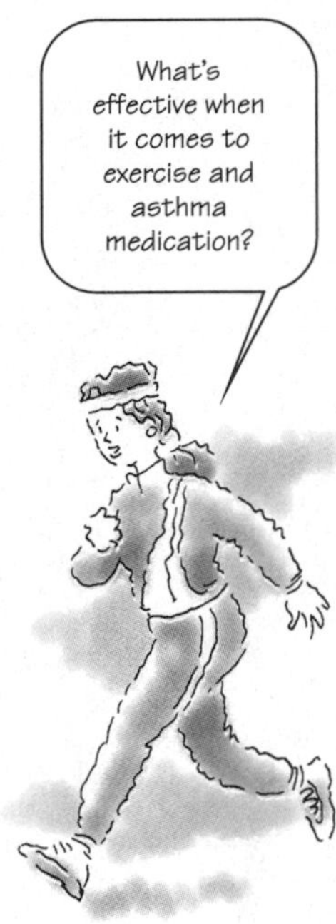

What's effective when it comes to exercise and asthma medication?

141. An asthmatic client is being discharged on a new asthma medication. Teaching about cromolyn (Intal inhaler) is effective when the client makes which statement?

1. "I should use my inhaler no more than 1 hour before I exercise."
2. "I should use my inhaler whenever I feel an asthma attack coming on."
3. "I should stop taking steroids if I need a dose of my inhaler."
4. "I should avoid gargling and rinsing my mouth after using my inhaler."

141. 1. The client should verbalize the need to use the inhaler no more than 1 hour before exercise when indicated for exercise-induced asthma. Cromolyn is contraindicated during an acute asthma attack. A client who is taking steroids should continue to take them during cromolyn therapy, if appropriate. Gargling and rinsing the mouth after cromolyn administration can reduce mouth dryness.

NP: Evaluation; CN: Health promotion and maintenance; CNS: Prevention and early detection of disease; CL: Analysis

142. Sputum analysis is ordered when a client with pneumonia expectorates green sputum. Which guideline should the nurse include in the teaching plan?

1. Fluids will be restricted the night before the test.
2. The client will be asked to take several deep abdominal breaths and then to take one more breath, bend forward, and cough into the provided sterile container.
3. If bronchoscopy is required for specimen collection, the client will have no oral intake for 12 hours before the procedure.
4. After bronchoscopy, the client will receive a drink of water.

142. 2. If the specimen will be collected by expectoration, the client should be instructed to take several deep abdominal breaths; when he's ready to cough, he should take one more deep abdominal breath, bend forward, and cough into the provided sterile container. He should be instructed to drink plenty of fluids the night before the test. If the specimen will be collected during bronchoscopy, the client should fast for 6 hours before the procedure. After bronchoscopy, he's observed for possible complications. He can have liquids when his gag reflex returns.

NP: Planning; CN: Physiological integrity; CNS: Reduction of risk potential; CL: Application

143. A 57-year-old client is admitted with acute bronchitis. During the admission interview, he tells the nurse he's allergic to bananas. Based on this statement, he may also have an allergy to which of the following?

1. Iodine-containing drugs
2. Cephalosporins
3. Penicillins
4. Latex

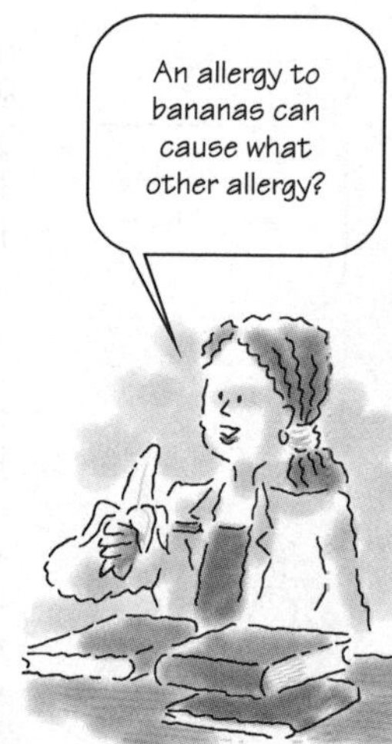

An allergy to bananas can cause what other allergy?

143. 4. Clients who are allergic to certain cross-reactive foods—including apricots, avocados, bananas, cherries, chestnuts, grapes, kiwis, passion fruit, peaches, and tomatoes—may also be allergic to latex. When exposed to latex, they may have an allergic response similar to the one these foods produce. Clients with allergies to shellfish may be allergic to iodine-containing drugs. Hypersensitivity reactions to cephalosporins are more common in clients with penicillin allergy. There's no link between food allergies and penicillin.

NP: Assessment; CN: Safe, effective care environment; CNS: Safety and infection control; CL: Application

144. The care plan for a 42-year-old client with deep vein thrombosis (DVT) includes monitoring the client for complications. Which of the following pulmonary complications is the client most at risk for developing?

1. Pulmonary embolism
2. Pneumothorax
3. Pulmonary edema
4. Pneumonia

144. 1. The most common etiology of pulmonary embolism is thromboembolism from a distant site, particularly from deep veins of the legs and pelvis (90% to 95%). Moreover, the immobilization used to treat DVT is an additional clinical risk factor for pulmonary embolism. Although immobility also places the client at risk for pneumonia, the risk isn't as great for this client. Pneumothorax and pulmonary edema aren't complications of DVT.

NP: Assessment; CN: Physiological integrity; CNS: Reduction of risk potential; CL: Application

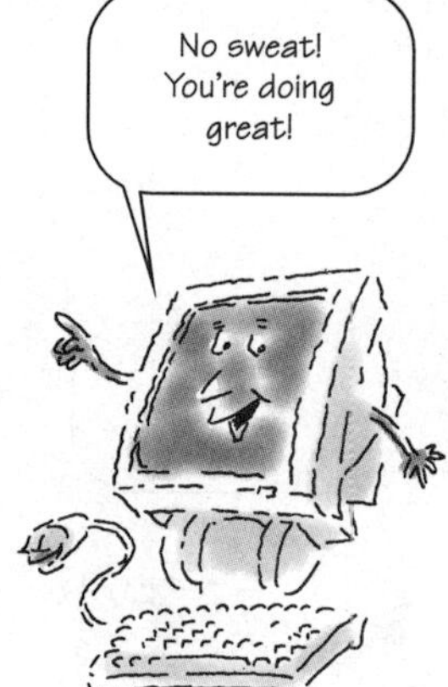

No sweat! You're doing great!

145. A 20-year-old client with cystic fibrosis is being discharged with a high-frequency chest wall oscillating vest. Which statement by the client indicates that she understands how to use the vest?

1. "I'll wear the vest for 5 minutes each time a treatment is due."
2. "I'll lie down to use the vest."
3. "I'll require help in applying the vest."
4. "I can be in any position to use the vest."

145. 4. The vest system doesn't require special positioning or breathing to be effective. In most cases, treatments last 15 to 20 minutes and clients can manage therapy without any assistance.

NP: Evaluation; CN: Physiological integrity; CNS: Basic care and comfort; CL: Analysis

146. To obtain an arterial blood sample from a client's radial artery, which of the following should the nurse do first?

1. Perform Allen's test.
2. Place a rolled towel under the client's wrist.
3. Clean the puncture site with an alcohol or povidone-iodine pad.
4. Palpate the artery with the index and middle fingers of one hand.

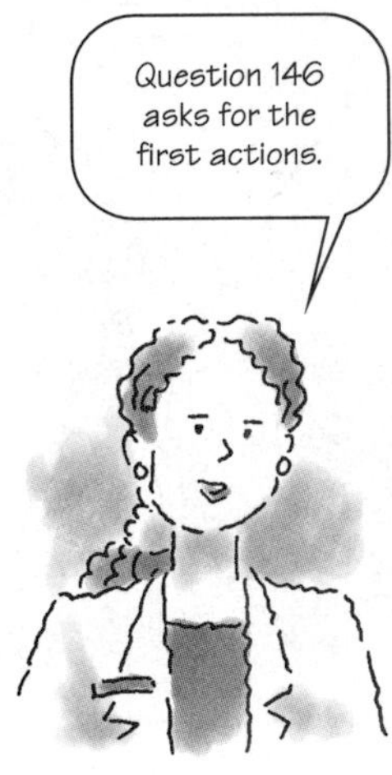
Question 146
asks for the
first actions.

146. 1. First perform Allen's test to assess circulation. Next, wash your hands, put on gloves, and place a rolled towel under the client's wrist for support. Then locate the artery and palpate it for a strong pulse. Next, clean the puncture site with an alcohol or povidone-iodine pad. Then palpate the artery with the index and middle fingers of one hand while holding the syringe over the puncture site with the other hand. Holding the needle bevel at a 30- to 45-degree angle, puncture the skin and arterial wall in one smooth motion, watch for blood backflow in the syringe, and fill it to the 5-ml mark. After collecting the sample, press a gauze pad over the puncture site for at least 5 minutes.

NP: Implementation; CN: Physiological integrity; CNS: Reduction of risk potential; CL: Application

147. After receiving radiation treatment for lung cancer, a client complains that he has lost his appetite. The nurse should provide which instruction?

1. "Drink plenty of fluids."
2. "Eat hot meats with spices to improve the taste."
3. "Limit activities immediately before and after meals."
4. "Consume food high in calories."

147. 4. The client should consume high-calorie foods whenever he can eat, to help compensate for the times when he can't eat. Consuming large amounts of fluids creates a feeling of fullness, which can limit food intake. Hot meats tend to cause taste aversions during radiation therapy. Activity increases the appetite

NP: Implementation; CN: Physiological integrity; CNS: Reduction of risk potential; CL: Application

148. Three days after an abdominal aortic aneurysm repair, a client develops a pulmonary embolus. Which nursing diagnosis takes priority?

1. Ineffective tissue perfusion (cardiopulmonary)
2. Impaired physical mobility
3. Ineffective airway clearance
4. Risk for aspiration

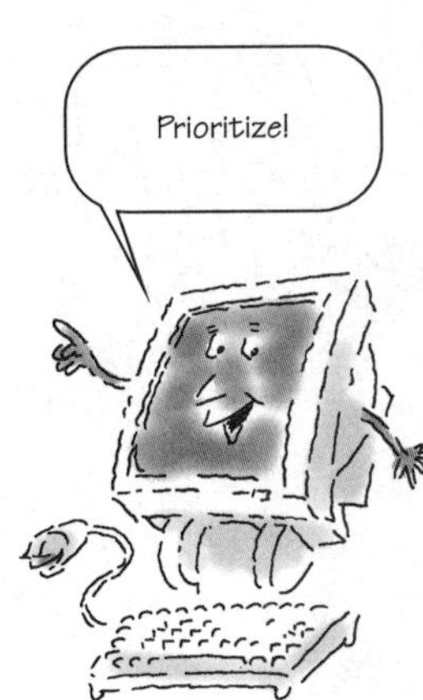
Prioritize!

148. 1. Pulmonary embolus occurs when a thrombus lodges in a branch of the pulmonary artery, partially or totally occluding it. The lung is adequately ventilated but can't be perfused, resulting in impaired cardiopulmonary tissue perfusion. Although impaired physical mobility is an appropriate nursing diagnosis for this client, it doesn't take priority over ineffective tissue perfusion (cardiopulmonary). A pulmonary embolus doesn't increase secretions, so ineffective airway clearance isn't an appropriate diagnosis. It also doesn't place the client at risk for aspiration.

NP: Analysis; CN: Physiological integrity; CNS: Physiological adaptation; CL: Analysis

149. After experiencing an anxiety attack, a client comes to the emergency department complaining of dizziness and light-headedness. Arterial blood gas (ABG) analysis reveals a pH of 7.62, $Paco_2$ of 22 mm Hg, Pao_2 of 96 mm Hg, and HCO_3^- of 24 mEq/L. Which of the following actions should the nurse take?

1. Do nothing; these ABG values are normal.
2. Encourage the client to breathe into a paper bag.
3. Notify the physician and prepare to give sodium bicarbonate.
4. Notify the physician and prepare to give supplemental oxygen.

149. 2. These ABG values reveal respiratory alkalosis (elevated pH, decreased $Paco_2$, and normal Pao_2 and HCO_3^- levels), so the client is most likely hyperventilating from anxiety. Breathing into a paper bag can stop the hyperventilation by increasing carbon dioxide. Doing nothing or giving sodium bicarbonate could worsen respiratory alkalosis. The client has a normal Pao_2 level and doesn't need supplemental oxygen.

NP: Implementation; CN: Physiological integrity; CNS: Reduction of risk potential; CL: Analysis

150. After the nurse teaches a group of police officers about the spread of tuberculosis (TB), which of the following statements by an officer indicates that teaching has been effective?

1. "I could get TB by being in close proximity for a brief time with someone who has the disease."
2. "I could get TB if I inhale infected droplets when an infected individual coughs."
3. "I could get TB if I search the home of someone infected with TB."
4. "I could get TB if I come in contact with blood from an infected person."

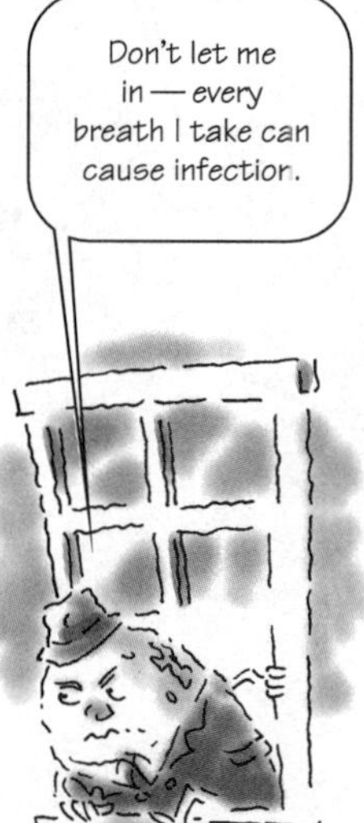

Don't let me in — every breath I take can cause infection.

150. 2. TB isn't a highly contagious disease. Infection typically occurs from inhaling infected droplets after a person with TB coughs. Transmission usually requires close, frequent, prolonged contact. Human immunodeficiency virus — not TB — is spread through contact with an infected person's blood.

NP: Evaluation; CN: Safe, effective care environment; CNS: Safety and infection control; CL: Analysis

151. A client receives midazolam (Versed), 2 mg I.V., as sedation before bronchoscopy. Five minutes after he receives the drug, his respiratory rate drops to 4 breaths/minute. Which of the following agents should the nurse administer to reverse the effects of midazolam?

1. Naloxone (Narcan)
2. Protamine sulfate
3. Phentolamine (Regitine)
4. Flumazenil (Romazicon)

151. 4. Flumazenil reverses the effects of benzodiazepines such as midazolam. Naloxone is used to reverse opioids, such as morphine. Protamine sulfate reverses the effects of heparin. Phentolamine is injected into the tissues to reverse the damaging effects of a dopamine (Intropin) infiltration.

NP: Implementation; CN: Physiological integrity; CNS: Pharmacological and parenteral therapies; CL: Application

152. The physician places an order in the computer for the nurse to change the client's chest drainage system from suction to gravity drainage. How should the nurse proceed?

1. Detach the tubing from the suction port to provide a vent.
2. Clamp the client drainage tube.
3. Question the physician's order.
4. Turn off the suction source and leave the tubing connected.

152. 1. When the suction source is turned off, the drainage system should be opened to the atmosphere so intrapleural air can escape from the system. Detaching the tubing from the suction port provides an exit vent for the air and, thus, reduces the risk of tension pneumothorax. Clamping the tube may cause air to accumulate in the pleural space, rapidly leading to tension pneumothorax. There's no need to question the order.

NP: Implementation; CN: Physiological integrity; CNS: Physiological adaptation; CL: Application

153. A client with cancer develops pleural effusion. During chest auscultation, which of the following breath sounds should the nurse expect to hear?

1. Crackles
2. Rhonchi
3. Diminished breath sounds
4. Wheezes

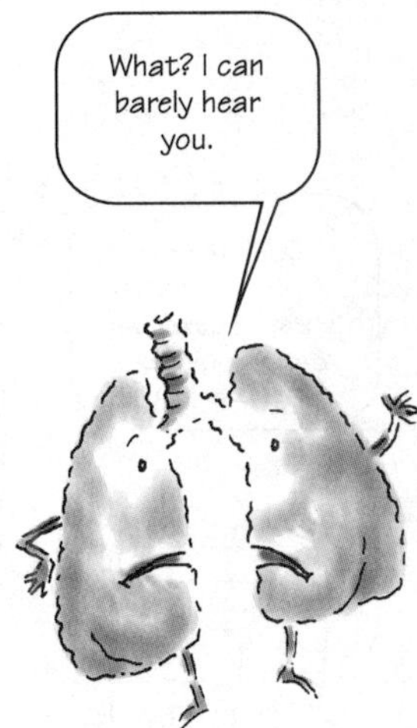
What? I can barely hear you.

153. 3. In pleural effusion, fluid accumulates in the pleural space, impairing transmission of normal breath sounds. Because of the acoustic mismatch, breath sounds are diminished. Crackles (short explosive or popping sounds) commonly accompany atelectasis, interstitial fibrosis, and left-sided heart failure. Rhonchi (low-pitched sounds with a snoring quality) suggest secretions in the large airways. Wheezes (high-pitched, hissing sounds) result from narrowed airways, as in asthma, chronic obstructive pulmonary disease, or bronchitis.

NP: Assessment; CN: Physiological integrity; CNS: Physiological adaptation; CL: Application

154. All health care workers must undergo annual tuberculosis testing. The employee-health nurse who performs annual purified protein derivative (PPD) testing instructs the staff that their results must be read within how many hours after administration?

1. 6 to 12 hours
2. 12 to 24 hours
3. 24 to 48 hours
4. 48 to 72 hours

154. 4. To ensure accurate results, a PPD test must be read 48 to 72 hours after administration.

NP: Planning; CN: Safe, effective care environment; CNS: Safety and infection control; CL: Application

155. A 79-year-old client suddenly develops pulmonary edema. The physician prescribes furosemide (Lasix), 40 mg I.V., and use of a nonrebreather mask. Which oxygen concentrations does this mask deliver?

1. 60% to 80%
2. 80% to 100%
3. 36%
4. 44%

155. 2. The nonrebreather mask delivers oxygen concentrations of 80% to 100%. It's reserved for emergency situations. A partial rebreather mask delivers concentrations of 60% to 80%. A nasal cannula delivers oxygen at flow rates of 1 to 6 L/minute. A flow rate of 4 L/minute delivers an oxygen concentration of 36%; a rate of 6 L/minute delivers an oxygen concentration of 44%.

NP: Implementation; CN: Physiological integrity; CNS: Physiological adaptation; CL: Application

156. A nurse passes by a neighbor's swimming pool and notices an adult at the bottom of the pool. She immediately calls for help and tries to rescue the person. When she reaches him, he's unresponsive and breathless. How should the nurse proceed?

1. By opening the airway and beginning rescue breathing immediately
2. By immobilizing the cervical spine
3. By starting chest compressions
4. By performing abdominal thrust

156. 1. The nurse should open the airway and begin rescue breathing immediately—while still in the water, if possible. Immobilizing the cervical spine won't provide the needed oxygenation. Chest compressions should be delivered only if circulation is absent. Performing abdominal thrust in an attempt to remove water from the lungs would delay the start of rescue breathing.

NP: Implementation; CN: Physiological integrity; CNS: Physiological adaptation; CL: Application

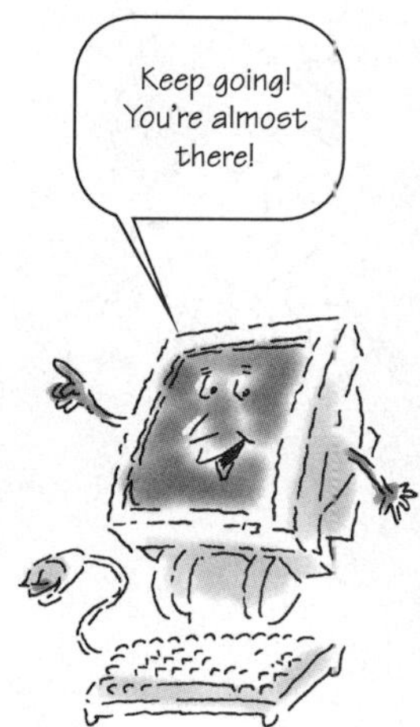
Keep going! You're almost there!

157. A client with newly diagnosed chronic obstructive pulmonary disease (COPD) presents to the clinic for a routine examination. The nurse teaches him strategies for preventing airway irritation and infection. Which statement by the client indicates that teaching was successful?

1. "I should avoid enclosed, crowded areas during the summer."
2. "I'm glad I only need to get the flu vaccine."
3. "I should use products with aerosol sprays."
4. "I should avoid using powders."

157. 4. A client with COPD should verbalize the need to avoid exposure to powders, dusts, and smoke from cigarettes, pipes, and cigars. He should stay indoors when the humidity, temperature, and pollen counts are high; avoid enclosed, crowded areas during cold and flu season; and avoid aerosol sprays. He should obtain immunizations against pneumococcal pneumonia as well as influenza.

NP: Evaluation; CN: Health promotion and maintenance; CNS: Prevention and early detection of disease; CL: Analysis

158. A client with lung cancer has developed syndrome of inappropriate antidiuretic hormone (SIADH). Which of the following interventions should the client's care plan include?

1. Increased oral fluid intake
2. Rapid correction of hyponatremia
3. Massive I.V. fluid administration
4. Restriction of fluid intake

158. 4. Restriction of fluid intake to 800 to 1,000 ml daily is essential to maintain normal sodium levels. To avoid the possibility of inducing brain damage, the serum sodium concentration shouldn't be raised too rapidly.

NP: Planning; CN: Physiological integrity; CNS: Reduction of risk potential; CL: Application

159. A 56-year-old client is scheduled for a right pneumonectomy for lung cancer in the morning. When the nurse enters the client's room, she finds him anxiously pacing around the room. Which response by the nurse is most appropriate?

1. "I need to listen to your lungs now."
2. "I'm sure you'll breeze through your surgery tomorrow."
3. "You seem upset, would you like to talk?"
4. "You should try to calm down, you'll upset your family when they come to visit."

160. Theophylline is prescribed for a client with chronic bronchitis. Which substance increases the elimination of theophylline leading to subtherapeutic levels of the drug?

1. Caffeine-containing beverages
2. Oral contraceptives
3. Corticosteroids
4. Marijuana

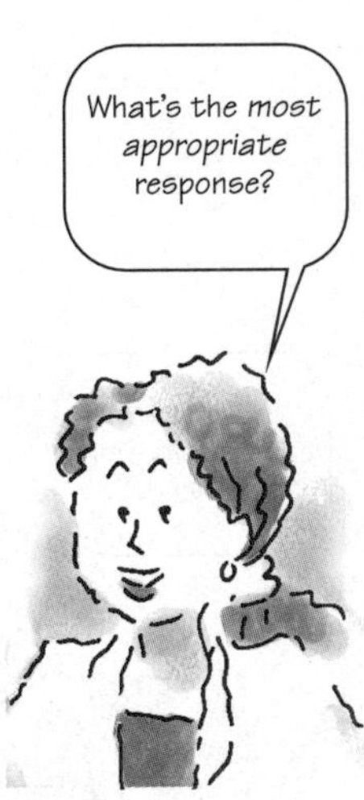

159. 3. The most appropriate response is to acknowledge the client's anxiety and provide an opportunity for the client to verbalize his feelings. Verbalization is therapeutic for the client and listening by the nurse helps allay the client's anxiety. Proceeding with the routine doesn't offer the client the opportunity to express his feelings. Offering false reassurance isn't therapeutic. Telling the client to calm down minimizes his feelings of anxiety.

NP: Implementation; CN: Psychosocial integrity; CNS: Coping and adaptation; CL: Application

160. 4. Smoking cigarettes or marijuana increases theophylline elimination decreasing its serum concentrations and effectiveness. Drinking beverages that contain caffeine may result in additive adverse reactions to theophylline or signs and symptoms of toxicity. Oral contraceptives and corticosteroids may increase theophylline levels leading to toxicity.

NP: Assessment; CN: Physiological integrity; CNS: Pharmacological and parenteral therapies; CL: Application

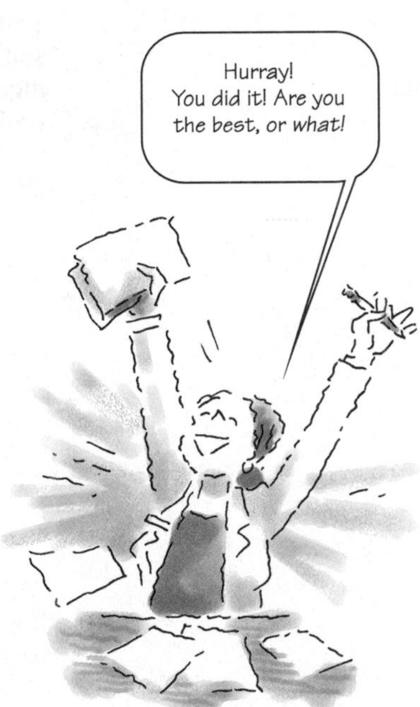

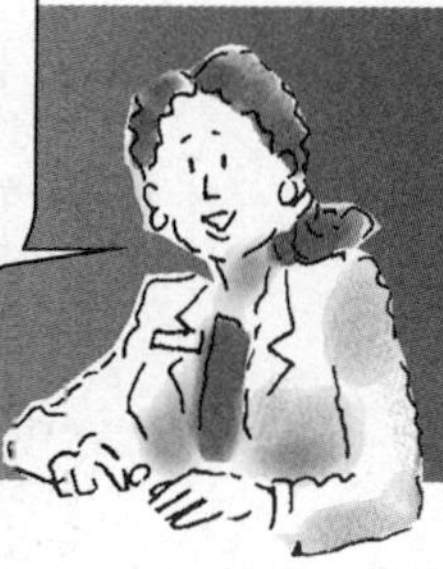

Chapter 6 Neurosensory disorders

1. An elderly client had a stroke and can only see the nasal visual field on one side and the temporal portion on the opposite side. Which of the following terms correctly describes this condition?

1. Astereognosis
2. Homonymous hemianopia
3. Oculogyric crisis
4. Receptive aphasia

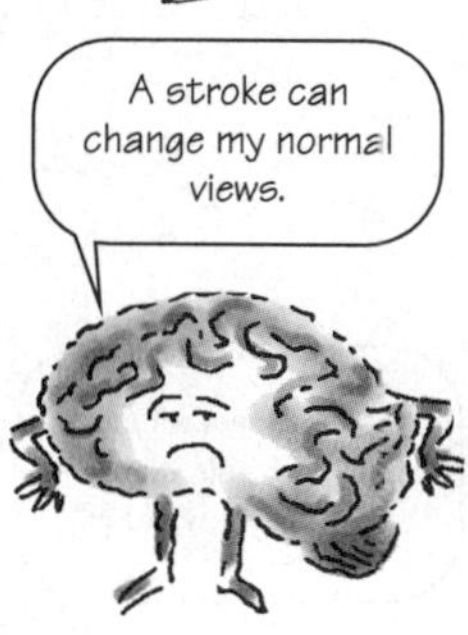

A stroke can change my normal views.

1. 2. Homonymous hemianopia describes the loss of visual field on the nasal side and the opposite temporal side due to damage of the optic nerves. Astereognosis is the inability to identify common objects through touch. Oculogyric crisis, a fixed position of the eyeballs that can last for minutes or hours, occurs in response to antipsychotic medications. Receptive aphasia is the inability to understand words or word meaning.

NP: Assessment; CN: Physiological integrity; CNS: Physiological adaptation; CL: Application

2. A client had an embolic stroke. Which of the following conditions places a client at risk for thromboembolic stroke?

1. Atrial fibrillation
2. Bradycardia
3. Deep vein thrombosis (DVT)
4. History of myocardial infarction (MI)

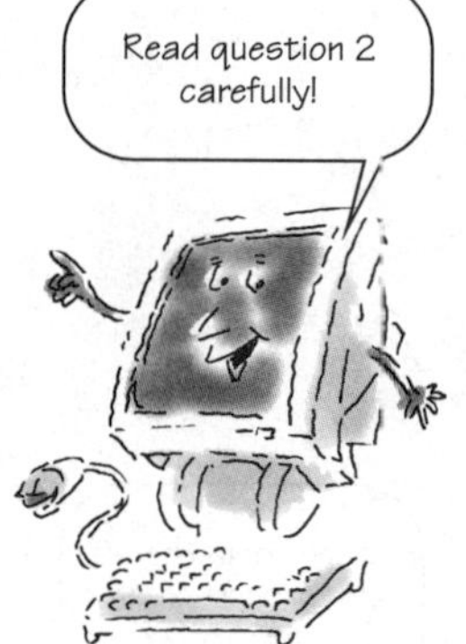

Read question 2 carefully!

2. 1. Atrial fibrillation occurs with the irregular and rapid discharge from multiple ectopic atrial foci that causes quivering of the atria without atrial systole. This asynchronous atrial contraction predisposes to mural thrombi, which may embolize, leading to a stroke. Bradycardia, DVT, or past MI won't lead to arterial embolization.

NP: Planning; CN: Physiological integrity; CNS: Physiological adaptation; CL: Application

3. A heparin infusion at 1,500 units/hour is ordered for a 65-year-old client with a stroke in evolution. The infusion contains 25,000 units of heparin in 500 ml of saline solution. How many milliliters per hour should be given?

1. 15 ml/hour
2. 30 ml/hour
3. 45 ml/hour
4. 50 ml/hour

3. 2. An infusion prepared with 25,000 units of heparin in 500 ml of saline solution yields 50 units of heparin per milliliter of solution. The equation is set up as 50 units times X (the unknown quantity) equals 1,500 units/hour; X equals 30 ml/hour.

NP: Implementation; CN: Physiological integrity; CNS: Pharmacological and parenteral therapies; CL: Application

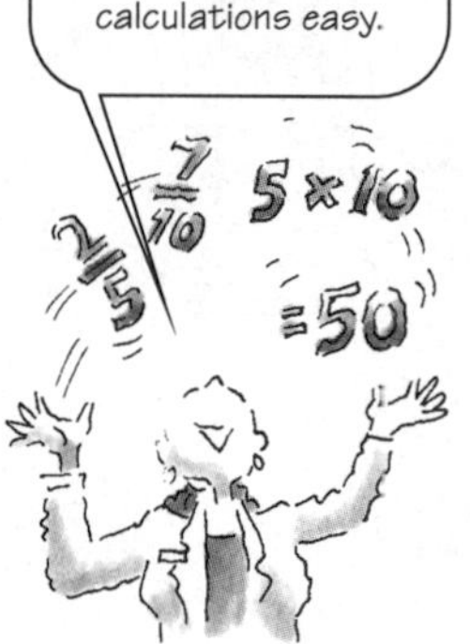

4. Which of the following medications may be prescribed to prevent a thromboembolic stroke?

1. Acetaminophen
2. Streptokinase
3. Ticlopidine
4. Methylprednisolone

4. 3. Ticlopidine inhibits platelet aggregation by interfering with adenosine diphosphate release in the coagulation cascade and is used to prevent thromboembolic stroke. Aspirin, not acetaminophen, interferes with platelet aggregation. Streptokinase is a medication used with evolving myocardial infarctions and dissolves clots. Methylprednisolone is a steroid with anticoagulant properties.

NP: Planning; CN: Physiological integrity; CNS: Pharmacological and parenteral therapies; CL: Application

5. To maintain airway patency during a stroke in evolution, which of the following nursing interventions is appropriate?

1. Thicken all dietary liquids.
2. Restrict dietary and parenteral fluids.
3. Place the client in the supine position.
4. Have tracheal suction available at all times.

5. 4. Because of a potential loss of gag reflex and potential altered level of consciousness, the client should be kept in Fowler's or a semiprone position with tracheal suction available at all times. Thickening dietary liquids isn't done until the gag reflex returns or the stroke has evolved and the deficit can be assessed. Unless heart failure is present, restricting fluids isn't indicated.

NP: Implementation; CN: Physiological integrity; CNS: Reduction of risk potential; CL: Application

6. For a client with a stroke, which of the following criteria must be fulfilled before the client is fed?

1. The gag reflex returns.
2. Speech returns to normal.
3. Cranial nerves III, IV, and VI are intact.
4. The client swallows small sips of water without coughing.

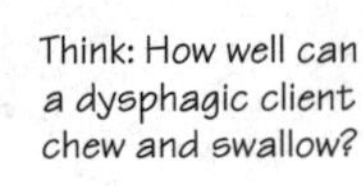

Think: How well can a dysphagic client chew and swallow?

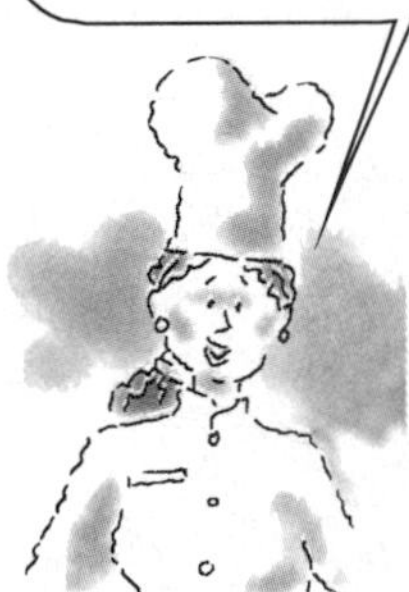

6. 1. An intact gag reflex shows a properly functioning cranial nerve IX (glossopharyngeal). Speech may be normal while the gag reflex is absent. Cranial nerves III, IV, and VI evaluate eye movement and accommodation. A nurse shouldn't offer food or fluids without assessing for intact gag reflexes.

NP: Planning; CN: Physiological integrity; CNS: Reduction of risk potential; CL: Application

7. Which of the following diets would be least likely to lead to aspiration in a client who had a stroke with residual dysphagia?

1. Clear liquid
2. Full liquid
3. Mechanical soft
4. Thickened liquid

7. 4. Thickened liquids are easiest to form into a bolus and swallow. Clear and full liquids are amorphous and can't easily form a bolus. A mechanical soft diet may be too hard to chew and too dry to swallow when dysphagia is present.

NP: Planning; CN: Physiological integrity; CNS: Reduction of risk potential; CL: Application

8. A 77-year-old client had a thromboembolic right stroke; his left arm is swollen. Which of the following conditions may cause swelling after a stroke?

1. Elbow contracture secondary to spasticity
2. Loss of muscle contraction decreasing venous return
3. Deep vein thrombosis (DVT) due to immobility of the ipsilateral side
4. Hypoalbuminemia due to protein escaping from an inflamed glomerulus

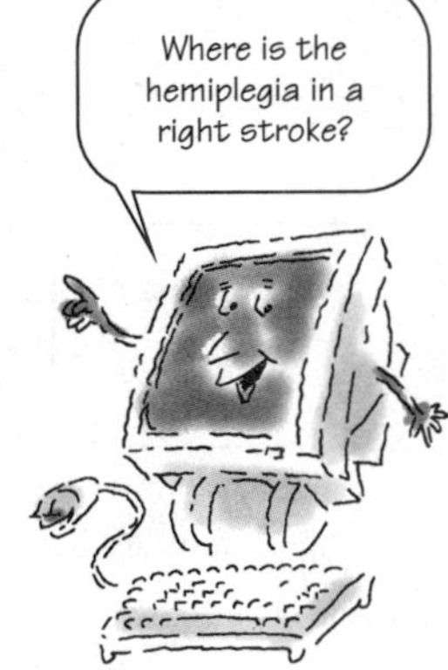

Where is the hemiplegia in a right stroke?

8. 2. In clients with hemiplegia or hemiparesis, loss of muscle contraction decreases venous return and may cause swelling of the affected extremity. Contractures, or bony calcifications, may occur with a stroke, but don't appear with swelling. DVT may develop in clients with a stroke but is more likely to occur in the lower extremities. A stroke isn't linked to protein loss.

NP: Planning; CN: Physiological integrity; CNS: Physiological adaptation; CL: Analysis

9. After a brain stem infarction, a nurse would observe for which of the following conditions?

1. Aphasia
2. Bradypnea
3. Contralateral hemiplegia
4. Numbness and tingling to the face or arm

9. 2. The brain stem contains the medulla and the vital cardiac, vasomotor, and respiratory centers. A brain stem infarction leads to vital sign changes such as bradypnea. Aphasia, contralateral hemiplegia, and numbness or tingling in the face or arm may occur with a stroke.

NP: Assessment; CN: Physiological integrity; CNS: Physiological adaptation; CL: Application

10. Which of the following conditions is a risk factor for the development of cataracts in a 40-year-old client?

1. History of frequent streptococcal throat infections
2. Maternal exposure to rubella during pregnancy
3. Increased intraocular pressure
4. Prolonged use of steroidal anti-inflammatory agents

10. 4. Prolonged use of steroidal anti-inflammatory agents is a risk factor for cataracts. The other risk factors don't contribute to the development of cataracts.

NP: Assessment; CN: Health promotion and maintenance; CNS: Prevention and early detection of disease; CL: Application

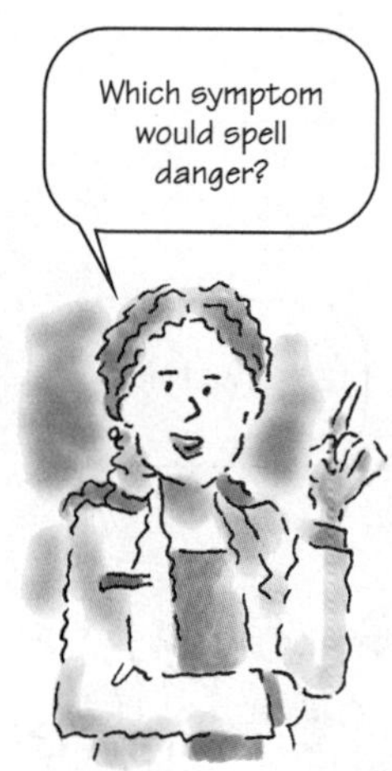
Which symptom would spell danger?

11. A client who had cataract surgery should be told to call his physician if he has which of the following conditions?

1. Blurred vision
2. Eye pain
3. Glare
4. Itching

11. 2. Pain shouldn't be present after cataract surgery. The client should be told the other symptoms might be present.

NP: Implementation; CN: Physiological integrity; CNS: Physiological adaptation; CL: Comprehension

12. Clear fluid is draining from the nose of a client who had a head trauma 3 hours ago. This may indicate which of the following conditions?

1. Basilar skull fracture
2. Cerebral concussion
3. Cerebral palsy
4. Sinus infection

12. 1. Clear fluid draining from the ear or nose of a client may mean a cerebrospinal fluid leak, which is common in basilar skull fractures. Concussion is associated with a brief loss of consciousness, cerebral palsy is associated with nonprogressive paralysis present since birth, and sinus infection is associated with facial pain and pressure with or without nasal drainage.

NP: Assessment; CN: Physiological integrity; CNS: Physiological adaptation; CL: Analysis

13. A 19-year-old client with a mild concussion is discharged from the emergency department. Before discharge, he complains of a headache. When offered acetaminophen, his mother tells the nurse the headache is severe and she would like her son to have something stronger. Which of the following responses by the nurse is appropriate?

1. "Your son had a mild concussion, acetaminophen is strong enough."
2. "Aspirin is avoided because of the danger of Reye's syndrome in children or young adults."
3. "Narcotics are avoided after a head injury because they may hide a worsening condition."
4. "Stronger medications may lead to vomiting, which increases the intracranial pressure (ICP)."

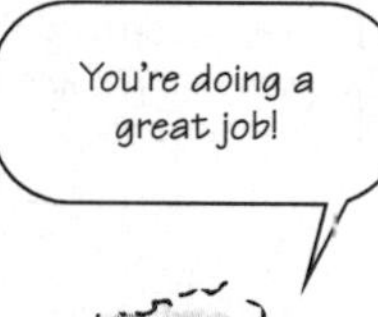
You're doing a great job!

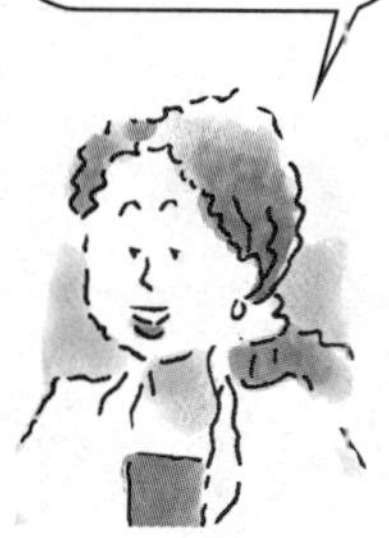

13. 3. Narcotics may mask changes in the level of consciousness that indicate increased ICP and shouldn't be given. Saying acetaminophen is strong enough ignores the mother's question and therefore isn't appropriate. Aspirin is contraindicated in conditions that may have bleeding, such as trauma, and for children or young adults with viral illnesses due to the danger of Reye's syndrome. Stronger medications may not necessarily lead to vomiting but will sedate the client, thereby masking changes in his level of consciousness.

NP: Implementation; CN: Physiological integrity; CNS: Reduction of risk potential; CL: Application

14. A client admitted to the hospital with a subarachnoid hemorrhage has complaints of severe headache, nuchal rigidity, and projectile vomiting. The nurse knows lumbar puncture (LP) would be contraindicated in this client in which of the following circumstances?

1. Vomiting continues.
2. Intracranial pressure (ICP) is increased.
3. The client needs mechanical ventilation.
4. Blood is anticipated in the cerebrospinal fluid (CSF).

14. 2. Sudden removal of CSF results in pressures lower in the lumbar area than the brain and favors herniation of the brain; therefore, LP is contraindicated with increased ICP. Vomiting may be caused by reasons other than increased ICP; therefore, LP isn't strictly contraindicated. An LP may be performed on clients needing mechanical ventilation. Blood in the CSF is diagnostic for subarachnoid hemorrhage and was obtained before signs and symptoms of increased ICP.

NP: Planning; CN: Physiological integrity; CNS: Physiological adaptation; CL: Application

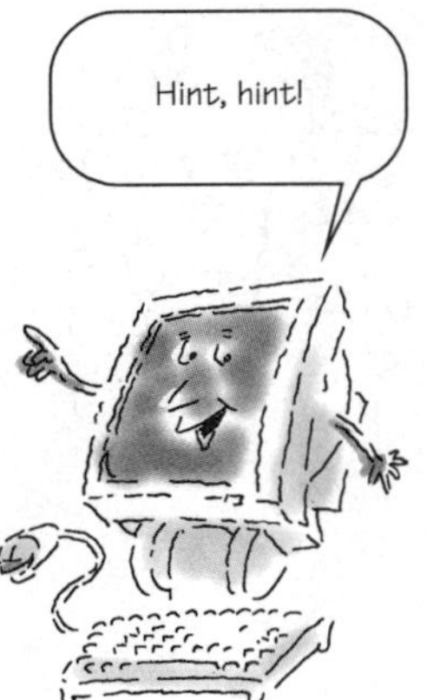

Hint, hint!

15. A client with head trauma develops a urine output of 300 ml/hour, dry skin, and dry mucous membranes. Which of the following nursing interventions is the most appropriate to perform immediately?

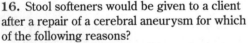

1. Evaluate urine specific gravity.
2. Anticipate treatment for renal failure.
3. Provide emollients to the skin to prevent breakdown.
4. Slow the I.V. fluids and notify the physician.

15. 1. Urine output of 300 ml/hour may indicate diabetes insipidus, which is failure of the pituitary to produce antidiuretic hormone. This may occur with increased intracranial pressure and head trauma; the nurse evaluates for low urine specific gravity, increased serum osmolarity, and dehydration. There's no evidence that the client is experiencing renal failure. Providing emollients to prevent skin breakdown is important, but doesn't need to be performed immediately. Slowing the rate of I.V. fluid would contribute to dehydration when polyuria is present.

NP: Evaluation; CN: Physiological integrity; CNS: Physiological adaptation; CL: Analysis

16. Stool softeners would be given to a client after a repair of a cerebral aneurysm for which of the following reasons?

1. To stimulate the bowel due to loss of nerve innervation
2. To prevent straining, which increases intracranial pressure (ICP)
3. To prevent the Valsalva maneuver, which may lead to bradycardia
4. To prevent constipation when osmotic diuretics are used

16. 2. Straining when having a bowel movement, sneezing, coughing, and suctioning may lead to increased ICP and should be avoided when potential increased ICP exists. Stool softeners don't stimulate the bowel and aren't used in combination with osmotic diuretics. Although the Valsalva maneuver may lead to bradycardia and reflex tachycardia, this rationale doesn't apply to this client.

NP: Planning; CN: Physiological integrity; CNS: Reduction of risk potential; CL: Application

Knowing why you do something can help prevent errors.

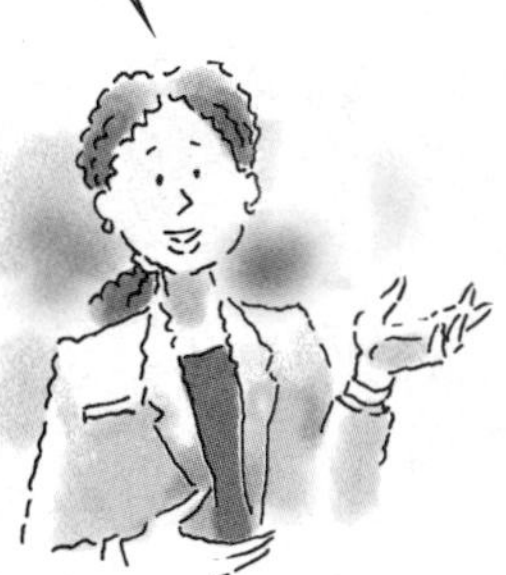

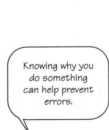

17. A client with a subdural hematoma becomes restless and confused, with dilation of the ipsilateral pupil. The physician orders mannitol for which of the following reasons?

1. To reduce intraocular pressure
2. To prevent acute tubular necrosis
3. To promote osmotic diuresis to decrease intracranial pressure (ICP)
4. To draw water into the vascular system to increase blood pressure

17. 3. Mannitol promotes osmotic diuresis by increasing the pressure gradient, drawing fluid from intracellular to intravascular spaces. Although mannitol is used for all the reasons described, the reduction of ICP in this client is of concern.

NP: Planning; CN: Physiological integrity; CNS: Pharmacological and parenteral therapies; CL: Knowledge

18. A client with a subdural hematoma was given mannitol to decrease intracranial pressure (ICP). Which of the following results would best show the mannitol was effective?

1. Urine output increases.
2. Pupils are 8 mm and nonreactive.
3. Systolic blood pressure remains at 150 mm Hg.
4. Blood urea nitrogen (BUN) and creatinine levels return to normal.

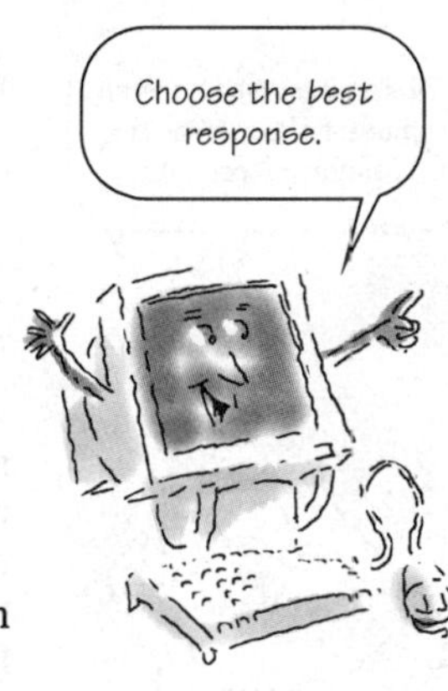
Choose the best response.

18. 1. Mannitol promotes osmotic diuresis by increasing the pressure gradient in the renal tubules. Fixed and dilated pupils are symptoms of increased ICP or cranial nerve damage. No information is given about abnormal BUN and creatinine levels or that mannitol is being given for renal dysfunction or blood pressure maintenance.

NP: Evaluation; CN: Physiological integrity; CNS: Physiological adaptation; CL: Application

19. When evaluating an arterial blood gas from a client with a subdural hematoma, the nurse notes the $Paco_2$ is 30 mm Hg. Which of the following responses best describes this result?

1. Appropriate; lowering carbon dioxide (CO_2) reduces intracranial pressure (ICP)
2. Emergent; the client is poorly oxygenated
3. Normal
4. Significant; the client has alveolar hypoventilation

19. 1. A normal $Paco_2$ value is 35 to 45 mm Hg. CO_2 has vasodilating properties; therefore, lowering $Paco_2$ through hyperventilation will lower ICP caused by dilated cerebral vessels. Oxygenation is evaluated through Pao_2 and oxygen saturation. Alveolar hypoventilation would be reflected in an increased $Paco_2$.

NP: Evaluation; CN: Physiological integrity; CNS: Physiological adaptation; CL: Analysis

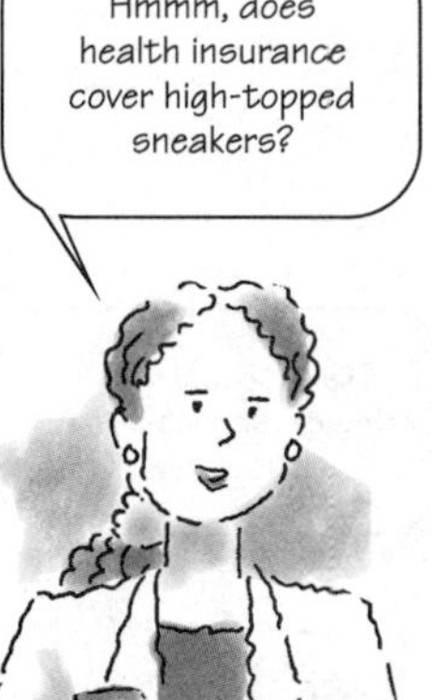
Hmmm, does health insurance cover high-topped sneakers?

20. Which of the following nursing interventions should be used to prevent foot drop and contractures in a client recovering from a subdural hematoma?

1. High-topped sneakers
2. Low-dose heparin therapy
3. Physical therapy consultation
4. Sequential compression device

20. 1. High-topped sneakers are used to prevent foot drop and contractures in neurologic clients. Low-dose heparin therapy and sequential compression boots will prevent deep vein thrombosis. Although a consultation with physical therapy is important to prevent foot drop, a nurse may use high-topped sneakers independently.

NP: Implementation; CN: Physiological integrity; CNS: Reduction of risk potential; CL: Application

21. A client who had a transsphenoidal hypophysectomy should be watched carefully for hemorrhage, which may be shown by which of the following signs?

1. Bloody drainage from the ears
2. Frequent swallowing
3. Guaiac-positive stools
4. Hematuria

21. 2. Frequent swallowing after brain surgery may indicate fluid or blood leaking from the sinuses into the oropharynx. Blood or fluid draining from the ear may indicate a basilar skull fracture, guaiac-positive stools indicate GI bleeding, and hematuria may result from cystitis or other urologic complications.

NP: Assessment; CN: Physiological integrity; CNS: Physiological adaptation; CL: Analysis

22. After a hypophysectomy, vasopressin is given I.M. for which of the following reasons?

1. To treat growth failure
2. To prevent syndrome of inappropriate antidiuretic hormone (SIADH)
3. To reduce cerebral edema and lower intracranial pressure
4. To replace antidiuretic hormone (ADH) normally secreted from the pituitary

22. 4. After hypophysectomy, or removal of the pituitary gland, the body can't synthesize ADH. Somatropin or growth hormone, not vasopressin is used to treat growth failure. SIADH results from excessive ADH secretion. Mannitol or corticosteroids are used to decrease cerebral edema.

NP: Implementation; CN: Physiological integrity; CNS: Pharmacological and parenteral therapies; CL: Application

23. Which of the following values is considered normal for intracranial pressure (ICP)?
1. 0 to 15 mm Hg
2. 25 mm Hg
3. 35 to 45 mm Hg
4. 120/80 mm Hg

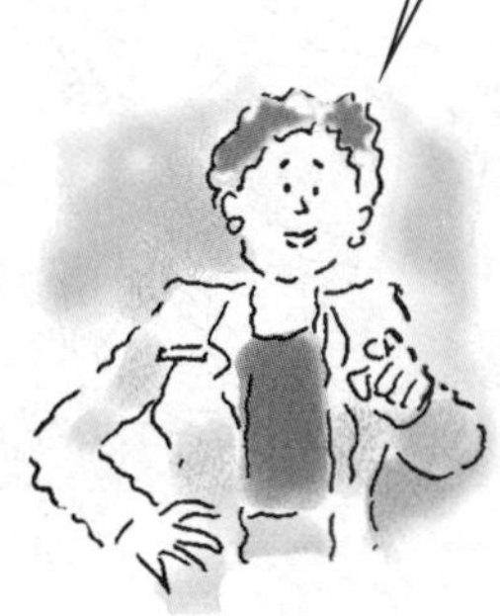

Be familiar with normal values to recognize an abnormal result.

23. 1. Normal ICP is 0 to 15 mm Hg.
NP: Assessment; CN: Physiological integrity; CNS: Physiological adaptation; CL: Comprehension

24. A 33-year-old client undergoes an L4-L5 laminectomy. Which of the following methods would be best to prevent skin breakdown and hypostatic pneumonia?
1. Apply an alternating air mattress to the bed.
2. Use a foam wedge when propping the client on his side.
3. Logroll the client with assistance, if necessary, to keep his back in alignment.
4. Teach the client to reach for the side rail with his dominant hand to pull himself onto his side.

24. 3. Turning the client as a unit by logrolling is necessary to prevent stress on the intradiskal area. An air mattress will help prevent skin breakdown, but the client must be turned to prevent stasis of pulmonary secretions. A foam wedge will maintain the client's position but not prevent breakdown. Having the client reach out will cause lordosis of the spine.
NP: Implementation; CN: Physiological integrity; CNS: Reduction of risk potential; CL: Application

25. Voiding small frequent amounts of urine after a lumbar laminectomy may indicate which of the following conditions?
1. Diabetes insipidus
2. Diabetic ketoacidosis
3. Urine retention
4. Urinary tract infection (UTI)

25. 3. Swelling or pressure on the peripheral nerves controlling micturition, anesthesia, or use of an indwelling urinary catheter may lead to urine retention with overflow of small frequent amounts of urine. Diabetes insipidus and diabetic ketoacidosis are shown by polyuria. UTI may be shown by dysuria and small frequent amounts of voided urine, but would be less likely in this situation.
NP: Evaluation; CN: Physiological integrity; CNS: Basic care and comfort; CL: Analysis

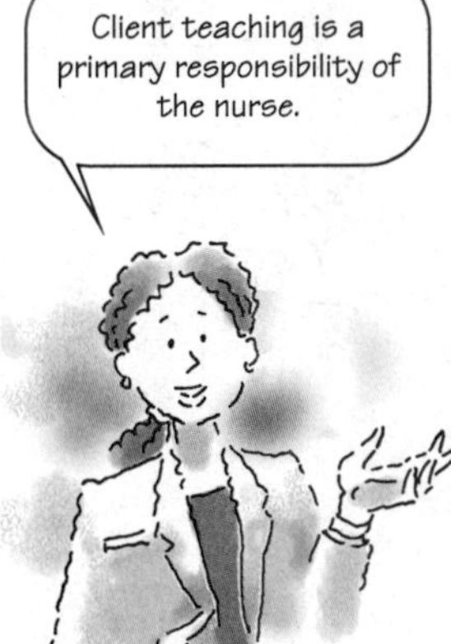

Client teaching is a primary responsibility of the nurse.

26. A client with lower back pain and a herniated nucleus pulposus should be taught that strengthening which of the following muscles after laminectomy will prevent lower back pain?
1. Abdominal
2. Diaphragm
3. Gluteus
4. Rectus femoris

26. 1. Strengthening abdominal muscles will support the back, preventing lower back pain. Strengthening the diaphragm, the gluteus, or the rectus femoris won't prevent lower back pain.
NP: Planning; CN: Physiological integrity; CNS: Reduction of risk potential; CL: Application

27. When preparing a client with suspected herniated nucleus pulposus for myelography, which of the following nursing interventions should be done before the test?
1. Question the client about allergy to iodine.
2. Mark distal pulses on the foot in indelible ink.
3. Assess and document pain along the sciatic nerve.
4. Tell the client he may be asked to cough or pant to clear the dye.

27. 1. A radiopaque dye, usually iodine-based, is instilled into the spinal canal to outline structures during myelography. Pain may be expected along the sciatic nerve with a herniated nucleus pulposus. During cardiac catheterization, a client is asked to cough or pant to clear the dye, and before cardiac catheterization or arteriogram, the nurse marks pedal pulses in ink.
NP: Planning; CN: Physiological integrity; CNS: Reduction of risk potential; CL: Application

28. A client is scheduled for chemonucleolysis with chymopapain to relieve the pain of a herniated disk. Which of the following factors should be assessed before the procedure?

1. Allergy to meat tenderizers
2. Allergy to shellfish
3. Ability to lie flat during the procedure
4. Range of motion on the affected side

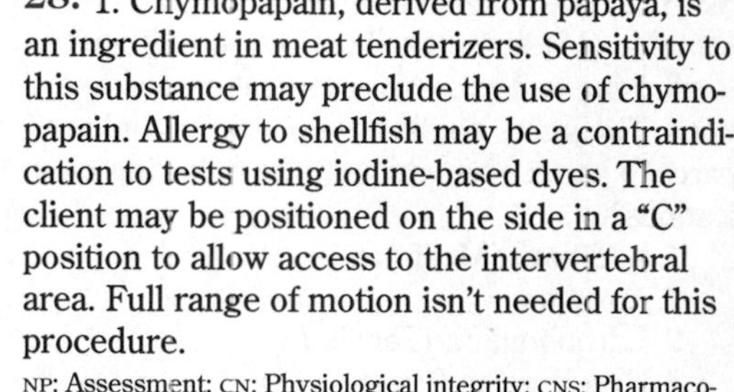

28. 1. Chymopapain, derived from papaya, is an ingredient in meat tenderizers. Sensitivity to this substance may preclude the use of chymopapain. Allergy to shellfish may be a contraindication to tests using iodine-based dyes. The client may be positioned on the side in a "C" position to allow access to the intervertebral area. Full range of motion isn't needed for this procedure.

NP: Assessment; CN: Physiological integrity; CNS: Pharmacological and parenteral therapies; CL: Application

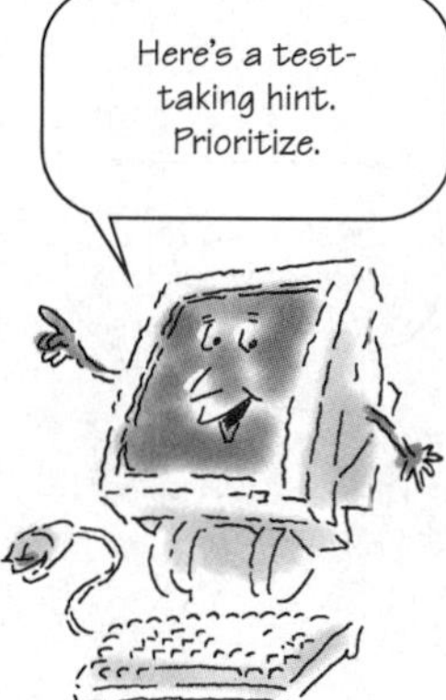

Here's a test-taking hint. Prioritize.

29. When prioritizing care, which of the following clients should the nurse assess **first**?

1. A 17-year-old client 24-hours postappendectomy
2. A 33-year-old client with a recent diagnosis of Guillain-Barré syndrome
3. A 50-year-old client 3 days postmyocardial infarction
4. A 50-year-old client with diverticulitis

29. 2. Guillain-Barré syndrome is characterized by ascending paralysis and potential respiratory failure. The order of client assessment should follow client priorities, with disorders of airway, breathing, and then circulation. There's no information to suggest the postmyocardial infarction client has an arrhythmia or other complication. There's no evidence to suggest hemorrhage or perforation for the remaining clients as a priority of care.

NP: Planning; CN: Safe, effective care environment; CNS: Management of care; CL: Analysis

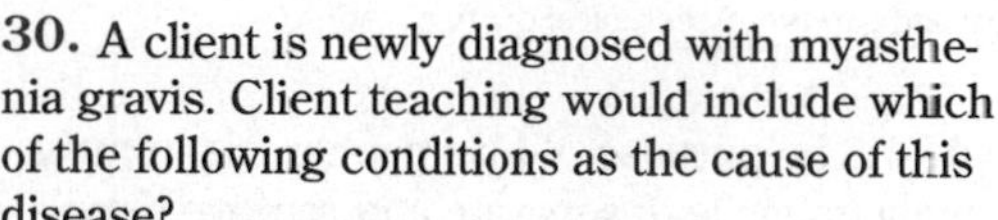

30. A client is newly diagnosed with myasthenia gravis. Client teaching would include which of the following conditions as the cause of this disease?

1. A postviral illness characterized by ascending paralysis
2. Loss of the myelin sheath surrounding peripheral nerves
3. Inability of basal ganglia to produce sufficient dopamine
4. Destruction of acetylcholine receptors causing muscle weakness

30. 4. Myasthenia gravis, an autoimmune disorder, is caused by the destruction of acetylcholine receptors. Guillain-Barré syndrome is a postviral illness characterized by ascending paralysis, multiple sclerosis is caused by loss of the myelin sheath, and Parkinson's disease is caused by the inability of basal ganglia to produce sufficient dopamine.

NP: Planning; CN: Health promotion and maintenance; CNS: Prevention and early detection of disease; CL: Comprehension

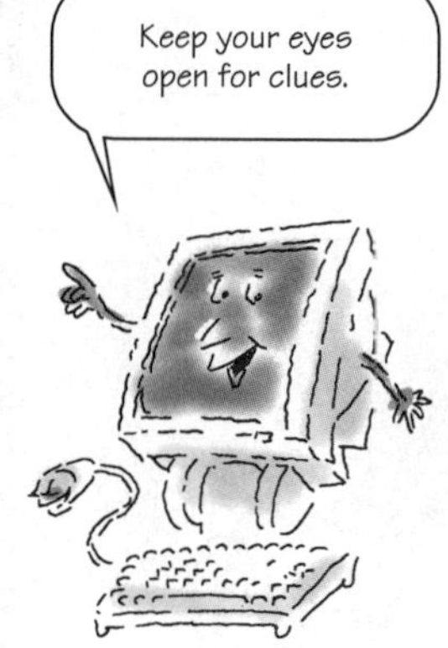

Keep your eyes open for clues.

31. Which of the following conditions is an **early** symptom commonly seen in myasthenia gravis?

1. Dysphagia
2. Fatigue improving at the end of the day
3. Ptosis
4. Respiratory distress

31. 3. Ptosis and diplopia are early signs of myasthenia gravis; dysphagia and respiratory distress occur later. Symptoms are typically milder in the morning and may be exacerbated by stress or lack of rest.

NP: Assessment; CN: Health promotion and maintenance; CNS: Prevention and early detection of disease; CL: Application

32. One hour after receiving pyridostigmine bromide (Mestinon), a client reports difficulty swallowing and excessive respiratory secretions. The nurse notifies the physician and prepares to administer which of the following medications?

1. Additional Mestinon
2. Atropine
3. Edrophonium (Tensilon)
4. Neostigmine (Prostigmin)

32. 2. These symptoms suggest cholinergic crisis or excessive acetylcholinesterase medication, typically appearing 45 to 60 minutes after the last dose of acetylcholinesterase inhibitor. Atropine, an anticholinergic drug, is used to antagonize acetylcholinesterase inhibitors. The other drugs are acetylcholinesterase inhibitors. Tensilon is used for the diagnosis and Mestinon and Prostigmin are used for the treatment of myasthenia gravis and would worsen these symptoms.

NP: Assessment; CN: Physiological integrity; CNS: Pharmacological and parenteral therapies; CL: Analysis

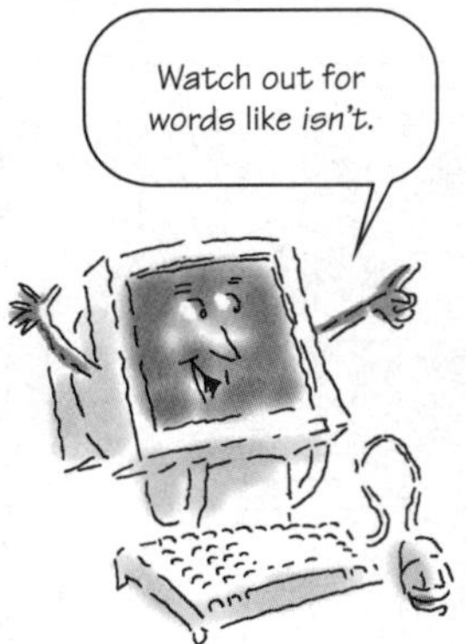
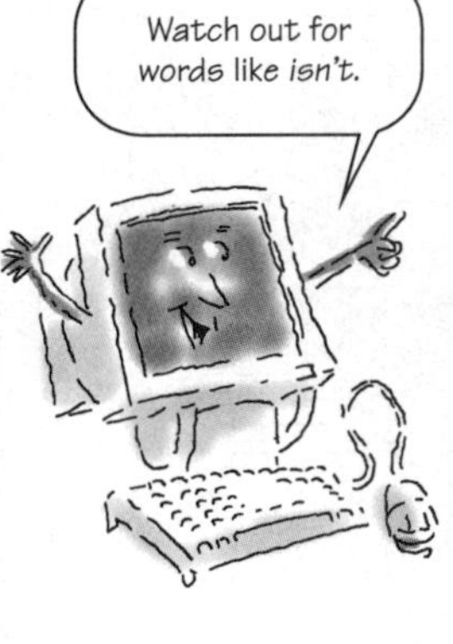
Watch out for
words like isn't.

33. A client with suspected myasthenia gravis is to undergo a Tensilon test. Tensilon is used to diagnose — but not treat — myasthenia gravis. Why isn't it used for treatment?

1. It isn't available in an oral form.
2. With repeated use, immunosuppression may occur.
3. Dry mouth and abdominal cramps may be intolerable adverse effects.
4. The short half-life of Tensilon makes it impractical for long-term use.

33. 4. The duration of action of Tensilon is 1 to 2 minutes, making it impractical for the long-term management of myasthenia gravis. Immunosuppression with repeated use is an adverse effect of steroid administration, a medication used to treat myasthenia gravis. Dry mouth and abdominal cramps are adverse effects of increased acetylcholine in the parasympathetic nervous system.

NP: Planning; CN: Physiological integrity; CNS: Pharmacological and parenteral therapies; CL: Application

34. A 20-year-old client with myasthenia gravis will undergo plasmapheresis. Which of the following actions describes the purpose of this procedure?

1. Preventing exacerbations during pregnancy
2. Removing T and B lymphocytes that attack acetylcholine receptors
3. Delivering acetylcholinesterase inhibitor directly into the bloodstream
4. Separating and removing acetylcholine receptor antibodies from the blood

34. 4. The purpose of plasmapheresis in myasthenia gravis is to separate and remove circulating acetylcholine receptor antibodies from the blood of clients refractory to the usual therapies or clients in crisis. Although stress, including pregnancy, may precipitate crisis, this isn't the purpose of the procedure. Plasmapheresis doesn't remove T and B lymphocytes, nor does it deliver acetylcholinesterase inhibitor directly into the bloodstream.

NP: Planning; CN: Physiological integrity; CNS: Pharmacological and parenteral therapies; CL: Application

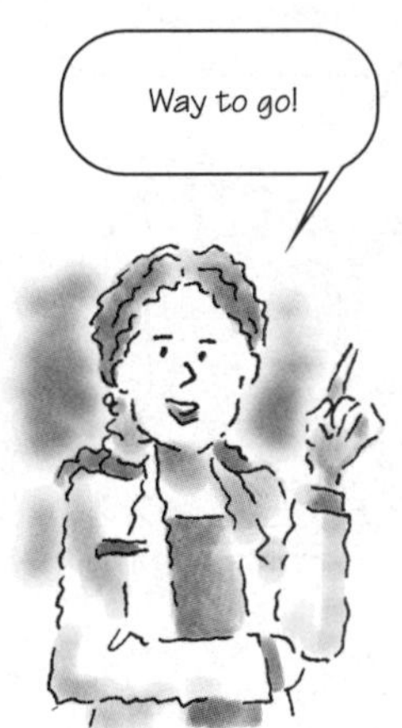
Way to go!

35. When assessing a client with glaucoma, a nurse expects which of the following findings?

1. Complaints of double vision
2. Complaints of halos around lights
3. Intraocular pressure of 15 mm Hg
4. Soft globe on palpation

35. 2. Complaints of halos around lights is a common finding in a client with glaucoma. Symptoms of glaucoma don't include double vision but can include loss of peripheral vision or blind spots, reddened sclera, firm globe, decreased accommodation, halos around lights, and occasional eye pain, but clients may be asymptomatic. Normal intraocular pressure is 10 to 21 mm Hg.

NP: Assessment; CN: Physiological integrity; CNS: Physiological adaptation; CL: Application

36. A client at the eye clinic is newly diagnosed with glaucoma. Client teaching includes the need to take his medication because noncompliance may lead to which of the following conditions?

1. Diplopia
2. Permanent vision loss
3. Progressive loss of peripheral vision
4. Pupillary constriction

36. 2. Without treatment, glaucoma may progress to irreversible blindness. Treatment won't restore visual damage, but will halt disease progression. Blurred or foggy vision, not diplopia, is typical in glaucoma. Central vision loss is typical in glaucoma. Miotics, which constrict the pupil, are used in the treatment of glaucoma to permit outflow of the aqueous humor.

NP: Implementation; CN: Physiological integrity; CNS: Pharmacological and parenteral therapies; CL: Application

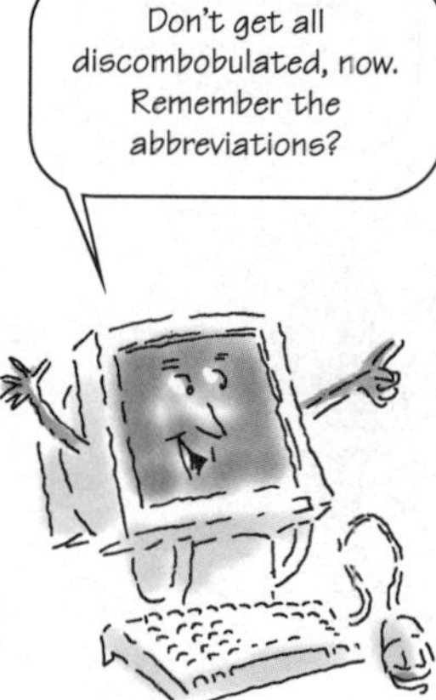

Don't get all discombobulated, now. Remember the abbreviations?

37. Pilocarpine, 2 gtt OU q.i.d., should be instilled according to which of the following procedures?

1. Two drops of the drug in both eyes four times daily
2. Two drops on the sclera of the left eye four times daily
3. Two drops over the lacrimal duct of the right eye four times daily
4. Two drops of the drug toward the nasal side of each conjunctival sac four times daily

37. 1. The abbreviation OU means both eyes, OS refers to the left eye, and OD to the right eye. Q.i.d. means four times daily and gtt means drops. Medications placed on the nasal side near the lacrimal duct will enter the nose and be ineffective.

NP: Implementation; CN: Physiological integrity; CNS: Pharmacological and parenteral therapies; CL: Application

38. When evaluating the extent of Parkinson's disease, a nurse observes for which of the following conditions?

1. Bulging eyeballs
2. Diminished distal sensation
3. Increased dopamine levels
4. Muscle rigidity

38. 4. Parkinson's disease is characterized by the slowing of voluntary muscle movement, muscular rigidity, and resting tremor. Bulging eyeballs (exophthalmos) occur in Graves disease. Diminished distal sensation doesn't occur in Parkinson's disease. Dopamine is deficient in this disorder.

NP: Assessment; CN: Physiological integrity; CNS: Physiological adaptation; CL: Application

39. Which of the following statements best describes the cause of Parkinson's disease?

1. Loss of the myelin sheath surrounding peripheral nerves
2. Degeneration of the substantia nigra, depleting dopamine
3. Bleeding into the brain stem, resulting in motor dysfunction
4. An autoimmune disorder that destroys acetylcholine receptors

39. 2. Parkinson's disease is caused by degeneration of the substantia nigra in the basal ganglia of the brain, where dopamine is produced and stored. This results in motor dysfunction. Loss of the myelin sheath around the peripheral nerves describes multiple sclerosis. Bleeding into the brain stem resulting in motor dysfunction describes a hemorrhagic stroke, and myasthenia gravis is an autoimmune disorder that destroys acetylcholine receptors.

NP: Analysis; CN: Physiological integrity; CNS: Physiological adaptation; CL: Comprehension

40. Which of the following clients would be most at risk for secondary Parkinson's disease caused by pharmacotherapy?

1. A 30-year-old client with schizophrenia taking chlorpromazine (Thorazine)
2. A 50-year-old client taking nitroglycerin tablets for angina
3. A 60-year-old client taking prednisone for chronic obstructive pulmonary disease
4. A 75-year-old client using naproxen for rheumatoid arthritis

40. 1. Phenothiazines such as Thorazine deplete dopamine, which may lead to tremor and rigidity (extrapyramidal effects). The other clients aren't at a greater risk for developing Parkinson's disease.

NP: Evaluation; CN: Physiological integrity; CNS: Pharmacological and parenteral therapies; CL: Application

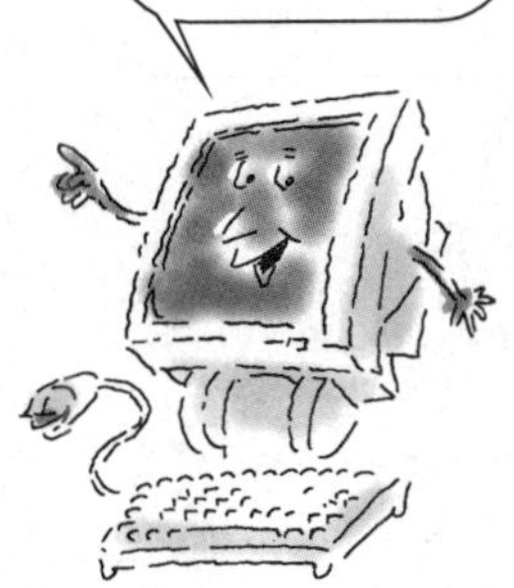

Read question 41 carefully to get the correct answer.

41. Which of the following symptoms occurs initially in Parkinson's disease?

1. Akinesia
2. Aspiration of food
3. Dementia
4. Pill rolling movements of the hand

41. 4. Early symptoms of Parkinson's disease include coarse resting tremors of the fingers and thumb. Akinesia and aspiration are late signs of Parkinson's disease. Dementia occurs in only 20% of the clients with Parkinson's disease.

NP: Assessment; CN: Health promotion and maintenance; CNS: Prevention and early detection of disease; CL: Application

42. To evaluate the effectiveness of levodopa-carbidopa (Sinemet), a nurse would watch for which of the following results?

1. Improved visual acuity
2. Decreased dyskinesia
3. Reduction in short-term memory
4. Lessened rigidity and tremor

42. 4. Levodopa-carbidopa increases the amount of dopamine in the central nervous system, allowing for more smooth, purposeful movements. The drug doesn't affect visual acuity and should improve dyskinesia and short-term memory.

NP: Evaluation; CN: Physiological integrity; CNS: Pharmacological and parenteral therapies; CL: Application

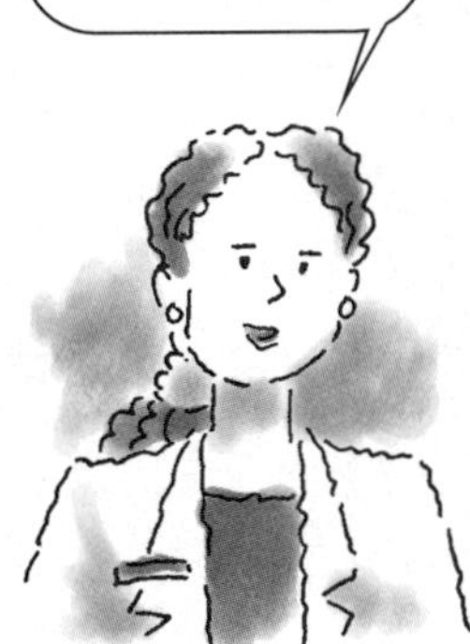

My mouth isn't dry anymore. But hmmm, that's odd. Now I'm transparent.

43. Two days after starting therapy with trihexyphenidyl (Artane), a client complains of a dry mouth. Which of the following nursing interventions would best relieve the client's dry mouth?

1. Offer the client ice chips and frequent sips of water
2. Withhold the drug and notify the physician
3. Change the client's diet to clear liquid until the symptoms subside
4. Encourage the use of supplemental puddings and shakes to maintain weight

43. 1. Trihexyphenidyl is an anticholinergic agent that causes blurred vision, dry mouth, constipation, and urine retention. There's no need to withhold the drug unless hypotension or tachyarrhythmia occurs. A clear liquid diet doesn't provide adequate nutrition and may be more difficult to swallow than thickened liquids if dysphagia is present; it isn't indicated at this time. Weight loss may occur with Parkinson's disease; however, the question relates to effects of trihexyphenidyl.

NP: Implementation; CN: Physiological integrity; CNS: Pharmacological and parenteral therapies; CL: Analysis

44. Which of the following anti-Parkinsonian drugs can cause drug tolerance or toxicity if taken for too long at one time?

1. Amantadine (Symmetrel)
2. Levodopa-carbidopa (Sinemet)
3. Pergolide (Permax)
4. Selegiline (Eldepryl)

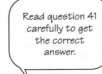

44. 2. Long-term therapy with levodopa-carbidopa can result in drug tolerance or toxicity, shown by confusion, hallucinations, or decreased drug effectiveness. The other drugs don't require that the client take a drug holiday.

NP: Evaluation; CN: Physiological integrity; CNS: Pharmacological and parenteral therapies; CL: Application

45. Which of the following clients would be most likely to develop multiple sclerosis (MS)?

1. A 20-year-old soccer player
2. A 35-year-old White female teacher
3. A 45-year-old, type A male smoker
4. A 50-year-old Black female with hypertension

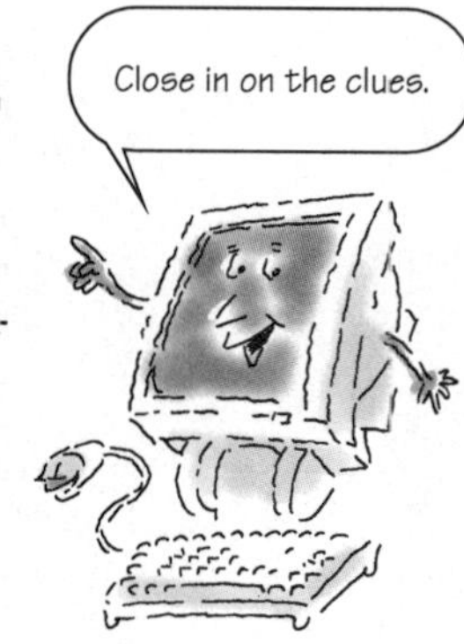

Close in on the clues.

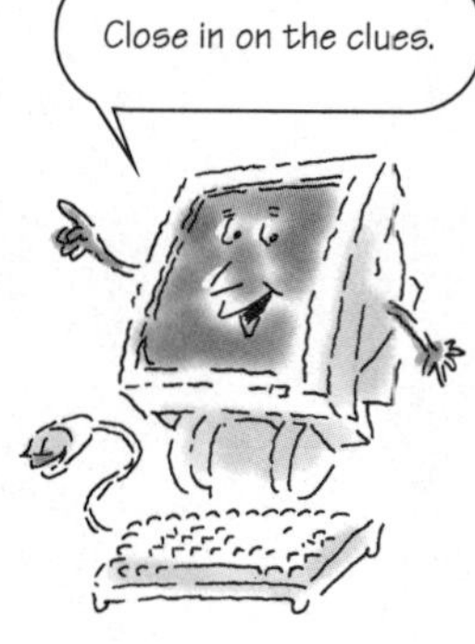

45. 2. MS is more common in White women ages 20 to 40 years, with a secondary onset between ages 40 to 60 years.

NP: Assessment; CN: Physiological integrity; CNS: Physiological adaptation; CL: Comprehension

46. Which of the following pathophysiologic processes are involved in multiple sclerosis (MS)?

1. Destruction of the brain stem and basal ganglia in the brain
2. Degeneration of the nucleus pulposus, causing pressure on the spinal cord
3. Chronic inflammation of rhizomes just outside the central nervous system
4. Development of demyelination of the myelin sheath, interfering with nerve transmission

46. 4. MS results from chronic progressive demyelination of the myelin sheath, interfering with nerve impulse transmission. The other processes don't describe MS.

NP: Assessment; CN: Physiological integrity; CNS: Physiological adaptation; CL: Comprehension

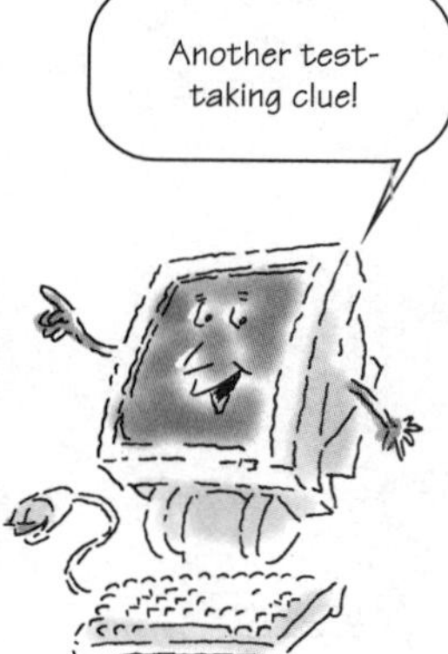

Another test-taking clue!

47. Which of the following symptoms usually occurs early in multiple sclerosis (MS)?

1. Diplopia
2. Grief
3. Hemiparesis
4. Recent memory loss

47. 1. Early symptoms of MS include slurred speech and diplopia. Paralysis is a late symptom. Although depression and a short attention span may occur, dementia is rarely associated with MS.

NP: Assessment; CN: Physiological integrity; CNS: Physiological adaptation; CL: Application

48. Which of the following measures would be included in teaching for the client with multiple sclerosis (MS) to avoid exacerbation of the disease?

1. Patching the affected eye
2. Sleeping 8 hours each night
3. Taking hot baths for relaxation
4. Drinking 1.5 to 2 L of fluid daily

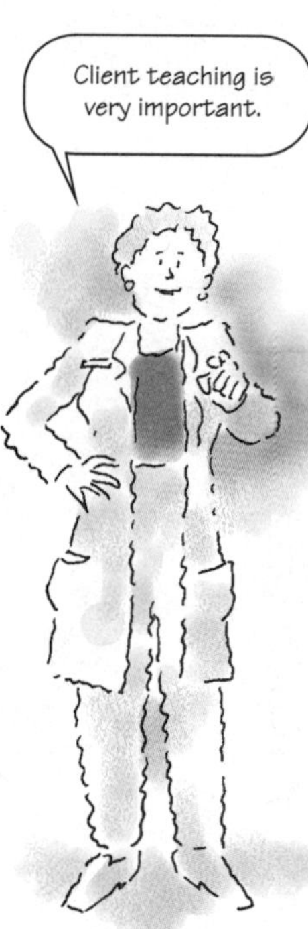

Client teaching is very important.

48. 2. MS is exacerbated by exposure to stress, fatigue, and heat. Clients should balance activity with rest. Patching the affected eye may result in improvement in vision and balance but won't prevent exacerbation of the disease. Adequate hydration will help prevent urinary tract infections secondary to a neurogenic bladder.

NP: Implementation; CN: Physiological integrity; CNS: Reduction of risk potential; CL: Application

49. Which of the following conditions or activities may exacerbate multiple sclerosis (MS)?

1. Pregnancy
2. Range-of-motion (ROM) exercises
3. Swimming
4. Urine retention

49. 1. Pregnancy, stress, fatigue, and heat may exacerbate MS. Exercise to maintain ROM is encouraged; swimming is particularly effective due to weightlessness and the cooling of nerves. Urine retention is common due to neurogenic bladder but doesn't lead to the exacerbation of symptoms.

NP: Implementation; CN: Physiological integrity; CNS: Reduction of risk potential; CL: Application

50. A client with suspected multiple sclerosis (MS) undergoes a lumbar puncture. Which of the following abnormalities is typically found in the cerebrospinal fluid (CSF) of clients with MS?

1. Blood or increased red blood cells
2. Elevated white blood cells (WBCs) or pus
3. Increased glucose concentrations
4. Increased protein levels

51. Which of the following terms describes involuntary, jerking, rhythmic movements of the eyes?

1. Diplopia
2. Exophthalmos
3. Nystagmus
4. Oculogyric crisis

52. Which of the following nursing interventions takes priority for the client having a tonic-clonic seizure?

1. Maintaining a patent airway
2. Timing the duration of the seizure
3. Noting the origin of seizure activity
4. Inserting a padded tongue blade to prevent the client from biting his tongue

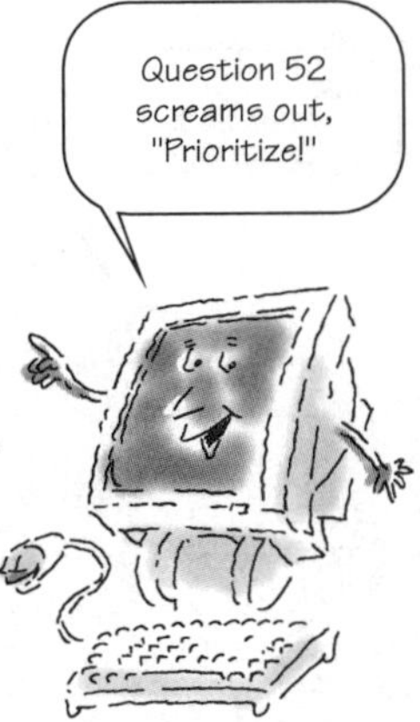
Question 52
screams out,
"Prioritize!"

53. A client recalls smelling an unpleasant odor before his seizure. Which of the following terms describes to this?

1. Atonic seizure
2. Aura
3. Icterus
4. Postictal experience

54. A client with new-onset seizures of unknown cause is started on phenytoin (Dilantin), 750 mg I.V. now and 100 mg P.O. t.i.d. Which of the following statements best describes the purpose of the loading dose?

1. To ensure that the drug reaches the cerebrospinal fluid
2. To prevent the need for surgical excision of the epileptic focus
3. To reduce secretions in case another seizure occurs
4. To more quickly attain therapeutic levels

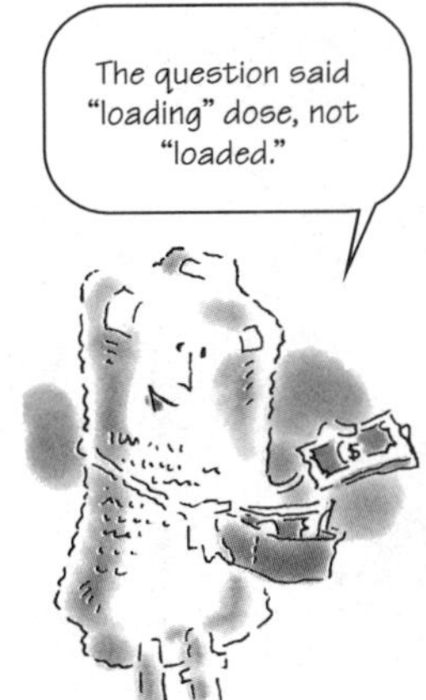
The question said
"loading" dose, not
"loaded."

50. 4. Elevated gamma globulin fraction in CSF without an elevated level in the blood occurs in MS. WBCs or pus indicate infection. Blood may be found with trauma or subarachnoid hemorrhage. Increased glucose concentration is a nonspecific finding indicating infection or subarachnoid hemorrhage.

NP: Assessment; CN: Physiological integrity; CNS: Physiological adaptation; CL: Analysis

51. 3. Nystagmus refers to jerking movements of the eye. Diplopia means double vision. Exophthalmos refers to bulging eyeballs, seen in Graves disease. Oculogyric crisis involves deviation of the eyes.

NP: Assessment; CN: Health promotion and maintenance; CNS: Prevention and early detection of disease; CL: Application

52. 1. The priority during and after a seizure is to maintain a patent airway. Timing the seizure activity and noting the origin of motor dysfunction are done, but not first. Nothing should be placed in the client's mouth during a seizure because teeth may be dislodged or the tongue pushed back, further obstructing the airway.

NP: Implementation; CN: Physiological integrity; CNS: Reduction of risk potential; CL: Application

53. 2. An aura occurs in some clients as a warning before a seizure. The client may experience a certain smell, a vision such as flashing lights, or a sensation. Atonic seizure or drop attack refers to an abrupt loss of muscle tone. Icterus refers to jaundice. Postictal experience occurs after a seizure, during which the client may be confused, somnolent, fatigued, and may need to sleep.

NP: Implementation; CN: Physiological integrity; CNS: Physiological adaptation; CL: Application

54. 4. A loading dose of phenytoin and other drugs is given to reach therapeutic levels more quickly; maintenance dosing follows. A loading dose of phenytoin can be oral or parenteral. Surgical excision of an epileptic focus is considered when seizures aren't controlled with anticonvulsant therapy. Phenytoin doesn't reduce secretions.

NP: Implementation; CN: Physiological integrity; CNS: Pharmacological and parenteral therapies; CL: Application

NP: Nursing process CN: Client needs category CNS: Client needs subcategory CL: Cognitive level

55. Which of the following adverse effects may occur during phenytoin (Dilantin) therapy?
1. Dry mouth
2. Furry tongue
3. Somnolence
4. Tachycardia

55. 3. Adverse effects of phenytoin include sedation, drowsiness, gingival hyperplasia, blood dyscrasia, and toxicity. The others symptoms aren't adverse effects of phenytoin.
NP: Implementation; CN: Physiological integrity; CNS: Pharmacological and parenteral therapies; CL: Application

56. Which of the following symptoms may occur with a phenytoin level of 32 mg/dl?
1. Ataxia and confusion
2. Sodium depletion
3. Tonic-clonic seizure
4. Urinary incontinence

56. 1. A therapeutic phenytoin level is 10 to 20 mg/dl. A level of 32 mg/dl indicates phenytoin toxicity. Symptoms of toxicity include confusion and ataxia. Phenytoin doesn't cause hyponatremia, seizure, or urinary incontinence. Incontinence may occur during or after a seizure.
NP: Evaluation; CN: Safe, effective care environment; CNS: Management of care; CL: Analysis

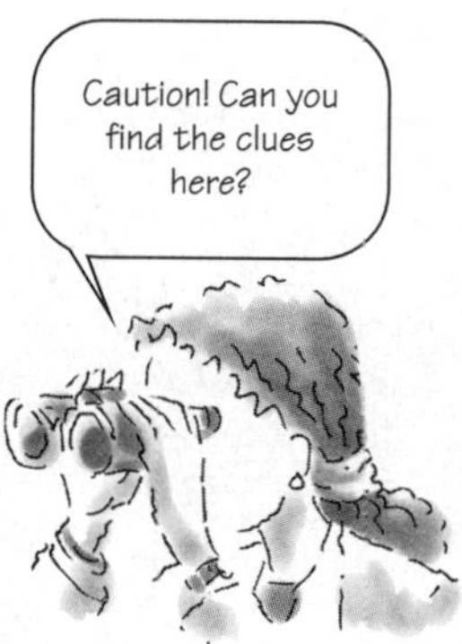

Caution! Can you find the clues here?

57. Which of the following precautions must be taken when giving phenytoin (Dilantin) to a client with a nasogastric (NG) tube for feeding?
1. Check the phenytoin level after giving the drug to check for toxicity.
2. Elevate the head of the bed before giving phenytoin through the NG tube.
3. Give phenytoin 1 hour before or 2 hours after NG tube feedings to ensure absorption.
4. Verify proper placement of the NG tube by placing the end of the tube in a glass of water and observing for bubbles.

57. 3. Nutritional supplements and milk interfere with the absorption of phenytoin, decreasing its effectiveness. Phenytoin levels are checked before giving the drug and the drug is withheld for elevated levels to avoid compounding toxicity. The head of the bed is elevated when giving all drugs or solutions and isn't specific to phenytoin administration. The nurse verifies NG tube placement by checking for stomach contents before giving drugs and feedings.
NP: Implementation; CN: Physiological integrity; CNS: Pharmacological and parenteral therapies; CL: Application

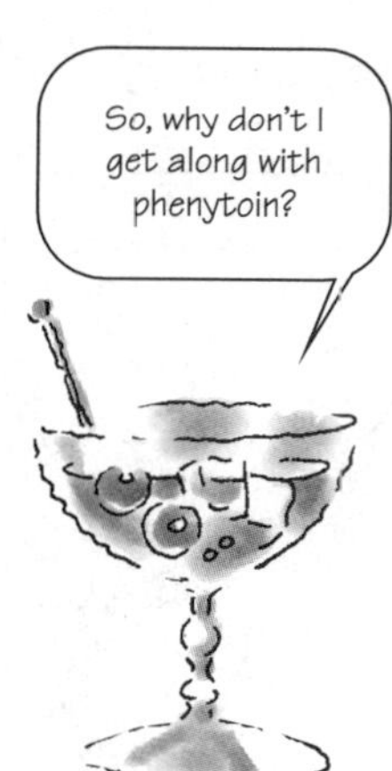

So, why don't I get along with phenytoin?

58. What's the most important concern for clients who drink alcohol while taking phenytoin?
1. Alcohol increases phenytoin activity.
2. Alcohol raises the seizure threshold.
3. Alcohol impairs judgment and coordination.
4. Alcohol decreases the effectiveness of phenytoin.

58. 4. Alcohol decreases phenytoin activity, diminishing its effectiveness. Although alcohol also reduces the seizure threshold and impairs judgement and coordination, these effects aren't the primary concern.
NP: Implementation; CN: Physiological integrity; CNS: Pharmacological and parenteral therapies; CL: Application

59. When assessing vital signs in a client with a seizure disorder, which of the following measures is used?
1. Checking for a pulse deficit
2. Checking for pulsus paradoxus
3. Taking an axillary instead of oral temperatures
4. Checking the blood pressure for an auscultatory gap

59. 3. To reduce the risk of injury, the nurse should take an axillary temperature or use a metal thermometer when taking an oral temperature to prevent injury if a seizure occurs. Pulse deficit occurs in an arrhythmia. Pulsus paradoxus may occur with cardiac tamponade. An auscultatory gap occurs in hypertension.
NP: Implementation; CN: Physiological integrity; CNS: Reduction of risk potential; CL: Application

60. A client in status epilepticus arrives at the emergency department. The family is interviewed to determine the cause of this problem. Which of the following events may have predisposed the client to this condition?

1. Abruptly stopping anticonvulsant therapy
2. Airplane travel
3. Exposure to sunlight
4. Recent upper respiratory infection

60. 1. Status epilepticus (seizures not responsive to usual therapies) occurs with the abrupt cessation of anticonvulsant drugs or ethanol intake. The other options don't cause status epilepticus.

NP: Evaluation; CN: Safe, effective care environment; CNS: Management of care; CL: Analysis

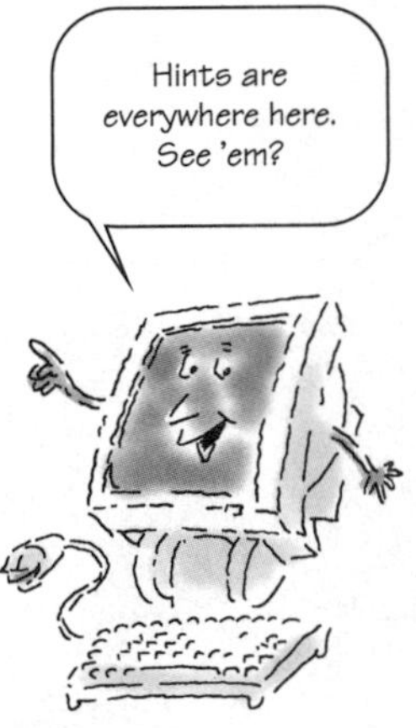

Hints are everywhere here. See 'em?

61. A client comes to the emergency department after hitting his head in a motor vehicle accident. He's alert and oriented. Which of the following nursing interventions should be done first?

1. Assess full range of motion (ROM) to determine the extent of injuries.
2. Call for an immediate chest X-ray.
3. Immobilize the client's head and neck.
4. Open the airway with the head-tilt chin-lift maneuver.

61. 3. All clients with a head injury are treated as if a cervical spine injury is present until X-rays confirm their absence. ROM would be contraindicated at this time. There is no indication the client needs a chest X-ray. The airway doesn't need to be opened since the client appears alert and not in respiratory distress. In addition, the head-tilt chin-lift maneuver wouldn't be used until cervical spine injury is ruled out.

NP: Implementation; CN: Physiological integrity; CNS: Reduction of risk potential; CL: Application

62. A client with a C6 spinal injury would most likely have which of the following symptoms?

1. Aphasia
2. Hemiparesis
3. Paraplegia
4. Tetraplegia

62. 4. Tetraplegia (quadriplegia) occurs as a result of cervical spine injuries. Aphasia refers to difficulty expressing or understanding spoken words. Hemiparesis describes weakness of one side of the body. Paraplegia occurs as a result of injury to the thoracic cord and below.

NP: Assessment; CN: Physiological integrity; CNS: Physiological adaptation; CL: Application

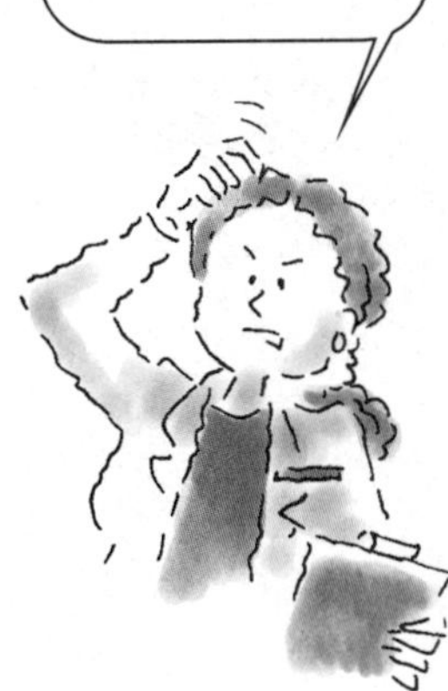

Let's see, what do all three of these brain areas have in common?

63. A client with damage to the hippocampus, amygdala, and fornix would have dysfunction in which of the following areas?

1. Emotions
2. Higher thought levels
3. Muscle synergy
4. Vital functions

63. 1. The hippocampus, amygdala, and fornix make up the limbic system, which regulates emotions. Higher thought level refers to the cortex. Muscle synergy is regulated by the cerebellum. The midbrain, pons, medulla oblongata, and reticular formation regulate vital functions.

NP: Assessment; CN: Safe, effective care environment; CNS: Management of care; CL: Knowledge

64. A 30-year-old client is admitted to the progressive care unit with a C5 fracture from a motorcycle accident. Which of the following assessments would take priority?
1. Bladder distention
2. Neurologic deficit
3. Pulse oximetry readings
4. The client's feelings about the injury

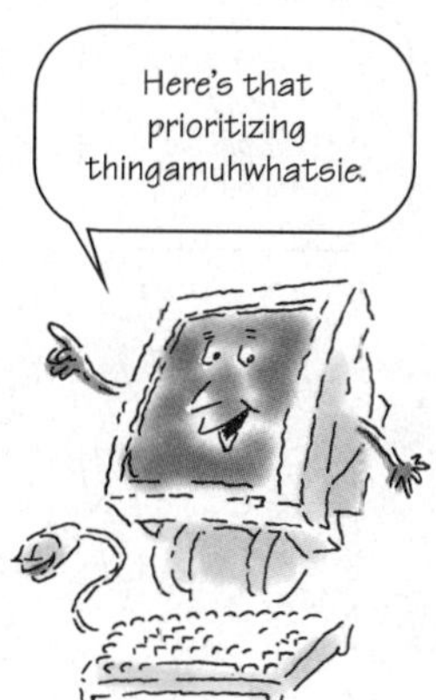

Here's that prioritizing thingamuhwhatsie.

64. 3. After a spinal cord injury, ascending cord edema may cause a higher level of injury. The diaphragm is innervated at the level of C4, so assessment of adequate oxygenation and ventilation is necessary. Although the other options would be necessary at a later time, observation for respiratory failure is the priority.
NP: Implementation; CN: Safe, effective care environment; CNS: Management of care; CL: Application

65. While in the emergency department, a client with C8 quadriplegia develops a blood pressure of 80/44 mm Hg, pulse of 48 beats/minute, and respiratory rate of 18 breaths/minute. The nurse suspects which of the following conditions?
1. Autonomic dysreflexia
2. Hemorrhagic shock
3. Neurogenic shock
4. Pulmonary embolism

65. 3. Symptoms of neurogenic shock include hypotension, bradycardia, and warm, dry skin due to loss of adrenergic stimulation below the level of the lesion. Hypertension, bradycardia, flushing, and sweating of the skin are seen with autonomic dysreflexia. Hemorrhagic shock presents with anxiety, tachycardia, and hypotension; this wouldn't be suspected without an injury. Pulmonary embolism presents with chest pain, hypotension, hypoxemia, tachycardia, and hemoptysis; this may be a later complication of spinal cord injury due to immobility.
NP: Assessment; CN: Health promotion and maintenance; CNS: Prevention and early detection of disease; CL: Analysis

66. A client is admitted with a spinal cord injury at the level of T12. He has limited movement of his upper extremities. Which of the following medications would be used to control edema of the spinal cord?
1. Acetazolamide (Diamox)
2. Furosemide (Lasix)
3. Methylprednisolone (Solu-Medrol)
4. Sodium bicarbonate

66. 3. High doses of methylprednisolone are used within 24 hours of spinal cord injury to reduce cord swelling and limit neurological deficit. The other drugs aren't indicated in this circumstance.
NP: Planning; CN: Physiological integrity; CNS: Pharmacological and parenteral therapies; CL: Application

67. A 22-year-old client with quadriplegia is apprehensive and flushed, with a blood pressure of 210/100 mm Hg and heart rate of 50 beats/minute. Which of the following nursing interventions should be done first?
1. Place the client flat in bed.
2. Assess patency of the indwelling urinary catheter.
3. Give one sublingual nitroglycerin tablet.
4. Raise the head of the bed immediately to 90 degrees.

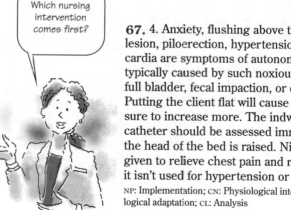

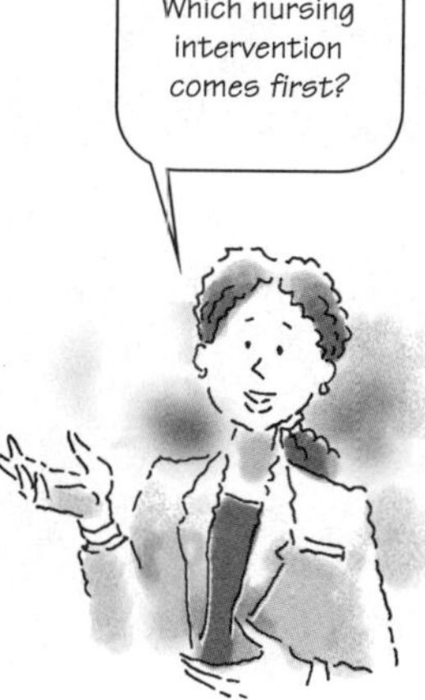

Which nursing intervention comes first?

67. 4. Anxiety, flushing above the level of the lesion, piloerection, hypertension, and bradycardia are symptoms of autonomic dysreflexia, typically caused by such noxious stimuli as a full bladder, fecal impaction, or decubitus ulcer. Putting the client flat will cause the blood pressure to increase more. The indwelling urinary catheter should be assessed immediately after the head of the bed is raised. Nitroglycerin is given to relieve chest pain and reduce preload; it isn't used for hypertension or dysreflexia.
NP: Implementation; CN: Physiological integrity; CNS: Physiological adaptation; CL: Analysis

68. A client with paraplegia from a T10 injury, is getting ready to transfer to a rehabilitation hospital. When a nurse offers to assist him, the client throws his suitcase on the floor and says, "You don't want to help me." Which of the following responses would be the most appropriate for the nurse to give?

1. "You know I want to help you, I offered."
2. "I'll pick these things up for you and come back later."
3. "You seem angry today. Going to rehab may be scary."
4. "When you get to rehab, they won't let you behave like a spoiled brat."

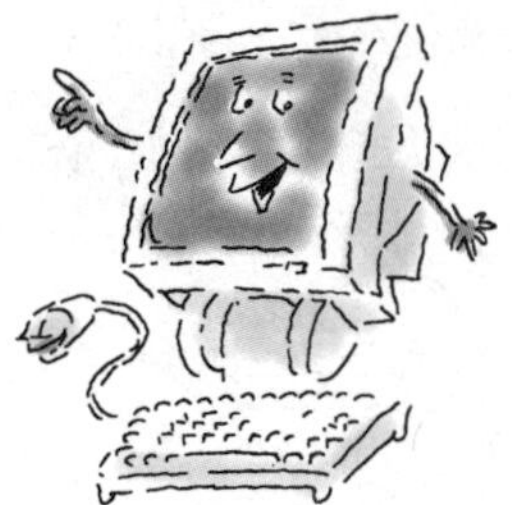

Choose the most therapeutic response.

68. 3. The nurse should always focus on the feelings underlying a particular action. Options 1 and 4 are confrontational. Offering to pick up the client's belongings doesn't deal with the situation and assumes he can't do it alone.

NP: Implementation; CN: Psychosocial integrity; CNS: Psychosocial adaptation; CL: Application

69. A client with a cervical spine injury has Gardner-Wells tongs inserted for which of the following reasons?

1. To hasten wound healing
2. To immobilize the surgical spine
3. To prevent autonomic dysreflexia
4. To hold bony fragments of the skull together

69. 2. Gardner-Wells, Vinke, and Crutchfield tongs immobilize the spine until surgical stabilization is accomplished. Tongs don't hasten wound healing, prevent autonomic dysreflexia, or hold bony fragments of the skull together.

NP: Implementation; CN: Physiological integrity; CNS: Physiological adaptation; CL: Comprehension

70. When a client with a halo vest is discharged from the hospital, which of the following instructions should the nurse give the client and family?

1. "Don't use the wheelchair while the halo vest is in place."
2. "Clean the pin sites with povidone-iodine and apply water-soluble lubricant."
3. "Keep the wrench that opens the vest attached to the client at all times."
4. "Perform range-of-motion exercises to the neck and shoulders four times daily."

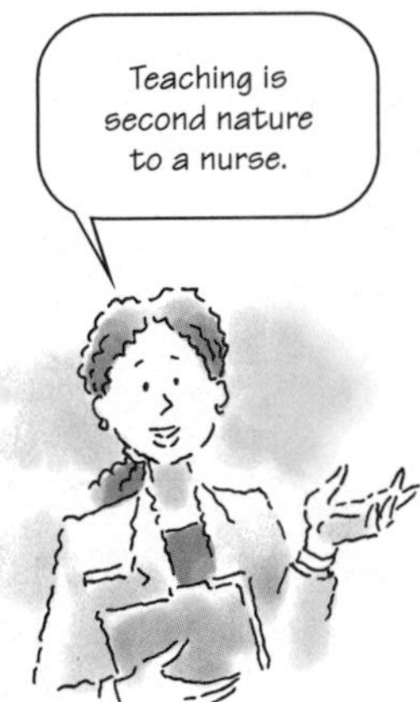

Teaching is second nature to a nurse.

70. 3. The wrench must be attached at all times to remove the vest in case the client needs cardiopulmonary resuscitation. The vest is designed to improve mobility; the client may use a wheelchair. The pins are cleaned with peroxide and povidone-iodine. The purpose of the vest is to immobilize the neck; range-of-motion exercises to the neck are prohibited but should be performed to other areas.

NP: Implementation; CN: Physiological integrity; CNS: Reduction of risk potential; CL: Application

71. Which of the following statements best describes the purpose of a Harrington rod?

1. It immobilizes the surgical spine.
2. It permits ambulation.
3. It stabilizes the knee joints.
4. It stabilizes the thoracolumbar spine.

71. 4. A Harrington rod is implanted to stabilize the thoracolumbar spine and provide upright posture. Harrington rods don't immobilize the spine, permit ambulation, or stabilize knee joints.

NP: Planning; CN: Safe, effective care environment; CNS: Management of care; CL: Comprehension

72. Which of the following interventions describes an appropriate bladder program for a client in rehabilitation for spinal cord injury?
1. Insert an indwelling urinary catheter to straight drainage.
2. Schedule intermittent catheterization every 2 to 4 hours.
3. Perform a straight catheterization every 8 hours while awake.
4. Perform Credé's maneuver to the lower abdomen before the client voids.

72. 2. Intermittent catheterization should begin every 2 to 4 hours early in treatment. When residual volume is less than 400 ml, the schedule may advance to every 4 to 6 hours. Indwelling catheters may predispose the client to infection and are removed as soon as possible. Credé's maneuver is applied after voiding to enhance bladder emptying.
NP: Implementation; CN: Physiological integrity; CNS: Basic care and comfort; CL: Application

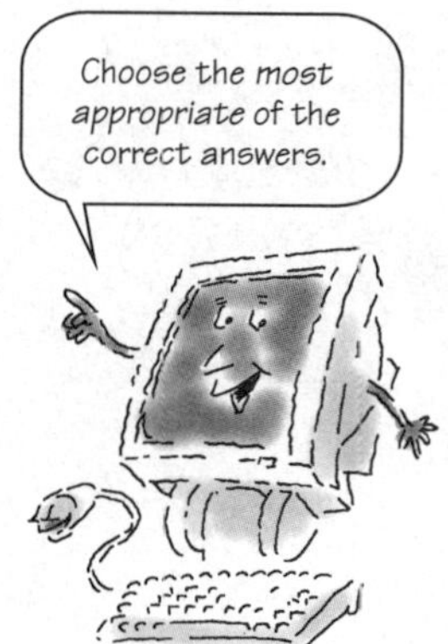

Choose the most appropriate of the correct answers.

73. A 46-year-old client with breast cancer complains of back pain and difficulty moving her legs. Which of the following nursing interventions is the most appropriate?
1. Notify the physician.
2. Position the client on her side, and prop her with a foam wedge.
3. Ask the physician for a physical therapy consultation.
4. Give acetaminophen, and reassure the client the pain will disappear soon.

73. 1. Symptoms of back pain and neurologic deficits may be symptoms of metastasis. The physician should be notified. Repositioning the client, physical therapy, or acetaminophen may help the pain but may delay evaluation and treatment.
NP: Implementation; CN: Health promotion and maintenance; CNS: Prevention and early detection of disease; CL: Analysis

74. A client was admitted to the hospital because of a transient ischemic attack secondary to atrial fibrillation. He would be given which of the following medications to prevent further neurologic deficit?
1. Digoxin (Lanoxin)
2. Diltiazem (Cardizem)
3. Heparin
4. Quinidine gluconate (Quinaglute Dura-Tabs)

74. 3. Atrial fibrillation may lead to the formation of mural thrombi, which may embolize to the brain. Heparin will prevent further clot formation and prevent clot enlargement. The other drugs are used in the treatment and control of atrial fibrillation but won't affect clot formation.
NP: Implementation; CN: Physiological integrity; CNS: Pharmacological and parenteral therapies; CL: Application

75. A client is diagnosed with Ménière's disease. Which of the following nursing diagnoses would take priority for this client?
1. Ineffective tissue perfusion (cerebral)
2. Imbalanced nutrition: More than body requirements
3. Impaired social interaction
4. Risk for injury

75. 4. Ménière's disease results in dizziness so the client should be protected from falling. Ménière's disease doesn't alter cerebral tissue perfusion or directly affect nutrition. Although hearing loss may occur, causing impaired social interaction, this isn't a priority.
NP: Implementation; CN: Safe, effective care environment; CNS: Safety and infection control; CL: Application

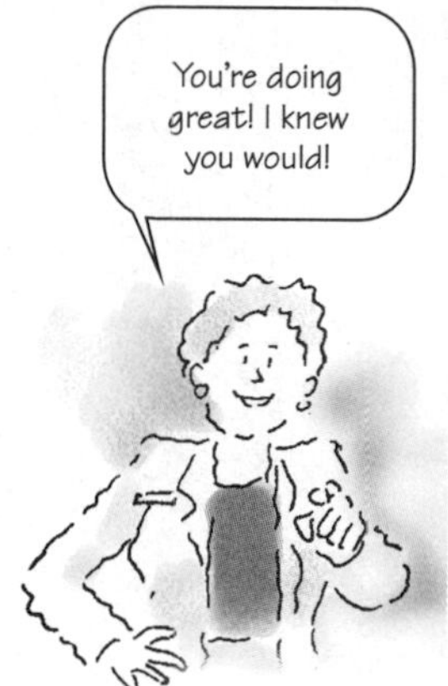

You're doing great! I knew you would!

76. Which of the following positions would be the most appropriate for a client who has undergone stapedectomy?
1. On the affected side
2. On the unaffected side
3. Prone
4. Sims'

76. 2. The client should be positioned with the operative ear up, on the unaffected side. Although Sims' position is a side-lying position, it doesn't consider which side is best for after ear surgery.
NP: Implementation; CN: Safe, effective care environment; CNS: Management of care; CL: Application

77. Which of the following symptoms would the nurse expect to find when assessing a client with Ménière's disease?

1. Epistaxis
2. Facial pain
3. Ptosis
4. Tinnitus

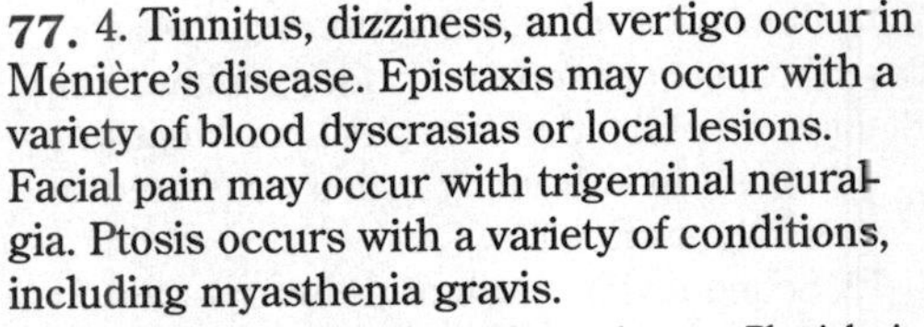

77. 4. Tinnitus, dizziness, and vertigo occur in Ménière's disease. Epistaxis may occur with a variety of blood dyscrasias or local lesions. Facial pain may occur with trigeminal neuralgia. Ptosis occurs with a variety of conditions, including myasthenia gravis.

NP: Assessment; CN: Physiological integrity; CNS: Physiological adaptation; CL: Application

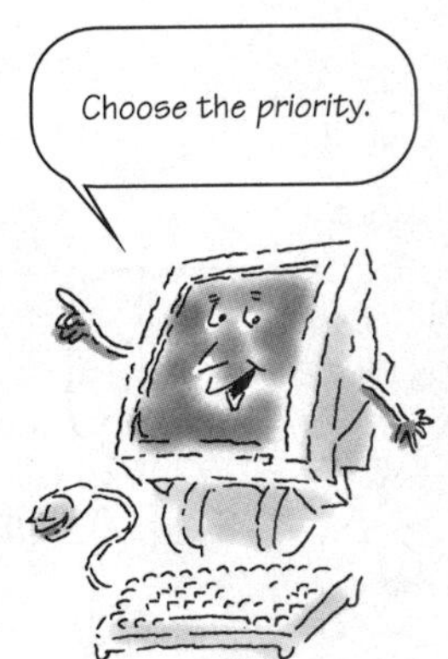
Choose the priority.

78. Which of the following nursing interventions has priority for an occupational nurse treating a client with a foreign body protruding from the eye?

1. Irrigate the eye with sterile saline.
2. Assess visual acuity with a Snellen chart.
3. Remove the foreign body with sterile forceps.
4. Patch both eyes until seen by the ophthalmologist.

78. 4. One or both eyes may be patched to prevent pain with extraocular movement or accommodation. Chemicals or small foreign bodies may be irrigated. Assessment of visual acuity isn't a priority, although it may be done after treatment. Protruding objects aren't removed by the nurse because the vitreous body may rupture.

NP: Implementation; CN: Safe, effective care environment CNS: Safety and infection control; CL: Application

79. A client with severe eye pain requests a prescription for the topical anesthetic the ophthalmologist instilled. A nurse explains these drugs shouldn't be used on an ongoing basis for which of the following reasons?

1. They are a way for pathogens to enter.
2. They cause dependence and rebound pain.
3. Damage could occur to the cornea due to lack of sensation.
4. The resulting blurred vision from mydriasis makes activity hazardous.

79. 3. Corneal damage may occur with the prolonged use of topical anesthetics. If the bottle isn't touched to the eye or lashes, the entry of pathogens should be limited. Dependence and rebound don't occur from topical anesthetics. Anesthetics don't cause mydriasis.

NP: Implementation; CN: Physiological integrity; CNS: Reduction of risk potential; CL: Application

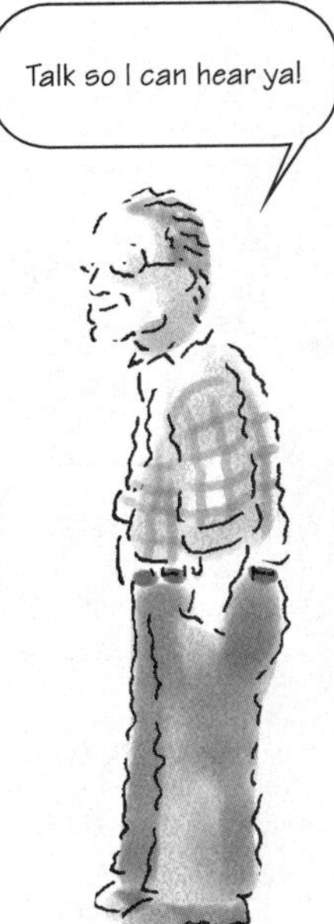
Talk so I can hear ya!

80. An 86-year-old client admitted to the hospital with chest pain is hearing impaired. Which of the following methods should be used when assessing the client?

1. Obtain an ear wick.
2. Shout into the better ear.
3. Lower your voice pitch while facing the client.
4. Ask the family to go home and get the client's hearing aid.

80. 3. Hearing loss in an elderly client typically involves the upper ranges; lowering the pitch of your voice and facing the client is essential for the client to use others means of understanding, such as lip reading, mood, and so on. An ear wick is used to allow medications to enter the ear canal. Shouting is typically in the upper ranges and could cause anxiety to an already anxious client. Alternate means of communication such as writing may also be used to assess chest pain while waiting for the family to bring the hearing aid from home.

NP: Assessment; CN: Physiological integrity; CNS: Basic care and comfort; CL: Application

81. A client is scheduled for magnetic resonance imaging (MRI) of the head. Which of the following areas is essential to assess before the procedure?

1. Food or drink intake within the past 8 hours
2. Metal fillings, prostheses, or a pacemaker
3. The presence of carotid artery disease
4. Voiding before the procedure

81. 2. Strong magnetic waves may dislodge metal in the client's body, causing tissue injury. Although the client may be told to restrict food for 8 hours, particularly if contrast is used, metal is an absolute contraindication for this procedure. Voiding beforehand would make the client more comfortable and better able to remain still during the procedure, but isn't essential for the test. Having carotid artery disease isn't a contraindication to having an MRI.

NP: Assessment; CN: Safe, effective care environment; CNS: Safety and infection control; CL: Application

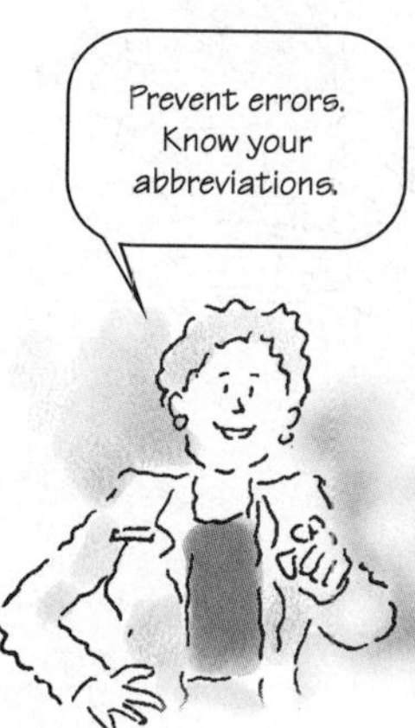

Prevent errors. Know your abbreviations.

82. When giving hydrocortisone, 1 gtt AU t.i.d., which of the following methods would the nurse use?

1. One drop into each ear three times daily
2. One drop into each eye three times daily
3. One drop of gold salts into each eye three times daily
4. Three drops into the right eye once daily

82. 1. A is the abbreviation for ears; O, for eyes; D, for right (*dexter* in Latin); and S, for left (*sinister* in Latin). AU refers to both ears. Although Au is the symbol for gold, gold isn't placed in the eye and isn't a correct option here.

NP: Implementation; CN: Physiological integrity; CNS: Pharmacological and parenteral therapies; CL: Comprehension

83. To properly instill eardrops in a 28-year-old client with otitis externa, which of the following methods is correct?

1. Pulling the pinna down and back
2. Pulling the pinna up and back
3. Pulling the tragus up and back
4. Separating the palpebral fissures with a clean gauze pad

83. 2. To straighten the ear canal of an adult, the pinna is pulled up and back. The other options aren't appropriate methods for preparing the ear to receive eardrops. The palpebral fissures are in the eye.

NP: Implementation; CN: Physiological integrity; CNS: Pharmacological and parenteral therapies; CL: Application

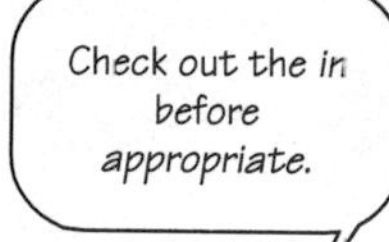

Check out the in before appropriate.

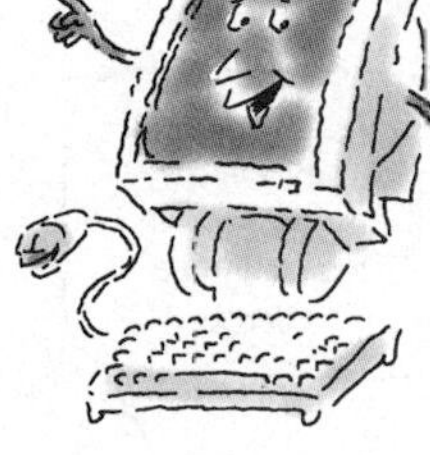

84. Which of the following instructions given to a client after cataract surgery is <u>in</u>appropriate?

1. "Avoid bending and straining"
2. "Avoid high-sodium foods to reduce intraocular pressure"
3. "Don't drive or sleep on the affected side"
4. "Don't use makeup on the affected eye"

84. 2. After cataract surgery, there's no need to restrict sodium. Using makeup, bending, straining, lifting, vomiting, and sleeping on the affected side may increase intraocular pressure and put strain on the sutures.

NP: Implementation; CN: Physiological integrity; CNS: Reduction of risk potential; CL: Application

85. Which of the following signs and symptoms of increased intracranial pressure (ICP) after head trauma would appear first?

1. Bradycardia
2. Large amounts of very dilute urine
3. Restlessness and confusion
4. Widened pulse pressure

85. 3. The earliest symptom of increased ICP is a change in mental status. Bradycardia, widened pulse pressure, and bradypnea occur later. The client may void large amounts of very dilute urine if there's damage to the posterior pituitary.

NP: Assessment; CN: Physiological integrity; CNS: Physiological adaptation; CL: Application

86. A client admitted to the emergency department for head trauma is diagnosed with an epidural hematoma. The underlying cause of epidural hematoma is usually related to which of the following conditions?

1. Laceration of the middle meningeal artery
2. Rupture of the carotid artery
3. Thromboembolism from a carotid artery
4. Venous bleeding from the arachnoid space

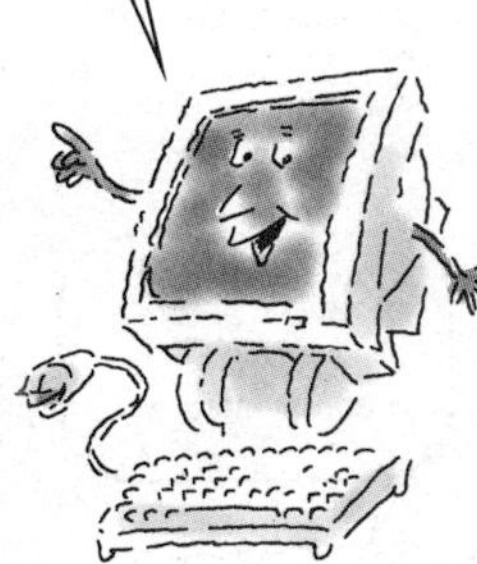

The word usually helps you choose between more than one correct answer.

86. 1. Epidural hematoma or extradural hematoma is usually caused by laceration of the middle meningeal artery. An embolic stroke is a thromboembolism from a carotid artery that ruptures. Venous bleeding from the arachnoid space is usually observed with subdural hematoma.

NP: Planning; CN: Physiological integrity; CNS: Physiological adaptation; CL: Comprehension

87. A 23-year-old client has been hit on the head with a baseball bat. The nurse notes clear fluid draining from his ears and nose. Which of the following nursing interventions should be done first?

1. Position the client flat in bed.
2. Check the fluid for dextrose with a dipstick.
3. Suction the nose to maintain airway patency.
4. Insert nasal and ear packing with sterile gauze.

87. 2. Clear liquid from the nose (rhinorrhea) or ear (otorrhea) can be determined to be cerebral spinal fluid or mucus by the presence of dextrose. Placing the client flat in bed may increase intracranial pressure and promote pulmonary aspiration The nose wouldn't be suctioned because of the risk for suctioning brain tissue through the sinuses. Nothing is inserted into the ears or nose of a client with a skull fracture because of the risk of infection.

NP: Assessment; CN: Physiological integrity; CNS: Physiological adaptation; CL: Analysis

88. When discharging a client from the emergency department after a head trauma, the nurse teaches the guardian to observe for a lucid interval. Which of the following statements best describes a lucid interval?

1. An interval when the client's speech is garbled
2. An interval when the client is alert but can't recall recent events
3. An interval when the client is oriented but then becomes somnolent
4. An interval when the client has a "warning" symptom, such as an odor or visual disturbance

88. 3. A lucid interval is described as a brief period of unconsciousness followed by alertness; after several hours, the client again loses consciousness. Garbled speech is known as dysarthria. An interval in which the client is alert but can't recall recent events is known as amnesia. Warning symptoms or auras typically occur before seizures.

NP: Implementation; CN: Health promotion and maintenance; CNS: Prevention and early detection of disease; CL: Comprehension

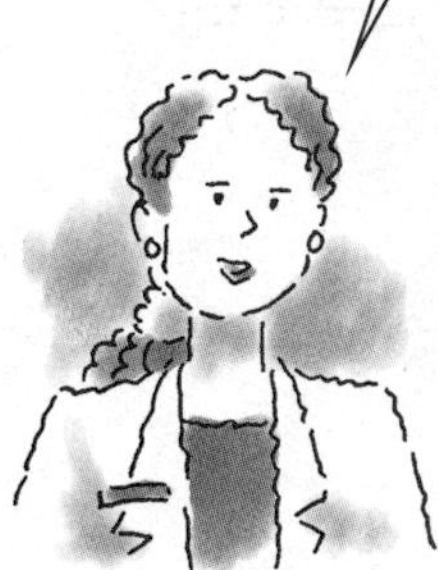

Teaching the family is as important as teaching the client.

89. When teaching the family of a client with C4 quadriplegia how to suction his tracheostomy, the nurse includes which of the following instructions?

1. Suction for 10 to 15 seconds at a time.
2. Regulate the suction machine to –300 cm suction.
3. Apply suction to the catheter during insertion only.
4. Pass the suction catheter into the opening of the tracheostomy tube ¾″ to 1¼″ (2 to 3 cm).

89. 1. Suction should be applied for 10 to 15 seconds at a time. Suction is regulated to 80 to 120 cm. Suction should be applied only during withdrawal of the catheter. When suctioning the trachea, the catheter is inserted 4″ to 6″ (10 to 15 cm) or until resistance is felt.

NP: Implementation; CN: Physiological integrity; CNS: Reduction of risk potential; CL: Application

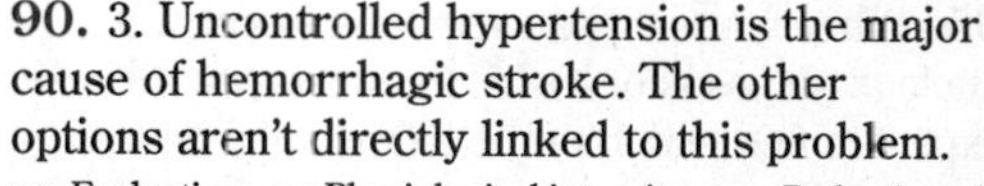

90. Which of the following conditions is a risk factor for hemorrhagic stroke?
1. Coronary artery disease
2. Diabetes
3. Hypertension
4. Recent viral infection

90. 3. Uncontrolled hypertension is the major cause of hemorrhagic stroke. The other options aren't directly linked to this problem.
NP: Evaluation; CN: Physiological integrity; CNS: Reduction of risk potential; CL: Application

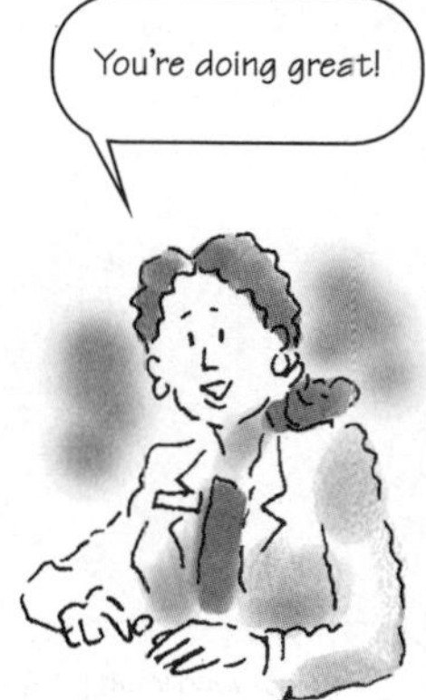
You're doing great!

91. An 86-year-old client with a stroke in evolution and a history of coronary artery disease is brought to the medical-surgical floor. His medications include heparin, isosorbide, and verapamil. Which of the following conditions should be avoided in a client with a stroke?
1. Dehydration
2. Hypocarbia
3. Hypotension
4. Tube feeding

91. 3. Isosorbide and verapamil can cause hypotension, which reduces brain perfusion and should be avoided in a client with a stroke. Dehydration would be inappropriate in this instance. Hypocarbia is used to reduce intracranial pressure through cerebral vasoconstriction. Nutrition may be delivered by tube when dysphagia exists.
NP: Planning; CN: Physiological integrity; CNS: Physiological adaptation; CL: Application

92. Which of the following clients on the rehabilitation unit is most likely to develop autonomic dysreflexia?
1. A client with brain injury
2. A client with herniated nucleus pulposus
3. A client with a high cervical spine injury
4. A client with a stroke

92. 3. Autonomic dysreflexia refers to uninhibited sympathetic outflow in clients with spinal cord injuries above the level of T10. The other clients aren't prone to dysreflexia.
NP: Planning; CN: Safe, effective care environment; CNS: Management of care; CL: Application

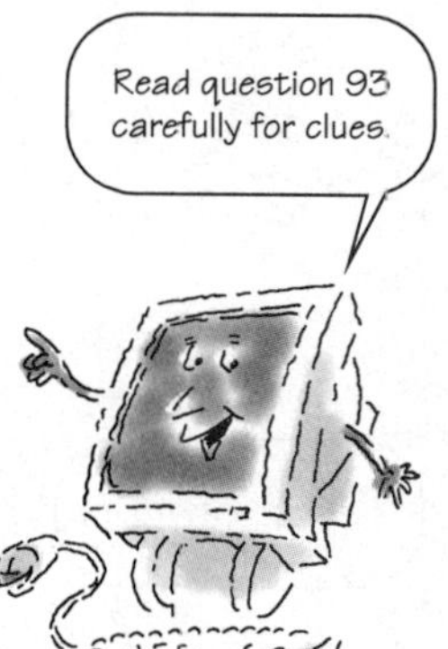
Read question 93 carefully for clues.

93. Which of the following conditions indicates that spinal shock is resolving in a client with C7 quadriplegia?
1. Absence of pain sensation in chest
2. Spasticity
3. Spontaneous respirations
4. Urinary continence

93. 2. Spasticity, the return of reflexes, is a sign of resolving shock. Spinal or neurogenic shock is characterized by hypotension, bradycardia, dry skin, flaccid paralysis, or the absence of reflexes below the level of injury. The absence of pain sensation in the chest doesn't apply to spinal shock. Spinal shock descends from the injury, and respiratory difficulties occur at C4 and above. Slight muscle contraction at the bulbocavernosus reflex occurs, but not enough for urinary continence.
NP: Assessment; CN: Physiological integrity; CNS: Physiological adaptation; CL: Application

94. When discharging a client from the hospital after a laminectomy, the nurse recognizes that the client needs further teaching when he makes which of the following statements?
1. "I'll sleep on a firm mattress."
2. "I won't drive for 2 to 4 weeks."
3. "When I pick things up, I'll bend my knees."
4. "I can't wait to pick up my granddaughter."

94. 4. Lifting more than 10 lb (4.5 kg) for several weeks after surgery is contraindicated. The other responses are appropriate.
NP: Evaluation; CN: Physiological integrity; CNS: Reduction of risk potential; CL: Analysis

95. When assessing a client with herniated nucleus pulposus of L4-L5, the nurse would expect to find which of the following signs and symptoms of spinal cord compression?

1. Lower back pain
2. Pain radiating across the buttocks
3. Positive Kernig's sign
4. Urinary incontinence

95. 4. Progressive neurological deficits at L4-L5, including worsening muscle weakness, paresthesia, and loss of bowel and bladder control, are symptoms of spinal cord compression. The other symptoms usually occur in clients with herniated nucleus pulposus.

NP: Planning; CN: Physiological integrity; CNS: Reduction of risk potential; CL: Analysis

96. A nurse assesses a client who has episodes of autonomic dysreflexia. Which of the following conditions can cause autonomic dysreflexia?

1. Headache
2. Lumbar spinal cord injury
3. Neurogenic shock
4. Noxious stimuli

96. 4. Noxious stimuli, such as a full bladder, fecal impaction, or a decubitus ulcer, may cause autonomic dysreflexia. A headache is a symptom of autonomic dysreflexia, not a cause. Autonomic dysreflexia is most commonly seen with injuries at T10 or above. Neurogenic shock isn't a cause of dysreflexia.

NP: Assessment; CN: Physiological integrity; CNS: Physiological adaptation; CL: Application

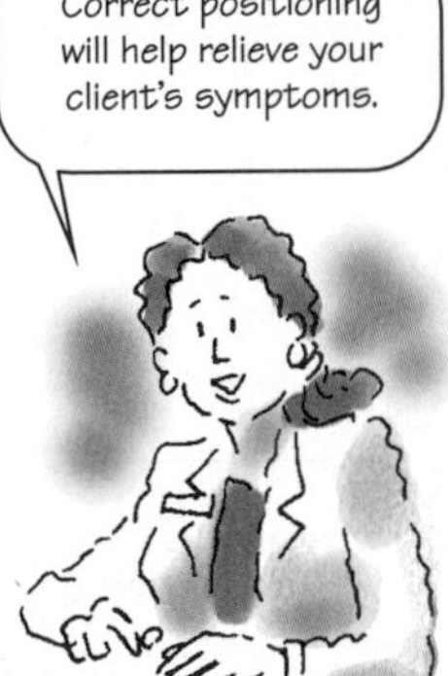

Correct positioning will help relieve your client's symptoms.

97. During an episode of autonomic dysreflexia in which the client becomes hypertensive, the nurse should perform which of the following interventions?

1. Elevate the client's legs.
2. Put the client flat in bed.
3. Put the bed in Trendelenburg's position.
4. Put the client in high Fowler's position.

97. 4. Putting the client in high Fowler's position will decrease cerebral blood flow, decreasing hypertension. Elevating the client's legs, putting the client flat in bed, or putting the bed in Trendelenburg's position places the client in positions that improve cerebral blood flow, worsening hypertension.

NP: Implementation; CN: Physiological integrity; CNS: Reduction of risk potential; CL: Application

98. A client recovering from a spinal cord injury has a great deal of spasticity. Which of the following medications may be used to control spasticity?

1. Hydralazine (Apresoline)
2. Baclofen (Lioresal)
3. Lidocaine (Xylocaine)
4. Methylprednisolone (Medrol)

98. 2. Baclofen is a skeletal muscle relaxant used to decrease spasms. Hydralazine is an antihypertensive and afterload reducing agent. Lidocaine is an antiarrhythmic and a local anesthetic agent. Methylprednisolone, an anti-inflammatory drug, is used to decrease spinal cord edema.

NP: Planning; CN: Physiological integrity; CNS: Pharmacological and parenteral therapies; CL: Application

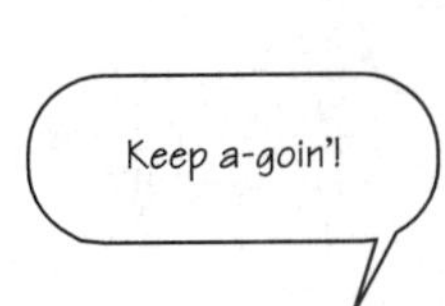

Keep a-goin'!

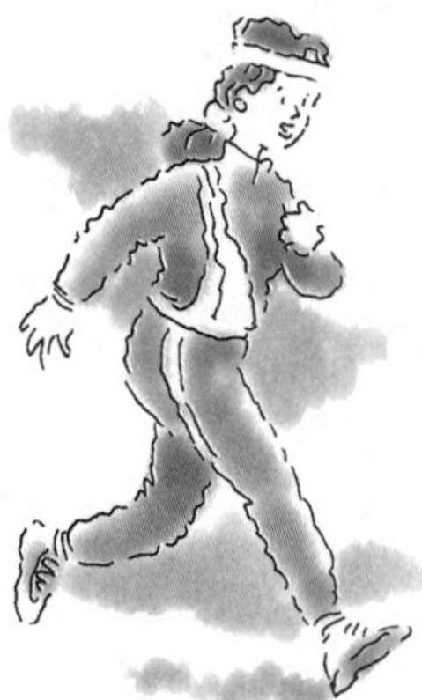

99. Client teaching for a client with Gardner-Wells tongs would include which of the following reasons for their use?

1. To reduce intracranial pressure (ICP)
2. To reduce dislocations and pain
3. To prevent deep vein thrombosis (DVT)
4. To improve neurologic outcome

99. 2. Gardner-Wells tongs are used to reduce dislocations, subluxations, pain, and spasm in cervical spinal cord injuries. They aren't used to reduce ICP, prevent DVT, or improve neurologic outcome.

NP: Implementation; CN: Physiological integrity; CNS: Reduction of risk potential; CL: Application

100. A client with a T1 spinal cord injury arrives at the emergency department with a blood pressure of 82/40 mm Hg; pulse, 34 beats/minute; dry skin, and flaccid paralysis of the lower extremities. Which of the following conditions would most likely be suspected?

1. Autonomic dysreflexia
2. Hypervolemia
3. Neurogenic shock
4. Sepsis

101. A client has a cervical spine injury at the level of C5. Which of the following conditions would the nurse anticipate during the acute phase?

1. Absent corneal reflex
2. Decerebrate posturing
3. Movement of only the right or left half of the body
4. The need for mechanical ventilation

102. When caring for a client with quadriplegia, which of the following nursing interventions takes priority?

1. Forcing fluids to prevent renal calculi
2. Maintaining skin integrity
3. Obtaining adaptive devices for more independence
4. Preventing atelectasis

103. A client with C7 quadriplegia is flushed and anxious and complains of a pounding headache. Which of the following symptoms would also be anticipated?

1. Decreased urine output or oliguria
2. Hypertension and bradycardia
3. Respiratory depression
4. Symptoms of shock

104. A client has a diagnosis of a stroke versus a transient ischemic attack (TIA). Which of the following statements shows the difference between a TIA and a stroke?

1. TIAs typically resolve in 24 hours.
2. TIAs may be hemorrhagic in origin.
3. TIAs may cause a permanent motor deficit.
4. TIAs may predispose the client to a myocardial infarction (MI).

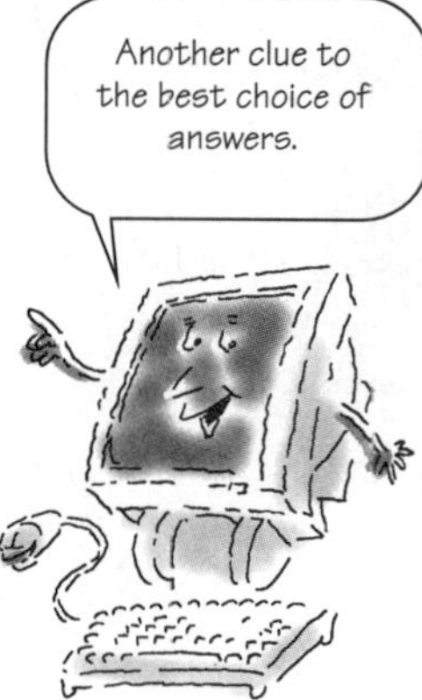

Another clue to the best choice of answers.

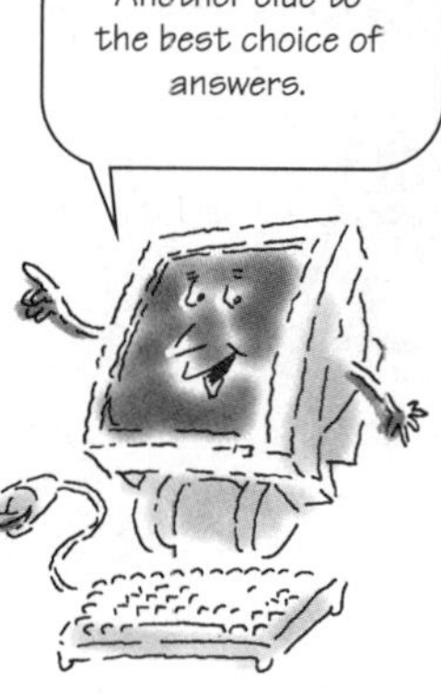

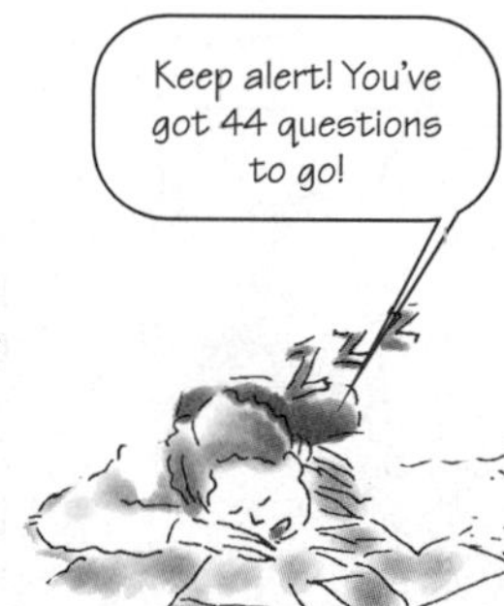

Keep alert! You've got 44 questions to go!

100. 3. Loss of sympathetic control and unopposed vagal stimulation below the level of the injury typically cause hypotension, bradycardia, pallor, flaccid paralysis, and warm, dry skin in the client in neurogenic shock. Hypervolemia is indicated by a rapid and bounding pulse and edema. Autonomic dysreflexia occurs after neurogenic shock abates. Signs of sepsis would include elevated temperature, increased heart rate, and increased respiratory rate.

NP: Assessment; CN: Physiological integrity; CNS: Physiological adaptation; CL: Analysis

101. 4. The diaphragm is stimulated by nerves at the level of C4. Initially, this client may need mechanical ventilation due to cord edema. This may resolve in time. Absent corneal reflexes, decerebrate posturing, and hemiplegia occur with brain injuries, not spinal cord injuries.

NP: Planning; CN: Physiological integrity; CNS: Physiological adaptation; CL: Application

102. 4. Clients with quadriplegia have paralysis or weakness of the diaphragm, abdominal, or intercostal muscles. Maintenance of airway and breathing take top priority. Although forcing fluids, maintaining skin integrity, and obtaining adaptive devices for more independence are all important interventions, preventing atelectasis has more priority.

NP: Planning; CN: Physiological integrity; CNS: Reduction of risk potential; CL: Application

103. 2. Hypertension, bradycardia, anxiety, blurred vision, and flushing above the lesion occur with autonomic dysreflexia due to uninhibited sympathetic nervous system discharge. The other options are incorrect.

NP: Assessment; CN: Physiological integrity; CNS: Physiological adaptation; CL: Analysis

104. 1. Symptoms of a TIA result from a transient lack of oxygen to the brain and usually resolve within 24 hours. Hemorrhage into the brain has the worst neurological outcome and isn't associated with a TIA. A permanent motor deficit doesn't result from a TIA. Unstable angina, not a TIA, may predispose the client to a future MI.

NP: Planning; CN: Physiological integrity; CNS: Physiological adaptation; CL: Comprehension

105. A client with a right stroke has a flaccid left side. Which of the following interventions would best prevent shoulder subluxation?
1. Splint the wrist.
2. Use an air splint.
3. Put the affected arm in a sling.
4. Perform range-of-motion exercises on the affected side.

105. 3. Due to the weight of the flaccid extremity, the shoulder may disarticulate. A sling will support the extremity. The other options won't support the shoulder.
NP: Planning; CN: Physiological integrity; CNS: Basic care and comfort; CL: Application

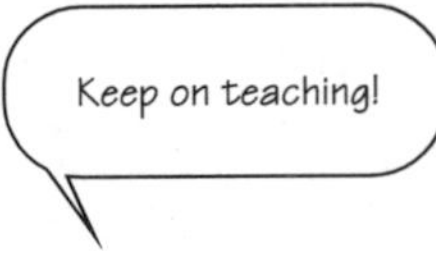

Keep on teaching!

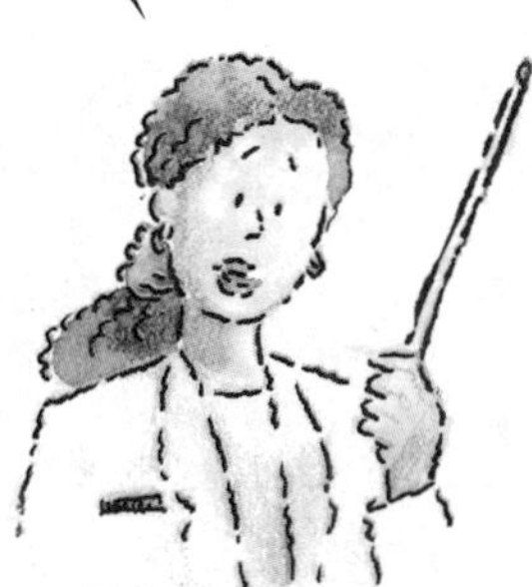

106. A 40-year-old paraplegic must perform intermittent catheterization of the bladder. Which of the following instructions should be given?
1. "Clean the meatus from back to front."
2. "Measure the quantity of urine."
3. "Gently rotate the catheter during removal."
4. "Clean the meatus with soap and water."

106. 4. Intermittent catheterization may be performed chronically with clean technique, using soap and water to clean the urinary meatus. The meatus is always cleaned from front to back in a woman, or in expanding circles working outward from the meatus in a man. It isn't necessary to measure the urine. The catheter doesn't need to be rotated during removal.
NP: Planning; CN: Physiological integrity; CNS: Basic care and comfort; CL: Application

107. Which of the following methods should be used to assess pupil accommodation?
1. Assessing for peripheral vision
2. Touching the cornea lightly with a wisp of cotton
3. Having the client follow an object upward, downward, obliquely, and horizontally
4. Observing for pupil constriction and convergence while focusing on an object coming toward the client

107. 4. Accommodation refers to convergence and constriction of the pupil while following a near object. Assessing for peripheral vision refers to visual fields. Touching the cornea lightly with a wisp of cotton describes assessment of the corneal reflex. Having the client follow an object upward, downward, obliquely, and horizontally refers to cardinal fields of gaze.
NP: Assessment; CN: Physiological integrity; CNS: Physiological adaptation; CL: Application

108. A client at the eye clinic reports difficulty seeing at night. This may result from which of the following nutritional deficiencies?
1. Vitamin A
2. Vitamin B_6
3. Vitamin C
4. Vitamin K

108. 1. Night blindness (nyctalopia) may be caused from a vitamin A deficiency or dysfunctional rod receptors. None of the other deficiencies lead to nyctalopia.
NP: Assessment; CN: Physiological integrity; CNS: Physiological adaptation; CL: Application

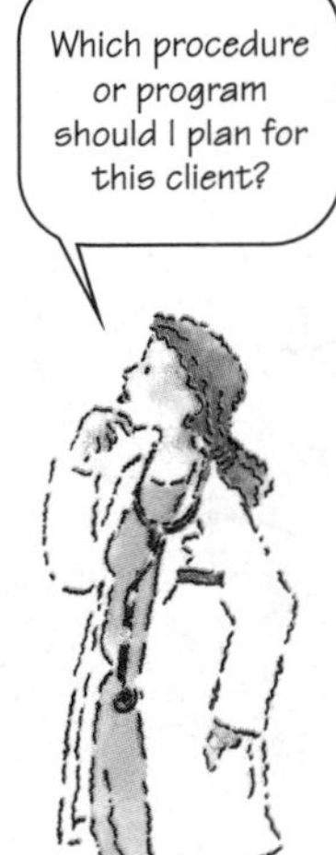

Which procedure or program should I plan for this client?

109. A client with a spinal cord injury has a neurogenic bladder. When planning for discharge, the nurse anticipates the client will need which of the following procedures or programs?
1. Intermittent catheterization program
2. Kock pouch
3. Transurethral prostatectomy
4. Ureterostomy

109. 1. Intermittent catheterization, starting with 2-hour intervals and increasing to 4- to 6-hour intervals, is used to manage neurogenic bladder. A Kock pouch is a type of urinary diversion. Transurethral prostatectomy is indicated for obstruction to urinary outflow by benign prostatic hyperplasia or for the treatment of cancer. An ileostomy or ureterostomy isn't necessary.
NP: Planning; CN: Physiological integrity; CNS: Basic care and comfort; CL: Application

119. A client underwent an enucleation of the right eye for a malignancy. Which of the following interventions will the nurse perform?

1. Instilling miotics as ordered to the affected eye
2. Teaching the client to clean the prosthesis in soap and water
3. Assessing reactivity of the pupils to light and accommodation
4. Teaching the client to prevent straining at stool leading to increased intraocular pressure

119. 2. Enucleation of the eye refers to surgical removal of the entire eye; therefore, the client needs instructions about the prosthesis. There are no activity restrictions or need for eye drops; however, prophylactic antibiotics may be used in the immediate postoperative period.

NP: Planning; CN: Physiological integrity; CNS: Physiological adaptation; CL: Application

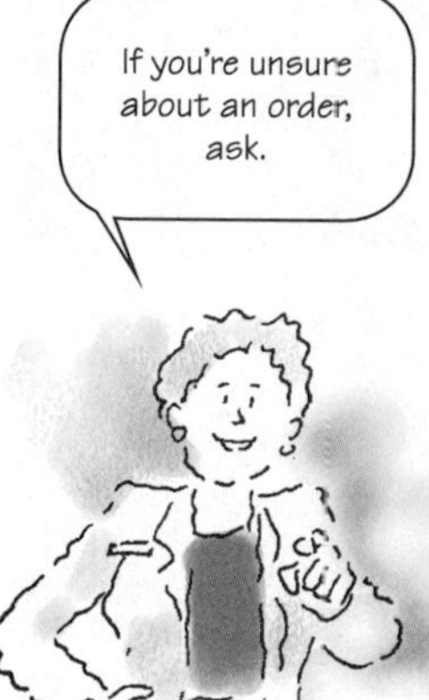

If you're unsure about an order, ask.

120. A nurse would question an order to irrigate the ear canal in which of the following circumstances?

1. Ear pain
2. Hearing loss
3. Otitis externa
4. Perforated tympanic membrane

120. 4. Irrigation of the ear canal is contraindicated with perforation of the tympanic membrane because solution entering the inner ear may cause dizziness, nausea, vomiting, and infection. The other conditions aren't contraindications to irrigation of the ear canal.

NP: Planning; CN: Physiological integrity; CNS: Reduction of risk potential; CL: Application

121. Which of the following interventions is essential when instilling Cortisporin suspension, 2 gtts AD?

1. Verifying the proper client and route
2. Warming the solution to prevent dizziness
3. Holding an emesis basin under the client's ear
4. Positioning the client in the semi-Fowler's position

121. 1. When giving medications, a nurse follows the five R's of medication administration: right client, right drug, right dose, right route, and right time. The drops may be warmed to prevent pain or dizziness, but this action isn't essential. An emesis basin would be used for irrigation of the ear. Put the client in the lateral position to prevent the drops from draining out for 5 minutes, not semi-Fowler's position.

NP: Planning; CN: Physiological integrity; CNS: Pharmacological and parenteral therapies; CL: Application

122. When teaching the client with Ménière's disease, which of the following instructions would a nurse give about vertigo?

1. "Report dizziness at once."
2. "Drive in daylight hours only."
3. "Get up slowly, turning the entire body."
4. "Change your position using the logroll technique."

122. 3. Turning the entire body, not the head, will prevent vertigo. Dizziness is expected but can be prevented with Ménière's disease. The client shouldn't drive as he may reflexively turn the wheel to correct for vertigo. Turning the client in bed slowly and smoothly will be helpful; logrolling isn't needed.

NP: Implementation; CN: Physiological integrity; CNS: Reduction of risk potential; CL: Application

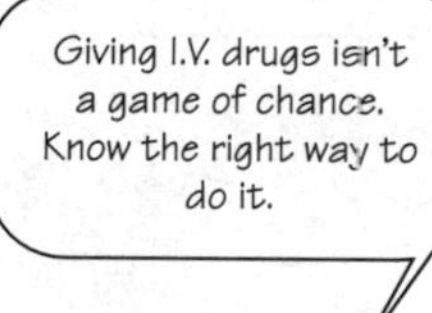

Giving I.V. drugs isn't a game of chance. Know the right way to do it.

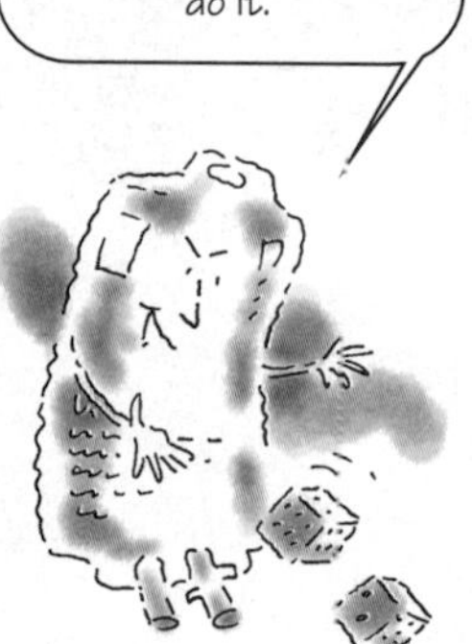

123. When giving I.V. phenytoin (Dilantin), which of the following methods should be used?

1. Administering rapidly
2. Withholding other anticonvulsants
3. Mixing the drug with saline solution only
4. Flushing the I.V. catheter with dextrose solution

123. 3. Phenytoin is compatible only with saline solutions; dextrose causes an insoluble precipitate to form. Phenytoin should be administered slowly (50 mg/minute). There's no need to withhold additional anticonvulsants.

NP: Implementation; CN: Physiological integrity; CNS: Pharmacological and parenteral therapies; CL: Application

124. An 18-year-old client was hit in the head with a baseball during practice. When discharging him to the care of his mother, the nurse gives which of the following instructions?

1. "Watch him for keyhole pupil for the next 24 hours."
2. "Expect profuse vomiting for 24 hours after the injury."
3. "Wake him every hour and assess his orientation to person, time, and place."
4. "Notify the physician immediately if he has a headache."

Instruct the client's mother about the care for her son's injury.

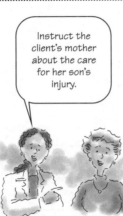

125. A client taking carbamazepine (Tegretol) should be monitored for which of the following potential complications?

1. Adult respiratory distress syndrome (ARDS)
2. Diplopia
3. Elevated levels of phenytoin (Dilantin)
4. Leukocytosis

126. For a client with damage to the caudate nucleus, putamen, and globus pallidus, which of the following conditions should be monitored?

1. Eye movement
2. Modulation of sounds
3. Motor movement
4. Muscle synergy

127. Nursing care of a client with damage to the thalamus, hypothalamus, and pineal gland would be based on knowing the client has problems in which of the following areas?

1. Seizure control
2. Identifying foreign agents
3. Difficulty regulating emotions
4. Initiating movements and maintaining temperature control and the sleep-awake cycle

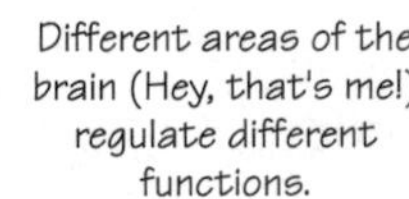

Different areas of the brain (Hey, that's me!) regulate different functions.

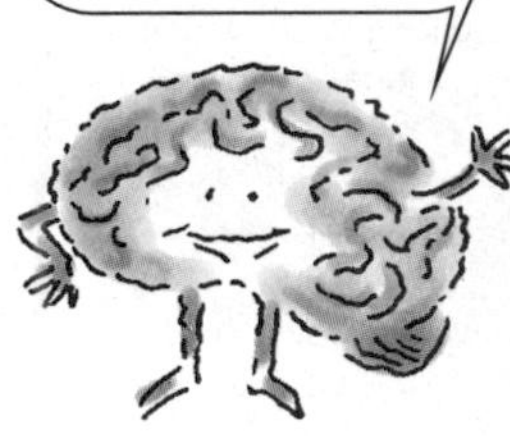

124. 3. Changes in level of consciousness (LOC) may indicate expanding lesions such as subdural hematoma; orientation and LOC are assessed frequently for 24 hours. A keyhole pupil is found after iridectomy. Profuse or projectile vomiting is a symptom of increased intracranial pressure and should be reported immediately. A slight headache may last for several days after concussion; severe or worsening headaches should be reported.

NP: Implementation; CN: Physiological integrity; CNS: Physiological adaptation; CL: Application

125. 2. Carbamazepine is more likely to cause diplopia, dizziness, ataxia, and a rash. ARDS isn't a complication of carbamazepine. Carbamazepine decreases blood levels of phenytoin and oral contraceptives; it also causes agranulocytosis because of the reduction in leukocytes.

NP: Analysis; CN: Physiological integrity; CNS: Pharmacological and parenteral therapies; CL: Comprehension

126. 3. Motor movement is regulated by the basal ganglia, which consists of the caudate nucleus, putamen, and globus pallidus. Eye movement is too vague because there are several cranial nerves responsible for various forms of eye movement. Modulation of sounds occurs from the occipital lobe. The cerebellum regulates muscle synergy.

NP: Planning; CN: Safe, effective care environment; CNS: Management of care; CL: Application

127. 4. The thalamus is the relay center of communication of sensory and motor information between the higher and lower regions of the brain. The hypothalamus regulates temperature control, and the pineal gland is important to the sleep-awake cycle. Seizure control is more related to neurotransmitter dysfunction. Identifying foreign agents is a function of the immune system. Regulating emotions is a function of the limbic system.

NP: Assessment; CN: Safe, effective care environment; CNS: Management of care; CL: Knowledge

128. Problems with memory and learning would relate to which of the following lobes?
1. Frontal
2. Occipital
3. Parietal
4. Temporal

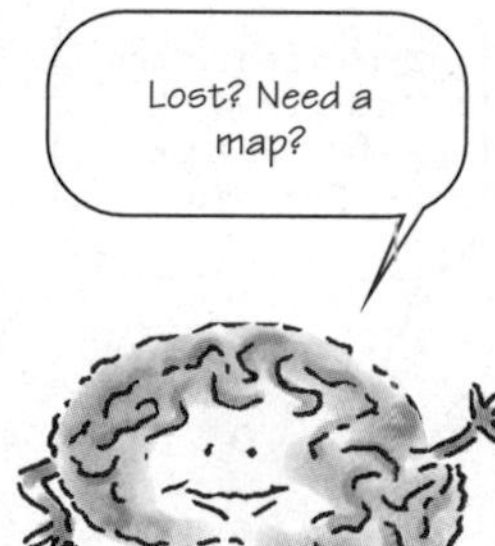
Lost? Need a map?

128. 4. The temporal lobe functions to regulate memory and learning problems because of the integration of the hippocampus. The frontal lobe primarily functions to regulate thinking, planning, and judgment. The occipital lobe functions to regulate vision. The parietal lobe primarily functions with sensory function.

NP: Analysis; CN: Physiological integrity; CNS: Physiological adaptation; CL: Knowledge

129. While cooking, your client couldn't feel the temperature of a hot oven. Which lobe could be dysfunctional?
1. Frontal
2. Occipital
3. Parietal
4. Temporal

129. 3. The parietal lobe regulates sensory function, which would include the ability to sense hot or cold objects. The frontal lobe regulates thinking, planning, and judgment, and the occipital lobe is primarily responsible for vision function. The temporal lobe regulates memory.

NP: Assessment; CN: Safe, effective care environment; CNS: Safety and infection control; CL: Knowledge

130. Which neurotransmitter is responsible for many of the functions of the frontal lobe?
1. Dopamine
2. Gamma-aminobutyric acid (GABA)
3. Histamine
4. Norepinephrine

130. 1. The frontal lobe primarily functions to regulate thinking, planning, and affect. Dopamine is known to circulate widely throughout this lobe, which is why it's such an important neurotransmitter in schizophrenia. GABA is widely circulated in the hippocampus and hypothalamus. Histamine is primarily found in the hypothalamus. Norepinephrine primarily functions with the hippocampal region not located in the frontal lobe.

NP: Analysis; CN: Physiological integrity; CNS: Physiological adaptation; CL: Knowledge

131. The nurse is discussing the purpose of an electroencephalogram (EEG) with the family of a client with massive cerebral hemorrhage and loss of consciousness. It would be most accurate for the nurse to tell family members that the test measures which of the following conditions?
1. Extent of intracranial bleeding
2. Sites of brain injury
3. Activity of the brain
4. Percent of functional brain tissue

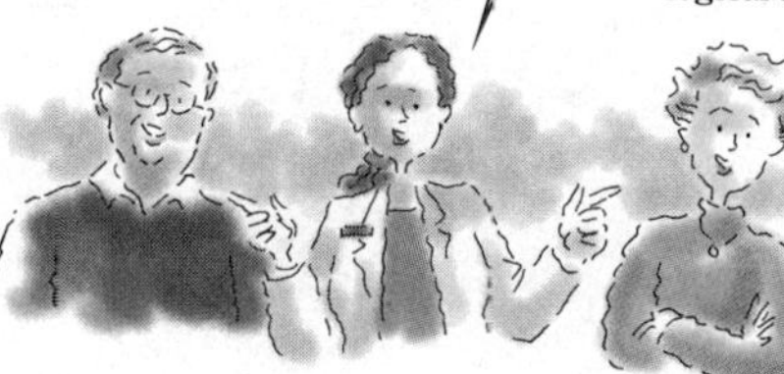
What should I be telling the family of a client about an EEG?

131. 3. An EEG measures the electrical activity of the brain. Extent of intracranial bleeding and location of the injury site would be determined by computerized tomography or magnetic resonance imaging. Percent of functional brain tissue would be determined by a series of tests.

NP: Implementation; CN: Physiological integrity; CNS: Physiological adaptation; CL: Comprehension

132. The nurse is teaching a client and his family about dietary practices related to Parkinson's disease. Which of the following signs and symptoms would be most important for the nurse to address?

1. Fluid overload and drooling
2. Aspiration and anorexia
3. Choking and diarrhea
4. Dysphagia and constipation

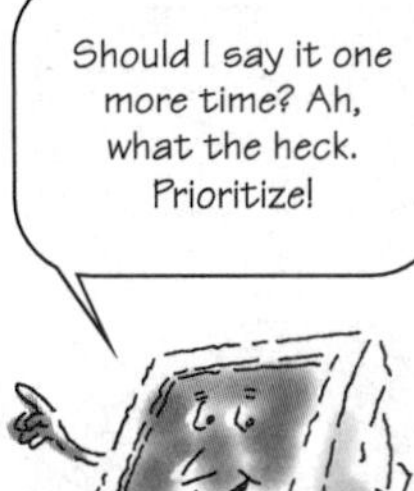

Should I say it one more time? Ah, what the heck. Prioritize!

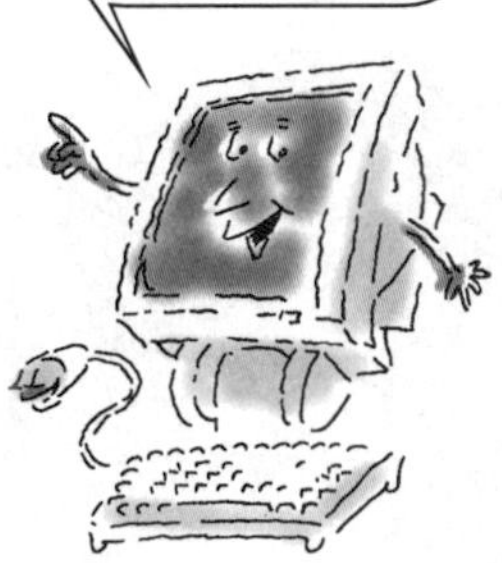

132. 4. The eating problems associated with Parkinson's disease include dysphagia, risk of choking, aspiration, and constipation. Fluid overload, anorexia, and diarrhea aren't problems specifically related to Parkinson's disease.

NP: Implementation; CN: Physiological integrity; CNS: Reduction of risk potential; CL: Analysis

133. In some clients with multiple sclerosis (MS), plasmapheresis diminishes symptoms. Plasmapheresis achieves this effect by removing which of the following blood components?

1. Catecholamines
2. Antibodies
3. Plasma proteins
4. Lymphocytes

133. 2. In plasmapheresis, antibodies are removed from the client's plasma. Antibodies attack the myelin sheath of the neuron causing the manifestations of MS. The treatment of MS with plasmapheresis isn't for the purpose of removing catecholamines, plasma proteins, or lymphocytes.

NP: Evaluation; CN: Physiological integrity; CNS: Physiological adaptation; CL: Comprehension

134. The nurse performs a neurologic assessment on a client complaining of headache and dizziness. Which assessment technique helps assess the motor function of cranial nerve VII?

1. Asking the client to clench his jaw
2. Testing the gag reflex by placing an applicator against the pharynx
3. Asking the client to frown, smile, and raise his eyebrows
4. Asking the client to swallow

134. 3. To assess the motor function of cranial nerve VII, the nurse should ask the client to frown, smile, and raise his eyebrows. If these facial expressions are symmetrical, motor function is intact. Jaw clenching is a test for cranial nerve V function. Testing the gag reflex by placing an applicator against the pharynx, and assessing swallowing ability are ways to evaluate cranial nerve IX function. Testing the gag reflex also helps assess cranial nerve X function.

NP: Assessment; CN: Health promotion and maintenance; CNS: Prevention and early detection of disease; CL: Application

135. An unconscious client is receiving mechanical ventilation. Which nursing diagnosis takes priority?

1. Ineffective airway clearance related to the inability to expectorate
2. Risk for impaired skin integrity related to immobility
3. Imbalanced nutrition: Less than body requirements related to inability to swallow
4. Dressing or grooming self-care deficit related to unconsciousness

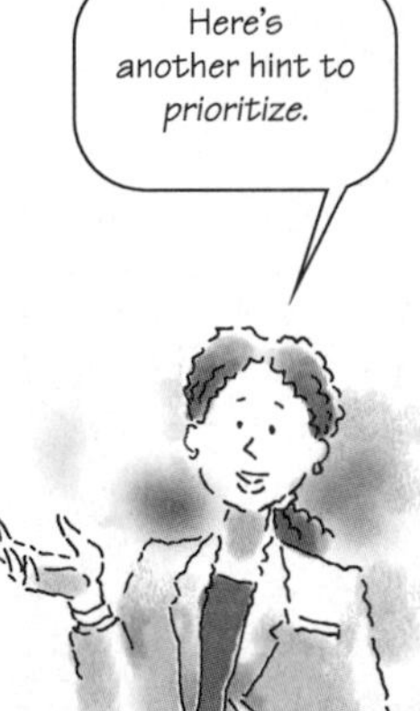

Here's another hint to prioritize.

135. 1. Ineffective airway clearance related to the inability to expectorate takes priority in an unconscious client. The other nursing diagnoses are appropriate but are less important than airway, breathing, and circulation.

NP: Analysis; CN: Physiological integrity; CNS: Physiological adaptation; CL: Application

136. An 18-year-old client is admitted with a closed head injury sustained in a motor vehicle accident. His intracranial pressure (ICP) shows an upward trend. Which intervention should the nurse perform first?

1. Reposition the client to avoid neck flexion.
2. Administer 1 g of mannitol (Osmitrol) I.V. as ordered.
3. Increase the ventilator's respiratory rate to 20 breaths/minute.
4. Administer 100 mg of pentobarbital (Nembutal) I.V. as ordered.

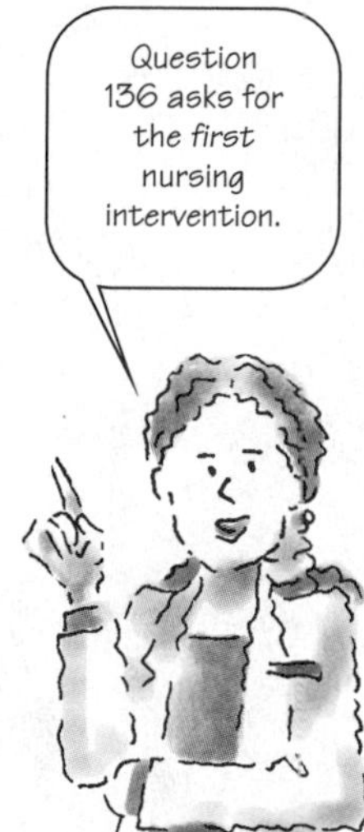

Question 136 asks for the first nursing intervention.

136. 1. The nurse should first attempt nursing interventions, such as repositioning the client to avoid neck flexion, which increases venous return and lowers ICP. If nursing measures prove ineffective, notify the physician, who may prescribe mannitol, pentobarbital, or hyperventilation therapy.

NP: Implementation; CN: Physiological integrity; CNS: Physiological adaptation; CL: Application

137. A client arrives at the emergency department after slipping on a patch of ice and hitting her head. A computed tomography scan of the head shows a collection of blood between the skull and dura mater. Which type of head injury does this finding suggest?

1. Subdural hematoma
2. Subarachnoid hemorrhage
3. Epidural hematoma
4. Contusion

137. 3. An epidural hematoma occurs when blood collects between the skull and dura mater. In a subdural hematoma, venous blood collects between the dura mater and arachnoid mater. In a subarachnoid hemorrhage, blood collects between the pia mater and arachnoid membrane. A contusion is a bruise on the brain's surface.

NP: Assessment; CN: Physiological integrity; CNS: Physiological adaptation; CL: Application

138. After falling 20′ (6 m), a 36-year-old construction worker sustains a C6 fracture with spinal cord transection. Which other findings should the nurse expect?

1. Quadriplegia with gross arm movement and diaphragmatic breathing
2. Quadriplegia and loss of respiratory function
3. Paraplegia with intercostal muscle loss
4. Loss of bowel and bladder control

138. 1. A client with a spinal cord injury at levels C5 to C6 has quadriplegia with gross arm movement and diaphragmatic breathing. Injuries at levels C1 to C4 lead to quadriplegia with total loss of respiratory function. Paraplegia with intercostal muscle loss occurs with injuries at T1 to L2. Injuries below L2 cause paraplegia and loss of bowel and bladder control.

NP: Assessment; CN: Physiological integrity; CNS: Physiological adaptation; CL: Application

139. A client with a subarachnoid hemorrhage is prescribed a 1,000-mg loading dose of phenytoin (Dilantin) I.V. Which consideration is most important when administering this dose?

1. Therapeutic drug levels should be maintained between 20 to 30 mg/ml.
2. Rapid phenytoin administration can cause cardiac arrhythmias.
3. Phenytoin should be mixed in dextrose in water before administration.
4. Phenytoin should be administered through an I.V. catheter in the client's hand.

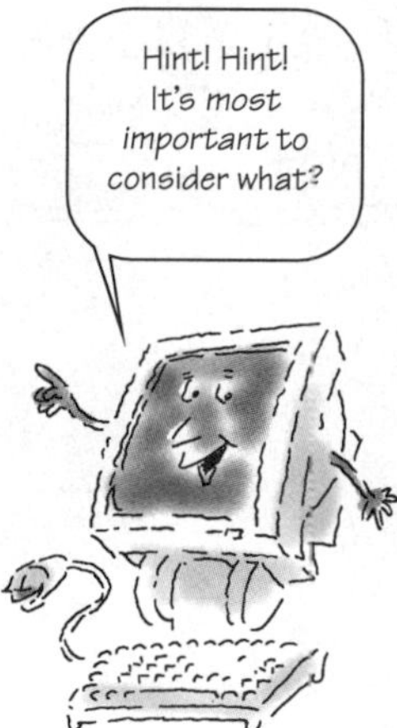

Hint! Hint! It's most important to consider what?

139. 2. Phenytoin I.V. shouldn't be given at a rate exceeding 50 mg/minute. Rapid administration can depress the myocardium, causing arrhythmias. Therapeutic drug levels range from 10 to 20 mg/ml. Phenytoin shouldn't be mixed in solution for administration. However, because it's compatible with normal saline solution, it can be injected through an I.V. line containing normal saline solution. When given through an I.V. catheter in the hand, phenytoin may cause purple glove syndrome.

NP: Implementation; CN: Physiological integrity; CNS: Pharmacological and parenteral therapies; CL: Application

140. The nurse is developing a discharge teaching plan for a client who has been prescribed phenytoin (Dilantin). Which instruction should the plan include?

1. "Take the drug on an empty stomach."
2. "You can consume alcoholic beverages in moderation."
3. "You can take any phenytoin brand because all brands are the same."
4. "Don't stop taking the drug except with medical supervision."

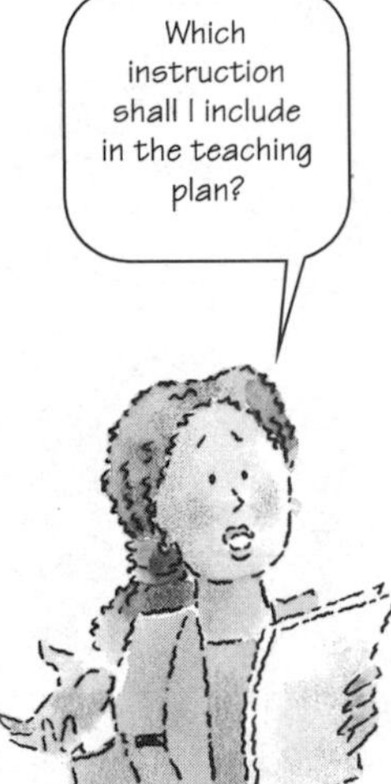

Which instruction shall I include in the teaching plan?

140. 4. Abrupt phenytoin withdrawal may trigger status epilepticus, so the client should be warned not to stop taking the drug unless the physician approves. Taking phenytoin with food minimizes GI distress. Alcoholic beverages can decrease the drug's effectiveness. Changing phenytoin brands may alter the therapeutic effect.

NP: Planning; CN: Physiological integrity; CNS: Pharmacological and parenteral therapies; CL: Application

141. A 20-year-old client who fell approximately 30′ (9 m) is unresponsive and breathless. A cervical spine injury is suspected. How should the first-responder open the client's airway for rescue breathing?

1. By inserting a nasopharyngeal airway
2. By inserting an oropharyngeal airway
3. By performing the jaw-thrust maneuver
4. By performing the head-tilt, chin-lift maneuver

141. 3. If the client has a suspected cervical spine injury, the jaw-thrust maneuver should be used to open the airway. If the tongue or relaxed throat muscles are obstructing the airway, a nasopharyngeal or oropharyngeal airway can be inserted; however, the client must have spontaneous respirations when the airway is open. The head-tilt, chin-lift maneuver requires neck hyperextension, which can worsen a cervical spine injury.

NP: Implementation; CN: Physiological integrity; CNS: Physiological adaptation; CL: Analysis

142. An 87-year-old client is admitted with a stroke. During the admission interview and assessment, his speech is slow, nonfluent, and labored. How should the nurse document this finding?

1. Receptive aphasia
2. Wernicke's aphasia
3. Expressive aphasia
4. Global aphasia

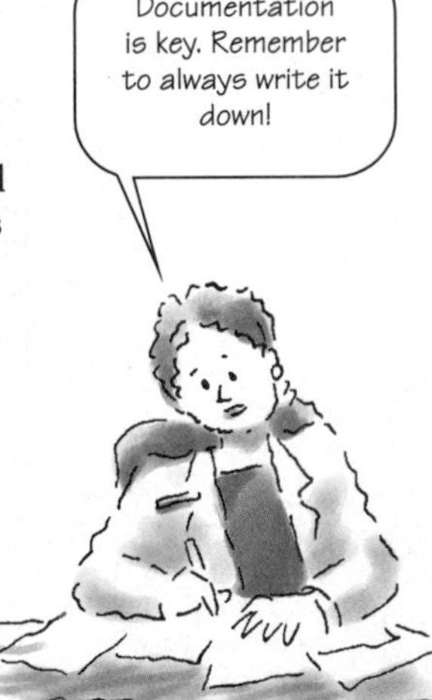

Documentation is key. Remember to always write it down!

142. 3. Expressive (Broca's) aphasia results from damage to Broca's area, located in the frontal lobe of the brain's dominant hemisphere. Typically, the client with expressive aphasia has difficulty expressing himself and his speech is slow, nonfluent, and labored; however, comprehension of written and verbal communication is intact. With receptive (Wernicke's) aphasia (which results from injury to Wernicke's area, located in the temporal lobe of the dominant hemisphere), the client can't comprehend written or verbal communication; his speech is normal but he conveys information poorly. With global aphasia— a combination of receptive and expressive aphasia—most of the brain's communication system is damaged. Global aphasia results from extensive damage to Broca's and Wernicke's areas.

NP: Assessment; CN: Physiological integrity; CNS: Physiological adaptation; CL: Application

143. The nurse is developing a teaching plan for a client who will undergo a stapedectomy for treatment of otosclerosis. Which point should the plan include?

1. Ringing in the ears is common after surgery.
2. Vertigo and dizziness are common after surgery.
3. Hearing should return immediately after surgery.
4. Excessive drainage is common after surgery.

143. 2. Vertigo is the most frequent complication of stapedectomy. The client should move slowly to avoid triggering or worsening vertigo and should ask for assistance with ambulation. Ringing in the ears (tinnitus) rarely follows this surgery and should be reported to the physician. Hearing typically decreases after surgery because of ear packing and tissue swelling, but commonly returns over the next 2 to 6 weeks. Usually, postoperative drainage and pain are minimal; excessive drainage should be reported.

NP: Planning; CN: Physiological integrity; CNS: Reduction of risk potential; CL: Application

144. A client has just been diagnosed with primary open-angle glaucoma and requires teaching about the disease. Which nursing diagnosis takes priority?

1. Risk for injury related to peripheral vision loss
2. Chronic pain related to increased intraocular pressure
3. Ineffective health maintenance related to medication adverse effects
4. Deficient knowledge related to new diagnosis of glaucoma

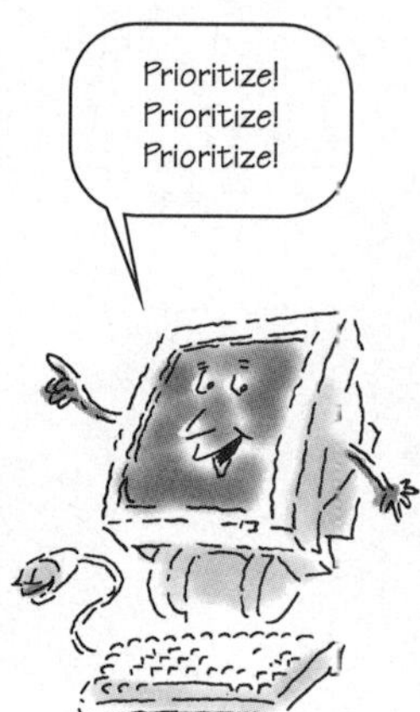
Prioritize!
Prioritize!
Prioritize!

144. 1. Risk for injury related to peripheral vision loss takes priority because open-angle glaucoma limits peripheral vision; the client risks injury from stumbling over peripheral objects that he can't see. Angle-closure glaucoma — not open-angle glaucoma — commonly causes acute pain. Primary open-angle glaucoma is an incurable disease that requires lifelong treatment; adverse effects of medications are common. Although ineffective health maintenance is an appropriate diagnosis for this client, safety takes priority. Deficient knowledge is appropriate for any client with a new diagnosis, but it takes lower priority than safety.

NP: Analysis; CN: Physiological integrity; CNS: Reduction of risk potential; CL: Comprehension

145. When teaching a client how to administer mydriatic agents, which instruction should the nurse provide?

1. "Your pupils will be small and your night vision will be diminished."
2. "Blurred vision is an adverse effect and you should report it to the physician immediately."
3. "Eye pain is common after administration."
4. "Compress the lacrimal sac for 1 minute after instillation."

145. 4. To prevent systemic absorption, the client should compress the lacrimal sac for 1 minute after instilling a mydriatic agent. The drug makes the pupils large and causes light sensitivity. Blurred vision is an expected effect of mydriatics and need not be reported immediately. The client should discontinue the drug if eye pain occurs.

NP: Implementation; CN: Physiological integrity; CNS: Pharmacological and parenteral therapies; CL: Application

146. A client with conjunctivitis wants to know how to avoid spreading the disease to her children. Teaching is effective when the client makes which of the following statements?

1. "I should cleanse the infected eye and then the uninfected eye, and then rinse my washcloth and wash the rest of my face."
2. "I can launder my washcloths and towels with those of others in my household as long as I use hot water."
3. "I should wash my hands before and after applying soaks to my eye."
4. "I shouldn't wipe the drainage from my eye."

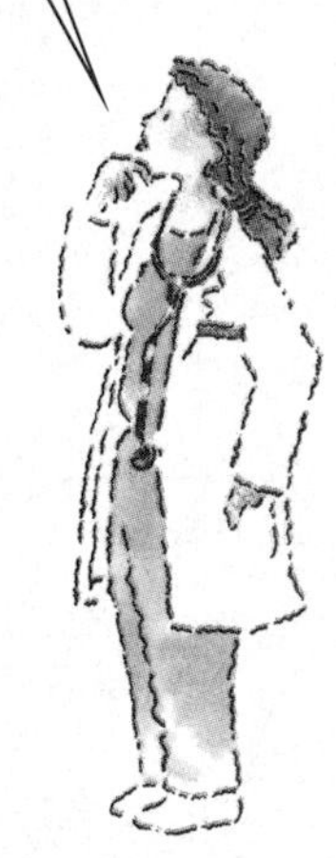

My teaching is effective only if the client understands.

146. 3. Measures that prevent the spread of conjunctivitis include washing the hands before and after applying soaks to the affected eye. The client should wash the uninfected eye first, then wash the infected eye, rinse the washcloth, and wash the rest of her face. Her washcloths, towels, and pillowcases should be laundered separately. She should use disposable tissues to wipe the drainage from the eye, dispose of used tissues in an appropriate container, and then wash her hands.

NP: Evaluation; CN: Safe, effective care environment; CNS: Safety and infection control; CL: Analysis

147. During a neurologic assessment, the nurse notes that the client's deep tendon reflexes (DTRs) are more brisk than average. How should these findings be documented?

1. 4+
2. 3+
3. 2+
4. 1+

147. 2. DTRs are graded and documented on a scale of 4 to 0. If these reflexes are very brisk or hyperactive, document them as 4+; if they're more brisk than average, document them as 3+. Document normal reflexes as 2+, a diminished response as 1+, and no response as 0.

NP: Implementation; CN: Health promotion and maintenance; CNS: Prevention and early detection of disease; CL: Application

148. A 35-year-old client with a subarachnoid hemorrhage undergoes cerebral angiography. Which action should the nurse take immediately after this procedure?

1. Assess for signs and symptoms of cerebral vasospasm.
2. Instruct the client to lie in a supine position for 4 hours after the procedure.
3. Check neurovascular status of the extremity distal to the insertion site.
4. Restrict the client's fluids to reduce cerebral edema.

148. 1. Cerebral vasospasm is a complication of cerebral angiography, so the nurse should assess for signs and symptoms of vasospasm (such as confusion, decreased level of consciousness, and agitation). The client should lie in a supine position for 8 hours and refrain from bending joints in the extremity used for puncture. The nurse should check vital signs and neurovascular status of the extremity every 15 minutes for 1 hour, then every half-hour for the next hour, and then every hour until stable. The nurse should give I.V. fluids as ordered to dilute the contrast dye in the client's circulation.

NP: Implementation; CN: Physiological integrity; CNS: Reduction of risk potential; CL: Application

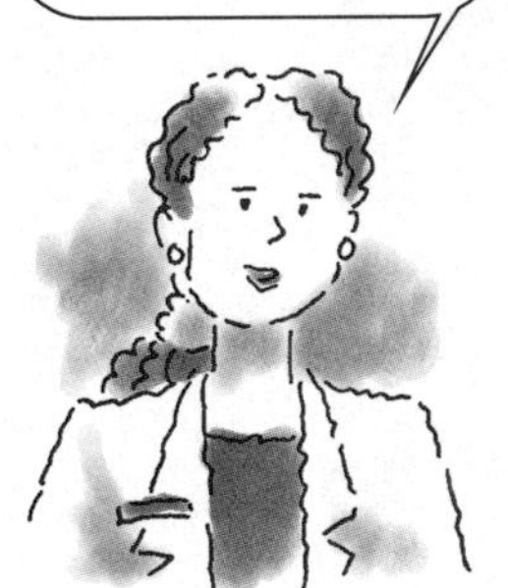

Congratulations! I absolutely, positively knew you could do it!

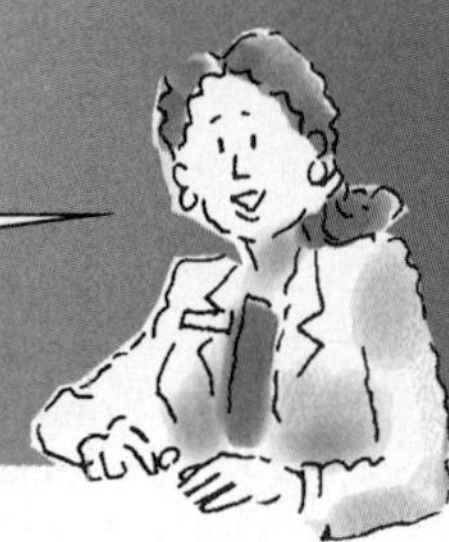

Here's a test that covers nursing care for clients with a disorder of the musculoskeletal system. So get moving! (Get it? Moving? Hmmm. I must be losing my touch.)

Chapter 7 Musculoskeletal disorders

1. Osteoblast activity is needed for which of the following functions?

1. Bone formation
2. Estrogen production
3. Hematopoiesis
4. Muscle formation

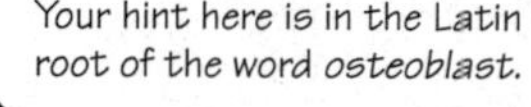

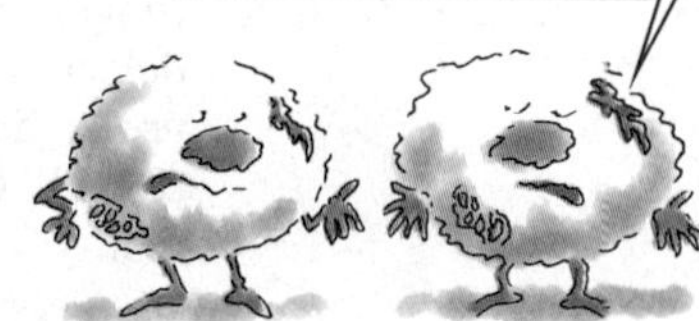

Your hint here is in the Latin root of the word *osteoblast*.

1. 1. Osteoblast activity is necessary for bone formation. Osteoblasts are bone-forming cells; they don't have a role in muscle formation. Estrogen is linked to calcium reuptake and building of bone tissue. Hematopoiesis is the production of red blood cells in the bone marrow.

NP: Assessment; CN: Physiological integrity; CNS: Physiological adaptation; CL: Knowledge

2. Which of the following conditions is the primary complication of osteoporosis?

1. Pain
2. Fractures
3. Hardening of the bones
4. Increased bone matrix and remineralization

3. Which of the following conditions is the cause of primary osteoporosis?

1. Alcoholism
2. Hormonal imbalance
3. Malnutrition
4. Osteogenesis imperfecta

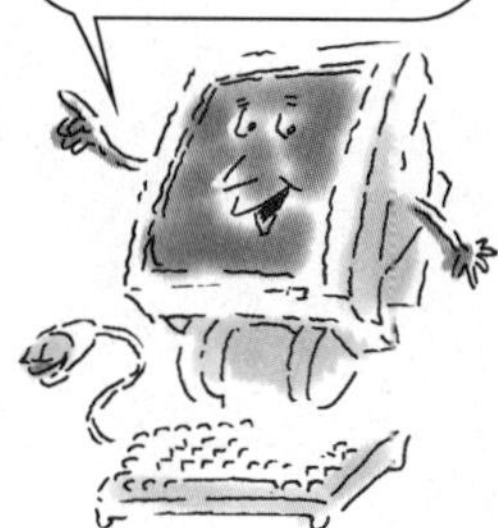

Watch out! In question 2, *primary* means *main* or *principal*. In question 3, it refers to a type of disease.

2. 2. The primary complication of osteoporosis is fractures. Bones soften, and there's a decrease in bone matrix and remineralization. Pain may occur, but fractures can be life threatening.

NP: Assessment; CN: Physiological integrity; CNS: Physiological adaptation; CL: Knowledge

3. 2. Hormonal imbalance, faulty metabolism, and poor dietary intake of calcium cause primary osteoporosis. Alcoholism, malnutrition, osteogenesis imperfecta, rheumatoid arthritis, liver disease, scurvy, lactose intolerance, hyperthyroidism, and trauma cause secondary osteoporosis.

NP: Assessment; CN: Physiological integrity; CNS: Physiological adaptation; CL: Knowledge

4. A 42-year-old woman just had a total hysterectomy. Is she at risk for osteoporosis?

1. No, because she still has her thyroid gland.
2. No, because she isn't at risk until she's older.
3. Yes, because she's still producing hormones.
4. Yes, because she's just had surgically induced menopause.

4. 4. Menopause at any age puts women at risk for osteoporosis because of the associated hormonal imbalance. This client's thyroid gland won't protect her from menopause. With her ovaries removed, she's no longer producing hormones.

NP: Assessment; CN: Physiological integrity; CNS: Physiological adaptation; CL: Comprehension

5. Primary prevention of osteoporosis includes which of the following measures?

1. Place items within reach of the client.
2. Install bars in the bathroom to prevent falls.
3. Maintain the optimal calcium intake, and use estrogen replacement therapy.
4. Use a professional alert system in the home in case a fall occurs when the client is alone.

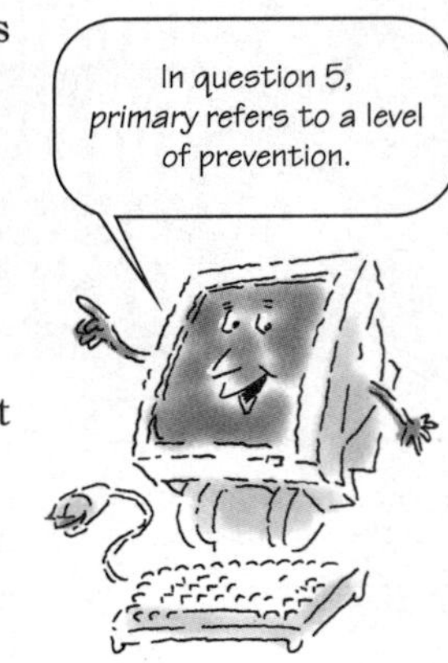

In question 5, primary refers to a level of prevention.

5. 3. Primary prevention of osteoporosis includes maintaining optimal calcium intake and using estrogen replacement therapy. Placing items within reach of the client, using a professional alert system in the home, and installing bars in bathrooms to prevent falls, are all secondary and tertiary prevention methods.

NP: Implementation; CN: Health promotion and maintenance; CNS: Prevention and early detection of disease; CL: Application

6. Which of the following mechanisms is believed to cause gout?

1. Overproduction of calcium
2. Underproduction of calcium
3. Overproduction of uric acid
4. Underproduction of uric acid

6. 3. Although the exact cause of primary gout remains unknown, it seems linked to a genetic defect in purine metabolism that causes overproduction of uric acid, retention of uric acid, or both. Gout isn't related to calcium production.

NP: Assessment; CN: Physiological integrity; CNS: Physiological adaptation; CL: Knowledge

7. In advanced gout, urate crystal deposits develop on the hands, knees, feet, forearms, ear, and Achilles tendon. Which of the following terms refers to these deposits?

1. Arthralgia
2. Gout nodules
3. Pinna
4. Tophi

7. 4. Urate crystal deposits are known as tophi. Arthralgia describes painful joints. Gout nodule is an incorrect term. The pinna is the outside of the ear.

NP: Assessment; CN: Physiological integrity; CNS: Physiological adaptation; CL: Knowledge

8. Which of the following phrases best explains the usual pattern of nonchronic gout?

1. Frequent painful attacks
2. Generally painful joints at all times
3. Painful attacks with pain-free periods
4. Painful attacks with less painful periods, but pain never subsides

8. 3. The usual pattern of gout involves painful attacks with pain-free periods. Chronic gout may lead to frequent attacks with persistently painful joints.

NP: Implementation; CN: Physiological integrity; CNS: Physiological adaptation; CL: Knowledge

9. A client has been prescribed a diet that limits purine-rich foods. Which of the following foods would the nurse teach him to avoid eating?

1. Bananas and dried fruits
2. Milk, ice cream, and yogurt
3. Wine, cheese, preserved fruits, meats, and vegetables
4. Anchovies, sardines, kidneys, sweetbreads, and lentils

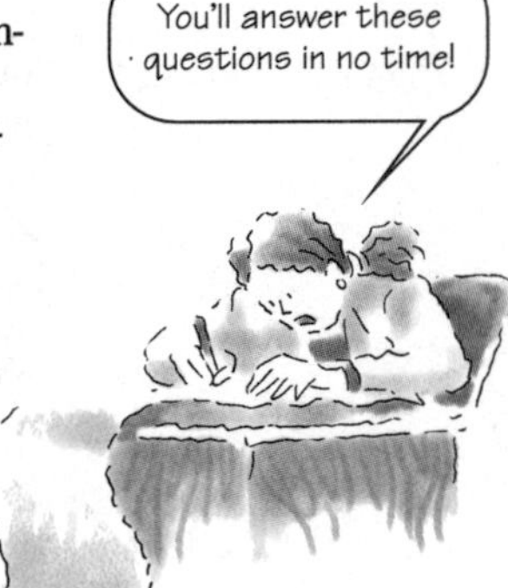

You'll answer these questions in no time!

9. 4. Anchovies, sardines, kidneys, sweetbreads, and lentils are high in purines. Bananas and dried fruits are high in potassium. Milk, ice cream, and yogurt are rich in calcium. Wine, cheese, preserved fruits, meats, and vegetables contain tyramine.

NP: Implementation; CN: Health promotion and maintenance; CNS: Prevention and early detection of disease; CL: Application

27. Clients in the late stages of osteoarthritis often use which of the following terms to describe joint pain?

1. Grating
2. Dull ache
3. Deep aching pain
4. Deep aching, relieved with rest

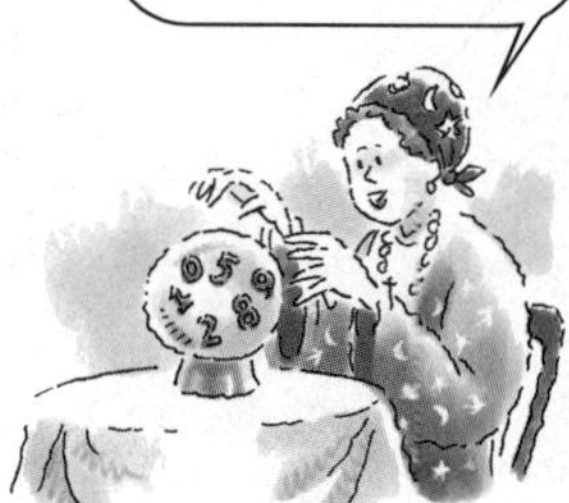
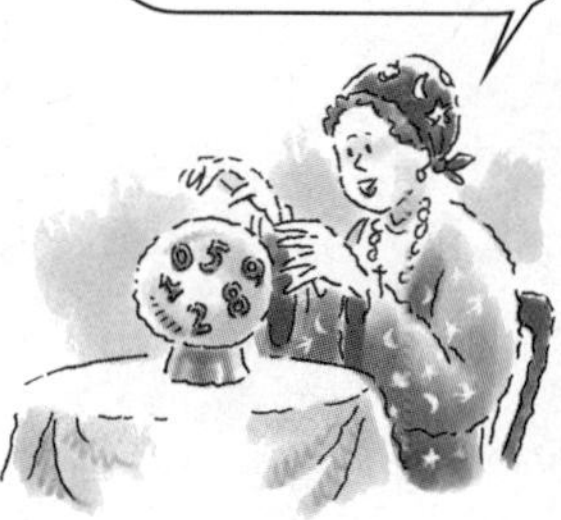

Ask your client about the pain; you don't need a crystal ball.

27. 1. In the late stages of osteoarthritis, the client often describes joint pain as grating. As the disease progresses, the cartilage covering the ends of bones is destroyed and bones rub against each other. Osteophytes, or bone spurs, may also form on the ends of bones. A dull ache and deep aching pain with or without relief with rest is often seen in the earlier stages of osteoarthritis.

NP: Assessment; CN: Physiological integrity; CNS: Physiological adaptation; CL: Analysis

28. A client uses a cane for assistance in walking. Which of the following statements is true about a cane or other assistive devices?

1. A walker is a better choice than a cane.
2. The cane should be used on the affected side.
3. The cane should be used on the unaffected side.
4. A client with osteoarthritis should be encouraged to ambulate without the cane.

28. 3. A cane should be used on the unaffected side. A client with osteoarthritis should be encouraged to ambulate with a cane, walker, or other assistive device as needed; their use takes weight and stress off joints.

NP: Implementation; CN: Physiological integrity; CNS: Physiological adaptation; CL: Application

29. Which of the following instructions about activity should be given to a client with osteoarthritis after he returns home?

1. "Learn to pace activity."
2. "Remain as sedentary as possible."
3. "Return to a normal level of activity."
4. "Include vigorous exercise in your daily routine."

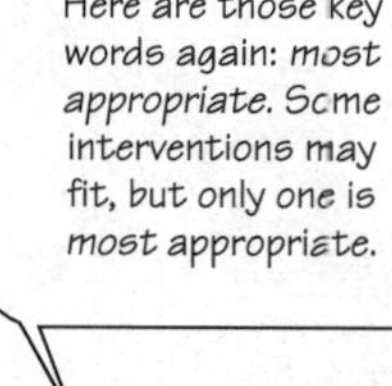

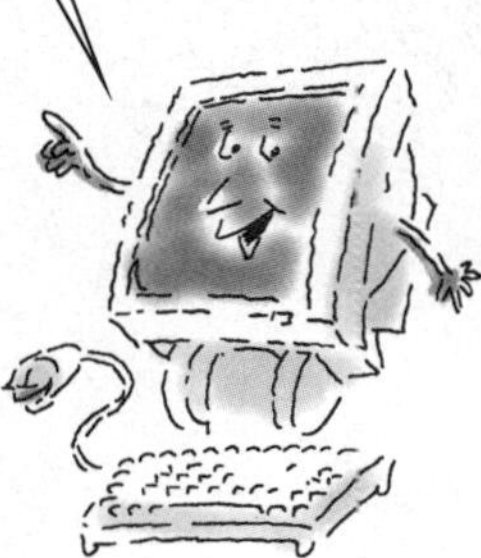

29. 1. A client with osteoarthritis should pace his activities and avoid overexertion. Overexertion can increase degeneration and cause pain. The client shouldn't become sedentary because he'll have a high risk of pneumonia and contractures.

NP: Planning; CN: Physiological integrity; CNS: Physiological adaptation; CL: Application

30. A client was prescribed an anti-inflammatory drug for osteoarthritis 5 days ago. He says the pain has decreased some but not completely. Which of the following nursing interventions would be the most appropriate?

1. Continue the present dose and offer other pain measures.
2. Notify the physician and suggest increasing the dose.
3. Notify the physician and suggest stopping the medication.
4. Notify the physician and suggest adding another medication.

30. 1. Anti-inflammatory medications may take 2 to 3 weeks for full benefits. If the client can tolerate the pain, continue on the medication and offer other pain measures, such as rest, massage, heat, or cold. Increasing, stopping or adding another medication aren't appropriate because the medication hasn't been taken long enough to show full benefit.

NP: Implementation; CN: Physiological integrity; CNS: Physiological adaptation; CL: Comprehension

31. A client is diagnosed with a herniated nucleus pulposus, or herniated disk. Which of the following statements about a herniated disk is correct?

1. The disk slips out of alignment.
2. The disk shatters, and fragments place pressure on nerve roots.
3. The nucleus tissue itself remains centralized, and the surrounding tissue is displaced.
4. The nucleus of the disk puts pressure on the anulus, causing pressure on the nerve root.

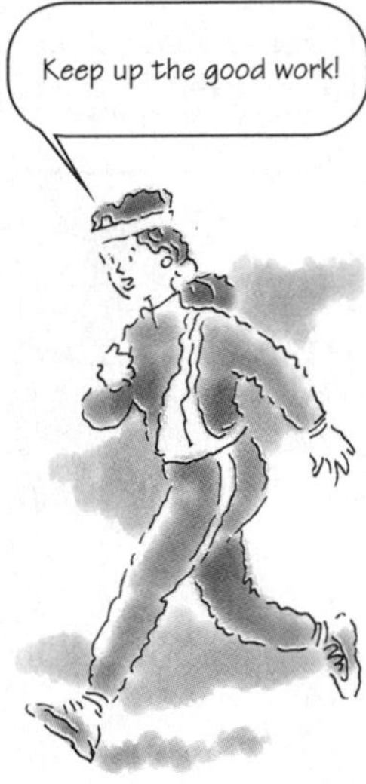

31. 4. With a herniated nucleus pulposus, or herniated disk, the nucleus of the disk puts pressure on the anulus, causing pressure on the nerve root. The disk itself doesn't slip, rupture, or shatter. The nucleus tissue usually moves from the center of the disk.

NP: Implementation; CN: Physiological integrity; CNS: Physiological adaptation; CL: Knowledge

32. Which of the following symptoms would occur with a herniated nucleus pulposus?

1. Pain, numbness, weakness, leg or foot pain
2. Shortness of breath, weakness, leg or foot pain
3. Inability to walk, shortness of breath, weakness, leg or foot pain
4. Unstable gait, disorientation, numbness, weakness, leg or foot pain

32. 1. Common symptoms of a herniated nucleus pulposus are pain, numbness, weakness, and leg or foot pain.

NP: Assessment; CN: Physiological integrity; CNS: Physiological adaptation; CL: Comprehension

33. Conservative treatment of a herniated nucleus pulposus would include which of the following measures?

1. Surgery
2. Bone fusion
3. Bed rest, pain medication, physiotherapy
4. Strenuous exercise, pain medication, physiotherapy

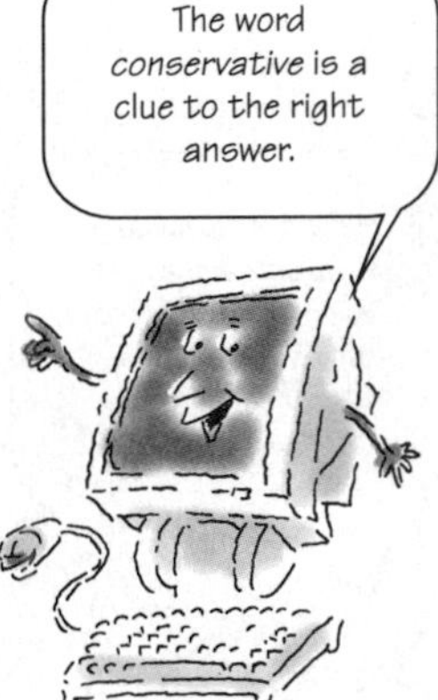

The word *conservative* is a clue to the right answer.

33. 3. Conservative treatment of a herniated nucleus pulposus may include bed rest, pain medication, and physiotherapy. Aggressive treatment may include surgery such as a bone fusion.

NP: Implementation; CN: Safe, effective care environment; CNS: Management of care; CL: Application

34. Closed spine surgery is a new technique to fix a herniated disk. Which of the following statements is true about closed spine surgery?

1. There is a greater associated risk.
2. Intense physical therapy is needed.
3. An endoscope is used to perform the surgery.
4. Recovery time is twice as long as with open spine surgery.

34. 3. Closed spine surgery uses endoscopy to fix a herniated disk. It's less risky than open surgery and has a shorter recovery time; it's commonly done as a same-day surgical procedure. Physical therapy may be less intensive or not needed at all.

NP: Implementation; CN: Physiological integrity; CNS: Physiological adaptation; CL: Knowledge

35. Which of the following descriptions best identifies the position of an intervertebral disk?
1. Encloses the anulus fibrosus
2. Surrounds the nucleus pulposus
3. Located between the vertebrae and the spinal column
4. Located between spinal nerves in the vertebral column

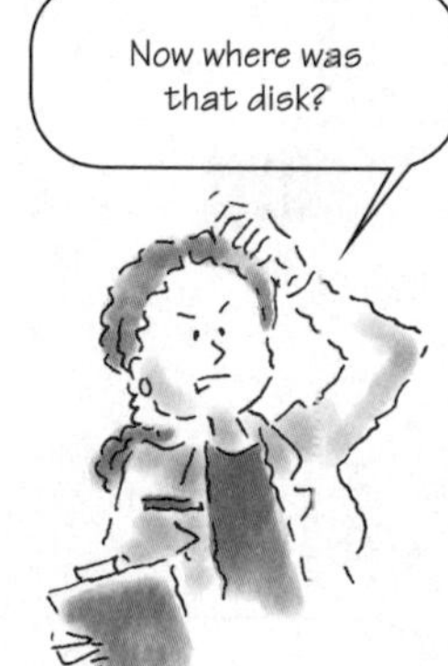

Now where was that disk?

35. 3. Intervertebral disks are between the vertebrae and the spinal column. The other answers are incorrect descriptions of vertebral disks.

NP: Assessment; CN: Physiological integrity; CNS: Physiological adaptation; CL: Knowledge

36. Herniation of a vertebral disk can occur under which of the following conditions?
1. Major trauma or stress
2. Minor trauma or stress
3. With a history of back problems
4. Either major or minor trauma or stress

36. 4. Herniation of a vertebral disk can occur with either major or minor trauma or stress. It can occur in anyone regardless of history.

NP: Assessment; CN: Physiological integrity; CNS: Physiological adaptation; CL: Knowledge

37. Which of the following areas of vertebral herniation is the most common?
1. L1-L2, L4-L5
2. L1-L2, L5-S1
3. L4-L5, L5-S1
4. L5-S1, S2-S3

37. 3. The most common areas of herniation are L4-L5, L5-S1.

NP: Assessment; CN: Physiological integrity; CNS: Physiological adaptation; CL: Knowledge

38. Which of the following tests may be used to diagnose a herniated nucleus pulposus?
1. Chest X-ray, magnetic resonance imaging (MRI), computed tomography (CT) scan
2. Lumbar puncture, chest X-ray, MRI, CT scan
3. Lumbar puncture, chest X-ray, myelography
4. Myelography, MRI, CT scan

38. 4. Tests used to diagnose a herniated nucleus pulposus include myelography, MRI, and CT scan. Chest X-ray and lumbar puncture aren't conclusive.

NP: Assessment; CN: Physiological integrity; CNS: Physiological adaptation; CL: Knowledge

39. Which of the following instructions would be included when teaching a client how to protect his back?
1. "Sleep on your side, and carry objects at arm's length."
2. "Sleep on your back, and carry objects at arm's length."
3. "Sleep on your side, and carry objects close to your body."
4. "Sleep on your back, and carry objects close to your body."

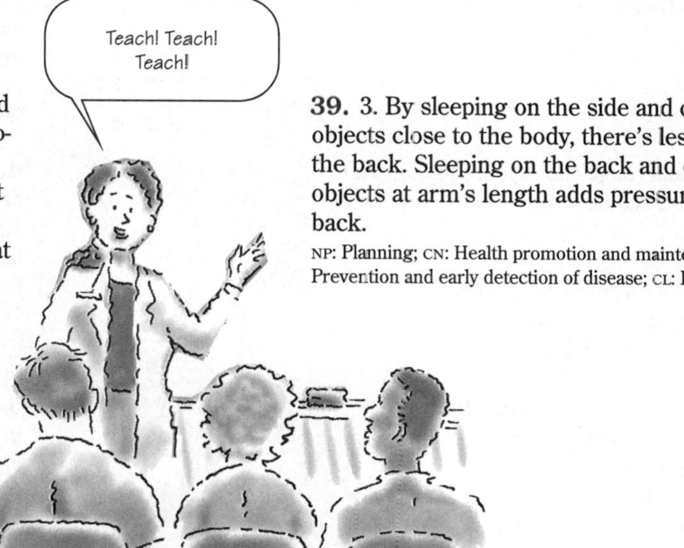

Teach! Teach! Teach!

39. 3. By sleeping on the side and carrying objects close to the body, there's less strain on the back. Sleeping on the back and carrying objects at arm's length adds pressure to the back.

NP: Planning; CN: Health promotion and maintenance; CNS: Prevention and early detection of disease; CL: Knowledge

40. Skeletal muscle relaxants may be used in the acute treatment of a herniated nucleus pulposus. Which of the following instructions should be included in client teaching?

1. "Change your position quickly to avoid dizziness."
2. "Double a missed dose to ensure proper muscle relaxation."
3. "Cough and cold medications are appropriate to take, if needed."
4. "Avoid activities that require alertness; muscle relaxants can cause drowsiness."

40. 4. Client teaching should include avoiding activities that require alertness; muscle relaxants can cause drowsiness. Tell the client to change position slowly to avoid dizziness. The client shouldn't double a missed dose or take cough and cold medications because this will increase the likelihood of adverse effects.

NP: Implementation; CN: Physiological integrity; CNS: Pharmacological and parenteral therapies; CL: Comprehension

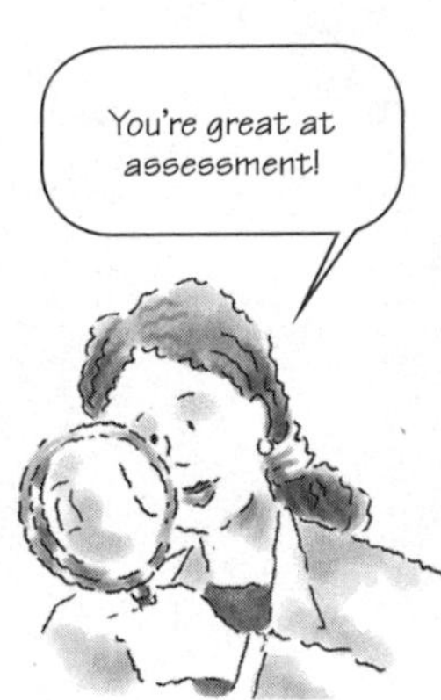
You're great at assessment!

41. A client with a recent fracture is suspected of having compartment syndrome. Assessment findings may include which of the following symptoms?

1. Body-wide decrease in bone mass
2. A growth in and around the bone tissue
3. Inability to perform active movement; pain with passive movement
4. Inability to perform passive movement; pain with active movement

41. 3. With compartment syndrome, the client can't perform active movement, and pain occurs with passive movement. Osteoporosis has a body-wide decrease in bone mass. A bone tumor shows growth in and around the bone tissue.

NP: Assessment; CN: Physiological integrity; CNS: Physiological adaptation; CL: Application

42. Compartment syndrome occurs under which of the following conditions?

1. Increase in scar tissue
2. Increase in bone mass
3. Decrease in bone mass
4. Hemorrhage into the muscle

42. 4. Compartment syndrome occurs when pressure within the muscle compartment, resulting from edema or bleeding, increases to the point of interfering with circulation. Crush injuries, burns, bites, and fractures requiring casts or dressings may cause this syndrome. It isn't a result of scar tissue or an increase or decrease in bone mass.

NP: Assessment; CN: Physiological integrity; CNS: Physiological adaptation; CL: Knowledge

43. The hemorrhage that occurs in compartment syndrome causes which of the following symptoms?

1. Edema
2. Decreased venous pressure
3. Increased venous circulation
4. Increased arterial circulation

43. 1. The hemorrhage in compartment syndrome causes edema, increased venous pressure, and decreased venous and arterial circulation.

NP: Assessment; CN: Physiological integrity; CNS: Physiological adaptation; CL: Comprehension

44. In compartment syndrome, how long would it take for tissue death to occur?

1. 2 to 4 hours
2. 6 to 8 hours
3. 24 hours
4. 72 hours

44. 1. Tissue death can occur in 2 to 4 hours in compartment syndrome.

NP: Assessment; CN: Physiological integrity; CNS: Physiological adaptation; CL: Knowledge

NP: Nursing process CN: Client needs category CNS: Client needs subcategory CL: Cognitive level

45. Treatment of compartment syndrome includes which of the following measures?

1. Amputation
2. Casting
3. Fasciotomy
4. Observation, no treatment is necessary

45. 3. Treatment of compartment syndrome includes fasciotomy, which involves cutting the fascia over the affected area to permit muscle expansion. Amputation and casting aren't treatments for compartment syndrome.

NP: Assessment; CN: Physiological integrity; CNS: Physiological adaptation; CL: Comprehension

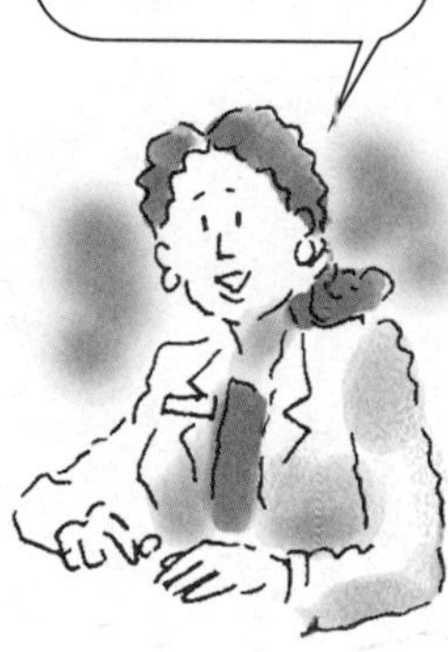

Here's a question your client with a similar problem is bound to ask.

46. A client is admitted to the emergency department with a foot fracture. Which of the following reasons explains why the foot is placed in a brace?

1. To act as a splint
2. To prevent infection
3. To allow for movement
4. To encourage direct contact

46. 1. The purpose of the brace is to act as a splint, maintain immobility, and prevent direct contact. A brace doesn't prevent infection.

NP: Implementation; CN: Physiological integrity; CNS: Reduction of risk potential; CL: Comprehension

47. After treatment of compartment syndrome, a client reports experiencing paresthesia. Which of the following symptoms would be seen with paresthesia?

1. Fever and chills
2. Change in range of motion
3. Pain and blanching
4. Numbness and tingling

47. 4. Paresthesia is described as numbness and tingling. It isn't associated with fever and chills or change in range of motion nor is it described as pain or blanching.

NP: Assessment; CN: Physiological integrity; CNS: Physiological adaptation; CL: Comprehension

48. Which of the following characteristics of the fascia can cause it to develop compartment syndrome?

1. It's highly flexible.
2. It's fragile and weak.
3. It's unable to expand.
4. It's the only tissue within the compartment.

48. 3. Compartment syndrome occurs because the fascia is unable to expand. It isn't flexible or weak. The compartment contains blood vessels and nerves.

NP: Assessment; CN: Physiological integrity; CNS: Physiological adaptation; CL: Comprehension

49. Compartment syndrome can occur from which of the following conditions?

1. Internal pressure
2. External pressure
3. Increased blood pressure
4. Internal and external pressure

49. 4. Compartment syndrome can occur from internal (bleeding) and external pressure (cast or dressing). Blood pressure isn't a cause of compartment syndrome.

NP: Assessment; CN: Physiological integrity; CNS: Physiological adaptation; CL: Knowledge

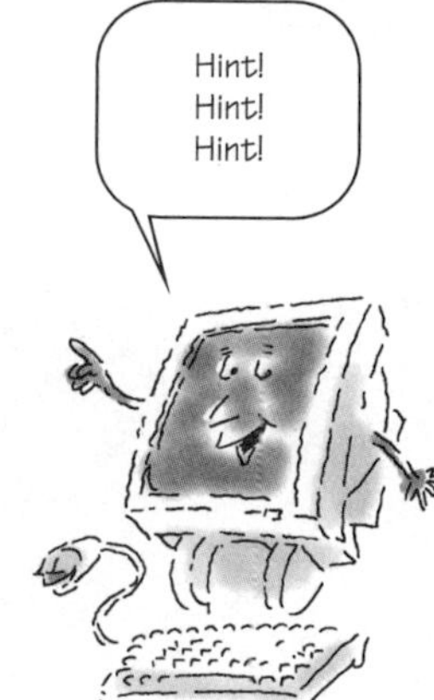

50. Which of the following symptoms is an early sign of compartment syndrome?

1. Heat
2. Paresthesia
3. Skin pallor
4. Swelling

50. 2. Paresthesia is the earliest sign of compartment syndrome. Pain, heat, and swelling are also signs but occur after paresthesia. Skin pallor isn't a sign of compartment syndrome.

NP: Assessment; CN: Physiological integrity; CNS: Physiological adaptation; CL: Knowledge

51. Which of the following symptoms are considered signs of a fracture?

1. Tingling, coolness, loss of pulses
2. Loss of sensation, redness, coolness
3. Coolness, redness, new site of pain
4. Redness, warmth, pain at the site of injury

51. 4. Signs of a fracture may include redness, warmth, numbness or loss of sensation, and new site of pain. Coolness, tingling, and loss of pulses are signs of a vascular problem.

NP: Assessment; CN: Physiological integrity; CNS: Physiological adaptation; CL: Application

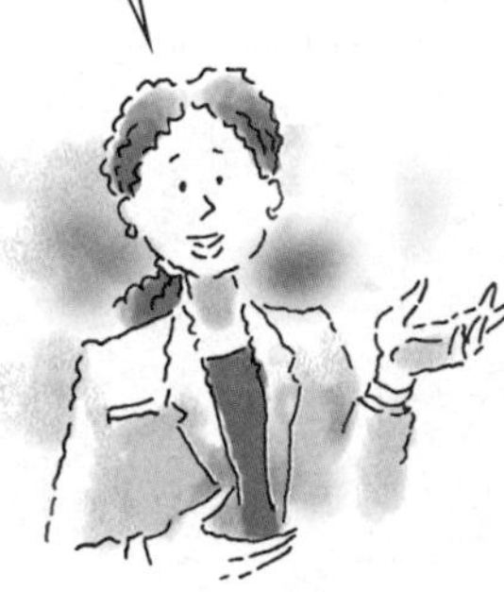

Knowing normal signs will alert you to what is wrong.

52. Which of the following areas would be included in a neurovascular assessment?

1. Orientation, movement, pulses, warmth
2. Capillary refill, movement, pulses, warmth
3. Orientation, pupillary response, temperature, pulses
4. Respiratory pattern, orientation, pulses, temperature

52. 2. A correct neurovascular assessment should include capillary refill, movement, pulses, and warmth. Neurovascular assessment involves nerve and blood supply to an area. Respiratory pattern, orientation, temperature, and pupillary response aren't part of a neurovascular examination.

NP: Assessment; CN: Physiological integrity; CNS: Physiological adaptation; CL: Application

53. Which of the following methods is the correct way to assess limb circumference?

1. Use a measuring tape.
2. Visually compare limbs bilaterally.
3. Check the client's medical history.
4. Follow the standardized chart for limb circumference.

53. 1. The right way to assess limb circumference is to use a measuring tape. Visual inspection and checking the past history are unreliable. There isn't a standardized chart for limb circumference.

NP: Assessment; CN: Health promotion and maintenance; CNS: Prevention and early detection of disease; CL: Knowledge

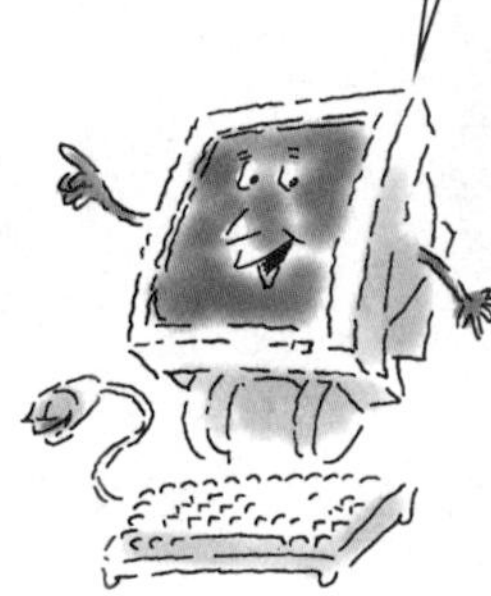

Question 54 asks you to prioritize your response.

54. If pulses aren't palpable, which of the following interventions should be performed first?

1. Check again in 1 hour.
2. Alert the nurse in charge immediately.
3. Verify the findings with Doppler ultrasonography.
4. Alert the physician immediately.

54. 3. If pulses aren't palpable, verify the assessment with Doppler ultrasonography. If pulses can't be found with Doppler ultrasonography, immediately notify the physician.

NP: Assessment; CN: Physiological integrity; CNS: Physiological adaptation; CL: Application

55. A client describes a foul odor from his cast. Which of the following responses or interventions would be the most appropriate?

1. Assess further because this may be a sign of infection.
2. Teach him proper cast care, including hygiene measures.
3. This is normal, especially when a cast is in place for a few weeks.
4. Assess further because this may be a sign of neurovascular compromise.

55. 1. A foul odor from a cast may be a sign of infection. The nurse needs to assess for fever, malaise and, possibly, an elevation in white blood cells. Odor from a cast is never normal, and it isn't a sign of neurovascular compromise, which would include decreased pulses, coolness, and paresthesia.

NP: Assessment; CN: Health promotion and maintenance; CNS: Prevention and early detection of disease; CL: Analysis

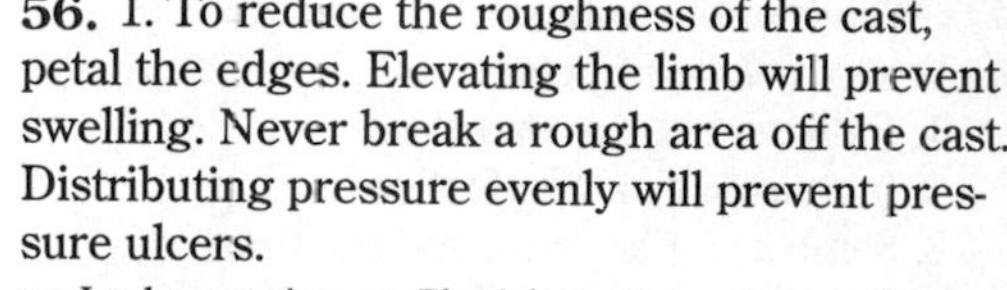

56. To reduce the roughness of a cast, which of the following measures should be used?
1. Petal the edges.
2. Elevate the limb.
3. Break off the rough area.
4. Distribute pressure evenly.

56. 1. To reduce the roughness of the cast, petal the edges. Elevating the limb will prevent swelling. Never break a rough area off the cast. Distributing pressure evenly will prevent pressure ulcers.
NP: Implementation; CN: Physiological integrity; CNS: Basic care and comfort; CL: Application

57. Elevating a limb with a cast will prevent swelling. Which of the following actions best describes how this is done?
1. Place the limb with the cast close to the body.
2. Place the limb with the cast at the level of the heart.
3. Place the limb with the cast below the level of the heart.
4. Place the limb with the cast above the level of the heart.

57. 4. To reduce swelling, place the limb with the cast above the level of the heart. To elevate a cast, the limb may need to be extended from the body. Placing it below or at the level of the heart won't reduce swelling.
NP: Implementation; CN: Physiological integrity; CNS: Physiological adaptation; CL: Application

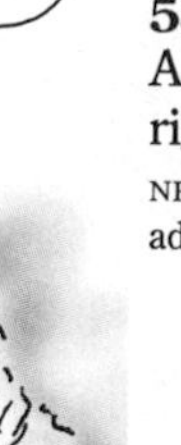

Your client depends on you to know the answers.

58. A client asks why a cast can't get wet. Which of the following responses would be the most appropriate?
1. A wet cast can cause a foul odor.
2. A wet cast will weaken or be destroyed.
3. A wet cast is heavy and difficult to maneuver.
4. It's all right to get the cast wet, just use a hair dryer to dry it off.

58. 2. A wet cast will weaken or be destroyed. A foul odor is a sign of infection. It's never all right to get a cast wet.
NP: Planning; CN: Physiological integrity; CNS: Physiological adaptation; CL: Knowledge

59. A client comes to the emergency department complaining of dull, deep bone pain unrelated to movement. Which of the following statements is correct to help decide if the bone pain is caused by a fracture?
1. These are classic symptoms of a fracture.
2. Fracture pain is sharp and related to movement.
3. Fracture pain is sharp and unrelated to movement.
4. Fracture pain is dull and deep and related to movement.

59. 2. Fracture pain is sharp and related to movement. Pain that's dull and deep and unrelated to movement isn't typical of a fracture.
NP: Assessment; CN: Health promotion and maintenance; CNS: Prevention and early detection of disease; CL: Analysis

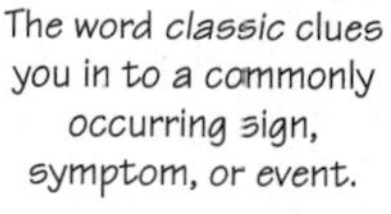

The word *classic* clues you in to a commonly occurring sign, symptom, or event.

60. Which of the following fractures is classic for occurring from trauma?
1. Brachial and clavicle
2. Brachial and humerus
3. Humerus and clavicle
4. Occipital and humerus

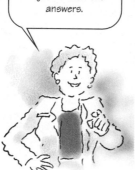

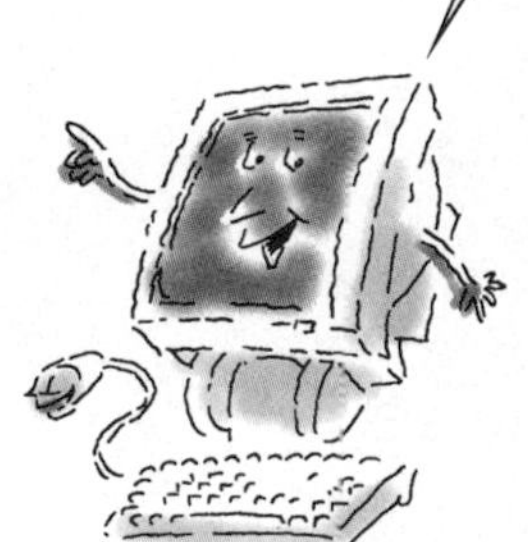

60. 3. Classic fractures that occur with trauma are those of the humerus and clavicle. The brachial and occipital bones aren't usually involved in a traumatic delivery.
NP: Assessment; CN: Physiological integrity; CNS: Physiological adaptation; CL: Knowledge

61. Which of the following characteristics applies to a closed fracture?
1. Extensive tissue damage
2. Increased risk of infection
3. Same as for a compound fracture
4. Intact skin over the fracture site

61. 4. A closed fracture maintains intact skin over the fracture site. An open fracture has extensive tissue damage, an increased risk of infection, and is also known as a compound fracture

NP: Assessment; CN: Physiological integrity; CNS: Physiological adaptation; CL: Knowledge

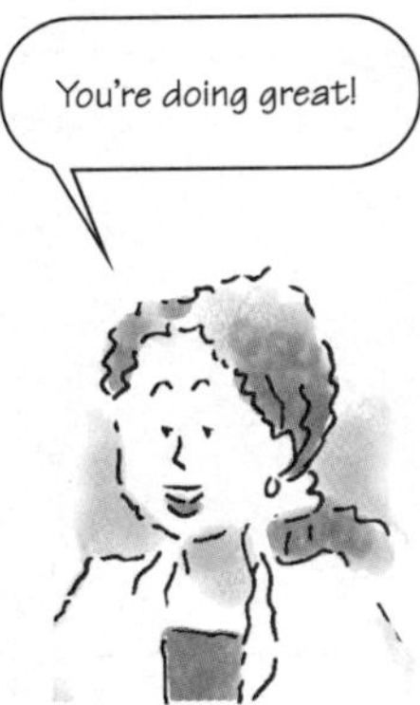

62. A client is put in traction before surgery. Which of the following reasons for the traction is correct?
1. Prevents skin breakdown
2. Aids in turning the client
3. Helps the client become active
4. Prevents trauma and overcomes muscle spasms

62. 4. Traction prevents trauma and overcomes muscle spasms. Traction doesn't prevent skin breakdown, help in turning the client, or help the client become active.

NP: Implementation; CN: Physiological integrity; CNS: Basic care and comfort; CL: Knowledge

63. When the fracture line is straight across the bone, the fracture is known as which of the following types?
1. Linear
2. Longitudinal
3. Oblique
4. Transverse

63. 4. A fracture line straight across the bone is called a transverse fracture. A linear fracture has an intact fracture line. A longitudinal fracture has a longitudinal fracture line. A fracture line at a 45-degree angle to the shaft of the bone is an oblique fracture.

NP: Assessment; CN: Physiological integrity; CNS: Physiological adaptation; CL: Knowledge

64. Which of the following fractures commonly occurs with such bone diseases as osteomalacia and Paget's disease?
1. Linear
2. Longitudinal
3. Oblique
4. Transverse

64. 4. A transverse fracture commonly occurs with such bone diseases as osteomalacia and Paget's disease. Linear, longitudinal, and oblique fractures generally occur with trauma.

NP: Assessment; CN: Physiological integrity; CNS: Physiological adaptation; CL: Knowledge

65. Which of the following fractures is commonly seen in the upper extremities and is related to physical abuse?
1. Longitudinal
2. Oblique
3. Spiral
4. Transverse

65. 3. Spiral fractures are commonly seen in the upper extremities and are related to physical abuse. Longitudinal and oblique fractures generally occur with trauma. A transverse fracture commonly occurs with such bone diseases as osteomalacia and Paget's disease.

NP: Assessment; CN: Physiological integrity; CNS: Physiological adaptation; CL: Knowledge

66. Which of the following mechanisms or conditions causes healing of a fracture?
1. Scar tissue
2. Displacement
3. Necrotic tissue formation
4. Formation of new bone tissue

66. 4. Healing of a fracture occurs by the formation of new bone tissue. Bone doesn't heal by forming scar tissue or necrotic tissue or by displacement.

NP: Assessment; CN: Physiological integrity; CNS: Physiological adaptation; CL: Knowledge

67. Which of the following conditions is a serious complication of a femoral shaft fracture?

1. Constipation
2. Decreased urine output
3. Hemorrhage
4. Pain

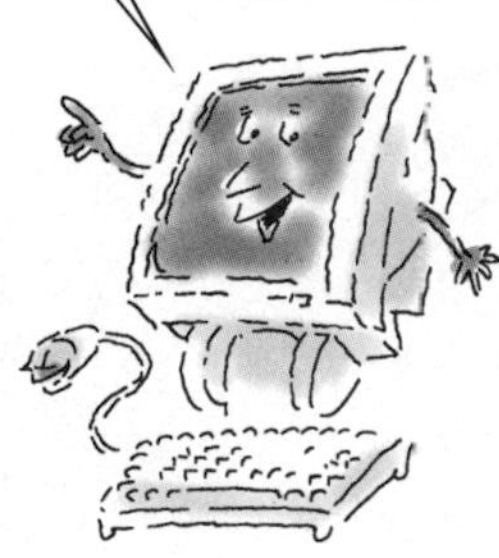

The word serious is a clue that should help you select the answer.

67. 3. Femoral shaft fractures may cause hemorrhage, with as much as 1,000 to 1,500 ml of blood loss. Constipation and decreased urine output aren't direct complications of a fracture. Pain may occur, but it can be controlled with analgesia.

NP: Assessment; CN: Physiological integrity; CNS: Reduction of risk potential; CL: Comprehension

68. Which of the following serious complications can occur with long bone fractures?

1. Bone emboli
2. Fat emboli
3. Platelet emboli
4. Serous emboli

68. 2. A serious complication of long bone fractures is the development of fat emboli. Bone or platelet emboli are rare occurrences. There aren't emboli known as serous emboli.

NP: Assessment; CN: Physiological integrity; CNS: Physiological adaptation; CL: Knowledge

69. Which of the following signs and symptoms can occur with fat emboli?

1. Tachypnea, tachycardia, shortness of breath, paresthesia
2. Paresthesia, bradypnea, bradycardia, petechial rash on chest and neck
3. Bradypnea, bradycardia, shortness of breath, petechial rash on chest and neck
4. Tachypnea, tachycardia, shortness of breath, petechial rash on chest and neck

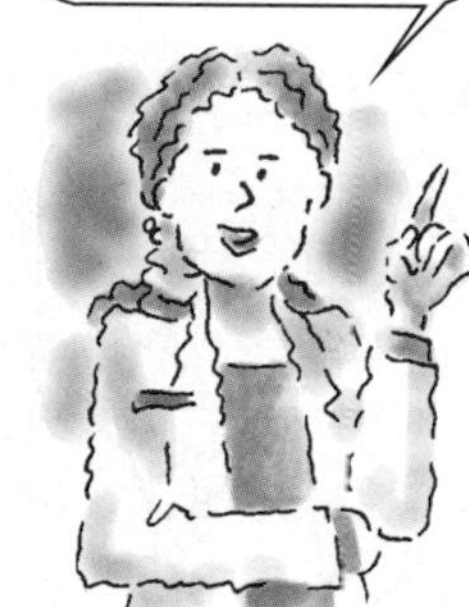

Assessment is a key skill for nurses in every field.

69. 4. Signs and symptoms of fat emboli include tachypnea, tachycardia, shortness of breath, and a petechial rash on the chest and neck. The fat molecules enter the venous circulation and travel to the lung, obstructing pulmonary circulation. Bradycardia, bradypnea, and paresthesia aren't usual symptoms.

NP: Assessment; CN: Health promotion and maintenance; CNS: Prevention and early detection of disease; CL: Knowledge

70. Treatment of a fat embolus may include which of the following therapies?

1. Albuterol, oxygen, I.V. fluids, steroids
2. Oxygen, I.V. fluids, steroids, antibiotics
3. Morphine, oxygen, I.V. fluids, antibiotics
4. Theophylline, morphine, oxygen, I.V. fluids

70. 2. Treatment of a fat embolus may include oxygen, I.V. fluids, steroids to counteract inflammation in the lungs and correct cerebral edema, and antibiotics to prevent infection. Albuterol, morphine, or theophylline aren't commonly used to treat fat emboli.

NP: Implementation; CN: Physiological integrity; CNS: Basic care and comfort; CL: Knowledge

71. A high-protein diet is ordered for a client recovering from a fracture. High protein is ordered for which of the following reasons?

1. Protein promotes gluconeogenesis.
2. Protein has anti-inflammatory properties.
3. Protein promotes cell growth and bone union.
4. Protein decreases pain medication requirements.

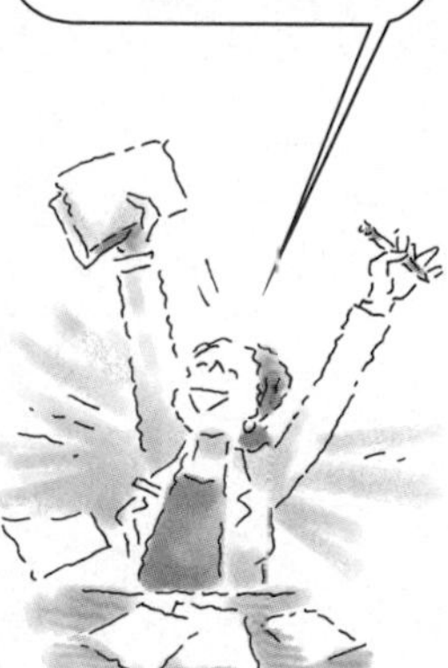

Wow! You've finished 71 questions! Outstanding!

71. 3. High-protein intake promotes cell growth and bone union. Protein doesn't promote gluconeogenesis, exert anti-inflammatory properties, or decrease pain medication requirements.

NP: Planning; CN: Physiological integrity; CNS: Basic care and comfort; CL: Application

72. Which of the following weights is commonly applied to an extremity for Buck's traction in an adult?
1. 1 to 2 lb
2. 1 to 5 lb
3. 5 to 7 lb
4. 8 to 10 lb

72. 3. The common weight used for Buck's traction in an adult is 5 to 7 lb.
NP: Implementation; CN: Safe, effective care environment; CNS: Management of care; CL: Knowledge

73. Which of the following types of traction is used for leg traction?
1. Bryant's traction
2. Buck's traction
3. Pelvic belt
4. Russell traction

73. 4. Russell's traction is used for leg traction. Bryant's traction is used for children who weigh less than 35 lb. Buck's traction is used for leg or arm traction. A pelvic belt is conservative treatment for lower back pain.
NP: Implementation; CN: Physiological integrity; CNS: Physiological adaptation; CL: Knowledge

74. Vitamin D intake is important in the healing of fractures for which of the following reasons?
1. It reduces the excretion of calcium and phosphorus.
2. It increases the excretion of calcium and phosphorus.
3. It reduces the absorption and use of calcium and phosphorus.
4. It increases the absorption and use of calcium and phosphorus.

74. 4. Vitamin D increases the absorption and use of calcium and phosphorus. It doesn't reduce the absorption or affect the excretion of calcium and phosphorus.
NP: Implementation; CN: Physiological integrity; CNS: Pharmacological and parenteral therapies; CL: Knowledge

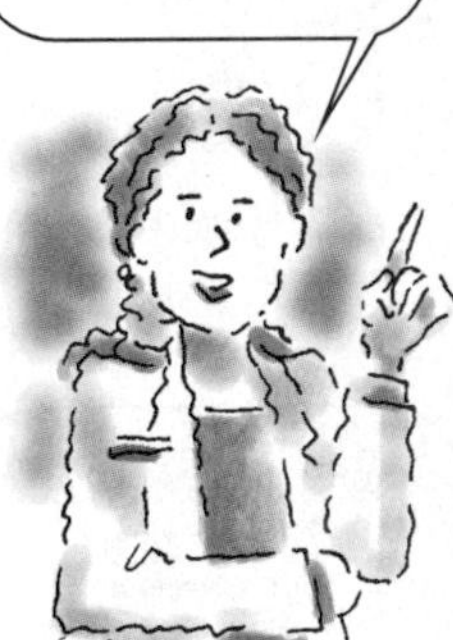

Placing the client in the correct position after this surgery is critical.

75. After surgical repair of a hip, which of the following positions is best for the client's legs and hips?
1. Abduction
2. Adduction
3. Prone
4. Subluxated

75. 1. After surgical repair of the hip, the desired position of the legs and hips is abduction. Adduction, prone, or subluxated positions don't keep the prosthesis within the acetabulum.
NP: Planning; CN: Physiological integrity; CNS: Reduction of risk potential; CL: Application

76. After a hip replacement, which of the following activity levels is usually ordered?
1. Bed rest
2. No restrictions
3. No weight bearing
4. Limited weight bearing

76. 4. After a hip replacement, the client's activity is usually ordered as limited weight bearing. The client is allowed to move with restrictions for approximately 2 to 3 months. The hip shouldn't be flexed more than 90 degrees. Abduction past the midline of the body is prohibited. Progressive weight bearing reduces the complications of immobility.
NP: Implementation; CN: Physiological integrity; CNS: Basic care and comfort; CL: Knowledge

77. Which of the following interventions would help prevent deep vein thrombosis (DVT) after hip surgery?
1. Bed rest
2. Egg crate mattress
3. Vigorous pulmonary care
4. Subcutaneous heparin and pneumatic compression boots

77. 4. To prevent DVT after hip surgery, subcutaneous heparin and pneumatic compression boots are used. Bed rest can cause DVT. Egg crate mattresses and pulmonary care don't prevent DVT.

NP: Analysis; CN: Health promotion and maintenance; CNS: Prevention and early detection of disease; CL: Application

78. Which of the following discharge instructions should be given to a client after surgery for repair of a hip fracture?
1. "Don't flex the hip more than 30 degrees, don't cross your legs, get help putting on your shoes."
2. "Don't flex the hip more than 60 degrees, don't cross your legs, get help putting on your shoes."
3. "Don't flex the hip more than 90 degrees, don't cross your legs, get help putting on your shoes."
4. "Don't flex the hip more than 120 degrees, don't cross your legs, get help putting on your shoes."

78. 3. Discharge instructions should include not flexing the hip more than 90 degrees, not crossing the legs, and getting help to put on shoes. These restrictions prevent dislocation of the new prosthesis.

NP: Planning; CN: Safe, effective care environment; CNS: Management of care; CL: Application

79. At the scene of an accident, which of the following interventions applies to a client with a suspected fracture?
1. Don't move the client.
2. Move the client to safety immediately.
3. Sit the client up to facilitate his airway.
4. Immobilize the extremity, and move the client to safety.

79. 4. At the scene of an accident, a client with a suspected fracture should have the extremity immobilized and be moved to safety. If the client is in a safe place, don't try to move him. Never try to sit the client up; this could make the fracture worse.

NP: Implementation; CN: Safe, effective care environment; CNS: Safety and infection control; CL: Application

80. Which of the following statements is true about fracture reduction?
1. All fractures can be reduced.
2. Fracture reduction restores alignment.
3. Nondisplaced fractures may be reduced.
4. Fracture reduction is usually performed with minimal discomfort.

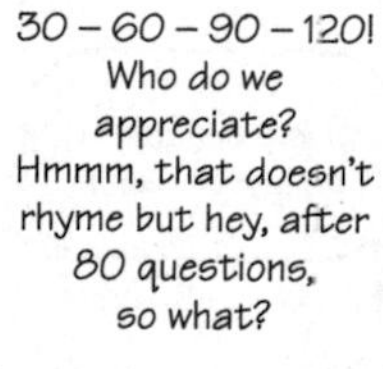
30 – 60 – 90 – 120!
Who do we
appreciate?
Hmmm, that doesn't
rhyme but hey, after
80 questions,
so what?

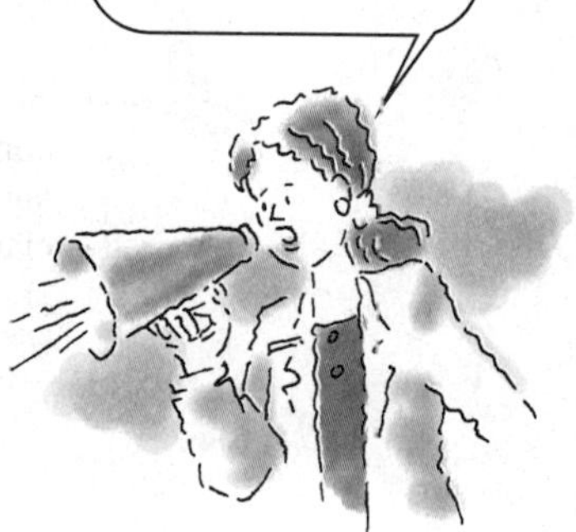

80. 2. Fracture reduction restores alignment. All fractures can't be reduced. Fracture reduction is usually painful. Nondisplaced fractures can't be reduced.

NP: Analysis; CN: Physiological integrity; CNS: Reduction of risk potential; CL: Knowledge

81. A client with a right hip fracture is complaining of left-sided leg pain and edema and has a positive Homans' sign. Which of the following conditions would show those symptoms?

1. Deep vein thrombosis (DVT)
2. Fat emboli
3. Infection
4. Pulmonary embolism

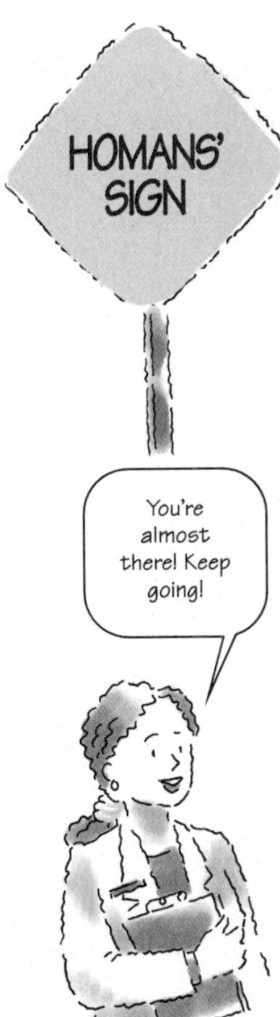

HOMANS' SIGN
You're almost there! Keep going!

81. 1. Unilateral leg pain and edema with a positive Homans' sign (not always present) might be symptoms of DVT. Symptoms of fat emboli include restlessness, tachypnea, and tachycardia and are more common in long-bone injuries. It's unlikely an infection would occur on the opposite side of the fracture without cause. Tachycardia, chest pain, and shortness of breath may be symptoms of a pulmonary embolism.

NP: Analysis; CN: Physiological integrity; CNS: Reduction of risk potential; CL: Knowledge

82. Which of the following nursing interventions is appropriate for a client in traction?

1. Assess the pin sites every shift and as needed.
2. Add and remove weights as the client wants.
3. Make sure the knots in the rope catch on the pulley.
4. Give range of motion to all joints, including those immediately proximal and distal to the fracture, every shift.

82. 1. Nursing care for a client in traction may include assessing pin sites every shift and as needed and making sure the knots in the rope don't catch on the pulley. Add and remove weights as the physician orders, and give range of motion to all joints except those immediately proximal and distal to the fracture every shift.

NP: Implementation; CN: Physiological integrity; CNS: Basic care and comfort; CL: Application

83. After helping the physician apply a cast, which of the following nursing interventions is included in the immediate cast care?

1. Rest the cast on the bedside table.
2. Dispose of the plaster water in the sink.
3. Support the cast with the palms of the hands.
4. Wait until the cast dries before cleaning the surrounding skin.

83. 3. After helping the physician apply a cast, support it with the palms of the hands; don't rest the cast on a hard or sharp surface. Dispose of the plaster water in a sink with a plaster trap or in a garbage bag. Clean the surrounding skin before the cast dries.

NP: Planning; CN: Safe, effective care environment; CNS: Management of care; CL: Comprehension

84. Synthetic casts take approximately how long to set?

1. Immediately
2. 20 minutes
3. 45 minutes
4. 2 hours

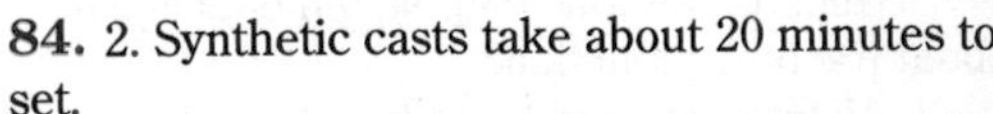

84. 2. Synthetic casts take about 20 minutes to set.

NP: Analysis; CN: Safe, effective care environment; CNS: Management of care; CL: Knowledge

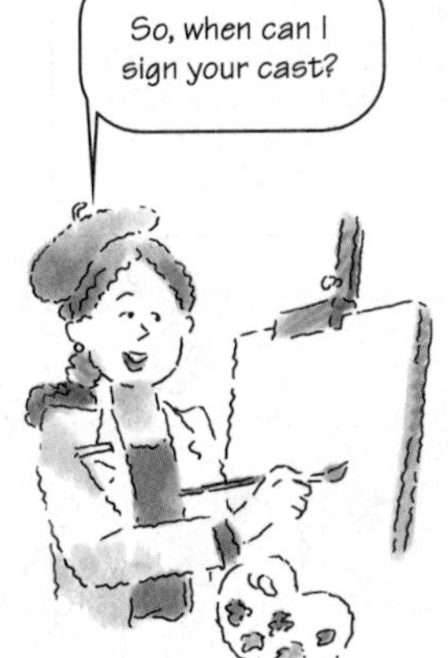

So, when can I sign your cast?

85. As a cast is drying, a client complains of heat from the cast. Which of the following interventions is the most appropriate?

1. Remove the cast immediately.
2. Explain this is a normal sensation.
3. Notify the physician.
4. Assess the client for other signs of infection.

85. 2. Normally as the cast dries, a client may complain of heat from the cast. Offer reassurance. Don't remove the cast or notify the physician. Heat from the cast isn't a sign of infection.

NP: Implementation; CN: Safe, effective care environment; CNS: Management of care; CL: Comprehension

86. To prevent foot drop in a leg with a cast, which of the following interventions is appropriate?

1. Encourage bed rest.
2. Support the foot with 45 degrees of flexion.
3. Support the foot with 90 degrees of flexion.
4. Place a stocking on the foot to provide warmth.

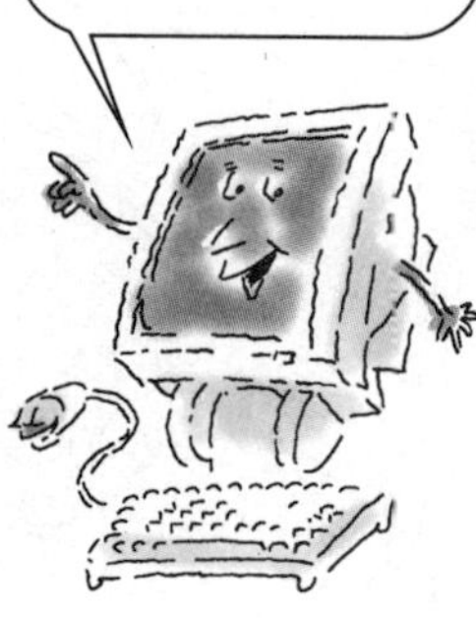

The word *prevent* is a hint. Look for a preventive measure, not a treatment.

86. 3. To prevent foot drop in a leg with a cast, the foot should be supported with 90 degrees of flexion. Bed rest can cause foot drop. Keeping the extremity warm won't prevent foot drop.

NP: Planning; CN: Health promotion and maintenance; CNS: Prevention and early detection of disease; CL: Comprehension

87. A client with a hip-spica cast should avoid gas-forming foods. Which of the following rationales best explains why?

1. To prevent flatus
2. To prevent diarrhea
3. To prevent constipation
4. To prevent abdominal distention

87. 4. A client with a hip-spica cast should avoid gas-forming foods to prevent abdominal distention. Gas-forming foods may cause flatus, but that isn't a reason to avoid them. Gas-forming foods generally don't cause diarrhea or constipation.

NP: Planning; CN: Physiological integrity; CNS: Reduction of risk potential; CL: Comprehension

88. Which of the following descriptions of touchdown weight bearing is correct?

1. Full weight bearing on the affected extremity
2. 30% to 50% weight bearing on the affected extremity
3. No weight on the extremity, but may touch the floor with it
4. No weight on the extremity, and keep it elevated at all times

88. 3. Touchdown weight bearing involves no weight on the extremity, but the client may touch the floor with the affected extremity. Full weight bearing allows for full weight to be put on the affected extremity. Partial weight bearing allows for 30% to 50% weight bearing on affected extremity. Non-weight bearing is no weight on the extremity.

NP: Implementation; CN: Safe, effective care environment; CNS: Management of care; CL: Knowledge

89. Which of the following interventions is the most effective way to prevent sports-related injuries?

1. Warming up
2. Pacing the activity
3. Building strength
4. Working with moderate intensity

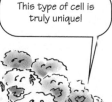

89. 1. The best way to prevent sports-related injuries is to warm up. Pacing the activity, building strength, and using moderate intensity are also prevention measures, but warming up is the most effective.

NP: Planning; CN: Safe, effective care environment; CNS: Management of care; CL: Knowledge

90. Which of the following tissues forms new tissue after an injury instead of scar tissue?

1. Bone tissue
2. Brain tissue
3. Kidney tissue
4. Liver tissue

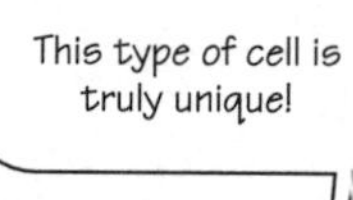

This type of cell is truly unique!

90. 1. Bone tissue regenerates; all other tissues form scar tissue after injury.

NP: Assessment; CN: Physiological integrity; CNS: Physiological adaptation; CL: Knowledge

91. Which of the following reactions is not an immune reaction to injury?
1. Tumor growth at a long-bone fracture
2. Swelling and redness at the site of a cut
3. Torn ligament with exudate below the torn ends
4. Necrotic tissue with mast cells at the fracture site

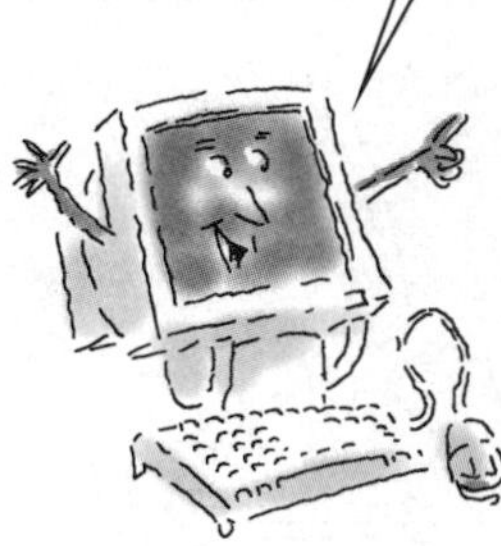

Watch out for negative verbs. Whenever you see one, double-check your answer.

91. 1. Tumor growth is the abnormal division and replication of cells that may result in fractures. The formation of exudate, swelling and redness at the site of an injury, and collection of mast cells at a fracture site, are all part of the immune response to injury.
NP: Assessment; CN: Physiological integrity; CNS: Physiological adaptation; CL: Analysis

92. Which of the following statements explains an open reduction of a fractured femur?
1. Traction will be used.
2. A cast will be applied.
3. Crutches will be used after surgery.
4. Some form of screw, plate, nail, or wire is usually used to maintain alignment.

92. 4. Open reduction means that the tissue must be surgically opened and the fractured bones realigned. To maintain proper alignment, a screw, plate, nail, or wire is inserted to prevent the bones from separating. Although traction may have been used before surgery, it won't be needed any longer once the fracture is reduced. A cast or crutches may be used after surgery, but the question asks specifically about the surgical procedure.
NP: Implementation; CN: Physiological integrity; CNS: Physiological adaptation; CL: Application

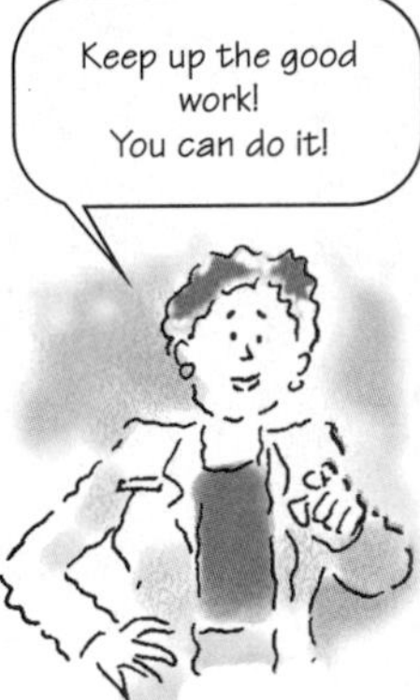

Keep up the good work!
You can do it!

93. Dislocation of the hip includes which of the following symptoms?
1. Pain relieved with pressure
2. Pain in the inguinal area, abnormal gait
3. Internal rotation of the knee, abduction of the leg
4. Pain in the hip, the thigh appears longer than the unaffected leg

93. 2. A dislocated hip will create problems with walking, and pain is often due to a pinched nerve in the joint. Pressure shouldn't be applied to a painful joint or fracture unless there's hemorrhage. The leg is usually adducted and shortened.
NP: Assessment; CN: Physiological integrity; CNS: Physiological adaptation; CL: Analysis

94. A 20-year-old client developed osteomyelitis 2 weeks after a fishhook was removed from his foot. Which of the following rationales best explains the expected long-term antibiotic therapy needed?
1. Bone has poor circulation.
2. Tissue trauma requires antibiotics.
3. Feet are normally more difficult to treat.
4. Fishhook injuries are highly contaminated.

94. 1. Bone has very poor blood circulation, making it difficult to treat an infection in the bone. This requires the long-term use of I.V. antibiotics to make sure the infection is cleared. Tissue trauma doesn't always require antibiotics, at least not long term. Feet aren't more difficult to treat than other parts of the body unless the client has a circulatory problem or diabetes mellitus. Fishhooks may not be any more contaminated than another instrument that caused an injury.
NP: Implementation; CN: Physiological integrity; CNS: Pharmacological and parenteral therapies; CL: Application

95. Degenerative joint disease, also commonly known as osteoarthritis, is a term describing which of the following conditions?
1. Noninflammatory joint disease
2. Immune-mediated joint disease
3. Joint inflammation after a viral infection
4. Joint inflammation related to systemic infections

95. 1. Degenerative joint disease is joint disease due to the wear and tear on joints and is often seen in athletes. It isn't immune-mediated, or inflammatory, or caused by systemic infections.
NP: Assessment; CN: Physiological integrity; CNS: Physiological adaptation; CL: Comprehension

96. Client education about gout includes which of the following information?
1. Good foot care will reduce complications.
2. Increased dietary intake of purine is needed.
3. Production of uric acid in the kidney affects joints.
4. Uric acid crystals cause inflammatory destruction of the joint.

96. 4. The client needs to know that uric acid crystals collect in the joint of the great toe and cause inflammation. The kidney excretes uric acid, an end product of metabolism. A diet low in purines would be indicated. Good foot care doesn't affect the development of complications, but increasing water intake may help prevent urinary stone formation.
NP: Implementation; CN: Physiological integrity; CNS: Reduction of risk potential; CL: Application

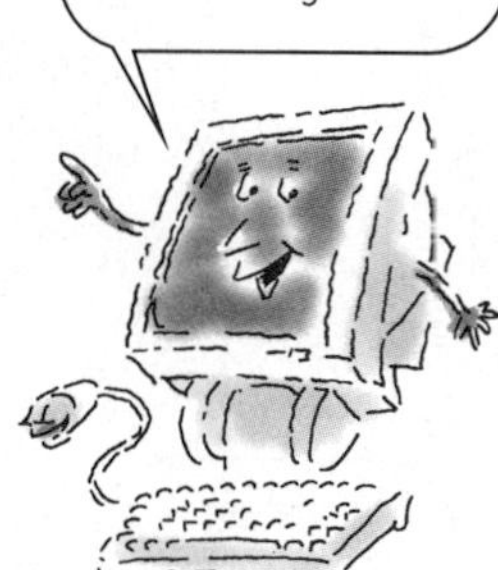

The words most commonly in questions 97 and 98 are clues to the answer. Am I right, or am I right?

97. If I.V. antibiotics don't eliminate osteomyelitis, which of the following treatments is most commonly used next?
1. Bone grafts
2. Hyperbaric oxygen therapy
3. Amputation of the extremity
4. Debridement of necrotic tissue

97. 4. The tissues may need to be debrided to eliminate necrotic tissue and allow new tissue to form. A bone graft would be done after debridement. Hyperbaric oxygen therapy is a new treatment modality that has been used in the successful treatment of osteomyelitis, but it isn't universally available. Amputation isn't indicated in the treatment of acute osteomyelitis.
NP: Assessment; CN: Physiological integrity; CNS: Physiological adaptation; CL: Comprehension

98. Osteomyelitis most commonly results from which of the following mechanisms?
1. Immune suppression
2. I.V. drug use
3. Surgery
4. Trauma

98. 4. Trauma is the most common event causing osteomyelitis. Individuals who are immunosuppressed may be at greater risk for osteomyelitis, but immunosuppression isn't a cause of osteomyelitis. I.V. drug use is more commonly associated with endocarditis. Surgery isn't likely to be a cause.
NP: Assessment; CN: Physiological integrity; CNS: Reduction of risk potential; CL: Comprehension

99. Nursing interventions to treat a musculoskeletal injury may include cold or heat therapy. Cold therapy decreases pain by which of the following actions?

1. Promotes analgesia and circulation
2. Numbs the nerves and dilates the vessels
3. Promotes circulation and reduces muscle spasms
4. Causes local vasoconstriction and prevents edema or muscle spasm

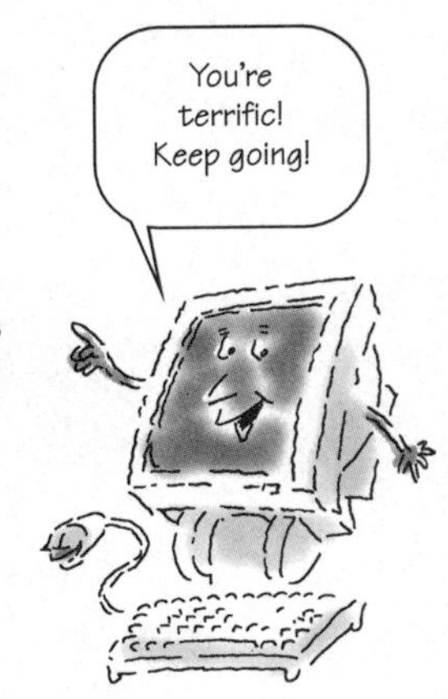
You're terrific! Keep going!

99. 4. Cold causes the blood vessels to constrict, which reduces the leakage of fluid into the tissues and prevents swelling and muscle spasms. Cold therapy may reduce pain by numbing the nerves and tissues. Heat therapy promotes circulation, enhances flexibility, reduces muscle spasms, and also provides analgesia.

NP: Implementation; CN: Physiological integrity; CNS: Basic care and comfort; CL: Comprehension

100. What discharge information should be given to a client with a cast?

1. "Use powder under the cast as needed."
2. "Itching under the cast indicates infection."
3. "Keep the extremity in a dependent position."
4. "Report fever and foul odors around the cast."

100. 4. Fever, foul odor, and warmth over a specific area of the cast after it's dry may be signs of infection. Itchy skin results from dry skin, and powder shouldn't be used. The extremity should be elevated for 24 to 48 hours.

NP: Implementation; CN: Health promotion and maintenance; CNS: Prevention and early detection of disease; CL: Application

101. Which of the following diagnoses would place a client at risk for traction-related complications?

1. Coronary artery disease
2. Diabetes mellitus
3. Hip fracture
4. Hypertension

101. 2. Because people with diabetes commonly have microvascular compromise and delayed wound healing, they need careful monitoring for early signs of skin breakdown. The other conditions don't increase the risk of traction-related complications.

NP: Evaluation; CN: Physiological integrity; CNS: Reduction of risk potential; CL: Analysis

102. A client complains that he experiences pain and numbness in his fingers when he types on a computer keyboard. Which action will help the nurse assess for Phalen's sign?

1. Having the client hold both hands above his head with his arms straight for 30 seconds
2. Having the client hold both wrists in acute flexion with the dorsal surfaces touching for 60 seconds
3. Tapping gently over the median nerve in the wrist
4. Having the client extend his wrists while the nurse provides resistance

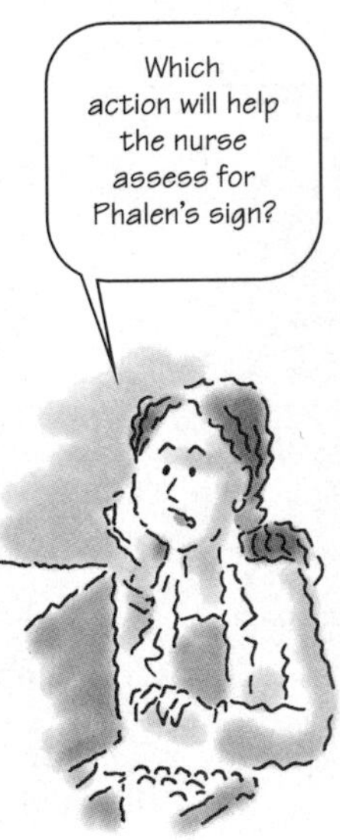
Which action will help the nurse assess for Phalen's sign?

102. 2. Acute wrist flexion places pressure on the inflamed median nerve, causing the pain and numbness of carpal tunnel syndrome (Phalen's sign). Holding the hands above the head with arms straight for 30 seconds isn't an assessment technique. Tapping gently over the median nerve tests for Tinel's sign, another sign of carpal tunnel syndrome. Placing the wrists in extension against resistance tests strength.

NP: Assessment; CN: Physiological integrity; CNS: Physiological adaptation; CL: Application

103. A client has a knee-high cast removed 6 weeks after suffering an ankle fracture. Palpation reveals a hard, nontender lump at the fracture site. How should the nurse interpret this finding?

1. Abnormal; the bone may have healed in misalignment, possibly from the short leg cast.
2. Abnormal; remodeling should have occurred by now, so the findings suggest malunion.
3. Normal; swelling and bruising may persist after a traumatic fracture.
4. Normal; callus formation normally occurs at this stage and may feel like a lump on the bone.

103. 4. Callus formation is a normal stage of bone repair. It's characterized by an overgrowth of bone that's reabsorbed gradually during the remodeling stage. This deformity is painless, whereas misalignment and malunion typically cause pain. Swelling and bruising should have disappeared by this time.

NP: Assessment; CN: Physiological integrity; CNS: Physiological adaptation; CL: Analysis

104. A client is being discharged from the emergency department after cast application for a tibial fracture. A serious complication of this injury is identified with the nursing diagnosis *Impaired gas exchange: Fat embolus related to long bone fracture.* Based on this diagnosis, which instruction should the nurse provide?

1. "Cough and deep breathe at least every 2 hours."
2. "Keep the leg elevated and apply ice for the first 24 to 48 hours."
3. "Call the physician at once if you experience apprehensiveness, shortness of breath, fever, or palpitations."
4. "Restrict your fluid intake to 1 L per day."

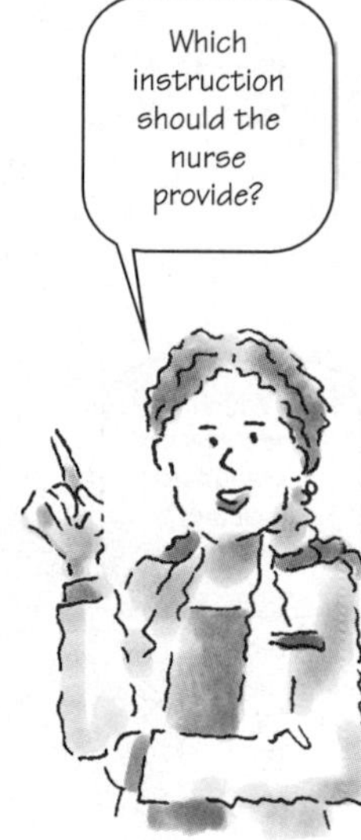
Which instruction should the nurse provide?

104. 3. Fat embolism is a complication of a long bone fracture. Signs and symptoms include apprehension, altered mental status, respiratory distress, tachycardia, tachypnea, fever, and petechiae over the neck, upper arms, and chest. Coughing and deep-breathing exercises as well as leg elevations with ice applications can help prevent other complications of a long bone fracture but have no effect on fat emboli. The client should also be instructed that drinking plenty of fluids to stay well hydrated will help him avoid embolic complications.

NP: Planning; CN: Physiological integrity; CNS: Reduction of risk potential; CL: Application

105. A client who's receiving acetaminophen for osteoarthritis complains of continuing pain. The physician prescribes rofecoxib (Vioxx). Which medication instruction should the nurse provide?

1. "Don't take the medication with dairy products."
2. "Report stomach upset to the physician."
3. "If you miss a dose, take a double dose the next day."
4. "Use a stool softener or fiber laxative daily to prevent constipation."

105. 2. GI irritation can be a precursor to GI bleeding and may necessitate a medication change. Dairy products help reduce GI irritation. The rofecoxib dose should never be doubled. Constipation isn't an adverse effect of this drug.

NP: Implementation; CN: Physiological integrity; CNS: Pharmacological and parenteral therapies; CL: Application

106. A client has an above-the-knee amputation 4 days after a traumatic injury. Which nursing diagnosis is most appropriate?

1. Risk for impaired skin integrity related to decreased peripheral circulation
2. Impaired gas exchange: Fat embolism related to surgical removal of bone and tissue
3. Acute pain: Phantom limb pain related to surgical removal of leg after traumatic injury
4. Decreased cardiac output: Shock related to decreased fluid volume

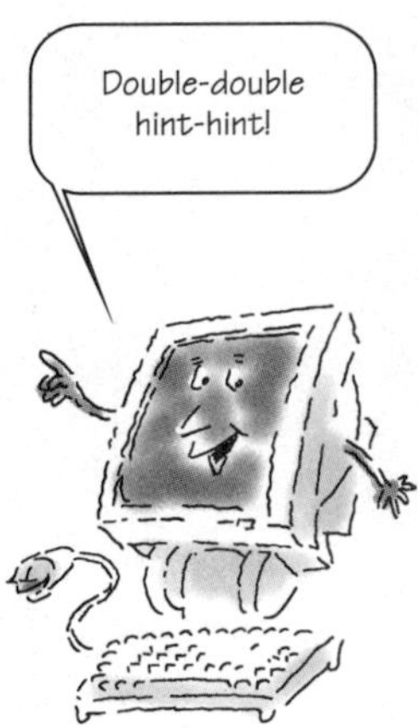
Double-double
hint-hint!

106. 3. Phantom limb pain is common after limb amputation and may be more severe with traumatic injury. Because the limb was severed traumatically rather than removed because of poor circulation, peripheral circulation should be adequate. Fat embolism is more typical with long bone fractures. The risk of shock is relatively low on the 4th postoperative day.
NP: Assessment; CN: Psychosocial integrity; CNS: Coping and adaptation; CL: Analysis

107. The nurse is assigned to care for a 70-year-old client with acute rheumatoid arthritis. Which of the following assessment findings will the nurse expect to find during the physical examination?

1. Tender, painful, stiff joints
2. Radial deviation of the distal phalanges
3. Heberden's nodes
4. Bouchard's nodes

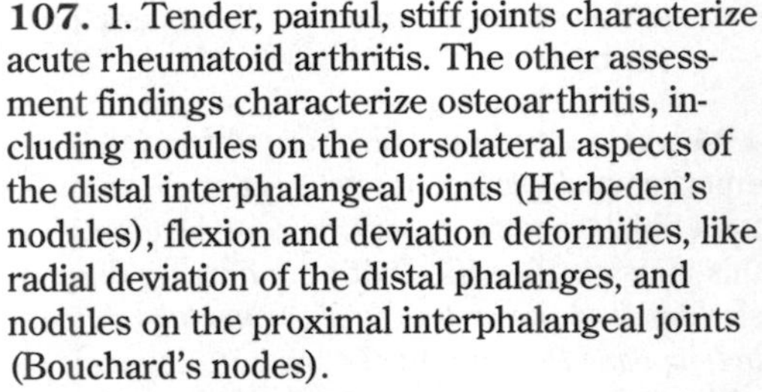

107. 1. Tender, painful, stiff joints characterize acute rheumatoid arthritis. The other assessment findings characterize osteoarthritis, including nodules on the dorsolateral aspects of the distal interphalangeal joints (Herbeden's nodules), flexion and deviation deformities, like radial deviation of the distal phalanges, and nodules on the proximal interphalangeal joints (Bouchard's nodes).
NP: Assessment; CN: Physiological integrity; CNS: Physiological adaptation; CL: Application

108. A client with lactose intolerance requires dietary teaching. Which of the following foods should the nurse advise him to eat to ensure adequate calcium intake?

1. Bananas and avocados
2. Beef liver and broccoli
3. Cheese and yogurt
4. Collard greens and spinach

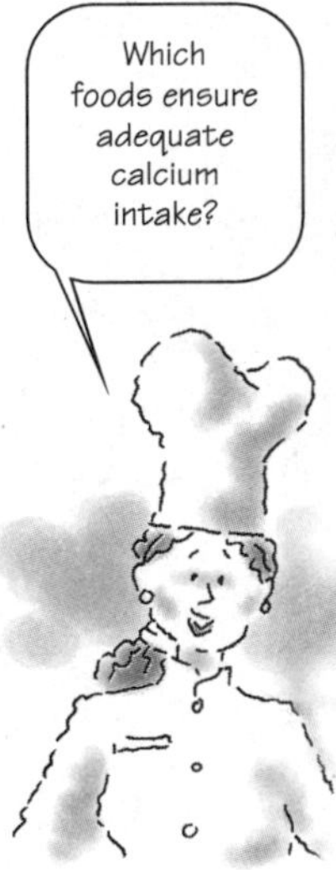
Which
foods ensure
adequate
calcium
intake?

108. 4. Dark green, leafy vegetables are the best nondairy sources of calcium. Bananas and avocados are good sources of vitamin K. Beef liver and broccoli supply iron. Cheese and yogurt are dairy products, which this client should avoid because of the lactose intolerance.
NP: Planning; CN: Health promotion and maintenance; CNS: Prevention and early detection of disease; CL: Application

109. An elderly client in a nursing home is particularly susceptible to bone loss. Which of the following can contribute to bone loss?

1. Calcium channel blockers
2. Chronic use of stool softeners
3. Decreased mobility
4. Lack of sunlight exposure

109. 4. Lack of sunlight exposure decreases absorption of vitamin D, which must be present for calcium to be absorbed from the small intestine. Calcium channel blockers don't affect serum calcium levels. Stool softeners don't increase peristalsis, so they don't impair calcium absorption. Decreased mobility is a result, not a cause, of bone loss.
NP: Planning; CN: Health promotion and maintenance; CNS: Growth and development through the life span; CL: Analysis

110. A client with a torn meniscus caused by a football injury arrives at the outpatient surgery clinic for an arthroscopic meniscectomy. Which teaching topic should the nurse cover at this time?

1. Exactly how the procedure will be performed
2. Avoidance of weight bearing for 2 weeks after the surgery
3. Postoperative exercises, such as straight-leg raising and quadriceps setting
4. The possibility of severe postoperative pain for 24 to 48 hours after surgery

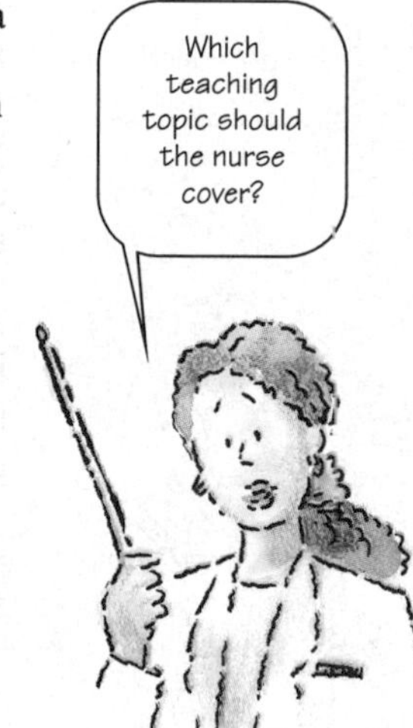

110. 3. The best time to teach about postoperative care is preoperatively. Straight-leg raising and quadriceps setting exercises help maintain the strength of the affected extremity. The physician, not the nurse, should explain the surgical procedure. Weight bearing may begin as soon as the day of surgery. Usually, pain is mild to moderate after arthroscopic surgery.

NP: Implementation; CN: Physiological integrity; CNS: Basic care and comfort; CL: Application

111. A client is ready to be discharged after arthroscopic knee surgery. Which instruction should the nurse provide?

1. "Ice and elevate the extremity for 12 hours after discharge."
2. "Infection isn't a potential problem because of the small incision size."
3. "Swelling and coolness of the joint and limb are normal right after surgery."
4. "Take acetaminophen with codeine every 4 hours as necessary for pain relief."

111. 4. Mild to moderate pain is normal after this type of surgery and can be relieved by oral narcotic analgesics. To minimize swelling, the client should ice and elevate the extremity for at least 24 hours after surgery. Infection is a potential problem after an invasive procedure. Swelling and coolness of the joint and limb may indicate complications from tourniquet use during surgery.

NP: Implementation; CN: Physiological integrity; CNS: Basic care and comfort; CL: Application

112. The nurse is counseling a perimenopausal client, age 50, about hormone replacement therapy (HRT). The client is at high risk for osteoporosis because of her family history, lactose intolerance, and small body frame. Which health history factor may contraindicate HRT?

1. History of breast cancer
2. Obesity
3. Smoking
4. Type II diabetes

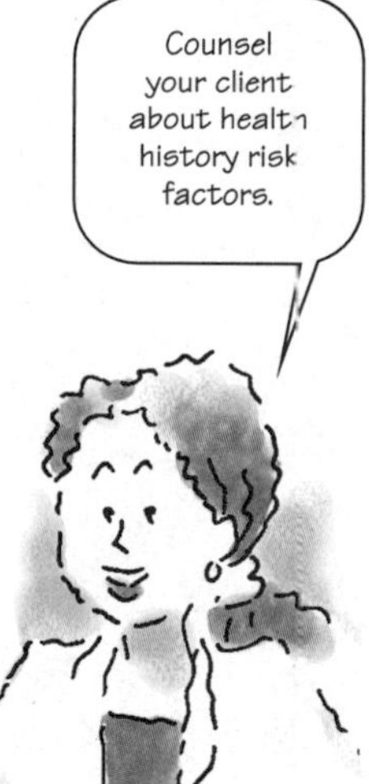

Counsel your client about health history risk factors.

112. 1. Studies show that estrogen in HRT may influence the development of breast and uterine cancers. Obesity, smoking, and type II diabetes haven't been found to significantly increase risks associated with HRT. Benefits of HRT may outweigh the risks.

NP: Planning; CN: Physiological integrity; CNS: Pharmacological and parenteral therapies; CL: Analysis

113. For a client diagnosed with Ewing's sarcoma, which test is *most* useful in determining the extent of metastasis?

1. Bone scan
2. Computerized tomography (CT) scan
3. Magnetic resonance imaging (MRI)
4. Positron emission tomography (PET)

113. 1. A bone scan views the entire skeletal structure, indicating areas of possible metastases. CT scan, MRI, and PET scan visualize only one body area at a time.

NP: Assessment; CN: Physiological integrity; CNS: Reduction of risk potential; CL: Application

114. An 80-year-old client with pneumonia is admitted to the hospital. Her past medical history includes chronic rheumatoid arthritis. Which of the following assessment findings will the nurse expect during the physical examination?

1. Flattened thenar eminence
2. Thickened plaque overlying the flexor tendon of the ring finger
3. Cystic swelling on the dorsum of the wrist
4. Swan neck deformity

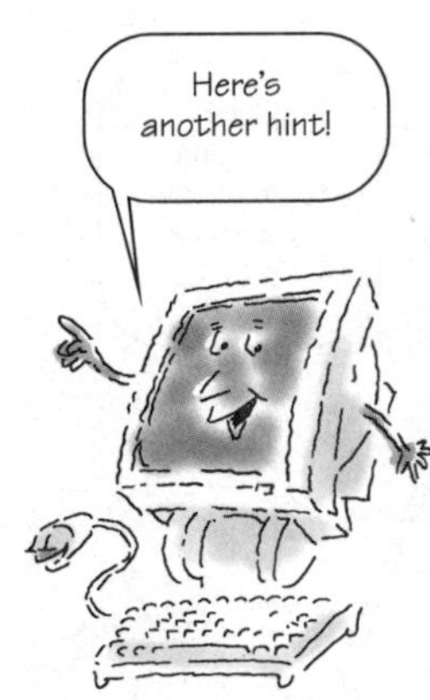
Here's
another hint!

114. 4. In chronic rheumatoid arthritis, the fingers may show hyperextension of the proximal interphalangeal joints with fixed flexion of the distal interphalangeal joints, referred to as swan neck deformities. Flattened thenar eminence characterizes thenar atrophy, a condition which suggests an ulnar nerve disorder. The first sign of a Dupuytren's contracture is a thickened plaque overlying the flexor tendon of the ring finger and possibly the little finger at the level of the distal palmar crease. Ganglia are cystic, round, usually nontender swellings located along tendon sheaths or joint capsules; ganglia frequently involve the dorsum of the wrist.

NP: Assessment; CN: Physiological integrity; CNS: Physiological adaptation; CL: Application

115. A 64-year-old client with complications related to metastatic cancer and complaints of back pain is admitted to the hospital. Which of the following assessment findings will the nurse expect during the physical examination?

1. A rounded thoracic convexity
2. A gibbus
3. Gentle concavities in the cervical and lumbar regions and a convexity in the thorax
4. An accentuation of the normal lumbar curve

115. 2. Gibbus is an angular deformity of collapsed vertebra and is frequently caused by metastatic cancer or tuberculosis of the spine. A rounded thoracic convexity, kyphosis, is common in aging, especially in women. Gentle curves of the normal spine include concavities in the cervical and lumbar regions and a convexity of the thorax. An accentuation of the normal lumbar curve, lordosis, frequently develops to compensate for the protuberant abdomen of pregnancy or marked obesity.

NP: Assessment; CNS: Physiological integrity; CNS: Physiological adaptation; CL: Application

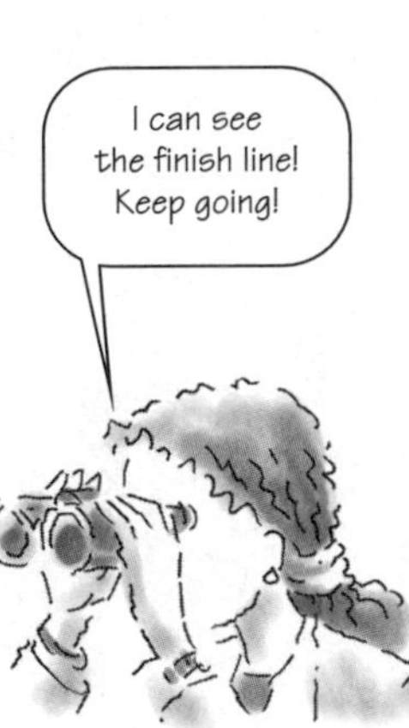
I can see
the finish line!
Keep going!

116. An elderly client with rheumatoid arthritis is being treated with prednisone (Deltasone). Which of the following can occur with long-term prednisone therapy?

1. Breast and uterine cancer
2. Osteoporosis and diabetes mellitus
3. Deep vein thrombosis (DVT), pulmonary embolus, and stroke
4. Weight loss and lactose intolerance

116. 2. Long-term prednisone therapy can increase the loss of calcium from bones, slow down the formation of new bone tissue (resulting in osteoporosis), and alter glucose metabolism (resulting in diabetes mellitus). Breast and uterine cancer, DVT, pulmonary embolus, stroke, weight loss, and lactose intolerance aren't common adverse effects of prednisone.

NP: Planning; CN: Physiological integrity; CNS: Pharmacological and parenteral therapies; CL: Analysis

117. A client with a femoral fracture is in skeletal traction. During the initial shift assessment, the nurse finds that the weight used in traction is heavier than specified by the nursing care plan. Which action should the nurse take first?

1. Ask the physician during rounds if the order for the weight was changed.
2. Assume that if the weight was changed, the physician ordered it.
3. Check the physician's orders to see if they include a weight change.
4. Remove the weight and replace it with the weight specified in the plan.

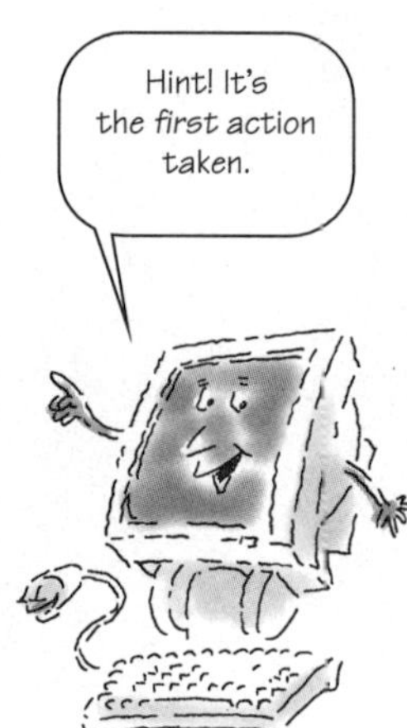
Hint! It's
the first action
taken.

117. 3. First, the nurse should check the physician's orders to see if a weight change was ordered. If it was, the nurse responsible for ensuring implementation of the care plan should investigate why the change wasn't incorporated in the plan.

NP: Evaluation; CN: Safe, effective care environment; CNS: Management of care; CL: Analysis

118. The nurse is assessing a client's response to skeletal traction applied to the lower extremity. Which finding would be considered normal?

1. Coolness and pallor below the fracture level
2. Erythema and swelling immediately around the pin insertion site
3. Moderate to severe muscle spasms around the fracture area
4. Serous drainage and crust formation at the pin insertion site

118. 4. Serous drainage around the pin insertion site is a normal finding; some institutions don't recommend crust removal because of its protective nature. A pale extremity may indicate arterial compromise. Erythema and swelling signal infection. Severe muscle spasms may indicate improper alignment of the body or traction.

NP: Assessment; CN: Physiological integrity; CNS: Reduction of risk potential; CL: Analysis

119. Which nursing diagnosis is appropriate for a client with diabetes who is placed in skeletal traction after a motor vehicle accident?

1. Imbalanced nutrition: less than body requirements related to malabsorption of nutrients
2. Risk for infection related to the skeletal pin
3. Risk for injury related to subluxation of the joint above the pin insertion site
4. Risk for autonomic dysreflexia

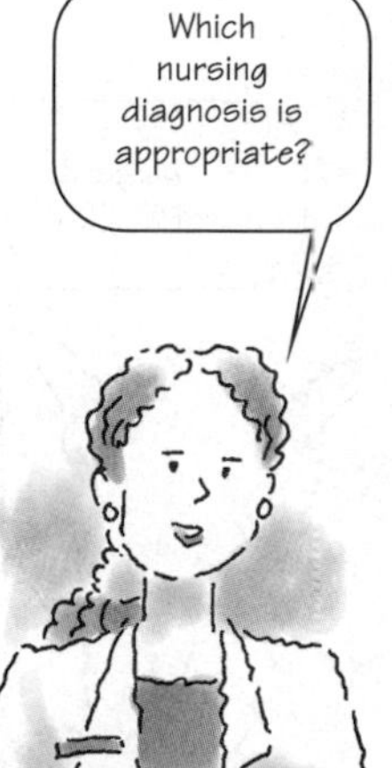
Which
nursing
diagnosis is
appropriate?

119. 2. This client has a significant risk of osteomyelitis secondary to the skeletal pin. A dangerous bone infection that's hard to eradicate, osteomyelitis should be prevented at all costs — especially in a client with diabetes, who is already prone to infection. Based on the information provided, the other nursing diagnoses aren't appropriate.

NP: Assessment; CN: Physiological integrity; CNS: Reduction of risk potential; CL: Analysis

120. A client in skeletal traction complains of pain even though he received an analgesic 1 hour ago. The nurse wants to offer an alternative pain-management measure. Which of the following can she implement within her scope of practice?

1. Acupressure and shiatsu
2. Hypnosis and therapeutic touch
3. Relaxation and imagery
4. Swedish massage and the Feldenkrais method

120. 3. Relaxation and imagery are effective adjuncts to pharmacologic pain management that the nurse can implement without a physician's order. Although the other therapies may promote pain management, they require special training or certification.

NP: Implementation; CN: Physiological integrity; CNS: Basic care and comfort; CL: Application

121. The nurse is preparing to change the dressing of a client 1 day after an open amputation of the right lower extremity. Which type of drainage should the nurse expect to find?

1. Little to no drainage on the staples
2. Sanguinous drainage contained with a two-layer 4″ × 4″ gauze dressing
3. Serous drainage contained with a two-layer 4″ × 4″ gauze dressing
4. Serosanguinous, purulent drainage soaking a large gauze dressing

121. 4. An open amputation is done when drainage of fluid and pus is expected. Because the client had surgery the previous day, serosanguinous drainage is expected. If the wound was surgically closed, drainage eventually would break open the suture line, disrupting the surgical incision. Initial drainage should be heavy. Staples aren't present after an open amputation.

NP: Assessment; CN: Physiological integrity; CNS: Reduction of risk potential: CL: Analysis

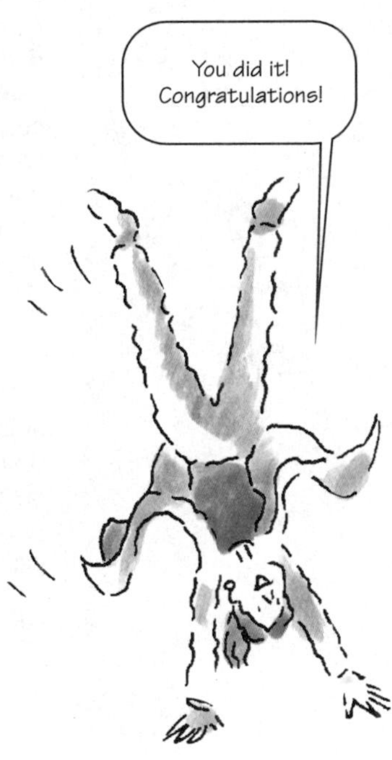
You did it!
Congratulations!

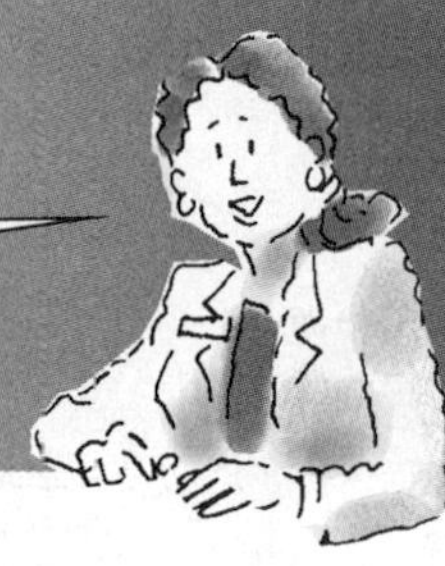

From hiatal hernias to diverticulitis to pancreatitis, this chapter covers all the GI disorders you could ask for, in one handy package. Gotta love it!

Chapter 8 Gastrointestinal disorders

1. Which of the following conditions can cause a hiatal hernia?

1. Increased intrathoracic pressure
2. Weakness of the esophageal muscle
3. Increased esophageal muscle pressure
4. Weakness of the diaphragmatic muscle

1. 4. A hiatal hernia is caused by weakness of the diaphragmatic muscle and increased intra-abdominal — not intrathoracic — pressure. This weakness allows the stomach to slide into the esophagus. The esophageal supports weaken, but esophageal muscle weakness or increased esophageal muscle pressure isn't a factor in hiatal hernia.

NP: Assessment; CN: Physiological integrity; CNS: Physiological adaptation; CL: Knowledge

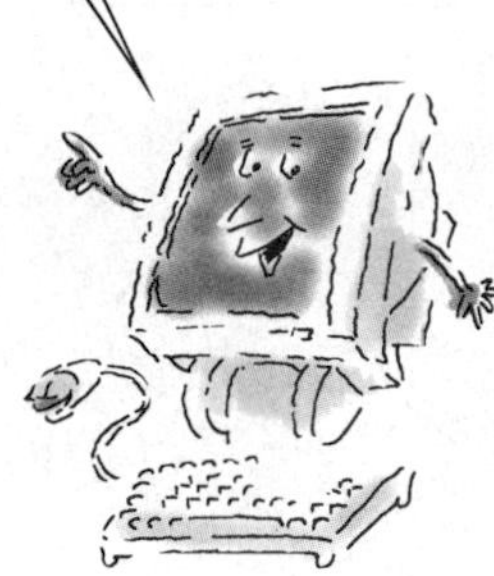

Read this question carefully. The answer refers to a cause.

2. Risk factors for the development of hiatal hernias are those that lead to increased abdominal pressure. Which of the following complications can cause increased abdominal pressure?

1. Obesity
2. Volvulus
3. Constipation
4. Intestinal obstruction

2. 1. Obesity may cause increased abdominal pressure that pushes the lower portion of the stomach into the thorax. A volvulus is a type of intestinal obstruction. Obstructions may complicate a rolling hiatal hernia, but they don't cause the hernia. Constipation has no effect on a hiatal hernia.

NP: Assessment; CN: Physiological integrity; CNS: Physiological adaptation; CL: Comprehension

3. Which of the following symptoms is common with a hiatal hernia?

1. Left arm pain
2. Lower back pain
3. Esophageal reflux
4. Abdominal cramping

3. 3. Esophageal reflux is a common symptom of hiatal hernia. This seems to be associated with chronic exposure of the lower esophageal sphincter to the lower pressure of the thorax, making it less effective. Left arm pain is a common symptom of heart attack. Lower back pain can be caused by lumbar strain. Abdominal cramping can be caused by intestinal infection.

NP: Assessment; CN: Physiological integrity; CNS: Physiological adaptation; CL: Comprehension

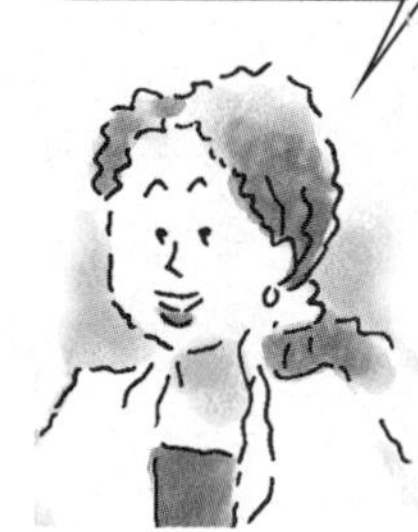

4. Which of the following tests can be performed to diagnose a hiatal hernia?

1. Colonoscopy
2. Lower GI series
3. Barium swallow
4. Abdominal X-ray series

4. 3. A barium swallow with fluoroscopy shows the position of the stomach in relation to the diaphragm. A colonoscopy and a lower GI series show disorders of the intestine. An abdominal X-ray series will show structural defects but not necessarily a hiatal hernia, unless it's sliding or rolling at the time of the X-ray.

NP: Implementation; CN: Health promotion and maintenance; CNS: Prevention and early detection of disease; CL: Comprehension

NP: Nursing process CN: Client needs category CNS: Client needs subcategory CL: Cognitive level

5. Which of the following complications is thought to be the most common cause of appendicitis?

1. A fecalith
2. Bowel kinking
3. Internal bowel occlusion
4. Abdominal wall swelling

5. 1. A fecalith is a fecal calculus, or stone, that occludes the lumen of the appendix and is the most common cause of appendicitis. Bowel wall swelling, kinking of the appendix, and external occlusion, not internal occlusion, of the bowel by adhesions can also be causes of appendicitis.

NP: Assessment; CN: Physiological integrity; CNS: Physiological adaptation; CL: Knowledge

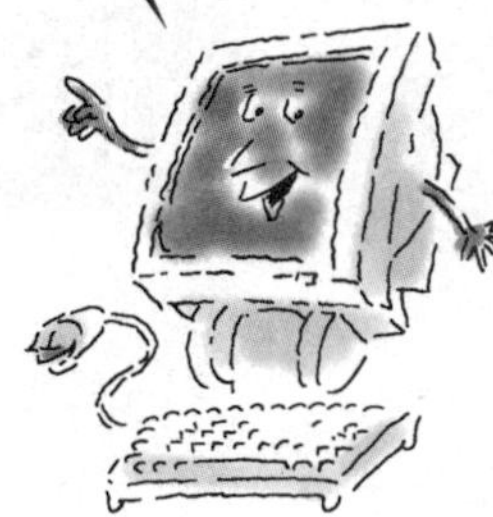

This question is a real pain in the .... side!

6. Which of the following terms best describes the pain associated with appendicitis?

1. Aching
2. Fleeting
3. Intermittent
4. Steady

6. 4. The pain begins in the epigastrium or periumbilical region, then shifts to the right lower quadrant and becomes steady. The pain may be moderate to severe.

NP: Assessment; CN: Physiological integrity; CNS: Physiological adaptation; CL: Knowledge

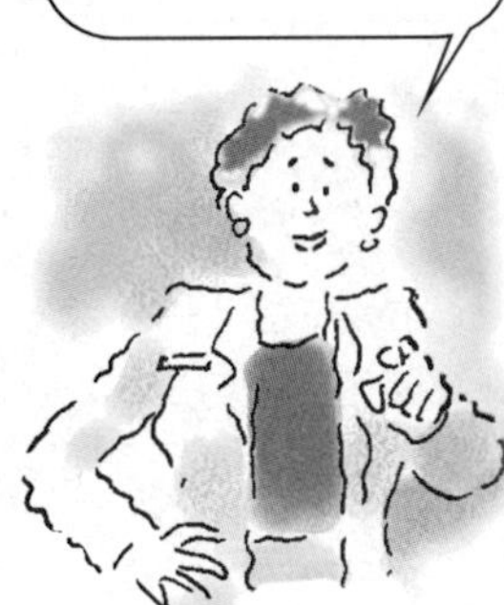

Before selecting a position, carefully note the difference between each!

7. Which of the following positions should a client with appendicitis assume to help relieve the pain?

1. Prone
2. Sitting
3. Supine, stretched out
4. Lying with legs drawn up

7. 4. Lying still with the legs drawn up toward the chest helps relieve tension on the abdominal muscles, which helps to reduce the amount of discomfort felt. Lying flat or sitting may increase the amount of pain experienced.

NP: Assessment; CN: Physiological integrity; CNS: Physiological adaptation; CL: Comprehension

8. Which of the following nursing interventions should be implemented to manage a client with appendicitis?

1. Assessing for pain
2. Encouraging oral intake of clear fluids
3. Providing discharge teaching
4. Assessing for symptoms of peritonitis

8. 4. The focus of care is to assess for peritonitis, or inflammation of the peritoneal cavity. Peritonitis is most commonly caused by appendix rupture and invasion of bacteria, which could be lethal. The client with appendicitis will have pain that should be controlled with analgesia. The nurse should discourage oral intake in preparation for surgery. Discharge teaching is important; however, in the acute phase, management should focus on minimizing preoperative complications and recognizing when such may be occurring.

NP: Implementation; CN: Physiological integrity; CNS: Reduction of risk potential; CL: Application

9. Which of the following definitions best describes gastritis?

1. Erosion of the gastric mucosa
2. Inflammation of a diverticulum
3. Inflammation of the gastric mucosa
4. Reflux of stomach acid into the esophagus

9. 3. Gastritis is an inflammation of the gastric mucosa that may be acute (often resulting from exposure to local irritants) or chronic (associated with autoimmune infections or atrophic disorders of the stomach). Erosion of the mucosa results in ulceration. Inflammation of a diverticulum is called diverticulitis; reflux of stomach acid is known as gastroesophageal reflux disease.

NP: Assessment; CN: Physiological integrity; CNS: Physiological adaptation; CL: Knowledge

NP: Nursing process CN: Client needs category CNS: Client needs subcategory CL: Cognitive level

10. Which of the following substances is most likely to cause gastritis?
1. Milk
2. Bicarbonate of soda, or baking soda
3. Enteric-coated aspirin
4. Nonsteroidal anti-inflammatory drugs

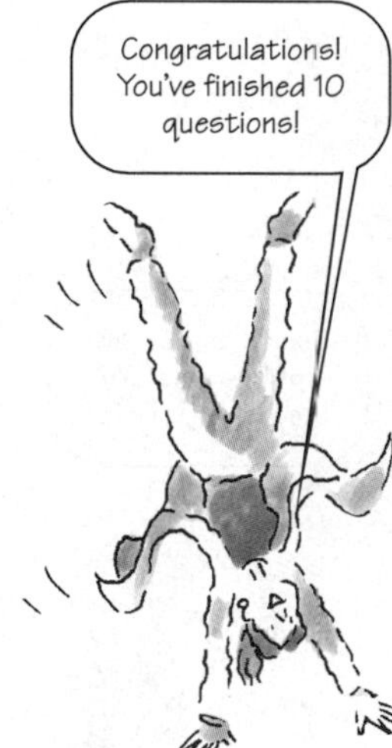

10. 4. Nonsteroidal anti-inflammatory drugs are a common cause of gastritis because they inhibit prostaglandin synthesis. Milk, once thought to help reduce gastritis, has little effect on the stomach mucosa. Bicarbonate of soda, or baking soda, may be used to neutralize stomach acid, but it should be used cautiously because it may lead to metabolic acidosis. Aspirin with enteric coating shouldn't contribute significantly to gastritis because the coating limits the aspirin's effect on the gastric mucosa.

NP: Assessment; CN: Physiological integrity; CNS: Reduction of risk potential; CL: Knowledge

11. Which of the following tasks should be included in the immediate postoperative management of a client who has undergone gastric resection?
1. Monitoring gastric pH to detect complications
2. Assessing for bowel sounds
3. Providing nutritional support
4. Monitoring for symptoms of hemorrhage

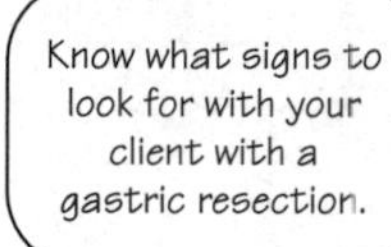

Know what signs to look for with your client with a gastric resection.

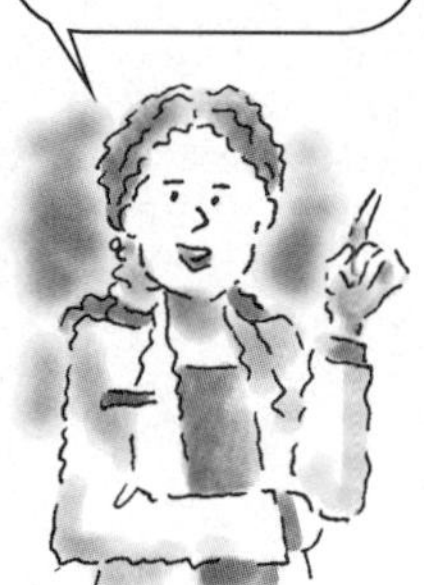

11. 4. The client should be monitored closely for signs and symptoms of hemorrhage, such as bright red blood in the nasogastric tube suction, tachycardia, or a drop in blood pressure. Gastric pH may be monitored to evaluate the need for histamine-2 receptor antagonists. Bowel sounds may not return for up to 72 hours postoperatively. Nutritional needs should be addressed soon after surgery.

NP: Assessment; CN: Physiological integrity; CNS: Reduction of risk potential; CL: Comprehension

12. Which of the following treatments should be included in the immediate management of acute gastritis?
1. Reducing work stress
2. Completing gastric resection
3. Treating the underlying cause
4. Administering enteral tube feedings

12. 3. Discovering and treating the cause of gastritis is the most beneficial approach. Reducing or eliminating oral intake until the symptoms are gone and reducing the amount of stress are important in the recovery phase. A gastric resection is only an option when serious erosion has occurred.

NP: Assessment; CN: Safe, effective care environment; CNS: Safety and infection control; CL: Comprehension

13. Which of the following risk factors can lead to chronic gastritis?
1. Young age
2. Antibiotic usage
3. Gallbladder disease
4. *Helicobacter pylori* infection

13. 4. *H. pylori* infection can lead to chronic atrophic gastritis. Chronic gastritis can occur at any age but is more common in older adults. It may be caused by conditions that allow reflux of bile acids into the stomach. Drugs such as nonsteroidal anti-inflammatory agents, not antibiotics, may cause gastritis. Chronic gastritis isn't related to gallbladder disease.

NP: Assessment; CN: Physiological integrity; CNS: Physiological adaptation; CL: Comprehension

14. Which of the following factors associates chronic gastritis with pernicious anemia?
1. Chronic blood loss
2. Inability to absorb vitamin B_{12}
3. Overproduction of stomach acid
4. Overproduction of vitamin B_{12}

14. 2. With gastritis, the stomach lining becomes thin and atrophic, decreasing stomach acid secretion (the source of intrinsic factor). This causes a reduction in the absorption of vitamin B_{12}, leading to pernicious anemia.
NP: Assessment; CN: Physiological integrity; CNS: Physiological adaptation; CL: Comprehension

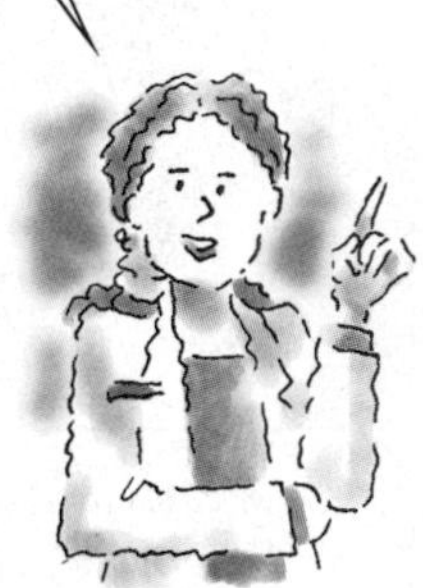

Read the first two options carefully. They're very similar.

15. Which of the following definitions best describes diverticulosis?
1. An inflamed outpouching of the intestine
2. A noninflamed outpouching of the intestine
3. The partial impairment of the forward flow of intestinal contents
4. An abnormal protrusion of an organ through the structure that usually holds it

15. 2. Diverticulosis involves a noninflamed outpouching of the intestine. Diverticulitis involves an inflamed outpouching. The partial impairment of forward flow of the intestine is an obstruction; abnormal protrusion of an organ is a hernia.
NP: Assessment; CN: Physiological integrity; CNS: Physiological adaptation; CL: Comprehension

16. Which of the following types of diets is implicated in the development of diverticulosis?
1. Low-fiber diet
2. High-fiber diet
3. High-protein diet
4. Low-carbohydrate diet

16. 1. Low-fiber diets have been implicated in the development of diverticula because these diets decrease the bulk in the stool and predispose the person to the development of constipation. A high-fiber diet is recommended to help prevent diverticulosis. A high-protein or low-carbohydrate diet has no effect on the development of diverticulosis.
NP: Assessment; CN: Health promotion and maintenance; CNS: Prevention and early detection of disease; CL: Comprehension

17. Which of the following mechanisms can facilitate the development of diverticulosis into diverticulitis?
1. Treating constipation with chronic laxative use, leading to dependence on the laxatives
2. Chronic constipation causing an obstruction, reducing forward flow of intestinal contents
3. Herniation of the intestinal mucosa, rupturing the wall of the intestine
4. Undigested food blocking the diverticulum, predisposing the area to bacterial invasion

17. 4. Undigested food can block the diverticulum, decreasing blood supply to the area and predisposing the area to the invasion of bacteria. Chronic laxative use is a common problem in elderly clients, but it doesn't cause diverticulitis. Chronic constipation can cause an obstruction — not diverticulitis. Herniation of the intestinal mucosa causes an intestinal perforation.
NP: Assessment; CN: Physiological integrity; CNS: Physiological adaptation; CL: Comprehension

18. Which of the following symptoms indicate diverticulosis?
1. No symptoms exist
2. Change in bowel habits
3. Anorexia and low-grade fever
4. Episodic, dull or steady midabdominal pain

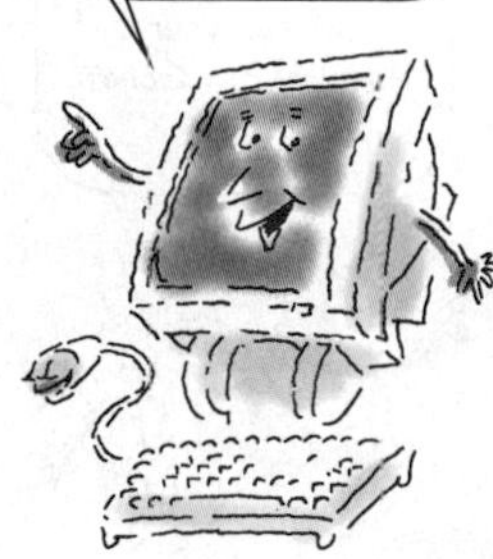

Be careful. This isn't a negative question, but the answer is tricky.

18. 1. Diverticulosis is an asymptomatic condition. The other choices are signs and symptoms of diverticulitis.

NP: Assessment; CN: Physiological integrity; CNS: Physiological adaptation; CL: Comprehension

19. Which of the following tests should be administered to a client suspected of having diverticulosis?
1. Abdominal ultrasound
2. Barium enema
3. Barium swallow
4. Gastroscopy

19. 2. A barium enema will cause diverticula to fill with barium and be easily seen on an X-ray. An abdominal ultrasound can tell more about structures, such as the gallbladder, liver, and spleen, than the intestine. A barium swallow and gastroscopy view upper GI structures.

NP: Planning; CN: Health promotion and maintenance; CNS: Prevention and early detection of disease; CL: Comprehension

20. Medical management of the client with acute diverticulitis should include which of the following treatments?
1. Reduced fluid intake
2. Increased fiber in diet
3. Administration of antibiotics
4. Exercises to increase intra-abdominal pressure

20. 3. Antibiotics are used to reduce the inflammation. The client typically isn't allowed anything orally until the acute episode subsides. Parenteral fluids are given until the client feels better; then it's recommended that the client drink eight 8-oz glasses of water per day and gradually increase fiber in the diet to improve intestinal motility. During the acute phase, activities that increase intra-abdominal pressure should be avoided to decrease pain and the chance of intestinal obstruction.

NP: Assessment; CN: Safe, effective care environment; CNS: Safety and infection control; CL: Comprehension

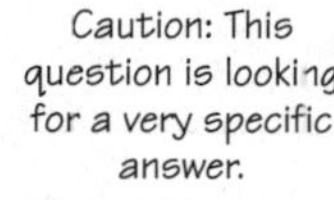

Caution: This question is looking for a very specific answer.

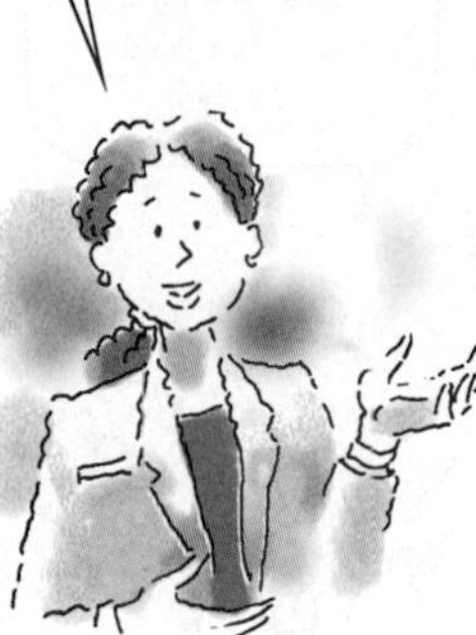

21. Crohn's disease can be described as a chronic relapsing disease. Which of the following areas of the GI system may be involved with this disease?
1. The entire length of the large colon
2. Only the sigmoid area
3. The entire large colon through the layers of mucosa and submucosa
4. The small intestine and colon; affecting the entire thickness of the bowel

21. 4. Crohn's disease can involve any segment of the small intestine, the colon, or both, affecting the entire thickness of the bowel. Answers 1 and 3 describe ulcerative colitis. Answer 2 is too specific and, therefore, not likely.

NP: Assessment; CN: Physiological integrity; CNS: Physiological adaptation; CL: Comprehension

22. Which area of the alimentary canal is the most common location for Crohn's disease?

1. Ascending colon
2. Descending colon
3. Sigmoid colon
4. Terminal ileum

22. 4. Studies have shown that the terminal ileum is the most common site for recurrence in clients with Crohn's disease. The other areas may be involved but aren't as common.

NP: Assessment; CN: Physiological integrity; CNS: Physiological adaptation; CL: Knowledge

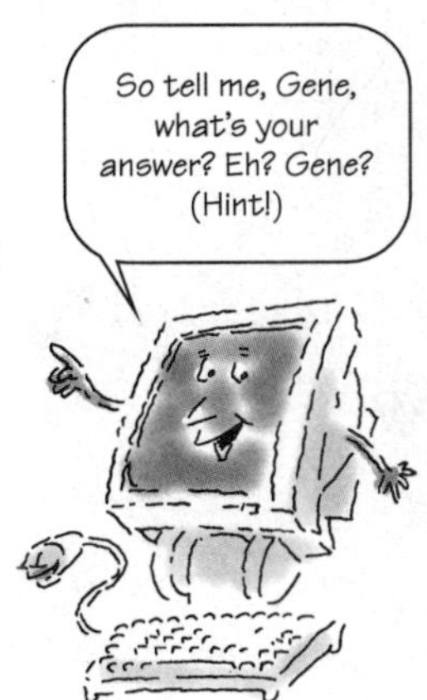

So tell me, Gene, what's your answer? Eh? Gene? (Hint!)

23. Which of the following factors is believed to be linked to Crohn's disease?

1. Constipation
2. Diet
3. Heredity
4. Lack of exercise

23. 3. Although the definitive cause of Crohn's disease is unknown, it's thought to be associated with infectious, immune, or psychological factors. Because it has a higher incidence in siblings, it may have a genetic cause.

NP: Assessment; CN: Health promotion and maintenance; CNS: Prevention and early detection of disease; CL: Comprehension

24. Which of the following factors is believed to cause ulcerative colitis?

1. Acidic diet
2. Altered immunity
3. Chronic constipation
4. Emotional stress

24. 2. Several theories exist regarding the cause of ulcerative colitis. One suggests altered immunity as the cause based on the extraintestinal characteristics of the disease, such as peripheral arthritis and cholangitis. Diet and constipation have no effect on the development of ulcerative colitis. Emotional stress may exacerbate the attacks but isn't believed to be the primary cause.

NP: Assessment; CN: Health promotion and maintenance; CNS: Prevention and early detection of disease; CL: Comprehension

25. Fistulas are most common with which of the following bowel disorders?

1. Crohn's disease
2. Diverticulitis
3. Diverticulosis
4. Ulcerative colitis

25. 1. The lesions of Crohn's disease are *transmural;* that is, they involve all thicknesses of the bowel. These lesions may perforate the bowel wall, forming fistulas with adjacent structures. Fistulas don't develop in diverticulitis or diverticulosis. The ulcers that occur in the submucosal and mucosal layers of the intestine in ulcerative colitis usually don't progress to fistula formation as in Crohn's disease.

NP: Assessment; CN: Physiological integrity; CNS: Physiological adaptation; CL: Comprehension

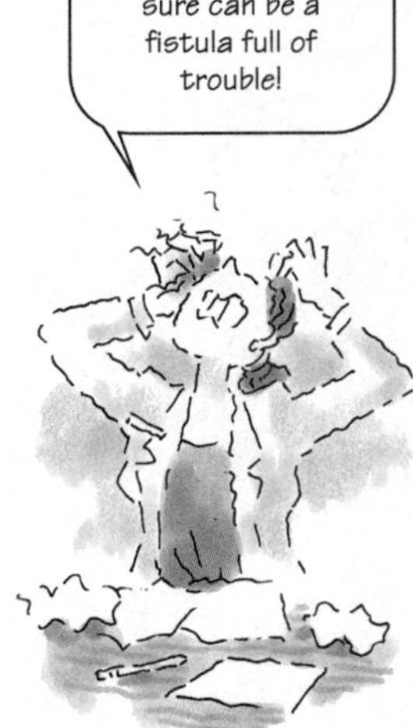

NCLEX questions sure can be a fistula full of trouble!

26. Which of the following areas is the most common site of fistulas in clients with Crohn's disease?

1. Anorectal
2. Ileum
3. Rectovaginal
4. Transverse colon

26. 1. Fistulas occur in all these areas, but the anorectal area is most common because of the relative thinness of the intestinal wall in this area.

NP: Assessment; CN: Physiological integrity; CNS: Physiological adaptation; CL: Comprehension

27. Which of the following associated disorders may a client with ulcerative colitis exhibit?
1. Gallstones
2. Hydronephrosis
3. Nephrolithiasis
4. Toxic megacolon

27. 4. Toxic megacolon is extreme dilation of a segment of the diseased colon caused by paralysis of the colon, resulting in complete obstruction. This disorder is associated with both Crohn's disease *and* ulcerative colitis. The other disorders are more commonly associated with Crohn's disease.

NP: Assessment; CN: Physiological integrity; CNS: Physiological adaptation; CL: Comprehension

28. Which of the following associated disorders may the client with Crohn's disease exhibit?
1. Ankylosing spondylitis
2. Colon cancer
3. Malabsorption
4. Lactase deficiency

28. 3. Because of the transmural nature of Crohn's disease lesions, malabsorption may occur with Crohn's disease. Ankylosing spondylitis and colon cancer are more commonly associated with ulcerative colitis. Lactase deficicency is caused by a congenital defect in which an enzyme isn't present.

NP: Assessment; CN: Physiological integrity; CNS: Physiological adaptation; CL: Comprehension

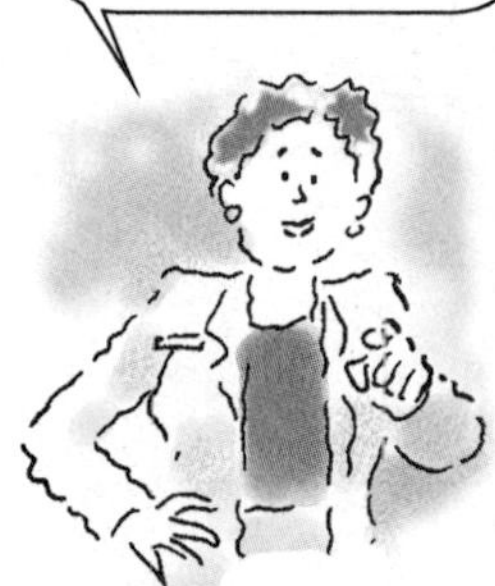

Many GI disorders have similar symptoms. Pay attention to which one the question is asking about.

29. Which of the following symptoms may be exhibited by a client with Crohn's disease?
1. Bloody diarrhea
2. Narrow stools
3. Nausea and vomiting
4. Steatorrhea

29. 4. Steatorrhea from malabsorption can occur with Crohn's disease. Nausea, vomiting, and bloody diarrhea are symptoms of ulcerative colitis. Narrow stools are associated with diverticular disease

NP: Assessment; CN: Health promotion and maintenance; CNS: Prevention and early detection of disease; CL: Comprehension

30. Which of the following symptoms is associated with ulcerative colitis?
1. Dumping syndrome
2. Rectal bleeding
3. Soft stools
4. Fistulas

30. 2. In ulcerative colitis, rectal bleeding is the predominant symptom. Soft stools are more commonly associated with Crohn's disease, in which malabsorption is more of a problem. Dumping syndrome occurs after gastric surgeries. Fistulas are associated with Crohn's disease.

NP: Assessment; CN: Health promotion and maintenance; CNS: Prevention and early detection of disease; CL: Knowledge

31. If a client had irritable bowel syndrome, which of the following diagnostic tests would determine if the diagnosis is Crohn's disease or ulcerative colitis?
1. Abdominal computed tomography (CT) scan
2. Abdominal X-ray
3. Barium swallow
4. Colonoscopy with biopsy

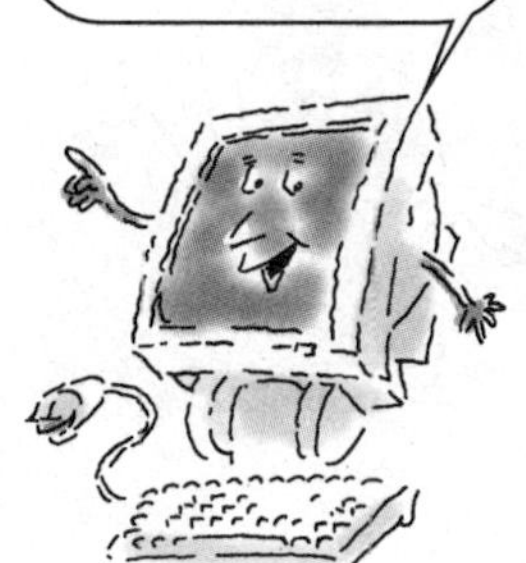

One of these tests can help you distinguish between two GI disorders.

31. 4. A colonoscopy with biopsy can be performed to determine the state of the colon's mucosal layers, presence of ulcerations, and level of cytologic involvement. An abdominal X-ray or a CT scan wouldn't provide the cytologic information necessary to diagnose which disease it is. A barium swallow doesn't involve the intestine.

NP: Assessment; CN: Physiological integrity; CNS: Physiological adaptation; CL: Comprehension

32. Which of the following interventions should be included in the medical management of Crohn's disease?

1. Increasing oral intake of fiber
2. Administering laxatives
3. Using long-term steroid therapy
4. Increasing physical activity

32. 3. Management of Crohn's disease may include long-term steroid therapy to reduce the extensive inflammation associated with the deeper layers of the bowel wall. Other management focuses on bowel rest (not increasing oral intake) and reducing diarrhea with medications (not giving laxatives). The pain associated with Crohn's disease may require bed rest, not an increase in physical activity.

NP: Implementation; CN: Physiological integrity; CNS: Basic care and comfort; CL: Application

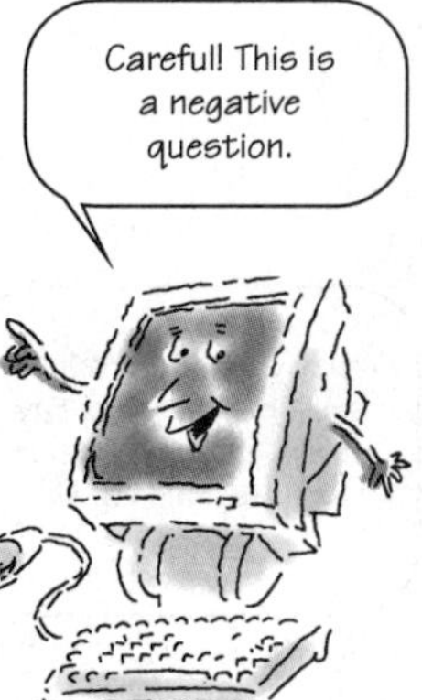
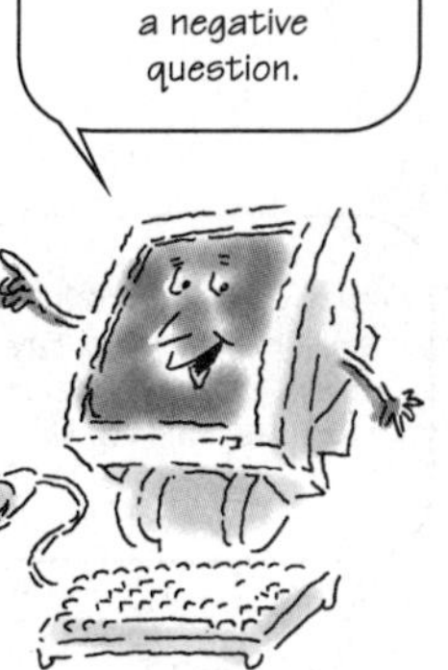
Careful! This is a negative question.

33. In a client with Crohn's disease, which of the following symptoms should not be a direct result of antibiotic therapy?

1. Decrease in bleeding
2. Decrease in temperature
3. Decrease in body weight
4. Decrease in the number of stools

33. 3. A decrease in body weight may occur during therapy due to inadequate dietary intake, but it isn't related to antibiotic therapy. Effective antibiotic therapy will be noted by a decrease in temperature, number of stools, and bleeding.

NP: Evaluation; CN: Physiological integrity; CNS: Pharmacological and parenteral therapies; CL: Comprehension

34. Surgical management of ulcerative colitis may be performed to treat which of the following complications?

1. Gastritis
2. Bowel herniation
3. Bowel outpouching
4. Bowel perforation

34. 4. Perforation, obstruction, hemorrhage, and toxic megacolon are common complications of ulcerative colitis that may require surgery. Herniation and gastritis aren't associated with irritable bowel diseases, and outpouching of the bowel wall is diverticulosis.

NP: Implementation; CN: Safe, effective care environment; CNS: Safety and infection control; CL: Comprehension

35. Which of the following medications is most effective for treating the pain associated with irritable bowel disease?

1. Acetaminophen
2. Opiates
3. Steroids
4. Stool softeners

35. 3. The pain of irritable bowel disease is caused by inflammation, which steroids can reduce. Stool softeners aren't necessary. Acetaminophen has little effect on the pain, and opiate narcotics won't treat its underlying cause.

NP: Assessment; CN: Physiological integrity; CNS: Pharmacological and parenteral therapies; CL: Comprehension

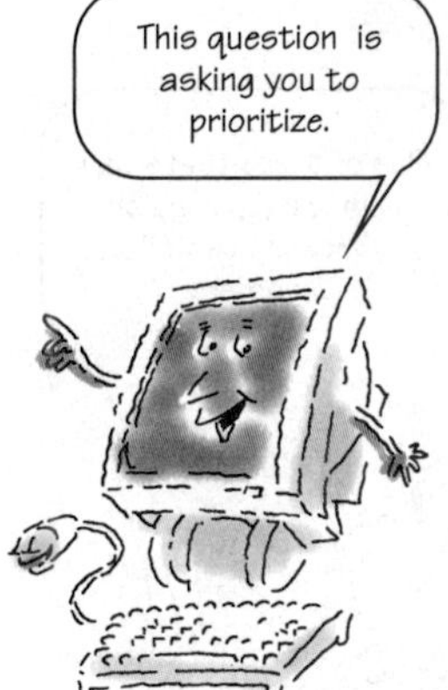
This question is asking you to prioritize.

36. During the first few days of recovery from ostomy surgery for ulcerative colitis, which of the following aspects should be the first priority of client care?

1. Body image
2. Ostomy care
3. Sexual concerns
4. Skin care

36. 2. Although all of these are concerns the nurse should address, being able to safely manage the ostomy is crucial for the client before discharge.

NP: Implementation; CN: Physiological integrity; CNS: Basic care and comfort; CL: Application

37. Colon cancer is most closely associated with which of the following conditions?

1. Appendicitis
2. Hemorrhoids
3. Hiatal hernia
4. Ulcerative colitis

37. 4. Chronic ulcerative colitis, granulomas, and familial polyposis seem to increase a person's chance of developing colon cancer. The other conditions listed have no known effect on colon cancer risk.

NP: Assessment; CN: Health promotion and maintenance; CNS: Prevention and early detection of disease; CL: Comprehension

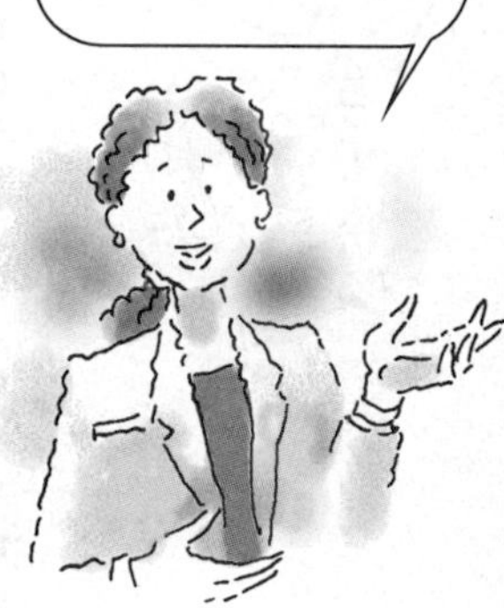

The NCLEX will test your understanding of the links between diet and disease.

38. Which of the following diets is most commonly associated with colon cancer?

1. Low-fiber, high-fat
2. Low-fat, high-fiber
3. Low-protein, high-carbohydrate
4. Low-carbohydrate, high-protein

38. 1. A low-fiber, high-fat diet reduces motility and increases the chance of constipation. The metabolic end-products of this type of diet are carcinogenic. A low-fat, high-fiber diet is recommended to help avoid colon cancer. Carbohydrates and protein aren't necessarily associated with colon cancer.

NP: Assessment; CN: Health promotion and maintenance; CNS: Prevention and early detection of disease; CL: Knowledge

39. Which of the following diagnostic tests should be performed annually after age 50 to screen for colon cancer?

1. Abdominal computed tomography (CT) scan
2. Abdominal X-ray
3. Colonoscopy
4. Fecal occult blood test

39. 4. Surface blood vessels of polyps and cancers are fragile and often bleed with the passage of stools. Abdominal X-ray and CT scan can help establish tumor size and metastasis. A colonoscopy can help to locate a tumor as well as polyps, which can be removed before they become malignant.

NP: Assessment; CN: Health promotion and maintenance; CNS: Prevention and early detection of disease; CL: Knowledge

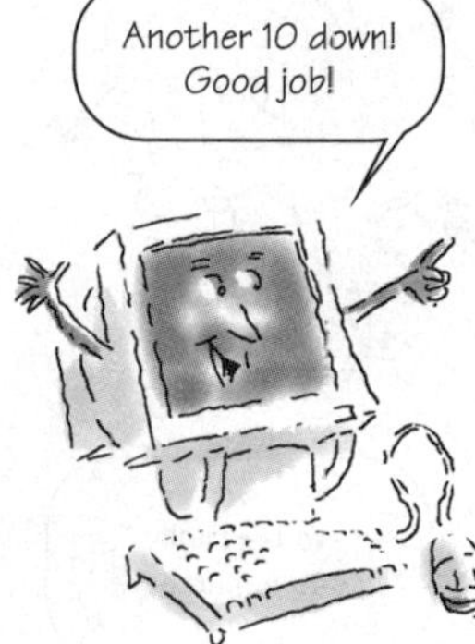

Another 10 down! Good job!

40. Radiation therapy is used to treat colon cancer before surgery for which of the following reasons?

1. Reducing the size of the tumor
2. Eliminating the malignant cells
3. Curing the cancer
4. Helping heal the bowel after surgery

40. 1. Radiation therapy is used to treat colon cancer before surgery to reduce the size of the tumor, making it easier to be resected. Radiation therapy isn't curative, can't eliminate the malignant cells (though it helps to define tumor margins), and could slow postoperative healing.

NP: Implementation; CN: Physiological integrity; CNS: Reduction of risk potential; CL: Comprehension

41. Which of the following symptoms is a client with colon cancer most likely to exhibit?

1. A change in appetite
2. A change in bowel habits
3. An increase in body weight
4. An increase in body temperature

41. 2. The most common complaint of the client with colon cancer is a change in bowel habits. The client may have anorexia, secondary abdominal distention, or weight loss. Fever isn't related to colon cancer.

NP: Assessment; CN: Physiological integrity; CNS: Basic care and comfort; CL: Application

42. A client has just had surgery for colon cancer. Which of the following disorders might this client develop?

1. Peritonitis
2. Diverticulosis
3. Partial bowel obstruction
4. Complete bowel obstruction

42. 1. Bowel spillage could occur during surgery, resulting in peritonitis. Complete or partial intestinal obstruction may occur *before* bowel resection. Diverticulosis doesn't result from surgery for colon cancer.
NP: Evaluation; CN: Physiological integrity; CNS: Physiological adaptation; CL: Application

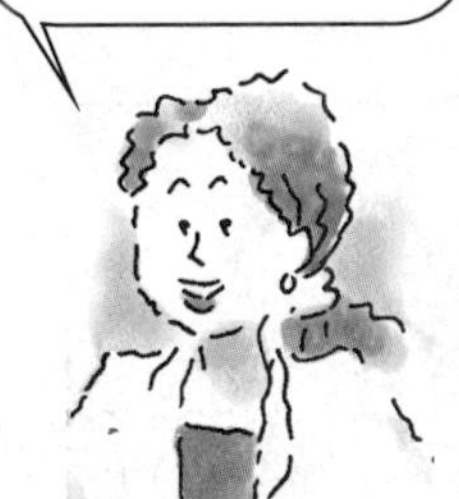

Again, make sure you read the question carefully and know what disorder is being addressed.

43. A client with gastric cancer may exhibit which of the following symptoms?

1. Abdominal cramping
2. Constant hunger
3. Feeling of fullness
4. Weight gain

43. 3. The client with gastric cancer may report a feeling of fullness in the stomach, but not enough to cause him to seek medical care. Abdominal cramping isn't associated with gastric cancer. Anorexia and weight loss (not increased hunger or weight gain) are common symptoms of gastric cancer.
NP: Assessment; CN: Physiological integrity; CNS: Physiological adaptation; CL: Comprehension

44. Which of the following diagnostic tests may be performed to determine if a client has gastric cancer?

1. Barium enema
2. Colonoscopy
3. Gastroscopy
4. Serum chemistry levels

44. 3. A gastroscopy will allow direct visualization of the tumor. A colonoscopy or a barium enema would help to diagnose *colon cancer*. Serum chemistry levels don't contribute data useful to the assessment of gastric cancer.
NP: Assessment; CN: Health promotion and maintenance; CNS: Prevention and early detection of disease; CL: Comprehension

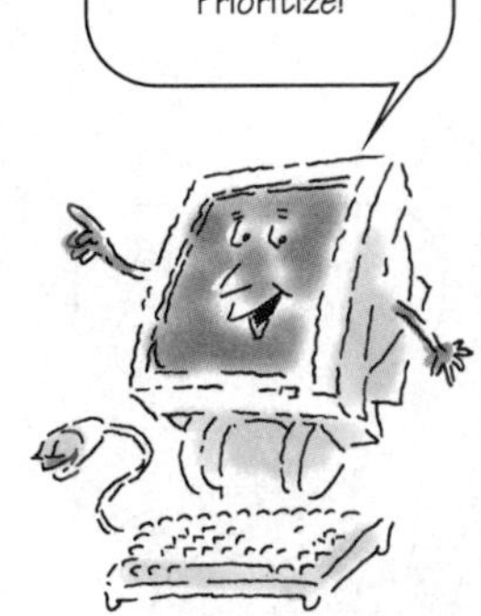

45. A client with gastric cancer can expect to have surgery for resection. Which of the following should be the nursing management priority for the preoperative client with gastric cancer?

1. Discharge planning
2. Correction of nutritional deficits
3. Prevention of deep vein thrombosis (DVT)
4. Instruction regarding radiation treatment

45. 2. Clients with gastric cancer commonly have nutritional deficits and may be cachectic. Discharge planning before surgery is important, but correcting the nutritional deficit is a higher priority. At present, radiation therapy hasn't been proven effective for gastric cancer, and teaching about it preoperatively wouldn't be appropriate. Prevention of DVT also isn't a high priority prior to surgery, though it assumes greater importance after surgery.
NP: Planning; CN: Physiological integrity; CNS: Basic care and comfort; CL: Application

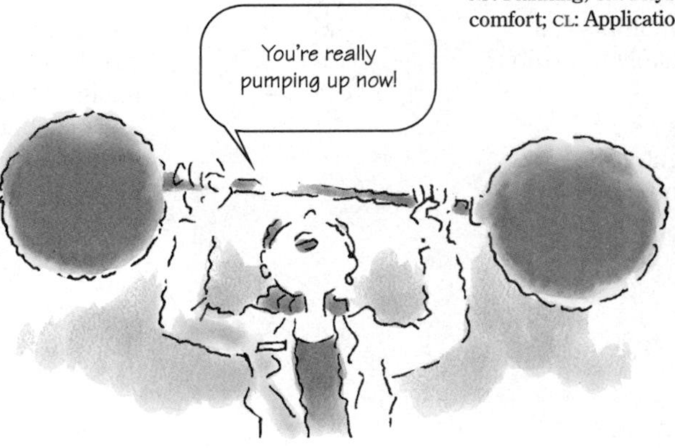

You're really pumping up now!

46. Care of the postoperative client after gastric resection should focus on which of the following problems?

1. Body image
2. Nutritional needs
3. Skin care
4. Spiritual needs

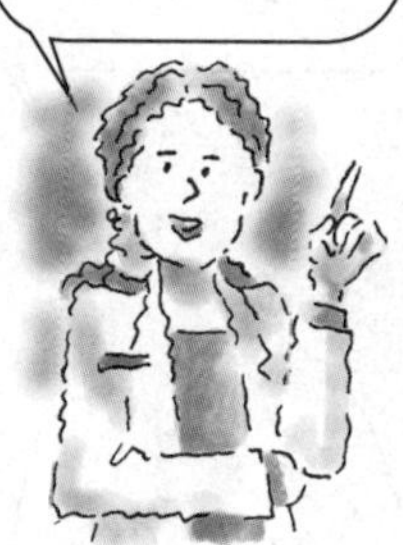

What's the key to the treatment of GI disorders in general?

46. 2. After gastric resection, a client may require total parenteral nutrition or jejunostomy tube feedings to maintain adequate nutritional status. Body image isn't much of a problem for this client because clothing can cover the incision site. Wound care of the incision site is necessary to prevent infection; otherwise the skin shouldn't be affected. Spiritual needs may be a concern, depending on the client, and should be addressed as the client demonstrates readiness to share concerns.

NP: Planning; CN: Physiological integrity; CNS: Basic care and comfort; CL: Comprehension

47. Which of the following complications of gastric resection should the nurse teach the client to watch for?

1. Constipation
2. Dumping syndrome
3. Gastric spasm
4. Intestinal spasms

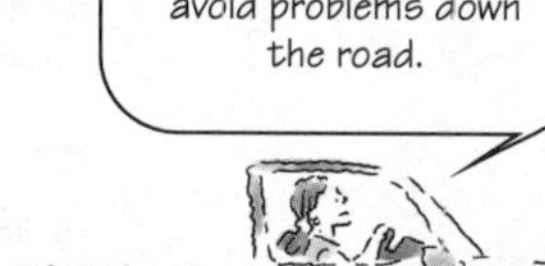

Knowing what to teach your patients can help avoid problems down the road.

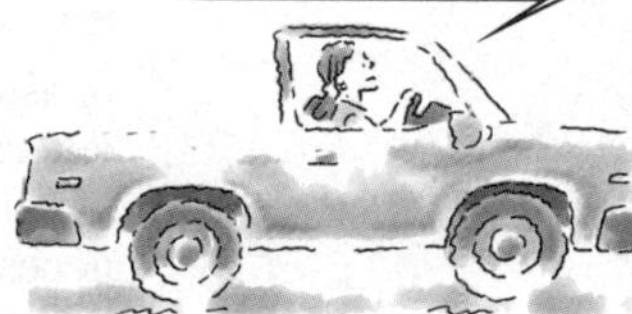

47. 2. Dumping syndrome is a problem that occurs postprandially after gastric resection because ingested food rapidly enters the jejunum without proper mixing and without the normal duodenal digestive processing. Diarrhea, not constipation, may also be a symptom. Gastric or intestinal spasms don't occur, but antispasmodics may be given to slow gastric emptying.

NP: Planning; CN: Health promotion and maintenance; CNS: Prevention and early detection of disease; CL: Application

48. A client with rectal cancer may exhibit which of the following symptoms?

1. Abdominal fullness
2. Gastric fullness
3. Rectal bleeding
4. Right upper quadrant pain

48. 3. Rectal bleeding is a common symptom of rectal cancer. Rectal cancer may be missed because other conditions such as hemorrhoids can cause rectal bleeding. Abdominal fullness may occur with colon cancer, gastric fullness may occur with gastric cancer, and right upper quadrant pain may occur with liver cancer.

NP: Assessment; CN: Physiological integrity; CNS: Physiological adaptation; CL: Comprehension

49. A client with which of the following conditions may be likely to develop rectal cancer?

1. Adenomatous polyps
2. Diverticulitis
3. Hemorrhoids
4. Peptic ulcer disease

49. 1. A client with adenomatous polyps has a higher risk for developing rectal cancer than others do. Clients with diverticulitis are more likely to develop colon cancer. Hemorrhoids don't increase the chance of any type of cancer. Clients with peptic ulcer disease have a higher incidence of gastric cancer.

NP: Assessment; CN: Health promotion and maintenance; CNS: Prevention and early detection of disease; CL: Analysis

50. Which of the following treatments is used for rectal cancer but not for colon cancer?
1. Chemotherapy
2. Colonoscopy
3. Radiation
4. Surgical resection

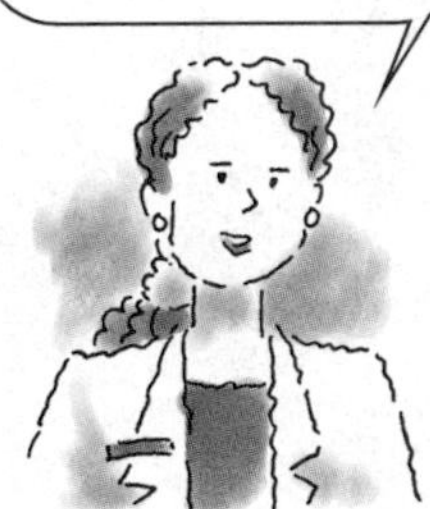

Be careful. The *not* in this question makes it seem like a negative question.

50. 3. A client with rectal cancer can expect to have radiation therapy in addition to chemotherapy and surgical resection of the tumor. A colonoscopy is performed to diagnose the disease. Radiation therapy isn't usually indicated in colon cancer.
NP: Implementation; CN: Safe, effective care environment; CNS: Management of care; CL: Comprehension

51. Which of the following symptoms may cause hemorrhoids?
1. Diarrhea
2. Diverticulosis
3. Portal hypertension
4. Rectal bleeding

51. 3. Portal hypertension and other conditions associated with persistently high intra-abdominal pressure such as pregnancy can lead to hemorrhoids. The passing of hard stool, not diarrhea, can aggravate hemorrhoids. Diverticulosis has no relationship to hemorrhoids. Rectal bleeding can be a symptom of hemorrhoids.
NP: Assessment; CN: Physiological integrity; CNS: Physiological adaptation; CL: Analysis

52. Which of the following assessments is most relevent with the diagnosis of hemorrhoids?
1. Abdominal assessment
2. Diet history
3. Digital rectal examination
4. Sexual history

52. 3. Digital rectal examination is important to assess for internal hemorrhoids and to determine if other causes of the pain and bleeding are present. Abdominal assessment isn't necessary for hemorrhoids. Diet history is relevant because constipation can worsen hemorrhoids, but it isn't as important to diagnosis as a digital rectal examination. Sexual history may also be relevant, but again, the history isn't as important as a digital rectal examination.
NP: Assessment; CN: Physiological integrity; CNS: Physiological adaptation; CL: Comprehension

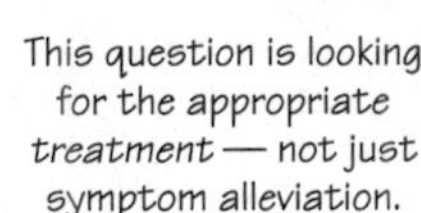

This question is looking for the appropriate *treatment* — not just symptom alleviation.

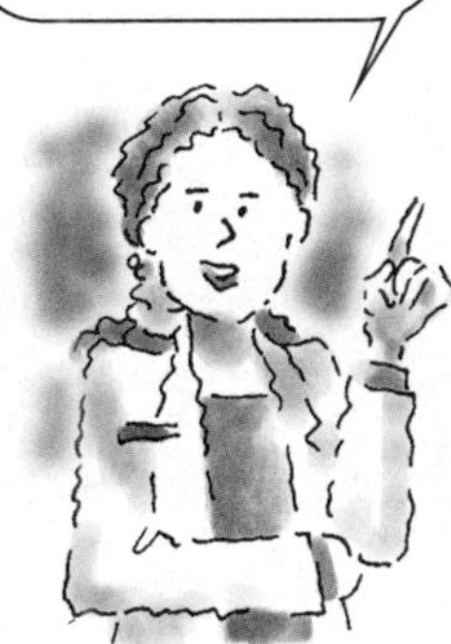

53. Medical management of hemorrhoids includes which of the following treatments?
1. Recommending a high-fiber diet
2. Applying cold to reduce swelling
3. Using astringent lotions to reduce swelling
4. Elevating the buttocks to reduce engorgement

53. 1. A high-fiber diet will add bulk to the stool and ease its passage through the rectum. Application of cold isn't recommended because it can cause injury to the tissue. Astringent lotions can be used to reduce pain, but they aren't a treatment. The buttocks should be elevated only when prolapsed hemorrhoids are present.
NP: Assessment; CN: Physiological integrity; CNS: Physiological adaptation; CL: Comprehension

54. Which of the following responses should the nurse offer to a client who asks why he's having a vagotomy to treat his ulcer?

1. To repair a hole in the stomach
2. To reduce the ability of the stomach to produce acid
3. To prevent the stomach from sliding into the chest
4. To remove a potentially malignant lesion in the stomach

55. Which of the following conditions is most likely to directly cause peritonitis?

1. Cholelithiasis
2. Gastritis
3. Perforated ulcer
4. Incarcerated hernia

56. Which of the following symptoms would a client in the early stages of peritonitis exhibit?

1. Abdominal distention
2. Abdominal pain and rigidity
3. Hyperactive bowel sounds
4. Right upper quadrant pain

57. Which of the following laboratory results would be expected in a client with peritonitis?

1. Partial thromboplastin time above 100 seconds
2. Hemoglobin level below 10 mg/dl
3. Potassium level above 5.5 mEq/L
4. White blood cell (WBC) count above 15,000/μl

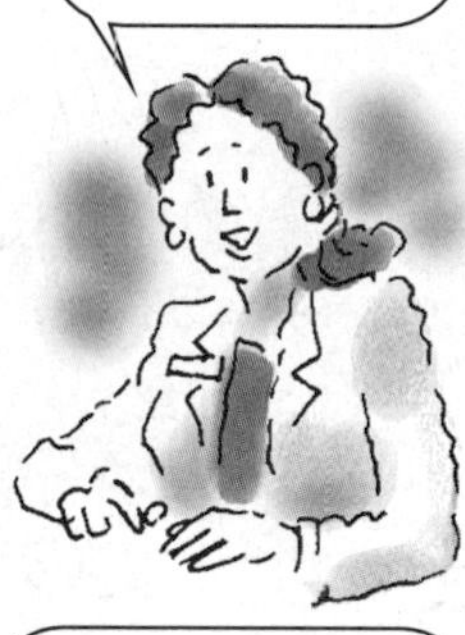

Client education is an important tool for obtaining compliance.

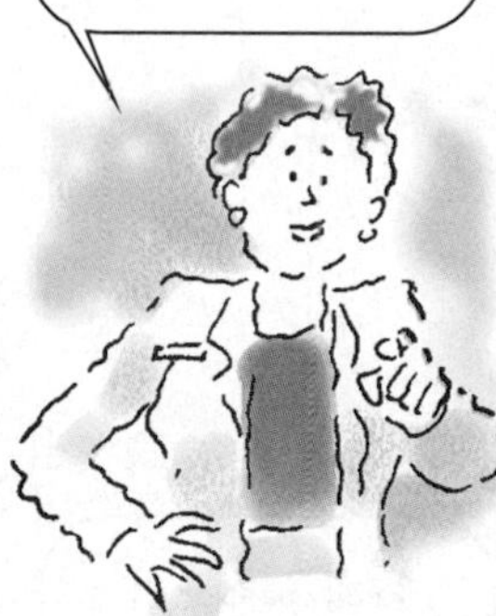

All of these complications can lead to peritonitis. Which one has the most direct causal effect?

54. 2. A vagotomy is performed to eliminate the acid-secreting stimulus to gastric cells. A perforation would be repaired with a gastric resection. Repair of hiatal hernia (fundoplication) prevents the stomach from sliding through the diaphragm. Removal of a potentially malignant tumor wouldn't reduce the entire acid-producing mechanism.

NP: Implementation; CN: Physiological integrity; CNS: Reduction of risk potential; CL: Application

55. 3. The most common cause of peritonitis is a perforated ulcer, which can pour contaminants into the peritoneal cavity, causing inflammation and infection within the cavity. The other conditions—cholelithiasis, gastritis, and incarcerated hernia—don't by themselves cause peritonitis. However, if cholelithiasis leads to rupture of the gall bladder, gastritis leads to erosion of the stomach wall, or an incarcerated hernia leads to rupture of the intestines, peritonitis may develop.

NP: Assessment; CN: Physiological integrity; CNS: Reduction of risk potential; CL: Application

56. 2. Abdominal pain causing rigidity of the abdominal muscles is characteristic of peritonitis. Abdominal distention may occur as a late sign but not early on. Bowel sounds may be normal or decreased but not increased. Right upper quadrant pain is characteristic of cholecystitis or hepatitis.

NP: Assessment; CN: Health promotion and maintenance; CNS: Prevention and early detection of disease; CL: Comprehension

57. 4. Because of infection, the client's WBC count will be elevated. A hemoglobin level below 10 mg/dl may occur from hemorrhage. A partial thromboplastin time longer than 100 seconds may suggest disseminated intravascular coagulation, a serious complication of septic shock. A potassium level above 5.5 mEq/L may suggest renal failure.

NP: Assessment; CN: Physiological integrity; CNS: Physiological adaptation; CL: Application

58. Which of the following therapies is <u>not</u> included in the medical management of a client with peritonitis?

1. Broad-spectrum antibiotics
2. Electrolyte replacement
3. I.V. fluids
4. Regular diet

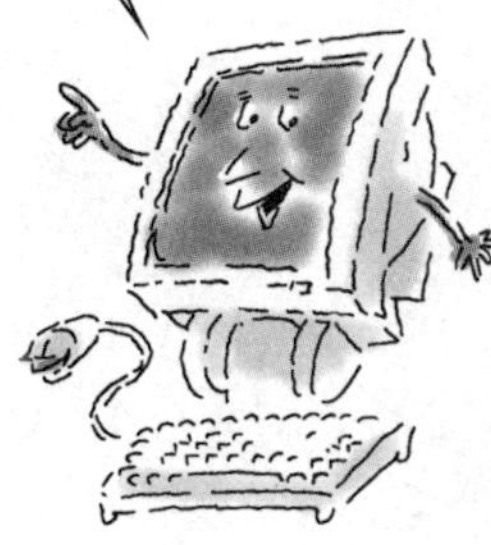

Watch it! This is another negative question.

58. 4. The client with peritonitis usually isn't allowed anything orally until the source of the peritonitis is confirmed and treated. The client also requires broad-spectrum antibiotics to combat the infection. I.V. fluids are given to maintain hydration and hemodynamic stability and to replace electrolytes.

NP: Implementation; CN: Safe, effective care environment; CNS: Management of care; CL: Knowledge

59. Which of the following aspects is the priority focus of nursing management for a client with peritonitis?

1. Fluid and electrolyte balance
2. Gastric irrigation
3. Pain management
4. Psychosocial issues

59. 1. Peritonitis can advance to shock and circulatory failure, so fluid and electrolyte balance is the priority focus of nursing management. Gastric irrigation may be needed periodically to ensure patency of the nasogastric tube. Although pain management is important for comfort and psychosocial care will address concerns such as anxiety, focusing on fluid and electrolyte balance will maintain hemodynamic stability.

NP: Planning; CN: Physiological integrity; CNS: Reduction of risk potential; CL: Analysis

60. Which of the following factors is most commonly associated with the development of pancreatitis?

1. Alcohol abuse
2. Hypercalcemia
3. Hyperlipidemia
4. Pancreatic duct obstruction

60. 1. Alcohol abuse is the major cause of acute pancreatitis in males, although gallbladder disease is more commonly implicated in women. Hypercalcemia, hyperlipidemia, and pancreatic duct obstruction are also causes of pancreatitis but occur less frequently.

NP: Assessment; CN: Physiological integrity; CNS: Reduction of risk potential; CL: Comprehension

61. Which of the following actions of pancreatic enzymes can cause pancreatic damage?

1. Utilization by the intestine
2. Autodigestion of the pancreas
3. Reflux into the pancreas
4. Clogging of the pancreatic duct

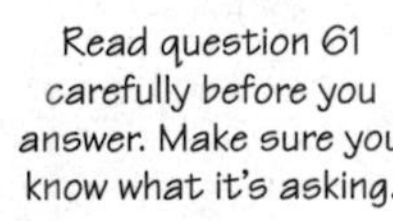

Read question 61 carefully before you answer. Make sure you know what it's asking.

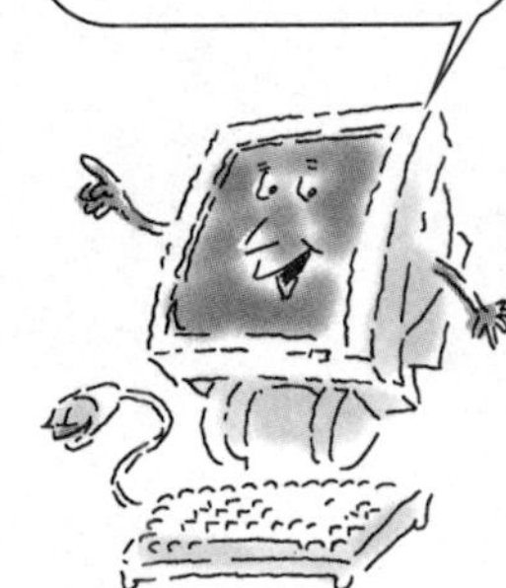

61. 2. In pancreatitis, pancreatic enzymes become activated and begin to autodigest the pancreas. The enzymes are activated but aren't used properly by the intestine. Reflux of bile into the pancreatic duct and clogging of the pancreatic duct may occur before autodigestion of the pancreas occurs.

NP: Assessment; CN: Physiological integrity; CNS: Physiological adaptation; CL: Knowledge

62. Which of the following laboratory tests is used to diagnose pancreatitis?

1. Lipase level
2. Hemoglobin level
3. Blood glucose level
4. White blood cell (WBC) count

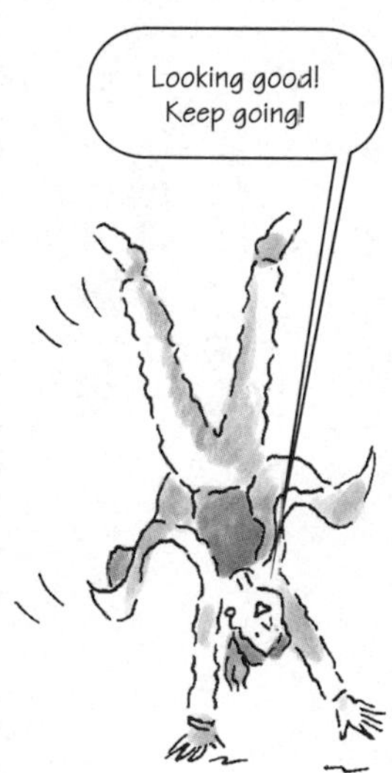

Looking good!
Keep going!

62. 1. Lipase is an enzyme secreted by the pancreas; when elevated, it's useful in diagnosing pancreatitis. Hemoglobin level can be low in pancreatitis, but there are other causes for this. The blood glucose level may be elevated with pancreatitis, but this factor isn't diagnostic. The WBC count may also be elevated in pancreatitis, but this symptom can be due to infection.

NP: Assessment; CN: Health promotion and maintenance; CNS: Prevention and early detection of disease; CL: Analysis

63. The client with pancreatitis may exhibit Cullen's sign on physical examination. Which of the following symptoms best describes Cullen's sign?

1. Jaundiced sclera
2. Pain that occurs with movement
3. Bluish discoloration of the left flank area
4. Bluish discoloration of the periumbilical area

63. 4. Cullen's sign is bluish discoloration of the periumbilical area from severe hemorrhagic pancreatitis. Pain with movement is a common finding with peritonitis. Turner's sign is the bluish discoloration of the left flank area, which can be present in peritonitis. Jaundiced sclera occurs with hepatitis.

NP: Assessment; CN: Health promotion and maintenance; CNS: Prevention and early detection of disease; CL: Analysis

64. Which of the following factors should be the focus of nursing management in a client with acute pancreatitis?

1. Dietary management
2. Fluid and electrolyte balance
3. Management of hypoglycemia
4. Pain control

64. 2. Acute pancreatitis is commonly associated with fluid isolation and accumulation in the bowel secondary to ileus or peripancreatic edema. Fluid and electrolyte loss from vomiting is a major concern. The priority is to manage the hypovolemia and restore the electrolyte balance. Pain control and dietary management are important concerns because a client with acute pancreatitis may have increased pain on eating and may not be allowed anything orally. Clients are at risk for hyperglycemia, not hypoglycemia.

NP: Implementation; CN: Physiological integrity; CNS: Physiological adaptation; CL: Comprehension

65. When admitting a client to the hospital with suspected acute pancreatitis, which of the following electrolyte disorders would not be expected?

1. Hyperglycemia
2. Hypernatremia
3. Hypocalcemia
4. Hypokalemia

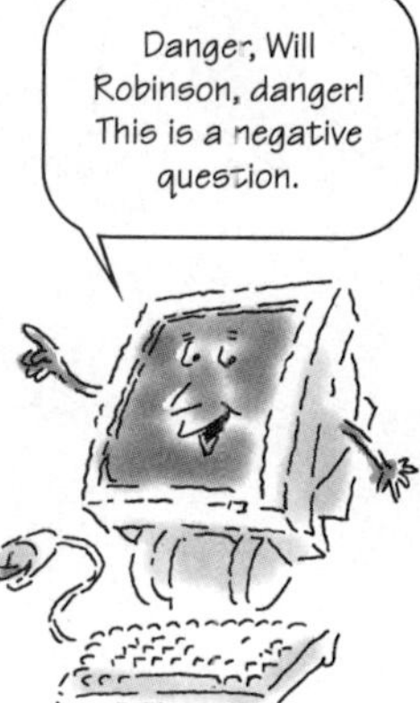

Danger, Will
Robinson, danger!
This is a negative
question.

65. 2. The client with acute pancreatitis may exhibit hypocalcemia due to the deposit of calcium in areas of fat necrosis. Hyperglycemia may occur due to reduced insulin production caused by islet of Langerhans involvement. Hypokalemia may occur because potassium is lost in emesis. Hyponatremia may occur for the same reason, but hypernatremia is unlikely.

NP: Assessment; CN: Physiological integrity; CNS: Physiological adaptation; CL: Analysis

66. If a gastric ulcer perforates, which of the following actions should not be included in the immediate management of the client?

1. Blood replacement
2. Antacid administration
3. Nasogastric (NG) tube suction
4. Fluid and electrolyte replacement

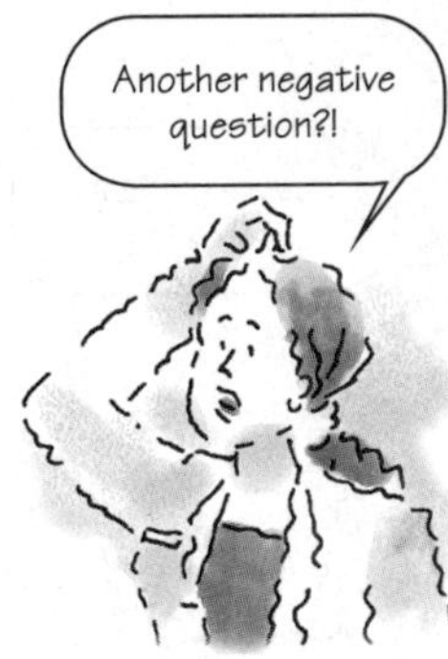
Another negative question?!

66. 2. Antacids aren't helpful in perforation. The client should be treated with antibiotics as well as fluid, electrolyte, and blood replacement. NG tube suction also should be performed to prevent further spillage of stomach contents into the peritoneal cavity.

NP: Planning; CN: Physiological integrity; CNS: Physiological adaptation; CL: Application

67. Which of the following symptoms would be unusual for the client with chronic pancreatitis to exhibit?

1. Abdominal pain
2. Diabetes mellitus
3. Hematochezia
4. Weight loss

67. 3. Hematochezia (blood in the stool) is unusual for a client with pancreatitis. The client is more likely to exhibit abdominal pain, diabetes mellitus, weight loss, and steatorrhea.

NP: Assessment; CN: Physiological integrity; CNS: Physiological adaptation; CL: Knowledge

68. In alcohol-related pancreatitis, which of the following interventions is the best way to reduce the exacerbation of pain?

1. Lying supine
2. Taking aspirin
3. Eating a low-fat diet
4. Abstaining from alcohol

68. 4. Abstaining from alcohol is imperative to reduce the injury to the pancreas; in fact, it may be enough to completely control pain. Lying supine usually aggravates the pain because it stretches the abdominal muscles. Taking aspirin can cause bleeding in hemorrhagic pancreatitis. During an attack of acute pancreatitis, the client usually isn't allowed to ingest anything orally.

NP: Planning; CN: Physiological integrity; CNS: Reduction of risk potential; CL: Application

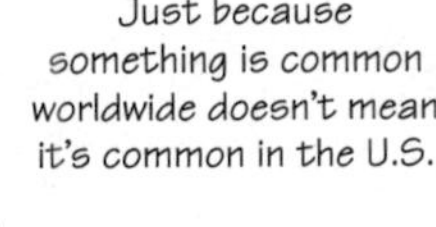
Just because something is common worldwide doesn't mean it's common in the U.S.

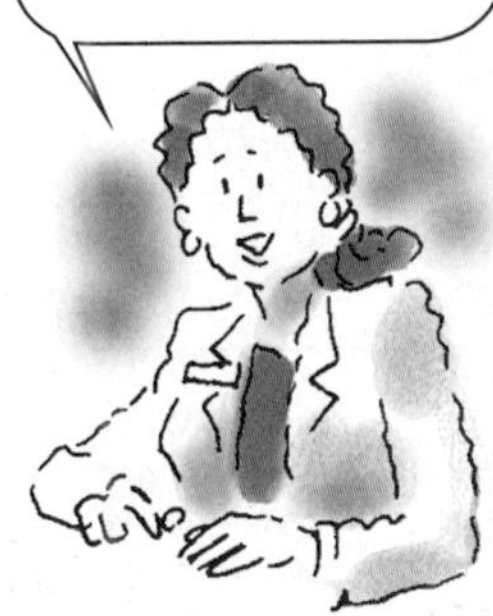

69. Which of the following types of cirrhosis is most common in the United States?

1. Biliary
2. Cardiac
3. Laënnec's
4. Postnecrotic

69. 3. Sixty-five percent of clients with cirrhosis in the United States have Laënnec's, or alcohol-related, cirrhosis. Postnecrotic cirrhosis is the most common form worldwide.

NP: Assessment; CN: Physiological integrity; CNS: Physiological adaptation; CL: Knowledge

70. Which of the following factors causes biliary cirrhosis?

1. Acute viral hepatitis
2. Alcohol hepatotoxicity
3. Chronic biliary inflammation or obstruction
4. Heart failure with prolonged venous hepatic congestion

70. 3. Chronic biliary inflammation or obstruction causes biliary cirrhosis. Acute viral hepatitis can cause postnecrotic cirrhosis. Alcohol hepatotoxicity is Laënnec's cirrhosis. Heart failure with prolonged venous hepatic congestion will cause cardiac cirrhosis.

NP: Assessment; CN: Physiological integrity; CNS: Physiological adaptation; CL: Comprehension

71. Which of the following findings would strongly indicate the possibility of cirrhosis?
1. Dry skin
2. Hepatomegaly
3. Peripheral edema
4. Pruritus

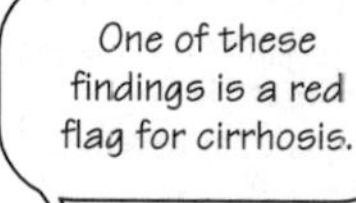
One of these findings is a red flag for cirrhosis.

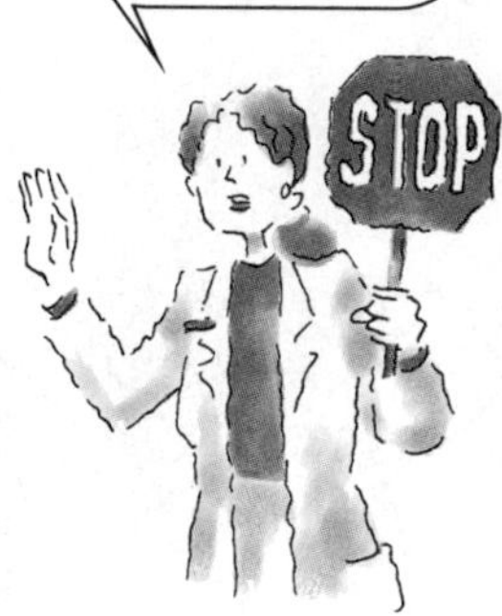

71. 2. The client with cirrhosis has a liver that is enlarged (hepatomegaly), fibrotic, and nodular, which makes it palpable. The client may develop dry skin, pruritus, and peripheral edema, but these symptoms may have other causes.

NP: Assessment; CN: Physiological integrity; CNS: Physiological adaptation; CL: Comprehension

72. Which of the following diagnostic tests helps determine a definitive diagnosis for cirrhosis?
1. Albumin level
2. Bromsulfophthalein dye excretion
3. Liver biopsy
4. Liver enzyme levels

72. 3. A liver biopsy can reveal the exact cause of the hepatomegaly. The albumin level will be low, but that can be caused by poor nutritional states. Liver enzymes may be elevated, but other liver conditions may cause these elevations. Bromsulfophthalein dye excretion may be reduced, but other hepatocirculatory disorders could also cause this.

NP: Assessment; CN: Physiological integrity; CNS: Physiological adaptation; CL: Comprehension

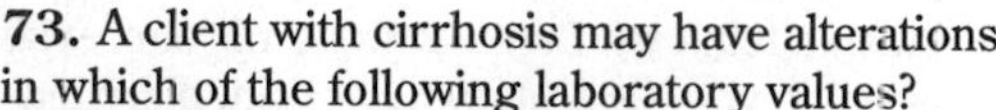

73. A client with cirrhosis may have alterations in which of the following laboratory values?
1. Carbon dioxide level
2. pH
3. Prothrombin time
4. White blood cell (WBC) count

73. 3. Clotting factors may not be produced normally when a client has cirrhosis, increasing the potential for bleeding. There's no associated change in carbon dioxide level or pH unless the client is developing other comorbidities, such as metabolic alkalosis. The WBC count can be elevated in acute cirrhosis but isn't always altered.

NP: Assessment; CN: Physiological integrity; CNS: Physiological adaptation; CL: Comprehension

74. Which of the following measures should the nurse focus on for the client with esophageal varices?
1. Recognizing hemorrhage
2. Controlling blood pressure
3. Encouraging nutritional intake
4. Teaching the client about varices

74. 1. Recognizing the rupture of esophageal varices, or hemorrhage, is the focus of nursing care because the client could succumb to this quickly. Controlling blood pressure is also important because it helps reduce the risk of variceal rupture. It is also important to teach the client what varices are and what foods he should avoid such as spicy foods.

NP: Planning; CN: Physiological integrity; CNS: Physiological adaptation; CL: Application

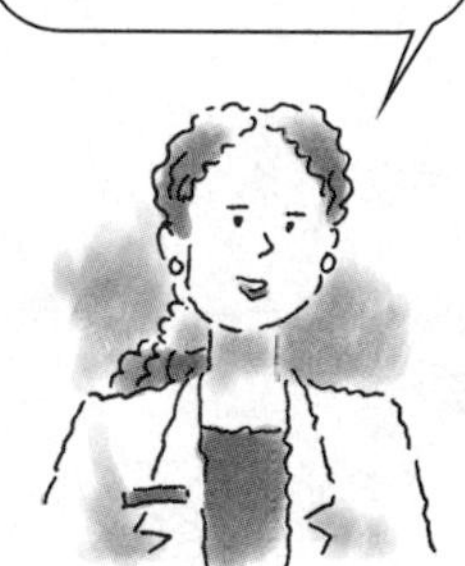
Give yourself a pat on the back! You've completed 75 questions!

75. Which of the following conditions is most likely to cause hepatitis?
1. Bacterial infection
2. Biliary dysfunction
3. Metastasis
4. Viral infection

75. 4. The most common types of hepatitis are those caused by viruses — hepatitis A, B, C, D, and E. Other types of hepatitis are alcoholic, toxic, and chronic. Bacterial infections rarely cause hepatitis, and biliary dysfunction isn't a cause. Liver metastasis from colon cancer causes liver cancer, not hepatitis.

NP: Assessment; CN: Health promotion and maintenance; CNS: Prevention and early detection of disease; CL: Knowledge

76. Which of the following factors can cause hepatitis A?

1. Blood contact
2. Blood transfusion
3. Contaminated shellfish
4. Sexual contact

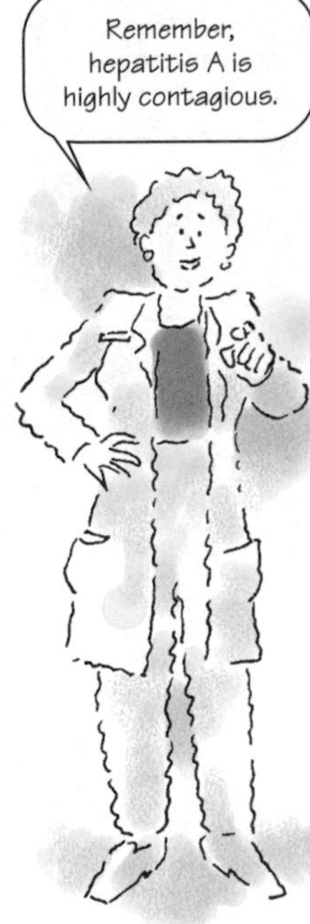

Remember, hepatitis A is highly contagious.

76. 3. Hepatitis A can be caused by infected water, milk, or food, especially shellfish from contaminated waters. Hepatitis B is caused by blood contact and sexual contact. Hepatitis C is usually caused by contact with infected blood, including blood transfusions.
NP: Assessment; CN: Health promotion and maintenance; CNS: Prevention and early detection of disease; CL: Knowledge

77. Mucosal barrier fortifiers are used in peptic ulcer disease management for which of the following indications?

1. To inhibit mucus production
2. To neutralize acid production
3. To stimulate mucus production
4. To stimulate hydrogen ion diffusion back into the mucosa

77. 3. The mucosal barrier fortifiers stimulate mucus production and prevent hydrogen ion diffusion back into the mucosa, resulting in accelerated ulcer healing. Antacids neutralize acid production.
NP: Implementation; CN: Physiological integrity; CNS: Pharmacological and parenteral therapies; CL: Comprehension

78. A client with viral hepatitis may exhibit which of the following symptoms?

1. Arthralgia
2. Excitability
3. Headache
4. Polyphagia

78. 1. Arthralgia is common in clients with viral hepatitis. Other symptoms of viral hepatitis include lethargy, flulike symptoms, anorexia, nausea and vomiting, abdominal pain, diarrhea, constipation, and fever. Excitability, headache, and polyphagia are *not* symptoms of viral hepatitis.
NP: Assessment; CN: Physiological integrity; CNS: Physiological adaptation; CL: Knowledge

79. The client who is developing hepatic encephalopathy may exhibit which of the following symptoms?

1. Asterixis
2. Good concentration
3. Increased energy
4. Talkativeness

79. 1. Asterixis, also known as liver flap, is commonly present in clients with hepatic encephalopathy. It can be easily elicited by applying a blood pressure cuff and noting if the flapping is present when the cuff is released. Lack of concentration, fatigue, and introversion are also symptoms of encephalopathy.
NP: Assessment; CN: Health promotion and maintenance; CNS: Prevention and early detection of disease; CL: Knowledge

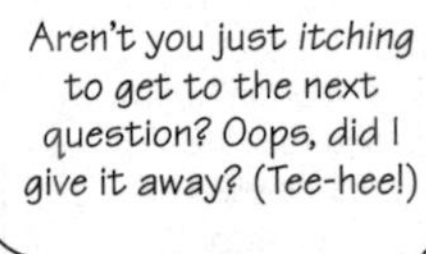

Aren't you just *itching* to get to the next question? Oops, did I give it away? (Tee-hee!)

80. Nursing interventions for the client with toxic hepatitis include which of the following actions?

1. Not allowing oral ingestion
2. Administering corticosteroids
3. Encouraging increased activity
4. Treating adverse effects

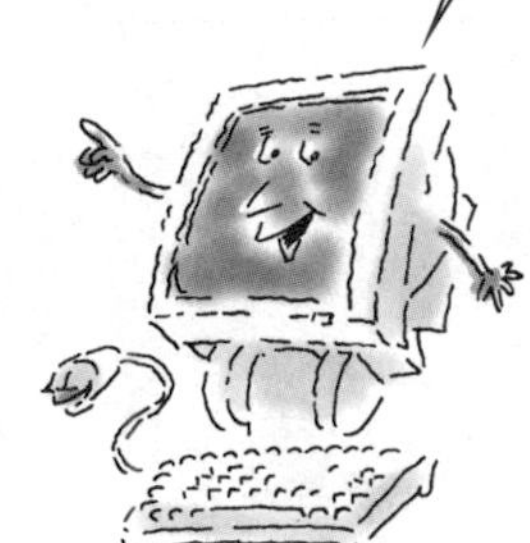

80. 4. Along with removal of the causative agent, alleviation of adverse effects, such as itching, is paramount to care of the client with toxic hepatitis. Other interventions include providing a high-calorie diet and promoting rest. Corticosteroids are rarely used in the care of the client with hepatitis.
NP: Assessment; CN: Safe, effective care environment; CNS: Management of care; CL: Comprehension

81. Which of the following tests is the most accurate for diagnosing liver cancer?
1. Abdominal ultrasound
2. Abdominal flat plate X-ray
3. Cholangiogram
4. Computed tomography (CT) scan

81. 4. A client with suspected liver cancer will likely undergo CT imaging to identify tumors. The results of a computed tomography scan are much more definitive than the findings of an X-ray or ultrasound. A cholangiogram evaluates the gallbladder, not the liver.

NP: Assessment; CN: Health promotion and maintenance; CNS: Prevention and early detection of disease; CL: Knowledge

82. Immediately after a liver biopsy, which of the following complications should the client be closely monitored for?
1. Abdominal cramping
2. Hemorrhage
3. Nausea and vomiting
4. Potential infection

82. 2. The liver is very vascular, and taking a biopsy could cause the client to hemorrhage. The client may experience some discomfort but typically not cramping. Nausea and vomiting may be present, and infection may occur but not immediately after the procedure.

NP: Assessment; CN: Physiological integrity; CNS: Reduction of risk potential; CL: Application

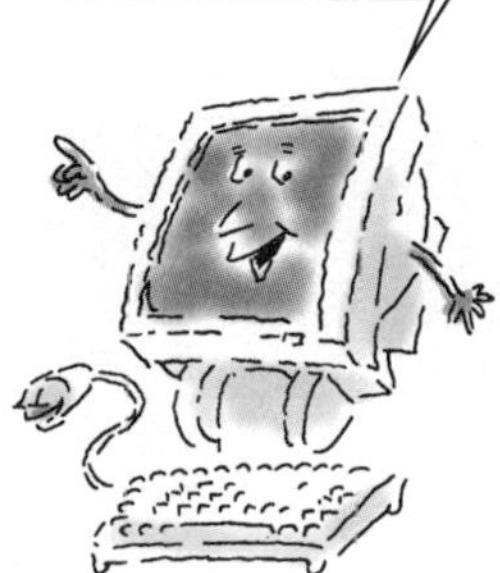

Coagulations! Oops! I meant congratulations! One less to go!

83. When a client who has a liver disorder is having an invasive procedure, the nurse helps assure safety by assessing the results of which of the following tests?
1. Coagulation studies
2. Liver enzyme levels
3. Serum chemistries
4. White blood cell count

83. 1. The liver produces coagulation factors. If the liver is affected negatively, production of these factors may be altered, placing the client at risk for hemorrhage. The other laboratory tests should also be monitored, but the results may not necessarily relate to the safety of the procedure.

NP: Planning; CN: Physiological integrity; CNS: Reduction of risk potential; CL: Analysis

84. Which of the following considerations has highest priority when preparing to administer a medication to a client with liver cancer?
1. Frequency of the medication
2. Purpose of the medication
3. Necessity of the medication
4. Metabolism of the medication

84. 4. Metabolism of medications by the liver will be altered in a client with liver cancer, so knowledge of how each medication is metabolized is essential. The other considerations are important but not as vital.

NP: Planning; CN: Physiological integrity; CNS: Reduction of risk potential; CL: Comprehension

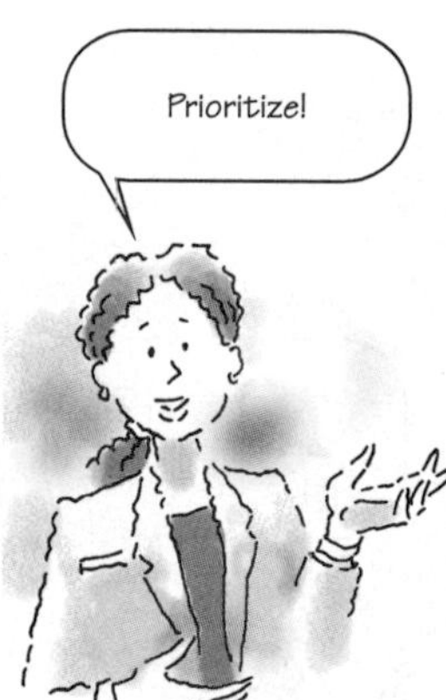

85. Which of the following procedures is likely to be most necessary for a client with a small tumor confined to one liver segment or lobe?
1. Chemotherapy only
2. Cryoablation or liver resection
3. Liver transplant
4. Radiation therapy only

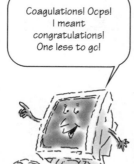

85. 2. If the tumor is confined and small, the best treatment would be cryoablation of the tumor or liver resection, removing the segment involved. Chemotherapy and radiation therapy may also be used to reduce the chance of cancerous hepatocytes from regrowing. Liver transplantation usually isn't indicated for liver cancer.

NP: Planning; CN: Physiological integrity; CNS: Physiological adaptation; CL: Application

86. When counseling a client in the ways to prevent cholecystitis, which of the following guidelines is most important?

1. Eat a low-protein diet
2. Eat a low-fat, low-cholesterol diet
3. Limit exercise to 10 minutes a day
4. Keep weight proportional to height

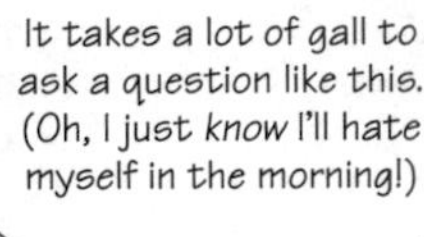

It takes a lot of gall to ask a question like this. (Oh, I just *know* I'll hate myself in the morning!)

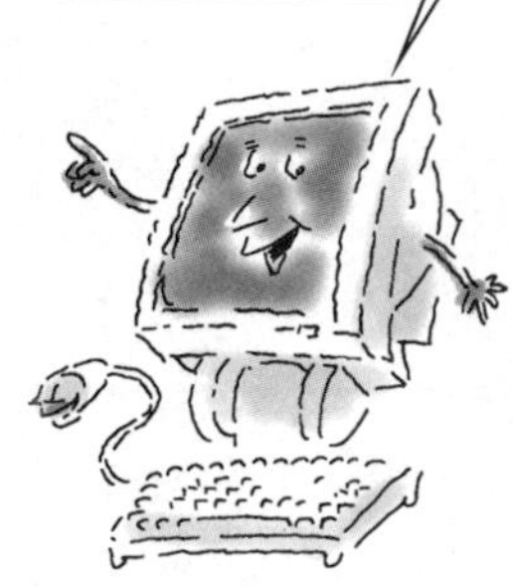

86. 4. Obesity is a known cause of gallstones, and maintaining a recommended weight will help to protect against gallstones. Excessive dietary intake of cholesterol is associated with the development of gallstones in many people. Dietary protein isn't implicated in cholecystitis. Liquid protein and low-calorie diets (with rapid weight loss of more than 5 lb [2.3 kg] per week) *are* implicated as the cause of some cases of cholecystitis. Regular exercise (30 minutes/three times a week) may help to reduce weight and improve fat metabolism. Reducing stress may reduce bile production, which may also indirectly decrease the chances of developing cholecystitis.

NP: Implementation; CN: Health promotion and maintenance; CNS: Prevention and early detection of disease; CL: Application

87. Which of the following symptoms best describes Murphy's sign?

1. Periumbilical ecchymosis exists
2. On deep palpation and release, pain is elicited
3. On deep inspiration, pain is elicited and breathing stops
4. Abdominal muscles are tightened in anticipation of palpation

87. 3. Murphy's sign is elicited when the client reacts to pain and stops breathing. It's a common finding in clients with cholecystitis. Periumbilical ecchymosis, Cullen's sign, is present in peritonitis. Pain on deep palpation and release is rebound tenderness. Tightening up abdominal muscles in anticipation of palpation is guarding.

NP: Assessment; CN: Physiological integrity; CNS: Physiological adaptation; CL: Knowledge

88. Which of the following tests is most commonly used to diagnose cholecystitis?

1. Abdominal computed tomography scan
2. Abdominal ultrasound
3. Barium swallow
4. Endoscopy

88. 2. An abdominal ultrasound can show if the gallbladder is enlarged, if gallstones are present, if the gallbladder wall is thickened, or if distention of the gallbladder lumen is present. An abdominal computed tomography scan can be used to diagnose cholecystitis, but it usually isn't necessary. A barium swallow looks at the stomach and the duodenum. Endoscopy looks at the esophagus, stomach, and duodenum.

NP: Assessment; CN: Health promotion and maintenance; CNS: Prevention and early detection of disease; CL: Comprehension

89. Which of the following factors should be the main focus of nursing management for a client hospitalized for acute cholecystitis?

1. Administration of antibiotics
2. Assessment for complications
3. Preparation for lithotripsy
4. Preparation for surgery

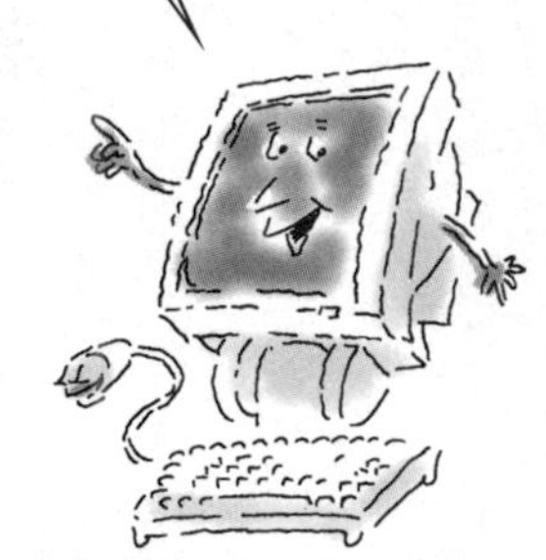

This question is asking you to prioritize again.

89. 2. The client with acute cholecystitis should *first* be monitored for perforation, fever, abscess, fistula, and sepsis. After assessment, antibiotics will be administered to reduce the infection. Lithotripsy is used for only a small percentage of clients. Surgery is usually done after the acute infection has subsided.

NP: Planning; CN: Physiological integrity; CNS: Reduction of risk potential; CL: Application

90. A client being treated for chronic cholecystitis should be given which of the following instructions?
1. Increase rest
2. Avoid antacids
3. Increase protein in diet
4. Use anticholinergics as prescribed

90. 4. Conservative therapy for chronic cholecystitis includes weight reduction by increasing physical activity, a low-fat diet, antacid use to treat dyspepsia, and anticholinergic use to relax smooth muscles and reduce ductal tone and spasm, thereby reducing pain.

NP: Implementation; CN: Physiological integrity; CNS: Pharmacological and parenteral therapies; CL: Comprehension

91. The client with a duodenal ulcer may exhibit which of the following findings on assessment?
1. Hematemesis
2. Malnourishment
3. Melena
4. Pain with eating

91. 3. The client with a duodenal ulcer may have bleeding at the ulcer site, which shows up as melena. The other findings are consistent with a gastric ulcer.

NP: Assessment; CN: Physiological integrity; CNS: Physiological adaptation; CL: Comprehension

92. Which of the following characteristics is associated with most stress ulcers?
1. A single, well-defined lesion
2. Increased gastric acid production
3. Decreased gastric mucosal blood flow
4. Increased blood flow to gastric mucosa

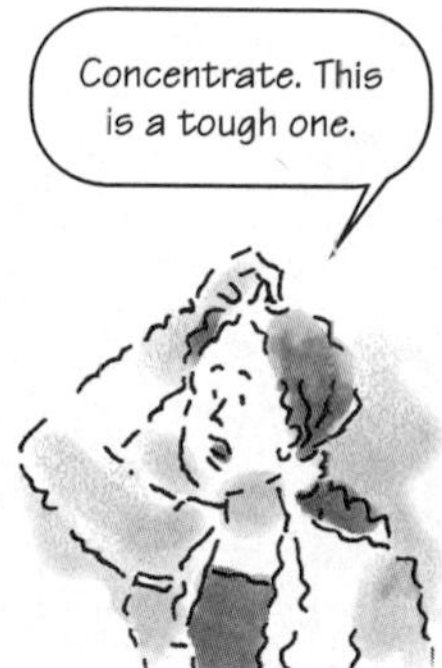
Concentrate. This is a tough one.

92. 3. Contrary to popular belief, overproduction of gastric acid is rarely the cause of stress ulcers. Rather, stress states decrease gastric mucosal blood flow, resulting in mucosal breakdown. Stress ulcers are usually more shallow and diffuse than peptic ulcers, which tend to be singular and well-defined.

NP: Assessment; CN: Physiological integrity; CNS: Physiological adaptation; CL: Comprehension

93. The pain of a duodenal ulcer can be distinguished from that of a gastric ulcer by which of the following characteristics?
1. Early satiety
2. Pain on eating
3. Dull upper epigastric pain
4. Pain on an empty stomach

93. 4. Pain on an empty stomach is relieved by taking food or antacids. The other symptoms are those of a gastric ulcer.

NP: Assessment; CN: Physiological integrity; CNS: Physiological adaptation; CL: Comprehension

94. Which of the following tests can be used to diagnose ulcers?
1. Abdominal X-ray
2. Barium swallow
3. Computed tomography (CT) scan
4. Esophagogastroduodenoscopy (EGD)

94. 4. The EGD can visualize the entire upper GI tract as well as allow for tissue specimens and electrocautery if needed. The barium swallow could locate a gastric ulcer. A CT scan and an abdominal X-ray aren't useful in the diagnosis of an ulcer.

NP: Assessment; CN: Health promotion and maintenance; CNS: Prevention and early detection of disease; CL: Knowledge

95. Which of the following best describes the method of action of medications, such as ranitidine (Zantac), which are used in the treatment of peptic ulcer disease?
1. Neutralize acid
2. Reduce acid secretions
3. Stimulate gastrin release
4. Protect the mucosal barrier

95. 2. Ranitidine is a histamine-2 receptor antagonist that reduces acid secretion by inhibiting gastrin secretion. Antacids neutralize acid, and mucosal barrier fortifiers protect the mucosal barrier.

NP: Assessment; CN: Physiological integrity; CNS: Pharmacological and parenteral therapies; CL: Knowledge

96. Which of the following laboratory values will the nurse interpret as confirming a client's diagnosis of pancreatitis?
1. Elevated amylase, elevated lipase, elevated serum glucose, and decreased serum calcium levels
2. Elevated amylase, elevated lipase, decreased serum glucose, and decreased serum calcium levels
3. Decreased amylase, decreased lipase, elevated serum glucose, and increased serum calcium levels
4. Decreased amylase, decreased lipase, decreased serum glucose, and increased serum calcium levels

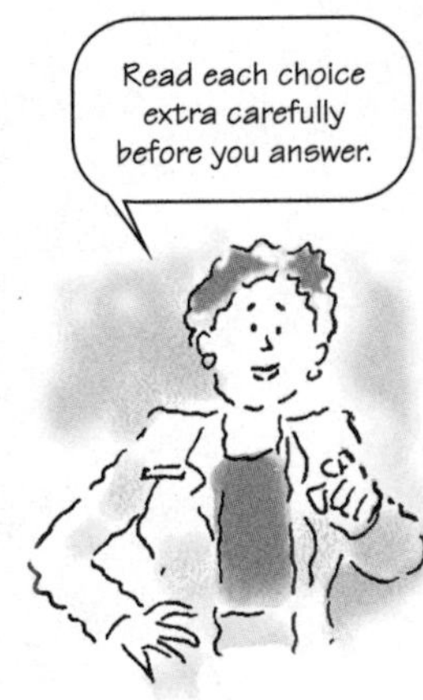

Read each choice extra carefully before you answer.

96. 1. Inflammation of the pancreas causes it to excrete pancreatic enzymes. The inflammation also causes a blockage of the ducts from the pancreas to the GI tract; therefore, the pancreatic enzymes are released into the blood, resulting in an elevation of amylase and lipase levels. Carbohydrate metabolism is impaired secondary to damage to pancreatic beta cells. This impairment causes the client to become hyperglycemic. As in many other disease processes, serum calcium level decreases because of the saponification of calcium by fatty acids in the area of the inflamed pancreas.
NP: Assessment; CN: Physiological integrity; CNS: Physiological adaptation; CL: Analysis

97. Which of the following instructions should the nurse give a client with pancreatitis during discharge teaching?
1. Consume high-fat meals
2. Consume low-calorie meals
3. Limit daily intake of alcohol
4. Avoid beverages that contain caffeine

97. 4. A client with pancreatitis must avoid foods or beverages that can cause a relapse of the disease. Caffeine must be avoided because it's a stimulant that will further irritate the pancreas. The client with pancreatitis must avoid all alcohol because chronic alcohol use is one of the causes of pancreatitis. The diet should be high in calories, especially carbohydrates, and low in fats.
NP: Implementation; CN: Physiological integrity; CNS: Reduction of risk potential; CL: Application

98. After a liver biopsy, the nurse should place the client in which of the following positions?
1. Left side-lying position, with the bed flat
2. Right side-lying position, with the bed flat
3. Left side-lying position, with the bed in semi-Fowler's position
4. Right side-lying position, with the bed in semi-Fowler's position

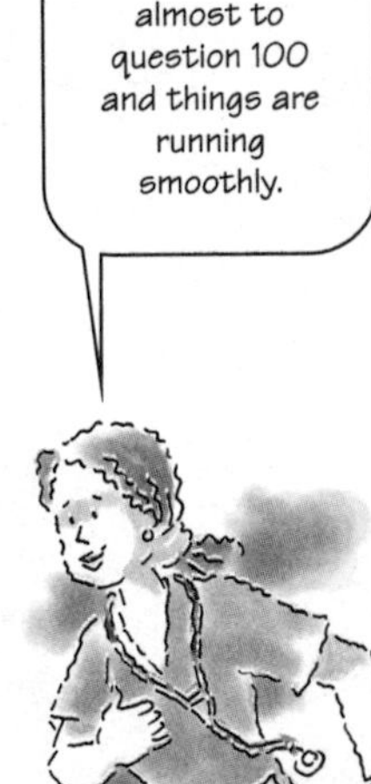

You're almost to question 100 and things are running smoothly.

98. 2. Lying the client on his right side with the bed flat will splint the biopsy site and minimize bleeding. The other positions won't do this and may cause increased bleeding at the site or internally.
NP: Implementation; CN: Physiological integrity; CNS: Reduction of risk potential; CL: Application

99. A client with irritable bowel syndrome is being prepared for discharge. Which of the following meal plans should the nurse give the client?
1. Low-fiber, low-fat
2. High-fiber, low-fat
3. Low-fiber, high-fat
4. High-fiber, high-fat

99. 2. The client with irritable bowel syndrome needs to be on a diet that contains at least 25 grams of fiber per day. Fatty foods are to be avoided because they may precipitate symptoms.
NP: Implementation; CN: Physiological integrity; CNS: Reduction of risk potential; CL: Application

100. A client presents to the emergency department, reporting that he has been vomiting every 30 to 40 minutes for the past 8 hours. Frequent vomiting puts him at risk for which of the following?
1. Metabolic acidosis and hyperkalemia
2. Metabolic acidosis and hypokalemia
3. Metabolic alkalosis and hyperkalemia
4. Metabolic alkalosis and hypokalemia

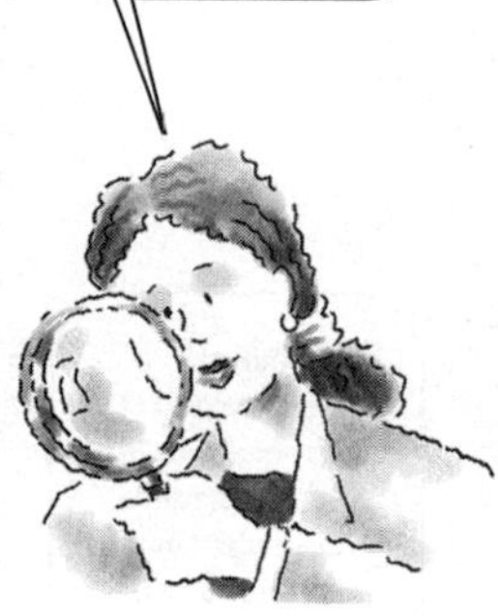

Closely examine the answers to question 100; it's easy to confuse them.

100. 4. Gastric acid contains large amounts of potassium, chloride, and hydrogen ions. Excessive loss of these substances, such as from vomiting, can lead to metabolic alkalosis and hypokalemia. It doesn't cause metabolic acidosis or hyperkalemia.
NP: Assessment; CN: Physiological integrity; CNS: Reduction of risk potential; CL: Application

101. Five days after undergoing surgery, a client develops a small-bowel obstruction. A Miller-Abbott tube is inserted for bowel decompression. Which nursing diagnosis takes priority?
1. Imbalanced nutrition: Less than body requirements
2. Acute pain
3. Deficient fluid volume
4. Excess fluid volume

101. 3. Fluid shifts to the site of the bowel obstruction, causing a fluid deficit in the intravascular spaces. If the obstruction isn't resolved immediately, the client may experience an imbalanced nutritional status (less than body requirements); however, deficient fluid volume takes priority. The client also may experience pain, but that nursing diagnosis is also of lower priority than deficient fluid volume.
NP: Analysis; CN: Physiological integrity; CNS: Physiological adaptation; CL: Analysis

102. A client presents to the clinic for a follow-up appointment after diagnostic tests show he has gastroesophageal reflux disease. Which instruction should the nurse provide?
1. "Lie down and rest after each meal."
2. "Avoid alcohol and caffeine."
3. "Drink 16 ounces of water with each meal."
4. "Eat three well-balanced meals every day."

102. 2. A client with gastroesophageal reflux disease should avoid alcohol, caffeine, and foods that increase acidity, all of which can cause epigastric pain. To further prevent reflux, the client should remain upright for 2 to 3 hours after eating; avoid eating for 2 to 3 hours before bedtime; avoid bending and wearing tight clothing; avoid drinking large fluid volumes with meals; and eat small, frequent meals to help reduce gastric acid secretion.
NP: Implementation; CN: Physiological integrity; CNS: Reduction of risk potential; CL: Application

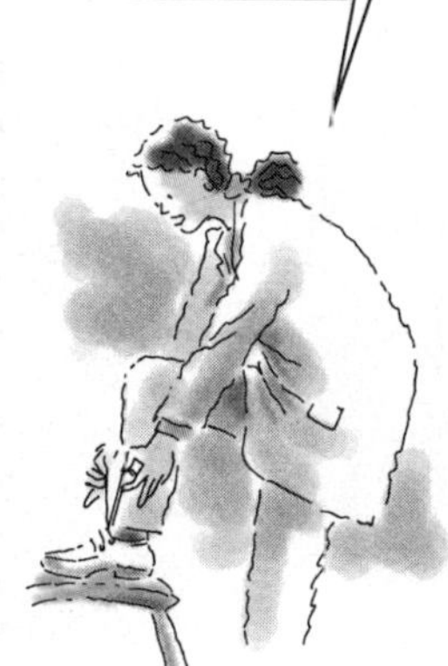

Exercise care in picking your answer. Oops, I just gave it away.

103. When teaching an elderly client how to prevent constipation, which of the following instructions should the nurse include?
1. "Drink six glasses of fluid each day."
2. "Avoid grain products and nuts."
3. "Add at least 4 grams of bran to your cereal each morning."
4. "Be sure to get regular exercise."

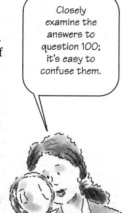

103. 4. Exercise helps prevent constipation. Fluids and dietary fiber promote normal bowel function. The client should drink eight to ten glasses of fluid per day. Although adding bran to cereal helps prevent constipation by increasing dietary fiber, the client should start with a small amount of bran and gradually increase the amount as tolerated to a maximum of 2 grams daily.
NP: Planning; CN: Health promotion and maintenance; CNS: Prevention and early detection of disease; CL: Application

104. In a client with diarrhea, which outcome indicates that fluid resuscitation is successful?

1. The client passes formed stools at regular intervals.
2. The client reports a decrease in stool frequency and liquidity.
3. The client exhibits firm skin turgor.
4. The client no longer experiences perianal burning.

104. 3. A client with diarrhea has a nursing diagnosis of ***Deficient fluid volume*** related to excessive fluid loss in stool. Expected outcomes include firm skin turgor, moist mucous membranes, and urine output of at least 30 ml/hour. The client also has a nursing diagnosis of ***Diarrhea,*** with expected outcomes of passage of formed stools at regular intervals and a decrease in stool frequency and liquidity. The client is at risk for impaired skin integrity related to irritation from diarrhea; expected outcomes for this diagnosis include absence of erythema in perianal skin and mucous membranes and absence of perianal tenderness or burning.

NP: Evaluation; CN: Physiological integrity; CNS: Basic care and comfort; CL: Analysis

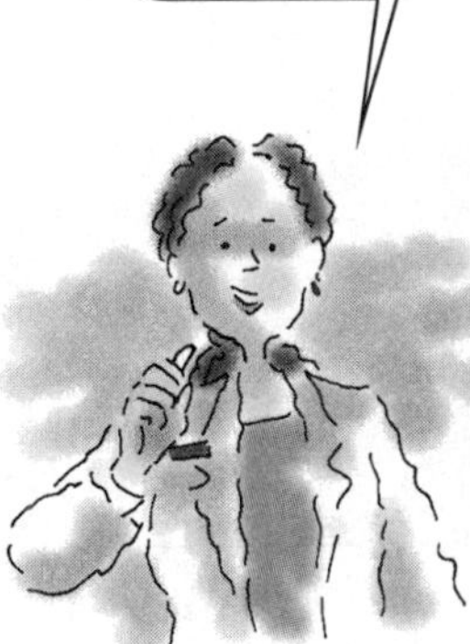

Eliminating the wrong answers can be as important as selecting the right one.

105. When teaching a community group about measures to prevent colon cancer, which instruction should the nurse include?

1. "Limit fat intake to 20% to 25% of your total daily calories."
2. "Include 15 to 20 grams of fiber in your daily diet."
3. "Get an annual rectal examination after age 35."
4. "Undergo sigmoidoscopy annually after age 50."

105. 1. To help prevent colon cancer, fats should account for no more than 20% to 25% of total daily calories and the diet should include 25 to 30 grams of fiber per day. A digital rectal examination isn't recommended as a stand-alone test for colorectal cancer. For colorectal cancer screening, the American Cancer Society advises clients over age 50 to have a flexible sigmoidoscopy every 5 years, yearly fecal occult blood tests, yearly fecal occult blood tests plus a flexible sigmoidoscopy every 5 years, a double-contrast barium enema every 5 years, or a colonoscopy every 10 years.

NP: Implementation; CN: Health promotion and maintenance; CNS: Prevention and early detection of disease; CL: Application

106. A 30-year-old client experiences weight loss, abdominal distention, crampy abdominal pain, and intermittent diarrhea after the birth of her second child. Diagnostic tests reveal gluten-induced enteropathy. Which foods must she eliminate from her diet permanently?

1. Milk and dairy products
2. Protein-containing foods
3. Cereal grains (except rice and corn)
4. Carbohydrates

106. 3. To manage gluten-induced enteropathy, the client must eliminate gluten, which means avoiding all cereal grains except rice and corn. In initial disease management, clients eat a high-calorie, high-protein diet with mineral and vitamin supplements to help normalize the nutritional status. Lactose intolerance is sometimes an associated problem, so milk and dairy products are limited until improvement occurs. Cereal grains are the only carbohydrates this client must eliminate.

NP: Implementation; CN: Physiological integrity; CNS: Basic care and comfort; CL: Application

107. After a right hemicolectomy for treatment of colon cancer, a 57-year-old client is reluctant to turn while on bed rest. Which action by the nurse would be appropriate?

1. Asking a coworker to help turn the client
2. Explaining to the client why turning is important
3. Allowing the client to turn when he's ready to do so
4. Telling the client that the physician's order states he must turn every 2 hours

107. 2. The appropriate action is to explain the importance of turning to avoid postoperative complications. Asking a coworker to help turn the client against his will would infringe on his rights. Allowing him to turn when he's ready would increase his risk for postoperative complications. Telling him he must turn because of the physician's orders would put him on the defensive and exclude him from participating in care decisions.

NP: Implementation; CN: Physiological integrity; CNS: Reduction of risk potential CL: Application

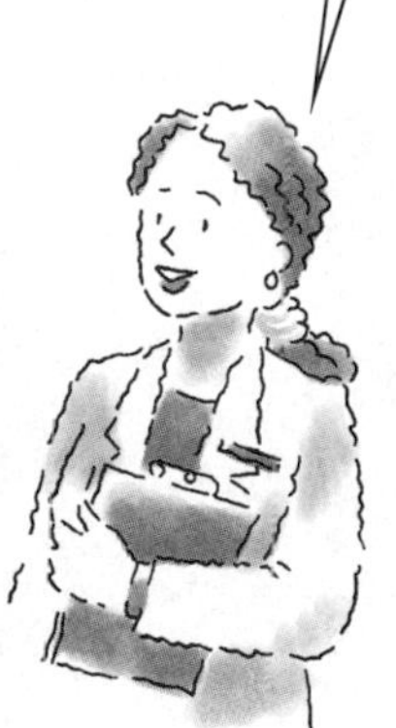

Take your time with this one. Good record keeping is a key factor in client care.

108. The nurse assists the physician during paracentesis. When documenting the procedure, which information should the nurse include?

1. Exactly what she did during the procedure
2. The reason for the procedure
3. The physician's name and the client's response to the procedure
4. Diagnostic tests performed before obtaining the specimen

108. 3. The nurse should document the date and time of the procedure, the physician's name, pertinent information about the procedure (including tests done on the specimen obtained), the client's response, and client teaching. Documentation should include response to her interventions during the procedure. The reason for the procedure doesn't need to be documented.

NP: Implementation; CN: Physiological integrity; CNS: Reduction of risk potential; CL: Analysis

109. A client has a percutaneous endoscopic gastrostomy tube inserted for tube feedings. Before starting a continuous feeding, the nurse should place the client in which position?

1. Semi-Fowler's
2. Supine
3. Reverse Trendelenburg
4. High Fowler's

109. 1. To prevent aspiration of stomach contents, the nurse should place the client in semi-Fowler's position. The supine and reverse Trendelenburg positions may cause aspiration. High-Fowler's position isn't necessary and may not be tolerated as well as semi-Fowler's.

NP: Implementation; CN: Physiological integrity; CNS: Reduction of risk potential; CL: Application

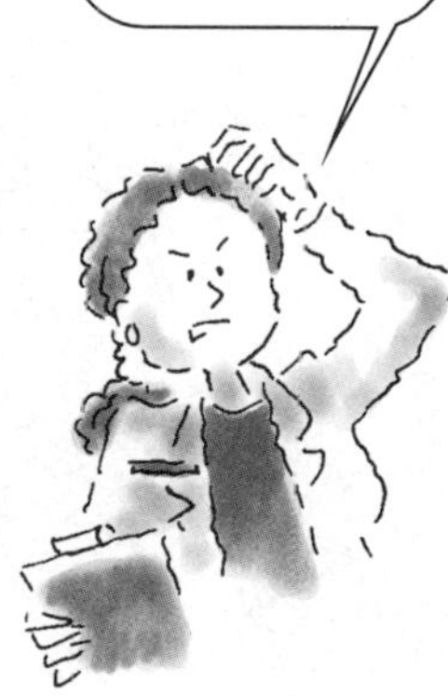

Knowing when to question orders is crucial for nurses and their clients.

110. An enema is prescribed for a client with suspected appendicitis. Which of the following actions should the nurse take?

1. Prepare 750 ml of irrigating solution warmed to 100° F (37.8° C).
2. Question the physician about the order.
3. Provide privacy and explain the procedure to the client.
4. Assist the client to left lateral Sims' position.

110. 2. Enemas are contraindicated in an acute abdominal condition of unknown origin (such as suspected appendicitis) as well as after recent colon or rectal surgery or myocardial infarction. The other answers are correct only when enema administration is appropriate. The nurse prepares the prescribed type and amount of irrigating solution; for an adult, the standard volume is 750 to 1,000 ml, warmed to 100° to 105° F (37.8° to 40.5°C). The nurse provides privacy and explains the procedure to the client, then washes her hands, puts on gloves, assists the client to a left lateral Sims' position, and follows the facility's specified procedure for enema administration.

NP: Implementation; CN: Safe, effective care environment; CNS: Safety and infection control; CL: Application

111. After a cholecystectomy, a client has a T-tube in place. When the client asks about the tube, the nurse should provide which instruction?

1. "The tube helps drain bile during the healing process."
2. "The tube will remain in place for about 5 days."
3. "We'll monitor the tube's patency and output every 8 hours."
4. "You'll have a feeling of fullness in your right upper abdomen while the tube is in place."

111. 1. A T-tube drains bile while healing occurs. Typically, it remains in place for 7 to 14 days after surgery. Tube patency and site condition are assessed hourly for the first 8 hours, and then every 4 hours. Right upper quadrant fullness and pain aren't normal; these symptoms indicate obstructed bile flow (as do chills, fever, tachycardia, nausea, jaundice, dark foamy urine, and clay-colored stools) and should be reported immediately.

NP: Implementation; CN: Physiological integrity; CNS: Reduction of risk potential; CL: Analysis

112. The nurse evaluates a client's readiness to learn about colostomy self-care. Which of the following behaviors best demonstrates that the client isn't ready to learn?

1. The client hasn't looked at the stoma.
2. The client verbalizes feeling slightly depressed about the colostomy.
3. The client asks questions about the colostomy.
4. The client asks how to care for the colostomy.

112. 1. A client who hasn't looked at the stoma may be in shock and disbelief, and isn't ready to learn about self-care. Although teaching won't be effective if the client is angry or depressed, a client who verbalizes slight depression may be ready to learn about colostomy self-care. Asking questions about the colostomy and its care indicates readiness to learn.

NP: Evaluation; CN: Psychosocial integrity; CNS: Coping and adaptation; CL: Analysis

113. Seven days after a gastrectomy, a client experiences tachycardia, palpitations, hypertension, diaphoresis, cramping, nausea, and diarrhea with meals. Based on these findings, the nurse should suspect which complication of gastrectomy?

1. Postprandial hypoglycemia
2. Dumping syndrome
3. Alkaline reflux gastritis
4. Acute gastric dilation

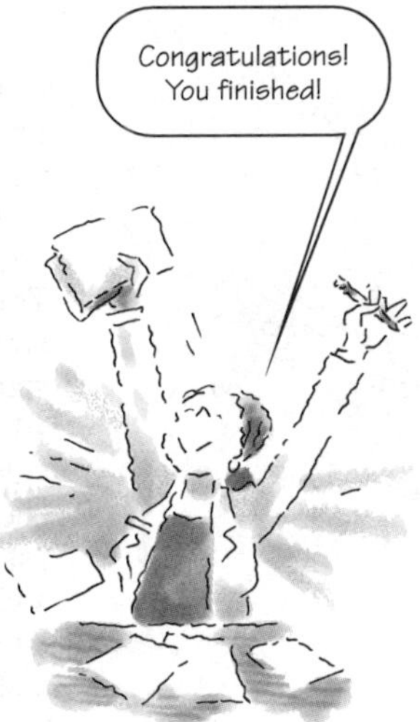
Congratulations!
You finished!

113. 2. Dumping syndrome, which can occur for 1 to 3 weeks after a gastrectomy, causes tachycardia, palpitations, syncope, hypertension, flushing, diaphoresis, bloating, cramping, diarrhea, and nausea with meals. Although the other answers are also complications of gastrectomy, they cause different symptoms. Postprandial hypoglycemia causes weakness, faintness, diaphoresis, hunger, nausea, anxiety, tremors, and palpitations 2 to 3 hours after eating. With alkaline reflux gastritis, expect nausea, vomiting, and persistent pain and epigastric burning worsening after meals. Acute gastric dilation leads to epigastric pain, a feeling of fullness, hiccups, gagging, tachycardia, and hypertension.

NP: Assessment; CN: Physiological integrity; CNS: Reduction of risk potential; CL: Analysis

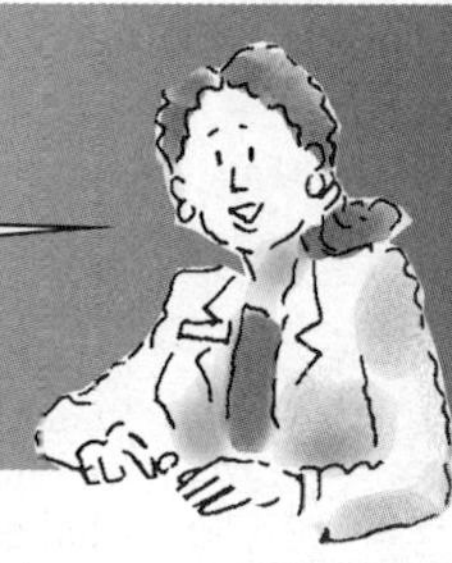

This chapter covers diabetes mellitus and other endocrine disorders, typically a difficult area for nursing students. Don't worry, though, I'll help you through all the tough spots.

Chapter 9 Endocrine disorders

1. Which of the following symptoms indicate hyperglycemia?
1. Polydipsia, polyuria, and weight loss
2. Weight gain, tiredness, and bradycardia
3. Irritability, diaphoresis, and tachycardia
4. Diarrhea, abdominal pain, and weight loss

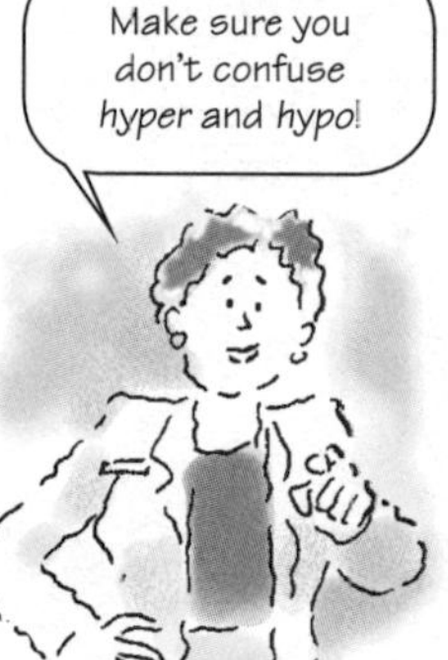

Make sure you don't confuse hyper and hypo!

1. 1. Symptoms of hyperglycemia include polydipsia, polyuria, and weight loss. Weight gain, tiredness, and bradycardia are symptoms of hypothyroidism. Irritability, diaphoresis, and tachycardia are symptoms of hypoglycemia. Symptoms of Crohn's disease include diarrhea, abdominal pain, and weight loss.

NP: Analysis; CN: Physiological integrity; CNS: Reduction of risk potential; CL: Knowledge

2. A client presents with diaphoresis, palpitations, jitters, and tachycardia approximately 1½ hours after taking his regular morning insulin. Which of the following treatments is appropriate for this client?
1. Check blood glucose level and administer carbohydrates.
2. Give nitroglycerin and perform an electrocardiogram (ECG).
3. Check pulse oximetry and administer oxygen therapy.
4. Restrict salt, administer diuretics, and perform a paracentesis.

2. 1. The client is experiencing symptoms of hypoglycemia. Checking the blood glucose level and administering carbohydrates will elevate blood glucose. Giving insulin will further lower blood glucose. ECG and nitroglycerin are treatments for myocardial infarction. Administering oxygen won't help correct the low blood glucose level. Restricting salt, administering diuretics, and performing a paracentesis are treatments for ascites.

NP: Assessment; CN: Physiological integrity; CNS: Physiological adaptation; CL: Comprehension

3. Which of the following nursing considerations must be taken into account for a client with type 1 diabetes mellitus on the morning of surgery?
1. The client should take one-half of his usual daily insulin.
2. The client should receive an oral antidiabetic agent.
3. The client should receive an I.V. insulin infusion.
4. The client should take his full daily insulin dose with no dextrose infusion.

3. 1. If the client takes his full daily dose of insulin when he isn't allowed anything orally before surgery, he'll become hypoglycemic. One-half the insulin dose will provide all that is needed. Clients with type 1 diabetes don't take oral antidiabetic agents. I.V. insulin infusions aren't standard for routine surgery; they're used in the management of clients undergoing stressful procedures, such as transplants or coronary artery bypass surgery.

NP: Planning; CN: Physiological integrity; CNS: Physiological adaptation; CL: Comprehension

NP: Nursing process CN: Client needs category CNS: Client needs subcategory CL: Cognitive level

4. Which of the following types of diabetes is controlled primarily through diet, exercise, and oral antidiabetic agents?
1. Diabetes insipidus
2. Diabetic ketoacidosis
3. Type 1 diabetes mellitus
4. Type 2 diabetes mellitus

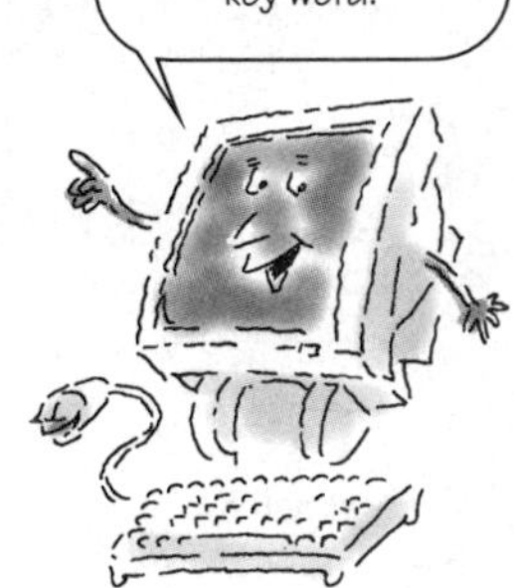

Read this question carefully. *Controlled* is the key word.

4. 4. Type 2 diabetes mellitus is controlled primarily through diet, exercise, and oral antidiabetic agents. Diet and exercise are important in type 1 diabetes mellitus, but blood glucose levels are controlled by insulin injections in that disorder. Desmopressin acetate, a long-acting vasopressin given intranasally, is the treatment of choice for diabetes insipidus. Treatment for diabetic ketoacidosis includes restoration of fluid volume, electrolyte management, reversal of acidosis, and control of blood glucose.
NP: Analysis; CN: Physiological integrity; CNS: Reduction of risk potential; CL: Knowledge

5. Which of the following nursing interventions should be taken for a client who complains of nausea and vomits 1 hour after taking his morning glyburide (DiaBeta)?
1. Give glyburide again.
2. Give subcutaneous insulin and monitor blood glucose.
3. Monitor blood glucose closely, and look for signs of hypoglycemia.
4. Monitor blood glucose, and assess for symptoms of hyperglycemia.

5. 3. When a client who has taken an oral antidiabetic agent vomits, the nurse would monitor glucose and assess him frequently for signs of hypoglycemia. Most of the medication has probably been absorbed. Therefore, repeating the dose would further lower glucose levels later in the day. Giving insulin also will lower glucose levels, causing hypoglycemia. The client wouldn't have hyperglycemia if the glyburide was absorbed.
NP: Assessment; CN: Physiological integrity; CNS: Pharmacological and parenteral therapies; CL: Analysis

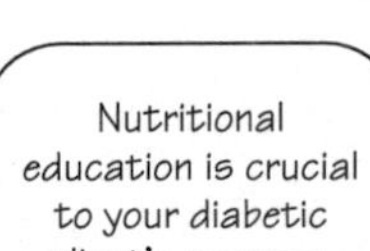

Nutritional education is crucial to your diabetic client's recovery.

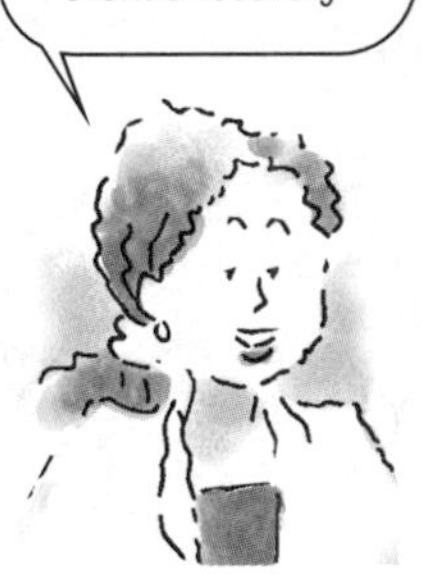

6. When teaching a newly diagnosed diabetic client about diet and exercise, it's important to include which of the following aspects?
1. Use of fiber laxatives and bulk-forming agents
2. Management of fluid, protein, and electrolytes
3. Reduction of calorie intake before exercising
4. Caloric goals, food consistency, and physical activity

6. 4. Diabetic clients must be taught the relationship among caloric goals, consistency of food composition, and physical activity. Management of fluids, proteins, and electrolytes is important for a client with acute renal failure. Fiber laxatives and bulk-forming agents are treatments for constipation. The diabetic client may need to intake additional calories before exercising.
NP: Planning; CN: Health promotion and maintenance; CNS: Prevention and early detection of disease; CL: Comprehension

7. Which of the following chronic complications is associated with diabetes mellitus?
1. Dizziness, dyspnea on exertion, and angina
2. Retinopathy, neuropathy, and coronary artery disease
3. Leg ulcers, cerebral ischemic events, and pulmonary infarcts
4. Fatigue, nausea, vomiting, muscle weakness, and cardiac arrhythmias

7. 2. Retinopathy, neuropathy, and coronary artery disease are all chronic complications of diabetes mellitus. Dizziness, dyspnea on exertion, and angina are symptoms of aortic valve stenosis. Hyperparathyroidism causes fatigue, nausea, vomiting, muscle weakness, and cardiac arrhythmias. Leg ulcers, cerebral ischemic events, and pulmonary infarcts are complications of sickle cell anemia.
NP: Analysis; CN: Physiological integrity; CNS: Reduction of risk potential; CL: Knowledge

8. Rotating injection sites when administering insulin prevents which of the following complications?
1. Insulin edema
2. Insulin lipodystrophy
3. Insulin resistance
4. Systemic allergic reactions

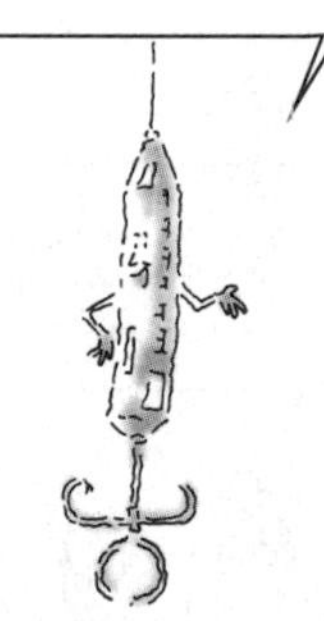

Rotating injection sites is important for preventing complications.

8. 2. Insulin lipodystrophy produces fatty masses at the injection sites, causing unpredictable absorption of insulin injected into these sites. Insulin edema is generalized retention of fluid, sometimes seen after normal blood glucose levels are established in a client with prolonged hyperglycemia. Insulin resistance occurs mostly in overweight clients and is due to insulin binding with antibodies, decreasing the amount of absorption. Systemic allergic reactions range from hives to anaphylaxis; rotating injection sites won't prevent these.

NP: Planning; CN: Health promotion and maintenance; CNS: Prevention and early detection of disease; CL: Comprehension

9. Which of the following tests allows a rapid measurement of glucose in whole blood?
1. Capillary blood glucose test
2. Serum ketone test
3. Serum T_4 test
4. Urine glucose test

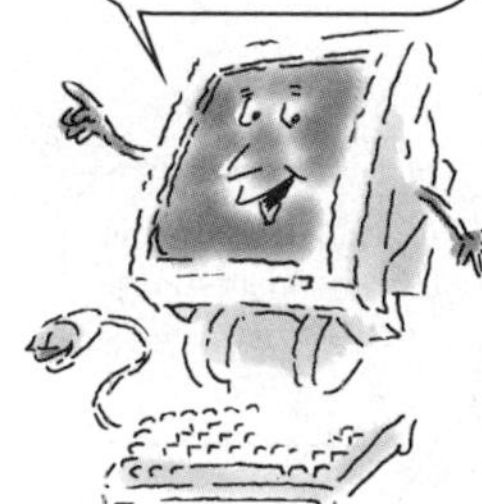

This question is asking for the best test for a specific indication.

9. 1. A capillary blood glucose test is a rapid test used to show blood glucose levels. A urine glucose test monitors glucose levels in urine and is influenced by both glucose and water excretion. Therefore, results correlate poorly with blood glucose levels. A serum T_4 test is used to diagnosis thyroid disorders. A serum ketone test is used to document diabetic ketoacidosis by titration and may allow determination of serum ketone concentration. Most of the time, however, neither serum ketone levels nor T_4 levels are useful in determining blood glucose levels.

NP: Evaluation; CN: Physiological integrity; CNS: Reduction of risk potential; CL: Comprehension

10. How long does the peak effect last for Novolin NPH, an intermediate-acting insulin?
1. 15 minutes to 1 hour
2. 2 to 6 hours
3. 6 to 16 hours
4. 14 to 26 hours

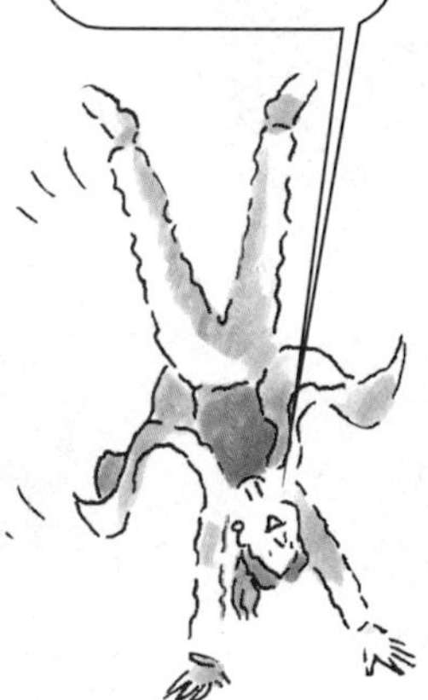

10. 3. Novolin NPH has a peak effect of 6 to 16 hours. The peak effect of rapid-acting insulin is 2 to 6 hours. Long-acting insulin has a peak effect of 14 to 26 hours. The onset of rapid-acting insulin is 15 minutes to 1 hour.

NP: Assessment; CN: Physiological integrity; CNS: Pharmacological and parenteral therapies; CL: Knowledge

11. The hormones triiodothyronine (T_3) and thyroxine (T_4) affect which of the following body processes?
1. Blood glucose level and glycogenolysis
2. Growth and development as well as metabolic rate
3. Growth of bones, muscles, and other organs
4. Bone resorption, calcium absorption, and blood calcium levels

11. 2. T_3 and T_4 are thyroid hormones that affect growth and development as well as metabolic rate. Bone resorption and increased calcium absorption are the principle effects of parathyroid hormone. Glucagon raises blood glucose levels and stimulates glycogenolysis. The growth hormone somatotrophin affects the growth of bones, muscles, and other organs.

NP: Analysis; CN: Physiological integrity; CNS: Physiological adaptation; CL: Knowledge

12. The nurse should anticipate administration of which of the following medications to a client with hypothyroidism?
1. Dexamethasone
2. Lactulose
3. Levothyroxine
4. Lidocaine

12. 3. Levothyroxine, a synthetic form of the thyroid hormone T_4, is the medication of choice for treating hypothyroidism. Dexamethasone is a steroid and an antithyroid medication. Lactulose is used to produce an osmotic diarrhea, resulting in an acidic diarrhea. Lidocaine is used to treat ventricular arrhythmias.
NP: Implementation; CN: Physiological integrity; CNS: Pharmacological and parenteral therapies; CL: Knowledge

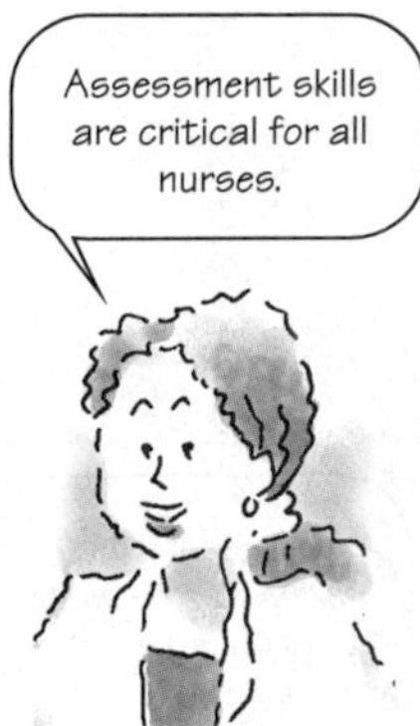

Assessment skills are critical for all nurses.

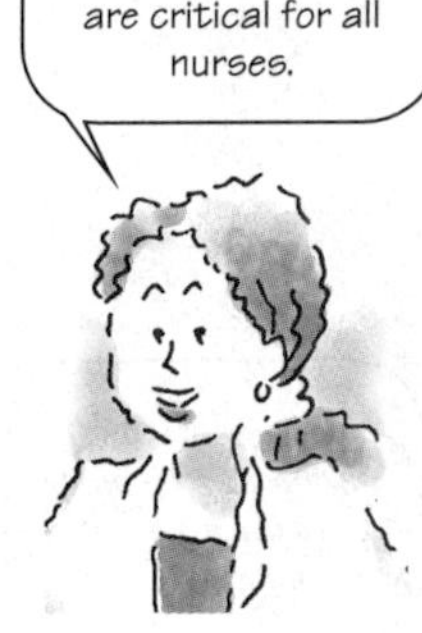

13. The thyroid gland is properly palpated by which of the following actions?
1. Have the client flex his neck onto his chest and cough while the nurse palpates the anterior neck with her fingertips.
2. Place hands around the client's neck, with the thumbs in the front of the neck, and gently massage the anterior neck.
3. Encircle the client's neck with both hands, have the client slightly extend his neck, and ask him to swallow.
4. Have the client hyperextend his neck and take slow, deep inhalations while the nurse palpates the neck with her fingertips.

13. 3. This is the correct method for palpating the thyroid gland. As the client swallows, the gland is palpated for enlargement as the tissue rises and falls. Having the client flex his neck wouldn't allow for palpation. Massaging the area or checking during inhalation doesn't allow for the movement of tissue that swallowing provides.
NP: Assessment; CN: Physiological integrity; CNS: Reduction of risk potential; CL: Analysis

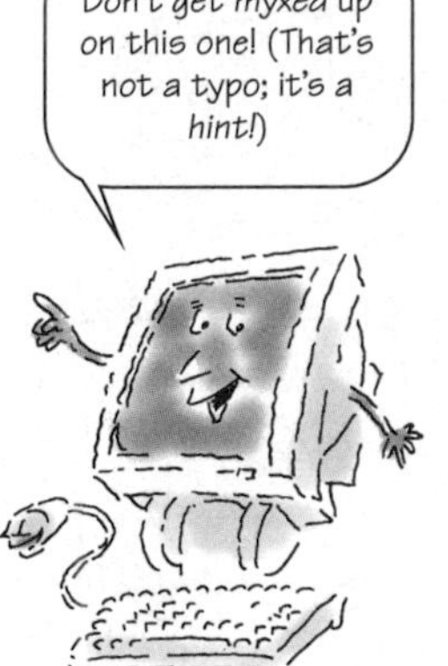

Don't get myxed up on this one! (That's not a typo; it's a hint!)

14. A client with hypothyroidism who experiences trauma, emergency surgery, or severe infection is at risk for developing which of the following conditions?
1. Hepatitis B
2. Malignant hyperthermia
3. Myxedema coma
4. Thyroid storm

14. 3. Myxedema coma represents the most severe form of hypothyroidism. The client develops severe hypothermia and hypoglycemia and becomes comatose. Myxedema coma can be precipitated by narcotics, stress (such as surgery), trauma, and infections. The client would be hypothermic, not hyperthermic. Thyroid storm is a complication of hyperthyroidism. Hepatitis B is a virus and isn't caused by thyroid disorders.
NP: Assessment; CN: Physiological integrity; CNS: Pharmacological and parenteral therapies; CL: Application

15. Which of the following potentially serious complications may occur when treating hypothyroidism?
1. Acute hemolytic reaction
2. Angina or cardiac arrhythmia
3. Retinopathy
4. Thrombocytopenia

15. 2. Precipitation of angina or cardiac arrhythmia is a potentially serious complication of hypothyroidism treatment, especially in the elderly or clients with underlying heart disease. Acute hemolytic reaction is a complication of blood transfusions. Retinopathy is usually a complication of diabetes mellitus. Thrombocytopenia is defined as a platelet count of less than 150,000/µl and doesn't result from treating hypothyroidism.
NP: Evaluation; CN: Physiological integrity; CNS: Reduction of risk potential; CL: Comprehension

16. What tests should be ordered if hypothyroidism is suspected?

1. Liver function tests
2. Hemoglobin A_{1C}
3. T_4 and thyroid-stimulating hormone
4. 24-hour urine free cortisol measurement

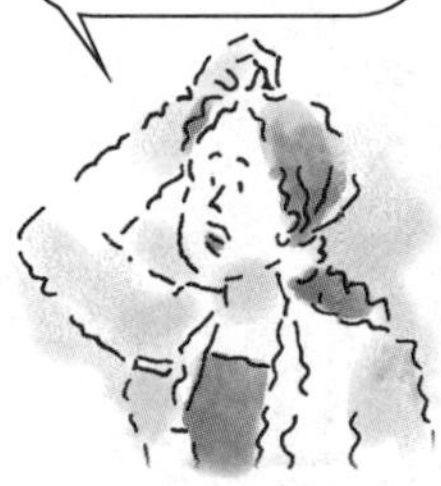

Know which test to order to ensure a proper diagnosis.

16. 3. Levels of thyroid-stimulating hormone and T_4 should be measured if hypothyroidism is suspected. Hemoglobin A_{1C} measurement is used to assess hyperglycemia. Liver function tests are used to determine liver disease. As part of the screening process for Cushing's syndrome, a 24-hour urinary free cortisol measurement is completed.

NP: Planning; CN: Physiological integrity; CNS: Physiological adaptation; CL: Knowledge

17. A client with hypothyroidism may present with which of the following symptoms?

1. Polyuria, polydipsia, and weight loss
2. Heat intolerance, nervousness, weight loss, and hair loss
3. Coarsening of facial features and extremity enlargement
4. Tiredness, cold intolerance, weight gain, and constipation

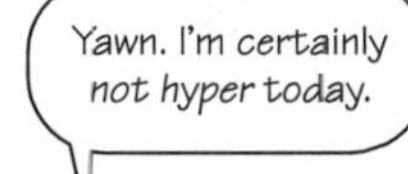

Yawn. I'm certainly not hyper today.

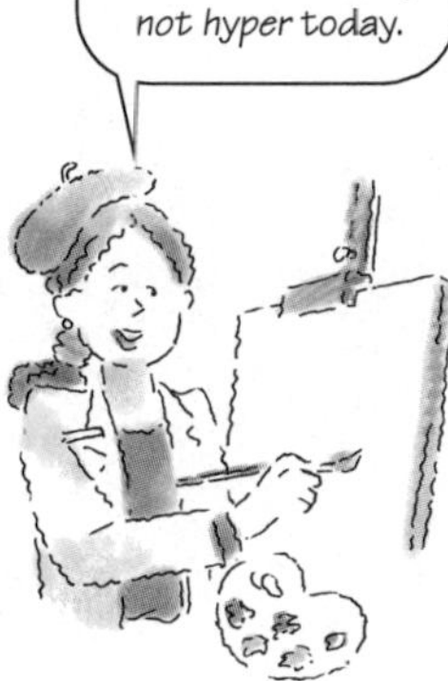

17. 4. Tiredness, cold intolerance, weight gain, and constipation are symptoms of hypothyroidism, secondary to a decrease in cellular metabolism. Polyuria, polydipsia, and weight loss are symptoms of type 1 diabetes mellitus. Hyperthyroidism has symptoms of heat intolerance, nervousness, weight loss, and hair loss. Coarsening of facial features and extremity enlargement are symptoms of acromegaly.

NP: Assessment; CN: Physiological integrity; CNS: Physiological adaptation; CL: Application

18. Which of the following groups of hormones are released by the medulla of the adrenal gland?

1. Epinephrine and norepinephrine
2. Glucocorticoids, mineralocorticoids, and androgens
3. Thyroxine, triiodothyronine, and calcitonin
4. Insulin, glucagon, and somatostatin

18. 1. The medulla of the adrenal gland causes the release of epinephrine and norepinephrine. Glucocorticoids, mineralocorticoids, and androgens are released from the adrenal cortex. Thyroxine, triiodothyronine, and calcitonin are secreted by the thyroid gland. The islet cells of the pancreas secrete insulin, glucagon, and somatostatin.

NP: Analysis; CN: Physiological integrity; CNS: Physiological adaptation; CL: Knowledge

19. When a client is scheduled for a thyroid test, the nurse must determine if the client has taken any medication containing iodine, which would alter the test results. Which of the following medications contain iodine?

1. Acetaminophen and aspirin
2. Estrogen and amphetamines
3. Insulin and oral antidiabetic agents
4. Contrast media, topical antiseptics, and multivitamins

19. 4. Contrast media, topical antiseptics, and multivitamins contain iodine and can alter thyroid function test results. Estrogen and amphetamines don't contain iodine but may alter thyroid function test results. Insulin, oral antidiabetic agents, acetaminophen, and aspirin won't affect a thyroid test.

NP: Planning; CN: Physiological integrity; CNS: Pharmacological and parenteral therapies; CL: Knowledge

20. Which of the following disorders can cause a client to retain fluid and develop hyponatremia secondary to the inability to excrete dilute urine?

1. Thyrotoxic crisis
2. Diabetes insipidus
3. Primary adrenocortical insufficiency
4. Syndrome of inappropriate antidiuretic hormone secretion (SIADH)

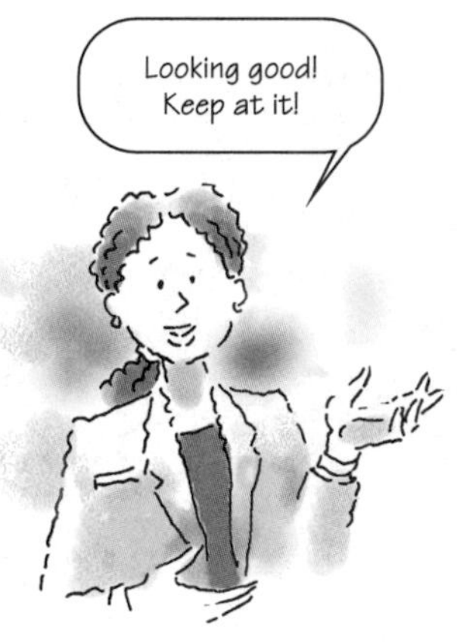

20. 4. SIADH is a condition in which the client has excessive levels of antidiuretic hormone (ADH) and can't excrete the dilute urine. Therefore, the client retains fluids. This disorder causes a dilutional hyponatremia. Diabetes insipidus creates an ADH deficiency, causing dilute urine and hypernatremia. Primary adrenocortical insufficiency (Addison's disease) is caused by deficiency of a cortical hormone. Thyrotoxic crisis occurs with severe hyperthyroidism.

NP: Analysis; CN: Physiological integrity; CNS: Reduction of risk potential; CL: Comprehension

21. Adrenal insufficiency develops secondary to inadequate secretion of which of the following pituitary hormones?

1. Corticotropin
2. Antidiuretic hormone (ADH)
3. Follicle-stimulating hormone (FSH)
4. Thyroid-stimulating hormone (TSH)

21. 1. Inadequate secretion of corticotropin from the pituitary gland results in adrenal insufficiency. ADH is secreted by the pituitary gland but doesn't affect the adrenal gland. FSH is also secreted by the pituitary gland but doesn't affect the adrenal gland; it stimulates the gonads. TSH is also secreted by the pituitary gland and stimulates the thyroid gland.

NP: Analysis; CN: Physiological integrity; CNS: Reduction of risk potential; CL: Knowledge

22. Which of the following conditions is caused by excessive secretion of vasopressin?

1. Thyrotoxic crisis
2. Diabetes insipidus
3. Primary adrenocortical insufficiency
4. Syndrome of inappropriate antidiuretic hormone secretion (SIADH)

22. 4. SIADH occurs as a result of excessive vasopressin. Diabetes insipidus is a deficiency of vasopressin. Adrenocortical insufficiency (Addison's disease) is caused by a deficiency of cortical hormones. Thyrotoxic crisis occurs with severe hyperthyroidism.

NP: Analysis; CN: Physiological integrity; CNS: Reduction of risk potential; CL: Knowledge

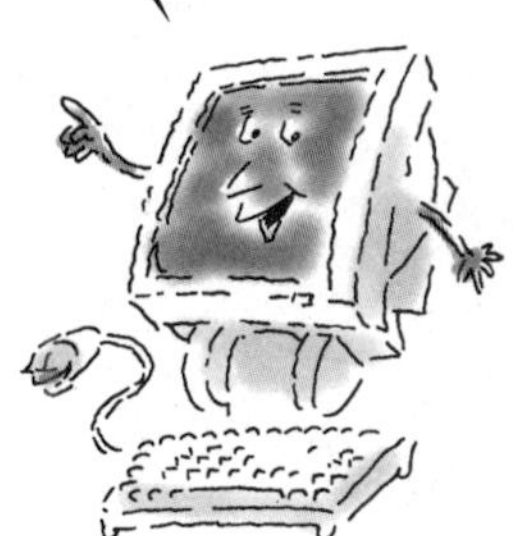

23. A client with muscle weakness, anorexia, dark pigmentation of the skin, and laboratory findings of low serum sodium and high potassium levels may be presenting with which of the following conditions?

1. Addison's disease
2. Cushing's syndrome
3. Diabetes insipidus
4. Thyrotoxic crisis

23. 1. The clinical picture of Addison's disease includes muscle weakness, anorexia, darkening of the skin's pigmentation, low sodium level, and high potassium level. Cushing's syndrome presents with obesity, "buffalo hump," "moonface," and thin extremities. Symptoms of diabetes insipidus include excretion of large volumes of dilute urine, leading to hypernatremia and dehydration. Thyrotoxic crisis can occur with severe hyperthyroidism.

NP: Assessment; CN: Physiological integrity; CNS: Physiological adaptation; CL: Comprehension

24. Head trauma, brain tumor, or surgical ablation of the pituitary gland can lead to which of the following conditions?

1. Addison's disease
2. Cushing's syndrome
3. Diabetes insipidus
4. Hypothyroidism

24. 3. The cause of diabetes insipidus is unknown, but it may be secondary to head trauma, brain tumors, or surgical ablation of the pituitary gland. Addison's disease is caused by a deficiency of cortical hormones, whereas Cushing's syndrome is an excess of cortical hormones. Hypothyroidism occurs when the thyroid gland secretes low levels of thyroid hormone.

NP: Analysis; CN: Physiological integrity; CNS: Physiological adaptation; CL: Comprehension

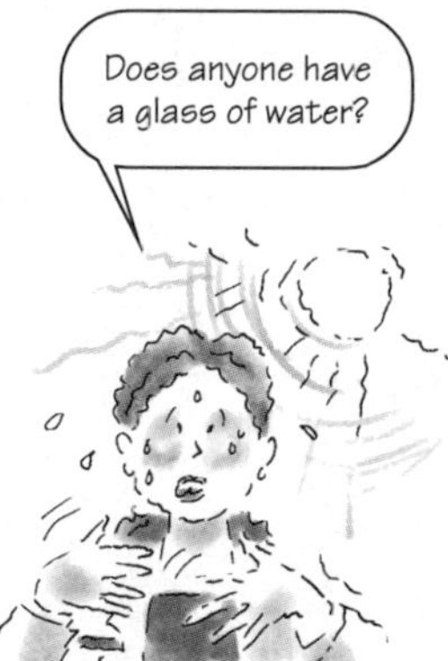
Does anyone have
a glass of water?

25. If fluid intake is limited in a client with diabetes insipidus, which of the following complications will he be at risk for developing?

1. Hypertension and bradycardia
2. Glucosuria and weight gain
3. Peripheral edema and hyperglycemia
4. Severe dehydration and hypernatremia

25. 4. A client with diabetes insipidus has high volumes of urine, even without fluid replacement. Therefore, limiting fluid intake will cause severe dehydration and hypernatremia. A client undergoing a fluid deprivation test may experience tachycardia and hypotension. A client with diabetes insipidus will usually experience weight loss, and his urine doesn't contain glucose. Diabetes insipidus has no effect on blood glucose. Therefore, the client wouldn't suffer from hyperglycemia. Peripheral edema isn't a symptom of diabetes insipidus.

NP: Assessment; CN: Physiological integrity; CNS: Physiological adaptation; CL: Comprehension

26. Adequate fluid replacement, vasopressin replacement, and correction of underlying intracranial pathology are objectives of therapy for which of the following disease processes?

1. Diabetes mellitus
2. Diabetes insipidus
3. Diabetic ketoacidosis
4. Syndrome of inappropriate antidiuretic hormone secretion (SIADH)

26. 2. Maintaining adequate fluid and replacing vasopressin are the main objectives in treating diabetes insipidus. An excess of vasopressin leads to SIADH, causing the client to retain fluid. Diabetic ketoacidosis is a result of severe insulin insufficiency. Diabetes mellitus doesn't involve vasopressin or an intracranial pathology but rather a disturbance in the production or use of insulin.

NP: Implementation; CN: Physiological integrity; CNS: Pharmacological and parenteral therapies; CL: Comprehension

27. Which of the following disorders is suggested by polydipsia and large amounts of waterlike urine with a specific gravity of 1.003?

1. Diabetes mellitus
2. Diabetes insipidus
3. Diabetic ketoacidosis
4. Syndrome of inappropriate antidiuretic hormone secretion (SIADH)

27. 2. Diabetes insipidus is characterized by a great thirst (polydipsia) and large amounts of waterlike urine, which has a specific gravity of 1.001 to 1.005. Diabetes mellitus presents with polydipsia, polyuria, and polyphagia, but the client also has hyperglycemia. Diabetic ketoacidosis presents with weight loss, polyuria, and polydipsia, and the client has a severe acidosis. A client with SIADH can't excrete a dilute urine; he retains fluid and develops a sodium deficiency.

NP: Assessment; CN: Physiological integrity; CNS: Physiological adaptation; CL: Analysis

28. Which of the following medications would be used to treat diabetes insipidus?

1. Desmopressin (DDAVP)
2. Glucocorticoids
3. Insulin
4. Oral antidiabetic agents

28. 1. Desmopressin, a synthetic vasopressin, is the medication of choice for treating diabetes insipidus. Glucocorticoids are hormones secreted by the adrenal gland, which isn't involved with diabetes insipidus. Insulin and oral antidiabetic agents are used to treat diabetes mellitus, a disorder of glucose metabolism.

NP: Implementation; CN: Physiological integrity; CNS: Pharmacological and parenteral therapies; CL: Knowledge

29. Diabetes insipidus is a disorder of which of the following glands?

1. Adrenal gland
2. Parathyroid gland
3. Pituitary gland
4. Thyroid gland

29. 3. Diabetes insipidus is a disorder of the posterior pituitary gland. The adrenal, thyroid, and parathyroid glands aren't involved.

NP: Analysis; CN: Physiological integrity; CNS: Reduction of risk potential; CL: Knowledge

30. A deficiency of which of the following hormones causes diabetes insipidus?

1. Androgen
2. Epinephrine
3. Norepinephrine
4. Vasopressin

30. 4. Clients with diabetes insipidus have a deficiency of vasopressin, the antidiuretic hormone. Epinephrine, norepinephrine, and androgen are hormones secreted by the adrenal gland and aren't related to diabetes insipidus.

NP: Analysis; CN: Physiological integrity; CNS: Physiological adaptation; CL: Knowledge

31. Which of the following tests is used to diagnose diabetes insipidus?

1. Capillary blood glucose test
2. Fluid deprivation test
3. Serum ketone test
4. Urine glucose test

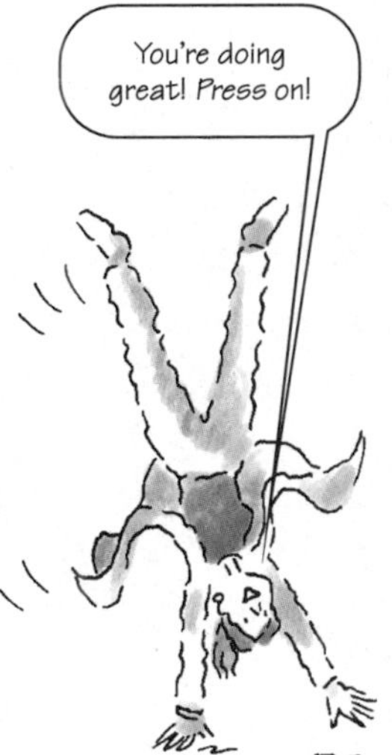
You're doing great! Press on!

31. 2. The fluid deprivation test involves withholding water for 4 to 18 hours and checking urine osmolarity periodically. Plasma osmolarity is also checked. A client with diabetes insipidus will have an increased serum osmolarity (of less than 300 mOsm/kg). Urine osmolarity won't increase. The capillary blood glucose test allows a rapid measurement of glucose in whole blood. The serum ketone test documents diabetic ketoacidosis. The urine glucose test monitors glucose levels in urine, but diabetes insipidus doesn't affect urine glucose levels.

NP: Evaluation; CN: Physiological integrity; CNS: Reduction of risk potential; CL: Analysis

32. Which of the following medical emergencies may occur when the client with Addison's disease develops acute hypotension, secondary to hypoadrenocorticism?
1. Addisonian crisis
2. Diabetic ketoacidosis
3. Myxedema
4. Thyrotoxic crisis

There's a hint built into the question on this one.

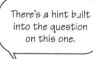

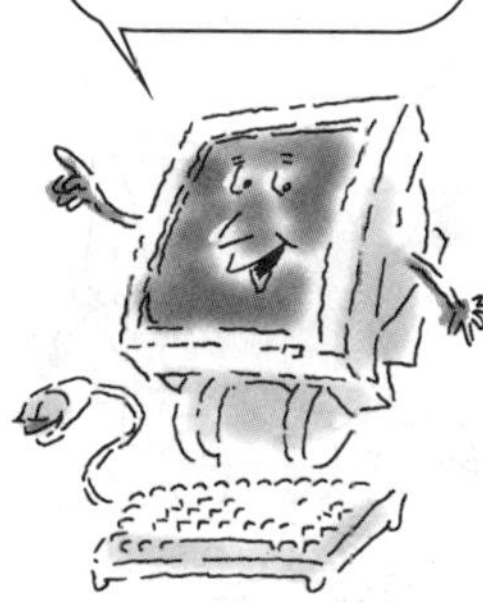

32. 1. As Addison's disease progresses, the client moves into an Addisonian crisis, a medical emergency marked by cyanosis, fever, and signs of shock. Diabetic ketoacidosis is a form of hyperglycemia. Myxedema is a form of severe hypothyroidism. Thyrotoxic crisis is a form of severe hyperthyroidism.
NP: Assessment; CN: Physiological integrity; CNS: Physiological adaptation; CL: Comprehension

33. Which of the following diseases is caused by a deficiency of cortical hormones?
1. Addison's disease
2. Cushing's syndrome
3. Diabetes mellitus
4. Diabetic ketoacidosis

33. 1. Addison's disease is caused by a deficiency of cortical hormones. Cushing's syndrome is the opposite of Addison's disease and includes excessive adrenocortical activity. Diabetes mellitus is a deficiency of insulin. Diabetic ketoacidosis is a state of severe hyperglycemia, causing acidosis.
NP: Analysis; CN: Physiological integrity; CNS: Physiological adaptation; CL: Knowledge

34. Laboratory findings indicating decreased levels of glucose and sodium and increased levels of potassium and white blood cells (WBCs) would correlate with which disease?
1. Addison's disease
2. Cushing's syndrome
3. Diabetes mellitus
4. Hypothyroidism

34. 1. Low levels of glucose and sodium, along with high levels of potassium and WBCs, are diagnostic of Addison's disease. Cushing's syndrome would have excessive levels of adrenocortical hormones. Diabetes mellitus would have increased blood glucose levels. Hypothyroidism would have low levels of thyroid hormone.
NP: Analysis; CN: Physiological integrity; CNS: Physiological adaptation; CL: Comprehension

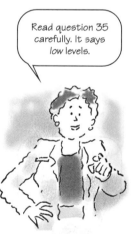

35. A client presenting with low levels of adrenocortical hormones in the blood or urine may have which of the following conditions?
1. Addison's disease
2. Cushing's syndrome
3. Hyperthyroidism
4. Hypopituitarism

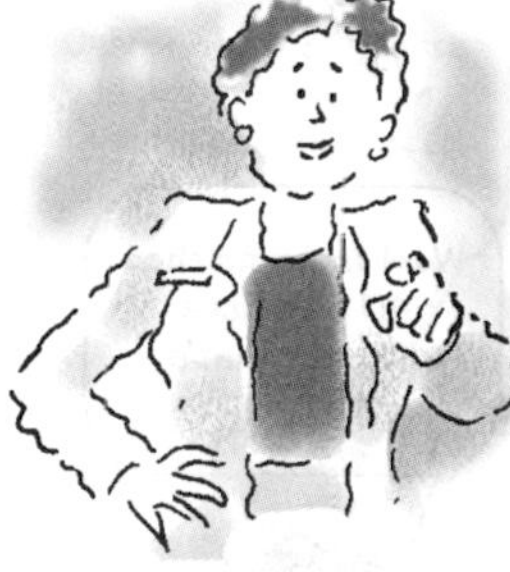

Read question 35 carefully. It says low levels.

35. 1. A definitive diagnosis of Addison's disease must have low levels of adrenocortical hormones. Cushing's syndrome would have *excessive* amounts of adrenocortical hormones. Hyperthyroidism has high levels of T_3 and T_4 (thyroxine and triiodothyronine). Lower pituitary hormone secretion levels are consistent with hypopituitarism.
NP: Assessment; CN: Physiological integrity; CNS: Physiological adaptation; CL: Comprehension

36. Hydrocortisone given I.V. is the proper treatment for which of the following diseases?
1. Addison's disease
2. Cushing's syndrome
3. Hyperthyroidism
4. Hypoparathyroidism

36. 1. I.V. hydrocortisone is the proper treatment for Addison's disease because it replaces the glucocorticoid deficiency. Cushing's syndrome has excessive amounts of glucocorticoids. Hyperthyroidism and hypoparathyroidism aren't treated with hydrocortisone.
NP: Implementation; CN: Physiological integrity; CNS: Pharmacological and parenteral therapies; CL: Knowledge

45. Treatment for Cushing's syndrome may involve removal of one of the adrenal glands, which could cause a temporary state of which of the following conditions?

1. Hyperkalemia
2. Adrenal insufficiency
3. Excessive adrenal hormone
4. Syndrome of inappropriate antidiuretic hormone secretion (SIADH)

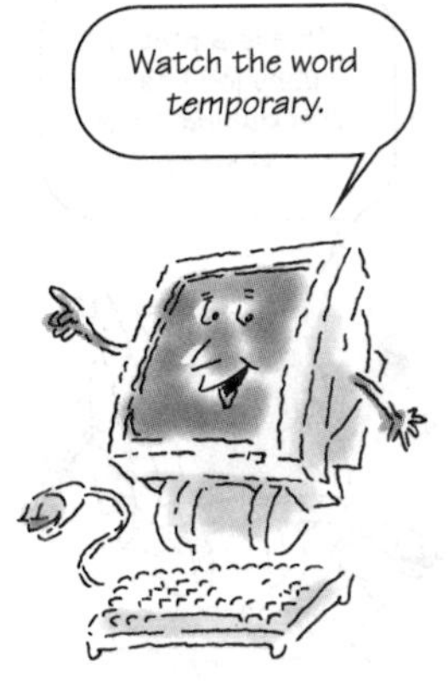

Watch the word temporary.

45. 2. Removing a major source of adrenal hormones may cause a state of temporary adrenal insufficiency, requiring short-term replacement therapy. When both adrenal glands are removed, the client requires lifelong hormone replacement. A client with Cushing's syndrome would have a low — not high — potassium level. The client wouldn't have excessive adrenal hormone if all or part of the adrenal glands were removed. SIADH doesn't involve the adrenal gland; it involves the pituitary gland.

NP: Implementation; CN: Physiological integrity; CNS: Physiological adaptation; CL: Comprehension

46. Which of the following nursing diagnoses is appropriate for a client with Cushing's syndrome?

1. Risk for infection
2. Deficient fluid volume
3. Acute pain with movement
4. Functional urinary incontinence

46. 1. Clients with Cushing's syndrome have an increased susceptibility to injury or infection, secondary to the immunosuppression caused by excessive cortisol. Fluid volume deficit, related to inadequate adrenal hormones, is common in clients with Addison's disease. Pain and functional incontinence aren't common in Cushing's syndrome.

NP: Planning; CN: Physiological integrity; CNS: Reduction of risk potential; CL: Application

47. Which of the following nursing interventions should be performed for a client with Cushing's syndrome?

1. Suggest clothing or bedding that is cool and comfortable.
2. Suggest consumption of high-carbohydrate and low-protein foods.
3. Explain that physical changes are a result of excessive corticosteroids.
4. Explain the rationale for increasing salt and fluid intake in times of illness, increased stress, and very hot weather.

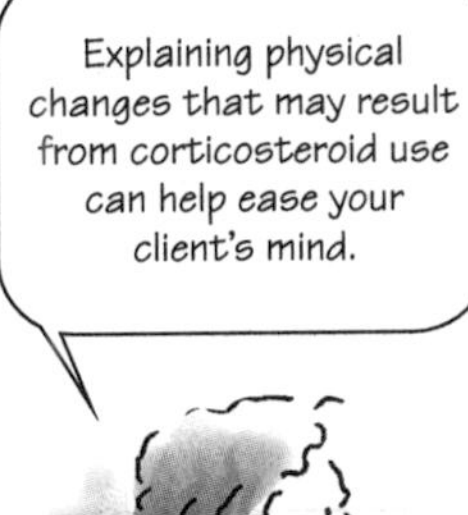

Explaining physical changes that may result from corticosteroid use can help ease your client's mind.

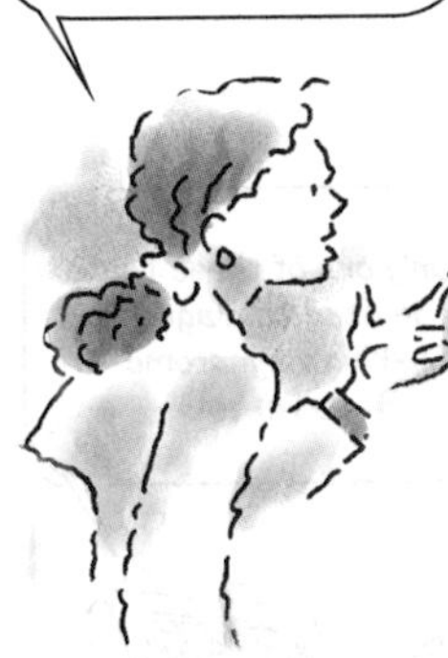

47. 3. Clients with Cushing's syndrome have physical changes related to excessive corticosteroids. Clients with hyperthyroidism are heat intolerant and must have comfortable, cool clothing and bedding. Clients with Cushing's syndrome should have a high-protein, not low-protein, diet. Clients with Addison's disease must increase sodium intake and fluid intake in times of stress to prevent hypotension.

NP: Evaluation; CN: Physiological integrity; CNS: Physiological adaptation; CL: Application

48. Which of the following disease processes is caused by an absence of insulin or inadequate amount of insulin, resulting in hyperglycemia and leading to a series of biochemical disorders?

1. Diabetes insipidus
2. Hyperaldosteronism
3. Diabetic ketoacidosis
4. Hyperosmolar hyperglycemic nonketotic syndrome (HHNS)

48. 3. Diabetic ketoacidosis is caused by inadequate amounts of insulin or absence of insulin, and leads to a series of biochemical disorders. Diabetes insipidus is caused by a deficiency of vasopressin. Hyperaldosteronism is an excess in aldosterone production, causing sodium and fluid excesses and hypertension. HHNS is a coma state in which hyperglycemia and hyperosmolarity dominate.

NP: Assessment; CN: Physiological integrity; CNS: Physiological adaptation; CL: Knowledge

49. A client who is insulin-dependent fails to take insulin regularly; he is at risk for which of the following complications?
1. Diabetic ketoacidosis
2. Hypoglycemia
3. Pancreatitis
4. Respiratory failure

49. 1. A client who fails to regularly take his insulin is at risk for hyperglycemia, which could lead to diabetic ketoacidosis. Hypoglycemia wouldn't occur because the lack of insulin would lead to increased levels of sugar in the blood. A client with chronic pancreatitis may develop diabetes (secondary to the pancreatitis), but insulin-dependent diabetes mellitus doesn't lead to pancreatitis. Respiratory failure isn't related to insulin levels.
NP: Evaluation; CN: Physiological integrity; CNS: Physiological adaptation; CL: Application

50. A client with diabetes presents with polyphagia, polydipsia, and oliguria; he also complains of headache, malaise, and some visual changes. Assessment shows signs of dehydration. Which of the following diagnoses could be made?
1. Diabetes insipidus
2. Diabetic ketoacidosis
3. Hypoglycemia
4. Syndrome of inappropriate antidiuretic hormone secretion (SIADH)

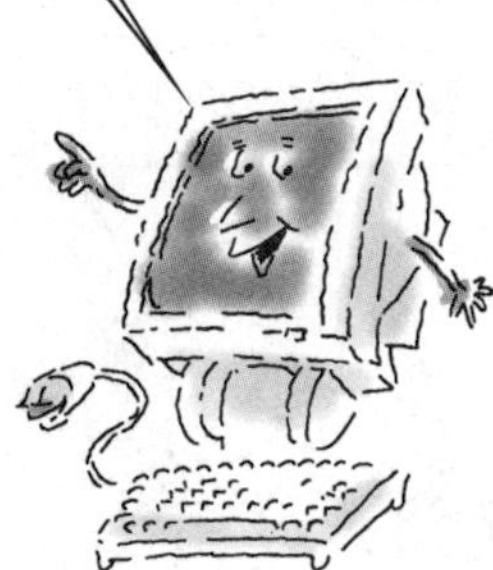

Good going! You're really charging through these questions!

50. 2. Early manifestations of diabetic ketoacidosis include polydipsia, polyphagia, and polyuria. As the client dehydrates and loses electrolytes, this condition often leads to oliguria, malaise, and visual changes. Diabetes insipidus may result in dehydration but not polyphagia and polydipsia. Symptoms of hypoglycemia include diaphoresis, tachycardia, and nervousness. A client with SIADH is unable to excrete a dilute urine, causing hypernatremia.
NP: Assessment; CN: Physiological integrity; CNS: Physiological adaptation; CL: Application

51. The thyroid gland is located in which of the following areas of the body?
1. Upper abdomen
2. Inferior aspect of the brain
3. Upper portion of the kidney
4. Lower neck, anterior to the trachea

51. 4. The thyroid gland is in the lower neck, anterior to the trachea. The pancreas is in the upper abdomen. The pituitary gland is located in the inferior aspect of the brain. The adrenal glands are attached to the upper portion of the kidneys.
NP: Assessment; CN: Health promotion and maintenance; CNS: Prevention and early detection of disease; CL: Knowledge

52. The thyroid gland produces which of the following groups of hormones?
1. Amylase, lipase, and trypsin
2. Triiodothyronine (T_3), thyroxine (T_4), and calcitonin
3. Glucocorticoids, mineralocorticoids, and androgens
4. Vasopressin, oxytocin, and thyroid-stimulating hormone (TSH)

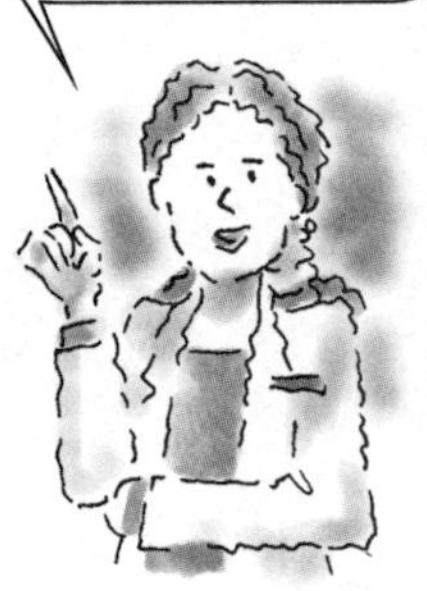

Do you know which glands produce which hormones? Here's a chance to test your knowledge.

52. 2. T_3, T_4, and calcitonin are all secreted by the thyroid gland. Amylase, lipase, and trypsin are enzymes produced by the pancreas that aid in digestion. Glucocorticoids, mineralocorticoids, and androgens are produced by the adrenal gland. The pituitary gland secretes vasopressin, oxytocin, and TSH.
NP: Assessment; CN: Health promotion and maintenance; CNS: Prevention and early detection of disease; CL: Knowledge

53. Secretion of thyroid-stimulating hormone (TSH) by which of the following glands controls the rate at which thyroid hormone is released?
1. Adrenal gland
2. Parathyroid gland
3. Pituitary gland
4. Thyroid gland

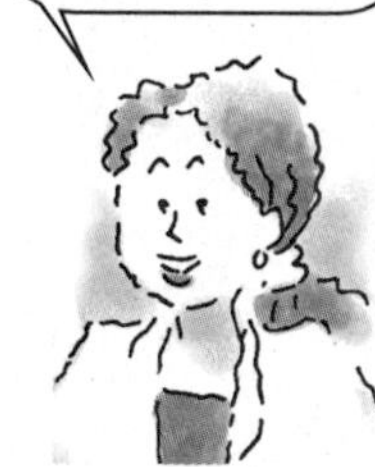

TSH is a trophic hormone with a target gland.

53. 3. By secretion of TSH, the pituitary gland controls the rate of thyroid hormone released. The adrenal gland isn't involved with the thyroid gland. The parathyroid gland secretes parathyroid hormones, depending on the levels of calcium and phosphorus in the blood. The thyroid gland secretes thyroid hormone but doesn't control how much is released.
NP: Analysis; CN: Physiological integrity; CNS: Physiological adaptation; CL: Knowledge

54. Which of the following treatments can be used for hyperthyroidism?
1. Cholelithotomy
2. Irradiation of the thyroid
3. Administration of oral thyroid hormones
4. Whipple procedure

54. 2. Irradiation, involving administration of the ^{131}I, destroys the thyroid gland and thereby treats hyperthyroidism. Oral thyroid hormones are the treatment for hypothyroidism. Cholelithotomy is used to treat gallstones. The Whipple procedure is a surgical treatment for pancreatic cancer.
NP: Analysis; CN: Physiological integrity; CNS: Pharmacological and parenteral therapies; CL: Knowledge

55. Which of the following group of symptoms of hyperthyroidism is most commonly found in elderly clients?
1. Depression, apathy, and weight loss
2. Palpitations, irritability, and heat intolerance
3. Cold intolerance, weight gain, and thinning hair
4. Numbness, tingling, and cramping of extremities

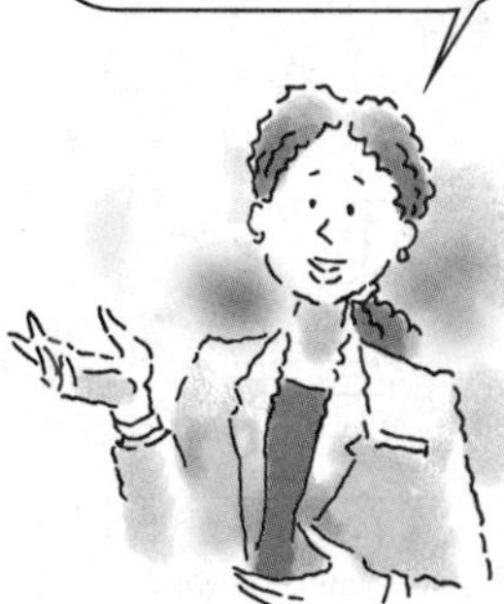

Elderly clients are different from other clients. Be aware of age-related symptoms.

55. 1. Most elderly clients present with depression, apathy, and weight loss, which are typical signs and symptoms of hyperthyroidism. Palpitations, irritability, and heat intolerance can be present with hyperthyroidism, but these aren't typical symptoms in elderly clients. Cold intolerance, weight gain, and thinning hair are some of the signs of hypothyroidism. Numbness, tingling, and cramping of extremities are symptoms of hypocalcemia, which may be a symptom of hypoparathyroidism.
NP: Assessment; CN: Physiological integrity; CNS: Physiological adaptation; CL: Application

56. Which of the following forms of severe hyperthyroidism is life threatening and produces high fever, extreme tachycardia, and altered mental status?
1. Hepatic coma
2. Thyroid storm
3. Myxedema coma
4. Hyperosmolar hyperglycemic nonketotic syndrome (HHNS)

56. 2. Thyroid storm is a form of severe hyperthyroidism that can be precipitated by stress, injury, or infection. Hepatic coma occurs in clients with profound liver failure. Myxedema coma is a rare disorder characterized by hypoventilation, hypotension, hypoglycemia, and hypothyroidism. HHNS occurs in clients with type 2 diabetes mellitus who are dehydrated and have severe hyperglycemia.
NP: Analysis; CN: Physiological integrity; CNS: Physiological adaptation; CL: Knowledge

57. Hyperthyroidism is commonly known as which of the following disorders?
1. Addison's disease
2. Buerger's disease
3. Cushing's syndrome
4. Graves' disease

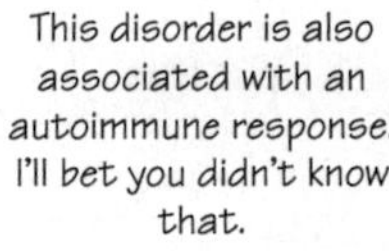

This disorder is also associated with an autoimmune response. I'll bet you didn't know that.

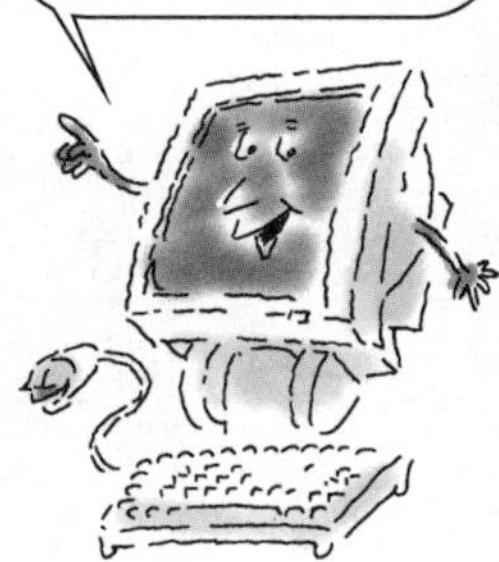

57. 4. Hyperthyroidism is known as Graves' disease. Addison's disease is a deficiency of cortical hormones. Cushing's syndrome is an excess of cortical hormones. Buerger's disease is a recurring inflammation of blood vessels in the upper and lower extremities.
NP: Assessment; CN: Physiological integrity; CNS: Physiological adaptation; CL: Knowledge

58. Excessive output of thyroid hormone from abnormal stimulation of the thyroid gland is the etiology of which condition?
1. Hyperparathyroidism
2. Hypoparathyroidism
3. Hyperthyroidism
4. Hypothyroidism

58. 3. Excessive output of thyroid hormone is the etiology of hyperthyroidism. Hyperparathyroidism is overproduction of parathyroid hormone, characterized by bone calcification or renal calculi. Hypoparathyroidism is inadequate secretion of parathyroid hormone that occurs after interruption of the blood supply or surgical removal of the parathyroid. Hypothyroidism is slow production of thyroid hormone.
NP: Assessment; CN: Physiological integrity; CNS: Physiological adaptation; CL: Knowledge

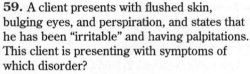

59. A client presents with flushed skin, bulging eyes, and perspiration, and states that he has been "irritable" and having palpitations. This client is presenting with symptoms of which disorder?
1. Hyperthyroidism
2. Myocardial infarction (MI)
3. Pancreatitis
4. Type 1 diabetes mellitus

59. 1. Signs and symptoms of hyperthyroidism include nervousness, palpitations, irritability, bulging eyes, heat intolerance, weight loss, and weakness. MI usually presents with chest pain that may radiate to arms, back, or neck and shortness of breath. Pancreatitis presents with severe abdominal pain and back tenderness. Type 1 diabetes mellitus presents with polyuria, polydipsia, and weight loss.
NP: Assessment; CN: Physiological integrity; CNS: Physiological adaptation; CL: Comprehension

60. Which of the following hormones is secreted by the anterior pituitary gland?
1. Corticotropin
2. Antidiuretic hormone
3. Cortisol
4. Oxytocin

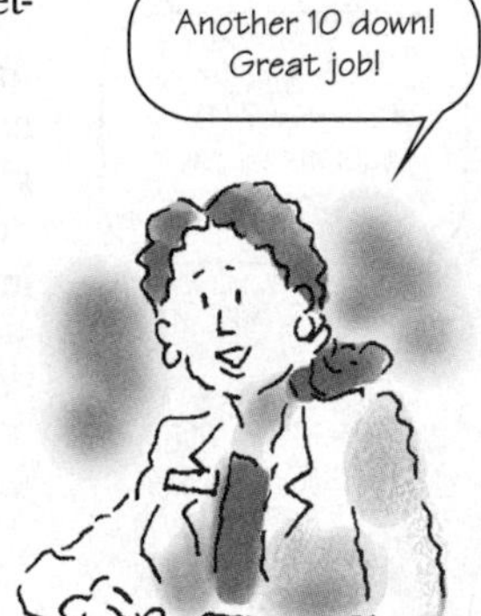

Another 10 down! Great job!

60. 1. Corticotropin is secreted by the anterior pituitary gland. Antidiuretic hormone and oxytocin are secreted by the posterior pituitary gland. Cortisol is secreted by the adrenal glands.
NP: Assessment; CN: Physiological integrity; CNS: Physiological adaptation; CL: Knowledge

61. A client is brought into the emergency department with a brain stem contusion. Two days after admission, the client has a large amount of urine and a serum sodium level of 155 mEq/dl. Which of the following conditions may be developing?

1. Myxedema coma
2. Diabetes insipidus
3. Type 1 diabetes mellitus
4. Syndrome of inappropriate antidiuretic hormone secretion (SIADH)

61. 2. Two leading causes of diabetes insipidus are hypothalamic or pituitary tumors and closed head injuries. Myxedema coma is a form of hypothyroidism. Type 1 diabetes mellitus isn't caused by a brain injury. A client with SIADH would have hyponatremia; this client's sodium level was 155 mEq/dl, which is above normal levels of 135 to 145 mEq/dl.

NP: Analysis; CN: Physiological integrity; CNS: Physiological adaptation; CL: Application

62. Which of the following conditions could be diagnosed in a client with serum ketones and a serum glucose level above 300 mg/dl?

1. Diabetes insipidus
2. Diabetic ketoacidosis
3. Hypoglycemia
4. Somogyi phenomenon

62. 2. Clients with serum ketones and serum glucose levels above 300 mg/dl could be diagnosed with diabetic ketoacidosis. Diabetes insipidus is an overproduction of antidiuretic hormone and doesn't create ketones in the blood. Hypoglycemia causes low blood glucose levels. The Somogyi phenomenon is rebound hyperglycemia following an episode of hypoglycemia.

NP: Assessment; CN: Physiological integrity; CNS: Physiological adaptation; CL: Knowledge

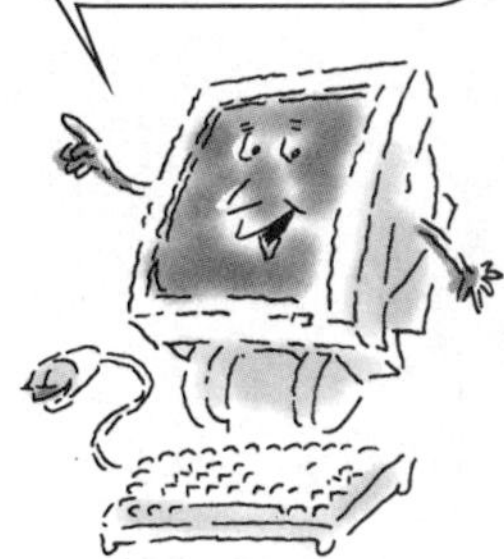

Before you answer, make sure you know which disorder the question is asking you to treat.

63. Objectives for treating diabetic ketoacidosis (DKA) include administration of which of the following treatments?

1. Glucagon
2. Blood products
3. Glucocorticoids
4. Insulin and I.V. fluids

63. 4. A client with DKA would receive insulin to lower glucose and I.V. fluids to correct hypotension. Blood products aren't needed to correct DKA. Glucagon is given to treat hypoglycemia; DKA involves hyperglycemia. Glucocorticoids aren't needed because the adrenal glands aren't involved.

NP: Implementation; CN: Physiological integrity; CNS: Pharmacological and parenteral therapies; CL: Application

64. Which of the following methods of insulin administration would be used in the initial treatment of hyperglycemia in a client with diabetic ketoacidosis?

1. Subcutaneous
2. Intramuscular
3. I.V. bolus only
4. I.V. bolus, followed by continuous infusion

64. 4. An I.V. bolus of insulin is given initially to control the hyperglycemia; followed by a continuous infusion, titrated to control blood glucose. After the client is stabilized, subcutaneous insulin is given. Insulin is never given intramuscularly.

NP: Implementation; CN: Physiological integrity; CNS: Pharmacological and parenteral therapies; CL: Application

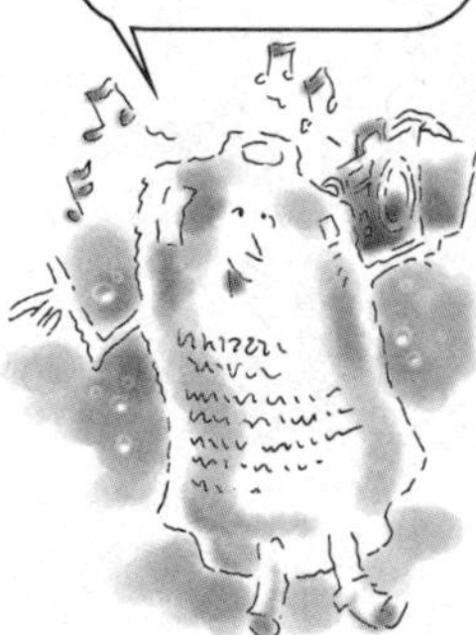

Isn't life a bolus full of cherries? (They told me to say that!)

83. Which of the following terms is used to describe the carpopedal spasm caused by occluding the blood flow of an arm for 3 minutes with a blood pressure cuff?
1. Negative Chvostek's sign
2. Positive Chvostek's sign
3. Negative Trousseau's sign
4. Positive Trousseau's sign

83. 4. A Trousseau's sign is positive when a carpopedal spasm is induced by occluding the blood flow of an arm for 3 minutes using a blood pressure cuff. Chvostek's sign is positive when a sharp tapping over the facial nerve, in front of the parotid gland and anterior to the ear, causes the mouth, nose, and eye to twitch.
NP: Evaluation; CN: Physiological integrity; CNS: Reduction of risk potential; CL: Comprehension

84. After undergoing a thyroidectomy, a client develops hypocalcemia and tetany. Which of the following medications should the nurse anticipate administering?
1. Calcium gluconate
2. Potassium chloride
3. Sodium bicarbonate
4. Sodium phosphorus

84. 1. Immediate treatment for a client who develops hypocalcemia and tetany after thyroidectomy is calcium gluconate. Potassium chloride and sodium bicarbonate aren't indicated. Sodium phosphorus wouldn't be given because phosphorus levels are already elevated.
NP: Planning; CN: Physiological integrity; CNS: Pharmacological and parenteral therapies; CL: Application

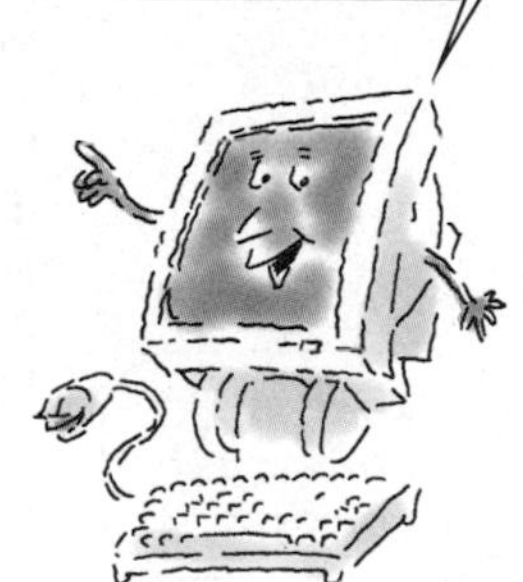

I can't believe we had the gall to ask you this question! (Oooh, that one hurt.)

85. Which of the following disorders may cause acute pancreatitis?
1. Gallstones
2. Crohn's disease
3. High gastric acid levels
4. Low thyroid hormone level

85. 1. Gallstones may cause obstruction and swelling at the ampulla of Vater, preventing flow of pancreatic juices into the duodenum and leading to pancreatitis. Gallbladder obstruction and alcoholism are the major causes of acute pancreatitis. Crohn's disease usually involves the terminal ileum and wouldn't affect the pancreas. Low thyroid hormone levels and high gastric acid levels aren't related to an acute pancreatitis attack.
NP: Analysis; CN: Physiological integrity; CNS: Physiological adaptation; CL: Comprehension

86. Severe abdominal pain in the midepigastric region, back tenderness, nausea, and vomiting are symptoms of which of the following conditions?
1. Acute pancreatitis
2. Crohn's disease
3. Hypophysectomy
4. Pheochromocytoma

86. 1. Severe abdominal pain in the midepigastric region, back tenderness, nausea, and vomiting are due to irritation of the pancreas. A client with Crohn's disease would have abdominal pain, but the pain would be in the lower quadrant; the client would also have diarrhea. Hypophysectomy is removal of the pituitary gland. Pheochromocytoma is a benign tumor of the adrenal medulla.
NP: Assessment; CN: Physiological integrity; CNS: Physiological adaptation; CL: Knowledge

87. Which of the following organs can become inflamed from autodigestion by the enzymes it produces, principally trypsin?
1. Adrenal gland
2. Appendix
3. Kidney
4. Pancreas

87. 4. Acute pancreatitis stems from the digestion of the pancreas by the very enzymes it produces, especially trypsin. The kidney, adrenal gland, and appendix don't produce enzymes.
NP: Assessment; CN: Physiological integrity; CNS: Physiological adaptation; CL: Knowledge

88. An acute pancreatitis attack may be more severe when combined with which of the following factors?

1. Bowel movement
2. Cold weather
3. A heavy meal
4. Hot weather

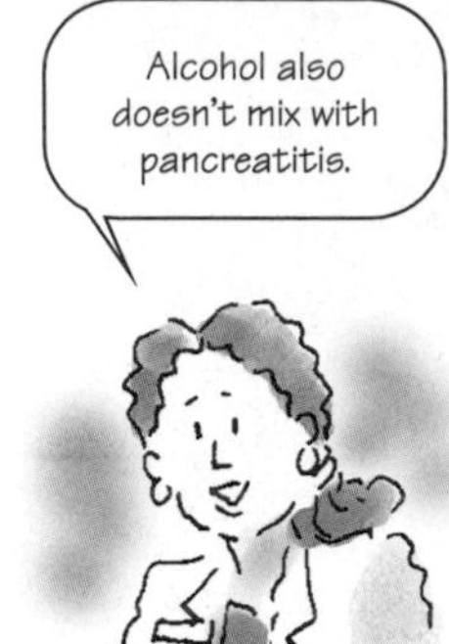

Alcohol also doesn't mix with pancreatitis.

88. 3. An acute pancreatitis attack may be more severe after a heavy meal or alcohol ingestion. Eating a heavy meal triggers the need for digestive enzymes, which are trapped in the pancreas. Bowel movements aren't related to the pancreas. Cold and heat intolerance are related to thyroid disorders.

NP: Assessment; CN: Physiological integrity; CNS: Physiological adaptation; CL: Knowledge

89. If a pancreatitis attack has been brought on by gallstones or gallbladder disease, a client may require reinforcement about the need to follow which of the following types of diets?

1. High-calorie, high-protein diet
2. High-fiber diet, encouraging fluid intake
3. Low-fat diet, avoiding heavy meals
4. Diet high in protein, calcium, and vitamin D

89. 3. A client who survives an acute pancreatitis attack caused by gallstones or gallbladder disease requires reinforcement to maintain a low-fat diet and to avoid heavy meals. A high-calorie, high-protein diet is appropriate for clients with hyperthyroidism. A diet high in fiber, encouraging fluid intake, is recommended for constipation. A client with Cushing's syndrome should follow a diet high in protein, calcium, and vitamin D.

NP: Implementation; CN: Physiological integrity; CNS: Reduction of risk potential; CL: Application

90. Which of the following disorders is an inflammatory disease characterized by progressive anatomic and functional destruction of the pancreas?

1. Acute pancreatitis
2. Addison's disease
3. Chronic pancreatitis
4. Graves' disease

90. 3. Chronic pancreatitis is an inflammatory disease characterized by progressive anatomic and functional destruction of the pancreas. Acute pancreatitis is a digestion of the pancreas by the enzymes it produces. Addison's disease is a deficiency of adrenocortical hormones. Graves' disease is another name for hyperthyroidism.

NP: Assessment; CN: Physiological integrity; CNS: Physiological adaptation; CL: Knowledge

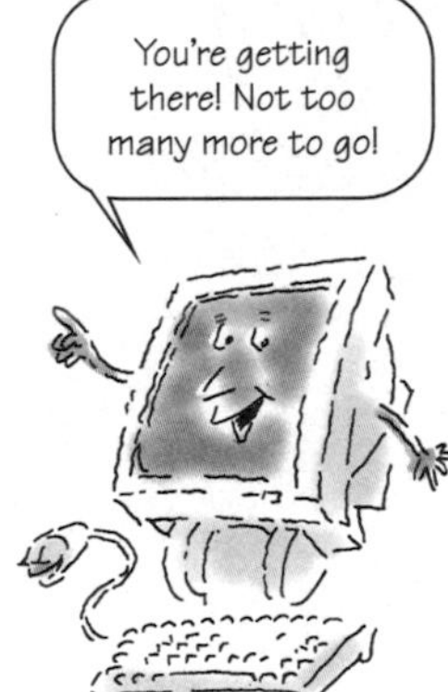

You're getting there! Not too many more to go!

91. A client is in diabetic ketoacidosis, secondary to infection. As the condition progresses, which of the following symptoms might the nurse see?

1. Kussmaul's respirations and a fruity odor on the breath
2. Shallow respirations and severe abdominal pain
3. Decreased respirations and increased urine output
4. Cheyne-Stokes respirations and foul-smelling urine

91. 1. Coma and severe acidosis are ushered in with Kussmaul's respirations (very deep but not labored respirations) and a fruity odor on the breath (acidemia). Shallow respirations and severe abdominal pain may be symptoms of pancreatitis. Decreased respirations and increased urine output aren't symptoms related to acidemia. Cheyne-Stokes respirations and foul-smelling urine don't result from diabetic ketoacidosis.

NP: Assessment; CN: Physiological integrity; CNS: Physiological adaptation; CL: Application

92. Which of the following parameters is measured with the dexamethasone suppression test?

1. The amount of dexamethasone in the system
2. Cortisol levels after the system is challenged
3. Changes in certain body chemicals, which are altered in depression
4. Cortisol levels before and after the system is challenged with a synthetic steroid

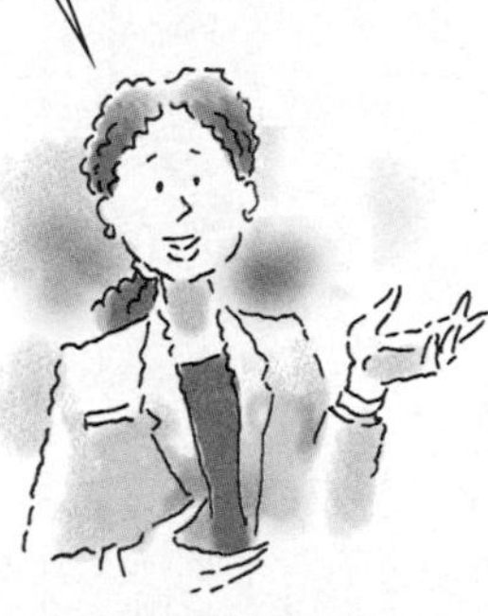

Make sure you read all choices before you answer this one. Some are similar, but only one is correct.

92. 4. The dexamethasone suppression test measures cortisol levels before and after the system is challenged with a synthetic steroid. The dexamethasone suppression test doesn't measure dexamethasone. Dexamethasone is used to challenge the cortisol level.

NP: Planning; CN: Health promotion and maintenance; CNS: Prevention and early detection of disease; CL: Knowledge

93. Clients with insulin-dependent diabetes mellitus may require which of the following changes to their daily routine during periods of infection?

1. No changes
2. Less insulin
3. More insulin
4. Oral antidiabetic agents

93. 3. During periods of infection or illness, insulin-dependent clients may need even more insulin to compensate for increased blood glucose levels. The other options are incorrect.

NP: Assessment; CN: Physiological integrity; CNS: Pharmacological and parenteral therapies; CL: Application

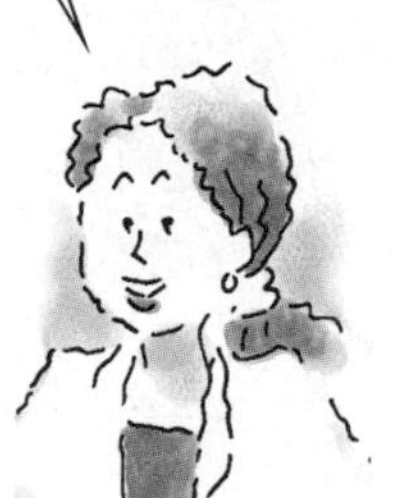

Think of the causes of each of these conditions before answering.

94. Which of the following disorders is characterized by a sudden drop in blood glucose, followed by rebound hyperglycemia caused by the gradual and excessive administration of insulin?

1. Diabetes insipidus
2. Diabetic ketoacidosis
3. Somogyi phenomenon
4. Hyperosmolar hyperglycemic nonketotic syndrome (HHNS)

94. 3. The Somogyi phenomenon is characterized by a sudden fall in blood glucose, followed by a rebound hyperglycemia caused by the gradual excessive administration of insulin. Diabetes insipidus isn't related to insulin administration. Diabetic ketoacidosis and HHNS aren't characterized by this phenomenon.

NP: Assessment; CN: Physiological integrity; CNS: Pharmacological and parenteral therapies; CL: Comprehension

95. Which of the following fasting blood glucose levels, if found on two or more occasions, may lead to a diagnosis of diabetes mellitus in a nonpregnant adult?

1. Below 60 mg/dl
2. Below 100 mg/dl
3. Above 120 mg/dl
4. Above 140 mg/dl

95. 4. Based on the American Diabetes Association guidelines, fasting blood glucose of 140 mg/dl or more, on at least two occasions, is indicative of diabetes mellitus. Often, random blood glucose and glucose tolerance tests are done before making a definitive diagnosis.

NP: Analysis; CN: Physiological integrity; CNS: Physiological adaptation; CL: Knowledge

96. Which of the following terms is used to describe a usually benign tumor of the adrenal medulla?

1. Apical aneurysm
2. Endemic goiter
3. Pheochromocytoma
4. Ulcerogenic tumor

96. 3. A pheochromocytoma is a usually benign tumor of the adrenal medulla. An apical aneurysm isn't a tumor and is located in the heart. An endemic goiter is an iodine-deficient enlargement of the thyroid gland. Ulcerogenic tumors are located in the islets of Langerhans (part of the pancreas).

NP: Assessment; CN: Physiological integrity; CNS: Physiological adaptation; CL: Knowledge

97. Tumors of the adrenal medulla usually produce which of the following symptoms?

1. Carpopedal spasm
2. Hyperglycemia
3. Hypertension
4. "Moonface"

97. 3. Tumors of the adrenal medulla usually produce hypertension because they release excessive amounts of epinephrine and norepinephrine. Carpopedal spasm occurs as a result of hypocalcemia. Hyperglycemia is a result of low insulin levels. Clients with Cushing's syndrome usually have a "moonface."

NP: Assessment; CN: Physiological integrity; CNS: Physiological adaptation; CL: Comprehension

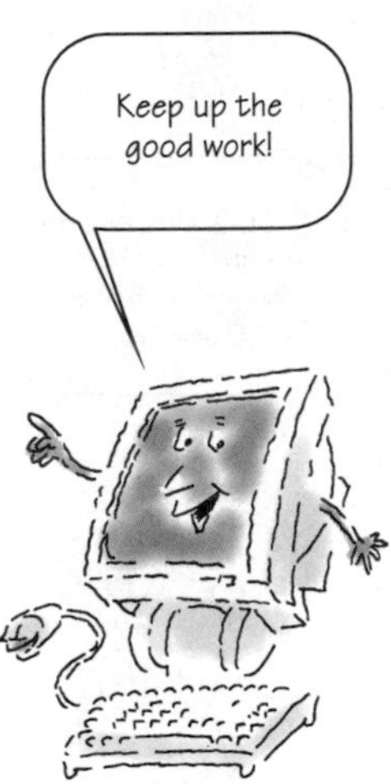

98. Which of the following adverse effects is related to corticosteroid therapy?

1. Hyponatremia
2. Hypoglycemia
3. Change in metabolism
4. Change in pituitary secretions

98. 3. A major adverse effect of corticosteroid therapy is a slowing of metabolism. This therapy also produces hyperglycemia and hypernatremia. Changes in pituitary secretions aren't affected by corticosteroid therapy.

NP: Assessment; CN: Physiological integrity; CNS: Pharmacological and parenteral therapies; CL: Comprehension

99. Which of the following conditions contributes to hyperparathyroidism?

1. Chronic renal failure
2. Thyroidectomy
3. Elevated serum calcium level
4. Steroid use

99. 1. Because failing kidneys can't convert vitamin D, the serum calcium level declines, causing hyperparathyroidism from increased release of parathyroid hormones. Thyroidectomy may lead to hypoparathyroidism if the parathyroid is also removed during surgery. Hyperparathyroidism may cause serum calcium levels to rise. Steroid use induces calcium to leave bone, suppressing parathyroid hormone.

NP: Analysis; CN: Physiological integrity; CNS: Physiological adaptation; CL: Analysis

100. A previously healthy 70-year-old male client has a serum glucose level of 1,200 mg/dl, a normal serum bicarbonate level, and urine free from acetone. The nurse should suspect the client has which condition?

1. Diabetic ketoacidosis
2. Diabetes insipidus
3. Hyperglycemic hyperosmolar nonketotic coma
4. Syndrome of inappropriate antidiuretic hormone

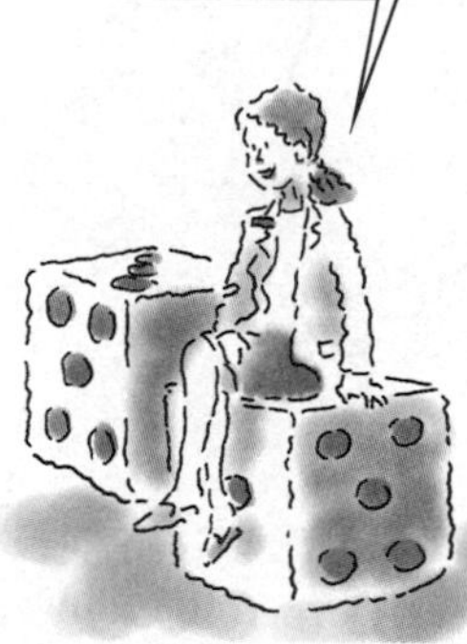

Always note
the stated age.
It can influence

100. 3. Elderly clients are at risk for developing a hyperosmolar state as their taste preferences shift to softer, higher-carbohydrate foods. The urine free from acetone indicates that the client isn't experiencing breakdown of fats and proteins, so the nurse shouldn't suspect ketoacidosis. The client's laboratory values don't indicate a disturbance in the production, secretion, or use of antidiuretic hormone, which would result in diabetes insipidus or syndrome of inappropriate antidiuretic hormone.

NP: Analysis; CN: Physiological integrity; CNS: Physiological adaptation; CL: Analysis

101. A client with Addison's disease is receiving a maintenance dose of steroids. Which topic should the nurse include in discharge teaching?

1. Importance of restricting fluids
2. Watching for signs of hypoglycemia
3. Taking steroids exactly as prescribed
4. Adjusting steroid doses based on dietary intake and exercise

101. 3. A client with Addison's disease needs more steroids than the body produces. Taking a lower dose may trigger an addisonian crisis; taking a higher dose increases the effects of potassium depletion, hyperglycemia, and fluid retention, leading to a life-threatening situation. Fluid restriction isn't desirable and could cause dehydration. Steroids tend to increase, not decrease, blood sugar. Steroid doses aren't adjusted for diet and exercise, although the client may need to administer insulin and adjust insulin doses.

NP: Planning; CN: Physiological integrity; CNS: Pharmacological and parenteral therapies; CL: Comprehension

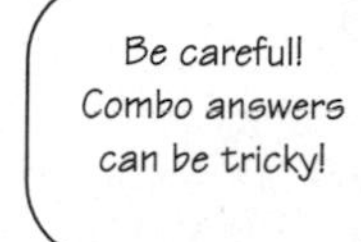

Be careful!
Combo answers
can be tricky!

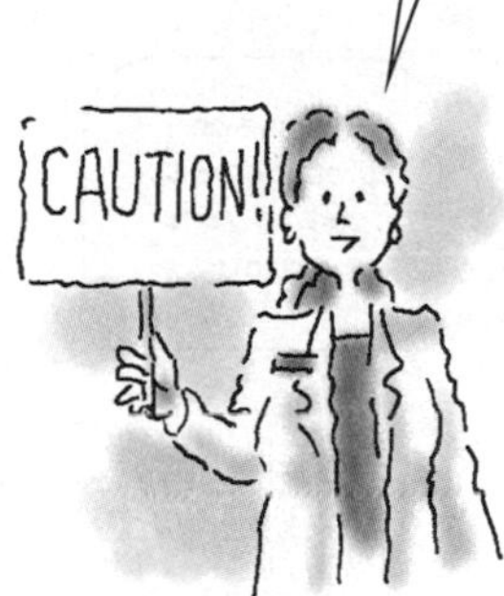

CAUTION!

102. A client is being treated for adrenal crisis (addisonian crisis). Which laboratory values are *most* important to monitor?

1. Serum bicarbonate and sodium
2. Serum glucose and ketones
3. Serum sodium and potassium
4. Serum calcium and magnesium

102. 3. If steroid replacement therapy is inadequate, sodium loss and potassium retention persist. If the steroid dose is too high, sodium and water are retained, and large amounts of potassium are excreted. Steroid replacement can affect glucose, but the replacement doesn't have as great an impact on ketones, bicarbonate, calcium, or magnesium as it does on sodium and potassium.

NP: Assessment; CN: Physiological integrity; CNS: Pharmacological and parenteral therapies; CL: Analysis

103. A client newly diagnosed with diabetic ketoacidosis has a serum glucose level of 485 mg/dl. After treatment, the serum glucose level drops to 185 mg/dl, and the cardiac monitor starts to show ventricular ectopic beats. Which of the following is the *most probable* cause of the arrhythmia?

1. Decreased serum chloride level
2. Decreased serum potassium level
3. Elevated serum glucose level
4. Elevated serum sodium level

103. 2. Correction of an elevated serum glucose level may alter the serum potassium level, predisposing the client to arrhythmias. Serum chloride and sodium changes are more likely to contribute to an altered level of consciousness, whereas elevated serum glucose contributes to long-term effects of diabetes mellitus, such as coronary artery disease, hypertension, and peripheral vascular disease.

NP: Analysis; CN: Physiological integrity; CNS: Physiological adaptation; CL: Analysis

104. When teaching a diabetic client about exchange diets, the nurse should state that which of the following is a suitable exchange for 1 cup of strawberries?

1. One small orange
2. 2 oz of raisins
3. 1 cup of applesauce
4. One slice of whole grain bread

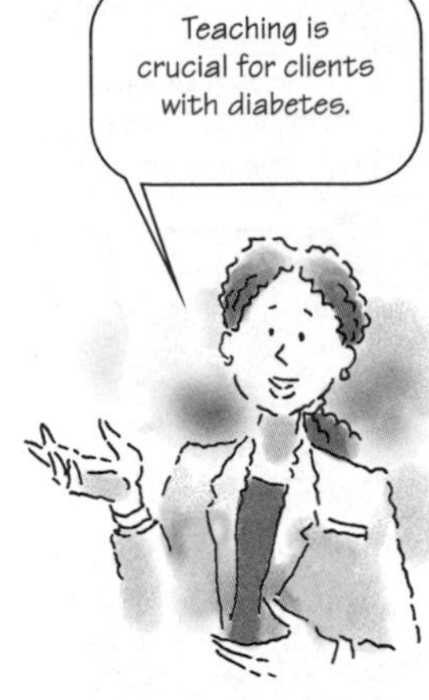

Teaching is crucial for clients with diabetes.

104. 1. One small orange is a suitable exchange for 1 cup of strawberries, with similar carbohydrate, calorie, vitamin, and water content. Raisins are a concentrated source of carbohydrates. One cup of applesauce is equivalent to two fruit servings. One slice of whole grain bread provides complex carbohydrates, whereas fruit exchanges provide simple carbohydrates.

NP: Implementation; CN: Physiological integrity; CNS: Basic care and comfort; CL: Application

105. An unemployed client with no health insurance hasn't filled her prescriptions for some time. According to her roommate, the client has been "getting sicker by the day." Which problem suggests the client isn't taking her prescribed levothyroxine (Synthroid)?

1. Diarrhea and vomiting
2. Rapid heart rate
3. Warm, dry, flushed skin
4. Temperature of 94° F (34.4° C)

105. 4. Levothyroxine is prescribed for hypothyroidism, which causes a hypodynamic state; failure to maintain levothyroxine therapy can lead to a low body temperature. The other problems indicate a hypermetabolic state; although the client may also experience these, they stem from infection and dehydration.

NP: Analysis; CN: Physiological integrity; CNS: Physiological adaptation; CL: Application

106. A client with newly diagnosed diabetes mellitus is ready for discharge. Discharge teaching must include which of the following?

1. Foot care and the need for a high-calorie diet
2. How to balance diet, exercise, and medication
3. Fasting before health care maintenance visits
4. Avoiding all carbohydrates and drinking 2 qt (2 L) of water daily

106. 2. With type 1, type 2, or gestational diabetes mellitus, balancing diet, exercise, and medication are essential to diabetes control. High-calorie and non-carbohydrate diets are contraindicated in diabetes. While fasting may reduce the serum glucose level temporarily, glycosylated hemoglobin tests show the effectiveness of long-term diabetes control.

NP: Planning; CN: Physiological integrity; CNS: Physiological adaptation; CL: Application

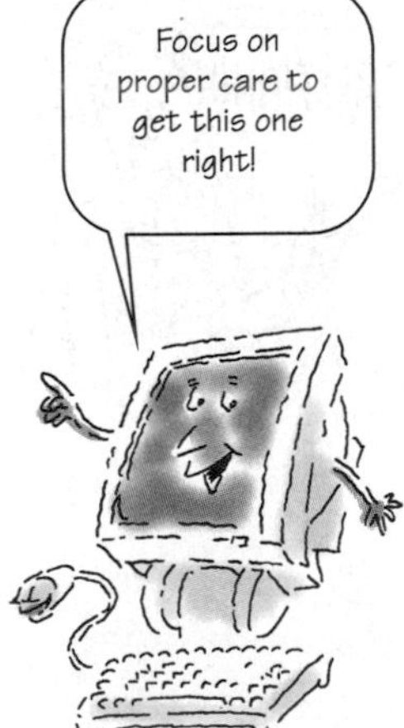

Focus on proper care to get this one right!

107. Which statement indicates that a client with diabetes understands proper foot care?

1. "I'll call for a physician's appointment if my feet start to ache."
2. "I'll rotate insulin injection sites from my left foot to my right foot."
3. "I'll go barefoot around the house to avoid pressure areas on my feet."
4. "I'll wear cotton socks with well-fitting shoes."

107. 4. Cotton socks wisk moisture away from the skin, helping to prevent fungal infections; proper shoe fit helps avoid pressure areas. Aching isn't a common sign of foot problems; however, a tingling sensation in the feet indicates neurovascular changes. Injecting insulin into the foot may lead to infection. Going barefoot can cause injury.

NP: Implementation; CN: Safe, effective care environment; CNS: Safety and infection control; CL: Analysis

108. A 17-year-old client with diabetes has a decreased level of consciousness, with a finger-stick glucose level of 39. Her family reports that she has been skipping meals in an effort to lose weight. Which nursing intervention is most appropriate?
1. Placing a Salem sump tube and providing tube feedings
2. Administering a 500-ml bolus of normal saline solution
3. Administering 1 ampule of 50% dextrose solution
4. Calling the physician for orders

108. 3. Administering 50% dextrose solution helps preserve and restore the client's physiologic integrity. Providing a feeding is appropriate only in a less urgent situation; during the time it takes to insert a nasogastric tube, administer a feeding, and wait for digestion to occur, the client may suffer permanent brain damage and seizures from severe hypoglycemia. A blood pressure drop wasn't mentioned; a bolus of normal saline solution would correct only the client fluid status, not her glucose level. Calling the physician would delay treatment at a time when rapid intervention is crucial.

NP: Implementation; CN: Physiological integrity; CNS: Pharmacological and parenteral therapies; CL: Application

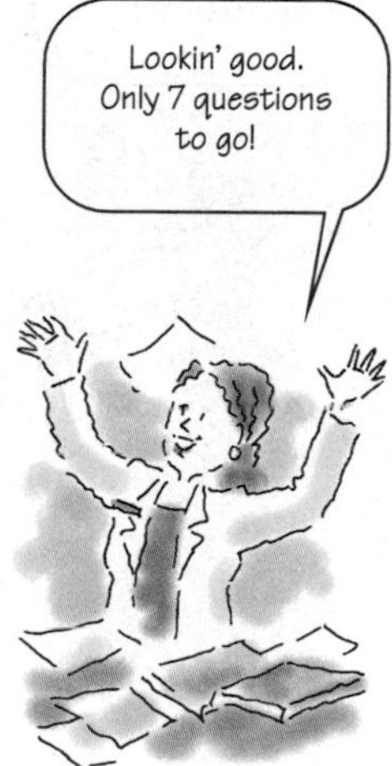

Lookin' good.
Only 7 questions to go!

109. A client is admitted to the telemetry floor with a diagnosis of pancreatitis. Which nursing intervention is appropriate?
1. Providing generous servings at mealtime
2. Reserving one antecubital site for a PICC
3. Providing a glass of wine with each meal because the client wasn't admitted to treat alcoholism
4. Serving coffee with breakfast to help clear the client's mind

109. 2. Pancreatitis treatment commonly involves resting the GI tract; use of a PICC enables the client to receive long-term total parenteral nutrition. Alcohol and caffeine stimulate the pancreas, increase pain, and may lead to a pseudocyst, with eventual rupture resulting in peritonitis.

NP: Implementation; CN: Physiological integrity; CNS: Pharmacological and parenteral therapies; CL: Application

110. A client is diagnosed with Cushing's disease. Which statement indicates that she understands her disease?
1. "My blood sugar is high only because I produce too much cortisone, so I don't need to watch my diet."
2. "I don't like fruits and vegetables, and potassium isn't that important to me."
3. "Because I'm susceptible to infection and heal poorly, I should get a Pneumovax (pneumococcal vaccine)."
4. "I'll continue to teach ice skating when I get out of the hospital."

110. 3. The client's concern about preventing disease shows an understanding of the body's response to elevated steroid levels. Elevated serum glucose or decreased serum potassium levels could lead to life-threatening health crises. With elevated steroid levels, minerals leave the bones, making the bones more fragile; a minor spill when walking or skating could cause long-bone or compression fractures.

NP: Evaluation; CN: Health promotion and maintenance; CNS: Prevention and early detection of disease; CL: Application

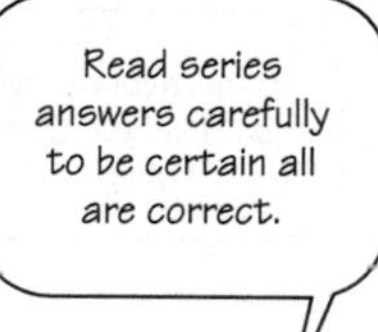

Read series answers carefully to be certain all are correct.

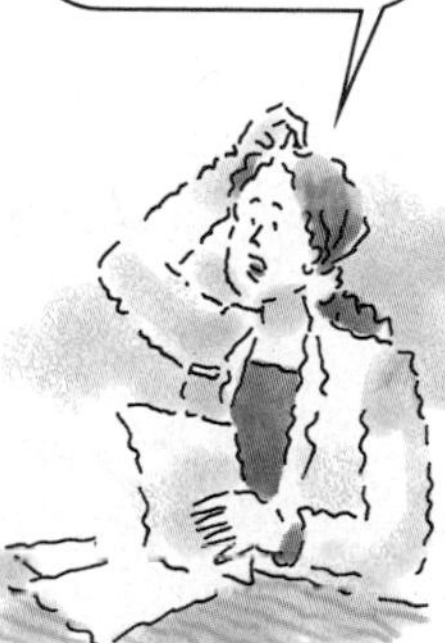

111. The most common signs and symptoms of hypothyroidism include which of the following?
1. Increased body temperature, tachycardia, and fatigue
2. Tachycardia, pitting, and facial edema
3. Facial edema, weight gain, and diarrhea
4. Cold intolerance, swollen hands and feet, and mental sluggishness

111. 4. Hypothyroidism slows the metabolic rate and mental responses, causing edema, decreased body temperature, and slower respiratory and heart rates. Hyperthyroidism causes increased body temperature, tachycardia, and fatigue. Tachycardia, pitting, and facial edema suggest a cardiac problem. Diarrhea and facial edema suggest hyperthyroidism.

NP: Assessment; CN: Physiological integrity; CNS: Physiological adaptation; CL: Analysis

112. A client with hypothyroidism is receiving liotrix (Thyrolar). With effective treatment, which assessment signs should be expected?

1. Diuresis and a decrease in the heart rate and blood pressure
2. Diuresis and an increase in the heart and respiratory rates
3. Weigh loss, increased blood pressure, and a decreased heart rate
4. Decreased respiratory rate and dehydration

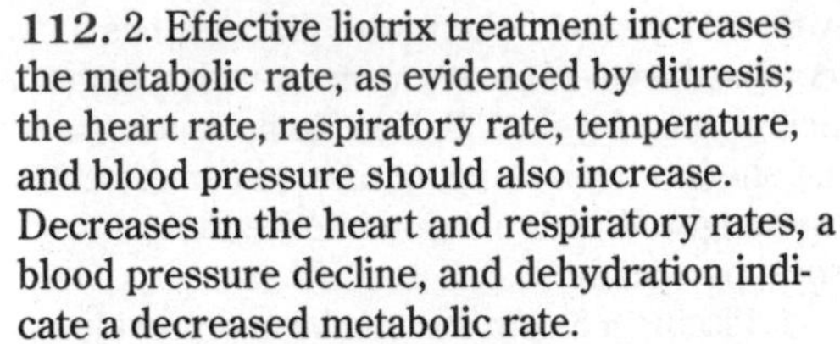

112. 2. Effective liotrix treatment increases the metabolic rate, as evidenced by diuresis; the heart rate, respiratory rate, temperature, and blood pressure should also increase. Decreases in the heart and respiratory rates, a blood pressure decline, and dehydration indicate a decreased metabolic rate.

NP: Analysis; CN: Physiological integrity; CNS: Pharmacological and parenteral therapies; CL: Analysis

113. A client with hyperthyroidism experiences a rapid decrease in level of consciousness (LOC). The physician prepares to perform a lumbar puncture. During this procedure, which action takes highest priority for the nurse?

1. Establishing I.V. access
2. Administering conscious sedation
3. Keeping the client from moving during the procedure
4. Monitoring oxygen saturation and maintaining a patent airway

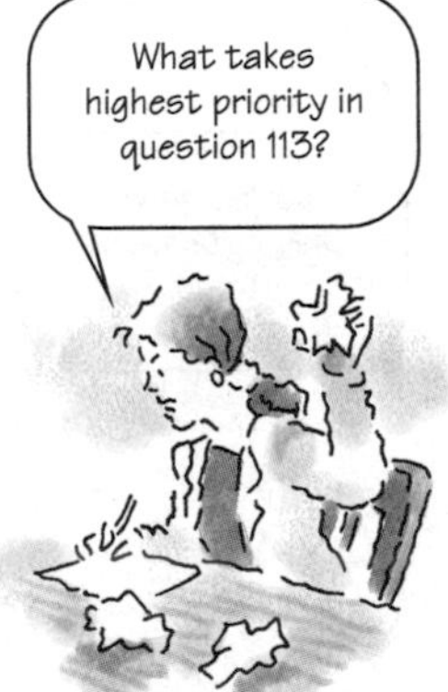
What takes highest priority in question 113?

113. 4. Because thyroid enlargement may cause airway obstruction, monitoring the client and maintaining a patent airway (that is, positioning the client to avoid obstruction, suctioning, and providing supplemental oxygen as needed) take top priority. I.V. access for emergency medications should be established in a client with a decreased LOC. Keeping the client from moving is important, but it has a lower priority. Sedation isn't desirable because of the client's decreased LOC.

NP: Implementation; CN: Safe, effective care environment; CNS: Safety and infection control; CL: Application

114. A 28-year-old female client with hyperthyroidism complains of her "ugly" appearance and asks, "Will I always look so terrible?" What is the nurse's best response?

1. "Makeup can help your protruding eyes seem less noticeable."
2. "Your appearance doesn't matter. It's what's inside that counts."
3. "With treatment, the fluid buildup behind your eyes will decrease."
4. "If you cut back on fluids, the swelling behind your eyes will go down."

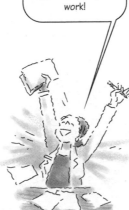

114. 3. Over time, swelling behind the eyes decreases, reducing the eyes' bulging appearance. Although makeup can improve the client's appearance, it's more important for the nurse to emphasize that fluid buildup will abate. Obviously, appearance does matter to this client, or she wouldn't have asked the nurse about it. Restricting fluids is inappropriate because a hyperthyroid client is hypermetabolic and can become dehydrated quickly.

NP: Analysis; CN: Psychosocial integrity; CNS: Coping and adaptation; CL: Application

115. A client with hyperthyroidism asks the nurse why he must take beta-adrenergic blockers. Which statement correctly describes the purpose of beta-adrenergic blockers for this client?

1. "Beta-adrenergic blockers protect the heart from damage."
2. "Beta-adrenergic blockers reduce blood pressure."
3. "Beta-adrenergic blockers will eliminate your headaches."
4. "Beta-adrenergic blockers slow the growth of the thyroid."

115. 1. By slowing the heart rate, beta-adrenergic blockers reduce myocardial oxygen demand and protect the heart from ischemia. Blood pressure reduction may be undesirable because hypermetabolic clients are frequently dehydrated. Although beta-adrenergic blockers are used to manage migraine, that isn't their most important use in this client. Beta-adrenergic blockers have no direct effect on thyroid growth.

NP: Planning; CN: Physiological integrity; CNS: Pharmacological and parenteral therapies; CL: Analysis

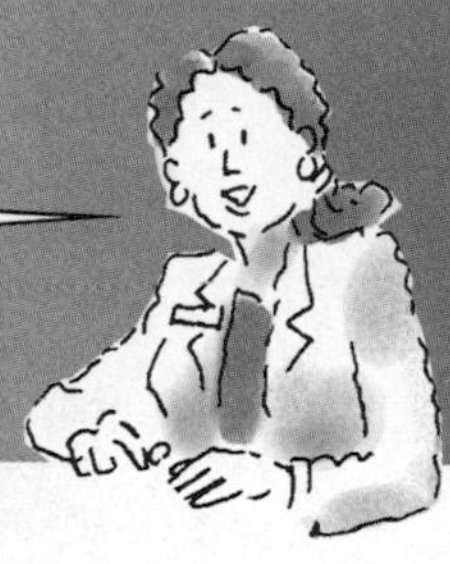

Chapter 10 Genitourinary disorders

1. Which of the following statements best explains why it's important to empty the bowel before treatment with intracavitary radiation for cancer of the cervix?

1. Feces in the bowel increase the risk for ileus.
2. An empty bowel allows the applicator to be positioned with little or no discomfort.
3. Bowel movements increase the risk for inadvertent contamination of the vagina and urethra.
4. Pressure changes in the pelvis associated with bowel movements can alter the position of the applicator and the radiation source.

2. A physician tells a client to return 1 week after treatment to have a repeat culture done to verify the cure. This order would be appropriate for a woman with which of the following conditions?

1. Genital warts
2. Genital herpes
3. Gonorrhea
4. Syphilis

3. Which of the following clients is at greatest risk for having a false-positive Venereal Disease Research Laboratory (VDRL) result?

1. An alcoholic
2. A narcotics addict
3. A transfusion recipient
4. A breast-feeding mother

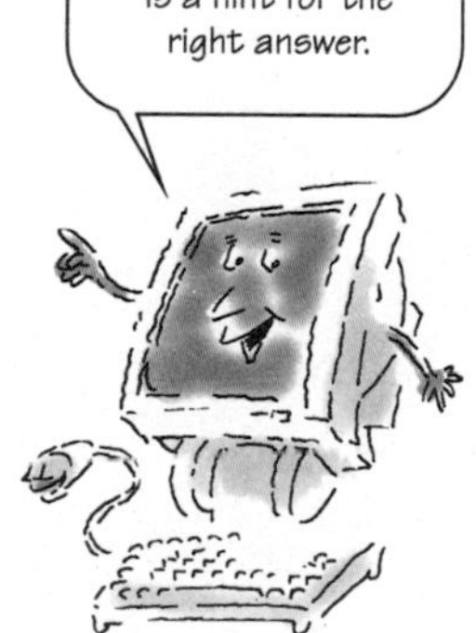

The word *greatest* is a hint for the right answer.

1. 4. A position change of the radioactive implant could deliver more radiation to healthy tissue and less to the malignant lesion. This increases the risk of injury to healthy tissue and decreases the effectiveness of treatment on the cancer. Feces in the bowel increase the likelihood of a bowel movement, which can change the position of the applicator and radiation source. Feces in the bowel don't increase the risk for ileus or inadvertant contamination of the vagina and urethra from a bowel movement. Applicators are usually inserted under anesthesia in the operating room.

NP: Planning; CN: Physiological integrity; CNS: Reduction of risk potential; CL: Comprehension

2. 3. Gonococcal infections can be completely eliminated by drug therapy. This is documented by a negative culture 4 to 7 days after therapy is finished. Genital warts aren't curable and are identified by appearance, not culture. The diagnosis of syphilis is by darkfield microscopy or serologic tests. Genital herpes isn't curable and is identified by the appearance of the lesions or cytologic studies.

NP: Planning; CN: Physiological integrity; CNS: Physiological adaptation; CL: Application

3. 2. The VDRL test is a nontreponemal test used to check for the presence of reagins in the client's serum. It isn't specific for syphilis, so false-positive results occur for a variety of reasons, most often in clients with chronic infection, autoimmune disease, and narcotics addiction. History of transfusion, alcoholism, or breast-feeding alone don't constitute a risk of a false-positive VDRL result.

NP: Assessment; CN: Physiological integrity; CNS: Physiological adaptation; CL: Comprehension

4. Which of the following statements made by a client with a chlamydial infection indicates understanding of the potential complications?

1. "I'm glad I'm not pregnant; I'd hate to have a malformed baby from this disease."
2. "I hope this medicine works before this disease gets into my urine and destroys my kidneys."
3. "If I had known a diaphragm would put me at risk for this, I would have taken birth control pills."
4. "I need to treat this infection so it doesn't spread into my pelvis because I want to have children some day."

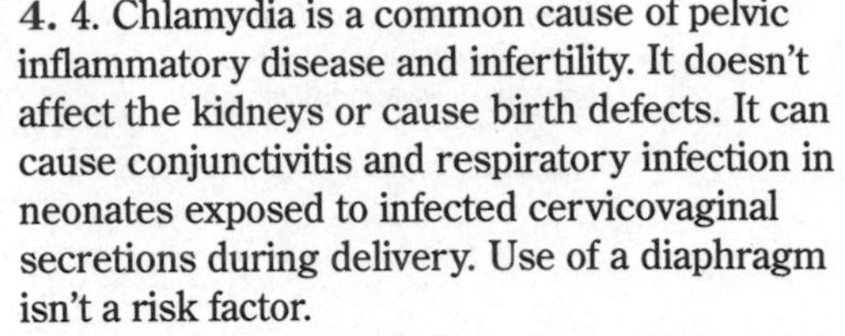

4. 4. Chlamydia is a common cause of pelvic inflammatory disease and infertility. It doesn't affect the kidneys or cause birth defects. It can cause conjunctivitis and respiratory infection in neonates exposed to infected cervicovaginal secretions during delivery. Use of a diaphragm isn't a risk factor.

NP: Evaluation; CN: Physiological integrity; CNS: Reduction of risk potential; CL: Application

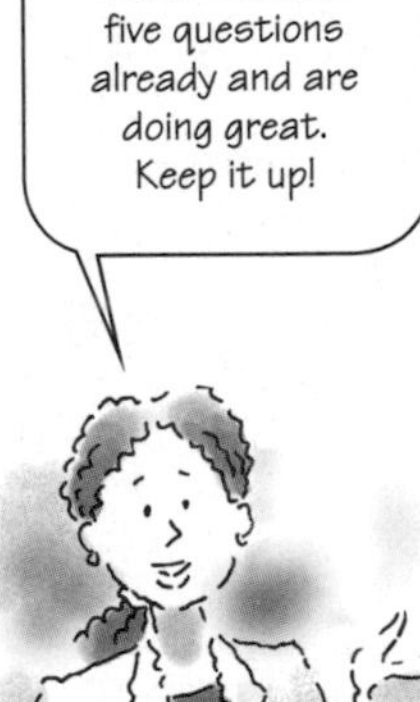

You've finished five questions already and are doing great. Keep it up!

5. Which of the following comfort measures can be recommended to a client with genital herpes?

1. Wear loose cotton underwear.
2. Apply a water-based lubricant to the lesions.
3. Rub rather than scratch in response to an itch.
4. Pour hydrogen peroxide and water over the lesions.

5. 1. Wearing loose cotton underwear promotes drying and helps avoid irritation of the lesions. The use of hydrogen peroxide and water on lesions isn't recommended. The use of lubricants is contraindicated because they can prolong healing time and increase the risk of secondary infection. Lesions shouldn't be rubbed or scratched because of the risk of tissue damage and additional infection. Cool, wet compresses can be used to soothe the itch.

NP: Implementation; CN: Physiological integrity; CNS: Basic care and comfort; CL: Comprehension

6. Giving instructions for breast self-examination is particularly important for clients with which of the following medical problems?

1. Cervical dysplasia
2. A dermoid cyst
3. Endometrial polyps
4. Ovarian cancer

6. 4. Clients with ovarian cancer are at increased risk for breast cancer. Breast self-examination supports early detection and treatment and is very important. There isn't a known relationship between breast cancer and cervical dysplasia, endometrial polyps, or dermoid cysts, so breast self-examination is no more or less important for these clients.

NP: Planning; CN: Health promotion and maintenance; CNS: Prevention and early detection of disease; CL: Application

7. On a follow-up visit after having a vaginal hysterectomy, a 32-year-old client has an elevated temperature and decreased hematocrit. Which of the following complications does this suggest?

1. Hematoma
2. Hypovolemia
3. Infection
4. Thromboembolism

7. 1. An elevated temperature and decreased hematocrit are signs of hematoma, a delayed complication of abdominal and vaginal hysterectomy. Symptoms of hypovolemia include increased hematocrit and hemoglobin values. Temperature is a classic sign of infection, but a decreased hematocrit isn't. Abrupt onset of fever is a symptom of thromboembolism, but other symptoms include dyspnea, chest pain, cough, hemoptysis, restlessness, and signs of shock.

NP: Evaluation; CN: Physiological integrity; CNS: Reduction of risk potential; CL: Application

8. Which of the following clients is at greatest risk for dehydration?

1. 48-year-old having intracavitary radiation for cancer of the cervix
2. 59-year-old 1 week after a radical vulvectomy
3. 67-year-old receiving adjuvant tamoxifen therapy for breast cancer
4. 72-year-old with a vesicovaginal fistula

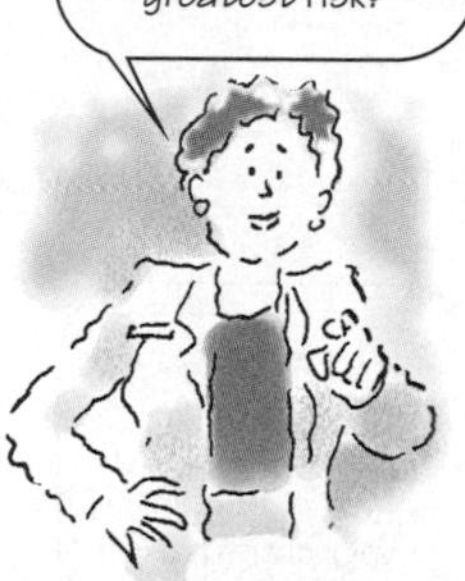

8. 1. Regardless of age, dehydration is a risk caused by fluid loss secondary to tissue destruction at the site of irradiation. Although urine may escape through the vagina as a result of a vesicovaginal fistula, it doesn't cause an unusual amount of urine or other fluid to be lost. After radical vulvectomy, wound drains are generally removed by postoperative day 4 or 5 and don't create a significant risk for dehydration. Tamoxifen therapy is unrelated to dehydration.

NP: Planning; CN: Physiological integrity; CNS: Physiological adaptation; CL: Application

9. In which of the following groups is it most important for the client to understand the importance of an annual Papanicolaou test?

1. Clients with a history of recurrent candidiasis
2. Clients with a pregnancy before age 20
3. Clients infected with the human papillomavirus (HPV)
4. Clients with a long history of oral contraceptive use

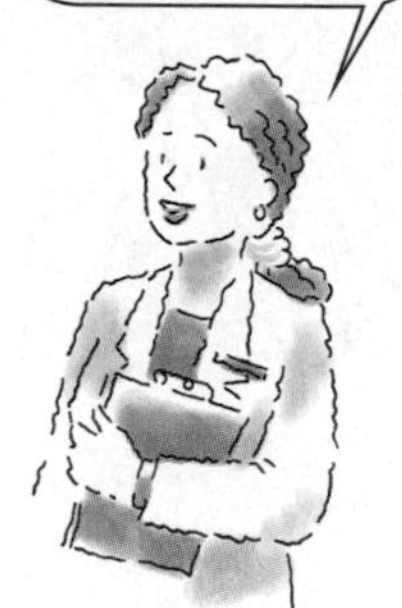

Nurses teach about prevention as well as about cure.

9. 3. HPV causes genital warts, which are associated with an increased incidence of cervical cancer. Recurrent candidiasis, use of oral contraceptives, and pregnancy before age 20 don't increase the risk of cervical cancer.

NP: Planning; CN: Health promotion and maintenance; CNS: Prevention and early detection of disease; CL: Application

10. Which of the following factors in a client's history indicates she's at risk for candidiasis?

1. Nulliparity
2. Menopause
3. Use of corticosteroids
4. Use of spermicidal jelly

10. 3. Small numbers of the fungus *Candida albicans* commonly are in the vagina. Because corticosteroids decrease host defense, they increase the risk of candidiasis. Candidiasis is rare before menarche and after menopause. The use of oral contraceptives, not spermicidal jelly, increases the risk of candidiasis. Pregnancy, not nulliparity, increases the risk for candidiasis.

NP: Assessment; CN: Health promotion and maintenance; CNS: Prevention and early detection of disease; CL: Application

11. Copious amounts of frothy, greenish vaginal discharge would be a symptom with which of the following infections?

1. Candidiasis
2. *Gardnerella vaginalis* vaginitis
3. Gonorrhea
4. Trichomoniasis

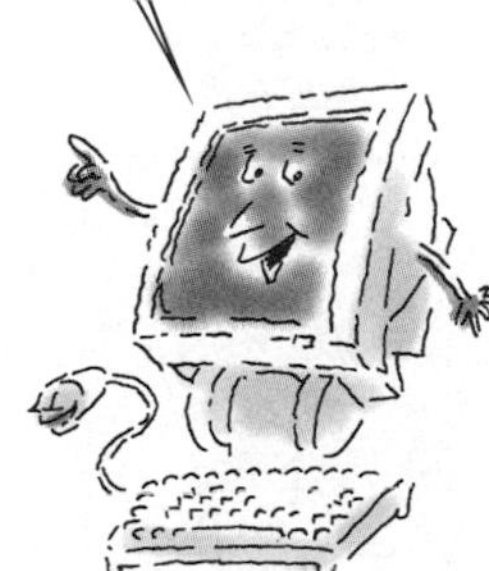

You've already finished 11 questions and are well on your way!

11. 4. The discharge associated with infection caused by *Trichomonas* organisms is homogenous, greenish gray, watery, and frothy or purulent. The discharge associated with infection due to *Gardnerella vaginalis* is thin and grayish white, with a marked fishy odor, while that associated with candidiasis is thick, white, and resembles cottage cheese in appearance. With gonorrhea, vaginal discharge is purulent when present but, in many women, gonorrhea is asymptomatic.

NP: Assessment; CN: Physiological integrity; CNS: Physiological adaptation; CL: Application

12. A 19-year-old woman reports an intermittent milky vaginal discharge. She isn't sexually active and doesn't report itching or burning. Which of the following factors is the most likely cause of the milky-appearing discharge?

1. Inadequate cleaning of the perineal area
2. Sensitivity to a feminine hygiene product
3. Normal fluctuation in estrogen and progesterone levels
4. Reaction to heat and moisture from wearing tight clothing

12. 3. Vaginal fluid is clear, milky, or cloudy, depending on the fluctuating levels of estrogen and progesterone. A milky-appearing vaginal discharge is normal and isn't associated with sensitivity, reaction to heat or moisture, or inadequate cleaning.

NP: Assessment; CN: Health promotion and maintenance; CNS: Growth and development through the life span; CL: Application

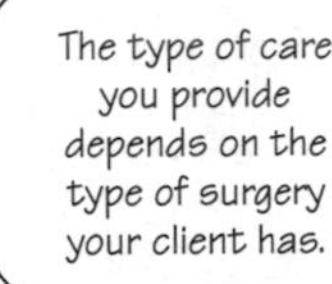

The type of care you provide depends on the type of surgery your client has.

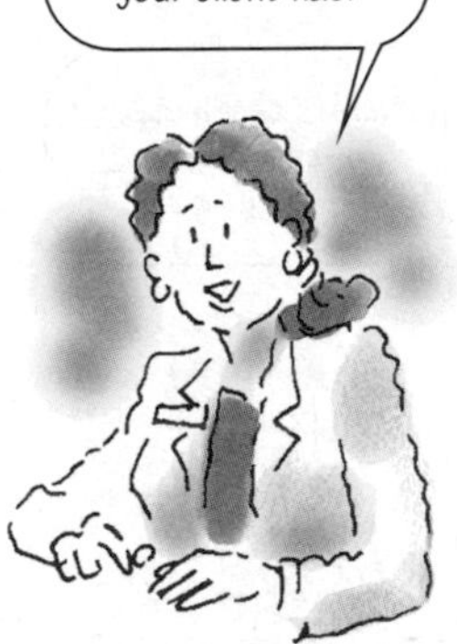

13. Which of the following nursing interventions is appropriate for a client who had breast reconstruction surgery?

1. Prevent hypothermia.
2. Maintain even pressure on the wound.
3. Position the client on the operative side.
4. Raise the client's arms over her head four times daily.

13. 1. Hypothermia causes a decrease in surface circulation. This can lead to ischemia of the skin or muscle graft and ultimately to tissue necrosis in clients who had breast reconstruction surgery. Because of the importance of maintaining good circulation, pressure on the breast wound must be avoided, so the client is positioned on the back or nonoperative side. Arms shouldn't be lifted above shoulder level for 4 to 6 weeks.

NP: Planning; CN: Physiological integrity; CNS: Reduction of risk potential; CL: Application

14. A client who had intracavitary radiation treatment for cancer of the cervix 1 month earlier reports small amounts of vaginal bleeding. This most likely represents which of the following conditions?

1. Recurrence of the carcinoma
2. Development of a rectovaginal fistula
3. Expected effect of the radiation therapy
4. Infection secondary to a change in vaginal flora

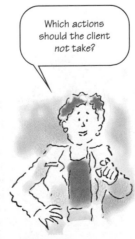

14. 3. After intracavitary radiation, some vaginal bleeding occurs for 1 to 3 months. Intermittent painless vaginal bleeding is a classic symptom of cervical cancer, but given the client's history, bleeding is more likely a result of the radiation than recurrent cancer. The passage of feces through the vagina, not vaginal bleeding, is a sign of rectovaginal fistula. Vaginal infections show various types of vaginal discharge but not vaginal bleeding.

NP: Evaluation; CN: Physiological integrity; CNS: Physiological adaptation; CL: Application

Which actions should the client not take?

15. A nurse enters the room of a client who had a left modified mastectomy 8 hours earlier. Which of the following observations indicates that the nursing assistant assigned to the client needs further instruction and guidance?

1. The client is squeezing a ball in her left hand.
2. The client is wearing a robe with elastic cuffs.
3. The client's affected arm is elevated on a pillow.
4. A blood pressure cuff is on the client's right arm.

15. 2. Elastic cuffs can contribute to the development of lymphedema and should be avoided. Blood pressure measurements in the affected arm also should be avoided. Simple exercises such as squeezing a ball help promote circulation and should be started as soon as possible after surgery. Elevation of the affected arm promotes venous and lymphatic return from the extremity.

NP: Evaluation; CN: Safe, effective care environment; CNS: Management of care; CL: Analysis

16. For which of the following symptoms should a client at risk for evisceration be monitored after an abdominal hysterectomy?

1. Tachycardia accompanied by a weak, thready pulse
2. Hypotension with a decreased level of consciousness
3. Shallow, rapid respirations and increasing vaginal drainage
4. Low-grade fever with increasing serosanguineous incisional drainage

16. 4. Signs of impending evisceration are low-grade fever and increasing serosanguineous drainage. Tachycardia; weak, thready pulse; shallow, rapid respirations; vaginal drainage; hypotension; and decreased level of consciousness after abdominal hysterectomy are all unrelated to impeding evisceration, although they may be associated with other serious problems such as shock.

NP: Planning; CN: Physiological integrity; CNS: Reduction of risk potential; CL: Comprehension

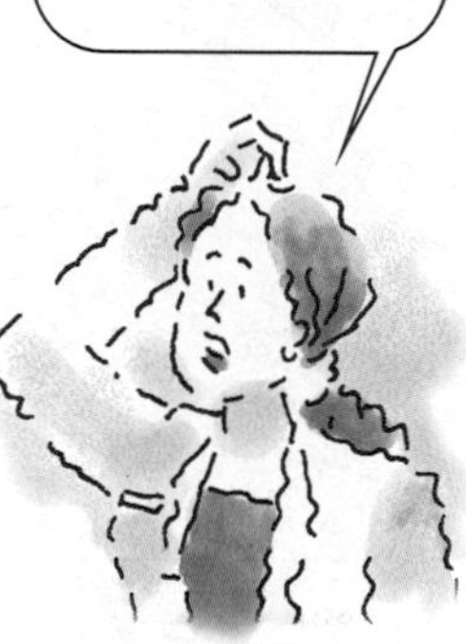

For what purpose are drugs that end with "one" given?

17. Which of the following findings indicates that oxycodone (Percodan) given to a client with breast cancer metastasized to the bone is exerting the desired effect?

1. Bone density is increased.
2. Pain is 0 to 2 on a 10-point scale.
3. Alphafetoprotein level is decreased.
4. Serum calcium level is within normal range.

17. 2. Oxycodone is an opioid analgesic used for alleviating severe pain, especially in terminal illness. If a client's pain has decreased to 0 to 2 on a 10-point scale (0 is no pain and 10 is the worst pain), the medication is working as desired. The drug doesn't directly affect bone density, serum calcium level, or alphafetoprotein level.

NP: Evaluation; CN: Physiological integrity; CNS: Pharmacological and parenteral therapies; CL: Analysis

18. Which of the following instructions should be given to a client with prostatitis who is receiving co-trimoxazole double strength (Bactrim-DS)?

1. Don't expect improvement of symptoms for 7 to 10 days.
2. Drink six to eight glasses of fluid daily while taking this medication.
3. If a sore mouth or throat develops, take the medication with milk or an antacid.
4. Use a sunscreen of at least SPF-15 with PABA to protect against drug-induced photosensitivity.

18. 2. Six to eight glasses of fluid daily are needed to prevent renal problems, such as crystalluria and stone formation. The symptoms should improve in a few days if the drug is effective. Sore throat and sore mouth are adverse effects that should be reported right away. The drug causes photosensitivity, but a PABA-free sunscreen should be used because PABA can interfere with the drug's action.

NP: Planning; CN: Physiological integrity; CNS: Pharmacological and parenteral therapies; CL: Application

19. Which of the following factors should be checked when evaluating the effectiveness of an alpha-adrenergic blocker given to a client with benign prostatic hyperplasia (BPH)?

1. Voiding pattern
2. Size of the prostate
3. Creatinine clearance
4. Serum testosterone level

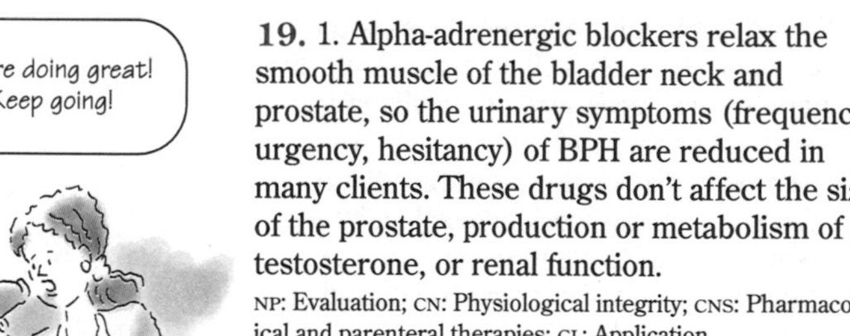

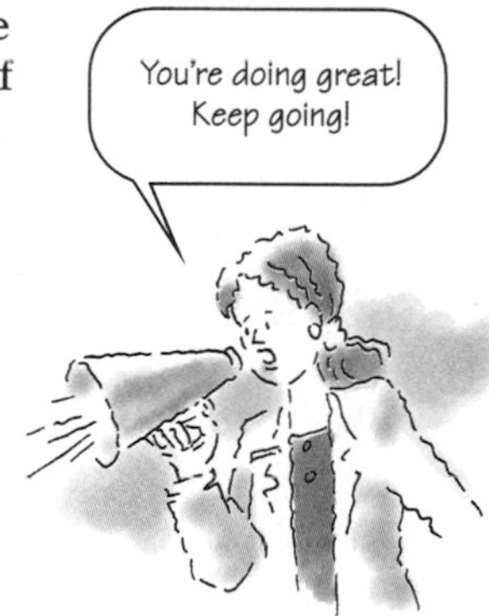

19. 1. Alpha-adrenergic blockers relax the smooth muscle of the bladder neck and prostate, so the urinary symptoms (frequency, urgency, hesitancy) of BPH are reduced in many clients. These drugs don't affect the size of the prostate, production or metabolism of testosterone, or renal function.

NP: Evaluation; CN: Physiological integrity; CNS: Pharmacological and parenteral therapies; CL: Application

20. A nursing diagnosis addressing risk for impaired tissue integrity would be most appropriate for which of the following clients?

1. A client with endometriosis
2. A client taking oral contraceptives
3. A client with a vaginal packing in place
4. A client having reconstructive breast surgery

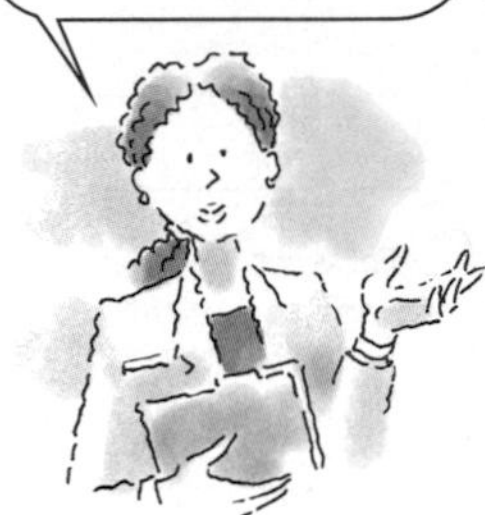

The appropriate nursing diagnosis helps everyone work toward the same goal.

20. 4. Reconstructive breast surgery places the client at risk for insufficient blood supply to the muscle graft and skin, which can lead to tissue necrosis. Endometriosis or oral contraceptives aren't generally associated with altered tissue perfusion. Pressure from vaginal packing can sometimes put pressure on the bladder neck and interfere with voiding.

NP: Planning; CN: Physiological integrity; CNS: Reduction of risk potential; CL: Analysis

21. A 27-year-old man arrives at the clinic with priapism. The nurse arranges for an immediate urologic consult because of the risk of which of the following conditions?

1. Disseminated intravascular coagulation
2. Hydronephrosis
3. Penile gangrene
4. Testicular atrophy

21. 3. Priapism is a condition in which the penis is persistently erect and painful. It's a urologic emergency because gangrene secondary to ischemia can result if venous drainage of the corpora cavernosa doesn't occur. Priapism doesn't cause disseminated intravascular coagulation, testicular atrophy, or hydronephrosis.

NP: Planning; CN: Physiological integrity; CNS: Reduction of risk potential; CL: Application

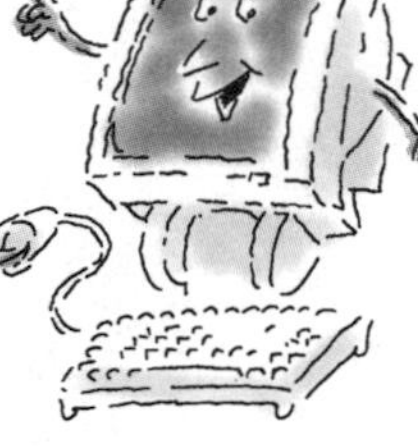

The words most important offer a hint!

22. Which of the following instructions is the most important to give women to decrease the risk of toxic shock syndrome?

1. Avoid douching.
2. Wear loose cotton underwear.
3. Use pads, not tampons, overnight.
4. Avoid sexual intercourse during menses.

22. 3. The cause of toxic shock syndrome is a toxin produced by *Staphylococcus aureus* bacteria. It occurs most often in menstruating women using tampons. Tampons, particularly when left in place for more than 8 hours (such as overnight), are believed to provide a good environment for growth of the bacteria, which then enter the bloodstream through breaks in the vaginal mucosa. Douching, use of loose cotton underwear, and sexual intercourse during menstruation have no direct association with toxic shock syndrome.

NP: Planning; CN: Health promotion and maintenance; CNS: Prevention and early detection of disease; CL: Comprehension

23. Which of the following responses is the most appropriate when a client asks what activity limitations are necessary after a dilatation and curettage procedure?

1. Tampons may be used during exercise.
2. Avoid strenuous work and sexual intercourse for at least 2 weeks.
3. Stay on bed rest for 3 days, then gradually resume normal activity.
4. Engage in activity as tolerated, and take a soaking tub bath each day to promote relaxation.

23. 2. Strenuous work, which can result in increased bleeding, should be avoided for 2 weeks to allow time for healing. Sexual intercourse should also be avoided for 2 weeks to allow healing and thus decrease the risk of infection. Overall activity should be gradually resumed, reaching preoperative levels in the 2-week period, but bed rest isn't necessary. Tampons and tub baths should be avoided for 1 week. No other restrictions are routinely necessary.

NP: Implementation; CN: Physiological integrity; CNS: Reduction of risk potential; CL: Application

24. Which of the following assessment findings is expected in a client receiving bicalutamide (Casodex) and leuprolide (Lupron) for advanced prostate cancer?
1. Abdominal distention
2. Acromegaly
3. Colicky pain
4. Scant facial hair

24. 4. Bicalutamide and leuprolide have an antiandrogenic effect. Because androgens are responsible for the development of the male genitalia and secondary male sex characteristics such as facial hair, low androgen levels can cause genital atrophy, scant facial hair, and breast enlargement. Abdominal distention, acromegaly, and colicky pain aren't caused by bicalutamide and leuprolide therapy.
NP: Evaluation; CN: Physiological integrity; CNS: Pharmacological and parenteral therapies; CL: Analysis

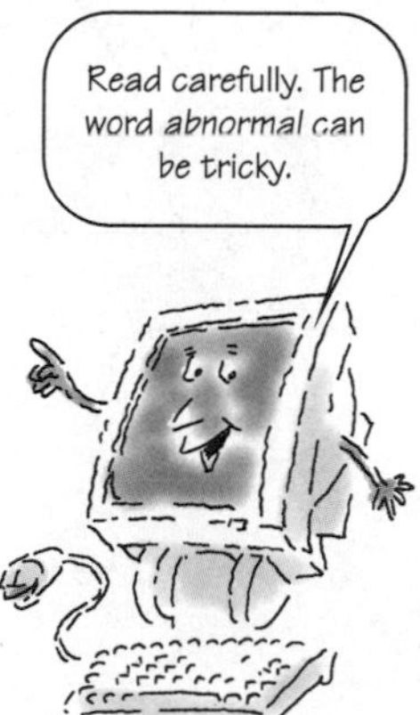

Read carefully. The word *abnormal* can be tricky.

25. Which of the following assessment findings is abnormal in a 72-year-old man?
1. Decreased sperm count
2. Small firm testes on palpation
3. History of slowed sexual response
4. Decreased plasma testosterone level

25. 1. Sperm continues to be produced despite the age-related degenerative changes that occur in the male reproductive system. Among the normal age-related changes are decreased size and increased firmness of the testes, decreased production of testosterone and progesterone, and a decrease in sexual potency.
NP: Assessment; CN: Physiological integrity; CNS: Physiological adaptation; CL: Application

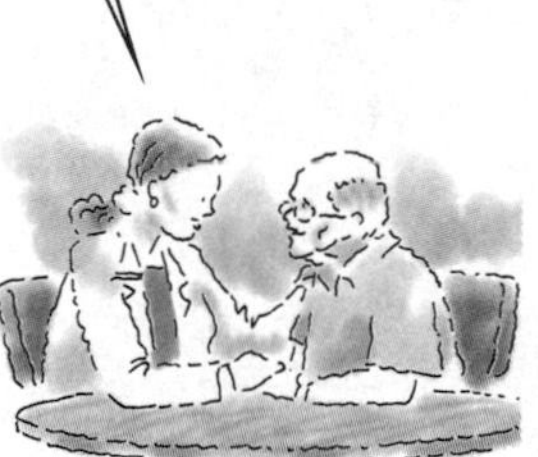

Client teaching includes making sure your client understands your instructions.

26. Which of the following comments made by a client being treated for chronic prostatitis indicates that self-care instructions need to be clarified?
1. "I miss not being able to have sex."
2. "I enjoy frequent soaking in a hot tub of water."
3. "Cutting down on coffee hasn't been as hard as I expected."
4. "I'm used to getting up and moving, not just sitting for long times."

26. 1. Ejaculation can aid in the treatment of chronic prostatitis by decreasing the retention of prostatic fluid. Coffee should be eliminated from the diet because it can increase prostate secretion. Warm sitz baths and not sitting for too long at a time promote comfort.
NP: Evaluation; CN: Physiological integrity; CNS: Physiological adaptation; CL: Application

27. Perineal pain in the absence of any observable cause is suggestive of which of the following conditions?
1. Endometriosis
2. Internal hemorrhoids
3. Prostatitis
4. Renal calculus

27. 3. Prostatitis can cause prostate pain, which is felt as perineal discomfort. Renal calculi typically produce flank pain. Hemorrhoids cause rectal pain and pressure. Endometriosis can cause pain low in the abdomen, deep in the pelvis, or in the rectal or sacrococcygeal area, depending on the location of the ectopic tissue.
NP: Assessment; CN: Health promotion and maintenance; CNS: Prevention and early detection of disease; CL: Comprehension

28. Which of the following assessment findings would be a cause for alarm in a client taking finasteride (Proscar)?
1. Azotemia
2. Breast enlargement
3. Decreased prostate size
4. Flushing

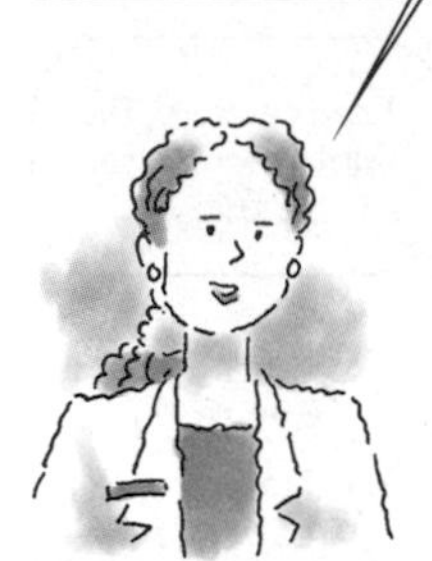

Which assessment finding is cause for alarm?

28. 1. Azotemia, a buildup of nitrogenous waste products in the blood, indicates impaired renal function. Proscar is prescribed for chronic urinary retention with large residual volumes secondary to benign prostatic hypertrophy. Azotemia in a client on finasteride therapy can indicate the drug isn't effective in relieving the urinary symptoms associated with benign prostatic hypertrophy or that an unrelated renal problem has occurred. Flushing, breast enlargement, and decrease in prostate size are expected effects of finasteride, an antiandrogenic agent.

NP: Assessment; CN: Physiological integrity; CNS: Pharmacological and parenteral therapies; CL: Application

29. Which of the following treatments is appropriate for a client with cervical polyps who has been treated with cryosurgery?
1. Daily douche
2. Oral antibiotics
3. Intravaginal antibiotic cream
4. Use of tampons for 72 hours

29. 3. Intravaginal antibiotic cream is often used to aid healing and prevent infection. Oral antibiotics are used for clients with acute cervicitis or perimetritis. Douching is generally avoided for 2 weeks, as is the use of tampons.

NP: Planning; CN: Physiological integrity; CNS: Reduction of risk potential; CL: Application

30. Which of the following interventions would **not** be correct for a woman having intracavitary radiation for cancer of the cervix?
1. Low-residue diet
2. Fowler's position when in bed
3. Indwelling urinary catheter to gravity drainage
4. Diphenoxylate and atropine (Lomotil) 2 mg four times daily

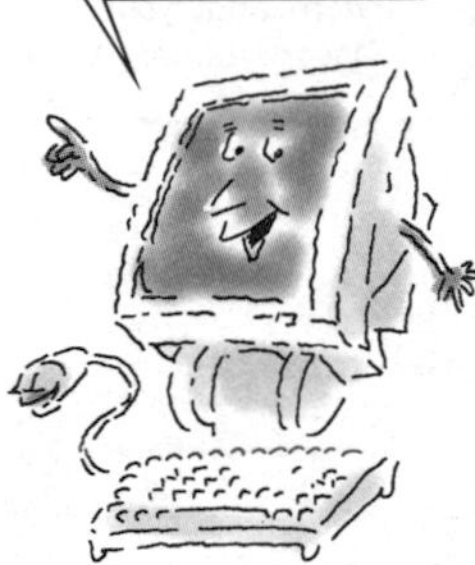

Careful! This question asks what is not correct!

30. 2. Clients having intracavitary radiation therapy are on strict bed rest, with the head of the bed elevated no more than 10 to 15 degrees to avoid displacing the radiation source. An order for Fowler's position when in bed is incorrect. An indwelling urinary catheter is used to prevent urine from distending the bladder and changing the position of tissues relative to the radiation source. A low-residue diet and diphenoxylate and atropine are used to prevent diarrhea during treatment.

NP: Planning; CN: Physiological integrity; CNS: Reduction of risk potential; CL: Analysis

31. Which of the following conditions of the female reproductive system generally requires the identification and treatment of sexual partners?
1. Bartholinitis
2. Candidiasis
3. *Chlamydia trachomatis* infection
4. Endometriosis

31. 3. Chlamydia is a common sexually transmitted disease requiring the treatment of all current sexual partners to prevent reinfection. Bartholinitis results from obstruction of a duct. Endometriosis occurs when endometrial cells are seeded throughout the pelvis and isn't a sexually transmitted disease. Candidiasis is a yeast infection that often occurs as a result of antibiotic use. Sexual partners may become infected, although men can usually be treated with over-the-counter products.

NP: Planning; CN: Health promotion and maintenance; CNS: Prevention and early detection of disease; CL: Application

32. Which of the following pieces of information should be given to a client taking metronidazole (Flagyl)?

1. Breathlessness and cough are common adverse effects.
2. Urine may develop a greenish tinge while the client is taking this drug.
3. Mixing this drug with alcohol causes severe nausea and vomiting.
4. Heart palpitations may occur and should be immediately reported.

32. 3. When mixed with alcohol, metronidazole causes a disulfiram-like effect involving nausea, vomiting, and other unpleasant symptoms. Urine may turn reddish brown, not greenish, from the drug. Cardiovascular or respiratory effects aren't associated with use of this drug.

NP: Planning; CN: Physiological integrity; CNS: Pharmacological and parenteral therapies; CL: Application

33. Which of the following symptoms is an adverse reaction of hydrocodone with acetaminophen that a client with metastatic prostate cancer should be instructed to report to the physician?

1. Blurred vision
2. Diarrhea
3. Unusual dreams
4. Vomiting

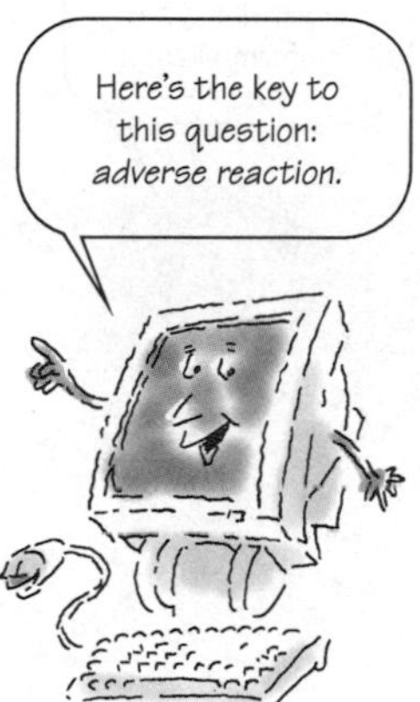

Here's the key to this question: adverse reaction.

33. 4. Vomiting is an adverse reaction to the drug that should be reported because it impairs the client's quality of life and places the client at risk for dehydration. Taking the medication with food may prevent vomiting. If not, other opiate analgesics may be better tolerated. Blurred vision and diarrhea aren't associated with the use of hydrocodone with acetaminophen. Unusual dreams are a common adverse effect but don't need to be reported unless bothersome to the client.

NP: Implementation; CN: Physiological integrity; CNS: Pharmacological and parenteral therapies; CL: Application

34. Which of the following interventions is appropriate for a client having hysterosalpingography?

1. Give the client a perineal pad to wear after the procedure.
2. Give the client nothing by mouth after midnight the night before the procedure.
3. Position the client in the knee-chest position during the procedure.
4. Keep the client in a dorsal recumbent position for 4 hours after the procedure.

34. 1. A perineal pad is needed after hysterosalpingography because the contrast medium may leak from the vagina for several hours and stain the clothing. The bowel needs to be cleaned before the procedure, but the client doesn't have to refrain from having anything by mouth after midnight. The procedure is performed with the client in the lithotomy position, and no special positioning is required after the procedure.

NP: Planning; CN: Physiological integrity; CNS: Basic care and comfort; CL: Application

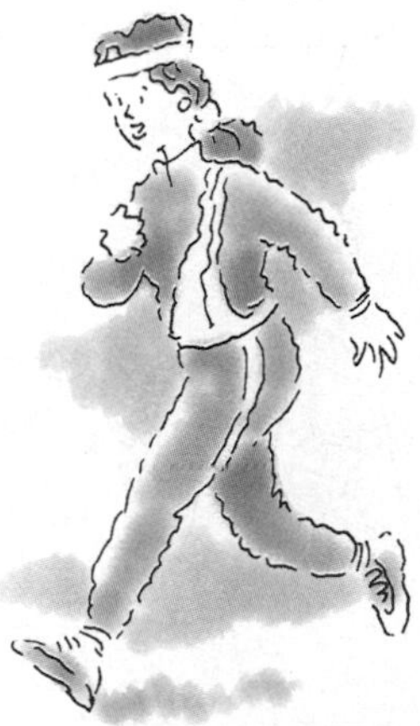

Keep going! You're doing an outstanding job!

35. Which of the following instructions apply to a vaginal irrigation?

1. Insert the nozzle about 3″ (8 cm) into the vagina.
2. Direct the tip of the nozzle toward the sacrum.
3. Instill the solution in a constant flow over 5 to 10 minutes.
4. Raise the solution at least 24″ (60 cm) above the client's hip level.

35. 2. The normal position of the vagina slants up and back toward the sacrum. Directing the tip of the nozzle toward the sacrum allows it to follow the normal slant of the vagina and minimizes tissue trauma. The nozzle should be inserted about 2″ (5 cm). The fluid can be instilled intermittently and, for best therapeutic results, over 20 to 30 minutes. The container should be no higher than 24″ above the client's hip level to avoid forcing fluid and bacteria through the cervical os into the uterus.

NP: Implementation; CN: Safe, effective care environment; CNS: Safety and infection control; CL: Comprehension

36. A 36-year-old man who has never had mumps reports that he was just notified that an 8-year-old child of a family with whom he stayed recently has been diagnosed with mumps. Which of the following treatments should the man receive?

1. I.V. antibiotics
2. Ice packs to the scrotum
3. Application of a scrotal support
4. Administration of gamma globulin

36. 4. Gamma globulin provides passive immunity to mumps. Antibiotic therapy is used in the treatment of bacterial orchitis. Ice and the use of a scrotal support are used as comfort measures in the treatment of orchitis.
NP: Planning; CN: Health promotion and maintenance; CNS: Prevention and early detection of disease; CL: Application

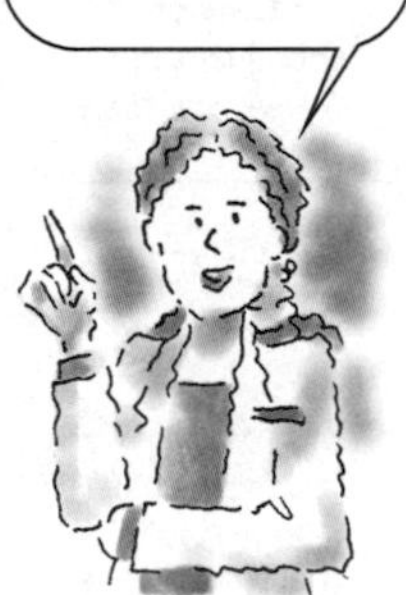

Look for signs that your client doesn't understand the information.

37. Which of the following statements by a man scheduled for a vasectomy indicates he needs further teaching about the procedure?

1. "If I decide I want a child, I'll just get a reversal."
2. "Amazing! I can make sperm but classify as sterile."
3. "I'm sure glad I made some deposits in the sperm bank."
4. "I can't believe I still have to worry about contraception after this surgery."

37. 1. Vasectomy procedures can be reversed but with varying degrees of success. Because of the variable success, a client can't be sure of reversibility and needs to consider vasectomy a permanent sterilization procedure when deciding to have it done. After vasectomy, the client remains fertile until sperm stored distal to the severed vas are evacuated. Once this occurs, sperm are still produced, but they don't enter the ejaculate and are absorbed by the body.
NP: Evaluation; CN: Physiological integrity; CNS: Physiological adaptation; CL: Application

38. Which of the following areas of client teaching should be stressed when the goal is preventing the development of phimosis in a 20-year-old uncircumcised man?

1. Proper cleaning of the prepuce
2. Importance of regular ejaculation
3. Technique of testicular self-examination
4. Proper hand washing before touching the genitals

38. 1. Proper cleaning of the preputial area to remove secretions is critical to the prevention of noncongenital phimosis. Hand washing is important in preventing the spread of infection, and testicular self-examination is important in the early detection and treatment of testicular cancer. Regular ejaculation can decrease the symptoms of chronic prostatitis, but it has no effect on the development of phimosis.
NP: Implementation; CN: Health promotion and maintenance; CNS: Prevention and early detection of disease; CL: Application

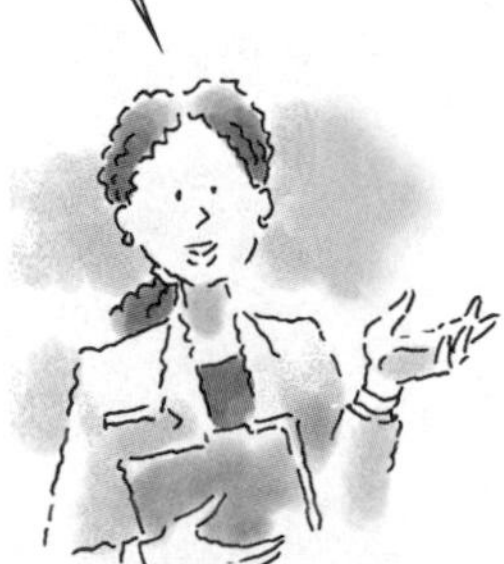

You can ease your client's worries through effective teaching efforts.

39. Which of the following statements should be included when teaching a client newly diagnosed with testicular cancer?

1. Testicular cancer isn't responsive to chemotherapy, but it's highly curative with surgery.
2. Radiation therapy is never used, so the unaffected testicle remains healthy.
3. Testicular self-examination is still important because there's increased risk for a second tumor.
4. Taking testosterone after orchiectomy prevents changes in appearance and sexual function.

39. 3. A history of a testicular malignancy puts the client at increased risk for a second tumor. Testicular self-examination allows for early detection and treatment and is critical. Radiation therapy is used on the retroperitoneal lymph nodes. Chemotherapy is added for clients who have evidence of metastasis after irradiation. Testosterone usually isn't needed because the unaffected testis usually produces sufficient hormone.
NP: Implementation; CN: Physiological integrity; CNS: Reduction of risk potential; CL: Application

40. Which of the following instructions should be given when teaching penile hygiene?
1. Use warm water without soap.
2. Dry all areas of the penis thoroughly.
3. Wash from the base of the shaft to the tip.
4. Avoid retracting the foreskin if not circumcised.

40. 2. Careful drying is essential to avoid maceration of the penis. To decrease the risk for genitourinary infection, wash the penis from the tip to the base to reduce the risk for introducing pathogens into the urethral meatus. Effective cleaning requires soap and thorough rinsing. It's also essential to remove secretions that accumulate under the foreskin because they can lead to inflammation and are associated with the development of penile cancer. The foreskin in uncircumcised men must be retracted for cleaning, then replaced to prevent paraphimosis.

NP: Implementation; CN: Health promotion and maintenance; CNS: Prevention and early detection of disease; CL: Comprehension

41. Which of the following statements shows the significance of a persistent elevation in alphafetoprotein level after orchiectomy for testicular cancer?
1. Fertility is maintained.
2. The cancer has recurred.
3. There is metastatic disease.
4. Testosterone levels are low.

41. 3. Alphafetoprotein is a tumor marker elevated in nonseminomatous malignancies of the testicle. Once the tumor is removed, the level should decrease. A persistent elevation after orchiectomy indicates tumor is present someplace outside the testicle that was removed. A recurrence of the cancer is indicated by a postsurgical decrease in alphafetoprotein level followed by an elevation as a new tumor starts to grow. The level of alphafetoprotein isn't related to fertility or testosterone level.

NP: Assessment; CN: Physiological integrity; CNS: Physiological adaptation; CL: Analysis

42. Which of the following discharge instructions should be given to a client after a prostatectomy?
1. Avoid straining at stool.
2. Report clots in the urine right away.
3. Soak in a warm tub daily for comfort.
4. Return to your usual activities in 3 weeks.

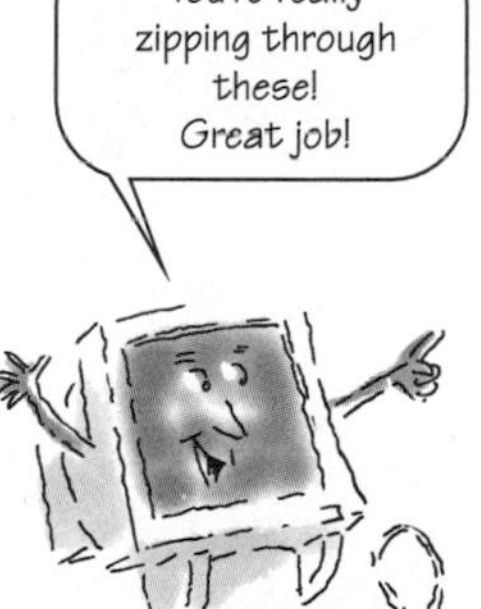

You're really zipping through these! Great job!

42. 1. Straining at stool after prostatectomy can cause bleeding. Small blood clots or pieces of tissue commonly are passed in the urine for up to 2 weeks postoperatively. Tub baths are prohibited because they cause dilation of pelvic blood vessels. Other activities are resumed based on the guidance of the physician. Sexual intercourse and driving are usually prohibited for about 3 weeks. Exercising and returning to work are usually prohibited for about 6 weeks.

NP: Implementation; CN: Physiological integrity; CNS: Reduction of risk potential; CL: Comprehension

43. After a biopsy of the prostate, which of the following symptoms should be reported?
1. Pain on ejaculation
2. Blood in the semen
3. Difficulty urinating
4. Temperature greater than 99°F (37.2° C)

43. 3. Difficulty urinating suggests urethral obstruction. Temperature more than 101°F (38.3° C) should be reported because it suggests infection. Blood in the semen is an expected finding for months, and discomfort on ejaculation is expected for weeks.

NP: Implementation; CN: Physiological integrity; CNS: Reduction of risk potential; CL: Comprehension

44. Two days after a transrectal biopsy of the prostate, a client calls the clinic to report his stool is streaked with blood. Which of the following responses is appropriate?

1. Tell the client to take a laxative.
2. Tell the client to come in for examination.
3. Reassure the client this is an expected occurrence.
4. Ask the client to collect a stool specimen for testing.

44. 3. After a transrectal prostatic biopsy, blood in the stool is expected for a number of days. Because blood in the stool is expected, testing the stool or examining the client isn't necessary. Stool softeners are prescribed if the client complains of constipation; straining at stool can precipitate bleeding, but laxatives generally aren't necessary. The client doesn't need to be seen at this time.

NP: Implementation; CN: Physiological integrity; CNS: Reduction of risk potential; CL: Application

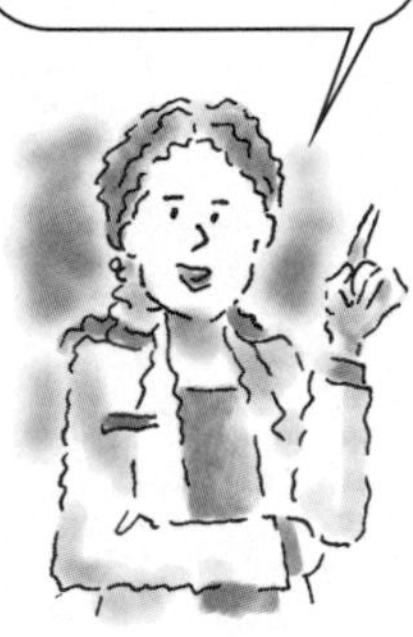

Teach your client the prodromal symptoms of an outbreak of genital herpes.

45. When assessing a client with a history of genital herpes, which of the following symptoms would indicate that an outbreak of lesions is imminent?

1. Headache and fever
2. Vaginal and urethral discharge
3. Dysuria and lymphadenopathy
4. Genital pruritus and paresthesia

45. 4. Pruritus and paresthesia as well as redness of the genital area are prodromal symptoms of recurrent herpes infection. These symptoms occur 30 minutes to 48 hours before the lesions appear. Headache and fever are symptoms of viremia associated with the primary infection. Dysuria and lymphadenopathy are local symptoms of primary infection that may also occur with recurrent infection. Vaginal and urethral discharge is also a local sign of primary infection.

NP: Assessment; CN: Physiological integrity; CNS: Physiological adaptation; CL: Comprehension

46. Which of the following instructions should be given to a woman newly diagnosed with genital herpes?

1. Obtain a Papanicolaou (Pap) test every year.
2. Have your partner use a condom when lesions are present.
3. Use a water-soluble lubricant for relief of pruritus.
4. Limit stress and emotional upset as much as possible.

46. 4. Stress, anxiety, and emotional upset seem to predispose to recurrent outbreaks of genital herpes. During an outbreak, creams and lubricants should be avoided because they may prolong healing. Sexual intercourse should be avoided during outbreaks, and a condom should used between outbreaks; it isn't known if the virus can be transmitted at this time. Because a relationship has been found between genital herpes and cervical cancer, a Pap test is recommended every 6 months.

NP: Implementation; CN: Physiological integrity; CNS: Physiological adaptation; CL: Application

47. Which of the following symptoms is consistent with primary syphilis?

1. A painless genital ulcer that appears about 3 weeks after unprotected sex
2. Copper-colored macules on the palms and soles after a brief fever
3. Patchy hair loss in red, broken skin involving the scalp, eyebrows, and beard area
4. One or more flat, wartlike papules in the genital area that are sensitive to the touch

47. 1. A painless genital ulcer is a symptom of primary syphilis. Macules on the palms and soles after fever are indicative of secondary syphilis, as is patchy hair loss. Wartlike papules are indicative of genital warts.

NP: Assessment; CN: Physiological integrity; CNS: Physiological adaptation; CL: Knowledge

48. A client is describing how she palpates her breasts for breast self-examination. Which of the following statements indicates the need for further teaching?

1. "I put lotion on my breasts before I begin to palpate them."
2. "I palpate both breasts standing up and then lying on my back."
3. "I'm careful to palpate under each arm and up to 2 inches below my collarbone."
4. "I start at the outer edge of the breast and work in to the nipple in smaller and smaller circles."

48. 3. Breast self-examination requires palpation of all breast tissue. This includes checking the area above the breast up to the collarbone and all the way over to the shoulder as well as the area between the breast and the underarm, including the underarm itself. Lotion or powder helps the fingers glide over the skin and facilitates palpation. Breasts need to be palpated in both erect and lying positions. Any pattern of palpation may be used in performing breast self-examination as long as each quadrant of the breast, tail, and axilla are examined.

NP: Evaluation; CN: Health promotion and maintenance; CNS: Prevention and early detection of disease; CL: Application

49. During a routine physical examination, a firm mass is palpated in the right breast of a 35-year-old woman. Which of the following findings or client history would suggest cancer of the breast as opposed to fibrocystic disease?

1. History of early menarche
2. Cyclic change in mass size
3. History of anovulatory cycles
4. Increased vascularity of the breast

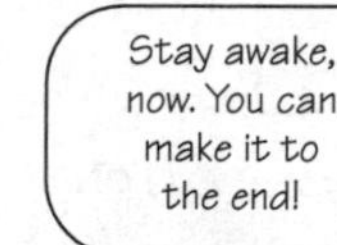

Stay awake, now. You can make it to the end!

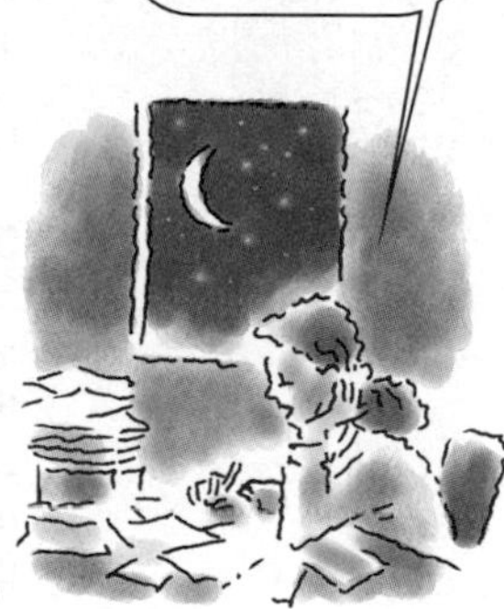

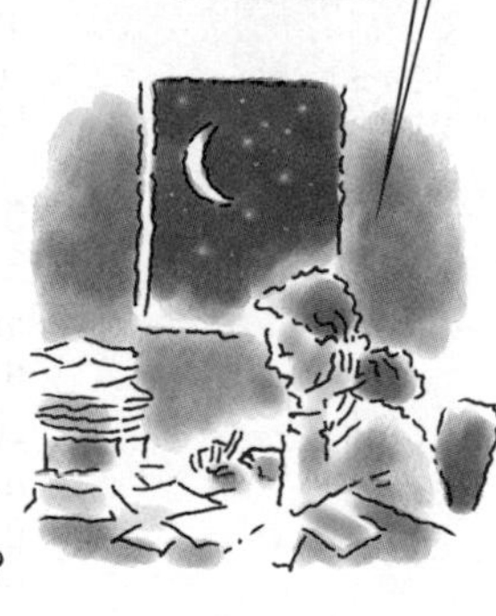

49. 4. Increase in breast size or vascularity is consistent with cancer of the breast. Early menarche as well as late menopause or a history of anovulatory cycles are associated with fibrocystic disease. Masses associated with fibrocystic disease of the breast are firm, most often located in the upper outer quadrant of the breast, and increase in size prior to menstruation. They may be bilateral in a mirror image and are typically well demarcated and freely moveable.

NP: Assessment; CN: Health promotion and maintenance; CNS: Prevention and early detection of disease; CL: Application

50. After which of the following procedures is a postoperative wound infection most likely?

1. Radical prostatectomy
2. Perineal prostatectomy
3. Suprapubic prostatectomy
4. Transurethral resection of the prostate (TURP)

50. 2. The incision in a perineal prostatectomy is close to the rectum, which normally contains gram-negative organisms that can cause infection if introduced into other areas of the body. Therefore, a perineal incision will become contaminated more often than either no external incision, as with TURP, or abdominal incisions, as with suprapubic or radical prostatectomy.

NP: Implementation; CN: Physiological integrity; CNS: Reduction of risk potential; CL: Application

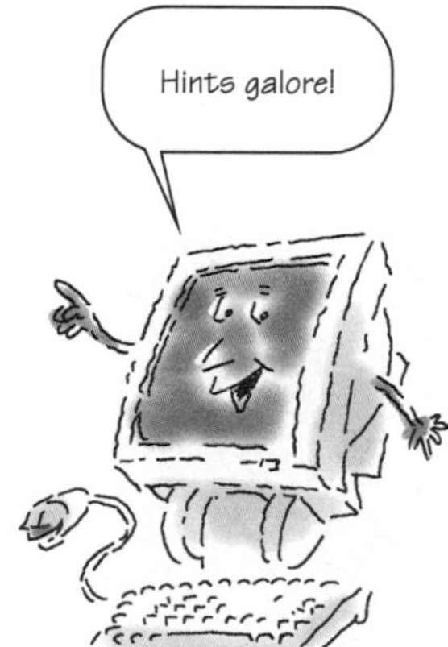

Hints galore!

51. Which of the following conditions is a common cause of prerenal acute renal failure?

1. Atherosclerosis
2. Decreased cardiac output
3. Prostatic hypertrophy
4. Rhabdomyolysis

51. 2. Prerenal refers to renal failure due to an interference with renal perfusion. Decreased cardiac output causes a decrease in renal perfusion, which leads to a lower glomerular filtration rate. Atherosclerosis and rhabdomyolysis are renal causes of acute renal failure. Prostatic hypertrophy would be an example of a postrenal cause of acute renal failure.

NP: Assessment; CN: Physiological integrity; CNS: Physiological adaptation; CL: Knowledge

52. A client admitted for acute pyelonephritis is about to start antibiotic therapy. Which of the following symptoms would be expected in this client?

1. Hypertension
2. Flank pain on the affected side
3. Pain that radiates toward the unaffected side
4. No tenderness with deep palpation over the costovertebral angle

52. 2. The client may complain of pain on the affected side because the kidney is enlarged and might have formed an abscess. Hypertension is associated with chronic pyelonephritis. The client would have tenderness with deep palpation over the costovertebral angle. Pain may radiate down the ureters or to the epigastrium.

NP: Analysis; CN: Physiological integrity; CNS: Physiological adaptation; CL: Knowledge

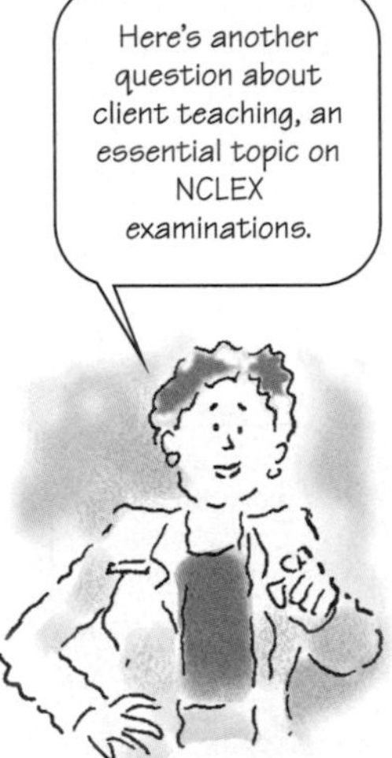

Here's another question about client teaching, an essential topic on NCLEX examinations.

53. Discharge instructions for a client treated for acute pyelonephritis should include which of the following statements?

1. Avoid taking any dairy products.
2. Return for follow-up urine cultures.
3. Stop taking the prescribed antibiotics when the symptoms subside.
4. Recurrence is unlikely because you've been treated with antibiotics.

53. 2. The client needs to return for follow-up urine cultures because bacteriuria may be present but asymptomatic. Pyelonephritis typically recurs as a relapse or new infection and frequently recurs within 2 weeks of completing therapy. Intake of dairy products won't contribute to pyelonephritis. Antibiotics need to be taken for the full course of therapy regardless of symptoms.

NP: Planning; CN: Health promotion and maintenance; CNS: Prevention and early detection of disease; CL: Comprehension

54. A client is complaining of severe flank and abdominal pain. A flat plate of the abdomen shows urolithiasis. Which of the following interventions is important?

1. Strain all urine.
2. Limit fluid intake.
3. Enforce strict bed rest.
4. Encourage a high-calcium diet.

54. 1. Urine should be strained for calculi and sent to the laboratory for analysis. Fluid intake of 3 to 4 qt (3 to 4 L)/day is encouraged to flush the urinary tract and prevent further calculi formation. A low-calcium diet is recommended to help prevent the formation of calcium calculi. Ambulation is encouraged to help pass the calculi through gravity.

NP: Implementation; CN: Physiological integrity; CNS: Reduction of risk potential; CL: Application

55. A client is receiving a radiation implant for the treatment of bladder cancer. Which of the following interventions is appropriate?

1. Flush all urine down the toilet.
2. Restrict the client's fluid intake.
3. Place the client in a semiprivate room.
4. Monitor the client for signs and symptoms of cystitis.

55. 4. Cystitis is the most common adverse reaction of clients undergoing radiation therapy; symptoms include dysuria, frequency, urgency, and nocturia. Clients with radiation implants require a private room. Urine of clients with radiation implants for bladder cancer should be sent to the radioisotopes laboratory for monitoring. It's recommended that fluid intake be increased.

NP: Assessment; CN: Physiological integrity; CNS: Reduction of risk potential; CL: Knowledge

56. A client has undergone a radical cystectomy and has an ileal conduit for the treatment of bladder cancer. Which of the following postoperative assessment findings must be reported to the physician immediately?

1. A red, moist stoma
2. A dusky-colored stoma
3. Urine output more than 30 ml/hour
4. Slight bleeding from the stoma when changing the appliance

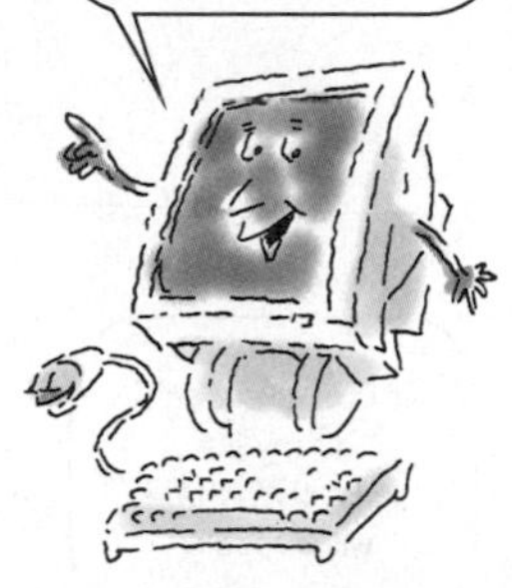

Question 56 asks you to prioritize responses according to which is most urgent.

56. 2. The stoma should be red and moist, indicating adequate blood flow. A dusky or cyanotic stoma indicates insufficient blood supply and is an emergency needing prompt intervention. Urine output less than 30 ml/hour or no urine output for more than 15 minutes should be reported. Slight bleeding from the stoma when changing the appliance may occur because the intestinal mucosa is fragile.

NP: Analysis; CN: Physiological integrity; CNS: Reduction of risk potential; CL: Comprehension

57. Which of the following instructions should be given to a client with an ileal conduit about skin care at the stoma site?

1. Change the appliance at bedtime.
2. Leave the stoma open to air while changing the appliance.
3. Clean the skin around the stoma with mild soap and water and dry it thoroughly.
4. Cut the faceplate or wafer of the appliance no more than 4 mm larger than the stoma.

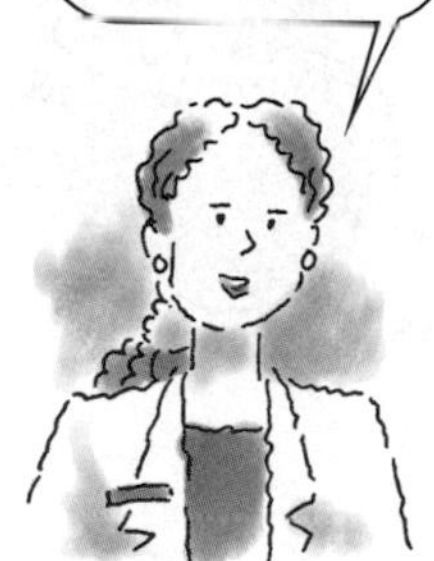

You're doing terrific! Keep up the good work!

57. 3. Cleaning the skin around the stoma with mild soap and water and drying it thoroughly helps keep the area clean from urine, which can irritate the skin. Change the appliance in the early morning when urine output is less to decrease the amount of urine in contact with the skin. The faceplate or wafer of the appliance shouldn't be more than 3 mm larger than the stoma to reduce the skin area in contact with urine. The stoma should be covered with a gauze pad when changing the appliance to prevent seepage of urine onto the skin.

NP: Implementation; CN: Physiological integrity; CNS: Basic care and comfort; CL: Knowledge

58. A client is diagnosed with cystitis. Client teaching aimed at preventing a recurrence should include which of the following instructions?

1. Bathe in a tub.
2. Wear cotton underpants.
3. Use a feminine hygiene spray.
4. Limit your intake of cranberry juice.

58. 2. Cotton underpants prevent infection because they allow for air to flow to the perineum. Women should shower instead of taking a tub bath to prevent infection. Feminine hygiene spray can act as an irritant. Cranberry juice helps prevent cystitis because it increases urine acidity; alkaline urine supports bacterial growth.

NP: Planning; CN: Health promotion and maintenance; CNS: Prevention and early detection of disease; CL: Application

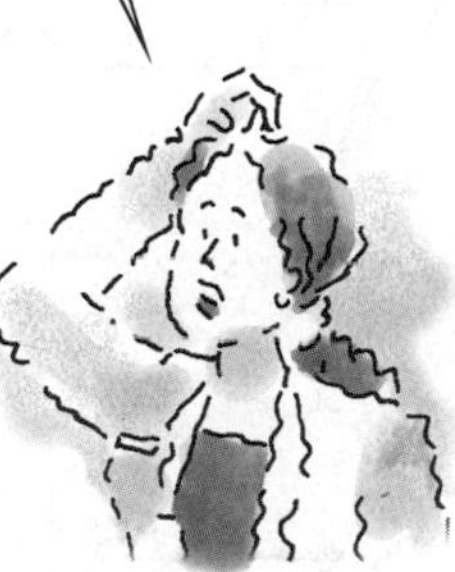

Here's a question straight from Nursing 101. Remember?

59. Care for an indwelling urinary catheter should include which of the following interventions?

1. Insert the catheter using clean technique.
2. Keep the drainage bag on the bed with the client.
3. Clean around the catheter at the meatus with soap and water.
4. Lay the drainage bag on the floor to allow for maximum drainage through gravity.

59. 3. It's important to clean around the meatus at the catheter site to decrease the chance of infection. The drainage bag shouldn't be placed on the floor because of the increased risk of infection due to microorganisms. It should hang on the bed in a dependent position. The catheter should be inserted using sterile technique. Keeping the drainage bag in the bed with the client causes backflow of urine into the urethra, increasing the chance of infection.

NP: Implementation; CN: Physiological integrity; CNS: Reduction of risk potential; CL: Comprehension

60. Which of the following methods should be used to collect a specimen for urine culture?
1. Have the client void in a clean container.
2. Clean the foreskin of the penis of uncircumcised men before specimen collection.
3. Have the client void into a urinal, and then pour the urine into the specimen container.
4. Have the client begin the stream of urine in the toilet and catch the urine in a sterile container midstream.

60. 4. Catching urine midstream reduces the amount of contamination by microorganisms at the meatus. Voiding in a urinal doesn't allow for an uncontaminated specimen because the urinal isn't sterile. When cleaning an uncircumcised male, the foreskin should be retracted, and the glans penis should be cleaned to prevent specimen contamination. Voiding in a clean container is done for a random specimen, not a clean-catch specimen for urine culture.
NP: Implementation; CN: Physiological integrity; CNS: Reduction of risk potential; CL: Knowledge

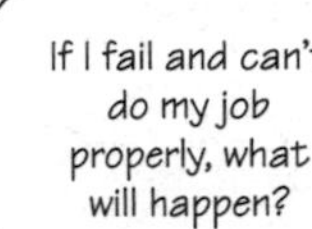

If I fail and can't do my job properly, what will happen?

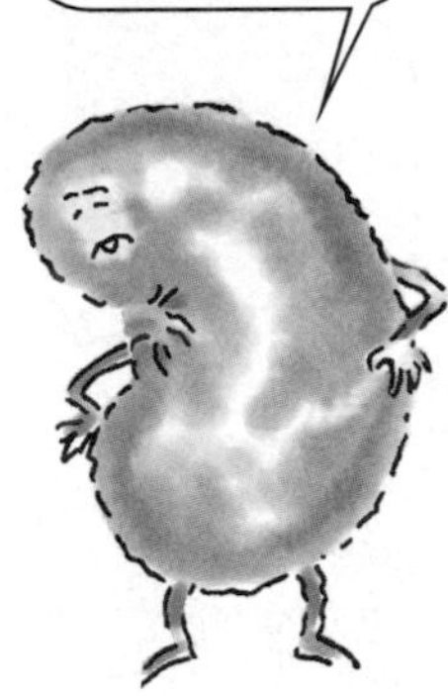

61. A client with a history of chronic renal failure is admitted to the unit with pulmonary edema after missing her dialysis treatment yesterday. Blood is drawn and sent for a chemistry analysis. Which of the following results is expected?
1. Alkalemia
2. Hyperkalemia
3. Hypernatremia
4. Hypokalemia

61. 2. The kidneys are responsible for excreting potassium. In renal failure, the kidneys are no longer able to excrete potassium, resulting in hyperkalemia. Hypokalemia is generally seen in clients undergoing diuresis. The kidneys are responsible for regulating the acid-base balance; in renal failure, acidemia would be seen. Generally, hyponatremia would be seen due to the dilutional effect of water retention.
NP: Assessment; CN: Physiological integrity; CNS: Physiological adaptation; CL: Comprehension

62. Dialysis allows for the exchange of particles across a semipermeable membrane by which of the following actions?
1. Osmosis and diffusion
2. Passage of fluid toward a solution with a lower solute concentration
3. Allowing the passage of blood cells and protein molecules through it
4. Passage of solute particles toward a solution with a higher concentration

62. 1. Osmosis allows for the removal of fluid from the blood by allowing it to pass through the semipermeable membrane to an area of high concentration (dialysate), and diffusion allows for passage of particles (electrolytes, urea, and creatinine) from an area of higher concentration to an area of lower concentration. Fluid passes to an area with a higher solute concentration. The pores of the semipermeable membrane are small, thus preventing the flow of blood cells and protein molecules through it.
NP: Planning; CN: Physiological integrity; CNS: Physiological adaptation; CL: Knowledge

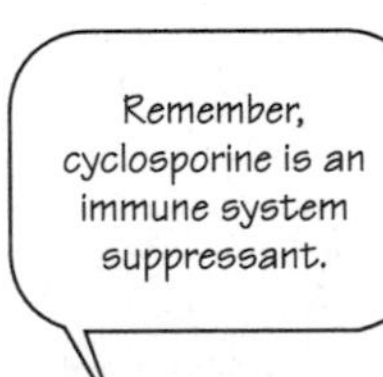

Remember, cyclosporine is an immune system suppressant.

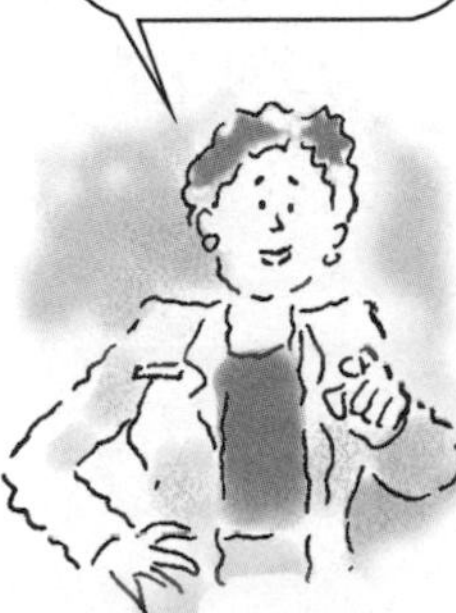

63. A client has just received a renal transplant and has started cyclosporine therapy to prevent graft rejection. Which of the following conditions is a major complication of this drug therapy?
1. Depression
2. Hemorrhage
3. Infection
4. Peptic ulcer disease

63. 3. Infection is the major complication to watch for in clients on cyclosporine therapy because it's an immunosuppressive drug. Depression may occur posttransplantation but not because of cyclosporine. Hemorrhage is a complication associated with anticoagulant therapy. Peptic ulcer disease is a complication of steroid therapy.
NP: Assessment; CN: Physiological integrity; CNS: Pharmacological and parental therapies; CL: Knowledge

64. A client received a kidney transplant 2 months ago. He's admitted to the hospital with the diagnosis of acute rejection. Which of the following assessment findings would be expected?

1. Hypotension
2. Normal body temperature
3. Decreased white blood cell (WBC) counts
4. Elevated blood urea nitrogen and creatinine levels

64. 4. In a client with acute renal graft rejection, evidence of deteriorating renal function is expected. The nurse would see elevated WBC counts and fever because the body is recognizing the graft as foreign and is attempting to fight it. The client would most likely have acute hypertension.

NP: Assessment; CN: Physiological integrity; CNS: Reduction of risk potential; CL: Analysis

65. A client is diagnosed with chronic renal failure and told she must start hemodialysis. Client teaching would include which of the following instructions?

1. Follow a high-potassium diet.
2. Strictly follow the hemodialysis schedule.
3. There will be few changes in your lifestyle.
4. Use alcohol on the skin to clean it due to integumentary changes.

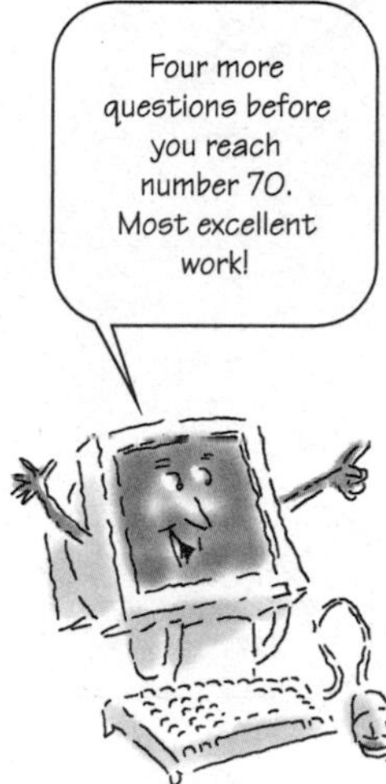

Four more questions before you reach number 70. Most excellent work!

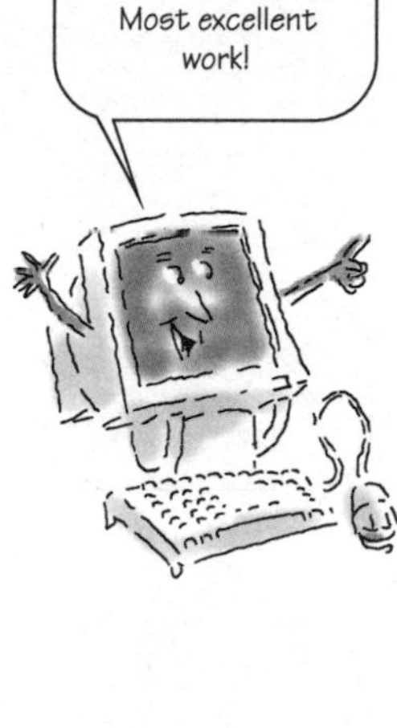

65. 2. To prevent life-threatening complications, the client must follow the dialysis schedule. Alcohol would further dry the client's skin more than it already is. The client should follow a low-potassium diet because potassium levels increase in chronic renal failure. The client should know hemodialysis is time-consuming and will definitely cause a change in current lifestyle.

NP: Planning; CN: Physiological integrity; CNS: Reduction of risk potential; CL: Comprehension

66. A client is to undergo a kidney transplantation with a living donor. Which of the following preoperative assessments is important?

1. Urine output
2. Signs of graft rejection
3. Signs and symptoms of infection
4. Client's support system and understanding of lifestyle changes

66. 4. The client undergoing a renal transplantation will need vigilant follow-up care and must adhere to the medical regimen. The client is most likely anuric or oliguric preoperatively, but postoperatively will require close monitoring of urine output to make sure the transplanted kidney is functioning optimally. While the client will always need to be monitored for signs and symptoms of infection, it's most important postoperatively due to the initiation of immunosuppressive therapy. Rejection can occur postoperatively.

NP: Assessment; CN: Psychosocial integrity; CNS: Coping and adaptation; CL: Application

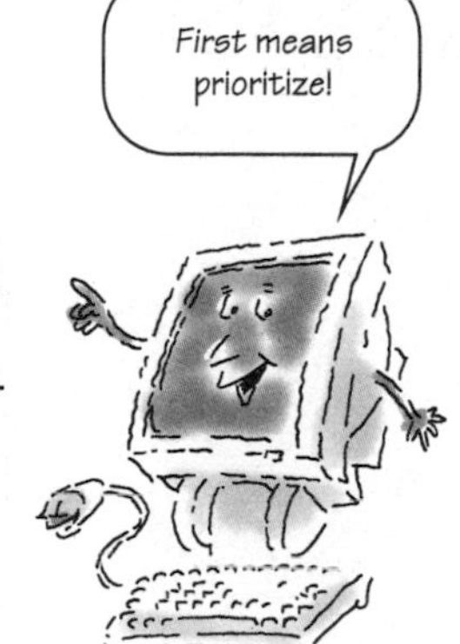

First means prioritize!

67. A client is undergoing peritoneal dialysis. The dialysate dwell time is completed, and the clamp is opened to allow the dialysate to drain. The nurse notes that drainage has stopped and only 500 ml has drained; the amount of dialysate instilled was 1,500 ml. Which of the following interventions would be done first?

1. Change the client's position.
2. Call the physician.
3. Check the catheter for kinks or obstruction.
4. Clamp the catheter and instill more dialysate at the next exchange time.

67. 3. The first intervention should be to check for kinks and obstructions because that could be preventing drainage. After checking for kinks, have the client change position to promote drainage. Don't give the next scheduled exchange until the dialysate is drained because abdominal distention will occur, unless the output is within the parameters set by the physician. If unable to get more output despite checking for kinks and changing the client's position, the nurse should then call the physician to determine the proper intervention.

NP: Implementation; CN: Physiological integrity; CNS: Reduction of risk potential; CL: Analysis

68. A client with receiving hemodialysis treatment arrives at the hospital with a blood pressure of 200/100 mm Hg, heart rate of 110 beats/minute, and a respiratory rate of 36 breaths/minute. Oxygen saturation in room air is 89%. He complains of shortness of breath, and +2 pedal edema is noted. His last hemodialysis treatment was yesterday. Which of the following interventions should be done first?

1. Administer oxygen.
2. Elevate the foot of the bed.
3. Restrict the client's fluids.
4. Prepare the client for hemodialysis.

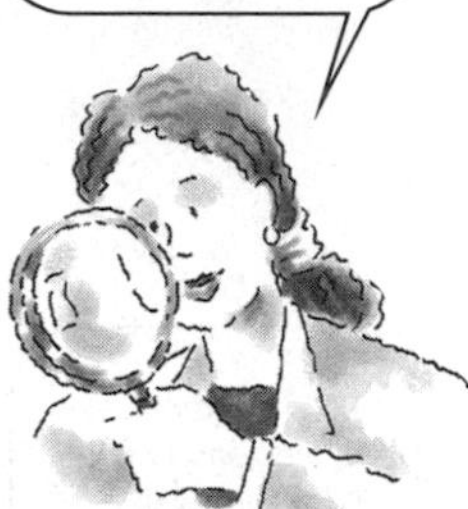

There's a lot of information given here. Look closely for the common patterns.

68. 1. Airway and oxygenation are always the first priority. Because the client is complaining of shortness of breath and his oxygen saturation is only 89%, the nurse needs to try to increase the Pao_2 by administering oxygen. The client is in pulmonary edema from fluid overload and will need to be dialyzed and have his fluids restricted, but the first intervention should be aimed at the immediate treatment of hypoxia. The foot of the bed may be elevated to reduce edema, but this isn't a priority.
NP: Implementation; CN: Physiological integrity; CNS: Physiological adaptation; CL: Analysis

69. A client with renal insufficiency is admitted with a diagnosis of pneumonia. He's being treated with I.V. antibiotics, which can be nephrotoxic. Which of the following laboratory values should be monitored closely?

1. Blood urea nitrogen (BUN) and creatinine levels
2. Arterial blood gas (ABG) levels
3. Platelet count
4. Potassium level

69. 1. BUN and creatinine levels should be monitored closely to detect elevations due to nephrotoxicity. ABG determinations are inappropriate for this situation. Platelets and potassium levels should be monitored according to routine.
NP: Assessment; CN: Physiological integrity; CNS: Reduction of risk potential; CL: Analysis

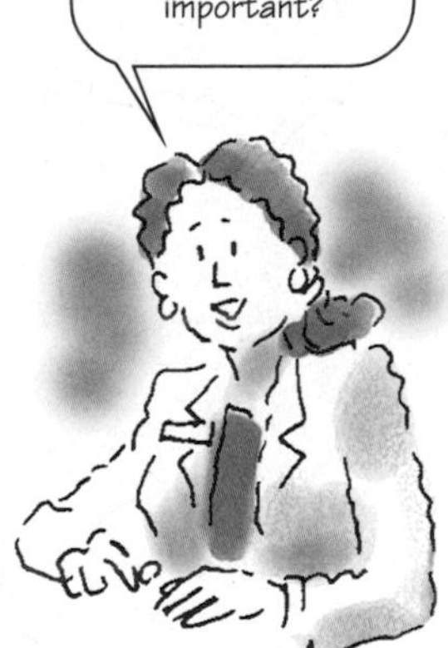

Lots to do, but what's the most important?

70. A client had transurethral prostatectomy for benign prostatic hypertrophy. He's currently being treated with a continuous bladder irrigation and is complaining of an increase in severity of bladder spasms. Which of the following interventions should be done first?

1. Administer an oral analgesic.
2. Stop the irrigation and call the physician.
3. Administer a belladonna and opium suppository as ordered by the physician
4. Check for the presence of clots, and make sure the catheter is draining properly.

70. 4. Blood clots and blocked outflow of the urine can increase spasms. The irrigation shouldn't be stopped as long as the catheter is draining because clots will form. A belladonna and opium suppository should be given to relieve spasms but only *after* assessment of the drainage. Oral analgesics should be given if the spasms are unrelieved by the belladonna and opium suppository.
NP: Implementation; CN: Physiological integrity; CNS: Physiological adaptation; CL: Comprehension

71. Proper maintenance of a continuous bladder irrigation system includes which of the following interventions?

1. Regulate irrigant flow to maintain red urine.
2. Regulate irrigant flow to maintain a good outflow of pink urine.
3. Maintain a slow flow rate of irrigant to prevent bladder distention.
4. Stop the irrigation if there is leakage of large amounts of urine around the catheter.

71. 2. The irrigant should be infused at a rate fast enough to maintain pink urine. Red urine indicates inadequate irrigation and possible clot formation. Bladder distention shouldn't occur as long as the system is draining properly and no clots are obstructing the outflow of urine. Leakage of urine around the catheter indicates clot formation on the catheter tip, needing manual irrigation. The irrigation shouldn't be stopped due to the potential for clot formation.
NP: Implementation; CN: Physiological integrity; CNS: Physiological adaptation; CL: Comprehension

72. A client has an indwelling urinary catheter, and urine is leaking from a hole in the collection bag. Which of the following nursing interventions would be most appropriate?

1. Cover the hole with tape.
2. Remove the catheter and insert a new one using sterile technique.
3. Disconnect the drainage bag from the catheter and replace it with a new bag.
4. Place a towel under the bag to prevent spillage of urine on the floor, which could cause the client to slip and fall.

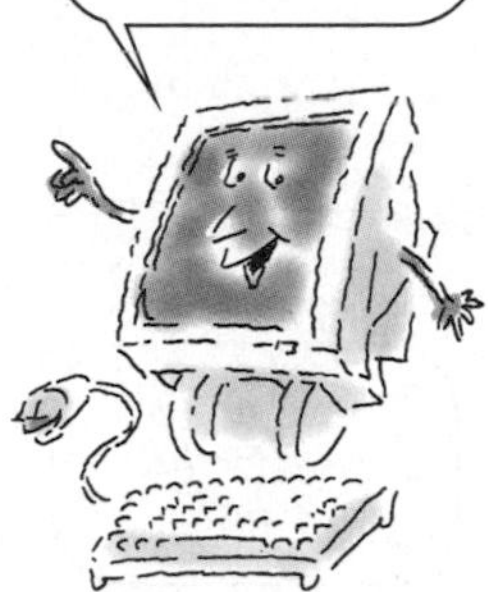

Here are those words: most appropriate. Don't you just love 'em?

72. 2. The system is no longer a closed system, and bacteria might have been introduced into the system, so a new sterile catheter should be inserted. Placing a towel under the bag and taping up the hole leave the system open, which increases the risk of infection. Replacing the drainage bag by disconnecting the old one from the catheter opens up the entire system and isn't recommended due to the increased risk of infection.

NP: Implementation; CN: Safe, effective care environment; CNS: Safety and infection control; CL: Analysis

73. A client is admitted with a diagnosis of hydronephrosis secondary to calculi. The calculi have been removed and postobstructive diuresis is occurring. Which of the following interventions should be done?

1. Take vital signs every 8 hours.
2. Weigh the client every other day.
3. Assess the urine output every shift.
4. Monitor the client's electrolyte levels.

73. 4. Postobstructive diuresis seen in hydronephrosis can cause electrolyte imbalances; laboratory values must be checked so electrolytes can be replaced as needed. Vital signs should initially be taken every 30 minutes for the first 4 hours and then every 2 hours. Urine output needs to be assessed hourly. The client's weight should be taken daily to assess fluid status more closely.

NP: Assessment; CN: Physiological integrity; CNS: Reduction of risk potential; CL: Analysis

74. A client is admitted with severe nausea, vomiting, and diarrhea and is hypotensive. She's noted to have severe oliguria with elevated blood urea nitrogen (BUN) and creatinine levels. The physician will most likely write an order for which of the following treatments?

1. Force oral fluids.
2. Give furosemide 20 mg I.V.
3. Start hemodialysis after a temporary access is obtained.
4. Start I.V. fluid of normal saline solution bolus followed by a maintenance dose.

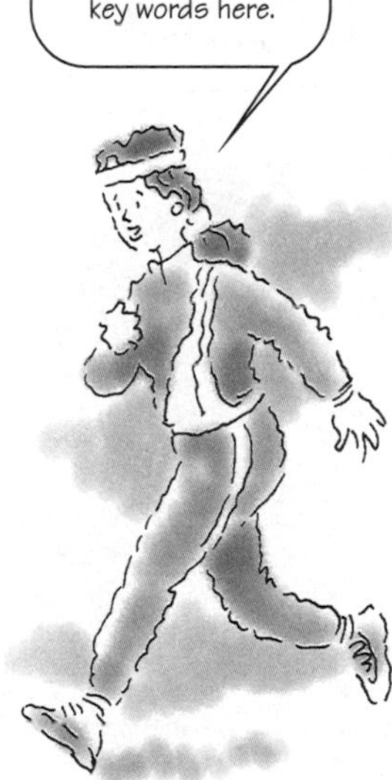

Most and likely are key words here.

74. 4. The client is prerenal secondary to hypovolemia. I.V. fluids should be given to rehydrate the client, urine output should increase, and the BUN and creatinine levels will normalize. The client wouldn't be able to tolerate oral fluids due to the nausea, vomiting, and diarrhea. The client isn't fluid overloaded, and her urine output won't increase with furosemide. The client won't need dialysis because the oliguria and increased blood urea nitrogen and creatinine levels are due to dehydration.

NP: Planning; CN: Physiological integrity; CNS: Physiological adaptation; CL: Analysis

75. A client has a history of chronic renal failure and receives hemodialysis treatments three times a week through an arteriovenous (AV) fistula in the left arm. Which of the following interventions is included in this client's care?

1. Keep the AV fistula site dry.
2. Keep the AV fistula wrapped in gauze.
3. Take the blood pressure in the left arm.
4. Assess the AV fistula for a bruit and thrill.

75. 4. Assessment of the AV fistula for bruit and thrill is important because, if not present, it indicates a nonfunctioning fistula. No blood pressures or venipunctures should be taken in the arm with the AV fistula. When not being dialyzed, the AV fistula site may get wet. Immediately after a dialysis treatment, the access site is covered with adhesive bandages.

NP: Implementation; CN: Physiological integrity; CNS: Physiological adaptation; CL: Application

76. Inflammation, incomplete bladder emptying, and anxiety may cause urinary frequency. Which of the following factors is also associated with urinary frequency?

1. Dehydration
2. Imipramine use
3. Opiate analgesics
4. Pressure from abdominal masses

76. 4. Abdominal masses may cause pressure on the bladder, reducing the capacity of the bladder (such as a pregnant uterus) or a urinary tract infection. Imipramine and narcotic analgesics can cause urinary retention, not frequency, and dehydration usually results in diminished output.

NP: Assessment; CN: Physiological integrity; CNS: Physiological adaptation; CL: Knowledge

77. A woman who reports painful urination during or after voiding might have a problem in which of the following locations?

1. Bladder
2. Kidneys
3. Ureters
4. Urethra

77. 1. Pain during or after voiding indicates a bladder problem, usually infection. Kidney and ureter pain would be in the flank area, and problems of the urethra would cause pain at the external orifice that's often felt at the start of voiding.

NP: Assessment; CN: Health promotion and maintenance; CNS: Prevention and early detection of disease; CL: Knowledge

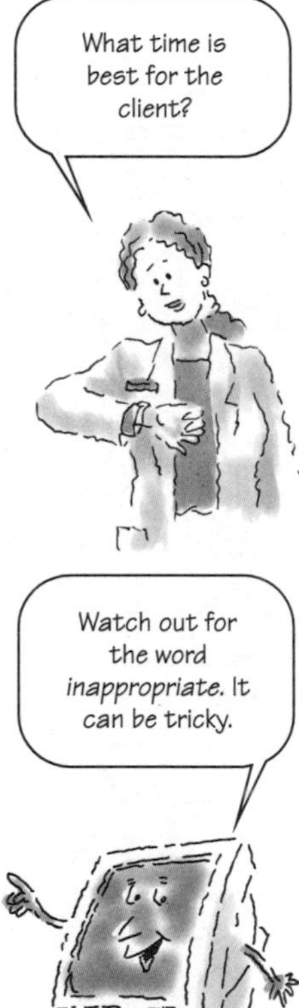

What time is best for the client?
Watch out for the word *inappropriate*. It can be tricky.

78. What is the best time of day to give diuretics?

1. Anytime
2. Bedtime
3. Morning
4. Noon

78. 3. A diuretic given in the morning has time to work throughout the day. Diuretics given at nighttime will cause the client to get up to go to the bathroom frequently, interrupting sleep.

NP: Implementation; CN: Physiological integrity; CNS: Pharmacological and parenteral therapies; CL: Application

79. Which of the following interventions would be inappropriate to help a client with postoperative urinary retention?

1. Give a diuretic.
2. Pour warm water over the perineum.
3. Consider inserting a bladder catheter.
4. Place the client in a sitting or semi-Fowler position.

79. 1. Urinary retention reflects bladder distention from urine. A diuretic isn't necessary. Sitting upright and pouring water over the perineum may help the client void. If these measures aren't successful, the nurse should consider inserting a bladder catheter to drain the bladder. This procedure needs an order from the primary health care provider.

NP: Planning; CN: Physiological integrity; CNS: Basic care and comfort; CL: Application

80. Which of the following factors may place a surgical client at risk for urinary retention?

1. Dehydration
2. History of smoking
3. Duration of surgery
4. Anticholinergic medication before surgery

80. 4. Anticholinergic medications, such as atropine and scopolamine, may cause urinary retention, particularly for the client who has surgery in the pelvic area (inguinal hernia, hysterectomy). Dehydration, smoking, and duration of surgery aren't risk factors for retention, although opiate analgesics are risk factors.

NP: Planning; CN: Physiological integrity; CNS: Reduction of risk potential; CL: Comprehension

81. Which type of catheter is generally used for the client with urine retention?

1. Coudé
2. Indwelling urinary
3. Straight
4. Three-way

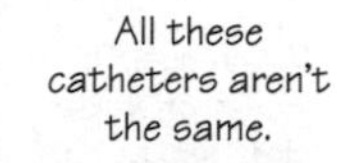

All these catheters aren't the same.

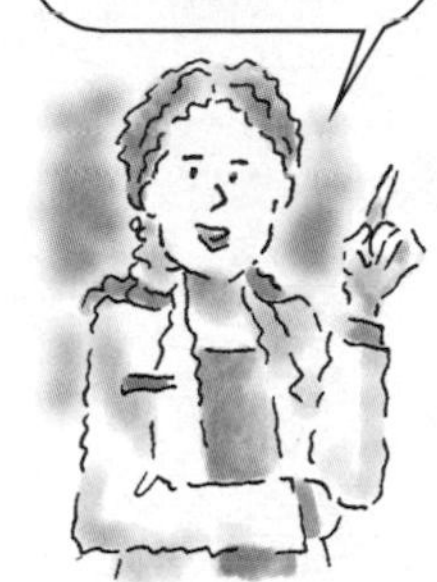

81. 3. Urine retention is usually a temporary problem that requires insertion of a straight catheter. The other catheters are used for longer-term bladder problems. A three-way catheter is used for clients who need bladder irrigation such as after a prostate resection. A catheter coudé is used only when it's difficult to insert a standard catheter, usually because of an enlarged prostate.

NP: Implementation; CN: Physiological integrity; CNS: Basic care and comfort; CL: Comprehension

82. An 80-year-old man reports urine retention. Which of the following factors may contribute to this client's problem?

1. Benign prostatic hyperplasia (BPH)
2. Diabetes
3. Diet
4. Hypertension

82. 1. BPH is common among elderly men and often results in urine retention, frequency, dribbling, and difficulty starting the urine stream. Diet, hypertension, and diabetes usually don't affect urine retention. Diabetes can cause renal failure.

NP: Assessment; CN: Physiological integrity; CNS: Reduction of risk potential; CL: Application

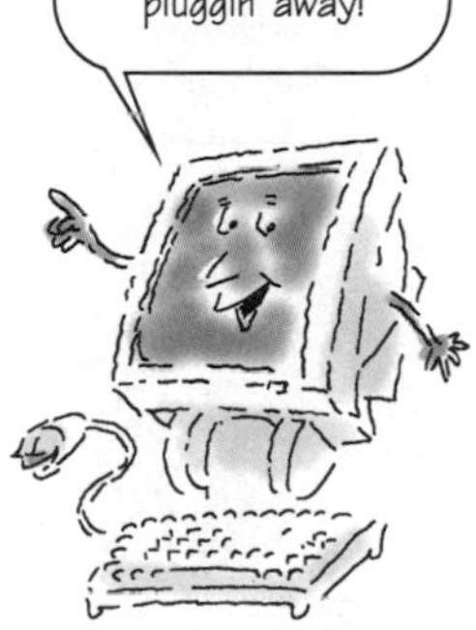

You're doing a great job! Keep pluggin' away!

83. Serum creatinine levels provide the most accurate picture of renal function for which of the following reasons?

1. Serum creatinine is rapidly reabsorbed by the renal tubules.
2. A slow urine flow through the kidneys increases creatinine level.
3. Serum creatinine levels indicate a decrease in glomerular filtration.
4. Serum creatinine levels are related to the rate of urine flow through the kidneys.

83. 3. Creatinine is filtered by the glomeruli and isn't reabsorbed by the renal tubules. A defect in glomerular filtration would cause an increase in serum creatinine level. Urea is rapidly reabsorbed by renal tubules and is related to the rate of urine flow through the kidneys. A slow urine flow can cause an increase in the blood urea nitrogen level without renal disease.

NP: Assessment; CN: Physiological integrity; CNS: Reduction of risk potential; CL: Knowledge

84. A urologic client undergoes excretory urography to evaluate which of the following areas?

1. Kidney function
2. Kidneys, ureters, and bladder
3. Abnormalities of the lower urinary tract
4. Abnormalities of the upper urinary tract

84. 2. Excretory urography identifies calculi or masses and helps diagnose other anomalies of the upper and lower urinary tract (kidney, ureters, urethra, bladder).

NP: Implementation; CN: Health promotion and maintenance; CNS: Prevention and early detection of disease; CL: Comprehension

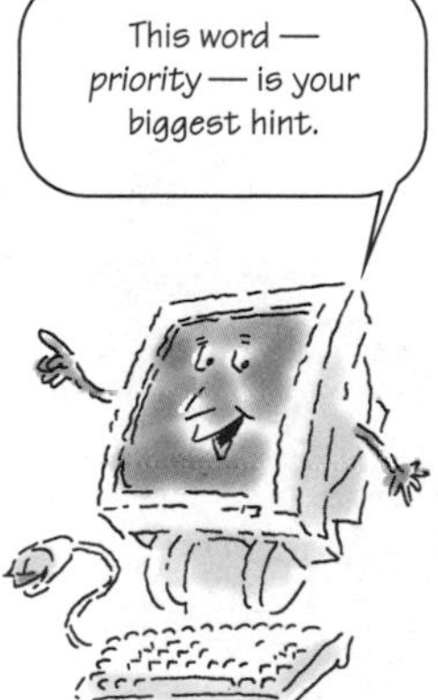

This word — *priority* — is your biggest hint.

85. A client is injected with radiographic contrast medium and immediately shows signs of dyspnea, flushing, and pruritis. Which of the following interventions should take priority?

1. Check vital signs.
2. Make sure the airway is patent.
3. Apply a cold pack to the I.V. site.
4. Call the physician.

85. 2. The client is showing symptoms of an allergy to the iodine in the contrast medium. The first action is to make sure the client's airway is patent. If compromised, call a cardiac arrest code. Checking vital signs and calling for the physician are important nursing actions but should follow making sure the airway is patent. A cold pack isn't indicated.

NP: Implementation; CN: Physiological integrity; CNS: Physiological adaptation; CL: Application

86. An 80-year-old man is admitted for a cystoscopy with biopsy of the bladder. After getting a history, surgery is postponed. Which of the following reasons would *not* be cause to postpone this client's surgery?

1. The client is on an anticoagulant.
2. The client has a urinary tract infection.
3. The client might have carcinoma of the bladder.
4. The client reports chest pain at rest for the past 3 days.

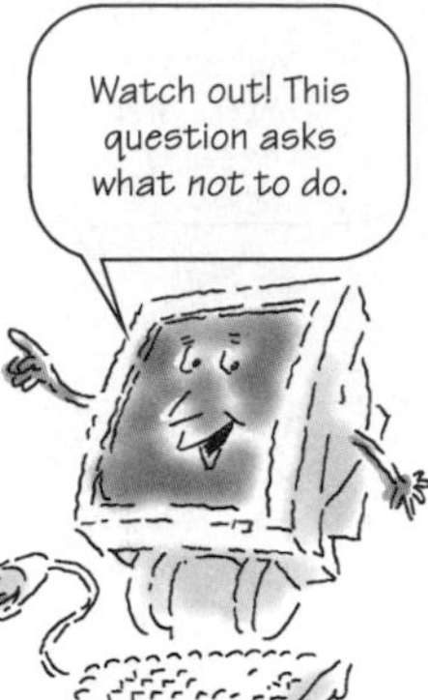

Watch out! This question asks what not to do.

86. 3. Suspected bladder carcinoma is probably the reason for the planned biopsy. Bladder biopsies shouldn't be done when an active urinary tract infection is present because sepsis may result. Chest pain at rest may indicate myocardial ischemia and would be an indication to postpone the biopsy until it can be further investigated. Anticoagulants should be discontinued for 3 to 5 days before the procedure.
NP: Implementation; CN: Physiological integrity; CNS: Reduction of risk potential; CL: Analysis

87. Unless there are postoperative complications, a cystoscopy client is discharged to home within 24 hours. Which of the following instructions is given at discharge?

1. Expect bloody urine for about a week.
2. Drink 8 to 10 glasses of water every 8 hours.
3. Try to urinate frequently, and measure your output.
4. Check the color, consistency, and amount of urine in the indwelling urinary catheter bag every 4 to 8 hours.

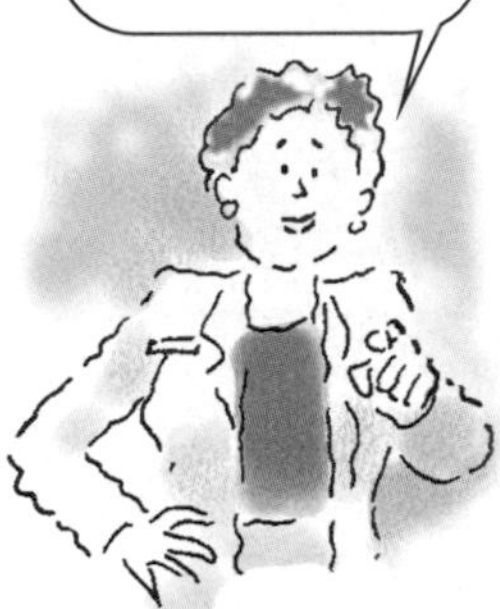

What would your client do without your professional, comprehensive teaching?

87. 3. The bladder needs to be emptied frequently, and output should be measured to make sure the bladder is emptying. Large amounts of fluids help flush microorganisms out of the body, but 8 to 10 glasses every 8 hours may not be reasonable. Also, clients don't tend to think in time periods, so instructions should be given per day. The client may not have an indwelling urinary catheter. Blood in the urine isn't normal except for small amounts during the first 24 hours after the procedure.
NP: Implementation; CN: Physiological integrity; CNS: Reduction of risk potential; CL: Application

88. Before a renal biopsy, which of the following information is most important to tell the physician?

1. The client signed a consent form.
2. The client understands the procedure.
3. The client has normal urinary elimination.
4. The client regularly takes aspirin or nonsteroidal anti-inflammatory drugs (NSAIDs).

88. 4. Aspirin and NSAIDs cause increased bleeding times and often result in hemorrhaging when biopsies are performed. It's the physician's responsibility to make sure the client understands the procedure, which is needed for informed consent. It isn't necessary to report that the client has normal urinary elimination.
NP: Implementation; CN: Physiological integrity; CNS: Reduction of risk potential; CL: Application

89. Kegel exercises are used to gain control of bladder function in women with stress incontinence and some men after prostate surgery. Which of the following instructions would help the client perform these exercises?

1. Completely empty the bladder.
2. Do the exercise 200 times a day.
3. Sit or stand with your legs together.
4. Drink small amounts of fluid frequently.

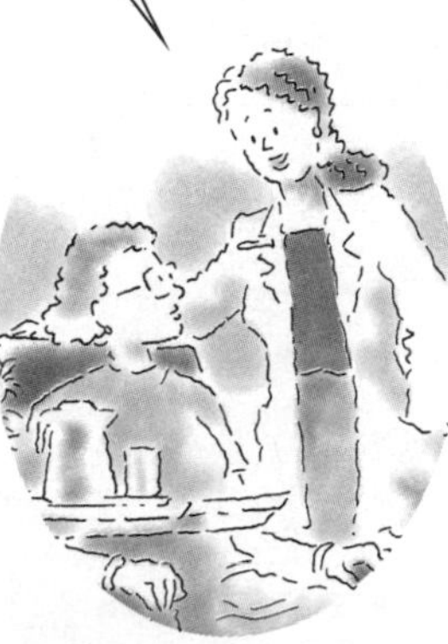

Kegel exercises can help the client gain bladder control.

89. 2. Exercises begin with tightening and relaxing the vagina, rectum, and urethra four or five times during each session and gradually increasing to 25 times for each session. The client stops the flow of urine during urination to practice holding the flow. Standing or sitting with the legs apart facilitates the exercise. Clients should drink plenty of fluids to prevent urinary problems.
NP: Evaluation; CN: Physiological integrity; CNS: Physiological adaptation; CL: Application

NP: Nursing process CN: Client needs category CNS: Client needs subcategory CL: Cognitive level

90. Which of the following instructions is given to clients with chronic pyelonephritis?
1. Stay on bed rest for up to 2 weeks.
2. Use analgesia on a regular basis for up to 6 months.
3. Have a urine culture every 2 weeks for up to 6 months.
4. You may need antibiotic treatment for several weeks or months.

90. 4. Chronic pyelonephritis can be a long-term condition and requires close monitoring to prevent permanent damage to the kidneys. Analgesia and bed rest may be used during the acute stage but usually aren't required long-term. A urine culture is done 2 weeks after stopping antibiotics to make sure the infection has been eradicated.

NP: Implementation; CN: Physiological integrity; CNS: Reduction of risk control; CL: Application

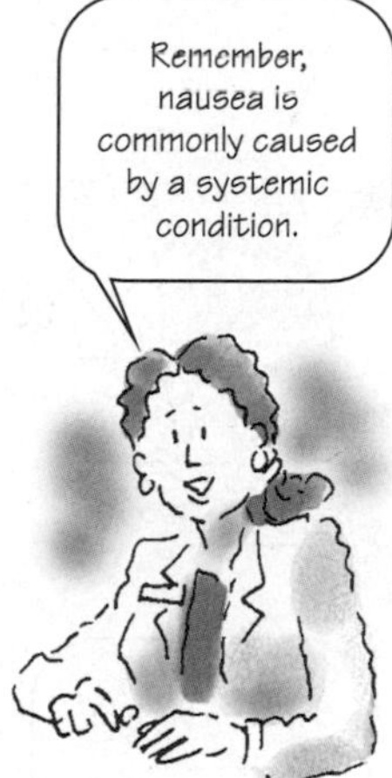

Remember, nausea is commonly caused by a systemic condition.

91. Which of the following factors causes the nausea associated with renal failure?
1. Oliguria
2. Gastric ulcers
3. Electrolyte imbalance
4. Accumulation of metabolic wastes

91. 4. Although clients with renal failure can develop stress ulcers, the nausea is usually related to the poisons of metabolic wastes that accumulate when the kidneys are unable to eliminate them. The client has electrolyte imbalances and oliguria, but these don't directly cause nausea.

NP: Assessment; CN: Physiological integrity; CNS: Physiological adaptation; CL: Comprehension

92. Which of the following clients is at greatest risk for developing acute renal failure?
1. A dialysis client who gets influenza
2. A teenager who has an appendectomy
3. A pregnant woman who has a fractured femur
4. A client with diabetes who has a heart catheterization

92. 4. Clients with diabetes are prone to renal insufficiency and renal failure. The contrast used for heart catheterization must be eliminated by the kidneys, which further stresses them and may produce acute renal failure. A teenager who has an appendectomy and a pregnant woman who fractures a femur aren't at increased risk for renal failure. A dialysis client already has end-stage renal disease and wouldn't develop acute renal failure.

NP: Assessment; CN: Health promotion and maintenance; CNS: Prevention and early detection of disease; CL: Analysis

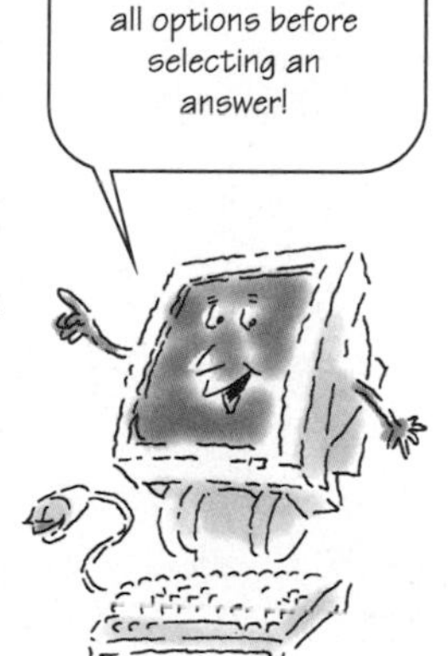

Carefully consider all options before selecting an answer!

93. Which of the following interventions would be done for a client with urinary calculus?
1. Save any calculi larger than 0.25 cm.
2. Strain the urine, limit oral fluids, give pain medications.
3. Encourage fluid intake, strain the urine, give pain medications.
4. Insert an indwelling urinary catheter, check intake and output, give pain medications.

93. 3. Encourage fluid intake, and strain all urine, saving all calculi, including "flecks." Give pain medications because renal calculi are painful. Indwelling urinary catheters aren't usually needed.

NP: Planning; CN: Physiological integrity; CNS: Basic care and comfort; CL: Application

94. Which of the following interventions is inappropriate for a client on hemodialysis?

1. Palpate for a thrill on the arm with the fistula.
2. Auscultate for a bruit on the arm with the fistula.
3. Report the absence of a thrill or bruit on the arm with the fistula.
4. Take the blood pressure, or start an I.V. on the arm with the fistula.

95. A client has passed a renal calculus. The nurse sends the specimen to the laboratory so it can be analyzed for which of the following factors?

1. Antibodies
2. Type of infection
3. Composition of calculus
4. Size and number of calculi

96. Which of the following symptoms indicate acute rejection of a transplanted kidney?

1. Edema, nausea
2. Fever, anorexia
3. Weight gain, pain at graft site
4. Increased white blood cell count, pain with voiding

97. Adverse reactions of prednisone therapy include which of the following conditions?

1. Acne and bleeding gums
2. Sodium retention and constipation
3. Mood swings and increased temperature
4. Increased blood glucose levels and decreased wound healing

98. Steroids, such as prednisone and methylprednisolone, are used to suppress the inflammatory immune response following a kidney transplant. Which of the following pieces of information should be given to a client with a transplant?

1. Alopecia may occur.
2. Orthostatic hypotension is common.
3. Cholesterol levels may become elevated.
4. Blood glucose levels may become elevated.

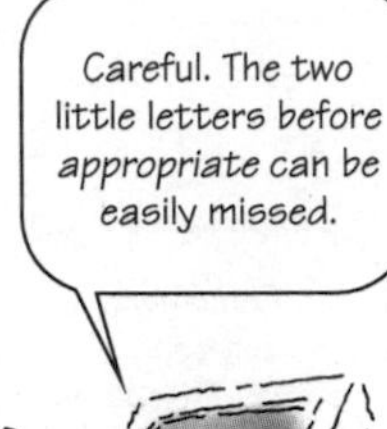

Careful. The two little letters before appropriate can be easily missed.

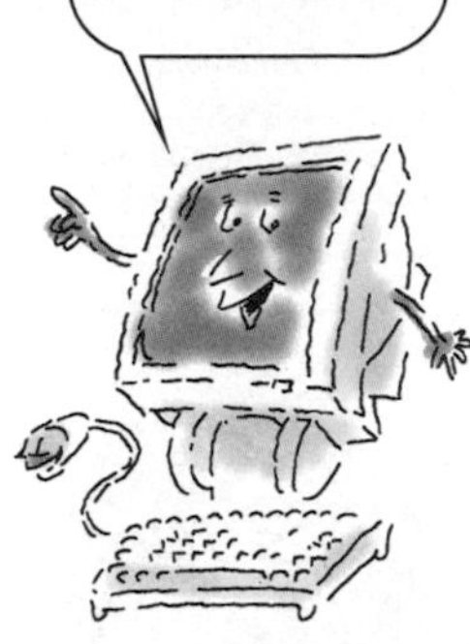

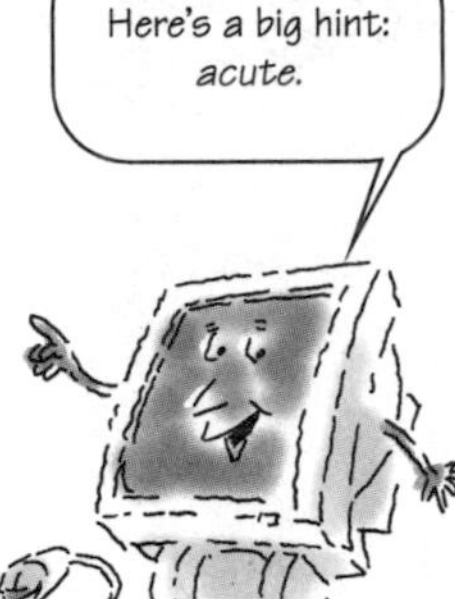

Here's a big hint: acute.

94. 4. The nurse would palpate for a thrill and auscultate for a bruit on the arm with a fistula, but no procedures (I.V. access, blood pressure, or blood draw) should be done on the arm with a fistula because it could damage the fistula. The absence of a thrill or bruit should be reported promptly to the physician because it indicates an occlusion.

NP: Implementation; CN: Physiological integrity; CNS: Reduction of risk potential; CL: Application

95. 3. The calculus should be analyzed for composition to determine appropriate interventions such as dietary restrictions. Calculi don't result from infections. The size and number of calculi aren't relevant, and they don't contain antibodies.

NP: Evaluation; CN: Physiological integrity; CNS: Reduction of risk potential; CL: Application

96. 3. Pain at the graft site and weight gain indicate the transplanted kidney isn't functioning and possibly is being rejected. Transplant clients typically have edema, anorexia, fever, and nausea before transplantation, so those symptoms may not indicate rejection.

NP: Evaluation; CN: Health promotion and maintenance; CNS: Prevention and early detection of disease; CL: Analysis

97. 4. Steroid use tends to increase blood glucose levels, particularly in clients with diabetes and borderline diabetes. Steroids also contribute to poor wound healing and may cause acne, mood swings, and sodium and water retention. Steroids don't affect thermoregulation, bleeding tendencies, or constipation.

NP: Evaluation; CN: Physiological integrity; CNS: Pharmacological and parenteral therapies; CL: Analysis

98. 4. Steroids may increase blood glucose levels but don't increase cholesterol levels. Hirsutism may occur, but not alopecia. Hypertension is common, not orthostatic hypotension. Weight gain is often reported, not weight loss.

NP: Implementation; CN: Physiological integrity; CNS: Pharmacological and parenteral therapies; CL: Analysis

99. The nurse suspects that a client with polyuria is experiencing water diuresis. Which laboratory value suggests water diuresis?

1. High urine specific gravity
2. High urine osmolarity
3. Normal to low urine specific gravity
4. Elevated urine pH

99. 3. Water diuresis causes low urine specific gravity, low urine osmolarity, and a normal to elevated serum sodium level. High specific gravity indicates dehydration. Hypernatremia signals acidosis and shock. Elevated urine pH can result from potassium deficiency, a high-protein diet, or uncontrolled diabetes.

NP: Assessment; CN: Physiological integrity; CNS: Physiological adaptation; CL: Application

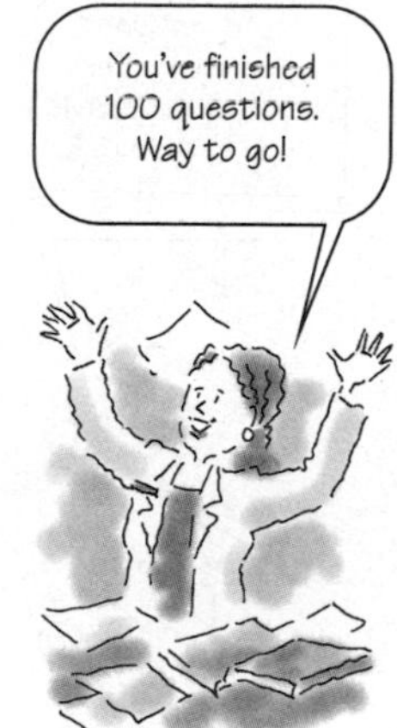

You've finished 100 questions. Way to go!

100. A client is diagnosed with genitourinary tuberculosis, which can infect the kidney, ureter, bladder, testes, and epididymis. Which statement about genitourinary tuberculosis is true?

1. It isn't infectious and can't be passed from one person to another.
2. It can't be passed sexually from partner to partner.
3. It's a late manifestation of respiratory tuberculosis.
4. It's an early manifestation of an autoimmune disorder.

100. 3. Genitourinary tuberculosis is usually a late manifestation of respiratory tuberculosis and can occur if the disease spreads through the bloodstream from the lungs. Bacillus in the urine is infectious, and urine should be handled cautiously. A condom should be used during sex to prevent spread of the infection.

NP: Implementation; CN: Physiological integrity; CNS: Physiological adaptation; CL: Knowledge

101. A client is diagnosed with prostate cancer. Which test is used to monitor progression of this disease?

1. Serum creatinine
2. Complete blood count (CBC)
3. Prostate specific antigen (PSA)
4. Serum potassium

101. 3. The PSA test is used to monitor prostate cancer progression; higher PSA levels indicate a greater tumor burden. Serum creatinine levels may suggest blockage from an enlarged prostate. CBC is used to diagnose anemia and polycythemia. Serum potassium levels identify hypokalemia and hyperkalemia.

NP: Evaluation; CN: Physiological integrity; CNS: Physiological adaptation; CL: Knowledge

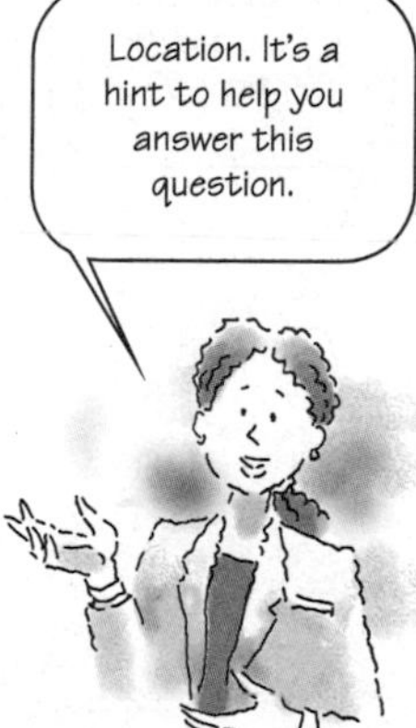

Location. It's a hint to help you answer this question.

102. When teaching a client about cystitis, the nurse explains that females are more prone to the disorder than males. Which of the following explains a female's increased susceptibility?

1. Higher estrogen levels
2. Inadequate fluid intake
3. Urethral proximity to the rectum
4. Continuous nature of the mucosa

102. 3. In females, the urethra and rectum are in close proximity, posing a greater risk for urethral contamination with feces after a bowel movement. Decreased estrogen levels may reduce vaginal and urethral lubrication, increasing the chance of irritation during coitus. Males and females can have equivalent fluid intake. The mucosa is continuous in both males and females.

NP: Implementation; CN: Physiological integrity; CNS: Physiological adaptation; CL: Application

103. A client presents with a possible urinary tract infection. Which of the following should the nurse assess first?

1. Urine clarity
2. Urine specific gravity
3. Urine acetone
4. Urine odor

103. 1. First, the nurse should assess urine clarity; cloudy urine usually indicates drainage, which may reflect infection. Urine specific gravity yields information about fluid balance. Neither urine acetone nor urine odor indicates infection.

NP: Assessment; CN: Health promotion and maintenance; CNS: Prevention and early detection of disease; CL: Comprehension

104. A 70-year old male client is diagnosed with secondary syphilis. Which finding should the nurse expect during assessment?

1. Chronic bone and joint irritation
2. Tender lymphadenopathy
3. Generalized rash on the palms and soles
4. Personality changes and mental confusion

Take assessment questions seriously. They play a noticeable role in the NCLEX.

104. 3. In secondary syphilis, a maculopapular nonpruritic rash appears on the palms and soles. Chronic bone and joint irritation aren't related to secondary syphilis. During the second stage of syphilis, nontender lymphadenopathy occurs. Personality changes occur during the late stage of syphilis.

NP: Assessment; CN: Physiological integrity; CNS: Basic care and comfort; CL: Knowledge

105. Which medication is most likely to be prescribed for a client with gonorrhea?

1. Penicillin (Penicillin G)
2. Azithromycin (Zithromax)
3. Ciprofloxacin (Cipro)
4. Trichloroacetic acid

105. 3. Ciprofloxacin, ceftrizoxime (Cefizox), cefixime (Suprax), ofloxacin (Floxin), and doxycycline (Vibramycin) are the drugs of choice for treating gonorrhea. Penicillin is used to treat syphilis. Azithromycin is used for chlamydial infection. Topical trichloroacetic acid is used for HPV.

NP: Implementation; CN: Physiological integrity; CNS: Pharmacological and parenteral therapies; CL: Application

106. In a client with renal failure, which assessment finding may indicate hypocalcemia?

1. Headache
2. Serum calcium level of 5 mEq/L
3. Increased blood coagulation
4. Diarrhea

106. 4. In renal failure, calcium absorption from the intestine declines, leading to increased smooth muscle contractions, causing diarrhea. CNS changes in renal failure rarely cause headache. A serum calcium level of 5 mEq/L indicates hypercalcemia. As renal failure progresses, bleeding tendencies increase.

NP: Assessment; CN: Health promotion and maintenance; CN: Prevention and early detection of disease; CL: Application

107. A 27-year-old client, who became paraplegic after a swimming accident, is experiencing autonomic dysreflexia. Which condition is the most common cause of autonomic dysreflexia?

1. Upper respiratory infection
2. Incontinence
3. Bladder distention
4. Diarrhea

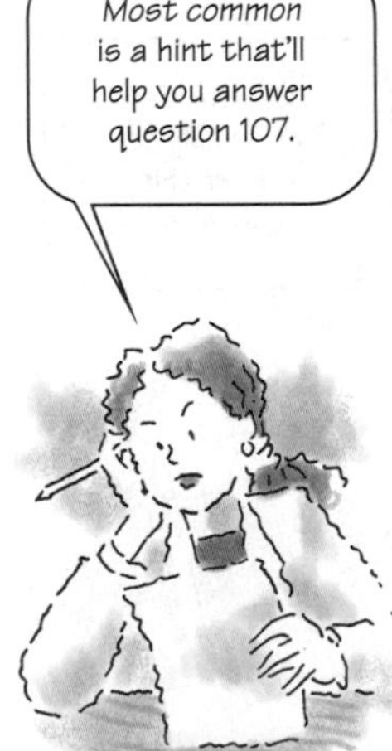
Most common is a hint that'll help you answer question 107.

107. 3. Autonomic dysreflexia is a potentially life-threatening complication of spinal cord injury, occuring from obstruction of the urinary system or bowel. Incontinence and diarrhea don't result in obstruction of the urinary system or bowel, respectively. An upper respiratory infection could obstruct the respiratory system, but not the urinary or bowel system.

NP: Assessment; CN: Safe, effective care environment; CNS: Safety and infection control; CL: Comprehension

NP: Nursing process CN: Client needs category CNS: Client needs subcategory CL: Cognitive level

108. When teaching a client how to prevent recurrences of acute glomerulonephritis, which instruction should the nurse include?

1. "Avoid physical activity."
2. "Strain all urine."
3. "Seek early treatment for respiratory infection."
4. "Monitor urine specific gravity every day."

108. 3. Hemolytic streptococci are common in throat infections and can cause an immune reaction that causes glomerular damage. Therefore, the client should seek early treatment for respiratory infection. Avoiding physical activity may promote urination but doesn't prevent recurrence of glomerulonephritis. Straining all urine helps identify renal calculi that have passed through the urine. Daily monitoring or urine specific gravity helps assess hydration status but doesn't aid in glomerulonephritis prevention.

NP: Implementation; CN: Physiological integrity; CNS: Reduction of risk potential; CL: Analysis

109. After radical prostatectomy for prostate cancer, a client has an indwelling catheter removed. He then begins to have periods of incontinence. During the postoperative period, which intervention should be implemented first?

1. Kegel exercises
2. Fluid restriction
3. Artificial sphincter use
4. Self-catheterization

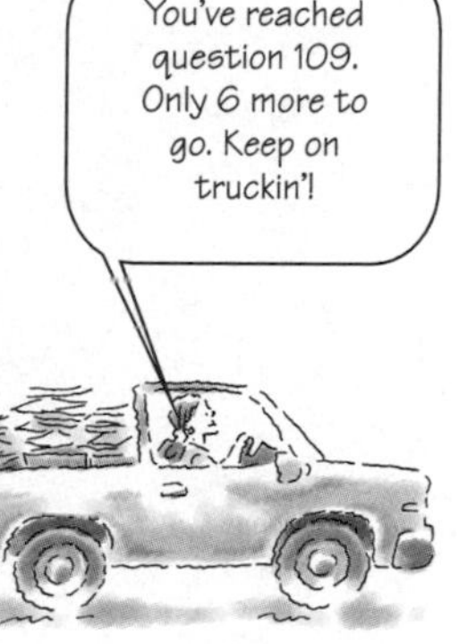

You've reached question 109. Only 6 more to go. Keep on truckin'!

109. 1. Kegel exercises are noninvasive and are recommended as the initial intervention for incontinence. Fluid restriction is useful for a client with increased detrusor contraction related to acidic urine. Artificial sphincter use isn't a primary intervention for post-prostatectomy incontinence. Self-catheterization may be used as a temporary measure but isn't a primary intervention.

NP: Implementation; CN: Physiological integrity; CNS: Physiological adaptation; CL: Application

110. When providing discharge teaching for a client with uric acid calculi, the nurse should include an instruction to avoid which type of diet?

1. Low-calcium
2. Low-oxalate
3. High-oxalate
4. High-purine

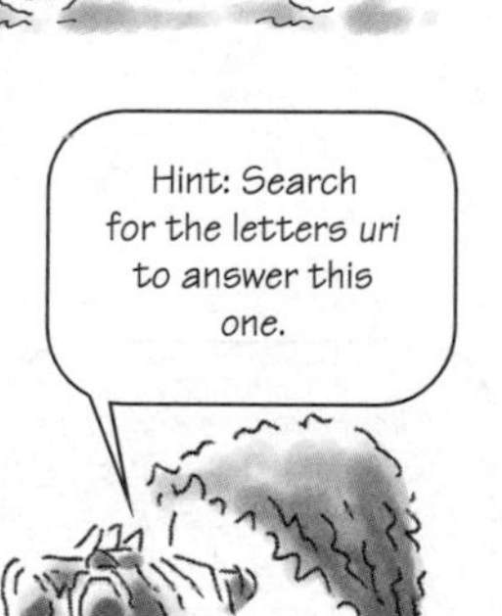

Hint: Search for the letters uri to answer this one.

110. 4. To control uric acid calculi, the client should follow a low-purine diet, which excludes high-purine foods such as organ meats. A low-calcium diet decreases the risk for oxalate renal calculi. Oxalate is an essential amino acid and must be included in the diet. A low-oxalate diet is used to control calcium or oxalate calculi.

NP: Implementation; CN: Physiological integrity; CNS: Reduction of risk potential; CL: Application

111. A 25-year-old male is admitted to the medical-surgical unit with a diagnosis of nephritic syndrome. Which of the following is a hallmark of this syndrome?

1. Osmotic diuresis
2. Edema
3. Hypolipidemia
4. Hyperproteinemia

111. 2. Edema is a hallmark of nephrosis. Edema may occur slowly, appearing first around the eyes and ankles and later becoming generalized. In osmotic diuresis, urine output is clear and increased; in nephritic syndrome, urine output may be dark and decreased. Nephritic syndrome may cause hypolipidemia and hypoproteinemia, but these aren't characteristic of nephrosis.

NP: Assessment; CN: Physiological integrity; CNS: Physiological adaptation; CL: Knowledge

112. A client has a history of renal calculi and must collect a 24-hour urine specimen. Which instruction should the nurse give regarding the first morning voiding?

1. "Save the first morning specimen in a jug, and save every specimen after that for the next 24 hours."
2. "Save the first morning specimen in a jug, and save every specimen except the last one in the jug for the next 24 hours."
3. "Discard the first morning specimen, and save every specimen except the last one in the jug for the next 24 hours."
4. "Discard the first morning specimen, and save every specimen after that in the jug for the next 24 hours."

112. 4. For 24-hour urine specimen collection, the client voids immediately after waking up, notes the time of voiding, discards the voided specimen, and then saves every subsequently voided specimen for the next 24 hours in a specimen jug kept on ice. At the end of 24 hours, the client voids and saves that specimen in the jug. The other instructions are incorrect.
NP: Implementation; CN: Physiological integrity; CNS: Reduction of risk potential; CL: Application

113. For a client with a nephrostomy tube, which of the following is expected during the postoperative period?

1. Frank bleeding at the insertion site for 3 to 4 hours
2. No urine output in the nephrostomy tube for the first 24 hours
3. Urine drainage on the dressing
4. A clamped indwelling urinary catheter

113. 3. Urine drainage on the dressing is common after insertion of a nephrostomy tube. Although the operative site may be blood-tinged, frank bleeding shouldn't appear. Because the nephrostomy tube was inserted to ensure the flow of urine, urine output should appear in the tube. The indwelling urinary catheter shouldn't be clamped.
NP: Assessment; CN: Physiological integrity; CNS: Reduction of risk potential; CL: Application

114. When preparing a care plan for a client with glomerulonephritis, the nurse should give top priority to which intervention?

1. Monitoring fluid status
2. Increasing the client's sodium intake
3. Providing high-protein snacks
4. Monitoring for hypokalemia

114. 1. A client with glomerulonephritis is at risk for fluid overload because the kidneys aren't working properly. Sodium should be restricted because of the risk of fluid overload and hypertension. Proteins should be monitored because of nitrogen retention and elevated blood urea nitrogen levels associated with this condition. This client is at risk for hyperkalemia, not hypokalemia.
NP: Planning; CN: Physiological integrity CNS: Physiological adaptation; CL: Application

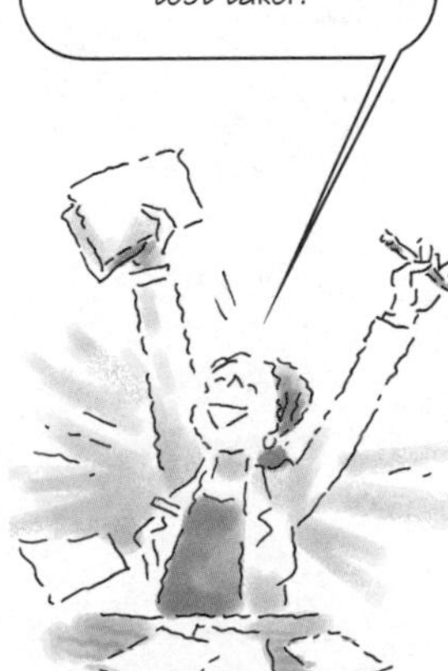
You're at the end of chapter 10! You've proven to be a careful and skillful test taker!

115. A client makes an appointment for her first pelvic examination and Papanicolaou test. After the nurse provides teaching about the examination and the tests to be performed, which client statement suggests the need for further instructions?

1. "I'll have a test for chlamydia."
2. "I'll have my blood drawn to check my white blood cell (WBC) count."
3. "I'll be asked about my obstetric history."
4. "I'll have a test for gonorrhea."

115. 2. Blood is drawn to check the WBC count only if the client has signs or symptoms of infection. During a pelvic examination, tests for chlamydia and gonorrhea are usually performed, and the client is asked about her obstetric history.
NP: Evaluation; CN: Health promotion and maintenance; CNS: Prevention and early detection of disease; CL: Application

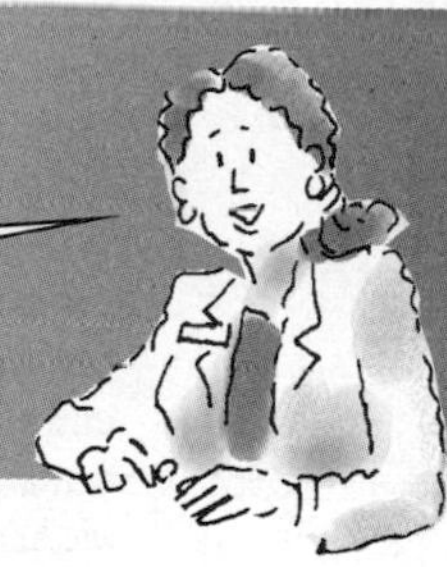

Chapter 11 Integumentary disorders

1. Adequate nutrition is essential for a burn client. Which of the following statements is correct about the nutritional needs of a burn client?

1. The client needs 100 cal/kg throughout hospitalization.
2. The hypermetabolic state after a burn injury contributes to poor healing.
3. A cool environment decreases caloric demand.
4. Maintaining a hypermetabolic rate decreases the client's risk of infection.

1. 2. A burn injury causes a hypermetabolic state resulting in protein and lipid catabolism that affects wound healing. Calories need to be 1½ to 2 times the basal metabolic rate, with at least 1.5 to 2 g/kg of body weight of protein daily. High metabolic rates increase the risk of infection. An environmental temperature within normal range lets the body function efficiently and devote caloric expenditure to healing and normal physiologic processes. If the temperature is too warm or too cold, the body gives energy to warming or cooling, which takes away from energy used for tissue repair.

NP: Analysis; CN: Physiological integrity; CNS: Basic care and comfort; CL: Knowledge

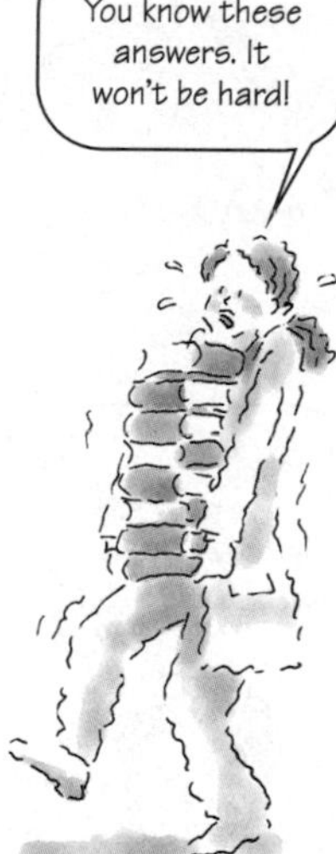

You know these answers. It won't be hard!

2. Which of the following characteristics is correct for a deep partial-thickness burn?

1. Pain and redness
2. Minimal damage to the epidermis
3. Necrotic tissue through all layers of skin
4. Necrotic tissue through most of the dermis

2. 4. A deep partial-thickness burn causes necrosis of the epidermal and dermal layers. Necrosis through all skin layers is seen with full-thickness injuries. Redness and pain are characteristics of a superficial injury. Superficial burns cause slight epidermal damage. With deep burns, the nerve fibers are destroyed and the client doesn't feel pain in the affected area.

NP: Analysis; CN: Physiological integrity; CNS: Physiological adaptation; CL: Knowledge

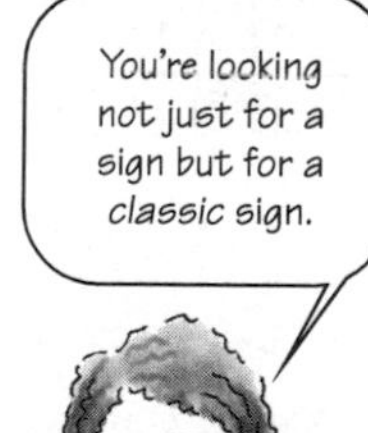

You're looking not just for a sign but for a classic sign.

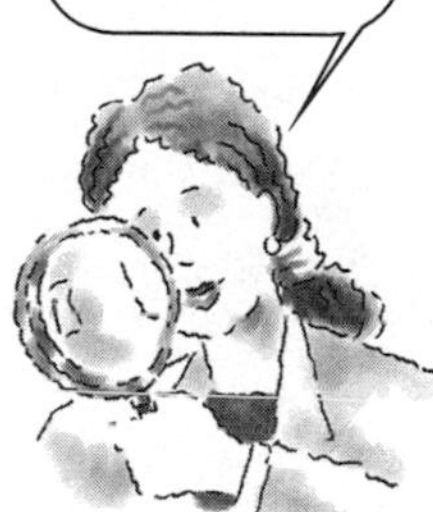

3. Which of the following characteristics is a classic sign of a bite from a brown recluse spider?

1. Bull's-eye rash
2. Painful rash around a necrotic lesion
3. Herald patch of oval lesions
4. Line of papules and vesicles that appear 1 to 3 days after exposure

3. 2. Necrotic, painful rashes are associated with the bite of a brown recluse spider. A bull's-eye rash located primarily at the site of the bite is a classic sign of Lyme disease. A herald patch — a slightly raised, oval lesion about 2 to 6 cm in diameter and appearing anywhere on the body — is indicative of pityriasis rosea. A linear, papular, vesicular rash is characteristic of exposure to poison ivy.

NP: Assessment; CN: Physiological integrity; CNS: Physiological adaptation; CL: Knowledge

4. Which of the following instructions should be observed when administering a Mantoux test?

1. Use the deltoid muscle.
2. Rub the site to help absorption.
3. Read the results within 72 hours.
4. Read the results by checking for a rash.

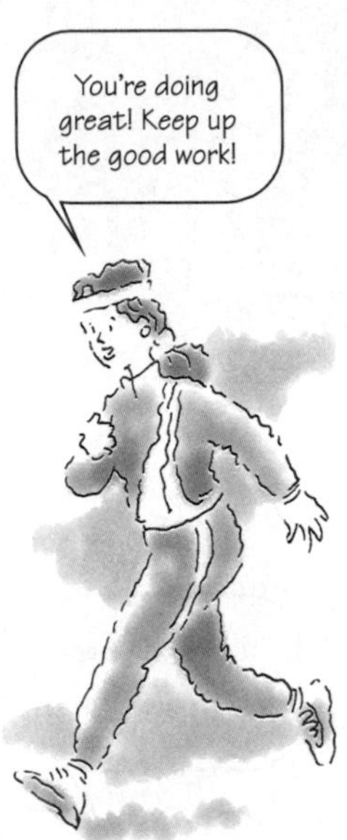
You're doing great! Keep up the good work!

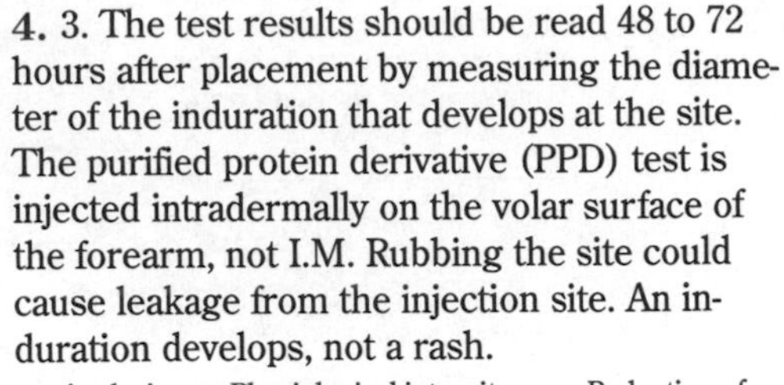

4. 3. The test results should be read 48 to 72 hours after placement by measuring the diameter of the induration that develops at the site. The purified protein derivative (PPD) test is injected intradermally on the volar surface of the forearm, not I.M. Rubbing the site could cause leakage from the injection site. An induration develops, not a rash.
NP: Analysis; CN: Physiological integrity; CNS: Reduction of risk potential; CL: Knowledge

5. A woman is worried she might have lice. Which of the following assessment findings is associated with this infestation?

1. Diffuse pruritic wheals
2. Oval white dots stuck to the hair shafts
3. Pain, redness, and edema with an embedded stinger
4. Pruritic papules, pustules, and linear burrows of the finger and toe webs

5. 2. Nits, the eggs of lice, are seen as white oval dots. Diffuse itching wheals are associated with an allergic reaction. Bites from honeybees are associated with a stinger, pain, and redness. Pruritic papules, vesicles, and linear burrows are diagnostic for scabies.
NP: Assessment; CN: Physiological integrity; CNS: Physiological adaptation; CL: Knowledge

6. A bite from a large dog will cause which of the following types of injuries?

1. Abrasion
2. Crush injury
3. Fracture
4. Puncture wound

6. 2. The bite of a large dog can exert between 150 to 400 psi of pressure, causing a crush injury, not a fracture. A bite from a small animal such as a cat will cause puncture wounds. An abrasion is caused by friction.
NP: Analysis; CN: Physiological integrity; CNS: Physiological adaptation; CL: Knowledge

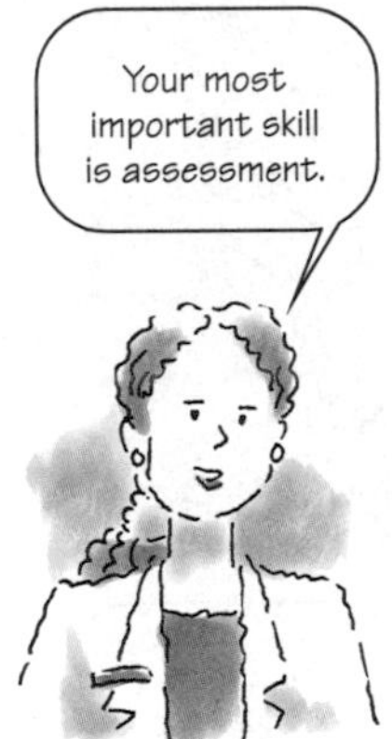
Your most important skill is assessment.

7. The distribution of lesions on the skin can help determine which of the following factors?

1. Disease
2. Type of lesion
3. Color of the lesion
4. Arrangement of the lesion

7. 1. The distribution of lesions can help diagnose the illness, as with herpes zoster. The arrangement, type, and color are specific characteristics used along with the distribution in describing lesions.
NP: Analysis; CN: Health promotion and maintenance; CNS: Prevention and early detection of disease; CL: Knowledge

8. A client arrives at the office of his physician complaining of several palpable elevated masses. Which of the following terms accurately describes these masses?

1. Erosions
2. Macules
3. Papules
4. Vesicles

8. 3. Papules are elevated up to 0.5 cm, and nodules and tumors are masses elevated more than 0.5 cm. Erosions are characterized as loss of the epidermis layer. Macules and patches are nonpalpable, flat changes in skin color. Fluid-filled lesions are vesicles and pustules.
NP: Analysis; CN: Health promotion and maintenance; CNS: Prevention and early detection of disease; CL: Knowledge

NP: Nursing process CN: Client needs category CNS: Client needs subcategory CL: Cognitive level

9. Which of the following adverse reactions may be caused by the use of isotretinoin (Accutane)?

1. Birth defects
2. Nausea and vomiting
3. Vaginal yeast infection
4. Gram-negative folliculitis

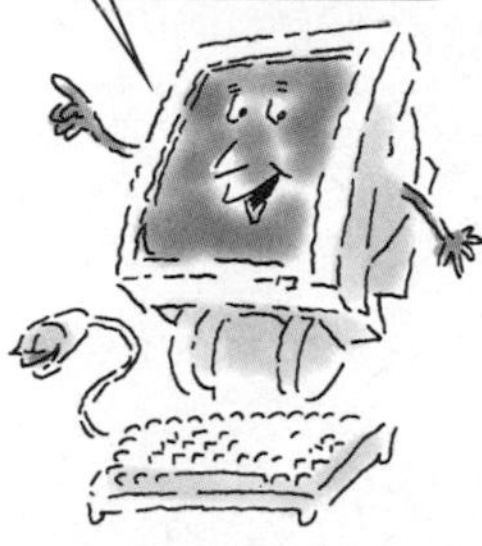

Questions about adverse reactions are common on NCLEX examinations. Better bone up on 'em!

9. 1. Even small amounts of Accutane are associated with severe birth defects. Most female clients are also prescribed oral contraceptives. Clindamycin phosphate (Cleocin T Gel), another medicine used in the treatment of acne, can cause both diarrhea and gram-negative folliculitis. Tetracycline is associated with yeast infections.

NP: Analysis; CN: Health promotion and maintenance; CNS: Growth and development through the life span; CL: Knowledge

10. A client complains of small, red, pruritic dots between his fingers and toes. Which of the following conditions is the most likely diagnosis?

1. Contusion
2. Herpes zoster
3. Scabies
4. Varicella

10. 3. Scabies are seen as linear burrows between the fingers and toes caused by a mite. Contusions don't have small pruritic dots. The varicella zoster virus causes herpes zoster, characterized by papulovesicular lesions that erupt along a dermatome, usually with hyperesthesia, pain, and tenderness. The papulovesicular lesions of varicella are distributed over the trunk, face, and scalp and don't follow a dermatome.

NP: Assessment; CN: Physiological integrity; CNS: Physiological adaptation; CL: Knowledge

11. Which of the following instructions is given to a client taking nystatin (Mycostatin) oral solution?

1. Take the drug right after meals.
2. Take the drug right before meals.
3. Mix the drug with small amounts of food.
4. Take half the dose before and half after meals.

11. 1. Nystatin oral solution should be swished around the mouth after eating for the best contact with mucous membranes. Taking the drug before or with meals doesn't allow for the best contact with the mucous membranes.

NP: Implementation; CN: Physiological integrity; CNS: Pharmacological and parenteral therapies; CL: Application

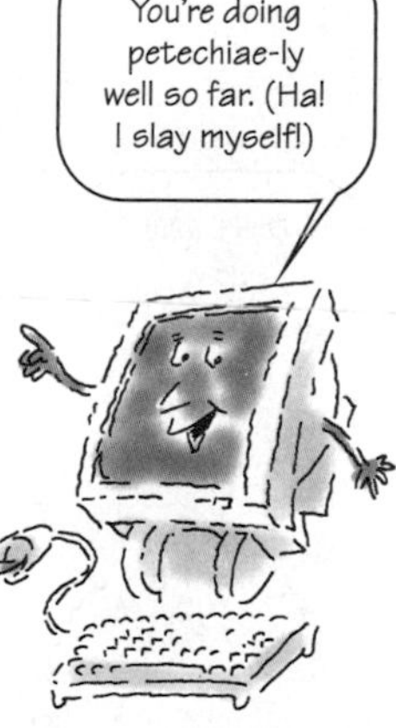

You're doing petechiae-ly well so far. (Ha! I slay myself!)

12. A client is examined and found to have pinpoint, pink-to-purple, nonblanching macular lesions 1 to 3 mm in diameter. Which of the following terms best describes these lesions?

1. Ecchymosis
2. Hematoma
3. Petechiae
4. Purpura

12. 3. Petechiae are small macular lesions 1 to 3 mm in diameter. Ecchymosis is a purple-to-brown bruise, macular or papular, and varied in size. A hematoma is a collection of blood from ruptured blood vessels more than 1 cm in diameter. Purpura are purple macular lesions larger than 1 cm.

NP: Assessment; CN: Physiological integrity; CNS: Physiological adaptation; CL: Knowledge

13. A client has a rash consisting of scattered lesions on various parts of the body. Which of the following types of rash is this?

1. Annular
2. Confluent
3. Diffuse
4. Linear

13. 3. A diffuse rash usually has widely distributed scattered lesions. An annular rash is ring shaped. Confluent lesions are touching or adjacent to each other. Linear rashes are lesions arranged in a line.

NP: Assessment; CN: Physiological integrity; CNS: Physiological adaptation; CL: Knowledge

14. Which of the following terms best describes hair loss in small round areas on the scalp?

1. Alopecia
2. Amblyopia
3. Exotropia
4. Seborrhea

14. 1. Alopecia is the correct term for thinning hair loss. Exotropia and amblyopia are eye disorders. Seborrhea is a chronic inflammatory dermatitis that occurs in infants.

NP: Analysis; CN: Physiological integrity; CNS: Physiological adaptation; CL: Knowledge

15. Which of the following conditions or factors is a cause of atopic dermatitis?

1. Bacteria
2. Fungus
3. Heredity
4. Virus

15. 3. Atopic dermatitis is a hereditary disorder associated with a family history of asthma, allergic rhinitis, or atopic dermatitis. Atopic dermatitis isn't a bacterial, fungal, or viral infection.

NP: Analysis; CN: Physiological integrity; CNS: Physiological adaptation; CL: Knowledge

16. A client has rough papules on the soles of his feet that are sometimes painful when he walks. Which of the following terms best describes this condition?

1. Filiform wart
2. Flat wart
3. Plantar wart
4. Venereal wart

16. 3. Plantar warts are rough papules commonly found on the soles of the feet. Filiform warts are long, spiny projections from the skin surface. Flat warts are flat-topped, smooth-surfaced lesions. Venereal warts appear on the genital mucosa and are confluent papules with rough surfaces.

NP: Assessment; CN: Physiological integrity; CNS: Physiological adaptation; CL: Knowledge

17. A client reports circular lesions on his neck. Which of the following conditions is the most likely explanation?

1. Candidiasis
2. Molluscum contagiosum
3. Tinea corporis
4. Tinea pedis

17. 3. Tinea corporis, or ringworm, is a flat scaling papular lesion with raised borders. Candidiasis is a fungal infection of the skin or mucous membranes commonly found in the oral, vaginal, and intestinal mucosal tissue. Molluscum contagiosum is a viral skin infection with small, red, papular lesions. Tinea pedis is a superficial fungal infection on the feet, commonly called athletes' foot, that causes itching and sweating and a foul odor.

NP: Analysis; CN: Physiological integrity; CNS: Physiological adaptation; CL: Knowledge

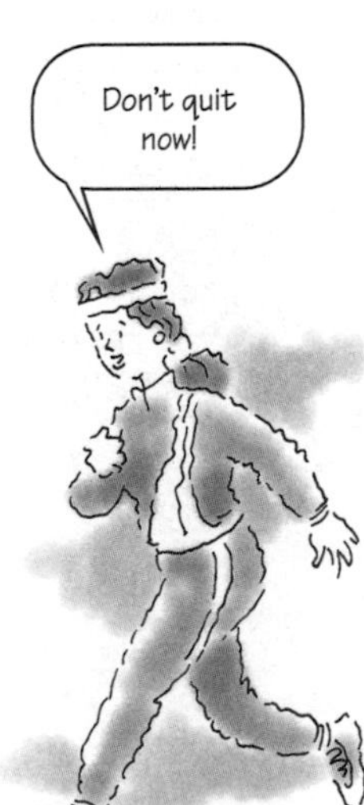

18. A client has thick, discolored nails with splintered hemorrhages, easily separated from the nail bed. There are also "ice pick" pits and ridges. Which of the following terms best describes these symptoms?

1. Paronychia
2. Psoriasis
3. Seborrhea
4. Scabies

18. 2. Psoriasis, a chronic skin disorder with an unknown cause, shows these characteristic skin changes. A paronychia is a bacterial infection of the nail bed. Seborrhea is a chronic inflammatory dermatitis known as cradle cap. Scabies are mites that burrow under the skin, generally between the webbing of the fingers and toes.

NP: Assessment; CN: Physiological integrity; CNS: Physiological adaptation; CL: Knowledge

37. Which of the following water temperatures is correct for a bed bath?

1. 97° to 100° F (36.1° to 37.8° C)
2. 100° to 110° F (37.8° to 43.3° C)
3. 110° to 115° F (43.3° to 46.1° C)
4. 115° to 120° F (46.1° to 48.9° C)

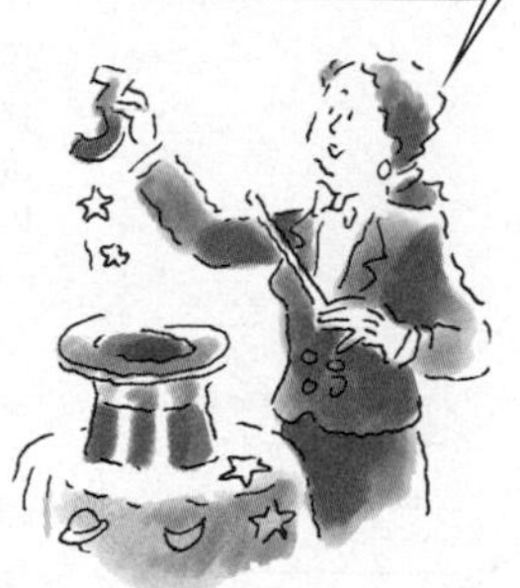

And the correct temperature is...

37. 3. The client should be protected from becoming chilled. The water temperature should be 110° to 115° F to compensate for evaporative body cooling during and after the bath. Water temperature the same as body temperature, slightly cooler, or slightly warmer will eventually cool, which could cause discomfort and increase evaporative body cooling. Water of 115° to 120° F would be too hot and put the client at risk for burns or discomfort. Water should always be tested with a bath thermometer.

NP: Planning; CN: Physiological integrity; CNS: Basic care and comfort; CL: Knowledge

38. A client received burns to his entire back and left arm. Using the Rule of Nines, the nurse calculates that he has sustained burns to which of the following percentages of his body?

1. 9%
2. 18%
3. 27%
4. 36%

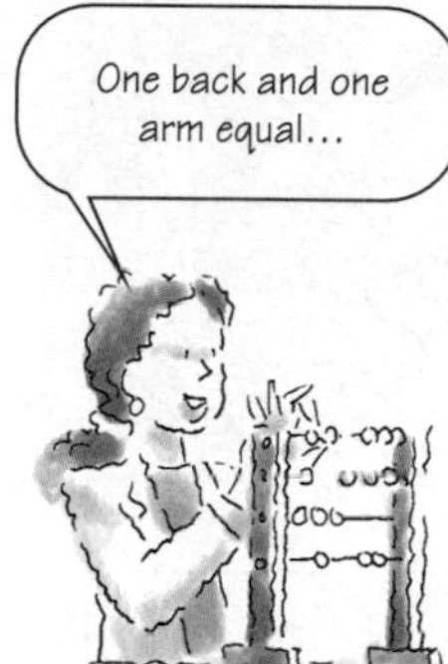

One back and one arm equal...

38. 3. According to the Rule of Nines, the posterior trunk, anterior trunk, and legs are each 18% of the total body surface. The head, neck, and arms are each 9% of total body surface, and the perineum is 1%. In this case, the client received burns to his back (18%) and one arm (9%), totaling 27% of his body.

NP: Assessment; CN: Physiological integrity; CNS: Reduction of risk potential; CL: Application

39. Which of the following techniques will maintain surgical asepsis?

1. Change the sterile field after sterile water is spilled on it.
2. Put on sterile gloves; then open a container of sterile saline.
3. Place a sterile dressing ½″ (1.3 cm) from the edge of the sterile field.
4. Clean the wound with a circular motion, moving from outer circles toward the center.

39. 1. A sterile field is considered contaminated when it becomes wet. Moisture can act as a wick, allowing microorganisms to contaminate the field. The outside of containers such as sterile saline bottles aren't sterile. The containers should be opened before sterile gloves are put on, and the solution poured over the sterile dressings placed in a sterile basin. Wounds should be cleaned from the most contaminated area to the least contaminated area, for example, from the center outward. The outer inch of a sterile field isn't considered sterile.

NP: Implementation; CN: Safe, effective care environment; CNS: Safety and infection control; CL: Application

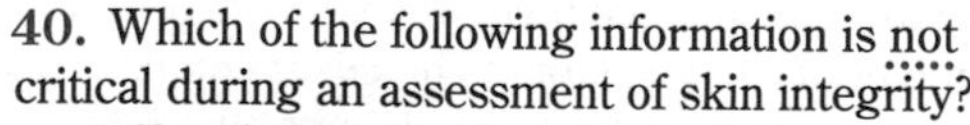

40. Which of the following information is not critical during an assessment of skin integrity?

1. Family history of pressure ulcers
2. Presence of existing pressure ulcers
3. Overall risk for developing pressure ulcers
4. Potential areas of pressure ulcer development

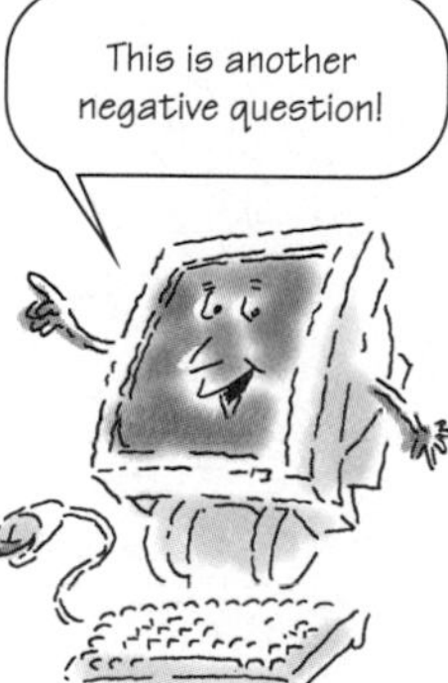

This is another negative question!

40. 1. Family history isn't important for the assessment of skin integrity. Areas already broken down need immediate treatment. Plans should be developed to avoid skin breakdown in areas at high risk. Certain clients are at high risk because of internal factors, such as malnutrition, cachexia, obesity, and diabetes.

NP: Assessment; CN: Physiological integrity; CNS: Reduction of risk potential; CL: Knowledge

41. Which of the following pieces of equipment for the wheelchair- or bed-bound client impedes circulation to the area it's meant to protect?

1. Waterbed
2. Ring or donut
3. Gel flotation pad
4. Polyurethane foam mattress

41. 2. Rings or donuts shouldn't be used because they restrict circulation. Foam mattresses evenly distribute pressure. Gel pads give with weight. The waterbed also distributes pressure over the entire surface.

NP: Implementation; CN: Physiological integrity; CNS: Reduction of risk potential; CL: Application

42. Which of the following interventions is inappropriate for the treatment of a postoperative wound evisceration?

1. Give prophylactic antibiotics as ordered.
2. Have the client drink as much fluid as possible.
3. Explain to the client what's happening and give support.
4. Cover the protruding internal organs with sterile gauze moistened with sterile saline.

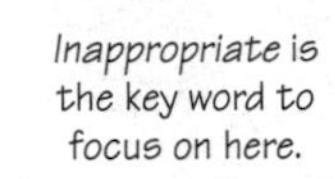

Inappropriate is the key word to focus on here.

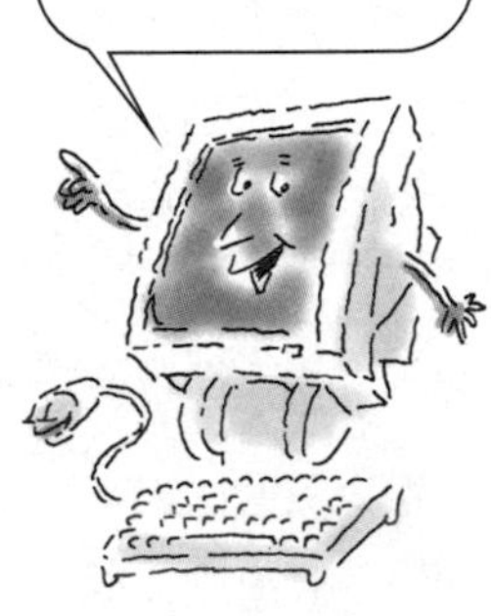

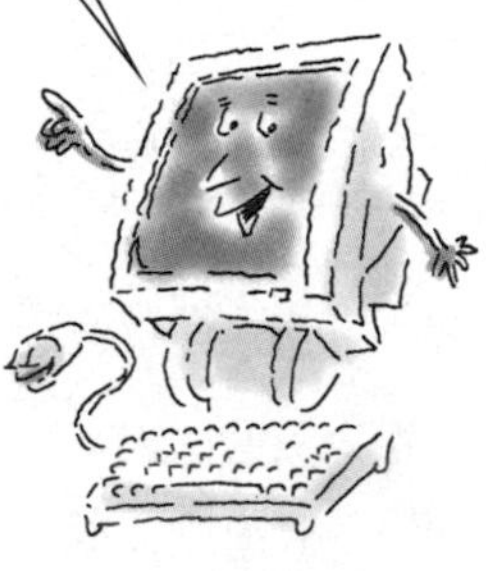

42. 2. Evisceration requires emergency surgery. The nurse should place the client on nothing-by-mouth status immediately. Evisceration is a frightening situation for any client. While the nurse works quickly to get the client treated, providing support that will reduce the client's anxiety is important. Covering the wound with moistened gauze will prevent the organs from drying. Both the gauze and the saline must be sterile to reduce the risk for infection. Antibiotics will usually be ordered immediately and should be started as soon as possible.

NP: Implementation; CN: Physiological integrity; CNS: Physiological adaptation; CL: Application

43. Which of the following interventions is performed first when changing a dressing or giving wound care?

1. Put on gloves.
2. Wash hands thoroughly.
3. Slowly remove the soiled dressing.
4. Observe the dressing for the amount, type, and odor of drainage.

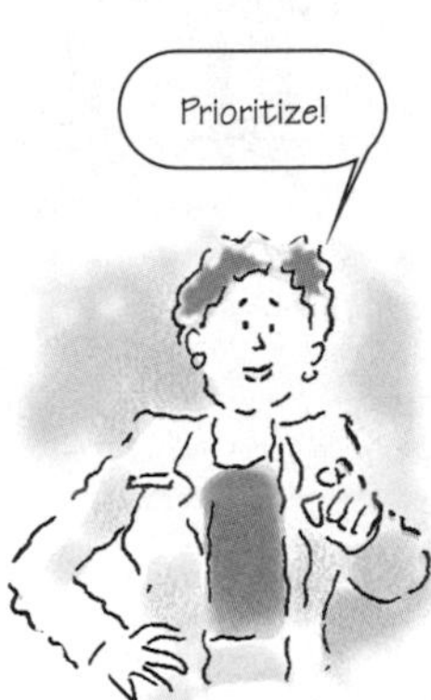

43. 2. The first thing the nurse must do is wash her hands. Putting on gloves, removing the dressing, and observing the drainage are all parts of the procedure of doing a dressing change.

NP: Implementation; CN: Physiological integrity; CNS: Basic care and comfort; CL: Application

44. When caring for a client who spends all or most of the time in bed, a turning schedule prevents the development of complications. Which of the following schedules is best for most clients?

1. Turn every half hour.
2. Turn every 1 to 2 hours.
3. Turn once every 8 hours.
4. Keep the client on his back as much as possible.

44. 2. Turning the client every 1 to 2 hours will prevent pressure areas from developing and help prevent atelectasis and other pulmonary complications. Turning every half hour is too frequent, and turning every 8 hours would make the client vulnerable to the development of complications. The client should spend time on his back according to the turning schedule. During that period, the head of the bed should be raised to prevent the client from aspirating.

NP: Planning; CN: Physiological integrity; CNS: Basic care and comfort; CL: Application

45. Which of the following instructions is most important when teaching a client about hypersensitivity skin test results?
1. Wash the sites daily with a mild soap.
2. Have the sites read on the correct date.
3. Keep the skin test areas moist with a mild lotion.
4. Stay out of direct sunlight until the tests are read.

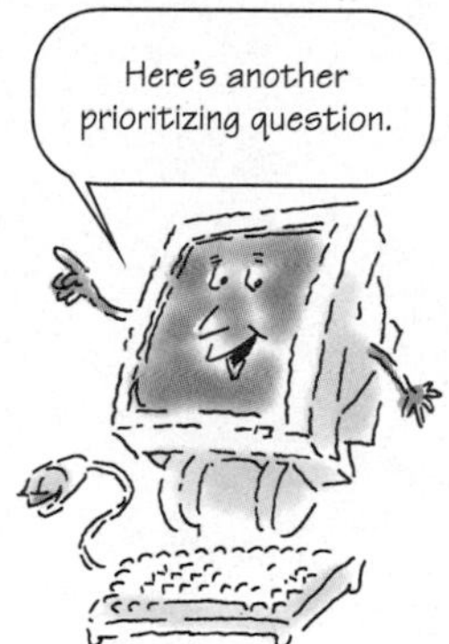
Here's another prioritizing question.

45. 2. An important facet of evaluating skin tests is to read the skin test results at the proper time. Evaluating the skin test too late or too early will give inaccurate and unreliable results. The sites should be kept dry. There is no need to wash the sites with soap, and direct sunlight isn't prohibited.
NP: Implementation; CN: Health promotion and maintenance; CNS: Prevention and early detection of disease; CL: Application

46. A client with disseminated herpes zoster is given I.V. hydrocortisone (Solu-Cortef). Which of the following serum chemistry values may be elevated as a result of this therapy?
1. Calcium
2. Glucose
3. Magnesium
4. Potassium

46. 2. Corticosteroids increase blood sugar and tend to lower serum potassium and calcium levels. Their effect on magnesium isn't substantial.
NP: Assessment; CN: Physiological integrity; CNS: Pharmacological and parenteral therapies; CL: Comprehension

47. A client has been admitted to the burn unit with extensive full-thickness burns. Which of the following considerations has priority?
1. Fluid status
2. Body image
3. Level of pain
4. Risk of infection

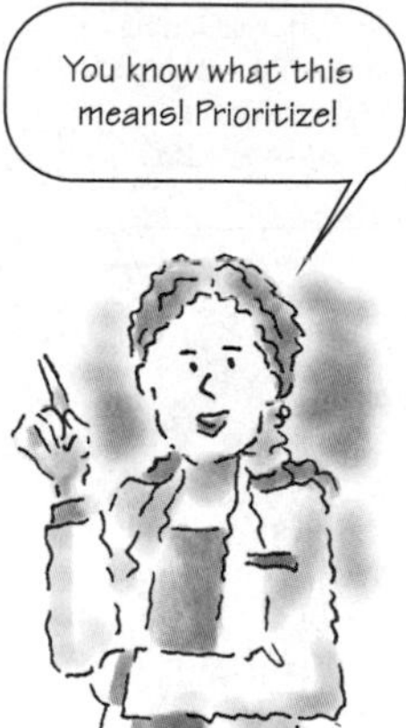
You know what this means! Prioritize!

47. 1. In early burn care, the client's greatest need is fluid resuscitation because of large-volume fluid loss through the damaged skin. Infection, body image, and pain are important concerns in the nursing care of a burn client but don't take precedence over fluid management in the early phase of burn care.
NP: Analysis; CN: Physiological integrity; CNS: Physiological adaptation; CL: Analysis

48. Which of the following characteristics is seen with deep partial-thickness burn wounds?
1. Blanching
2. Erythema
3. Eschar
4. Fluid-filled vesicles

48. 4. Fluid-filled vesicles are characteristic of deep partial-thickness skin destruction (also referred to as second-degree burns). Erythema and blanching on pressure are characteristic of partial-thickness skin destruction. Eschar is a manifestation of full-thickness skin destruction.
NP: Assessment; CN: Physiological integrity; CNS: Physiological adaptation; CL: Knowledge

49. A client with extensive burns has a new donor site. Which of the following considerations is important in positioning the client?
1. Make the site dependent.
2. Avoid pressure on the site.
3. Keep the site fully covered.
4. Allow ventilation of the site.

49. 2. A universal concern in the care of donor sites for burn care is to keep the site away from sources of pressure. Ventilation of the site and keeping the site fully covered are practices in some institutions but aren't hallmarks of donor site care. Placing the site in a position of dependence isn't a justified aspect of donor site care.
NP: Implementation; CN: Physiological integrity; CNS: Physiological adaptation; CL: Application

50. Prevention and early treatment of Lyme disease are crucial because which of the following complications can occur late in the disease?
1. Arthritis
2. Lung abscess
3. Renal failure
4. Sterility

50. 1. If Lyme disease goes untreated, arthritis, neurologic problems, and cardiac abnormalities may arise as late complications. Lung abscess, renal failure, and sterility aren't complications of Lyme disease.
NP: Analysis; CN: Physiological integrity; CNS: Reduction of risk potential; CL: Knowledge

51. A client is admitted with suspected malignant melanoma on his left shoulder. When performing the physical assessment, the nurse would expect to observe which of the following signs?
1. Brown birthmark that has lightened in color
2. Brown or black mole with red, white, or blue areas
3. Petechiae
4. Red birthmark that has recently become darker

51. 2. Melanomas have an irregular shape and lack uniformity in color. They may appear brown or black with red, white, or blue areas. Melanoma lesions don't appear as birthmarks that have changed color or as petechiae.
NP: Assessment; CN: Health promotion and maintenance; CNS: Prevention and early detection of disease; CL: Knowledge

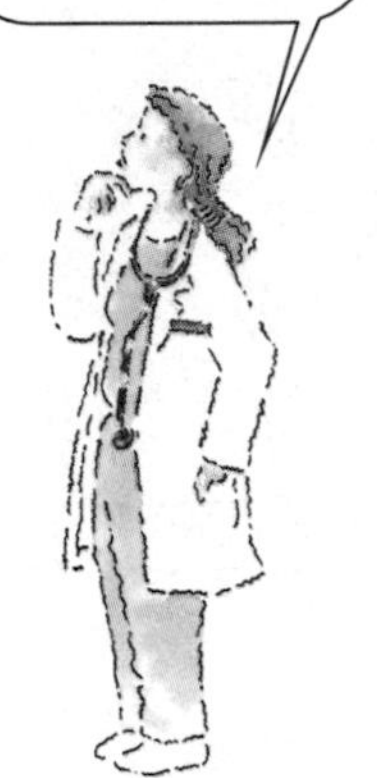

Scrutinize question 52 and its answers. Further teaching means you should find what skin does not do.

52. A nurse-educator is presenting a hygiene class to nursing students. Which statement by a student indicates the need for further teaching?
1. "The skin absorbs fluids."
2. "The skin serves as the body's first line of defense."
3. "The skin excretes waste products."
4. "The skin changes vitamin D to a form the body can use."

52. 4. The skin doesn't change vitamin D to a form the body can use. (The sun helps to convert vitamin D.) The skin absorbs fluids, serves as the body's first line of defense, and excretes waste products.
NP: Assessment; CN: Physiological integrity; CNS: Physiological adaptation; CL: Knowledge

53. Which of the following terms refers to the oil secreted by the skin?
1. Epidermis
2. Sebum
3. Follicle
4. Dermis

53. 2. Sebum is the oil secreted by the skin. The epidermis and dermis are skin layers. A follicle is a pouchlike depression from which a hair grows.
NP: Assessment; CN: Physiological integrity; CNS: Physiological adaptation; CL: Knowledge

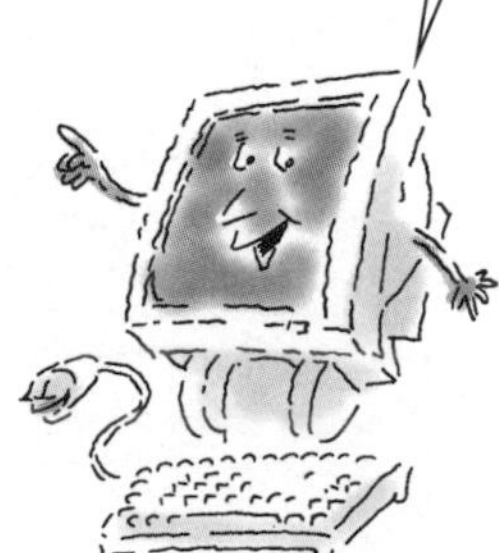

To answer question 54 correctly, zero in on the words *minimal scarring*.

54. During the late stages of healing, which intervention helps a burn wound to heal with minimal scarring?
1. Removing eschar from the skin
2. Applying continuous-compression wraps
3. Wearing clothing to protect the burn from the sun
4. Maintaining wound care irrigation

54. 2. Applying continuous-compression wraps aids skin healing and prevents hypertrophied tissue from forming. The other interventions are appropriate for the client with a burn wound but don't necessarily help minimize scarring.
NP: Implementation; CN: Physiological integrity; CNS: Reduction of risk potential; CL: Application

55. A client has an inflamed area on the right forearm that's causing considerable discomfort. The nurse should expect the physician to order which of the following treatments?

1. Warm, moist compresses
2. An elastic bandage
3. Hydrocortisone cream
4. Nonadherent dressing

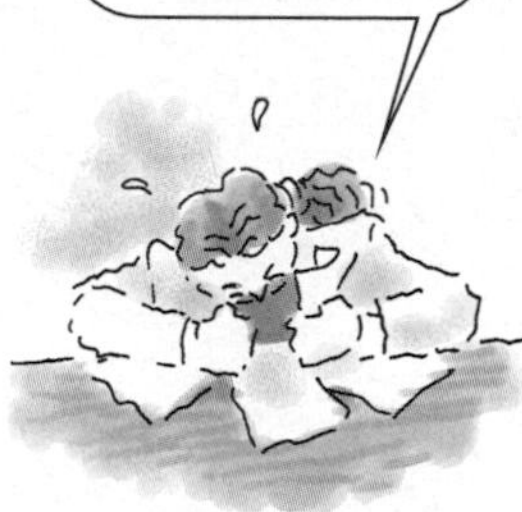

You've answered 55 questions! Don't despair. You're doing a great job!

55. 1. Warm, moist compresses increase circulation to the area, reducing discomfort and redness. An elastic bandage decompresses the area but doesn't ease inflammation. Hydrocortisone cream is useful on an inflamed area that itches. A nonadherent dressing doesn't relieve inflammation or pain.

NP: Implementation; CN: Physiological integrity; CNS: Basic care and comfort; CL: Application

56. An elderly client has a sore on the inside of her ankle that she says won't heal. After noting varicosities and coarse discoloration around the sore, the nurse should suspect which of the following?

1. Acute venous insufficiency
2. Chronic venous insufficiency
3. Acute arterial occlusive disease
4. Chronic arterial occlusive disease

56. 2. Classic signs of chronic venous insufficiency include skin discoloration (from blood extravasation in subcutaneous tissue) and stasis ulcers, usually found on the ankle's medial aspect. Acute or chronic arterial occlusive disease usually causes intermittent claudication and severe burning pain.

NP: Assessment; CN: Physiological integrity; CNS: Physiological adaptation; CL: Application

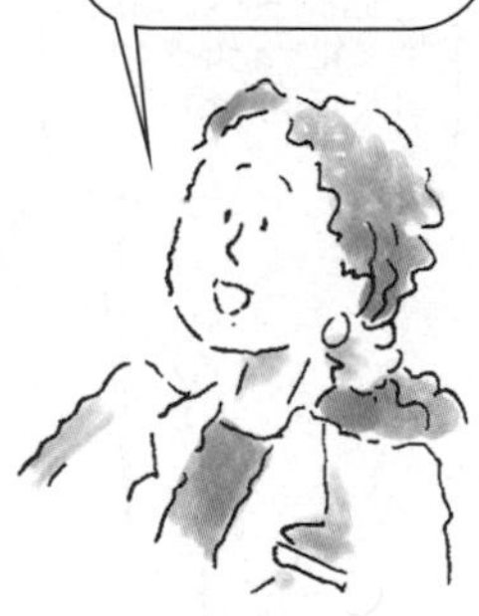

57. The nurse prepares a client for a shave biopsy of a skin lesion. Which point should not be included in the teaching plan?

1. How to care for the suture line
2. The need for pain relief
3. Explanation that scarring is minimal
4. How to care for the dressing

57. 1. A shave biopsy removes only the first or second layer of skin, causing a superficial wound with no suture line and minimal scarring. Pain relief and dressing care should be included in the teaching plan.

NP: Analysis; CN: Physiological integrity; CNS: Physiological adaptation; CL: Comprehension

58. The physician orders a wet-to-dry dressing for a client who has a pressure ulcer with infected, necrotic tissue. What's the rationale for this treatment?

1. To prevent extension of the infection
2. To debride the wound
3. To keep the wound moist
4. To reduce pain

58. 2. A wet-to-dry dressing placed over a necrotic area adheres to dead tissue and is debrided as the dressing is removed. Antibiotics, not dressings, help prevent extension of the infection. Keeping the wound moist would prevent the necessary debridement. The dressing has no analgesic effect.

NP: Implementation; CN: Physiological integrity; CNS: Physiological adaptation; CL: Application

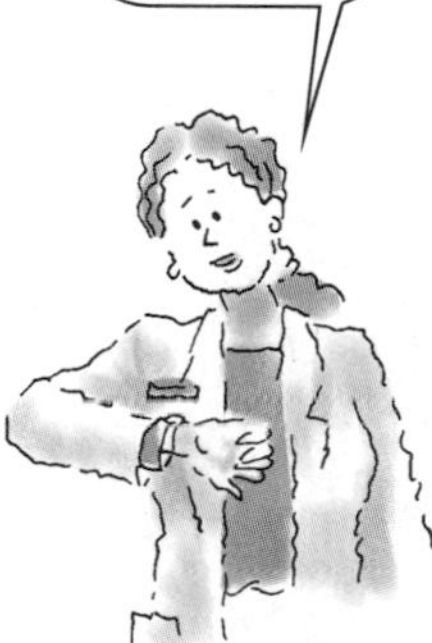

Observe the time in a question of this type.

59. A client has moist saline dressings applied to an open ulcer of the foot. Ten days after ulcer development, the wound should have which appearance?

1. Red, swollen tissue
2. Dry, crusted scab
3. Deep, wide keloid
4. Warm, painful tissue

59. 2. Ten days into healing, an ulcer should be at the end of the lag phase of healing, as indicated by a dry, crusted scab. Tissue is red, swollen, warm, or painful during the inflammatory phase, which occurs 2 to 7 days after the ulcer develops. A deep, wide keloid may appear 3 weeks to 2 years after ulcer development.

NP: Assessment; CN: Physiological integrity; CN: Physiological adaptation; CL: Application

60. When changing a dressing on a pressure ulcer, the nurse notes necrotic wound tissue. Which treatment should the nurse expect the physician to order?

1. Wound incision and drainage
2. Wound culturing
3. Wound debridement
4. Wound irrigation with an antiseptic

60. 3. For healing to occur, necrotic (dead) tissue must be removed from the wound; usually, this is done by debridement. Wound incision and drainage and wound culturing are done when infection is present or suspected. Wound irrigation with an antiseptic may damage sensitive tissue and prevent healing.
NP: Planning; CN: Physiological integrity; CNS: Physiological adaptation; CL: Application

61. After a traumatic injury, a client's wound heals and a smooth, pink, thickened, rubbery lesion forms over the wound. Which of the following should the nurse suspect?

1. Erosion
2. Fissure
3. Keloid
4. Abscess

61. 3. A keloid results from a defect in the healing process in which excess collagen develops at the healing site. Erosion refers to loss of part or all of the skin surface, usually from infection or pressure. A fissure is a slit in the wound. Abscess, which results from accumulation of purulent drainage, causes the wound to appear red, swollen, and tender.
NP: Analysis; CN: Physiological integrity; CNS: Physiological adaptation; CL: Comprehension

These questions aren't easy, but you're acing them anyway!

62. A client is diagnosed with urticaria. Which of the following describes the wheal that commonly accompanies urticaria?

1. Elevated, firm circumscribed lesion in the dermis, 1 to 2 cm in diameter
2. Flat, nonpalpable, irregularly shaped lesion, more than 1 cm in diameter
3. Transient, elevated, solid, firm, irregularly shaped area of cutaneous edema, with a variable diameter
4. Elevated, circumscribed lesion in the dermis or subcutaneous layer, filled with liquid or semisolid material

62. 3. A wheal is a transient, elevated, firm lesion of irregular shape and size. A nodule is an elevated lesion in the dermis with a diameter of 1 to 2 cm. A patch is a flat lesion with a diameter exceeding 1 cm. A cyst is an elevated, circumscribed lesion filled with liquid or semisolid material.
NP: Analysis; CN: Physiological integrity; CNS: Physiological adaptation; CL: Knowledge

63. A 70-year-old client who spilled hot coffee on his lap 3 days ago has multiple blisters. As the nurse provides care, two of the blisters break. Which action should the nurse take?

1. Remove the raised skin, because the blister has been compromised.
2. Wash the area vigorously with soap and water.
3. Apply alcohol to the area.
4. Clean the area with normal saline solution and cover it with a dressing.

63. 4. To maintain asepsis, the nurse should clean the area with normal saline solution and cover it with a dressing. Removing the raised skin would cause further skin damage. Washing the area vigorously with soap and water would damage the tissue and cause drying. Alcohol would dry out the tissue.
NP: Planning; CN: Safe, effective care environment; CNS: Safety and infection control; CL: Application

64. A client undergoes cryosurgery to remove a cancerous skin lesion. When assessing the wound a few days later, the nurse should expect to find which of the following?

1. Dry, itchy patches
2. Oozing and pain
3. Dryness, tenderness, and sutures
4. Swelling, blistering, and tenderness

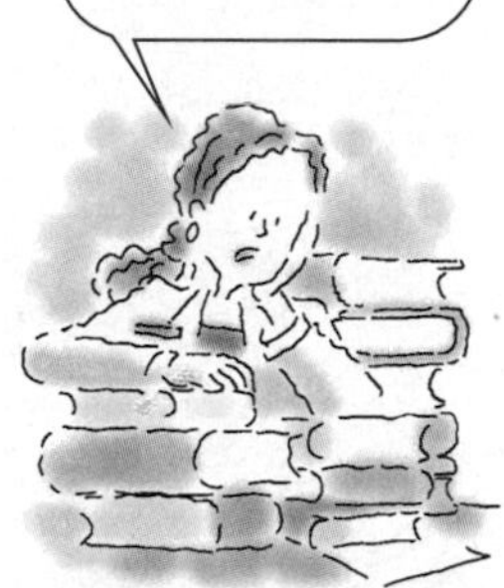

Know your assessment facts; they're critical in nursing and on the NCLEX.

64. 4. Cryosurgery leaves a wound resembling a burn, with swelling, blistering, and tenderness. Oozing and pain suggest an infection. The wound wouldn't be dry or itchy and wouldn't have sutures.

NP: Assessment; CN: Physiological integrity; CNS: Physiological adaptation; CL: Comprehension

65. A client with facial lacerations requires hospitalization for 1 week. During assessment, the nurse notes scabs on the wounds. This finding corresponds to which phase of wound healing?

1. Contraction phase
2. Inflammatory phase
3. Proliferative phase
4. Remodeling phase

65. 3. During the proliferative phase of wound healing, which lasts from the 4th to 21st day after injury, granulation tissue appears (scabs form) and the wound edges start to pull together. Contraction, the third phase of wound healing, may begin around the 7th day and involves a significant decrease in the wound surface. The inflammatory phase, the first healing phase, immediately follows the injury and lasts 4 to 6 days; it involves control of bleeding and release of chemicals needed for healing. The remodeling phase, the final phase, may lead to scar flattening and correction of any deformities that occurred during the third phase.

NP: Assessment; CN: Physiological integrity; CNS: Basic care and comfort; CL: Knowledge

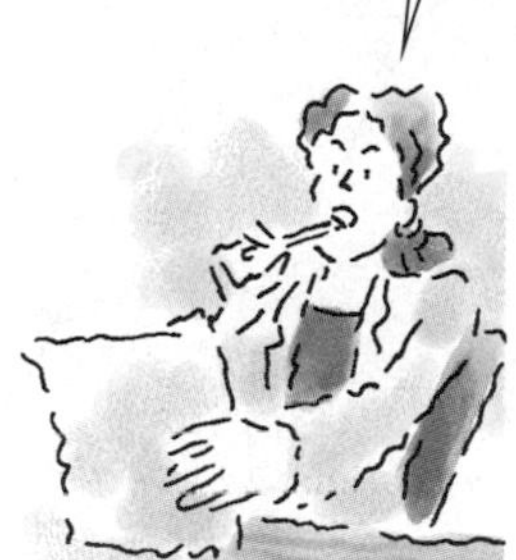

Looks like you've only got five more questions to go. Whew!

66. An 85-year-old woman who has spent a great deal of time outdoors tells the home health nurse that her skin is dry and itchy. Which instruction should the nurse provide?

1. "Soak in a bubble bath once per day."
2. "Bathe with antimicrobial soap once per day."
3. "Bathe with mild soap and water or with water only."
4. "Scrub the skin vigorously to remove dead skin cells."

66. 3. Bathing with mild soap and water or with water only can relieve skin itching and dryness. Bubble baths and antimicrobial soap can be very drying to an elderly person's sensitive skin. Scrubbing vigorously may worsen skin dryness.

NP: Assessment; CN: Physiological integrity; CNS: Basic care and comfort: CL: Comprehension

67. A client has a maculopapular rash on his trunk, which follows skin cleavage lines in a Christmas tree pattern. He reports that the rash started as a small lesion 4 days ago. What is the most likely cause of the rash?

1. Tinea corporis
2. Pityriasis rosea
3. Allergic reaction to a drug
4. Eczema

67. 2. Pityriasis rosea starts with a "herald patch" and then erupts in a Christmas tree pattern on the trunk. Tinea corporis is a skin infestation, usually seen as fine lines under the skin. Allergic reactions to drugs typically affect the entire body. Eczema is an erythematous papular rash typically affecting the antecubital and popliteal fossae.

NP: Assessment; CN: Physiological integrity; CNS: Physiological adaptation; CL: Knowledge

68. A 19-year-old client presents with second-degree sunburn on her face and both arms. Which intervention should the nurse implement **first**?

1. Administer analgesic medication as ordered.
2. Apply cold, moist towels to the burns.
3. Apply sterile, dry towels to the burns.
4. Apply vitamin A, D, and E ointment to the burns.

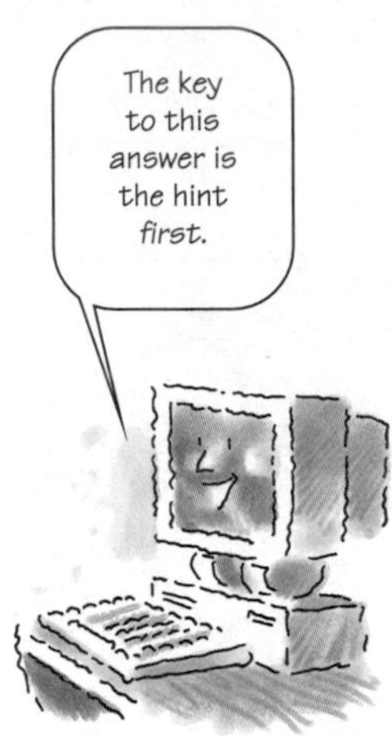

The key to this answer is the hint first.

68. 2. Cold, moist towels help stop the burning process. Analgesics should be administered as ordered after the burning process has been controlled. Dry towels would retain the heat and aren't used. Ointments are applied during the healing phase, but not initially.
NP: Implementation; CN: Physiological integrity; CNS: Basic care and comfort; CL: Application

69. For a client with a burn wound, which intervention decreases the chance of hypertrophied scarring during later stages of healing?

1. Removing all tissue in the wound area
2. Applying continuous pressure using elastic wraps
3. Wearing clothing to protect the burn from the sun
4. Maintaining wound dressing changes

69. 2. Using elastic wraps and bandages to apply continuous pressure during the early stages of wound healing can help prevent keloid scar formation. Removing tissue, especially eschar, promotes wound healing as do dressing changes, but neither directly decreases scar formation. Wearing clothing prevents sunburn but doesn't decrease scar formation.
NP: Implementation; CN: Physiological integrity; CNS: Physiological adaptation; CL: Application

70. A client sustains burns of the head, neck, right arm, right leg, anterior chest, and perineum. Based on the Rule of Nines, what's the total body surface area burned?

1. 34%
2. 54%
3. 55%
4. 35%

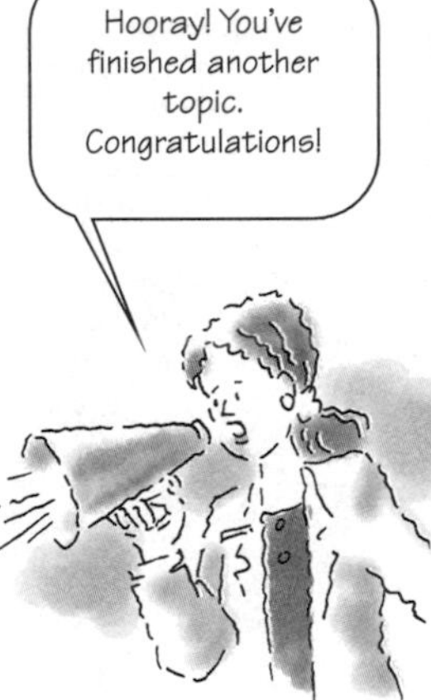

Hooray! You've finished another topic. Congratulations!

70. 3. According to the Rule of Nines, the head and neck account for 9% of body surface area; right arm, 9%; right leg, 18%; anterior chest, 18%; and perineum, 1%. These percentages total 55%.
NP: Assessment; CN: Physiological integrity; CNS: Physiological adaptation; CL: Application

71. A client suffers a second-degree burn on the entire surface of the upper left arm. Which nursing action is most important when assessing circulation?

1. Monitoring blood pressure in the left arm
2. Evaluating the strength of the left hand
3. Assessing capillary refill in the left hand
4. Measuring circumference of the left arm

71. 3. With a burn over the entire surface area of the left arm, the nurse must assess capillary refill in the left hand to check for the tourniquet effect (in which burn tissue surrounds the arm, and swelling and fluid decrease circulation to the distal part). Monitoring blood pressure in the left arm could damage the arm and decrease circulation. Evaluating hand strength is appropriate when assessing neuromuscular status, not circulation. Measuring arm circumference may be appropriate during a circulation check, but it's less important than assessing capillary refill.
NP: Implementation; CN: Physiological integrity; CNS: Physiological adaptation; CL: Application

Part III Care of the psychiatric client

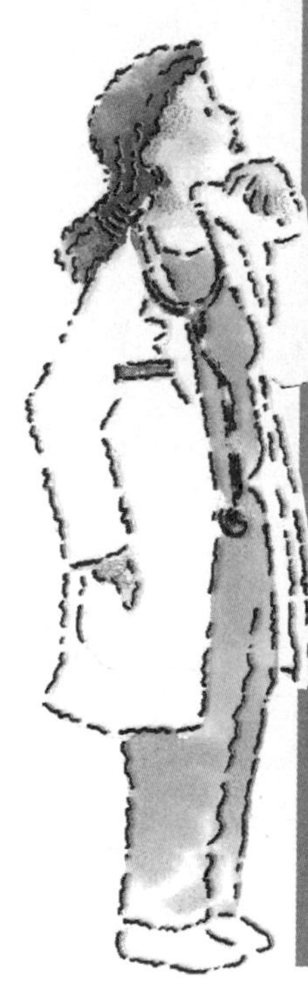

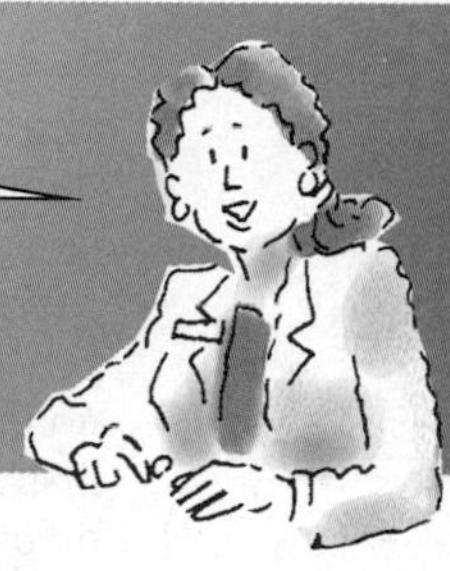
Before you take the tests
relating to psychiatric care,
take this test relating to tests
(and treatments, too) in
psychiatric care.

Chapter 12 Essentials of psychiatric care

1. A 50-year-old client is scheduled for electroconvulsive therapy (ECT). The nurse knows that ECT is most commonly prescribed for which of the following conditions?

1. Major depression
2. Antisocial personality disorder
3. Chronic schizophrenia
4. Somatoform disorder

1. 1. ECT is most commonly used for the treatment of major depression in clients who haven't responded to antidepressants or who have medical problems that contraindicate the use of antidepressants. ECT isn't commonly used for treatment of personality disorders. ECT doesn't appear to be of value to individuals with chronic schizophrenia and isn't the treatment of choice for clients with dissociative disorders.

NP: Analysis; CN: Safe, effective care environment; CNS: Management of care; CL: Knowledge

2. A patient with bipolar disorder becomes verbally aggressive in a group therapy session. Which of the following responses by the nurse would be best?

1. "You're behaving in an unacceptable manner, and you need to control yourself."
2. "If you continue to talk like that, no one will want to be around you."
3. "You're frightening everyone in the group. Leave the room immediately."
4. "Other people are disturbed by your profanity. I'll walk with you down the hall to help release some of that energy."

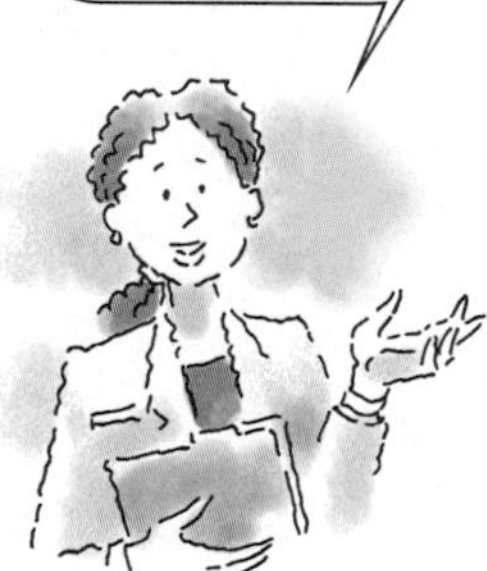
All of these
options might be
acceptable, but
which is best?

2. 4. This response informs the client that, although the behavior is unacceptable, the client is still worthy of help. The other responses indicate that the client is in control of the behavior.

NP: Implementation; CN: Safe, effective care environment; CNS: Management of care; CL: Application

3. A newly admitted client is extremely hostile toward a staff member she has just met, without apparent reason. According to Freudian theory, the nurse should suspect that the client is exhibiting which of the following phenomena?

1. Intellectualization
2. Transference
3. Triangulation
4. Splitting

3. 2. Transference is the unconscious assignment of negative or positive feelings evoked by a significant person in the client's past to another person. Intellectualization is a defense mechanism in which the client avoids dealing with emotions by focusing on facts. Triangulation refers to conflicts involving three family members. Splitting is a defense mechanism commonly seen in clients with personality disorders in which the world is perceived as all good or all bad.

NP: Assessment; CN: Psychosocial integrity; CNS: Psychosocial adaptation; CL: Analysis

4. Which intervention would be typical of a nurse using a cognitive-behavioral approach to a client experiencing low self-esteem?

1. Use of unconditional positive regard
2. Analysis of free associations
3. Classical conditioning
4. Examination of negative thought patterns

4. 4. Popular cognitive-behavioral approaches examine the validity of habitual patterns of thinking and belief systems that influence feelings and behaviors. Unconditional positive regard is a phrase from Carl Rogers's client-centered therapy and describes a supportive, nonjudgmental, neutral approach by a therapist. Analysis of free associations is characteristic of Freudian psychoanalysis. Classical conditioning is characteristic of a pure behavioral intervention.

NP: Implementation; CN: Safe, effective care environment; CNS: Management of care; CL: Application

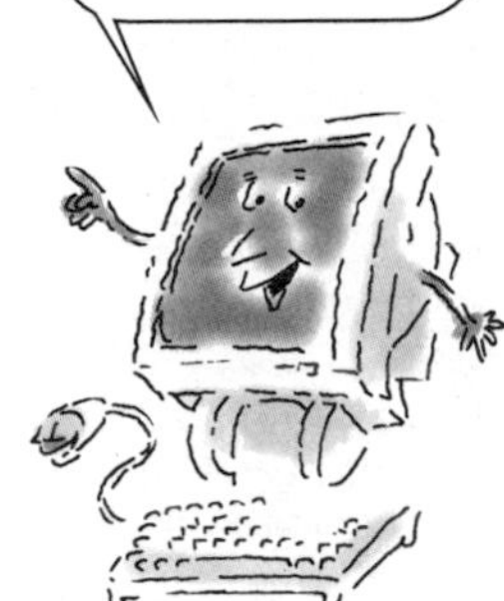

Isn't there a Yalom University somewhere? (Oops, I gave it away, didn't I? Shame!)

5. During group therapy, one client listening to another client's description of an abusive incident that occurred during childhood says, "I didn't think anyone else felt like I did as a child." The nurse recognizes this statement as a reflection of which of the following curative factors of group therapy, as identified by Yalom?

1. Altruism
2. Universality
3. Catharsis
4. Existential factors

5. 2. One of the 11 curative factors of group therapy identified by Yalom is universality, which assists group participants in recognizing common experiences and responses. This action helps reduce anxiety and allows other group members to provide support and understanding. Altruism, catharsis, and existential factors are other curative factors Yalom described but don't describe this particular incident. Altruism refers to finding meaning through helping others; catharsis is an open expression of previously suppressed feelings; and existential factors describe the recognition that one has control over the quality of one's life.

NP: Analysis; CN: Psychosocial integrity; CNS: Coping and adaptation; CL: Application

6. Which of the following statements best describes the key advantage of using groups in psychotherapy?

1. Decreases the focus on the individual
2. Fosters the physician-client relationship
3. Confronts individuals with their short-comings
4. Fosters a new learning environment

6. 4. In a group, the individual has the opportunity to learn that others have the same problems and needs. The group can also provide an arena where new methods of relating to others can be tried. Decreasing focus on the individual isn't a key advantage (and sometimes isn't an advantage at all). Groups don't, by themselves, foster the physician-client relationship, and they aren't always used to confront individuals.

NP: Evaluation; CN: Psychosocial integrity; CNS: Coping and adaptation; CL: Analysis

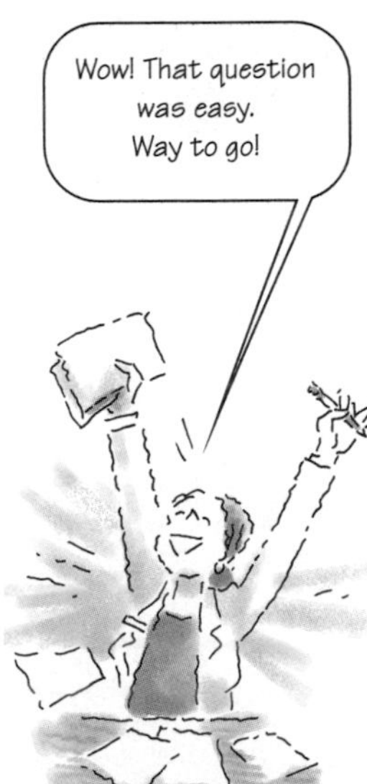

Wow! That question was easy. Way to go!

7. Which of the following therapies has been most strongly advocated for the treatment of posttraumatic stress disorder?

1. Electroconvulsive therapy (ECT)
2. Group therapy
3. Hypnotherapy
4. Individual therapy

7. 2. Group therapy has been especially effective with survivors of combat trauma. ECT, hypnotherapy, and individual therapy may be useful to this client, but these therapies aren't as strongly advocated as group therapy.

NP: Planning; CN: Safe, effective care environment; CNS: Management of care; CL: Knowledge

8. During a group therapy session, a teenage girl says she's fat and ugly and everybody makes fun of her. This statement reflects which common adolescent fear or anxiety?

1. Fear of the unknown
2. Fear of loss of respect, love, and emerging self-esteem
3. Anxiety related to guilt
4. Anxiety about body image and changes in physical appearance

8. 4. Anxiety about body image and changes in physical appearance is a common fear of adolescents. Fear of the unknown is associated with toddlerhood. Fear of loss of respect, love, and emerging self-esteem is associated with the school-age developmental phase. Anxiety related to guilt is also associated with the school-age-developmental phase.

NP: Assessment; CN: Psychosocial integrity; CNS: Psychosocial adaptation; CL: Comprehension

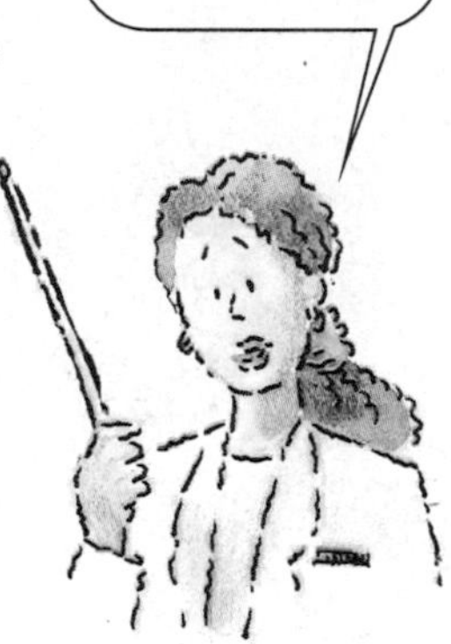

In psychiatric care, the nurse needs to recognize verbal as well as physical clues.

9. After telling the nurse to "pray for me," a client gives away personal possessions and shows a sudden calmness. The nurse recognizes that this behavior may signal which of the following?

1. Major depression
2. Panic attack
3. Suicidal ideation
4. Severe anxiety

9. 3. Verbal clues to suicidal ideation include such statements as "Pray for me," and "I won't be here when you get back." Nonverbal clues include giving away personal possessions, a sudden calmness, and risk-taking behaviors. The nurse should recognize the combination of these signs as indicating suicidal ideation—not depression, panic, or anxiety. Clients with major depression generally don't exhibit suicidal behavior until their outlook on their problems begins to improve (an improvement in behavior should raise suspicion, especially if accompanied by sudden calmness).

NP: Analysis; CN: Psychosocial integrity; CNS: Psychosocial adaptation; CL: Comprehension

10. A client recently lost a spouse. Which behavior indicates that the client is going through a normal stage of grieving?

1. The client starts using chemicals.
2. The client becomes an overachiever.
3. The client shows signs of hyperactivity.
4. The client shows a loss of warmth when interacting with others.

10. 4. Hostile reactions, such as loss of warmth when interacting with others, occur during normal grieving. Chemical use, overachieving, and hyperactivity commonly correlate with the roles and dynamics of an alcoholic family.

NP: Analysis; CN: Psychosocial integrity; CNS: Psychosocial adaptation; CL: Comprehension

11. Which of the following is classified as an Axis I disorder by the *Diagnostic and Statistical Manual of Mental Disorders,*Text Revision, *(DSM-IV-TR)?*

1. Obesity
2. Borderline personality disorder
3. Major depression
4. Hypertension

11. 3. The *DSM-IV-TR* classifies major depression as an Axis I disorder. Borderline personality disorder is an Axis II; obesity and hypertension, Axis III.

NP: Assessment; CN: Psychosocial integrity; CNS: Psychosocial adaptation; CL: Knowledge

12. The nurse is caring for a child with attention deficit hyperactivity disorder (ADHD). The *Diagnostic and Statistical Manual of Mental Disorders,* Text Revision *(DSM-IV-TR)* places this disorder on which axis?

1. Axis I
2. Axis II
3. Axis III
4. Axis IV

12. 1. ADHD, major depression, and disorder of written expression are on Axis I (for children). Neither Axis II nor III has diagnoses for children. Axis IV generally applies to sexual abuse disorders.

NP: Assessment; CN: Psychosocial integrity; CNS: Psychosocial adaptation; CL: Knowledge

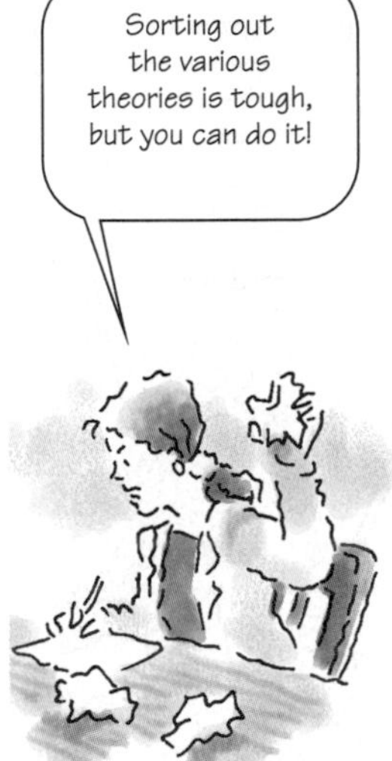

Sorting out the various theories is tough, but you can do it!

13. The psychiatric nurse practitioner uses theories of the behavioral theorist Jean Piaget in group and individual therapy. According to behavioral theories, symptoms represent which definition?

1. A response to anxiety arising from interpersonal relationships
2. Learned behaviors that are maintained because they're reinforced
3. Internal conflicts arising from early childhood trauma
4. A combination of past unresolved problems and current problems

13. 2. According to behavioral theorists, symptoms are learned behaviors maintained because they're reinforced. Social theorists (such as Sullivan, Maslow, and Rogers) view symptoms as a response to anxiety arising from interpersonal relationships. Psychological theorists (such as Freud and Jung) believe symptoms are internal conflicts arising from early childhood trauma and failure of developmental tasks; they also believe symptoms are a combination of unresolved problems and current problems.

NP: Analysis; CN: Psychosocial integrity; CNS: Psychosocial adaptation; CL: Knowledge

14. According to the psychological theorists, such as Freud and Jung, treatment of symptoms should involve which action?

1. Modifying behavior by manipulating the environment
2. Using desensitization
3. Uncovering past events
4. Using family therapy

14. 3. According to the psychological theorists, treatment of symptoms involves clarifying the meaning of events, uncovering past events, and using transference/countertransference. Behavioral theorists advocate modifying behavior by manipulating the environment and using desensitization. Social theorists treat symptoms using family therapy.

NP: Assessment; CN: Psychosocial integrity; CNS: Psychosocial adaptation; CL: Knowledge

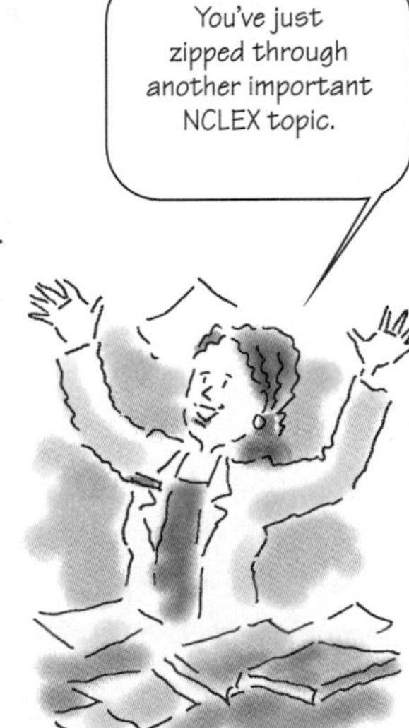

You've just zipped through another important NCLEX topic.

15. The nurse is teaching assertiveness techniques to a group of codependent clients. Of the following statements, which one is a therapeutic assertive response?

1. "You don't care about me."
2. "It was your mistake, but I forgive you."
3. "I feel you're frustrated with me."
4. "You're mad at me."

15. 3. Therapeutic assertive responses commonly begin with the word "I" or involve restating the message, reflecting the other person's feelings, or refocusing. The remaining responses place the point of reference on "you" and aren't assertive responses ("I") telling what the person actually feels, thinks, or believes.

NP: Analysis; CN: Psychosocial integrity; CNS: Psychosocial adaptation; CL: Application

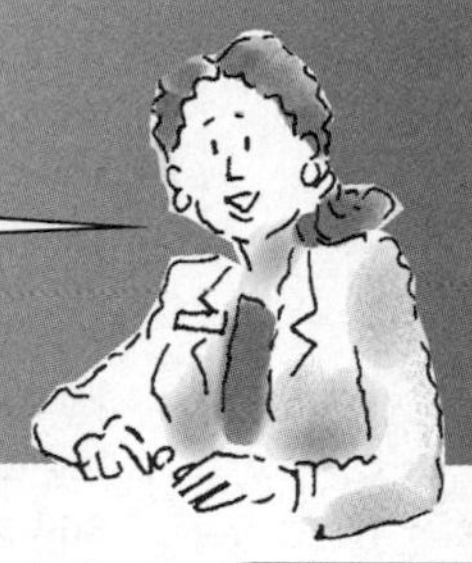

Can't remember much about a particular somatoform disorder? Type this address into your Internet browser: www.emedicine.com/. Then search for the disorder. Cool.

Chapter 13 Somatoform & sleep disorders

1. Which of the following statements is correct about clients who have somatoform disorders?
1. They usually seek medical attention.
2. They have organic pathologic disorders.
3. They regularly attend psychotherapy sessions without encouragement.
4. They're eager to discover the true reasons for their physical symptoms.

1. 1. A client with a somatization disorder usually seeks medical attention. These clients have a history of multiple physiological complaints without associated demonstrable organic pathologic causes. The expected behavior for this type of disorder is to seek treatment from several medical physicians for somatic complaints, not psychiatric evaluation.

NP: Assessment; CN: Health promotion and maintenance; CNS: Prevention and early detection of disease; CL: Knowledge

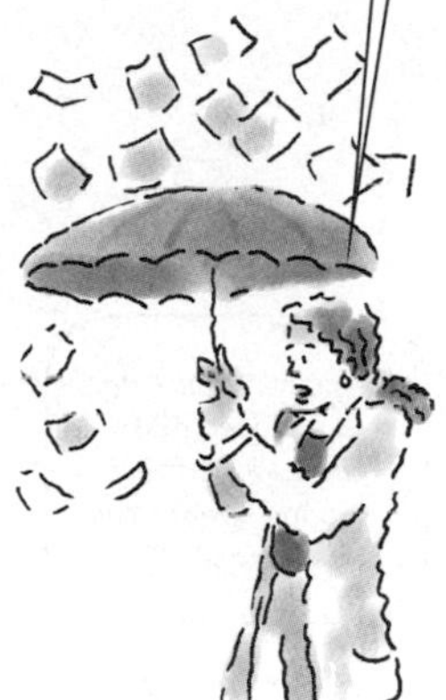

Not to worry. You'll finish these questions before you know it!

2. Which of the following statements is correct about the diagnosis of somatoform disorders?
1. The somatic complaints are limited to one organ system.
2. The event preceding the physical illness occurred recently.
3. They're physical conditions with organic pathologic causes.
4. They're disorders that occur in the absence of organic findings.

2. 4. The essential feature of somatoform disorders is a physical or somatic complaint without any demonstrable organic findings to account for the complaint. There are no known physiological mechanisms to explain the findings. Somatic complaints aren't limited to one organ system. The diagnostic criteria for somatoform disorders state that the client has a history of many physical complaints beginning before age 30 that occur over several years.

NP: Analysis; CN: Psychosocial integrity; CNS: Psychosocial adaptation; CL: Analysis

3. Which of the following rationales best explains the physical symptoms experienced by a client with a somatoform disorder?
1. The client complains of physical symptoms to cope with delusional thinking.
2. The client complains of physical symptoms to gain attention.
3. The client experiences physical symptoms in response to anxiety.
4. The client complains of physical symptoms that can be explained by a known physiologic cause.

3. 3. In a client with a somatofom disorder, physical symptoms are manifestations of psychological distress, such as anxiety and depression, that have no apparent physiologic cause. The physical symptoms enable the client to avoid unpleasant emotions, not seek individual attention. Somatic delusions are characteristic of schizophrenia.

NP: Analysis; CN: Psychosocial integrity; CNS: Coping and adaptation; CL: Analysis

4. Which of the following ego defense mechanisms describes the underlying dynamics of somatization disorder, according to the psychodynamic theory?

1. Repression of anger
2. Suppression of grief
3. Denial of depression
4. Preoccupation with pain

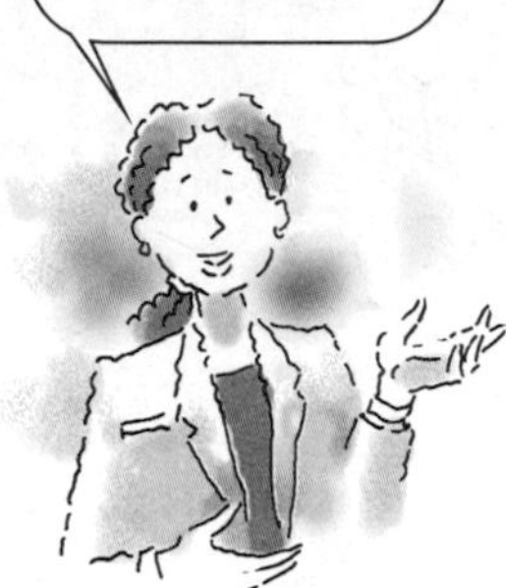

Remember, you're looking for a defense mechanism.

4. 1. One psychodynamic theory states that somatization is the transformation of aggressive and hostile wishes toward others into physical complaints. Repressed anger originating from past disappointments and unfilled needs for nurturing and caring are expressed by soliciting other people's concern and rejecting them as ineffective. Denial, suppression, and preoccupation aren't the defense mechanisms underlying the dynamics of somatization disorders.

NP: Analysis; CN: Psychosocial integrity; CNS: Coping and adaptation; CL: Knowledge

5. An 86-year-old client in an extended care facility is anxious most of the time and frequently complains of a number of vague symptoms that interfere with her ability to eat. These symptoms indicate which of the following disorders?

1. Conversion disorder
2. Hypochondriasis
3. Severe anxiety
4. Sublimation

5. 2. Complaints of vague physical symptoms that have no apparent medical causes are characteristic of clients with hypochondriasis. In many cases, the GI system is affected. Conversion disorders are characterized by one or more neurologic symptoms. The client's symptoms don't suggest severe anxiety. A client experiencing sublimation channels maladaptive feelings or impulses into socially acceptable behavior.

NP: Assessment; CN: Psychosocial integrity; CNS: Psychosocial adaptation; CL: Analysis

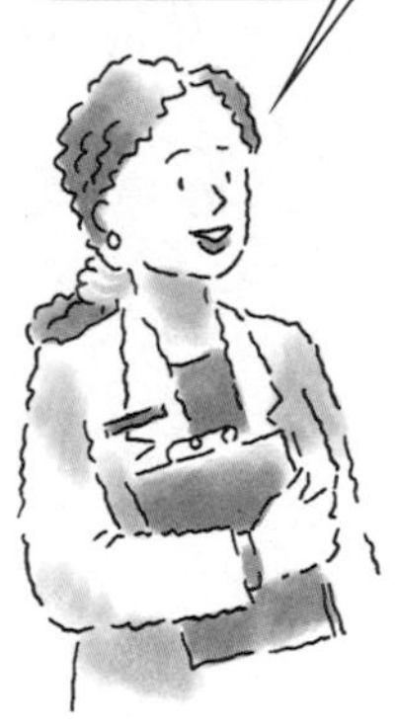

Accurate nursing diagnoses make sure all staff are working toward the same goal!

6. Which of the following nursing diagnoses is most appropriate for the disorder known as hypochondriasis?

1. Risk for injury
2. Anticipatory grieving
3. Risk for situational low self-esteem
4. Deficient diversional activity

6. 3. Hypochondriasis is a disorder manifested by fear, risk for situational low self-esteem, and feelings of worthlessness. Deficient diversional activity, anticipatory grieving, and risk for injury have no correlation to the disorder.

NP: Analysis; CN: Psychosocial integrity; CNS: Psychosocial adaptation; CL: Application

7. A college student frequently visited the health center during the past year with multiple vague complaints of GI symptoms before course examinations. Although physical causes have been eliminated, the student continues to express her belief that she has a serious illness. These symptoms are typical of which of the following disorders?

1. Conversion disorder
2. Depersonalization
3. Hypochondriasis
4. Somatization disorder

7. 3. Hypochondriasis in this case is shown by the client's belief that she has a serious illness, although pathologic causes have been eliminated. The disturbance usually lasts at least 6 months, and the GI system is commonly affected. Exacerbations are usually associated with identifiable life stressors such as, in this case, course examinations. Conversion disorders are characterized by one or more neurologic symptoms. Depersonalization refers to persistent, recurrent episodes of feeling detached from one's self or body. Somatoform disorders generally have a chronic course with few remissions.

NP: Assessment; CN: Psychosocial integrity; CNS: Psychosocial adaptation; CL: Analysis

25. A client is admitted for abrupt onset of paralysis in her left arm. Although no physiological cause has been found, the symptoms are exacerbated when she speaks of losing custody of her children in a recent divorce. These assessment findings are characteristic of which of the following disorders?

1. Body dysmorphic disorder
2. Conversion disorder
3. Delusional disorder
4. Malingering

25. 2. Conversion disorders are characterized by one or more neurologic symptoms associated with psychological conflict. The client doesn't have a delusion; this is the sole manifestation of a delusional disorder. Body dysmorphic disorder is an imagined belief that there's a defect in the appearance of all or part of the body. Malingering is the intentional production of symptoms to avoid obligations or obtain rewards.

NP: Assessment; CN: Psychosocial integrity; CNS: Psychosocial adaptation; CL: Analysis

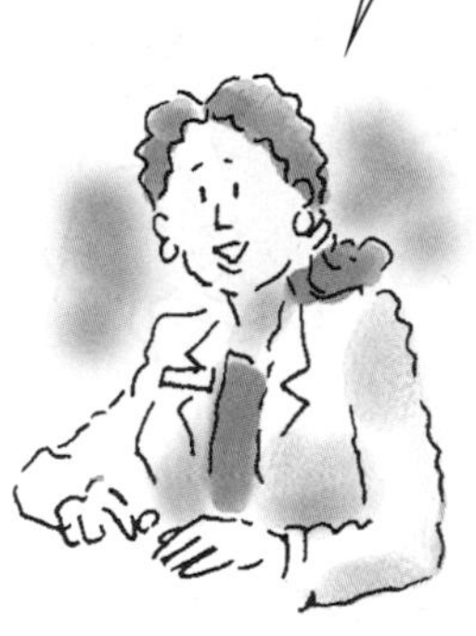

You're terrific at answering these questions!

26. A client has been diagnosed with conversion-disorder blindness. Which of the following statements best explains this manifestation?

1. The client is suppressing her true feelings.
2. The client's anxiety has been relieved through her physical symptoms.
3. The client is acting indifferent because she doesn't want to show her actual fear.
4. The client's needs are being met, so she doesn't need to be anxious.

26. 2. Conversion accomplishes anxiety reduction through the production of a physical symptom symbolically linked to an underlying conflict. The client isn't aware of the internal conflict. Hospitalization doesn't remove the source of the conflict.

NP: Analysis; CN: Psychosocial integrity; CNS: Psychosocial adaptation; CL: Analysis

27. A client with hypochondriasis complains of pain in her right side that she hasn't had before. Which of the following responses is the most appropriate?

1. "It's time for group therapy now."
2. "Tell me about this new pain you're having. You'll miss group therapy today."
3. "I'll report this pain to your physician. In the meantime, group therapy starts in 5 minutes. You must leave now to be on time."
4. "I'll call your physician and see if he'll order a new pain medication. Why don't you get some rest for now?"

27. 3. The amount of time focused on discussing physical symptoms should be decreased. Lack of positive reinforcement may help stop the maladaptive behavior. However, avoiding the statement all together demeans the client and doesn't address the underlying problem. Asking the client to further explain the pain emphasizes physical symptoms and prevents the client from attending group therapy. All physical complaints need to be evaluated for physiological causes by the physician.

NP: Implementation; CN: Psychosocial integrity; CNS: Coping and adaptation; CL: Application

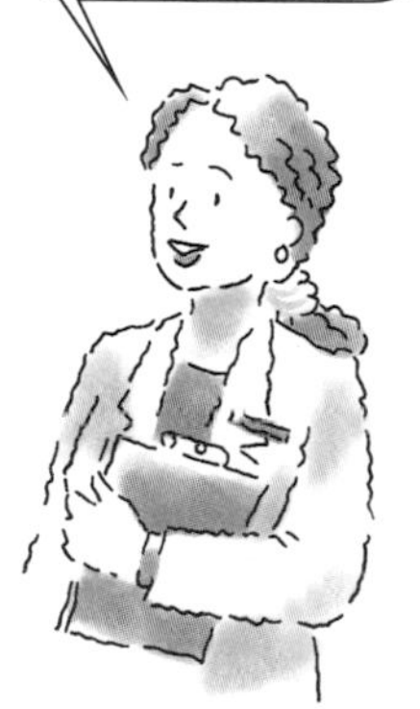

A client with a disorder of psychological origin may need the same interventions as one with a disorder of physical origin.

28. Which intervention would help a client with conversion-disorder blindness to eat?

1. Direct the client to independently locate items on the tray and feed himself.
2. See to the needs of the other clients in the dining room; then feed this client last.
3. Establish a "buddy" system with other clients who can feed the client at each meal.
4. Expect the client to feed himself after explaining the location of food on the tray.

28. 4. The client is expected to maintain some level of independence by feeding himself, while at the same time the nurse is supportive in a matter-of-fact way. Feeding the client leads to dependence.

NP: Implementation; CN: Psychosocial integrity; CNS: Coping and adaptation; CL: Application

37. Which of the following statements made by a client with a pain disorder shows the nurse that the goal of stress management was attained?

1. "My arm hurts."
2. "I enjoy being dependent on others."
3. "I don't really understand why I'm here."
4. "My muscles feel relaxed after that progressive relaxation exercise."

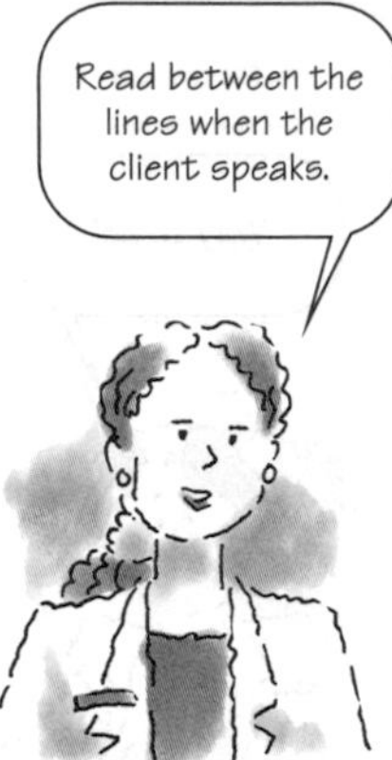

Read between the lines when the client speaks.

37. 4. The client is experiencing positive results from the relaxation exercise. All other responses alert the nurse that the client needs further interventions.

NP: Evaluation; CN: Physiological integrity; CNS: Physiological adaptation; CL: Evaluation

38. Pain disorders, such as headaches and musculoskeletal pain, are most frequently associated with which of the following groups?

1. Men
2. Women
3. Less educated population
4. Low socioeconomic population

38. 2. Pain disorders are more common in women than men. There isn't a high correlation of pain disorders with educational level or socioeconomic status.

NP: Assessment; CN: Physiological integrity; CNS: Physiological adaptation; CL: Knowledge

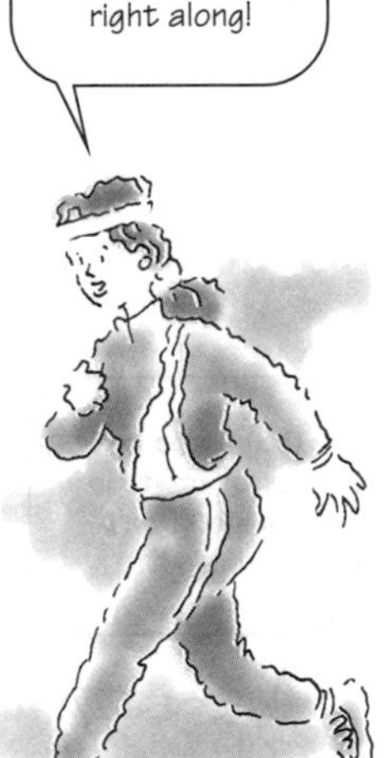

You're moving right along!

39. Which of the following descriptions best defines a somatoform pain disorder?

1. A preoccupation with pain in the absence of physical disease
2. A physical or somatic complaint without any demonstrable organic findings
3. A morbid fear or belief that one has a serious disease where none exists
4. One or more neurologic symptoms associated with psychological conflict or need

39. 1. Somatoform pain disorder is a preoccupation with pain in the absence of physical disease. A physical or somatic complaint refers to somatoform disorders in general. Neurologic symptoms are associated with conversion disorders. A morbid fear of serious illness is hypochondriasis.

NP: Assessment; CN: Psychosocial integrity; CNS: Coping and adaptation; CL: Knowledge

40. By which of the following processes does a client conceal the true motivations for his thoughts, actions, or feelings?

1. Displacement
2. Rationalization
3. Regression
4. Substitution

40. 2. Rationalization is a process by which an individual deals with emotional conflict or internal or external stressors by concealing the true motivations for his thoughts, actions, and feelings through the elaboration of reassuring or self-serving, but incorrect, explanations. This process isn't a defense mechanism related to pain disorders. Displacement, substitution, and regression are defense mechanisms that would be expected from a client with a pain disorder.

NP: Assessment; CN: Psychosocial integrity; CNS: Coping and adaptation; CL: Application

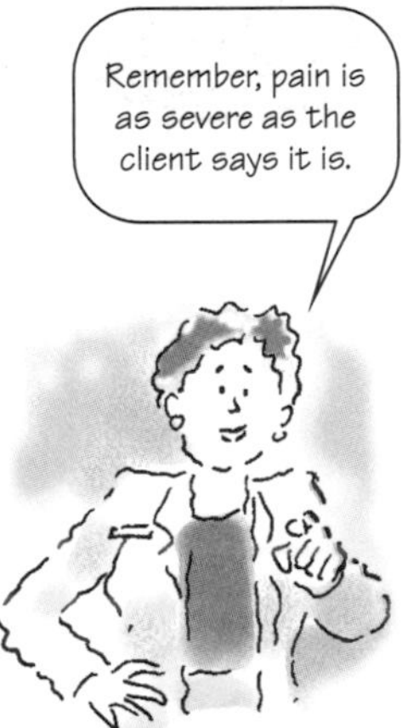

Remember, pain is as severe as the client says it is.

41. Which of the following nursing goals is appropriate for a client with a pain disorder?

1. The client will express less fear.
2. The client will increase independence.
3. The client will express relief from pain.
4. The client will adapt coping strategies to deal with stress.

41. 3. Relief of pain should be a priority for clients experiencing pain. The development of coping strategies would be beneficial for a client with a somatization disorder. Expression of less fear applies to a client with hypochondriasis. A focus on independence is appropriate for a client diagnosed with conversion disorder.

NP: Planning; CN: Physiological integrity; CNS: Physiological adaptation; CL: Application

42. Which of the following statements best defines malingering?

1. It's a preoccupation with pain in the absence of physical disease.
2. It's a voluntary production of a physical symptom for a secondary gain.
3. It's a morbid fear or belief that one has a serious disease where none exists.
4. It's associated with a psychological need or conflict in which the client shows one or more neurologic symptoms.

42. 2. Malingering is defined as a voluntary production of physical or psychological symptoms to accomplish a specific goal or secondary gain (avoidance of a specific situation such as a jail term or to obtain money). The other statements are associated with pain disorder, hypochondriasis, and conversion disorder, respectively.

NP: Assessment; CN: Health promotion and maintenance; CNS: Prevention and early detection of disease; CL: Comprehension

43. Based on a nursing diagnosis of ineffective coping for a client with somatoform pain disorder, which of the following nursing goals is most realistic?

1. The client will be free from injury.
2. The client will recognize sensory impairment.
3. The client will discuss beliefs about spiritual issues.
4. The client will verbalize absence or significant reduction of physical symptoms.

43. 4. Expression of feelings enables the client to ventilate emotions, which decreases anxiety and draws attention away from the physical symptoms. The client isn't experiencing a safety issue. Spiritual issues are related to spiritual distress, and no evidence exists to support that the client is having spiritual distress. There's also no apparent correlation with any sensory-perceptual alterations.

NP: Planning; CN: Physiological integrity; CNS: Basic care and comfort; CL: Analysis

44. Which of the following statements made by a client best meets the diagnostic criteria for pain disorder?

1. "I can't move my right leg."
2. "I'm having severe stomach and leg pain."
3. "I'm so afraid I might have human immunodeficiency virus."
4. "I'm having chest pain and pain radiating down my left arm that began more than 1 hour ago."

44. 2. The diagnostic criteria for pain disorders state that pain in one or more anatomic sites is the predominant focus of the clinical presentation and is of sufficient severity to warrant clinical attention. Hypochondriasis is a morbid fear or belief that one has a serious disease where none exists. A client with a conversion disorder can experience a motor neurologic symptom such as paralysis. Unremitting chest pain with radiation of pain down the left arm is symptomatic of a myocardial infarction.

NP: Assessment; CN: Psychosocial integrity; CNS: Psychosocial adaptation; CL: Application

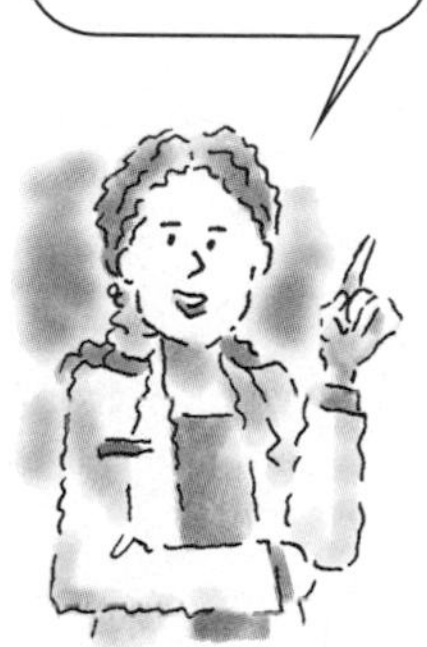
Remember, diagnostic criteria for psychological problems come from the latest edition of the *Diagnostic and Statistical Manual of Mental Disorders,* currently known as DSM-IV-TR.

45. Which of the following nursing diagnoses is appropriate for a client with somatoform pain disorder?

1. Interrupted family processes
2. Disturbed thought processes
3. Ineffective denial
4. Ineffective coping

45. 4. A somatoform pain disorder is closely associated with the client's inability to handle stress and conflict. Altered thought processes aren't directly correlated with this disorder. While interrupted family processes may be present, they aren't the primary focus.

NP: Analysis; CN: Psychosocial integrity; CNS: Psychosocial adaptation; CL: Application

46. Which of the following statements made by a nurse will help a client diagnosed with somatoform pain disorder become independent in self-care?

1. "I'll call you for all the group activities."
2. "I'll help you on a daily basis with your care."
3. "The staff will help you with your basic needs for today."
4. "We'll wait until you have no more pain before you participate in activities."

46. 3. Limited time in assisting a client will help the client develop independence. All other options would promote dependence on the staff.

NP: Implementation; CN: Safe, effective care environment; CNS: Management of care; CL: Application

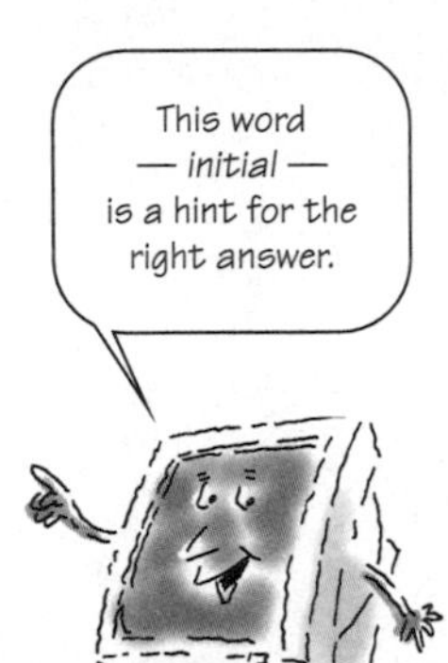
This word
— *initial* —
is a hint for the
right answer.

47. Which of the following initial therapeutic interventions is the most appropriate for a client diagnosed with ineffective coping related to a pain disorder?

1. Make an accurate assessment.
2. Promote expression of feelings.
3. Promote insight into the disorder.
4. Help the client develop alternative coping strategies.

47. 1. It's essential to accurately assess the client first before any interventions. Promoting insight and expression of feelings and helping the client develop coping strategies are appropriate interventions that can be implemented after the initial assessment.

NP: Implementation; CN: Psychosocial integrity; CNS: Psychosocial adaptation; CL: Application

48. A client with a somatoform pain disorder may obtain secondary gain. Which of the following statements refers to a secondary gain?

1. It brings some stability to the family.
2. It decreases the preoccupation with the physical illness.
3. It enables the client to avoid some unpleasant activity.
4. It promotes emotional support or attention for the client.

48. 4. Secondary gain refers to the benefits of the illness that allow the client to receive emotional support or attention. Primary gain enables the client to avoid some unpleasant activity. A dysfunctional family may disregard the real issue, although some conflict is relieved. Somatoform pain disorder is a preoccupation with pain in the absence of physical disease.

NP: Analysis; CN: Psychosocial integrity; CNS: Psychosocial adaptation; CL: Analysis

49. Which of the following nursing interventions is appropriate for a client diagnosed with a somatoform pain disorder?

1. Reinforce the client's behavior when it isn't focused on pain.
2. Allow the client to verbalize anxieties related to body image.
3. Allow the client to verbalize relief of fear related to the illness.
4. Assist the client in recovery of the lost or altered function of a body part.

49. 1. Help the client get attention and see himself as valuable without using pain. Fear of illness is related to hypochondriasis. Verbalization of anxieties related to body image may be beneficial in a client with body dysmorphic disorder. The recovery of a lost or altered function of a part is related to conversion disorders.

NP: Intervention; CN: Psychosocial integrity; CNS: Coping and adaptation; CL: Application

50. A nurse working in a psychiatric unit sees clients with a wide range of psychiatric diagnoses. What's the essential difference between dissociative disorders and somatoform disorders?

1. Dissociative disorders are related to childhood sexual abuse; somatoform disorders, to the environment.
2. Dissociative disorders are related to psychological factors; somatoform disorders, to stress.
3. Dissociative disorders involve memory or identity disruptions; somatoform disorders involve expression of psychological stress through somatic complaints.
4. Dissociative disorders are automatic; somatoform disorders are voluntary.

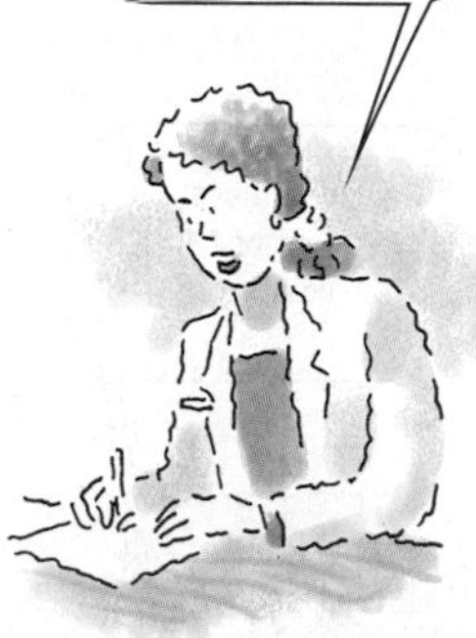

Take your time on diagnoses questions; they're important and you'll see lots of them on NCLEX.

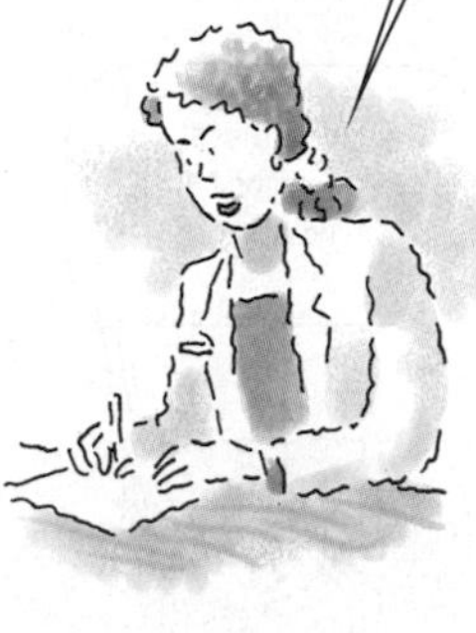

50. 3. Dissociative disorders involve memory lapses or identity disruptions, whereas somatoform disorders are manifested by somatic complaints related to psychological stress.

NP: Analysis; CN: Psychosocial integrity; CNS: Psychosocial adaptation; CL: Knowledge

51. A client with somatoform disorder experiences chronic headaches and fatigue. When her family helps her with housecleaning, she's experiencing which of the following?

1. Primary gain
2. Secondary gain
3. La belle indifference
4. Pain disorder

51. 2. Secondary gain is the receipt of extra care and support during an illness; it's an unintentionally sought benefit of an illness that might not be available otherwise. Primary gain refers to symbolic resolution of an unconscious conflict that decreases anxiety. La belle indifference is an indifferent attitude in situations where most people would be concerned. Pain disorder is a somatoform disorder in which pain is the dominant presenting symptom.

NP: Assessment; CN: Psychosocial integrity; CNS: Psychosocial adaptation; CL: Comprehension

52. A client with somatoform disorder states that her frequent headaches result from a brain tumor. However, a tumor hasn't shown up on diagnostic tests. The nurse identifies the client's form of somatization as which of the following?

1. Conversion disorder
2. Pain disorder
3. Hypochondriasis
4. Body dysmorphic disorder

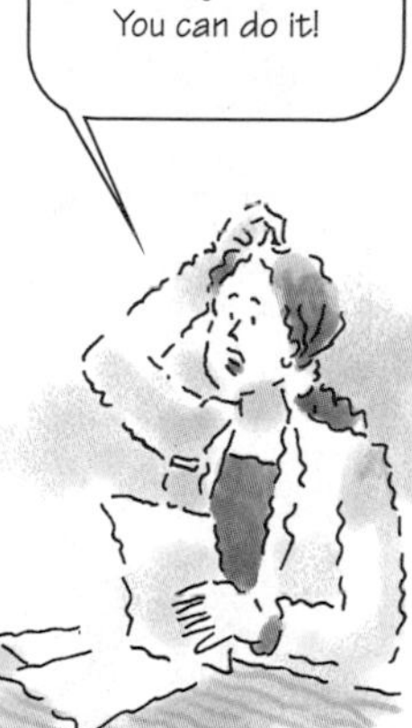

Have you sorted out the various forms of somatization? Don't try to rush. You can do it!

52. 3. In hypochondriasis, a physical symptom is interpreted as severe or life-threatening and causes exaggerated worry. In conversion disorder, the client loses a motor or sensory function but lacks appropriate concern about the loss. In pain disorder, pain is the dominant feature. In body dysmorphic disorder, the client is preoccupied with a perceived defect in appearance.

NP: Assessment; CN: Psychosocial integrity; CNS: Psychosocial adaptation; CL: Knowledge

53. The etiology of a somatoform disorder may involve which of the following?
1. Deficits in neurotransmitters
2. Traumatic childhood memories
3. Difficult learning experiences in elementary school
4. Negative personal assessments

53. 4. Clients with somatoform disorder commonly have low self-esteem and unmet dependency needs; the nurse should encourage positive self-coping statements when caring for these clients. Neurotransmitter deficits and difficult learning experiences aren't linked to somatoform disorders. Traumatic childhood memories are associated with dissociative, not somatoform, disorders.
NP: Analysis; CN: Psychosocial integrity; CNS: Psychosocial adaptation; CL: Comprehension

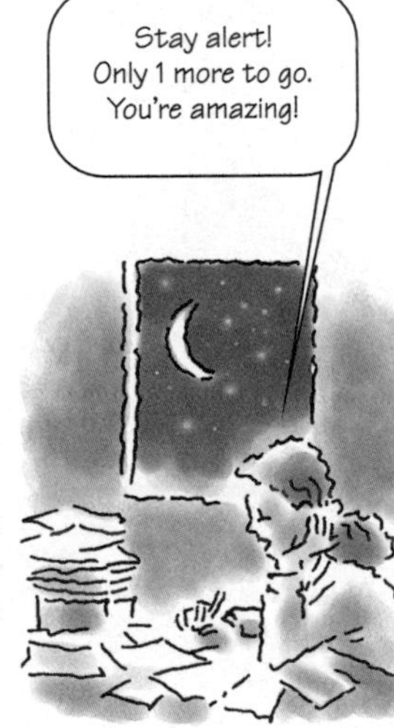

Stay alert!
Only 1 more to go.
You're amazing!

54. A 26-year-old client is diagnosed with somatoform disorder. When discussing the care plan with the client's husband, the nurse should give which instruction?
1. "Tell your wife that her symptoms are all in her head to force her to deal with reality."
2. "Tell your wife that her symptoms are an attempt to get attention and that you'll be more attentive."
3. "Accept the reality of the symptoms as your wife presents them, and don't dispute them."
4. "Realize that your wife is creating the symptoms on purpose."

54. 3. For a client with somatoform disorder, caregivers should accept the symptoms and avoid disputing them. The symptoms aren't contrived or all in the client's head. They're neither an attempt to get attention nor created "on purpose."
NP: Analysis; CN: Psychosocial integrity; CNS: Psychosocial adaptation; CL: Application

55. A client with a diagnosis of somatoform disorder has been admitted to the psychiatric unit and has difficulty breathing, numbness, and loss of movement in her left arm. She seems unusually calm and unconcerned about her loss. The nurse recognizes these symptoms as which of the following?
1. Conversion disorder
2. Hypochondriasis
3. Body dysmorphic disorder
4. Pain disorder

55. 1. Conversion disorder is characterized by loss of motor, sensory, or visceral functioning accompanied by the client's indifference to the loss. In hypochondriasis, the client interprets a physical symptom as severe or life-threatening and worries over it excessively. Body dysmorphic disorder is a preoccupation with a perceived defect in appearance. In pain disorder, pain is the dominant physical symptom.
NP: Analysis; CN: Psychosocial integrity; CNS: Psychosocial adaptation; CL: Application

Hooray for
you! You're the

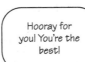

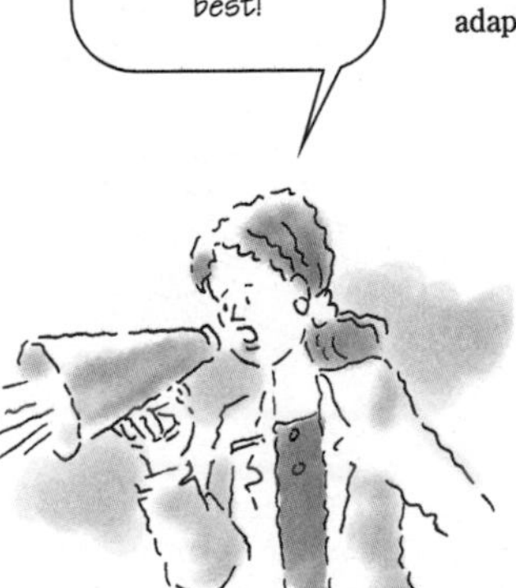

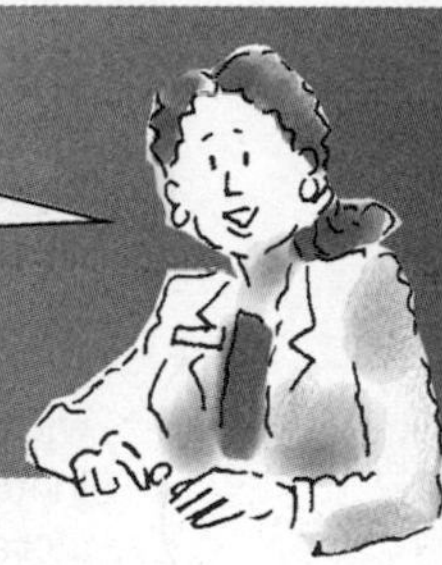

Want more information on anxiety and mood disorders to help you prepare for the NCLEX? Check out the Web site of the National Alliance for the Mentally Ill at www.nami.org/.

Chapter 14
Anxiety & mood disorders

1. Which of the following statements is typical of a client who experiences periodic panic attacks while sleeping?

1. "Yesterday, I sat up in bed and just felt so scared."
2. "I have difficulty sleeping because I'm so anxious."
3. "Sometimes I have the most wild and vivid dreams."
4. "When I drink beer, I fall asleep without any problems."

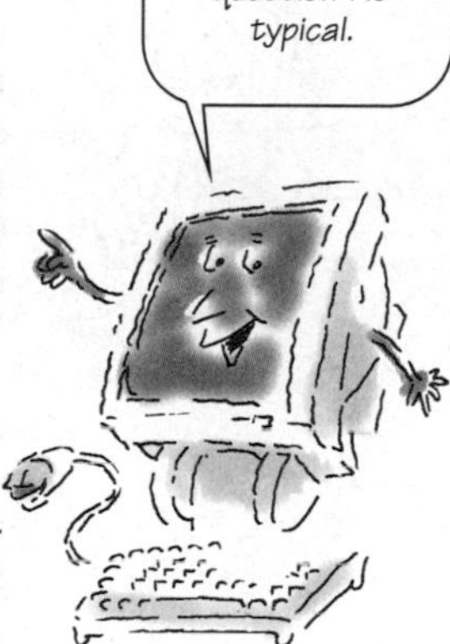

The key word in question 1 is typical.

2. A client with panic disorder should be monitored for the existence of which of the following other psychosocial problems?

1. Attention deficit hyperactivity disorder (ADHD)
2. Developmental disability
3. Dissociative behavior
4. Substance abuse

3. A client with a history of panic attacks who says, "I felt so trapped," right after an attack most likely has which of the following fears?

1. Loss of control
2. Loss of identity
3. Loss of memory
4. Loss of maturity

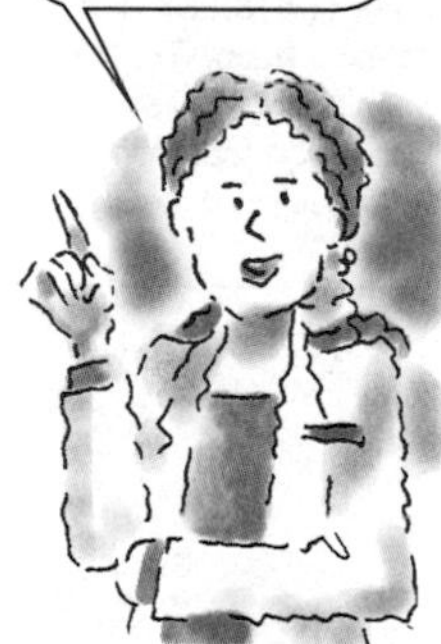

Question 3 doesn't ask for all possible answers, just the most likely one.

1. 1. A person who suffers a panic attack while sleeping experiences an abrupt awakening and feelings of fear. People with severe anxiety often have symptoms related to a sleep disorder; they wouldn't typically experience a sleep panic attack. A panic attack while sleeping often causes an inability to remember dreams. Intake of alcohol initially produces a drowsy feeling, but after a short period of time alcohol causes restless, fragmented sleep and strange dreams.

NP: Assessment; CN: Psychosocial integrity; CNS: Psychosocial adaptation; CL: Knowledge

2. 4. Studies show that more than one-third of people with panic disorders experience substance abuse. There is no relationship between panic disorder and ADHD. Developmental disabilities and dissociative behavior aren't associated with panic disorder.

NP: Assessment; CN: Psychosocial integrity; CNS: Coping and adaptation; CL: Knowledge

3. 1. People who fear loss of control during a panic attack often make statements about feeling trapped, getting hurt, or having little or no personal control over their situations. People who experience panic attacks don't tend to have memory impairment or loss of identity. People who have panic attacks also don't regress or become immature.

NP: Analysis; CN: Psychosocial integrity; CNS: Coping and adaptation; CL: Application

4. Which of the following problems would be reason for a client taking alprazolam (Xanax) for panic disorder to discontinue use of the drug?

1. Intermittent insomnia
2. Acute-angle glaucoma
3. Seizure disorder
4. Tartrazine hypersensitivity

4. 2. Acute-angle glaucoma is a medical problem that contraindicates the use of alprazolam. Alprazolam causes drowsiness and sedation, so sleep shouldn't be interrupted. Seizure disorder isn't a contraindication for the use of alprazolam. Tartrazine hypersensitivity is associated with yellow dye used in some convenience foods and isn't a contraindication for the use of alprazolam.

NP: Analysis; CN: Physiological integrity; CNS: Pharmacological and parenteral therapies; CL: Knowledge

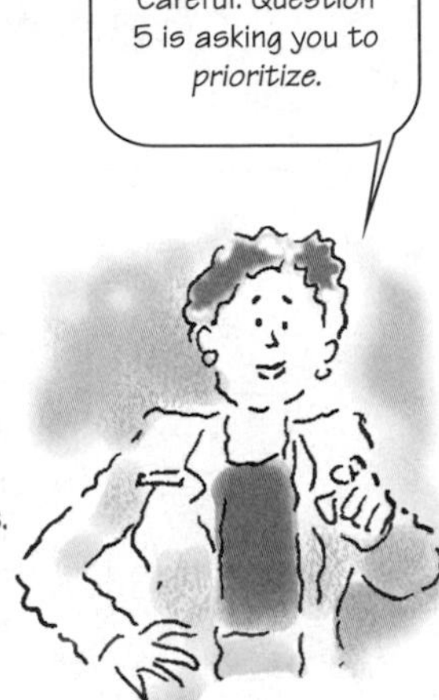

Careful. Question 5 is asking you to *prioritize.*

5. Which of the following nursing interventions is given priority in a care plan for a person having a panic disorder?

1. Tell the client to take deep breaths.
2. Have the client talk about the anxiety.
3. Encourage the client to verbalize feelings.
4. Ask the client about the cause of the attack.

5. 1. During a panic attack, the nurse should remain with the client and direct what's said toward changing the physiological response, such as taking deep breaths. During an attack, the client is unable to talk about anxious situations and isn't able to address feelings, especially uncomfortable feelings and frustrations. While having a panic attack, the client is also unable to focus on anything other than the symptoms, so the client won't be able to discuss the cause of the attack.

NP: Planning; CN: Psychosocial integrity; CNS: Psychosocial adaptation; CL: Knowledge

6. Which of the following instructions should the nurse include in a teaching session about panic disorder for clients and their families?

1. Identifying when anxiety is escalating
2. Determining how to stop a panic attack
3. Addressing strategies to reduce physical pain
4. Preventing the client from depending on others

6. 1. By identifying the presence of anxiety, it's possible to take steps to prevent its escalation. A panic attack can't be stopped. The nurse can take steps to assist the client safely through the attack. Later, the nurse can assist the client to alleviate the precipitating stressors. Clients who experience panic disorder don't tend to be in physical pain. The client experiencing a panic disorder may need to periodically depend on other people when having a panic attack.

NP: Planning; CN: Psychosocial integrity; CNS: Coping and adaptation; CL: Comprehension

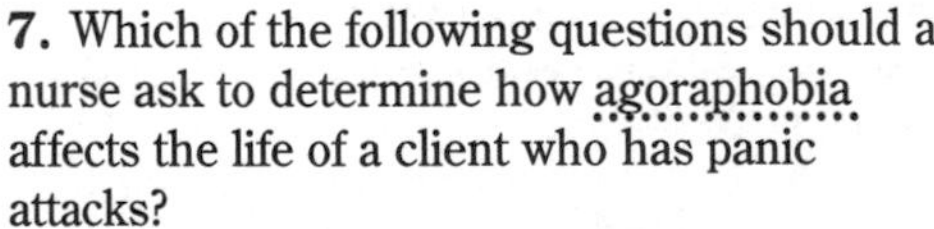

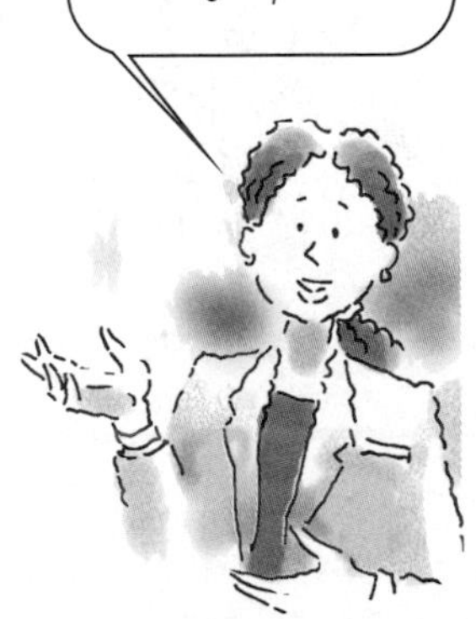

For the NCLEX, you should memorize the definitions of common fears such as *agoraphobia.*

7. Which of the following questions should a nurse ask to determine how agoraphobia affects the life of a client who has panic attacks?

1. How realistic are your goals?
2. Are you able to go shopping?
3. Do you struggle with impulse control?
4. Who else in your family has panic disorder?

7. 2. The client with agoraphobia often restricts himself to home and can't carry out normal socializing and life-sustaining activities. Clients with panic disorder are able to set realistic goals and tend to be cautious and reclusive rather than impulsive. Although there is a familial tendency toward panic disorder, information about client needs must be obtained to determine how agoraphobia affects the client's life.

NP: Planning; CN: Psychosocial integrity; CNS: Coping and adaptation; CL: Comprehension

8. Which of the following facts about the relationship between substance abuse and panic attacks would be helpful to a client considering lifestyle changes as part of a behavior modification program to treat his panic attacks?

1. Cigarettes can trigger panic episodes.
2. Fermented foods can cause panic attacks.
3. Hormonal therapy can induce panic attacks.
4. Tryptophan can predispose a person to panic attacks.

8. 1. Cigarettes are considered stimulants and can trigger panic attacks. None of the other options causes panic attacks.

NP: Implementation; CN: Psychosocial integrity; CNS: Psychosocial adaptation; CL: Comprehension

9. Which of the following interventions should the nurse initially implement when caring for a client with panic disorder?

1. Make the client role-play the panic attack.
2. Assist the client to develop an exercise program.
3. Teach the client to identify cognitive distortions.
4. Teach the client to identify sources of anxiety.

9. 4. The client must be aware of the connection between sources of anxiety and the symptoms of a panic attack. Role-playing a panic attack isn't useful. Role-playing coping strategies would be useful for the client. Later in treatment, the client can develop an exercise program as part of the overall plan to handle stress. Learning to identify cognitive distortions is a useful strategy to teach the client after he's begun to work on identifying sources of anxiety.

NP: Implementation; CN: Psychosocial integrity; CNS: Psychosocial adaptation; CL: Comprehension

10. Which of the following nursing interventions is appropriate for a client with panic disorder?

1. Identify childhood trauma.
2. Monitor nutritional intake.
3. Institute suicide precautions.
4. Monitor episodes of disorientation.

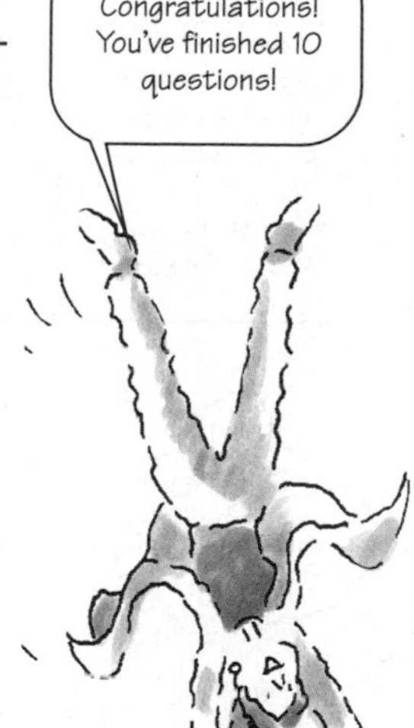
Congratulations! You've finished 10 questions!

10. 3. Clients with panic disorder are at risk for suicide. Childhood trauma is associated with posttraumatic stress disorder, ***not*** panic disorder. Nutritional problems don't typically accompany panic disorder. Clients aren't typically disoriented; they may have a temporary altered sense of reality, but that lasts only for the duration of the attack.

NP: Analysis; CN: Psychosocial integrity; CNS: Psychosocial adaptation; CL: Comprehension

11. A client diagnosed with panic disorder with agoraphobia is talking with the nurse about the progress made in treatment. Which of the following statements indicates a positive client response?

1. "I went to the mall with my friend last Saturday."
2. "I'm hyperventilating only when I have a panic attack."
3. "Today I decided that I can stop taking my medication."
4. "Last night I decided to eat more than a bowl of cereal."

11. 1. Clients with panic disorder tend to be socially withdrawn. Going to the mall is a sign of working on avoidance behaviors. Hyperventilation is a key symptom of panic disorder. Teaching breathing control is a major intervention for clients with panic disorder. The client taking medications for panic disorder, such as tricyclic antidepressants and benzodiazepines, must be weaned off these drugs. Most clients with panic disorder with agoraphobia don't have nutritional problems.

NP: Evaluation; CN: Psychosocial integrity; CNS: Psychosocial adaptation; CL: Analysis

12. Which of the following group therapy interventions would be of primary importance to a client with panic disorder?

1. Explore how secondary gains are derived from the disorder.
2. Discuss new ways of thinking and feeling about panic attacks.
3. Work to eliminate manipulative behavior used for meeting needs.
4. Learn the risk factors and other demographics associated with panic disorder.

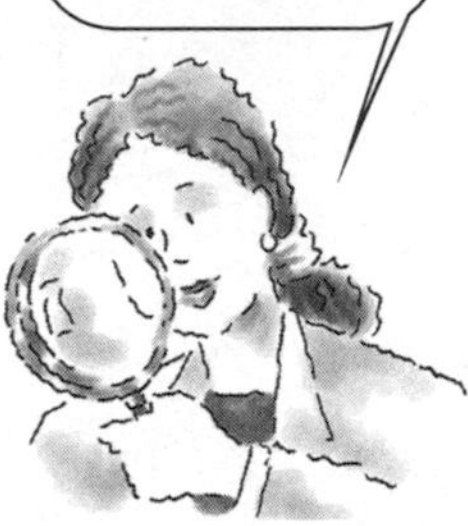

Question 12 wants you to focus on the intervention of primary importance.

12. 2. Discussing new ways of thinking and feeling about panic attacks can enable others to learn and benefit from a variety of intervention strategies. There are usually no secondary gains obtained from having a panic disorder. People with panic disorder aren't using the disorder as a way to manipulate others. Learning the risk factors could be accomplished in another format such as a psychoeducational program.

NP: Implementation; CN: Psychosocial integrity; CNS: Coping and adaptation; CL: Analysis

13. A client with social phobia should be observed for which of the following symptoms?

1. Self-harm
2. Poor self-esteem
3. Compulsive behavior
4. Avoidance of social situations

13. 4. Clients with social phobia avoid social situations for fear of being humiliated or embarrassed. They generally don't tend to be at risk for self-harm and usually don't demonstrate compulsive behavior. Not all individuals with social anxiety have low self-esteem.

NP: Assessment; CN: Psychosocial integrity; CNS: Coping and adaptation; CL: Knowledge

14. Which of the following statements is typical of a client with social phobia?

1. "Without people around, I just feel so lost."
2. "There is nothing wrong with my behavior."
3. "I like to be the center of attention."
4. "I know I can't accept that award for my brother."

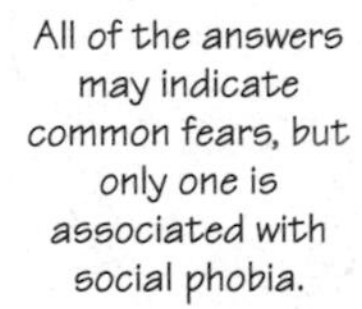

All of the answers may indicate common fears, but only one is associated with social phobia.

14. 4. People who have a social phobia usually undervalue themselves and their talents. They fear social gatherings and dislike being the center of attention. They tend to stay away from situations in which they may feel humiliated and embarrassed. They don't like to be in feared social situations or around many people. They're very critical of themselves and believe that others also will be critical.

NP: Assessment; CN: Psychosocial integrity; CNS: Coping and adaptation; CL: Application

15. Clients with a social phobia would most likely fear which of the following situations?

1. Dental procedures
2. Meeting strangers
3. Being bitten by a dog
4. Having a car accident

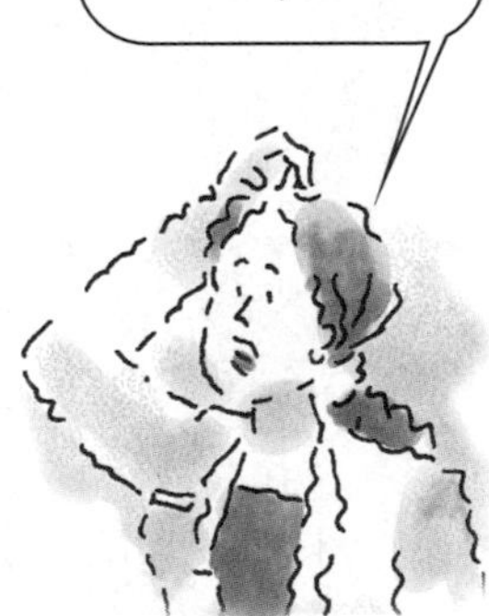

15. 2. Fear of meeting strangers is a common example of social phobia. Fears of having a dental procedure, being bitten by a dog, or having an accident are *not* social phobias.

NP: Assessment; CN: Psychosocial integrity; CNS: Coping and adaptation; CL: Knowledge

16. Which of the following factors would the nurse find most helpful in assessing a client for a blood-injection-injury phobia?
1. Episodes of fainting
2. Gregarious personality
3. Difficulty managing anger
4. Dramatic, overreactive personality

16. 1. Many people with a history of blood-injection-injury phobia report frequently fainting when exposed to this type of situation. All personality styles can develop phobias, so personality type doesn't provide information for assessing phobias. Information about a client's difficulty managing anger isn't related to a specific phobic disorder. Individuals with blood-injection-injury phobias aren't being dramatic or overreactive.

NP: Assessment; CN: Psychosocial integrity; CNS: Coping and adaptation; CL: Comprehension

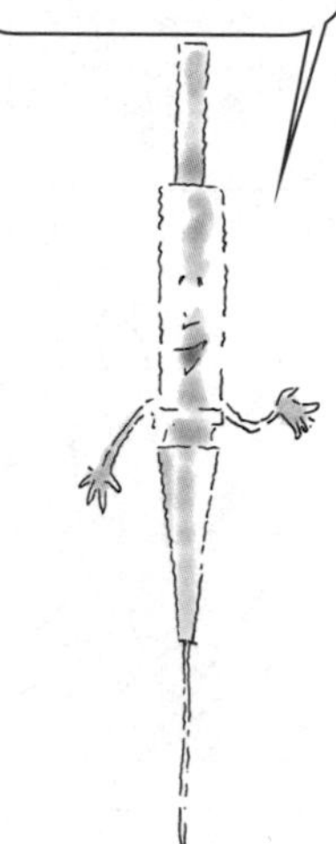

17. Which of the following individual counseling approaches should be used to assist a client with a phobic disorder?
1. Have the client keep a daily journal.
2. Help the client identify the source of the anxiety.
3. Teach the client effective ways to problem solve.
4. Develop strategies to prevent the client from using substances.

17. 2. By understanding the source of the anxiety, the client will understand how this anxiety has been displaced as a phobic response. Keeping a journal is an effective method in many situations; however, its use is limited in the treatment of phobias. Problem solving is a more useful technique for clients with obsessive-compulsive disorder than for clients with phobias. People with phobias don't tend to self-medicate like clients with other psychiatric disorders.

NP: Intervention; CN: Psychosocial integrity; CNS: Psychosocial adaptation; CL: Application

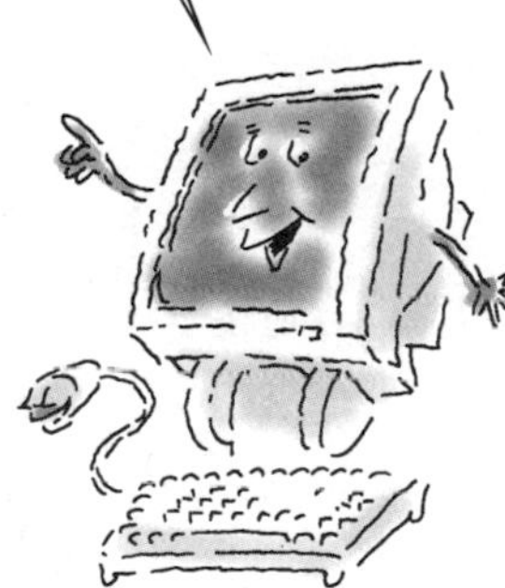
Along with
assessment, you
also need to
familiarize yourself
with common
treatments.

18. Which of the following behavior modification techniques is useful in the treatment of phobias?
1. Aversion therapy
2. Imitation or modeling
3. Positive reinforcement
4. Systematic desensitization

18. 4. Systematic desensitization is a common behavior modification technique successfully used to help treat phobias. Aversion therapy and positive reinforcement are *not* behavior modification techniques used with treatment of phobias. Imitation and modeling are social learning techniques, not behavior modification techniques.

NP: Implementation; CN: Psychosocial integrity; CNS: Psychosocial adaptation; CL: Application

19. Which of the following statements would be useful when teaching the client and family about phobias and the need for a strong support system?
1. The use of a family support system is only temporary.
2. The need to be assertive can be reinforced by the family.
3. The family needs to set limits on inappropriate behaviors.
4. The family plays a role in promoting client independence.

19. 4. The family plays a vital role in supporting the client in treatment and preventing the client from using the phobia to obtain secondary gains. Family support must be ongoing, not temporary. The family can be more helpful focusing on effective handling of anxiety, rather than focusing on developing assertiveness skills. People with phobias are already restrictive in their behavior; more restrictions aren't necessary.

NP: Implementation; CN: Psychosocial integrity; CNS: Psychosocial adaptation; CL: Analysis

20. Which of the following nursing interventions is of primary importance during the administration of paroxetine (Paxil) to a depressed client with a phobic disorder?

1. Monitor renal function.
2. Determine electrocardiogram (ECG) changes.
3. Assess for sleeping difficulties.
4. Observe for extrapyramidal symptoms.

20. 1. Clients with impaired renal function shouldn't take paroxetine. ECG changes aren't adverse effects of paroxetine. Other than a transient period of drowsiness occurring when the client begins to take the drug, sleep difficulties don't tend to be a problem. Extrapyramidal symptoms aren't seen with paroxetine.

NP: Implementation; CN: Physiological integrity; CNS: Pharmacological and parenteral therapies; CL: Comprehension

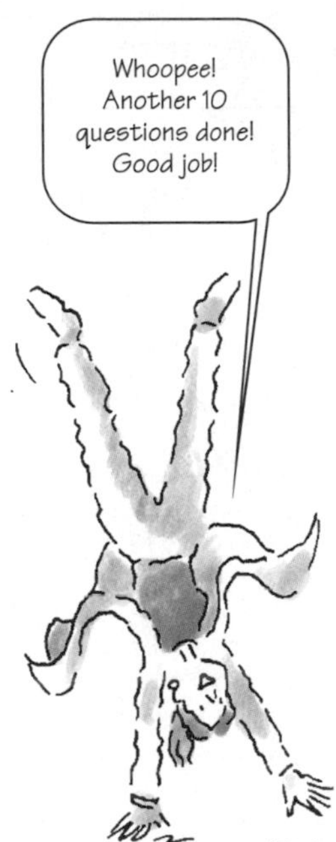

Whoopee! Another 10 questions done! Good job!

21. A client suspected of having posttraumatic stress disorder should be assessed for which of the following problems?

1. Eating disorder
2. Schizophrenia
3. Suicide
4. "Sundown" syndrome

21. 3. Clients who experience posttraumatic stress disorder are at high risk for suicide and other forms of violent behaviors. Eating disorders are possible but aren't a common complication of posttraumatic stress disorder. Clients with posttraumatic stress disorder don't usually have their extreme anxiety manifest itself as schizophrenia. "Sundown" syndrome is an increase in agitation accompanied by confusion. It's commonly seen in clients with dementia, not clients with posttraumatic stress disorder.

NP: Assessment; CN: Psychosocial integrity; CNS: Coping and adaptation; CL: Comprehension

22. Which of the following actions explains why tricyclic antidepressant medication is given to a client who has severe posttraumatic stress disorder?

1. It prevents hyperactivity and purposeless movements.
2. It increases the client's ability to concentrate.
3. It helps prevent experiencing the trauma again.
4. It facilitates the grieving process.

22. 3. Tricyclic antidepressant medication will decrease the frequency of reenactment of the trauma for the client. It will help memory problems and sleeping difficulties and will decrease numbing. The medication won't prevent hyperactivity and purposeless movements nor increase the client's concentration. No medication will facilitate the grieving process.

NP: Implementation; CN: Physiological integrity; CNS: Pharmacological and parenteral therapies; CL: Application

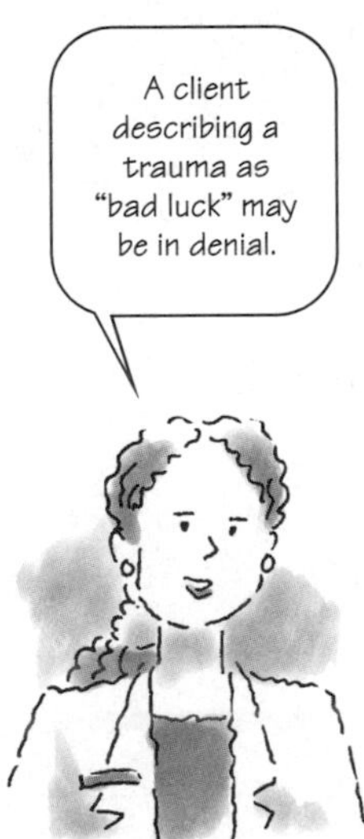

A client describing a trauma as "bad luck" may be in denial.

23. Which of the following nursing actions would be included in a care plan for a client with posttraumatic stress disorder who states that the experience was "bad luck"?

1. Encourage the client to verbalize the experience.
2. Assist the client in defining the experience as a trauma.
3. Work with the client to take steps to move on with life.
4. Help the client accept positive and negative feelings.

23. 2. The client must define the experience as traumatic to realize the situation wasn't under his personal control. Encouraging the client to verbalize the experience without first addressing the denial isn't a useful strategy. The client can move on with life only after acknowledging the trauma and processing the experience. Acknowledgment of the actual trauma and verbalization of the event should come *before* the acceptance of feelings.

NP: Planning; CN: Psychosocial integrity; CNS: Psychosocial adaptation; CL: Analysis

24. Which of the following instructions should the nurse include about relationships for the client with posttraumatic stress disorder?
1. Encourage the client to resume former roles as soon as possible.
2. Assess the client's discomfort when talking about feelings to family members.
3. Explain that avoiding emotional attachment protects against anxiety.
4. Warn the client that he'll have a tendency to be overdependent in relationships.

24. 3. The client may tend to avoid interpersonal relationships to protect himself against unrelieved anxiety. Because relationships tend to be avoided, the client won't express feelings to family members at this time and won't resume roles and responsibilities for a while. Clients with posttraumatic stress disorder don't tend to become overdependent in relationships but do tend to withdraw from them.
NP: Planning; CN: Psychosocial integrity; CNS: Psychosocial adaptation; CL: Application

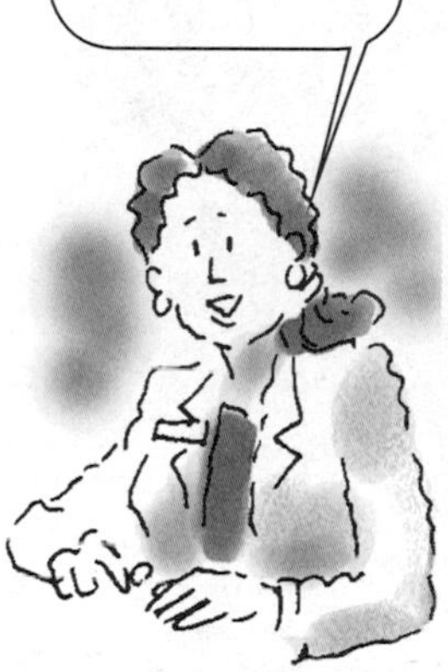

Caring for clients often means working with their families — a skill you can expect the NCLEX to test.

25. Which of the following approaches should the nurse use with the family when a posttraumatic stress disorder client states, "My family doesn't believe anything about posttraumatic stress disorder"?
1. Provide the family with information.
2. Teach the family about problem solving.
3. Discuss the family's view of the problem.
4. Assess for the presence of family violence.

25. 1. If the family can understand posttraumatic stress disorder, they can more readily participate in the client's care and be supportive. Learning problem-solving skills doesn't help clarify posttraumatic stress disorder. After being given information about posttraumatic stress disorder, the family can then ask questions and present its views. The family must first have information about posttraumatic stress disorder; then the discussion about violence to self or others can be addressed.
NP: Implementation; CN: Safe, effective care environment; CNS: Management of care; CL: Comprehension

26. While caring for a client with posttraumatic stress disorder, the family notices that loud noises cause a serious anxiety response. Which of the following explanations would help the family understand the client's response?
1. Environmental triggers can cause the client to react emotionally.
2. Clients often experience extreme fear about normal environmental stimuli.
3. After a trauma, the client can't respond to stimuli in an appropriate manner.
4. The response indicates that another emotional problem needs investigation.

26. 1. Repeated exposure to environmental triggers can cause the client to experience a hyperarousal state because there's a loss of physiological control of incoming stimuli. After experiencing a trauma, the client may have strong reactions to stimuli similar to those that occurred during the traumatic event. However, not *all* stimuli will cause an anxiety response. The client's anxiety response is typically seen after a traumatic experience and doesn't indicate the presence of another problem.
NP: Planning; CN: Psychosocial integrity; CNS: Coping and adaptation; CL: Application

27. Which of the following psychological symptoms would the nurse expect to find in a hospitalized client who is the only survivor of a train accident?
1. Denial
2. Indifference
3. Perfectionism
4. Trust

27. 1. Denial can act as a protective response. The client tends to be overwhelmed and disorganized by the trauma, not indifferent to it. Perfectionism is more commonly seen in clients with eating disorders, not in clients with posttraumatic stress disorder. Clients who have had a severe trauma often experience an inability to trust others.
NP: Assessment; CN: Psychosocial integrity; CNS: Coping and adaptation; CL: Comprehension

28. If a client suffering from posttraumatic stress disorder says, "I've decided to just avoid everything and everyone," the nurse might suspect the client is at greatest risk for which of the following behaviors?

1. Becoming homeless
2. Exhausting finances
3. Terminating employment
4. Using substances

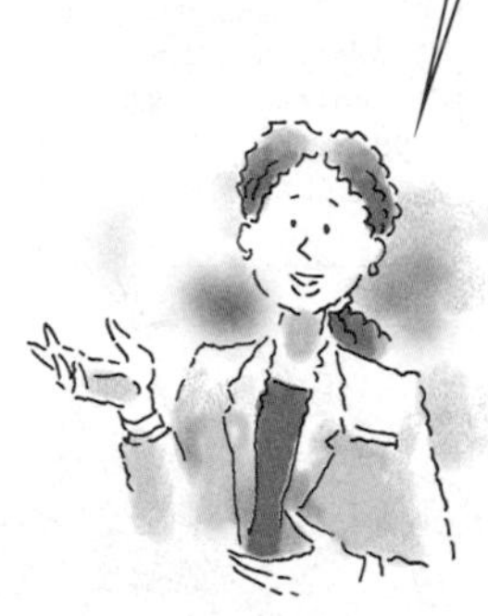

All of the answers may be possible risks, but you've got to choose the greatest risk.

29. Which of the following actions would be most appropriate when speaking with a client with posttraumatic stress disorder about the trauma?

1. Obtain validation of what the client says from another party.
2. Request that the client write down what's being said.
3. Ask questions to convey an interest in the details.
4. Listen attentively.

30. Which of the following client statements indicates an understanding of survivor guilt?

1. "I think I can see the purpose of my survival."
2. "I can't help but feel that everything is their fault."
3. "I now understand why I'm not able to forgive myself."
4. "I wish I could stop sabotaging my family relationships."

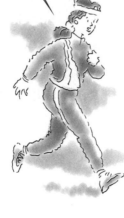

Thirty questions! You're well into the race now.

31. Which of the following nursing interventions would best help the client with posttraumatic stress disorder and his family handle interpersonal conflict at home?

1. Have the family teach the client to identify defensive behaviors.
2. Have the family discuss how to change dysfunctional family patterns.
3. Have the family agree not to tell the client what to do about problems.
4. Have the family arrange for the client to participate in social activities.

28. 4. The use of substances is a way for the client to deny problems and self-medicate distress. There are few homeless people with posttraumatic stress disorder as the cause of their homelessness. Most clients with posttraumatic stress disorder can manage money and maintain employment.

NP: Analysis; CN: Psychosocial integrity; CNS: Psychosocial adaptation; CL: Application

29. 4. An effective communication strategy for a nurse to use with a posttraumatic stress disorder client is listening attentively and staying with the client. There's no need to obtain validation about what the client says by asking for information from another party, asking the client to write what's being said, or distracting him by asking questions.

NP: Implementation; CN: Psychosocial integrity; CNS: Psychosocial adaptation; CL: Application

30. 3. Survivor guilt occurs when the person has almost constant thoughts about the other people who perished in the event. The survivor doesn't understand why he survived when a friend or loved one didn't. Blaming self, not others, is a component of survivor guilt. Survivor guilt and impaired interpersonal relationships are two different categories of responses to trauma.

NP: Evaluation; CN: Psychosocial integrity; CNS: Coping and adaptation; CL: Analysis

31. 2. Discussion of dysfunctional family patterns allows the family to determine why and how these patterns are maintained. Having family members point out the defensive behaviors of the client may inadvertently produce more defensive behavior. Families can be a source of support and assistance. Therefore, inflexible rules aren't useful to either the client or the family. The family shouldn't be encouraged to arrange social activities for the client. Social activities outside of the home don't help the family handle conflict within the home.

NP: Implementation; CN: Psychosocial integrity; CNS: Psychosocial adaptation; CL: Application

40. A client with generalized anxiety disorder is prescribed a benzodiazepine, but the client doesn't want to take the medication. Which of the following explanations by the client for this behavior would be most likely?

1. "I don't think the psychiatrist likes me."
2. "I want to solve my problems on my own."
3. "The voices tell me that I don't have to take the medication."
4. "I think my family gains by keeping me medicated."

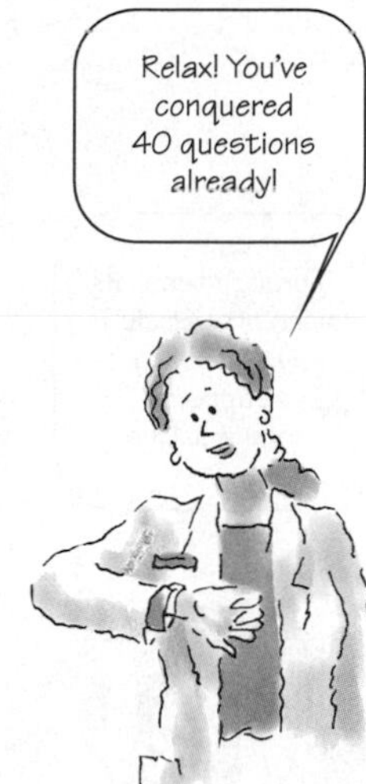

Relax! You've conquered 40 questions already!

40. 2. It's common for a client with generalized anxiety disorder to refuse to take medication because he believes that using a medication is a sign of personal weakness and that he can't solve problems by himself. Fear that the psychiatrist dislikes him reflects paranoid thinking that isn't usually seen in a client with generalized anxiety disorder. Auditory hallucinations and paranoia about the motives of friends and family members aren't characteristic of clients with generalized anxiety disorder.

NP: Analysis; CN: Psychosocial integrity; CNS: Coping and adaptation; CL: Analysis

41. Which of the following factors should the nurse consider when assisting the client with generalized anxiety disorder in verbalizing feelings?

1. The client may intellectualize the anxiety.
2. The client may regard the problem as genetic.
3. The client may decide that therapy isn't beneficial.
4. The client may believe only medications are useful.

41. 1. Clients who experience generalized anxiety disorder often need assistance acknowledging anxiety instead of denying or intellectualizing it. Although scientists believe that there may be a tendency for anxiety to be familial, the problem isn't regarded as genetic. A client who is unwilling to express feelings may not view therapy as helpful. The most effective treatment of generalized anxiety disorder combines psychotherapy and pharmacotherapy.

NP: Analysis; CN: Psychosocial integrity; CNS: Coping and adaptation; CL: Analysis

42. Which of the following statements by a 44-year-old client with a diagnosis of generalized anxiety disorder would convince the nurse that anxiety has been a long-standing problem?

1. "I was, and still am, an impulsive person."
2. "I've always been hyperactive, but not in useful ways."
3. "When I was in college, I never thought I would finish."
4. "All my life I've had intrusive dreams and scary nightmares."

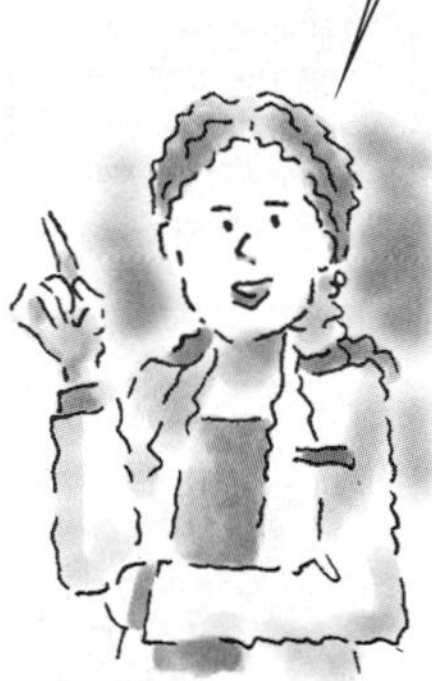

Certain psychological disorders tend to appear at particular ages — that's information to know for the NCLEX.

42. 3. For many people who have a generalized anxiety disorder, the age of onset is during young adulthood. The symptoms of impulsiveness and hyperactivity aren't commonly associated with a diagnosis of generalized anxiety disorder. Intrusive dreams and nightmares are associated with posttraumatic stress disorder rather than generalized anxiety disorder.

NP: Assessment; CN: Psychosocial integrity; CNS: Coping and adaptation; CL: Comprehension

43. Which of the following symptoms would the client with generalized anxiety disorder most likely display when assessed for muscle tension?

1. Difficulty sleeping
2. Restlessness
3. Strong startle response
4. Tachycardia

43. 2. Restlessness is a symptom associated with muscle tension. Difficulty sleeping and a strong startle response are considered symptoms of vigilance and scanning of the environment, not muscle tension. Tachycardia is classified as a symptom of autonomic hyperactivity, not muscle tension.

NP: Assessment; CN: Physiological integrity; CNS: Physiological adaptation; CL: Knowledge

44. Which of the following interventions should be given priority for a client with generalized anxiety disorder who is working to develop coping skills?

1. Determine whether the client has fears or obsessive thinking.
2. Monitor the client for overt and covert signs of anxiety.
3. Teach the client how to use effective communications skills.
4. Assist the client to identify coping mechanisms used in the past.

44. 4. To help a client develop effective coping skills, the nurse must know the client's baseline functioning. Determining whether the client has fears or obsessive thinking, monitoring for signs of anxiety, and teaching about effective communications skills are later priorities, not initial ones.

NP: Implementation; CN: Psychosocial integrity; CNS: Coping and adaptation; CL: Application

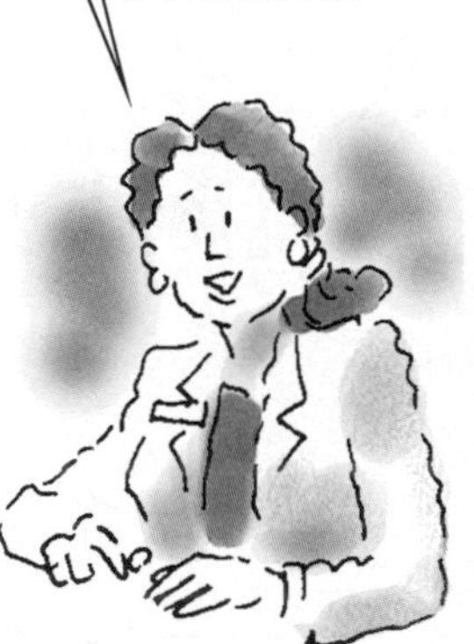

Thorough teaching plans often include ways to contact support organizations.

45. Which of the following instructions help the nurse deal with escalating client anxiety?

1. Explore feelings about current life stressors.
2. Discuss the need to flee from painful situations.
3. Have the client develop a realistic view of self.
4. Provide appropriate phone numbers for hotlines and clinics.

45. 4. By having information on hotlines and clinics, the client can pursue help when the anxiety is escalating. Discussion about current life stressors isn't useful when focusing on how best to handle the client's escalating anxiety. Fleeing from painful situations and discussing views of oneself aren't the best strategies; neither allows for problem solving.

NP: Implementation; CN: Psychosocial integrity; CNS: Psychosocial adaptation; CL: Knowledge

46. Which of the following instructions should the nurse include for the family of an adult client with generalized anxiety disorder?

1. Explain how the family can handle the confusion related to memory loss.
2. Teach the family not to take over for the client during periods of anxiety.
3. Teach the family how to cope with the client's sudden and unexpected travel behavior.
4. Have the family determine when and for what reasons the client should take medication.

46. 2. The family can be there for support, but they negate the client's ability to function if they take control of the situation and don't allow the client to use his own coping skills. A client who has confusion related to memory loss is often struggling with dissociative amnesia, not a generalized anxiety disorder. Sudden and unexpected travel behavior is a problem for families who have members with dissociative identity disorder, not generalized anxiety disorder. The client must handle and use medication as prescribed.

NP: Planning; CN: Psychosocial integrity; CNS: Coping and adaptation; CL: Comprehension

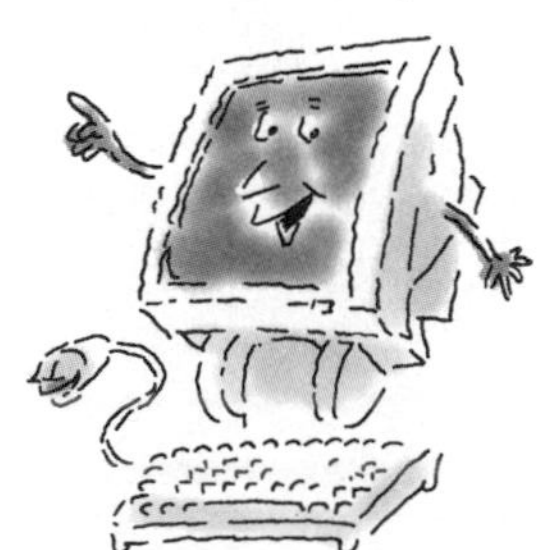

You should be familiar with the symptoms that discontinuing key medications may cause.

47. A client with a diagnosis of generalized anxiety disorder wants to stop taking his lorazepam (Ativan). Which of the following important facts should the nurse discuss with the client about discontinuing the medication?

1. Stopping the drug may cause depression.
2. Stopping the drug increases cognitive abilities.
3. Stopping the drug decreases sleeping difficulties.
4. Stopping the drug can cause withdrawal symptoms.

47. 4. Stopping antianxiety drugs such as benzodiazepines can cause the client to have withdrawal symptoms. Stopping a benzodiazepine doesn't tend to cause depression, increase cognitive abilities, or decrease sleeping difficulties.

NP: Implementation; CN: Physiological integrity; CNS: Pharmacological and parenteral therapies; CL: Application

48. Five days after running out of medication, a client taking clonazepam (Klonopin) says to the nurse, "I know I shouldn't have just stopped the drug like that, but I'm okay." Which of the following responses would be best?

1. "Let's monitor you for problems, in case something else happens."
2. "You could go through withdrawal symptoms for up to 2 weeks."
3. "You have handled your anxiety, and you now know how to cope with stress."
4. "If you're fine now, chances are you won't experience withdrawal symptoms."

48. 2. Withdrawal syndrome symptoms can appear after 1 or 2 weeks because the benzodiazepine has a long half-life. Looking for another problem unrelated to withdrawal isn't the nurse's best strategy. The act of discontinuing an antianxiety medication doesn't indicate that a client has learned to cope with stress. Every client taking medication needs to be monitored for withdrawal symptoms when the medication is stopped abruptly.

NP: Implementation; CN: Physiological integrity; CNS: Pharmacological and parenteral therapies; CL: Analysis

49. A client taking alprazolam (Xanax) reports light-headedness and nausea every day while getting out of bed. Which of the following actions should the nurse take to objectively validate this client's problem?

1. Take the client's blood pressure.
2. Monitor body temperature.
3. Teach the Valsalva maneuver.
4. Obtain a blood chemical profile.

49. 1. The nurse should take a blood pressure reading to validate orthostatic hypotension. A body temperature reading or chemistry profile won't yield useful information about hypotension. The Valsalva maneuver is performed to lower the heart rate and isn't an appropriate intervention.

NP: Implementation; CN: Physiological integrity; CNS: Reduction of risk potential; CL: Knowledge

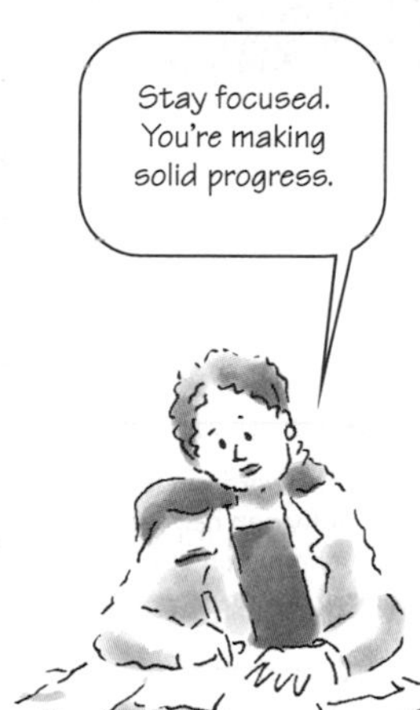
Stay focused. You're making solid progress.

50. A client with generalized anxiety disorder complains to the nurse about several other minor health problems. Which of the following concerns must the nurse keep in mind when preparing instructions for this client?

1. Clients may have a variety of somatic symptoms.
2. Clients undergo an alteration in their self-care skills.
3. Clients are prone to unhealthy binge eating episodes.
4. Clients will experience secondary gains from mental illness.

50. 1. Clients with anxiety disorders often experience somatic symptoms. They don't usually experience problems with self-care. Eating problems aren't a typical part of the diagnostic criteria for anxiety disorders. Not all clients obtain secondary gains from mental illness.

NP: Analysis; CN: Psychosocial integrity; CNS: Psychosocial adaptation; CL: Comprehension

51. Which of the following communication guidelines should the nurse use when talking with a client experiencing mania?

1. Address the client in a light and joking manner.
2. Focus and redirect the conversation as necessary.
3. Allow the client to talk about several different topics.
4. Ask only open-ended questions to facilitate conversation.

51. 2. To decrease stimulation, the nurse should attempt to redirect and focus the client's communication, not allow the client to talk about different topics. By addressing the client in a light and joking manner, the conversation may contribute to the client's feeling out of control. For a manic client, it's best to ask closed questions because open-ended questions may enable the client to talk endlessly, again possibly contributing to the client's feeling out of control.

NP: Analysis; CN: Psychosocial integrity; CNS: Psychosocial adaptation; CL: Comprehension

60. Which of the following facts does the nurse need to include when teaching the client with bipolar disorder and his family about the drug carbamazepine (Tegretol)?

1. The risk of losing hair is a problem for clients taking the drug.
2. Clients must be closely monitored for nephrogenic diabetes insipidus.
3. Hematologic toxicity and bone marrow depression are serious adverse effects.
4. To avoid toxic reactions, most other drugs shouldn't be taken concurrently.

61. Which of the following short-term goals is most appropriate for a client with bipolar disorder who is having difficulty sleeping?

1. Obtain medication for sleep.
2. Work on solving a problem.
3. Exercise before bedtime.
4. Develop a sleep ritual.

62. Which of the following topics should the nurse discuss with the family of a client with bipolar disorder if the family is distressed about the client's episodes of manic behavior?

1. Ways to protect self from client's behavior
2. How to proceed with an involuntary commitment
3. How to confront the client about the reckless behavior
4. When to safely increase medication during manic periods

63. Which of the following statements should the nurse explain to a client newly diagnosed with bipolar disorder who doesn't understand why frequent blood work is necessary while he is taking lithium?

1. Frequent lithium levels will help the primary care provider spot liver and renal damage early.
2. Frequent lithium levels will demonstrate whether the client is taking a high enough dosage.
3. Frequent lithium levels will indicate whether the drug passes through the blood-brain barrier.
4. Frequent lithium levels are unnecessary if the client takes the drug as ordered.

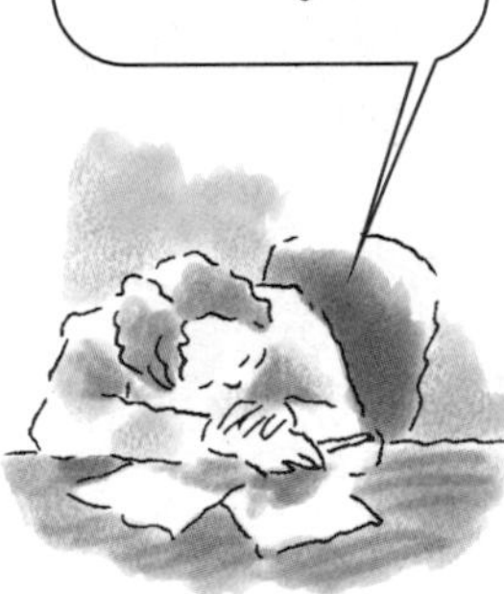

Remember, you're looking for the most appropriate sleep-related goal.

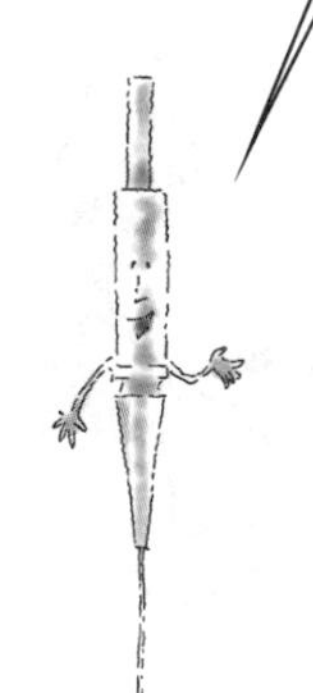

Monitoring blood levels helps ensure that adequate doses of lithium are being administered.

60. 3. The most dangerous adverse effect of carbamazepine is bone marrow depression. Other medications may be taken with carbamazepine. Hair loss doesn't occur in clients taking carbamazepine. Clients who take lithium, not carbamazepine, must be closely monitored for nephrogenic diabetes insipidus. The interactions of all drugs being taken must be monitored as some drugs can either increase or decrease the blood level of carbamazepine.

NP: Planning; CN: Physiological integrity; CNS: Pharmacological and parenteral therapies; CL: Comprehension

61. 4. A sleep ritual or nighttime routine helps the client to relax and prepare for sleep. Obtaining sleep medication is a temporary solution. Working on problem solving may excite the client rather than tire him. Exercise before retiring is inappropriate.

NP: Analysis; CN: Physiological integrity; CNS: Reduction of risk potential; CL: Knowledge

62. 1. Family members need to assess their needs and develop ways to protect themselves. Clients who have symptoms of impulsive or reckless behavior might not be candidates for hospitalization. Confronting the client during a manic episode may escalate the behavior. The family must never increase the dosage of prescribed medication without first consulting the primary health care provider.

NP: Implementation; CN: Safe, effective care environment; CNS: Safety and infection control; CL: Application

63. 2. Lithium levels determine whether an effective dose of lithium is being given to maintain a therapeutic level of the drug. The drug is contraindicated for clients with renal, cardiac, or liver disease. Lithium levels aren't drawn for the purpose of determining whether the drug passes through the blood-brain barrier. Taking the drug as ordered doesn't eliminate the need for blood work.

NP: Implementation; CN: Physiological integrity; CNS: Pharmacological and parenteral therapies; CL: Comprehension

64. What information is important to include in the nutritional counseling of a family with a member who has bipolar disorder?

1. If sufficient roughage isn't eaten while taking lithium, bowel problems will occur.
2. If the intake of carbohydrates increases, the lithium level will increase.
3. If the intake of calories is reduced, the lithium level will increase.
4. If the intake of sodium increases, the lithium level will decrease.

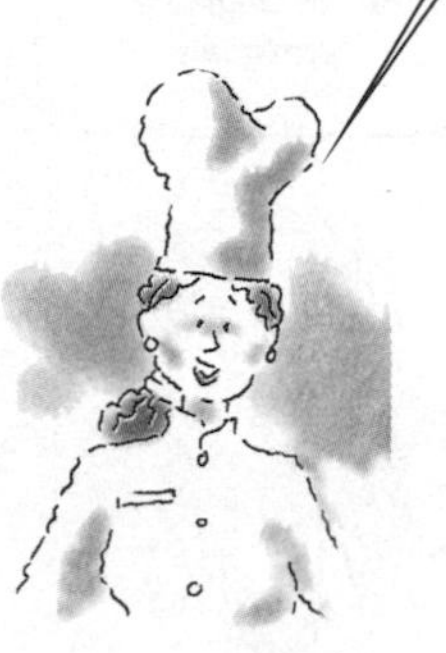

64. 4. Any time the level of sodium increases, such as with a change in dietary intake, the level of lithium will decrease. The intake of roughage and carbohydrates in the diet isn't related to the metabolism of lithium. Reducing the number of calories the client eats doesn't affect the lithium level in the body.

NP: Implementation; CN: Physiological integrity; CNS: Reduction of risk potential; CL: Analysis

65. Which of the following statements made by a client with bipolar disorder indicates that the nurse's teaching on coping strategies was effective?

1. "I can decide what to do to prevent family conflict."
2. "I can handle problems without asking for any help."
3. "I can stay away from my friends when I feel distressed."
4. "I can ignore things that go wrong instead of getting upset."

65. 1. The client should be focusing on his strengths and abilities to prevent family conflict. Not being able to ask for help is problematic and not a good coping strategy. Avoiding problems also isn't a good coping strategy. It's better to identify and handle problems as they arise. Ignoring situations that cause discomfort won't facilitate solutions or allow the client to demonstrate effective coping skills.

NP: Evaluation; CN: Psychosocial integrity; CNS: Coping and adaptation; CL: Analysis

66. Which of the following short-term goals would be given high priority for a client with depression admitted to the inpatient unit because of attempted suicide?

1. The client will seek out the nurse when feeling self-destructive.
2. The client will identify and discuss actual and perceived losses.
3. The client will learn strategies to promote relaxation and self-care.
4. The client will establish healthy and mutually caring relationships.

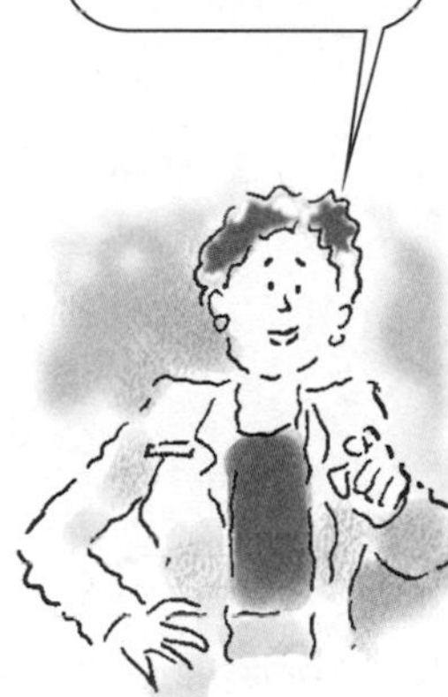

Question 66 is asking you to prioritize. Read it carefully.

66. 1. By seeking out the nurse when feeling self-destructive, the client can feel safe and begin to see that there are coping skills to assist in dealing with self-destructive tendencies. Discussion of losses also is important when dealing with feelings of depression, but the priority intervention is still to promote immediate client safety. Although relationship building and learning strategies to promote relaxation and self-care are important goals, safety is the priority intervention.

NP: Analysis; CN: Safe, effective care environment; CNS: Safety and infection control; CL: Comprehension

67. In conferring with the treatment team, the nurse should make which of the following recommendations for a client who tells the nurse that everyday thoughts of suicide are present?

1. A no-suicide contract
2. Weekly outpatient therapy
3. A second psychiatric opinion
4. Intensive inpatient treatment

67. 4. For a client thinking about suicide on a daily basis, inpatient care would be the best intervention. Although a no-suicide contract is an important strategy, this client needs additional care. The client needs a more intensive level of care than weekly outpatient therapy. Immediate intervention is paramount, not a second psychiatric opinion.

NP: Planning; CN: Safe, effective care environment; CNS: Safety and infection control; CL: Comprehension

68. Which of the following short-term goals should the nurse focus on for a client who makes statements about not deserving things?

1. Identify distorted thoughts.
2. Describe self-care patterns.
3. Discuss family relationships.
4. Explore communications skills.

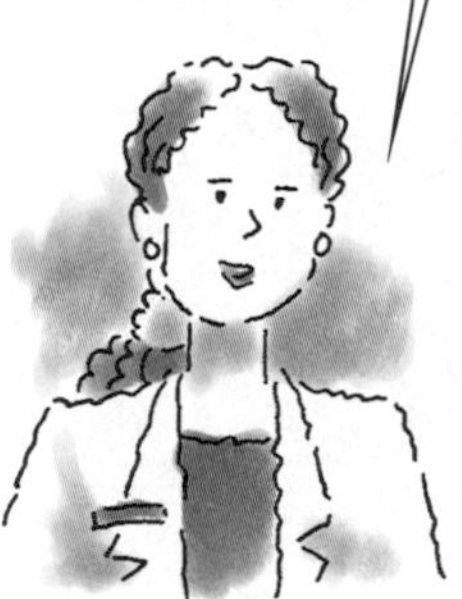
Note that question 68 asks about short-term goals, rather than long-term goals.

68. 1. It's important to identify distorted thinking because self-deprecating thoughts lead to depression. Self-care patterns don't necessarily reflect distorted thinking. Family relationships might not influence distorted thinking patterns. A form of communication called negative self-talk would be explored only after distorted thinking patterns were identified.
NP: Analysis; CN: Psychosocial integrity; CNS: Coping and adaptation; CL: Application

69. Which of the following interventions should be of primary importance to the nurse working with a client to modify the client's negative expectations?

1. Encourage the client to discuss spiritual matters.
2. Assist the client to learn how to problem-solve.
3. Help the client explore issues related to loss.
4. Have the client identify positive aspects of self.

69. 4. An important intervention used to counter negative expectations is to focus on the positive and have the client explore positive aspects of himself. Discussion of spiritual matters doesn't address the need to change negative expectations. Learning how to problem-solve won't modify the client's negative expectations. If the client dwells on the negative and focuses on loss, it will be natural to have negative expectations.
NP: Implementation; CN: Psychosocial integrity; CNS: Psychosocial adaptation; CL: Application

70. Which of the following intervention strategies is most appropriate to use with a client with depression who may be suicidal?

1. Speak to family members to ascertain whether the client is suicidal.
2. Talk to the client to determine whether the client is an attention seeker.
3. Arrange for the client to be placed on immediate suicidal precautions.
4. Ask a direct question such as, "Do you ever think about killing yourself?"

70. 4. The best approach to determining whether a client is suicidal is to ask about thoughts of suicide in a direct and caring manner. Assessing for attention-seeking behaviors doesn't deal directly with the problem. The client should be assessed directly, not through family members. Assessment must be performed before determining whether suicide precautions are necessary.
NP: Implementation; CN: Safe, effective care environment; CNS: Safety and infection control; CL: Knowledge

71. Which of the following instructions should the nurse include when teaching the family of a client with major depression?

1. Address how depression is a lifelong illness.
2. Explain that depression is an illness and can be treated.
3. Describe how depression masks a person's true feelings.
4. Teach how depression causes frequent disorganized thinking.

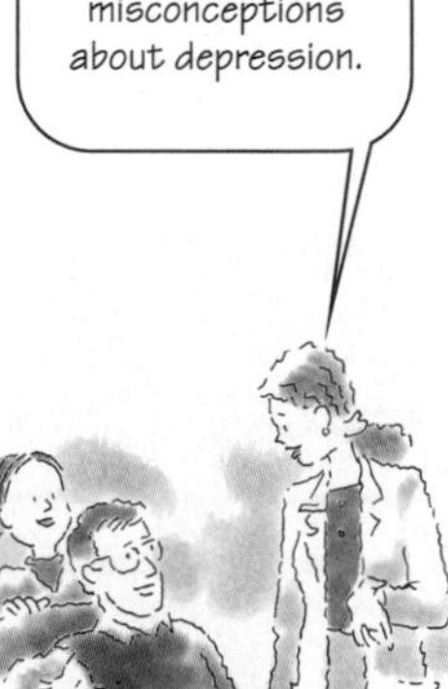
You may have misconceptions about depression.

71. 2. The nurse must help the family understand depression, its impact on the family, and recommended treatments. Depression doesn't need to be a lifelong illness. It's important to help families understand that depression can be successfully treated and that, in some situations, depression can reoccur during the life cycle. The feelings expressed by the client are genuine; they reflect cognitive distortions and disillusionment. Disorganized thinking is more commonly associated with schizophrenia rather than depression.
NP: Planning; CN: Psychosocial integrity; CNS: Psychosocial adaptation; CL: Application

72. A client with major depression asks why he is taking mirtazapine (Remeron) instead of imipramine hydrochloride (Tofranil). Which of the following explanations is most accurate?

1. The newer serotonin reuptake inhibitor drugs are better-tested drugs.
2. The serotonin reuptake inhibitors have few adverse effects.
3. The serotonin reuptake inhibitors require a low dose of antidepressant drug.
4. The serotonin reuptake inhibitors are as good as other antidepressant drugs.

72. 2. The serotonin reuptake inhibitors are drugs with few adverse effects and are unlikely to be toxic in an overdose. All drugs must be tested through a government-specified protocol. Comparison of two different types of antidepressant medications isn't useful. The final statement doesn't give the client helpful information.

NP: Implementation; CN: Physiological integrity; CNS: Pharmacological and parenteral therapies; CL: Analysis

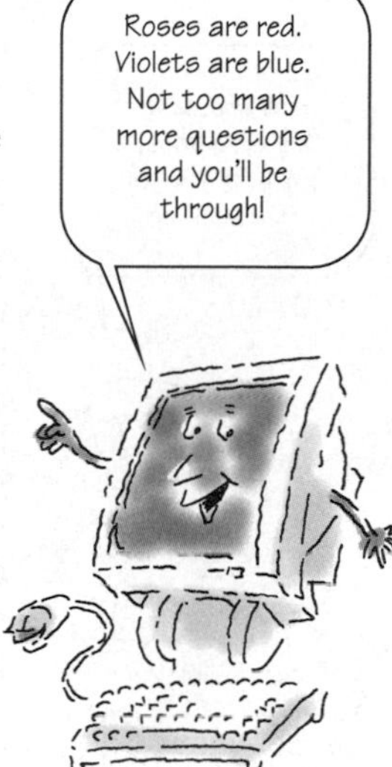
Roses are red.
Violets are blue.
Not too many
more questions
and you'll be
through!

73. Which of the following interventions is most likely to promote a positive sense of self in a client with depression whose goal is enhancing self-esteem?

1. Playing cards
2. Praying daily
3. Taking medication
4. Writing poetry

73. 4. Writing poetry or engaging in some other creative outlet will enhance self-esteem. Playing cards and praying don't necessarily promote self-esteem. Taking medication will decrease symptoms of depression after a blood level is established but it won't, by itself, promote self-esteem.

NP: Implementation; CN: Psychosocial integrity; CNS: Psychosocial adaptation; CL: Comprehension

74. An adolescent who is depressed and reported by his parents as having difficulty in school is brought to the community mental health center to be evaluated. Which of the following other health problems would the nurse suspect?

1. Anxiety disorder
2. Behavioral difficulties
3. Cognitive impairment
4. Labile moods

74. 2. Adolescents tend to demonstrate severe irritability and behavioral problems rather than simply a depressed mood. Anxiety disorder is more commonly associated with small children rather than with adolescents. Cognitive impairment is typically associated with delirium or dementia. Labile mood is more characteristic of a client with cognitive impairment or bipolar disorder.

NP: Analysis; CN: Psychosocial integrity; CNS: Coping and adaptation; CL: Analysis

75. Which of the following nursing interventions is most effective in lowering a client's risk of suicide?

1. Using a caring approach
2. Developing a strong relationship with the client
3. Establishing a suicide contract to ensure his safety
4. Encouraging avoidance of overstimulating activities

75. 3. Establishing a suicide contract with the client demonstrates that the nurse's concern for his safety is a priority and that his life is of value. When a client agrees to a suicide contract, it decreases his risk of a successful attempt. Caring alone ignores the underlying mechanism of the client's wish to commit suicide. Merely developing a strong relationship with the client isn't addressing the potential the client has for harming himself. Encouraging the client to stay away from activities could cause isolation, which would be detrimental to the client's well-being.

NP: Planning; CN: Safe, effective care environment; CNS: Safety and infection control; CL: Application

76. Which of the following mental disorders is associated with the gamma-aminobutyric acid (GABA) complex?
1. Alzheimer's disease
2. Anxiety
3. Depression
4. Posttraumatic stress disorder

76. 2. Anxiety is regulated by the amino acid GABA, which inhibits the excitability of the neurons and, as a result, regulates anxiety control. Alzheimer's disease has been associated with the dietary precursor acetylcholine. Depression and possibly posttraumatic stress disorder have been associated with norepinephrine, but not with GABA complex.
NP: Analysis; CN: Physiological integrity; CNS: Physiological adaptation; CL: Knowledge

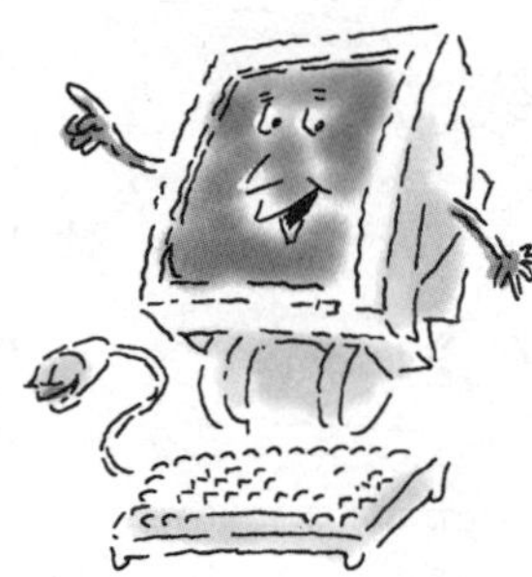

Think about what this drug does; it will help give you the answer.

77. Norepinephrine has been linked to posttraumatic stress disorder because it plays a role in which of the following activities?
1. Autonomic nervous system activity
2. Glutamate metabolism
3. Excitatory neurotransmitter inhibition
4. Pain regulation

77. 1. Norepinephrine has a major function in the autonomic nervous system. It's released by the sympathetic nervous system in response to stress, causing increased blood pressure and heart rate. Regulating pain isn't a function of norepinephrine. Norepinephrine doesn't function to inhibit excitatory neurotransmitter. Glutamate isn't implicated in the development of posttraumatic stress disorder, but in schizophrenia.
NP: Analysis; CN: Physiological integrity; CNS: Physiological adaptation; CL: Knowledge

78. Serotonin has been associated with depression because it plays which of the following roles?
1. It plays a role in cerebral functioning.
2. It has a proposed role in mood states.
3. It is found widely in the hippocampus.
4. It regulates the sleep and wakefulness cycle.

78. 2. Serotonin is widespread throughout the cortex and plays an important role in mood states that are implicated in depression. It's postulated that low levels of serotonin create abnormal levels of norepinephrine, causing depression. Although serotonin does play a role in cerebral functioning, this relationship isn't related to depression. Serotonin isn't found in the hippocampus. Serotonin doesn't regulate the sleep and wakefulness cycle.
NP: Analysis; CN: Physiological integrity; CN: Physiological adaptation; CL: Knowledge

79. A lack of dietary salt intake can have which of the following effects on lithium levels?
1. Decrease
2. Increase
3. Increase then decrease
4. No effect at all

79. 2. There is a direct relationship between the amount of salt and the plasma levels of lithium. Lithium plasma levels increase when there is a decrease in dietary salt. Increase in dietary salt causes the opposite effect of decreasing lithium plasma levels. It's important that the nurse monitor dietary sodium intake.
NP: Analysis; CN: Physiological integrity; CNS: Pharmacological and parenteral therapies; CL: Knowledge

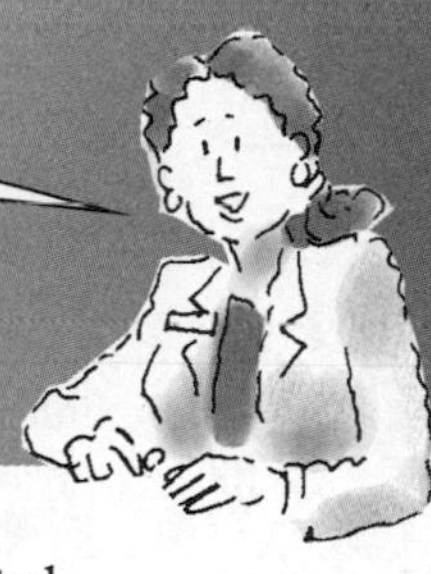

This chapter covers a host of cognitive disorders. Are your own cognitive powers ready? OK, let's go!

Chapter 15 Cognitive disorders

1. Which of the following disorders is related to dementia?

1. Alcohol withdrawal
2. Alzheimer's disease
3. Obsessive-compulsive disorder
4. Postpartum depression

1. 2. Dementia occurs in Alzheimer's disease and is generally progressive and deteriorating. The symptoms related to alcohol withdrawal result from alcohol intoxication. Effects of alcohol on the central nervous system include loss of memory, concentration, insight, and motor control. Obsessive-compulsive disorders are recurrent ideas, impulses, thoughts, or patterns of behavior that produce anxiety if resisted. Postpartum depression doesn't lead to dementia.

NP: Assessment; CN: Physiological integrity; CNS: Physiological adaptation; CL: Comprehension

2. A physician diagnoses a client with dementia of the Alzheimer's type. Which of the following statements about possible causes of this disorder is most accurate?

1. Alzheimer's disease is most commonly caused by cerebral abscess.
2. Chronic alcohol abuse plays a significant role in Alzheimer's disease.
3. Multiple small brain infarctions typically lead to Alzheimer's disease.
4. The cause of Alzheimer's disease is currently unknown.

2. 4. Several hypotheses suggest genetic factors, trauma, accumulation of aluminum, alterations in the immune system, or alterations in acetylcholine as contributing to the development of Alzheimer's disease, but the exact cause of Alzheimer's disease is unknown.

NP: Analysis; CN: Health promotion and maintenance; CNS: Prevention and early detection of disease; CL: Application

3. Of the following conditions that can cause a dementia similar to Alzheimer's disease, which is reversible?

1. Multiple sclerosis
2. Electrolyte imbalance
3. Multiple small brain infarctions
4. Human immunodeficiency virus infection

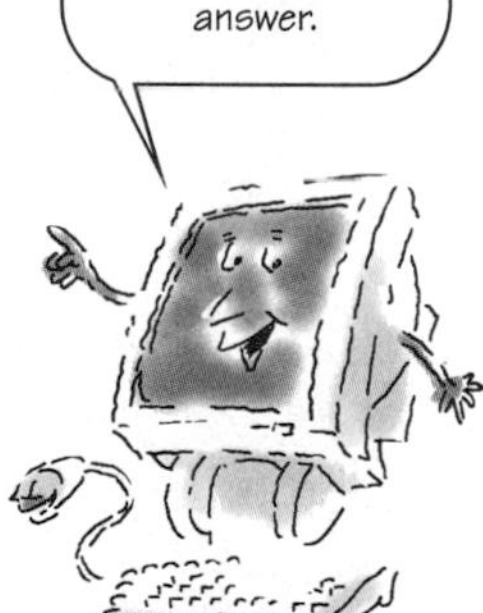

This word — *reversible* — clarifies the answer.

3. 2. Electrolyte imbalance is a correctable metabolic abnormality. The other conditions are irreversible.

NP: Analysis; CN: Physiological integrity; CNS: Physiological adaptation; CL: Application

4. In the early stages of Alzheimer's disease, which of the following symptoms is expected?
1. Dilated pupils
2. Rambling speech
3. Elevated blood pressure
4. Significant recent memory impairment

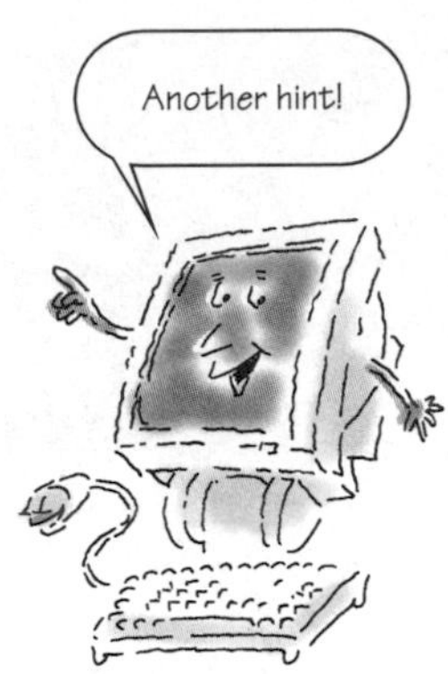

Another hint!

4. 4. Significant recent memory impairment, indicated by the inability to verbalize remembrances after several minutes to an hour, can be assessed in the early stages of Alzheimer's disease. Dilated pupils, increased blood pressure, and rambling speech are expected symptoms of delirium.

NP: Assessment; CN: Physiological integrity; CNS: Physiological adaptation; CL: Application

5. Which of the following pathophysiological changes in the brain causes the symptoms of Alzheimer's disease?
1. Glucose inadequacy
2. Atrophy of the frontal lobe
3. Degeneration of the cholinergic system
4. Intracranial bleeding in the limbic system

5. 3. Research related to Alzheimer's disease indicates that the enzyme needed to produce acetylcholine is dramatically reduced. The other pathophysiological changes don't cause the symptoms of Alzheimer's.

NP: Assessment; CN: Physiological integrity; CNS: Physiological adaptation; CL: Analysis

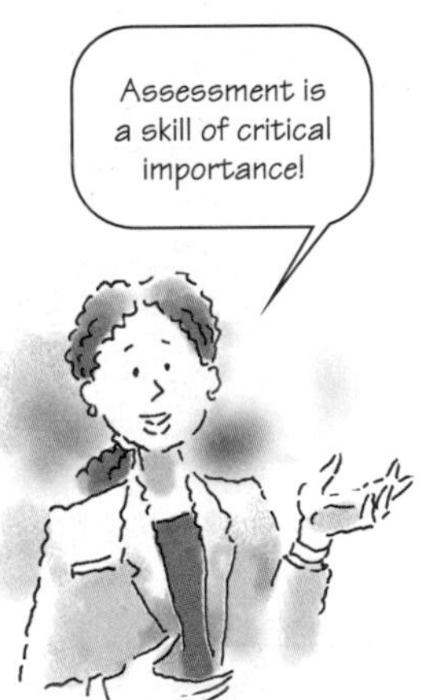

Assessment is a skill of critical importance!

6. Which of the following assessment findings shows impairment in abstract thinking and reasoning?
1. The client can't repeat a sentence.
2. The client has problems calculating simple problems.
3. The client doesn't know the name of the president of the United States.
4. The client can't find similarities and differences between related words or objects.

6. 4. Abstract thinking is assessed by noting similarities and differences between related words or objects. Not knowing the president of the United States is a deficiency in general knowledge. Not being able to do a simple calculation or repeat a sentence shows a client's inability to concentrate and focus on thoughts.

NP: Assessment; CN: Physiological integrity; CNS: Physiological adaptation; CL: Analysis

7. In addition to disturbances in cognition and orientation, a client with Alzheimer's disease may also show changes in which of the following areas?
1. Appetite
2. Energy levels
3. Hearing
4. Personality

7. 4. Personality change is common in dementia. There shouldn't be a remarkable change in appetite, energy level, or hearing.

NP: Assessment; CN: Physiological integrity; CNS: Physiological adaptation; CL: Application

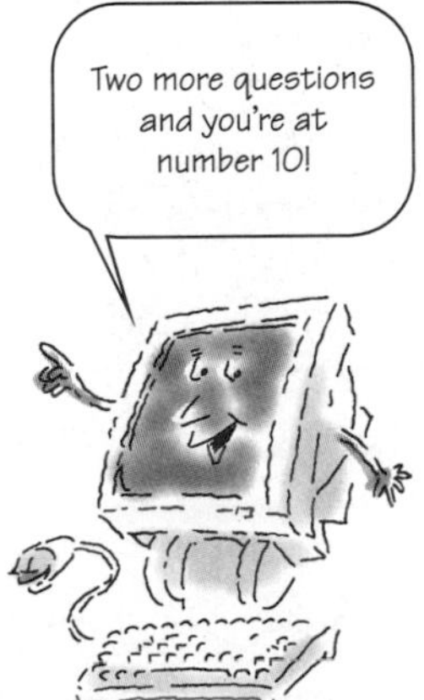

Two more questions and you're at number 10!

8. Which of the following interventions would help a client diagnosed with Alzheimer's disease perform activities of daily living?
1. Have the client perform all basic care without help.
2. Tell the client morning care must be done by 9 a.m.
3. Give the client a written list of activities he's expected to do.
4. Encourage the client, and give ample time to complete basic tasks.

8. 4. Clients with Alzheimer's disease respond to the affect of those around them. A gentle, calm approach is comforting and nonthreatening, and a tense, hurried approach may agitate the client. The client has problems performing independently. These expectations may lead to frustration.

NP: Implementation; CN: Safe, effective care environment; CNS: Management of care; CL: Application

9. Which of the following medications for Alzheimer's disease, approved by the Food and Drug Administration, is a moderately long-acting inhibitor of cholinesterase?

1. Bupropion (Wellbutrin)
2. Haloperidol (Haldol)
3. Tacrine (Cognex)
4. Triazolam (Halcion)

9. 3. Tacrine is used to improve cognition and functional autonomy in mild to moderate dementia of the Alzheimer's type. Wellbutrin is used for depression. Haldol is used for agitation, aggression, hallucinations, thought disturbances, and wandering. Halcion is used for sleep disturbances.

NP: Implementation; CN: Physiological integrity; CNS: Pharmacological and parenteral therapies; CL: Knowledge

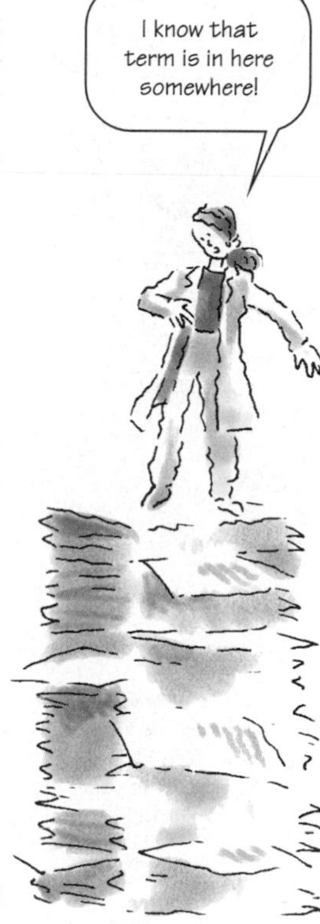

I know that term is in here somewhere!

10. A nurse places an object in the hand of a client with Alzheimer's disease and asks the client to identify the object. Which of the following terms represents the client's inability to name the object?

1. Agnosia
2. Aphasia
3. Apraxia
4. Perseveration

10. 1. Agnosia is the inability to recognize familiar objects. Aphasia is characterized by an impaired ability to speak. Apraxia refers to the client's inability to use objects properly. All three impairments usually occur in stage 3 of Alzheimer's disease. Perseveration is continued repetition of a meaningless word or phrase that occurs in stage 2 of Alzheimer's disease.

NP: Assessment; CN: Health promotion and maintenance; CNS: Prevention and early detection of disease; CL: Application

11. Which of the following nursing interventions will help a client with progressive memory deficit function in his environment?

1. Help the client do simple tasks by giving step-by-step directions.
2. Avoid frustrating the client by performing basic care routines for the client.
3. Stimulate the client's intellectual functioning by bringing new topics to the client's attention.
4. Promote the use of the client's sense of humor by telling jokes or riddles and discussing cartoons.

11. 1. Clients with cognitive impairment should do all the tasks they can. By receiving simple directions in a step-by-step fashion, the client can better process information and perform tasks. Clients with cognitive impairment may not be able to understand the joke or riddle, and cartoons may add to their confusion. Stimulation of intellect can be accomplished by discussing familiar topics with them; changes in topics may add to their confusion.

NP: Implementation; CN: Psychosocial integrity; CNS: Psychosocial adaptation; CL: Application

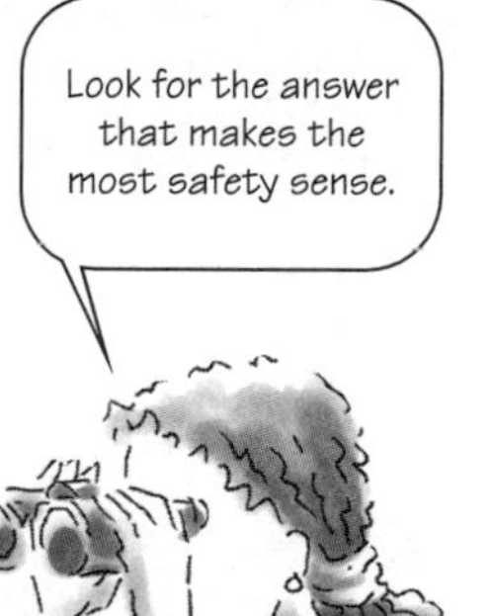

Look for the answer that makes the most safety sense.

12. Which of the following interventions is an important part of providing care to a client diagnosed with Alzheimer's disease?

1. Avoid physical contact.
2. Apply wrist and ankle restraints.
3. Provide a high level of sensory stimulation.
4. Monitor the client carefully.

12. 4. Whenever client safety is at risk, careful observation and supervision are of ultimate importance in avoiding injury. Applying restraints may cause agitation and combativeness. Physical contact is implemented during basic care. A high level of sensory stimulation may be too stimulating and distracting.

NP: Implementation; CN: Safe, effective care environment; CNS: Management of care; CL: Application

13. Which of the following nursing interventions is the most important in caring for a client diagnosed with Alzheimer's disease?

1. Make sure the environment is safe to prevent injury.
2. Make sure the client receives food she likes to prevent hunger.
3. Make sure the client meets other clients to prevent social isolation.
4. Make sure the client takes care of her daily physical care to prevent dependence.

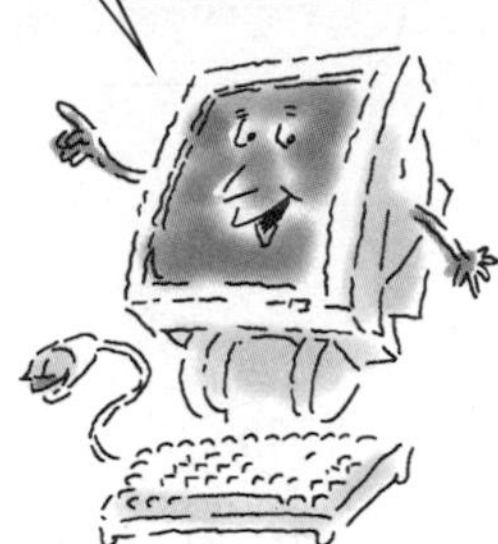

Question 13 asks you to prioritize.

13. 1. Providing client safety is the number one priority when caring for any client but particularly when a client is already compromised and at greater risk for injury.

NP: Implementation; CN: Safe, effective care environment; CNS: Safety and infection control; CL: Application

14. Which of the following medications is used to decrease the agitation, violence, and bizarre thoughts associated with dementia?

1. Diazepam (Valium)
2. Ergoloid (Hydergine)
3. Haloperidol (Haldol)
4. Tacrine (Cognex)

14. 3. Haloperidol is an antipsychotic that decreases the symptoms of agitation, violence, and bizarre thoughts. Diazepam is used for anxiety and muscle relaxation. Ergoloid is an adrenergic blocker used to block vascular headaches. Tacrine is used for improvement of cognition.

NP: Implementation; CN: Physiological integrity; CNS: Reduction of risk potential; CL: Application

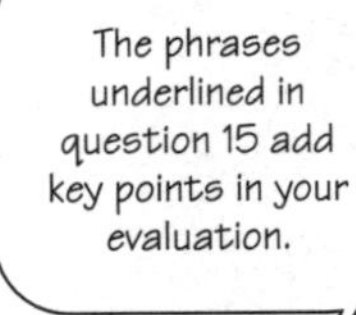

The phrases underlined in question 15 add key points in your evaluation.

15. A client diagnosed with Alzheimer's disease tells the nurse that today she has a luncheon date with her daughter, who is not visiting that day. Which of the following responses by the nurse would be most appropriate for this situation?

1. "Where are you planning on having your lunch?"
2. "You're confused and don't know what you're saying."
3. "I think you need some more medication, and I'll bring it to you."
4. "Today is Monday, March 8, and we'll be eating lunch in the dining room."

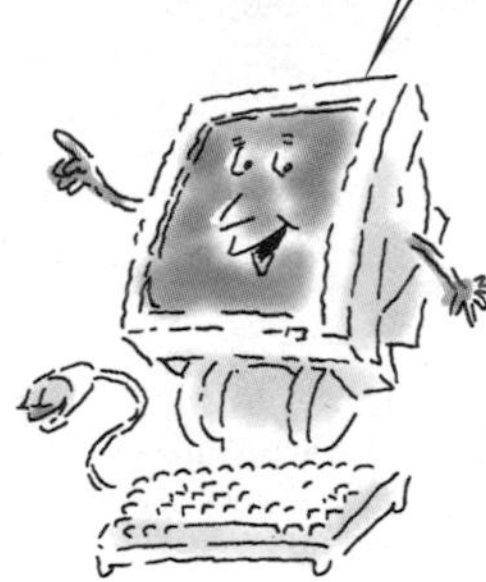

15. 4. The best nursing response is to reorient the client to the date and environment. Medication won't provide immediate relief for memory impairment. Confrontation can provoke an outburst.

NP: Implementation; CN: Psychosocial integrity; CNS: Psychosocial adaptation; CL: Application

16. Which of the following features is characteristic of cognitive disorders?

1. Catatonia
2. Depression
3. Feeling of dread
4. Deficit in cognition or memory

16. 4. Cognitive disorders represent a significant change in cognition or memory from a previous level of functioning. Catatonia is a type of schizophrenia characterized by periods of physical rigidity, negativism, excitement, and stupor. Depression is a feeling of sadness and apathy and is part of major depressive and other mood disorders. A feeling of dread is characteristic of an anxiety disorder.

NP: Assessment; CN: Physiological integrity; CNS: Physiological adaptation; CL: Application

17. Which of the following disorders is a degenerative disorder of cognition primarily associated with age or metabolic deterioration?
1. Delirium
2. Dementia
3. Neurosis
4. Psychosis

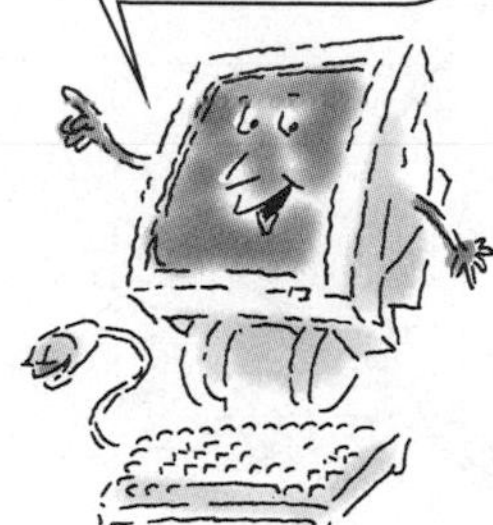

Another hint. Only one of the disorders is *degenerative*.

17. 2. Dementia is progressive and often associated with aging or underlying metabolic or organic deterioration. Delirium is characterized by abrupt, spontaneous cognitive dysfunction with an underling organic mental disorder. Neurosis and psychosis are psychological diagnoses.

NP: Assessment; CN: Physiological integrity; CNS: Physiological adaptation; CL: Knowledge

18. Which of the following characteristics best defines dementia?
1. Personal neglect in self-care
2. Poor judgment, especially in social situations
3. Memory loss occurring as a natural consequence of aging
4. Loss of intellectual abilities sufficient to impair the ability to perform basic care

18. 4. The ability to perform self-care is an important measure of the progression of dementia. Memory loss reflects underlying physical, metabolic, and pathologic processes. Personal neglect and poor judgment typically occur in dementia but aren't considered defining characteristics.

NP: Assessment; CN: Physiological integrity; CNS: Physiological adaptation; CL: Knowledge

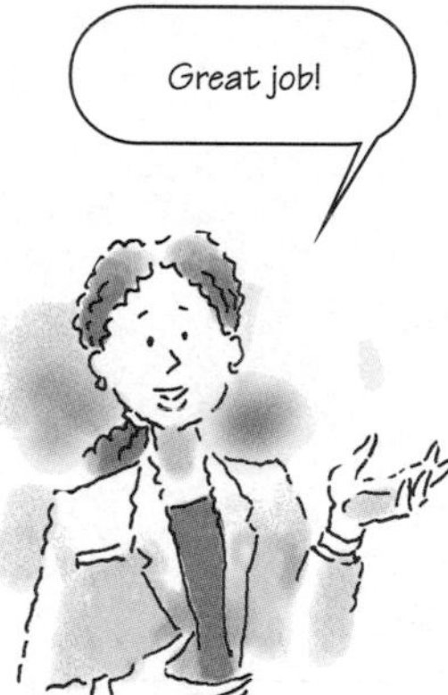

Great job!

19. Asking a client with a suspected dementia disorder to recall what she ate for breakfast would assess which of the following areas?
1. Food preferences
2. Recent memory
3. Remote memory
4. Speech

19. 2. Persons with dementia have difficulty in recent memory or learning, which may be a key to early detection. Assessing food preferences may be helpful in determining what the client likes to eat, but this assessment has no direct correlation in assessing dementia. Speech difficulties, such as rambling, irrelevance, and incoherence, may be related to delirium.

NP: Assessment; CN: Health promotion and maintenance; CNS: Prevention and early detection of disease; CL: Application

20. It's important to collect data for a definitive diagnosis of a dementia disorder to determine which of the following factors?
1. Prognosis
2. Genetic information
3. Degree of impairment
4. Implications for treatment

20. 4. The progression of biological impairment in the central nervous system is a function of the underlying pathologic states, so it's important to collect data and treat the underlying cause. The degree of impairment is necessary information for developing a care plan. Genetic information isn't relevant. Prognosis isn't the most important factor when making a diagnosis.

NP: Assessment; CN: Health promotion and maintenance; CNS: Prevention and early detection of disease; CL: Comprehension

21. Which of the following factors is considered a cause of vascular dementia?
1. Head trauma
2. Genetic factors
3. Acetylcholine alteration
4. Interruption of blood flow to the brain

21. 4. The cause of vascular dementia is directly related to an interruption of blood flow to the brain. Head trauma, genetic factors, and acetylcholine alteration are causative factors related to dementia of the Alzheimer's type.

NP: Analysis; CN: Physiological integrity; CNS: Physiological adaptation; CL: Comprehension

22. Which of the following factors is considered the most significant cause of vascular dementia?

1. Arterial hypertension
2. Hypoxia
3. Infection
4. Toxins

22. 1. Arterial hypertension, cerebral emboli, and cerebral thrombosis are causes of vascular dementia. Hypoxia, infection, and toxins are causes of delirium.

NP: Assessment; CN: Physiological integrity; CNS: Reduction of risk potential; CL: Knowledge

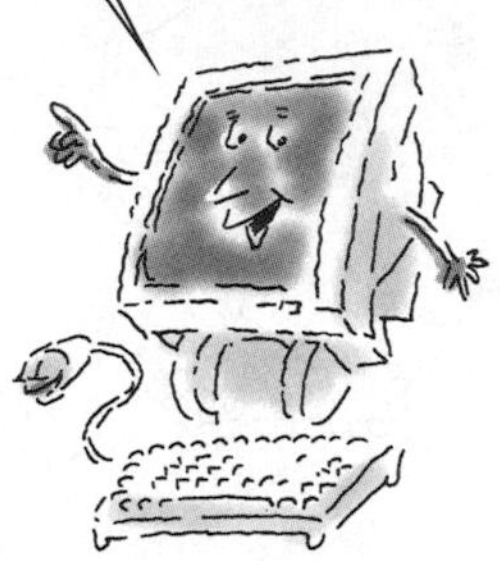

23. Which of the following assessment findings is expected for a client with vascular dementia?

1. Hypersomnolence
2. Insomnia
3. Restlessness
4. Small-stepped gait

23. 4. Focal neurologic signs commonly seen with vascular dementia include weakness of the limbs, small-stepped gait, and difficulty with speech. Insomnia, hypersomnolence, and restlessness are symptoms related to delirium.

NP: Assessment; CN: Physiological integrity; CNS: Physiological adaptation; CL: Application

24. In which of the following ways is vascular dementia different from Alzheimer's disease?

1. Vascular dementia has a more abrupt onset.
2. The duration of vascular dementia is usually brief.
3. Personality change is common in vascular dementia.
4. The inability to perform motor activities occurs in vascular dementia.

24. 1. Vascular dementia differs from Alzheimer's disease in that it has a more abrupt onset and runs a highly variable course. Personality change is common in Alzheimer's disease. The duration of delirium is usually brief. The inability to carry out motor activities is common in Alzheimer's disease.

NP: Analysis; CN: Health promotion and maintenance; CNS: Prevention and early detection of disease; CL: Analysis

25. A progression of symptoms that occurs in steps rather than a gradual deterioration indicates which type of dementia?

1. Alzheimer's dementia
2. Parkinson's dementia
3. Substance-induced dementia
4. Vascular dementia

25. 4. Vascular dementia differs from Alzheimer's disease in that vascular dementia has a more abrupt onset and progresses in steps. At times the dementia seems to clear up, and the individual shows fairly lucid thinking. Dementia of the Alzheimer's type has a slow onset with a progressive and deteriorating course. Dementia of Parkinson's sometimes resembles the dementia of Alzheimer's disease. Substance-induced dementia is related to the persisting effects of use of a substance.

NP: Assessment; CN: Physiological integrity; CNS: Physiological adaptation; CL: Analysis

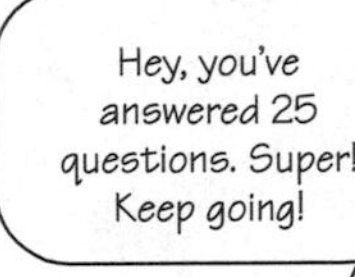

Hey, you've answered 25 questions. Super! Keep going!

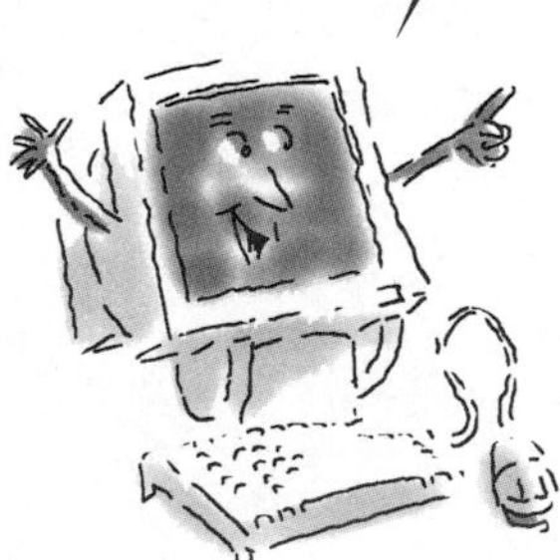

26. Which of the following cognitive disorders is characterized by a disturbance of consciousness and a change in cognition that develops rapidly over a short period?

1. Alzheimer's disease
2. Amnesia
3. Delirium
4. Dementia

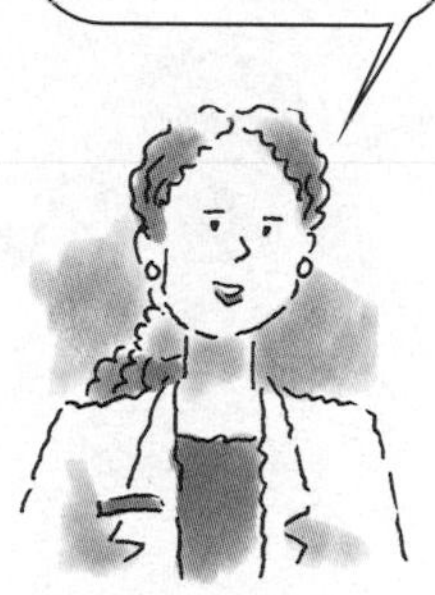

Which one of these conditions develops rapidly?

26. 3. One of the distinguishing characteristics of delirium is the development of symptoms over a short time, usually hours to days. Alzheimer's disease is a progressive dementia in which all known reversible causes are eliminated. Amnesia refers to recent short-term and long-term memory loss. Dementia is characterized by general impairment in intellectual functioning and occurs in a progressive, irreversible course.

NP: Assessment; CN: Physiological integrity; CNS: Physiological adaptation; CL: Knowledge

27. An elderly client has experienced memory and attention deficits that developed over a 3-day period. These symptoms are characteristic of which of the following disorders?

1. Alzheimer's disease
2. Amnesia syndrome
3. Delirium
4. Dementia

27. 3. Delirium is characterized by an abrupt onset of fluctuating levels of awareness, clouded consciousness, perceptual disturbances, and disturbed memory and orientation. Alzheimer's disease is a progressive dementia in which all known reversible causes are eliminated. Amnesia refers to recent short-term and long-term memory loss. Dementia is characterized by general impairment in intellectual functioning and occurs in a progressive, irreversible course.

NP: Assessment; CN: Physiological integrity; CNS: Physiological adaptation; CL: Application

28. Which of the following age-groups is at high risk for developing a state of delirium?

1. Adolescent
2. Elderly
3. Middle-aged
4. School-aged

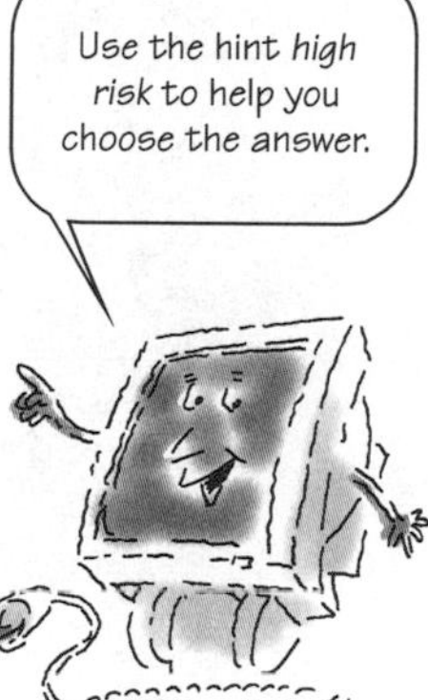

Use the hint *high risk* to help you choose the answer.

28. 2. The elderly population, because of normal physiological changes, is highly susceptible to delirium. All the other options are incorrect.

NP: Assessment; CN: Health promotion and maintenance; CNS: Prevention and early detection of disease; CL: Application

29. Which of the following nursing diagnoses is best for an elderly client experiencing visual and auditory hallucinations?

1. Interrupted family processes
2. Ineffective role performance
3. Impaired verbal communication
4. Disturbed sensory perception

29. 4. The client is experiencing visual and auditory hallucinations related to a sensory alteration. The other options don't address the hallucinations the client is experiencing.

NP: Analysis; CN: Health promotion and maintenance; CNS: Prevention and early detection of disease; CL: Application

30. Which of the following interventions is the most appropriate for clients with cognitive disorders?

1. Promote socialization.
2. Maintain optimal physical health.
3. Provide frequent changes in personnel.
4. Provide an overstimulating environment.

31. A newly admitted client diagnosed with delirium has a history of hypertension and anxiety. The client had been taking digoxin, furosemide (Lasix), and diazepam (Valium) for anxiety. This client's impairment may be related to which of the following conditions?

1. Infection
2. Metabolic acidosis
3. Drug intoxication
4. Hepatic encephalopathy

32. Which of the following environments is the most appropriate for a client experiencing sensory-perceptual alterations?

1. A softly lit room around the clock
2. A brightly lit room around the clock
3. Sitting by the nurses' desk while out of bed
4. A quiet, well-lit room without glare during the day and a darkened room for sleeping

33. As a nurse enters a client's room, the client says, "They're crawling on my sheets! Get them off my bed!" Which of the following assessments is the most accurate?

1. The client is experiencing aphasia.
2. The client is experiencing dysarthria.
3. The client is experiencing a flight of ideas.
4. The client is experiencing visual hallucinations.

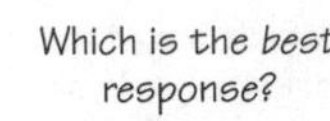

Which is the best response?

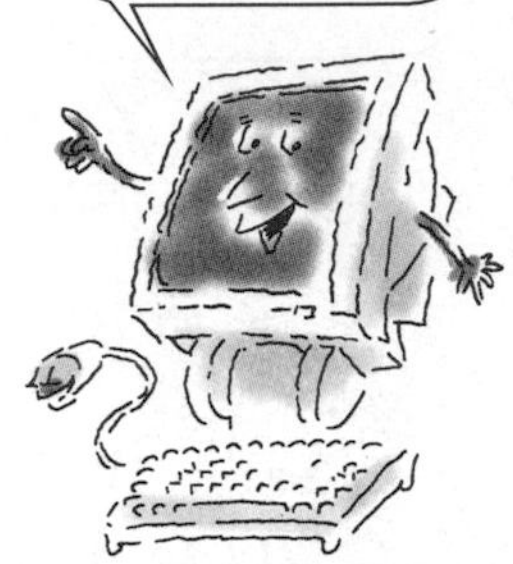

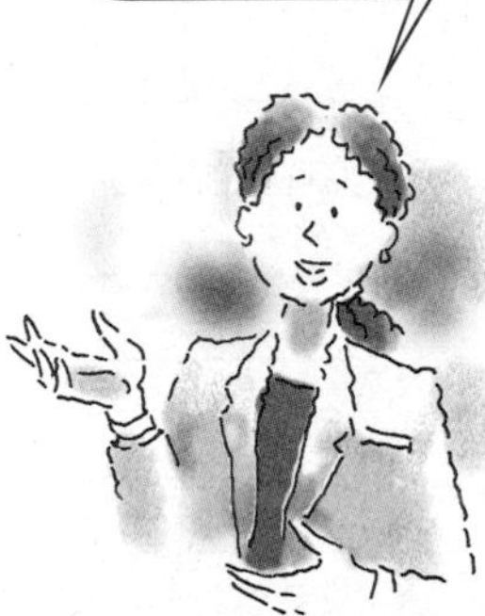

Your clients depend on you for meeting their environmental needs as well as their physical ones.

30. 2. A client's cognitive impairment may hinder self-care abilities. An overstimulating environment, frequent changes in staff members, and more socialization would only increase anxiety and confusion.

NP: Implementation; CN: Health promotion and maintenance; CNS: Prevention and early detection of disease; CL: Application

31. 3. This client was taking several medications that have a propensity for producing delirium; digoxin (a digitalis glycoside), furosemide (a thiazide diuretic), and diazepam (a benzodiazepine). Sufficient supporting data don't exist to suspect the other options as causes.

NP: Assessment; CN: Physiological integrity; CNS: Physiological adaptation; CL: Analysis

32. 4. A quiet, shadow-free environment produces the fewest sensory-perceptual distortions for a client with cognitive impairment associated with delirium.

NP: Implementation; CN: Safe, effective care environment; CNS: Safety and infection control; CL: Application

33. 4. The presence of a sensory stimulus correlates with the definition of a hallucination, which is a false sensory perception. Aphasia refers to a communications problem. Dysarthria is difficulty in speech production. Flight of ideas is rapid shifting from one topic to another.

NP: Assessment; CN: Health promotion and maintenance; CNS: Prevention and early detection of disease; CL: Application

42. During the early stages of amnesia, a client may use imaginary events to fill in memory gaps. Which of the following terms describes this process?
1. Confabulation
2. Delusions
3. Hypermnesia
4. Nihilism

42. 1. Confabulation is the fabrication of stories in response to questions about situations or events that aren't recalled. Delusion is a false belief maintained although contraindicated by social reality. Hypermnesia is the ability to recall material not ordinarily available to the memory process. Nihilism is feelings of nonexistence and hopelessness.

NP: Assessment; CN: Psychosocial integrity; CNS: Coping and adaptation; CL: Knowledge

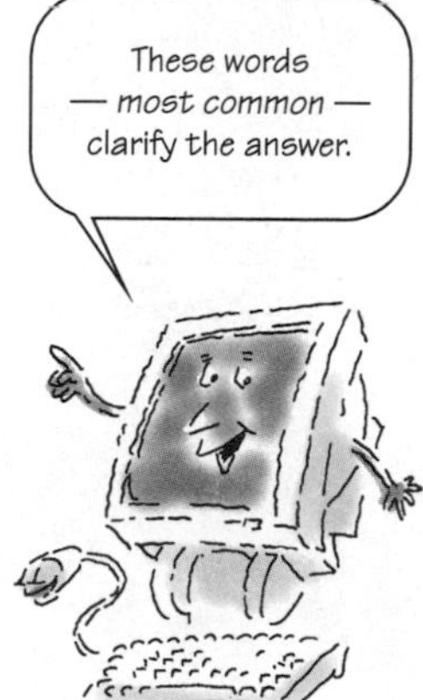

These words — most common — clarify the answer.

43. Which of the following factors or conditions is the most common cause of amnesic disorders?
1. Delirium
2. Metabolic factors
3. Organic factors
4. Thiamine deficiency related to alcohol abuse

43. 4. The most common cause is thiamine deficiency related to alcohol abuse. The diagnosis can't be made if amnesia occurs only during delirium. Both metabolic and organic factors can cause amnesic disorders, but they aren't the most common causes.

NP: Assessment; CN: Health promotion and maintenance; CNS: Prevention and early detection of disease; CL: Knowledge

44. Which of the following nursing diagnoses is appropriate for a client diagnosed with an amnesic disorder?
1. Anticipatory grieving related to loss of functional ability
2. Ineffective denial
3. Ineffective coping
4. Risk for injury related to impaired cognition

44. 4. Changes in cognitive ability place a client at high risk for injury. The client isn't aware of a loss and therefore doesn't grieve for it. The client isn't in denial but has an impaired ability to learn new information or to remember past information. The client isn't aware of a need to cope.

NP: Analysis; CN: Safe, effective care environment; CNS: Safety and infection control; CL: Analysis

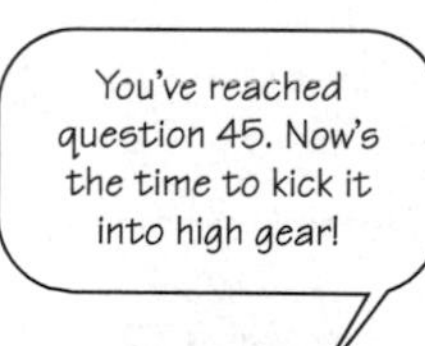

You've reached question 45. Now's the time to kick it into high gear!

45. Which of the following conditions indicates impairment in a client's ability to learn new information?
1. Anterograde amnesia
2. Korsakoff's syndrome
3. Retrograde amnesia
4. Wernicke's encephalopathy

45. 1. Anterograde amnesia refers to impairment in the ability to learn new information. Retrograde amnesia refers to inability to recall previously remembered knowledge. Korsakoff's syndrome is an amnesic syndrome caused by thiamine deficiency. Wernicke's encephalopathy is associated with Korsakoff's syndrome, in which the client experiences confusion, ataxia, and ophthalmoplegia.

NP: Assessment; CN: Physiological integrity; CNS: Physiological adaptation; CL: Knowledge

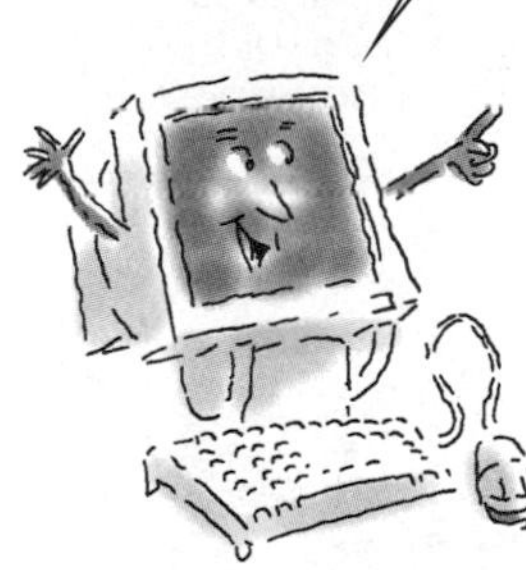

46. Which of the following medical conditions may be associated with an amnesic disorder?
1. Drug overdose
2. Cerebral anoxia
3. Medications (anticonvulsants)
4. Lead, mercury, and carbon dioxide toxins

46. 2. A variety of medical conditions are related to amnesic disorders, such as head trauma, cerebrovascular accident, cerebral neoplastic disease, herpes simplex, encephalitis, poorly controlled insulin-dependent diabetes, and cerebral anoxia. The other three options are substance induced.

NP: Assessment; CN: Physiological integrity; CNS: Physiological adaptation; CL: Application

47. Which of the following laboratory evaluations is an expected part of the initial workup for an amnesic disorder?
1. Angiography
2. Cardiac catheterization
3. Electrocardiography
4. Metabolic and endocrine tests

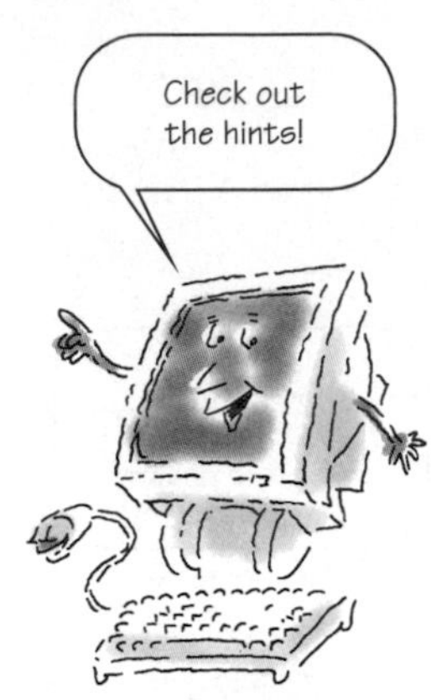
Check out
the hints!

47. 4. An amnesic disorder is caused by either physiological effects of a medical condition or effects of a substance, medication, or toxin, so metabolic and endocrine tests should be done. The other options are diagnostic tests related to the cardiovascular system.
NP: Assessment; CN: Health promotion and maintenance; CNS: Prevention and early detection of disease; CL: Application

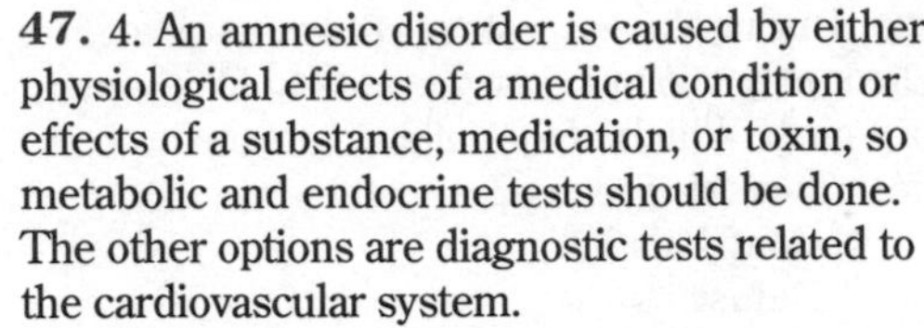

48. Which nursing intervention is appropriate for a client with memory impairment?
1. Speak to the client in a high-pitched tone.
2. Offer low-dose sedative-hypnotic drugs.
3. Ask a series of questions when obtaining information.
4. Identify yourself and look directly into the client's eyes.

48. 4. Clients with memory impairments need to reestablish the nurse's identification constantly. Asking a series of questions may create confusion; ask only one question at a time. A low-dose sedative-hypnotic medication may be used to promote rapid-eye-movement sleep. High-pitched tones may create more anxiety.
NP: Implementation; CN: Safe, effective care environment; CNS: Management of care; CL: Application

49. Transient global amnesia is generally associated with which of the following disorders?
1. Adjustment disorders
2. Cardiac anomalies
3. Cerebrovascular disease
4. Sleep disorders

49. 3. Transient global amnesia is usually associated with cerebrovascular disease that involves transient impairment in blood flow through the vertebrobasilar arteries. No correlation exists with the other options.
NP: Analysis; CN: Physiological integrity; CNS: Physiological adaptation; CL: Analysis

50. During conversation with a client, the nurse observes that he shifts from one topic to the next on a regular basis. Which of the following terms describes this disorder?
1. Flight of ideas
2 Concrete thinking
3 Ideas of reference
4. Loose associations

50. 4. Loose associations are conversations that constantly shift in topic. Concrete thinking implies highly definitive thought processes. Flight of ideas is characterized by conversation that's disorganized from the onset. Loose associations don't necessarily start in a disorganized way; the conversations can begin cogently, then become loose.
NP: Assessment; CN: Psychosocial integrity; CNS: Psychosocial adaptation; CL: Knowledge

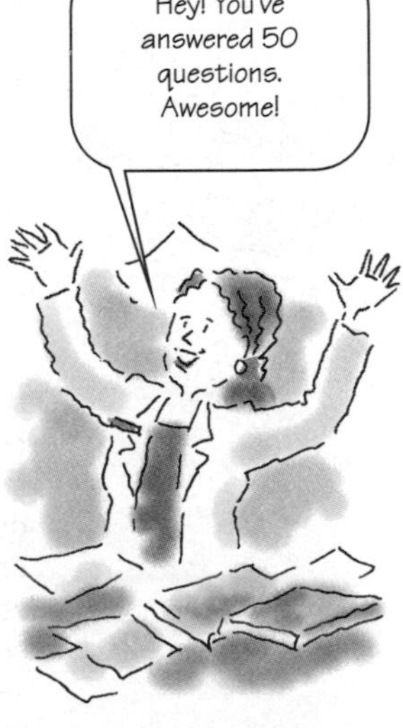
Hey! You've
answered 50
questions.
Awesome!

51. For a client with dementia, which assessment finding indicates worsening of dementia?

1. The client resists logical explanations.
2. The client stops redirecting negative energy.
3. The client stops maintaining a nondefensive position.
4. The client becomes increasingly agitated.

51. 4. A client with dementia who becomes increasingly agitated may be unable to perform expected tasks. Communication must be clear and concise; giving logical explanations is inappropriate. This client may revert to old ways of coping, and trying to change the client rarely proves successful; the nurse should try to decrease the source of negativity. The client with dementia is rarely defensive.

NP: Evaluation; CN: Safe, effective care environment; CNS: Management of care; CL: Analysis

52. For the family of a client with Alzheimer's disease, one goal is effective communication. Which outcome is successful for this goal?

1. Family members don't use humor with the client.
2. Family members speak to the client in a loud voice.
3. Family members give the client one-step commands.
4. Family members don't touch the client while speaking.

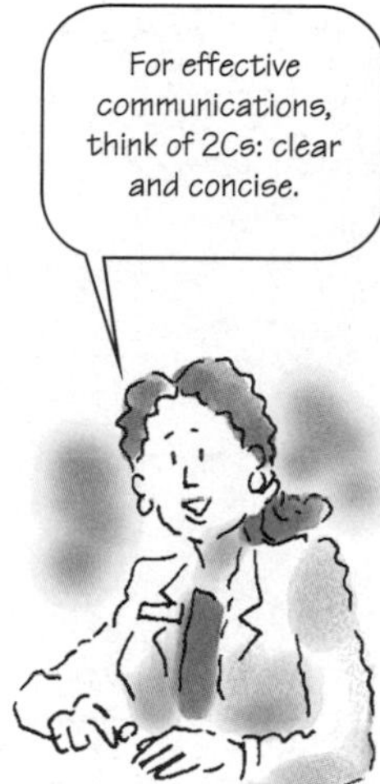

For effective communications, think of 2Cs: clear and concise.

52. 3. Giving one-step commands keeps communication simple, clear, concise, and pleasant. Humor must be used judiciously so as not to confuse the client. Speaking in a loud voice may be interpreted as shouting and cause agitation. Depending on the situation, the use of touch may be appropriate, helping to reassure and soothe the client.

NP: Evaluation; CN: Psychosocial integrity; CNS: Psychosocial adaptation; CL: Application

53. Immediately after visiting hours, the nurse identifies wandering behavior in a client with Alzheimer's disease. The client is showing which behavior?

1. The client may need to walk after eating a complete meal.
2. The client may feel tense because of an uncomfortable situation.
3. The client may be demonstrating several eccentric behaviors.
4. The client may have difficulty following directions.

53. 2. Tension and stress may cause a client with Alzheimer's disease to want to get away from an uncomfortable situation. Exercise is an important health promotion activity, but it doesn't help explain wandering behavior. Eccentric behaviors are rarely related to wandering. Many clients with dementia have difficulty following directions; however, wandering typically results from disorientation.

NP: Analysis; CN: Psychosocial integrity; CNS: Coping and adaptation; CL: Application

54. For a client with dementia who lives in a long-term care facility, which outcome takes the highest nursing care priority?

1. Maintaining the client's optimal level of functioning
2. Identifying coping methods the client can use to handle stress
3. Facilitating client conversation with five people each day
4. Having the client use physical activity to work off aggressive energy

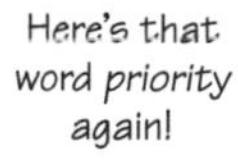

Here's that word priority again!

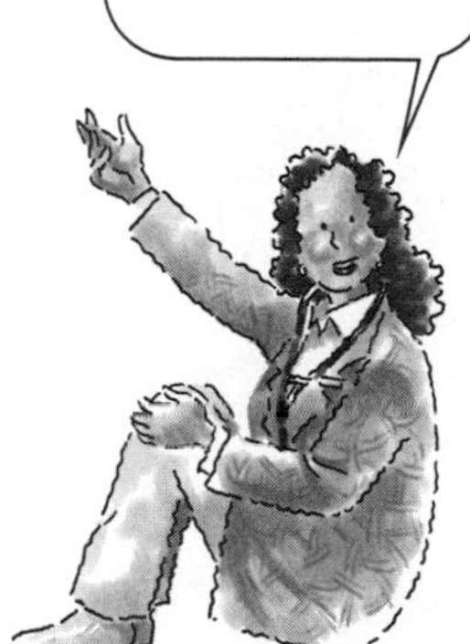

54. 1. The highest nursing care priority is to maintain the client's optimal level of functioning. Reducing the client's stress is the nurse's responsibility. Having a conversation with five people each day is unrealistic for this client. Expecting a client with dementia to use physical activity to decrease aggressive energy is also unrealistic.

NP: Analysis; CN: Safe, effective care environment; CNS: Management of care; CL: Application

55. The nurse teaches family caregivers of a dementia client how to take care of themselves. Which statement by a family member indicates effective teaching?

1. "It's difficult, but we keep telling Mother how important it is to write her memoirs."
2. "Today we decided to plan for a vacation and have the neighbors look in on Mom."
3. "Every evening we spend several hours talking about the problems we face."
4. "We've called community resources for respite care and asked for literature."

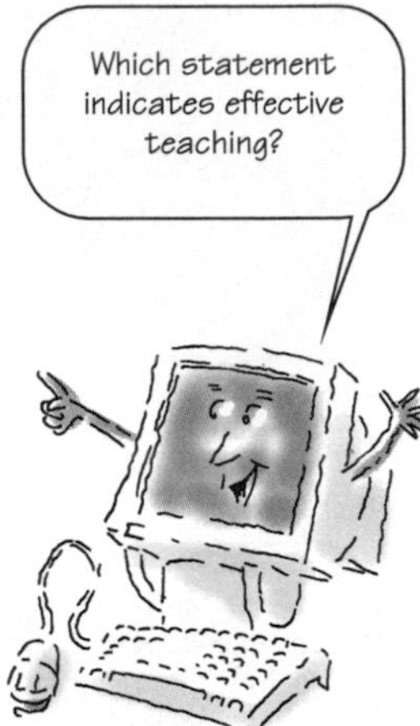

Which statement indicates effective teaching?

55. 4. Family members caring for a person with dementia must take care of themselves—for instance, by finding a respite service so they can take a break from their caregiving responsibilities. Clients with dementia aren't able to write memoirs. It isn't safe to leave a client with dementia home alone, with a neighbor overseeing from afar. Spending several hours each evening talking about problems uses too much time and energy; the family requires assistance with problem solving.

NP: Evaluation; CN: Safe, effective care environment; CNS: Management of care; CL: Application

56. Which intervention should the nurse use to keep a client with dementia oriented?

1. Administer medications at the same time each day.
2. Instruct the client to participate in self-care activities.
3. Place the client's personal possessions around the room.
4. Talk to the client about accepting the sick role.

56. 3. By placing the client's personal possessions around the room, the nurse promotes orientation and a sense of owning personal space. For therapeutic reasons, medications should be given at the same time each day; however, doing this doesn't promote client orientation. Participating in self-care activities won't orient the client. Talking to this client about accepting the sick role isn't appropriate.

NP: Implementation; CN: Safe, effective care environment; CNS: Management of care; CL: Knowledge

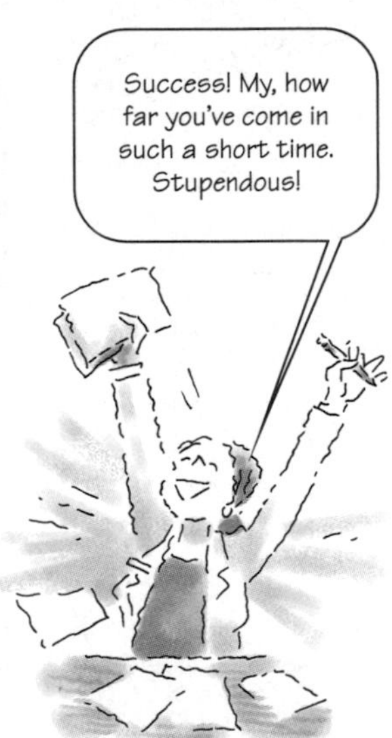

Success! My, how far you've come in such a short time. Stupendous!

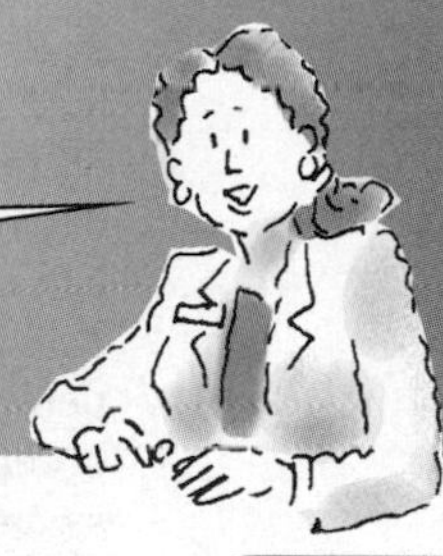

No, this chapter doesn't cover quirks of the rich and famous. It's all about mental disorders affecting the personality. Have a blast!

Chapter 16 Personality disorders

1. A client tells the nurse that her coworkers are sabotaging the computer. When the nurse asks questions, the client becomes argumentative. This behavior shows personality traits associated with which of the following personality disorders?

1. Antisocial
2. Histrionic
3. Paranoid
4. Schizotypal

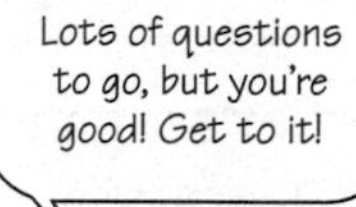

Lots of questions to go, but you're good! Get to it!

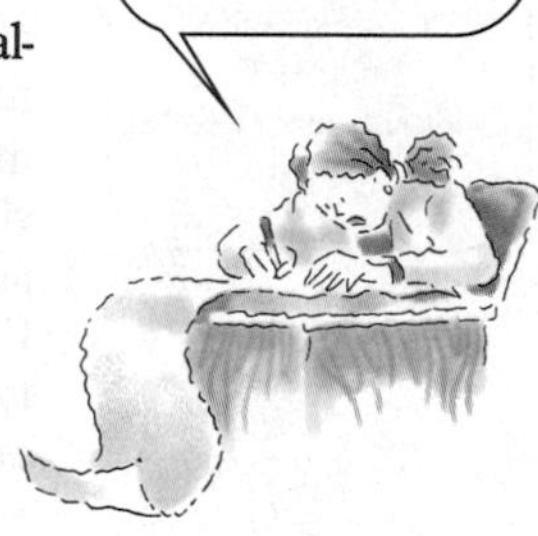

1. 3. Because of their suspiciousness, paranoid personalities ascribe malevolent activities to others and tend to be defensive, becoming quarrelsome and argumentative. Clients with antisocial personality disorder can also be antagonistic and argumentative but are less suspicious than paranoid personalities. Clients with a histrionic personality disorder are dramatic, not suspicious and argumentative. Clients with schizoid personality disorder are usually detached from others and tend to have eccentric behavior.

NP: Analysis; CN: Psychosocial integrity; CNS: Coping and adaptation; CL: Comprehension

2. A nurse notices that a client is mistrustful and shows hostile behavior. Which of the following types of personality disorder is associated with these characteristics?

1. Antisocial
2. Avoidant
3. Borderline
4. Paranoid

2. 4. Paranoid individuals have a need to constantly scan the environment for signs of betrayal, deception, and ridicule, appearing mistrustful and hostile. They expect to be tricked or deceived by others. The extreme suspiciousness is lacking in antisocial personalities, who tend to be more arrogant and self-assured despite their vigilance and mistrust. Individuals with avoidant personality disorders are guarded, fearing interpersonal rejection and humiliation. Clients with borderline personality disorders behave impulsively and tend to manipulate others.

NP: Analysis; CN: Psychosocial integrity; CNS: Coping and adaptation; CL: Knowledge

3. Which of the following traits is expected from a client with paranoid personality disorder?

1. The client can't follow limits set on behavior.
2. The client is afraid another person will inflict harm.
3. The client avoids responsibility for health care actions.
4. The client depends on others to make important decisions.

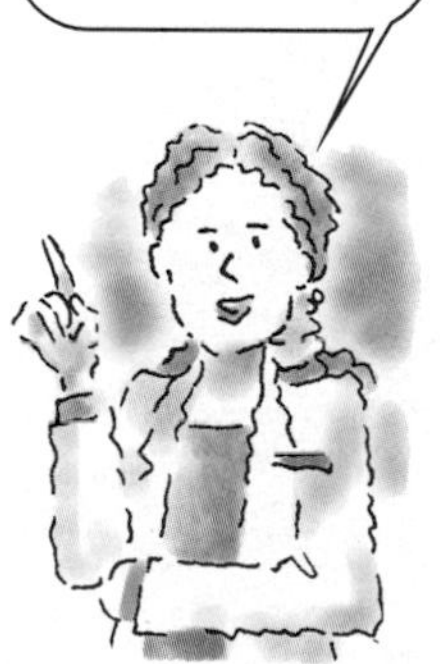

Understanding a client's traits will help you deal with him effectively.

3. 2. A client with paranoid personality disorder is afraid others will inflict harm. An individual with antisocial personality disorder won't be able to follow the limits set on behavior. An individual with an avoidant personality might avoid responsibility for health care because he tends to scan the environment for threatening things. A client with dependent personality disorder is likely to want others to make important decisions for him.

NP: Assessment; CN: Psychosocial integrity; CNS: Coping and adaptation; CL: Comprehension

NP: Nursing process CN: Client needs category CNS: Client needs subcategory CL: Cognitive level

4. Which of the following statements is typical for a client diagnosed with paranoid personality disorder?

1. "I understand you're to blame."
2. "I must be seen first; it's not negotiable."
3. "I see nothing humorous in this situation."
4. "I wish someone would select the outfit for me."

4. 3. Clients with paranoid personality disorder tend to be extremely serious and lack a sense of humor. Clients with borderline personality disorder tend to blame others for their problems. Clients with narcissistic personality disorders have a sense of self-importance and entitlement. Clients with dependent personality disorder want others to make their decisions.
NP: Assessment; CN: Psychosocial integrity; CNS: Coping and adaptation; CL: Analysis

5. Which of the following characteristics is expected for a client with paranoid personality disorder who receives bad news?

1. The client is overly dramatic after hearing the facts.
2. The client focuses on self to not become overanxious.
3. The client responds from a rational, objective point of view.
4. The client doesn't spend time thinking about the information.

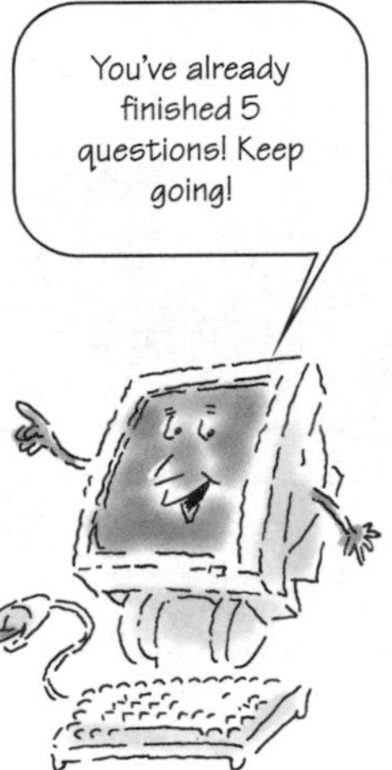
You've already finished 5 questions! Keep going!

5. 3. Clients with paranoid personality disorder are affectively restricted, appear unemotional, and appear rational and objective. Clients with histrionic personality disorder are overly dramatic in response to stress. Clients with narcissistic personality disorder focus on themselves and don't spend time thinking about bad news. Clients with an obsessive-compulsive personality disorder are preoccupied with the fear of becoming very anxious and losing control.
NP: Assessment; CN: Psychosocial integrity; CNS: Coping and adaptation; CL: Analysis

6. A nurse suspects a client has paranoid personality disorder. Which of the following findings confirms the nurse's suspicion?

1. Exhibitionism
2. Impulsiveness
3. Secretiveness
4. Self-destructiveness

6. 3. Clients with paranoid personality disorder tend to be secretive. Clients with histrionic personality disorder tend to be exhibitionists, and those with borderline personality disorder tend to be impulsive and self-destructive.
NP: Analysis; CN: Psychosocial integrity; CNS: Coping and adaptation; CL: Comprehension

7. Which of the following types of behavior is expected from a client diagnosed with paranoid personality disorder?

1. Eccentric
2. Exploitative
3. Hypersensitive
4. Seductive

7. 3. People with paranoid personality disorders are hypersensitive to perceived threats. Schizotypal personalities appear eccentric and engage in activities others find perplexing. Clients with narcissistic personality disorder are interpersonally exploitative to enhance themselves or indulge their own desires. A client with histrionic personality disorder can be extremely seductive when in search of stimulation and approval.
NP: Assessment; CN: Psychosocial integrity; CNS: Coping and adaptation; CL: Analysis

8. A client with paranoid personality disorder is discussing current problems with a nurse. Which of the following nursing interventions has priority in the care plan?

1. Have the client look at sources of frustration.
2. Have the client focus on ways to interact with others.
3. Have the client discuss the use of defense mechanisms.
4. Have the client clarify thoughts and beliefs about an event.

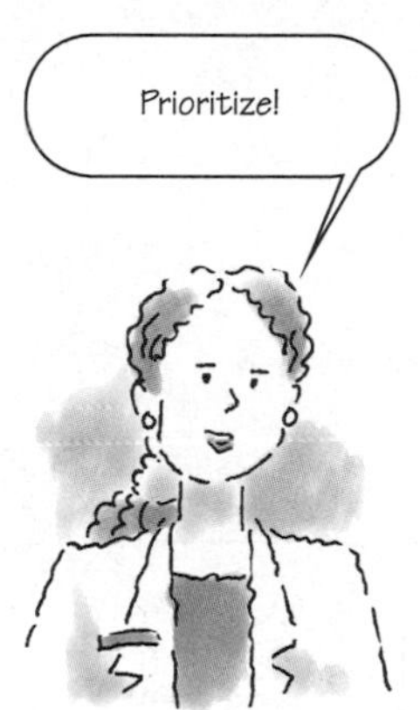

8. 4. Clarifying thoughts and beliefs helps the client avoid misinterpretations. Clients with a paranoid personality disorder tend to mistrust people and don't see interacting with others as a way to handle problems. They tend to be aggressive and argumentative rather than frustrated. The client's priority must be to interpret his thoughts and beliefs realistically, rather than discuss defensive mechanisms. A paranoid client will focus on defending self rather than acknowledging the use of defense mechanisms.
NP: Planning; CN: Psychosocial integrity; CNS: Psychosocial adaptation; CL: Analysis

9. A client with a paranoid personality disorder makes an inappropriate and unreasonable report to a nurse. Which of the following principles of good communication skills is important to use?

1. Use logic to address the client's concern.
2. Confront the client about the stated misperception.
3. Use nonverbal communication to address the issue.
4. Tell the client matter-of-factly that you don't share his interpretation.

9. 4. Telling the client you don't share his interpretation helps the client differentiate between realistic and emotional thoughts and conclusions. When the nurse uses logic to respond to a client's inappropriate statement, the nurse risks creating a power struggle with the client. The use of nonverbal communication will probably be misinterpreted and arouse the client's suspicion. It's unwise to confront a client with a paranoid personality disorder as the client will immediately become defensive.
NP: Analysis; CN: Psychosocial integrity; CNS: Psychosocial adaptation; CL: Analysis

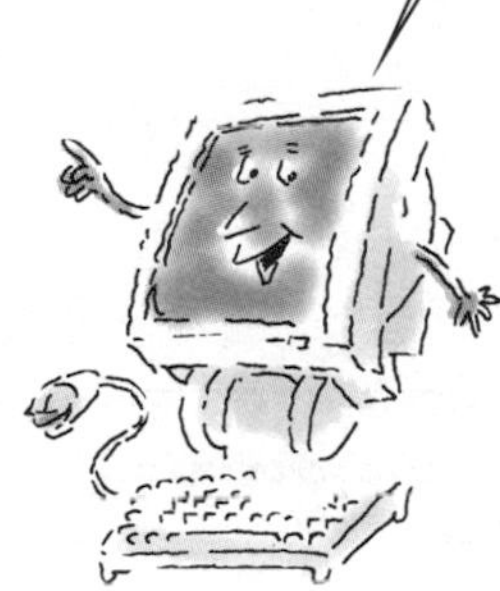

Identify and understand the key words before answering this question!

10. Which of the following short-term goals is most appropriate for the client with paranoid personality disorder who has impaired social skills?

1. Obtain feedback from other people.
2. Discuss anxiety-provoking situations.
3. Address positive and negative feelings about self.
4. Identify personal feelings that hinder social interaction.

10. 4. The client must address the feelings that impede social interactions before developing ways to address impaired social skills. Feedback can only be obtained after action is taken to improve or change the situation. Discussion of anxiety-provoking situations is important but doesn't help the client with impaired social skills. Addressing the client's positive and negative feelings about self won't directly influence impaired social skills.
NP: Analysis; CN: Psychosocial integrity; CNS: Psychosocial adaptation; CL: Application

11. Which of the following interventions is important for a client with paranoid personality disorder taking olanzapine (Zyprexa)?

1. Explain effects of serotonin syndrome.
2. Teach the client to watch for extrapyramidal adverse reactions.
3. Explain that the drug is less effective if the client smokes.
4. Discuss the need to report paradoxical effects such as euphoria.

11. 3. Olanzapine (Zyprexa) is less effective for clients who smoke cigarettes. Serotonin syndrome occurs with clients who take a combination of antidepressant medications. Olanzapine doesn't cause euphoria, and extrapyramidal adverse reactions aren't a problem. However, the client should be aware of adverse effects such as tardive dyskinesia.
NP: Implementation; CN: Physiological integrity; CNS: Pharmacological and parenteral therapies; CL: Application

12. Which of the following approaches should be used with a client with paranoid personality disorder who misinterprets many things the health care team says?

1. Limit interaction to activities of daily living.
2. Address only problems and causes of distress.
3. Explore anxious situations and offer reassurance.
4. Speak in simple messages without details.

12. 4. If the nurse speaks to the client with clear and simple messages, there's less chance information will be misinterpreted. Discussing complex topics creates a situation in which the client will have additional information to misinterpret. If the nurse addresses only problems and specific stressors, it will be difficult to establish a trust relationship. Interaction can't be limited because it will interfere with working on identified treatment goals.

NP: Implementation; CN: Psychosocial integrity; CNS: Psychosocial adaptation; CL: Application

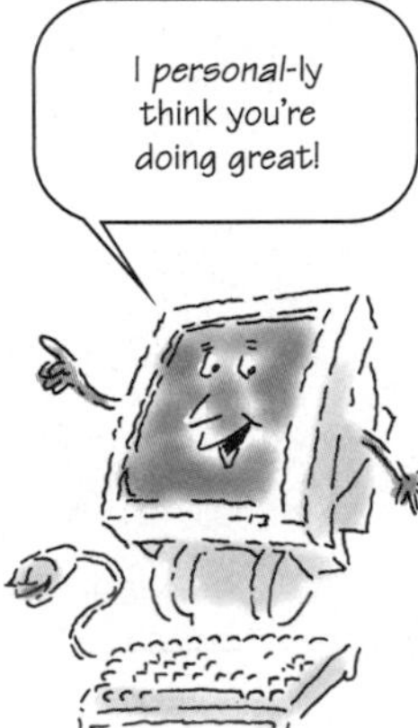

I personal-ly think you're doing great!

13. A client with paranoid personality disorder responds aggressively during a psychoeducational group to something another client said about him. Which of the following explanations is the most likely?

1. The client doesn't want to participate in the group.
2. The client took the statement as a personal criticism.
3. The client is impulsive and was acting out frustrations.
4. The client was attempting to handle emotional distress.

13. 2. Clients with paranoid personality disorder tend to be hypersensitive and take what other people say as a personal attack on their character. The client is driven by the suspicion that others will inflict harm. Group participation would be minimal because the client is directing energy toward emotional self-protection. Clients with a paranoid personality disorder tend to be rigid and guarded rather than expressive and acting out. The client with a paranoid personality disorder is acting to defend himself, not handle emotional distress.

NP: Analysis; CN: Psychosocial integrity; CNS: Psychosocial adaptation; CL: Analysis

14. A client with a paranoid personality disorder tells a nurse of his decision to stop talking to his wife. Which of the following areas should be assessed?

1. The client's doubts about the partner's loyalty
2. The client's need to be alone and have time for self
3. The client's decision to separate from the marital partner
4. The client's fears about becoming too much like the partner

14. 1. Clients with paranoid personality disorder are preoccupied with the loyalty or trustworthiness of people, especially family and friends. People commonly withdraw from a client with paranoid personality disorder due to the difficulty in maintaining a healthy relationship. The client's need to be alone and have time for self isn't related to the decision to stop talking to a partner. These clients focus on the belief that others will harm them, not that they may become like a marital partner.

NP: Analysis; CN: Psychosocial integrity; CNS: Coping and adaptation; CL: Application

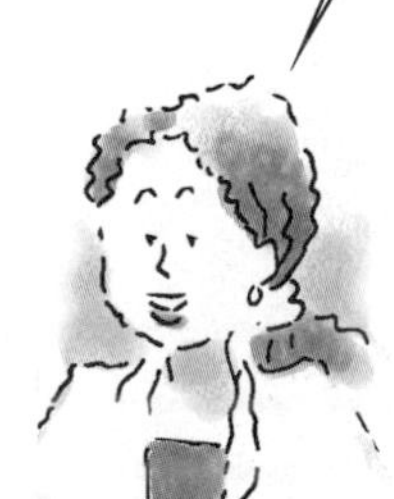

Try to establish a therapeutic relationship with the client.

15. Which of the following characteristics of a client with a paranoid personality disorder makes it **difficult** for a nurse to establish an interpersonal relationship?

1. Dysphoria
2. Hypervigilance
3. Indifference
4. Promiscuity

15. 2. Clients with paranoid personality disorder think others will harm, deceive, or exploit them in some way, and they're often guarded and ready to defend themselves from actual or perceived attacks. They don't tend to be dysphoric, indifferent, or promiscuous.

NP: Analysis; CN: Psychosocial integrity; CNS: Coping and adaptation; CL: Knowledge

16. The wife of a client diagnosed with paranoid personality disorder tells the client she wants a divorce. When discussing this situation with the couple, which of the following factors would help the nurse form a care plan for this couple?

1. Denied grief
2. Intense jealousy
3. Exploitation of others
4. Self-destructive tendencies

16. 2. Clients with paranoid personality disorder are often extremely suspicious and jealous and make frequent accusations of partners and family members. Clients with paranoid personality disorder don't tend to struggle with the denial of grief. Clients with narcissistic personality disorder tend to exploit other people. Clients with borderline personality disorder have self-destructive tendencies.

NP: Planning; CN: Psychosocial integrity; CNS: Psychosocial adaptation; CL: Comprehension

17. A client with a paranoid personality disorder tells a nurse that another nurse is out to get him. Which of the following actions by the nurse may cause this paranoid client distress?

1. Giving as-needed medication to another client
2. Taking the clients outside the unit for exercise
3. Checking vital signs of each person on the unit
4. Talking to another client in the corner of the lounge

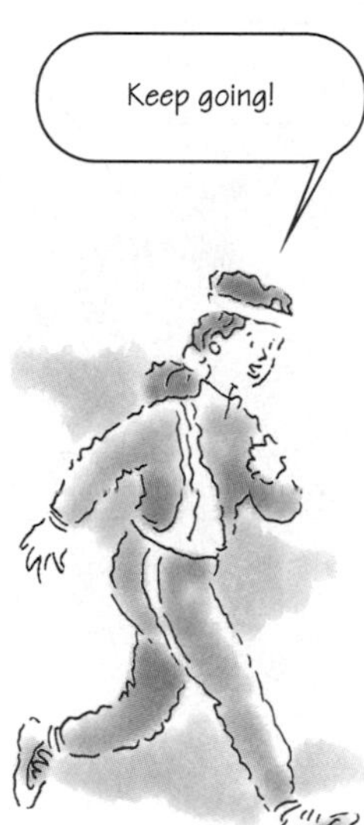

Keep going!

17. 4. Clients with paranoid personality disorder tend to interpret any discussion that doesn't include them as evidence of a plot against them. Giving medication to another client wouldn't alarm the client. Checking vital signs on each client on the unit or taking the clients outside for exercise probably wouldn't be seen as a threat to the client's well-being.

NP: Analysis; CN: Psychosocial integrity; CNS: Psychosocial adaptation; CL: Application

18. Which of the following statements made by a client with paranoid personality disorder shows that teaching about social relationships is effective?

1. "As long as I live, I won't abide by social rules."
2. "Sometimes I can see what causes relationship problems."
3. "I'll find out what problems others have so I won't repeat them."
4. "I don't have problems in social relationships; I never really did."

18. 2. Progress is shown when the client addresses behaviors that negatively impact relationships. Clients with paranoid personality disorder tend to have impaired social relationships and are very uncomfortable in social settings. Not recognizing the problem indicates the client is in denial. Knowing other people's problems isn't useful; the client must focus on his own issues. Clients with paranoid personality disorder struggle to understand and express their feelings about social rules.

NP: Evaluation; CN: Psychosocial integrity; CNS: Psychosocial adaptation; CL: Application

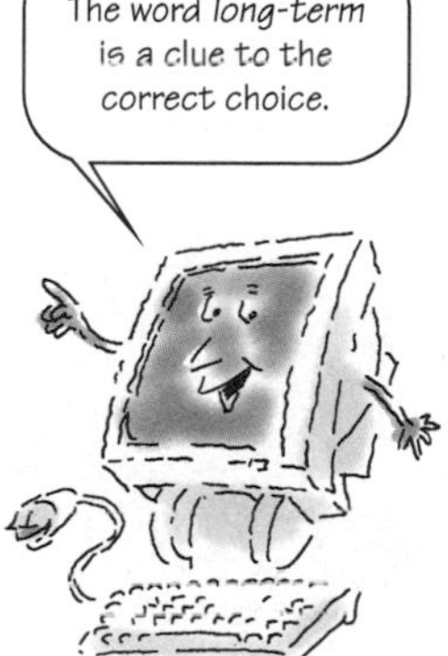

The word *long-term* is a clue to the correct choice.

19. Which of the following long-term goals is appropriate for a client with paranoid personality disorder who is trying to improve peer relationships?

1. The client will verbalize a realistic view of self.
2. The client will take steps to address disorganized thinking.
3. The client will become appropriately interdependent on others.
4. The client will become involved in activities that foster social relationships.

19. 4. An appropriate long-term goal is for the client to increase interactions and social skills and make the commitment to become involved with others on a long-term basis. A client with paranoid personality disorder won't allow himself to be interdependent on others. To verbalize a realistic view of self is a short-term goal. The client with a paranoid personality disorder doesn't tend to have disorganized thinking.

NP: Analysis; CN: Psychosocial integrity; CNS: Psychosocial adaptation; CL: Analysis

20. A family of a client with paranoid personality disorder is trying to understand the client's behavior. Which of the following interventions would help the family?

1. Help the family find ways to handle stress.
2. Explore the possibility of finding respite care.
3. Help the family manage the client's eccentric action.
4. Encourage the family to focus on the client's strength.

20. 3. The family needs to know how to handle the client's symptoms and eccentric behaviors. Focusing on the client's strengths is a positive action, but the family in this situation must learn how to manage the client's behavior. There's no need to find respite care for a client with a paranoid personality disorder. All people need to learn strategies for handling stress, but the focus must be on helping the family learn how to handle symptoms.

NP: Implementation; CN: Psychosocial integrity; CNS: Psychosocial adaptation; CL: Application

Therapeutic interventions must be appropriate for the client.

21. A client with antisocial personality disorder is trying to convince a nurse that he deserves special privileges and that an exception to the rules should be made for him. Which of the following responses is the most appropriate?

1. "I believe we need to sit down and talk about this."
2. "Don't you know better than to try to bend the rules?'
3. "What you're asking me to do for you is unacceptable."
4. "Why don't you bring this request to the community meeting?"

21. 3. These clients often try to manipulate the nurse to get special privileges or make exceptions to the rules on their behalf. By informing the client directly when actions are inappropriate, the nurse helps the client learn to control unacceptable behaviors by setting limits. By sitting down to talk about the request, the nurse is telling the client there's room for negotiation when there is none. The second option humiliates the client. The client's behavior is unacceptable and shouldn't be brought to a community meeting.

NP: Implementation; CN: Psychosocial integrity; CNS: Psychosocial adaptation; CL: Application

22. A client with antisocial personality disorder tells a nurse, "Life has been full of problems since childhood." Which of the following situations or conditions would the nurse explore in the assessment?

1. Birth defects
2. Distracted easily
3. Hypoactive behavior
4. Substance abuse

22. 4. Clients with antisocial personality disorder often engage in substance abuse during childhood. They don't have a higher incidence of birth defects than other people. They tend to be hyperactive, not hypoactive. Clients with antisocial personality disorder are often manipulative and are no more distracted from issues than others.

NP: Assessment; CN: Psychosocial integrity; CNS: Coping and adaptation; CL: Comprehension

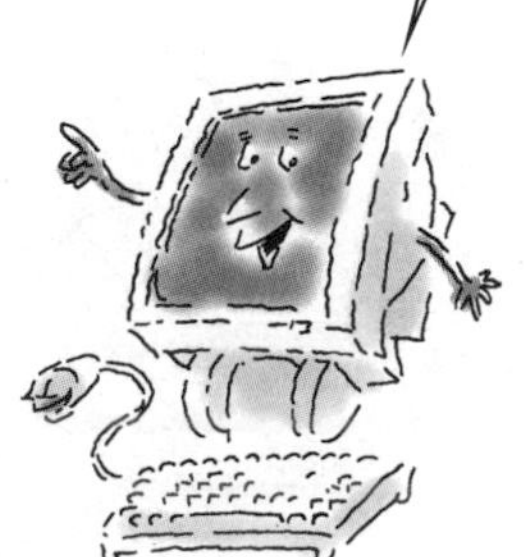

This is one of those further teaching questions. It asks you to identify a client behavior that signals the need for more teaching.

23. Which of the following behaviors by a client with antisocial personality disorder alerts a nurse to the need for teaching related to interaction skills?

1. Frequently crying
2. Having panic attacks
3. Avoiding social activities
4. Failing to follow social norms

23. 4. Failure to abide by social norms influences the client's ability to interact in a healthy manner with peers. Clients with antisocial personality disorders don't have frequent crying episodes or panic attacks. Avoiding social activities is more likely to be observed in avoidance personality style.

NP: Analysis; CN: Psychosocial integrity; CNS: Coping and adaptation; CL: Analysis

24. Which of the following behaviors is suspected when a client with antisocial personality disorder shows blatant disregard for the law?
1. Labeling self as bad
2. Resisting spiritual healing
3. Engaging in criminal behaviors
4. Successful manipulation of the legal system

24. 3. Clients with antisocial personality disorder tend to engage in a variety of criminal activities. They don't tend to label themselves as bad, and they have no interest in spiritual healing, no sense of remorse, and no inner need for forgiveness. They don't tend to successfully manipulate the legal system, but many of these clients are referred for treatment by the criminal justice system.
NP: Analysis; CN: Psychosocial integrity; CNS: Coping and adaptation; CL: Comprehension

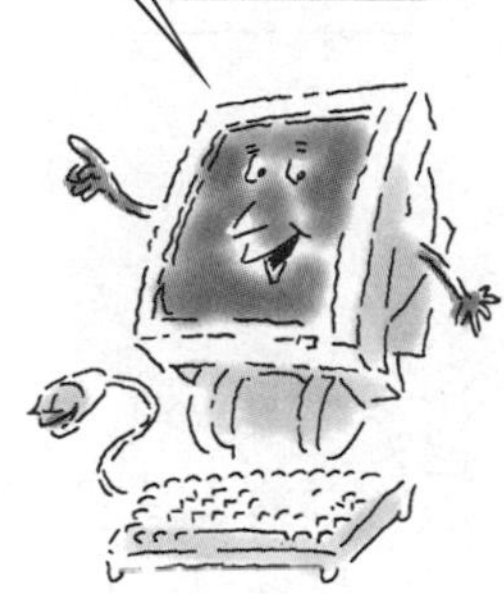

25. Which of the following interventions should be done first for a client who has an antisocial personality disorder and a history of polysubstance abuse?
1. Human immunodeficiency virus (HIV) testing
2. Electrolyte profile
3. Anxiety screening
4. Psychological testing

25. 1. A client who engages in high-risk behaviors such as polysubstance abuse should undergo HIV testing. This client would benefit from an entire chemistry profile as part of a complete medical examination, rather than a singular test for electrolytes. An anxiety screen isn't needed for a client with antisocial personality disorder. Information from psychological testing is valuable when developing a treatment but isn't an immediate concern.
NP: Planning; CN: Physiological integrity; CNS: Reduction of risk potential; CL: Application

26. Which of the following short-term goals is appropriate for a client with an antisocial personality disorder who acts out when distressed?
1. Develop goals for personal improvement.
2. Identify situations that are out of the client's control.
3. Encourage the client to identify traumatic life events.
4. Learn to express feelings in a nondestructive manner.

26. 4. By working on appropriate expression of feelings, the client learns how to talk about what's stressful, rather than hurt himself or others. The most pressing need is to learn to cope and talk about problems rather than act out. Developing goals for personal improvement is a long-term goal, not a short-term one. Although it's important to differentiate what is and isn't under the client's control, the most important goal for handling distress is to talk about feelings appropriately. The identification of traumatic life events will occur only after the client begins to express feelings appropriately.
NP: Analysis; CN: Safe, effective care environment; CNS: Safety and infection control; CL: Application

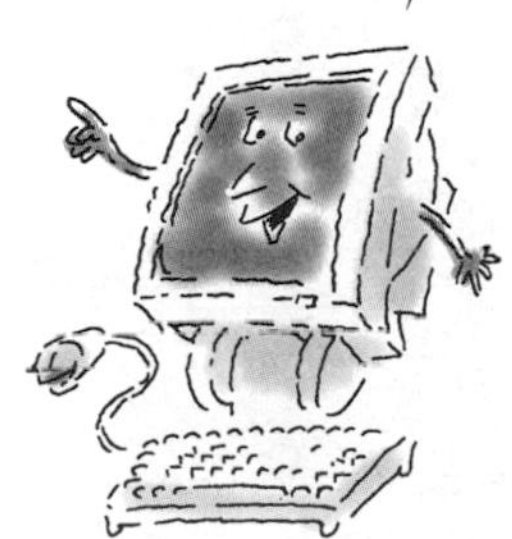

Read this question carefully. It seems to be asking you for a positive response, but it isn't.

27. A nurse notices other clients on the unit avoiding a client diagnosed with antisocial personality disorder. When discussing appropriate behavior in group therapy, which of the following comments is expected about this client by his peers?
1. Lack of honesty
2. Belief in superstitions
3. Show of temper tantrums
4. Constant need for attention

27. 1. Clients with antisocial personality disorder tend to engage in acts of dishonesty, shown by lying. Clients with schizotypal personality disorder tend to be superstitious. Clients with histrionic personality disorders tend to overreact to frustrations and disappointments, have temper tantrums, and seek attention.
NP: Analysis; CN: Psychosocial integrity; CNS: Coping and adaptation; CL: Application

28. During a family meeting for a client with antisocial personality disorder, which of the following statements is expected from an exasperated family member?

1. "Today I'm the enemy, but tomorrow I'll be a saint to him."
2. "When he's wrong, he never apologizes or even acts sorry."
3. "Sometimes I can't believe how he exaggerates about everything."
4. "There are times when his compulsive behavior is too much to handle."

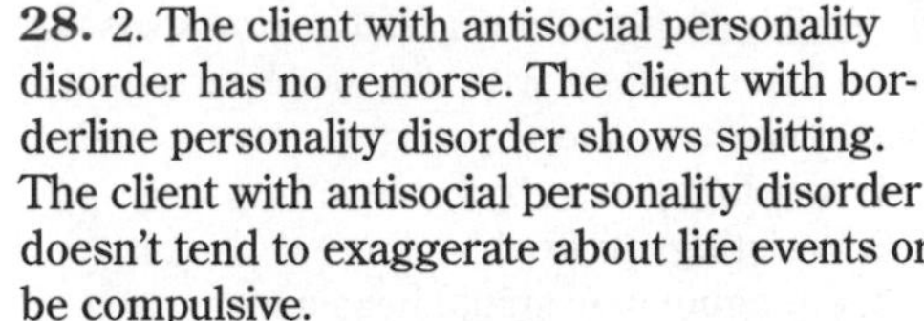

28. 2. The client with antisocial personality disorder has no remorse. The client with borderline personality disorder shows splitting. The client with antisocial personality disorder doesn't tend to exaggerate about life events or be compulsive.

NP: Analysis; CN: Psychosocial integrity; CNS: Coping and adaptation; CL: Analysis

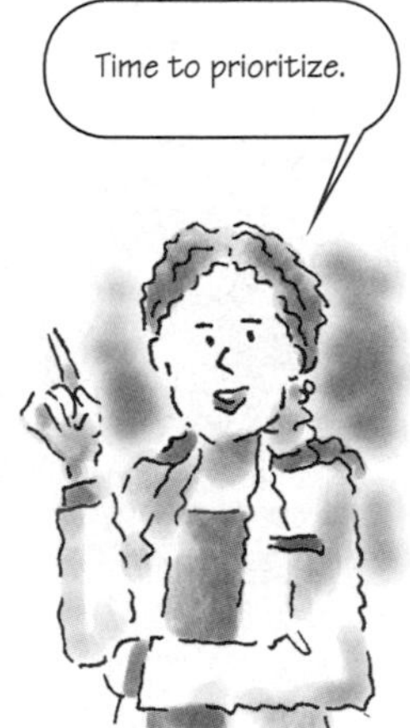

29. Which of the following goals is most appropriate for a client with antisocial personality disorder with a high risk for violence directed at others?

1. The client will discuss the desire to hurt others rather than act.
2. The client will be given something to destroy to displace the anger.
3. The client will develop a list of resources to use when anger escalates.
4. The client will understand the difference between anger and physical symptoms.

29. 1. By discussing the desire to be violent toward others, the nurse can help the client get in touch with the pain associated with the angry feelings. It isn't helpful to have the client destroy something. The client needs to talk about strong feelings in a nonviolent manner, not refer to a list of crisis references. Helping the client understand the relationship between feelings and physical symptoms can be done after discussing the desire to hurt others.

NP: Analysis; CN: Psychosocial integrity; CNS: Coping and adaptation; CL: Analysis

30. A client with antisocial personality disorder says, "I always want to blow things off." Which of the following responses is the most appropriate?

1. "Try to focus on what needs to be done and just do it."
2. "Let's work on considering some options and strategies."
3. "Procrastinating is a part of your illness that we'll work on."
4. "The best thing to do is decide on some useful goals to accomplish."

30. 2. By considering options or strategies, the client gains skills to overcome ineffective behaviors. The client tends to be irresponsible and needs guidance on what specifically to focus on to change behavior. Clients with an antisocial personality disorder don't tend to struggle with procrastination; instead, they show reckless and irresponsible behaviors. It's premature to decide on goals when the client needs to address the mental mind-set and work to change the irresponsible behavior.

NP: Implementation; CN: Psychosocial integrity; CNS: Psychosocial adaptation; CL: Analysis

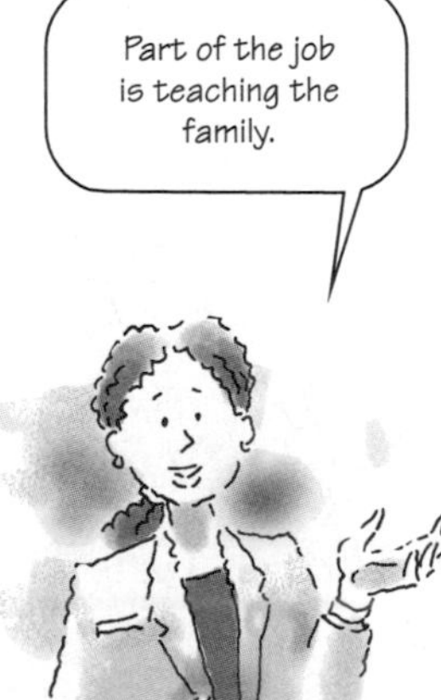

Part of the job is teaching the family.

31. Which of the following goals for the family of a client with antisocial disorder should the nurse stress in her teaching?

1. The family must assist the client to decrease ritualistic behavior.
2. The family must learn to live with the client's impulsive behavior.
3. The family must stop reinforcing inappropriate negative behavior.
4. The family must start to use negative reinforcement of the client's behavior.

31. 3. The family needs help learning how to stop reinforcing inappropriate client behavior. Negative reinforcement is an inappropriate strategy for the family to use to support the client. The family can set limits and reinforce consequences when the client shows shortsightedness and poor planning. Clients with antisocial personality disorder don't show ritualistic behaviors.

NP: Implementation; CN: Psychosocial integrity; CNS: Psychosocial adaptation; CL: Analysis

32. Which of the following nursing interventions has priority in the care plan for a client with antisocial personality disorder who shows defensive behaviors?

1. Help the client accept responsibility for his own decisions and behaviors.
2. Work with the client to feel better about himself by taking care of basic needs.
3. Teach the client to identify the defense mechanisms used to cope with distress.
4. Confront the client about the disregard of social rules and the feelings of others.

32. 1. Clients with antisocial personality disorder tend to blame other people for their behaviors and need to be taught how to take responsibility for their actions. Clients with antisocial personality disorder don't tend to have problems with self-care habits or meeting their basic needs. Clients with antisocial personality disorder will deny they're defensive or distressed. Most often, these clients feel justified with retaliatory behavior. To confront the client would only cause him to become even more defensive.

NP: Implementation; CN: Psychosocial integrity; CNS: Psychosocial adaptation; CL: Analysis

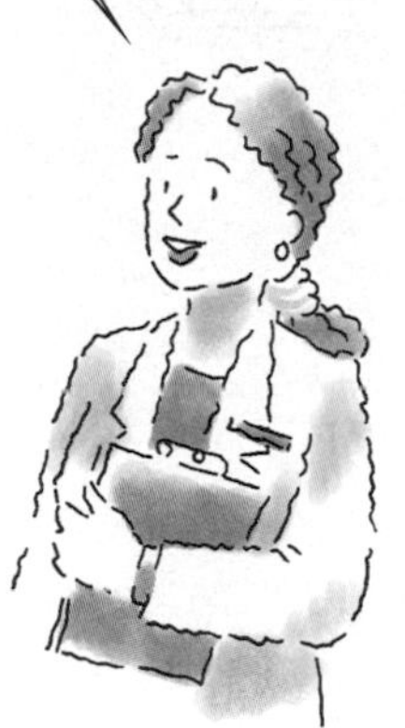

Staff must work together to help the client.

33. A client with antisocial personality disorder is trying to manipulate the health care team. Which of the following strategies is important for the staff to use?

1. Focus on how to teach the client more effective behaviors for meeting basic needs.
2. Help the client verbalize underlying feelings of hopelessness and learn coping skills.
3. Remain calm and don't emotionally respond to the client's manipulative actions.
4. Help the client eliminate the intense desire to have everything in life turn out perfectly.

33. 3. The best strategy to use with a client trying to manipulate staff is to stay calm and refrain from responding emotionally. Negative reinforcement of inappropriate behavior increases the chance it will be repeated. Later, it may be possible to address how to meet the client's basic needs. Clients with antisocial personality disorder don't tend to experience feelings of hopelessness or to desire life events to turn out perfectly. In most cases, these clients negate responsibility for their behavior.

NP: Implementation; CN: Psychosocial integrity; CNS: Psychosocial adaptation; CL: Analysis

34. A client with dependent personality disorder is working to increase self-esteem. Which of the following statements by the client shows teaching was successful?

1. "I'm not going to look just at the negative things about myself."
2. "I'm most concerned about my level of competence and progress."
3. "I'm not as envious of the things other people have as I used to be."
4. "I find I can't stop myself from taking over things others should be doing."

34. 1. As the client makes progress on improving self-esteem, self-blame and negative self-evaluations will decrease. Clients with dependent personality disorder tends to feel fragile and inadequate and would be extremely unlikely to discuss their level of competence and progress. These clients focus on self and aren't envious or jealous. Individuals with dependent personality disorders don't take over situations because they see themselves as inept and inadequate.

NP: Evaluation; CN: Psychosocial integrity; CNS: Psychosocial adaptation; CL: Application

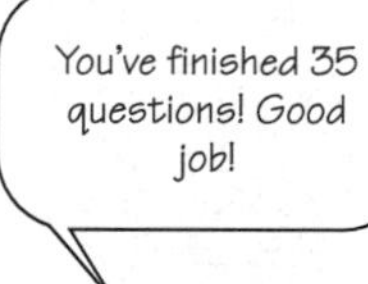

You've finished 35 questions! Good job!

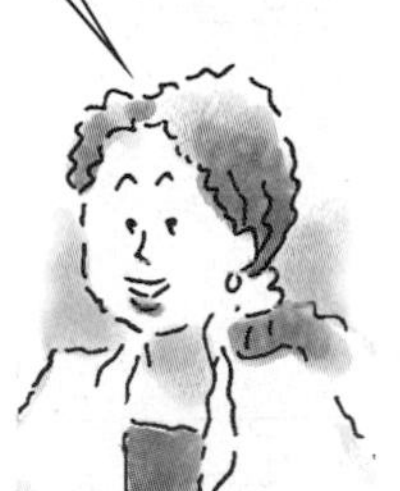

35. Which of the following characteristics or client histories substantiates a diagnosis of antisocial personality disorder?

1. Delusional thinking
2. Feelings of inferiority
3. Disorganized thinking
4. Multiple criminal charges

35. 4. Clients with antisocial personality disorder are often sent for treatment by the court after multiple crimes or for the use of illegal substances. Clients with antisocial personality disorder don't tend to have feelings of inferiority, delusional thinking, or disorganized thinking.

NP: Assessment; CN: Psychosocial integrity; CNS: Coping and adaptation; CL: Comprehension

36. A client with antisocial personality disorder talks about personal life changes that need to occur. Which of the following client statements shows group therapy is having a positive therapeutic effect?

1. "I'm not doing as bad as I thought I was."
2. "I wish I could believe I can change, but it's probably too late."
3. "I see all the problems, but I'm not sure there are good solutions."
4. "I'm finally learning how to live my life without living on the edge."

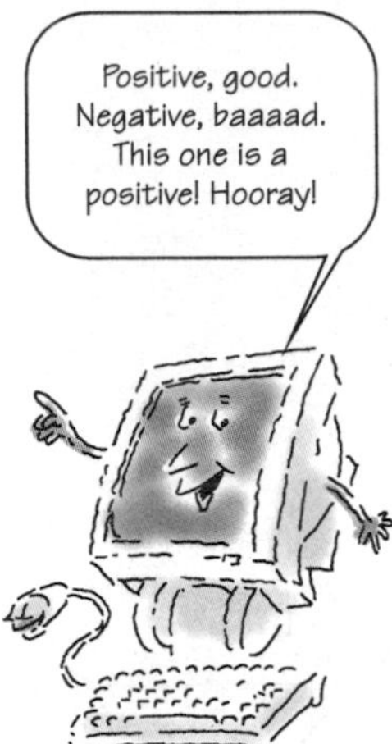

Positive, good. Negative, baaaad. This one is a positive! Hooray!

36. 4. The client is becoming aware of risky behaviors and how problematic these behaviors are. The first option indicates denial, and the client is somewhat defensive about making a change. The second option indicates defeat, and the client seems to feel stuck. The third option indicates problem identification but also uncertainty and ambivalence about the client's ability to change.

NP: Evaluation; CN: Psychosocial integrity; CNS: Psychosocial adaptation; CL: Analysis

37. Which of the following findings is consistent with a diagnosis of antisocial personality disorder?

1. Problematic work history
2. Struggle with severe anxiety
3. Severe physical health conditions
4. Being critical of positive feedback

37. 1. Clients with a diagnosis of antisocial personality disorder tend to have problems in their job roles and a poor work history. They don't have severe anxiety disorders or severe physical health problems and are able to accept positive feedback from others.

NP: Assessment; CN: Psychosocial integrity; CNS: Coping and adaptation; CL: Comprehension

38. A client with antisocial personality disorder is beginning to practice several socially acceptable behaviors in the group setting. Which of the following outcomes will result from this change?

1. Fewer panic attacks
2. Acceptance of reality
3. Improved self-esteem
4. Decreased physical symptoms

38. 3. When clients with antisocial personality disorder begin to practice socially acceptable behaviors, they also frequently experience a more positive sense of self. Clients with antisocial personality disorder don't tend to have panic attacks, somatic manifestations of their illness, or withdrawal or alteration in their perception of reality.

NP: Analysis; CN: Psychosocial integrity; CNS: Coping and adaptation; CL: Comprehension

39. A client with borderline personality disorder is admitted to the unit after slashing his wrist. Which of the following goals is most important after promoting safety?

1. Establish a therapeutic relationship with the client.
2. Identify whether splitting is present in the client's thoughts.
3. Talk about the client's acting out and self-destructive tendencies.
4. Encourage the client to understand why he blames others.

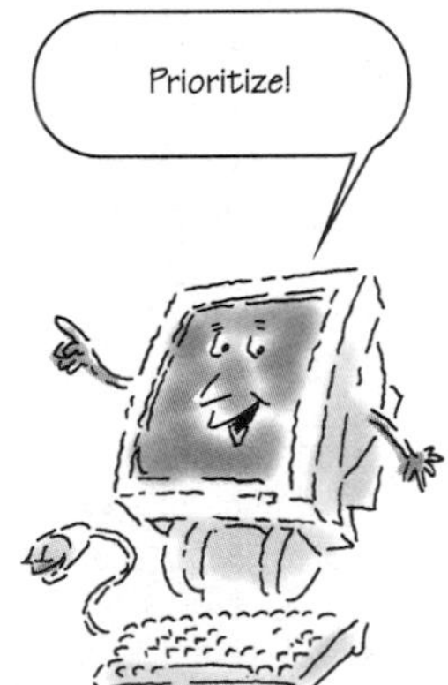

39. 1. After promoting client safety, the nurse establishes a rapport with the client to facilitate appropriate expression of feelings. At this time, the client isn't ready to address unhealthy behavior. A therapeutic relationship must be established before the nurse can effectively work with the client on self-destructive tendencies. A therapeutic relationship also must be established before working on the issue of splitting.

NP: Planning; CN: Psychosocial integrity; CNS: Psychosocial adaptation; CL: Comprehension

40. Which of the following nursing interventions is most appropriate in helping a client with a borderline personality disorder identify appropriate behaviors?

1. Schedule a family meeting.
2. Place the client in seclusion.
3. Formulate a behavioral contract.
4. Perform a mental status assessment.

40. 3. The use of a behavioral contract establishes a framework for healthier functioning and places responsibility for actions back on the client. Seclusion will reinforce the fears of abandonment of clients with borderline personality. Performing a mental status assessment or scheduling a family meeting won't help the client identify appropriate behaviors.

NP: Implementation; CN: Psychosocial integrity; CNS: Psychosocial adaptation; CL: Application

41. Which of the following statements is *typical* of a client with borderline personality disorder who has recurrent suicidal thoughts?

1. "I can't believe how everyone has suddenly stopped believing in me."
2. "I don't care what other people say, I know how badly I looked to them."
3. "I might as well check out since my boyfriend doesn't want me anymore."
4. "I won't stop until I've gotten revenge on all those people who blamed me."

41. 3. This statement is typical for the borderline personality disorder client who is suicidal and reflects the tendency toward all-or-nothing thinking. The first option indicates the client has experienced a credibility problem, the second option indicates the client is extremely embarrassed, and the last option indicates the client has antisocial personality disorder. None of these is a characteristic of borderline personality disorder.

NP: Assessment; CN: Safe, effective care environment; CNS: Safety and infection control; CL: Application

42. Which of the following findings is expected when taking a health history from a client with borderline personality disorder?

1. A negative sense of self
2. A tendency to be compulsive
3. A problem with communication
4. An inclination to be philosophical

42. 1. Clients with a borderline personality disorder have low self-esteem and a negative sense of self. They have little or no problem expressing themselves and communicating with others, and although they have a tendency to be impulsive, they aren't usually compulsive or philosophical.

NP: Assessment; CN: Psychosocial integrity; CNS: Coping and adaptation; CL: Comprehension

43. Which of the following characteristics or situations is indicated when a client with borderline personality disorder has a crisis?

1. Antisocial behavior
2. Suspicious behavior
3. Relationship problems
4. Auditory hallucinations

43. 3. Relationship problems can precipitate a crisis because they bring up issues of abandonment. Clients with borderline personality disorder aren't usually suspicious; they're more likely to be depressed or highly anxious. They don't have symptoms of antisocial behavior or auditory hallucinations.

NP: Analysis; CN: Psychosocial integrity; CNS: Coping and adaptation; CL: Analysis

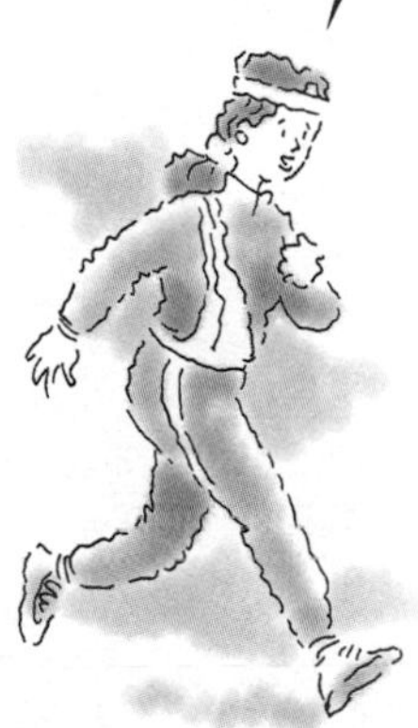

You're moving through these questions quite nicely. Keep plugging along!

44. Which of the following assessment findings is seen in a client diagnosed with borderline personality disorder?

1. Abrasions in various healing stages
2. Intermittent episodes of hypertension
3. Alternating tachycardia and bradycardia
4. Mild state of euphoria with disorientation

44. 1. Clients with borderline personality disorder tend to self-mutilate and have abrasions in various stages of healing. The other options don't tend to occur with this disorder.

NP: Assessment; CN: Psychosocial integrity; CNS: Coping and adaptation; CL: Application

45. Which of the following short-term goals is appropriate for a client with borderline personality disorder with low self-esteem?

1. Write in a journal daily.
2. Express fears and feelings.
3. Stop obsessive-compulsive behaviors.
4. Decrease dysfunctional family conflicts.

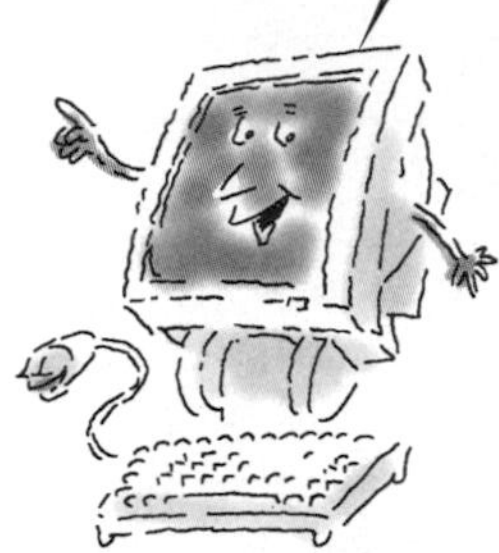

The key word clarifies the answer. Don't miss it!

45. 2. Acknowledging fears and feelings can help the client identify parts of himself that are uncomfortable, and he can begin to work on developing a positive sense of self. Writing in a daily journal isn't a short-term goal to enhance self-esteem. A client with borderline personality disorder doesn't struggle with obsessive-compulsive behaviors. Decreasing dysfunctional family conflicts is a long-term goal.

NP: Analysis; CN: Psychosocial integrity; CNS: Coping and adaptation; CL: Analysis

46. Which of the following interventions is important to include in a teaching plan for a family with a member diagnosed with borderline personality disorder?

1. Teach the family methods for handling the client's anxiety.
2. Explore how the family reinforces the sick role with the client.
3. Encourage the family to have the client express intense emotions.
4. Help the family put pressure on the client to improve current behavior.

46. 1. The family needs to learn how to handle the client's intense stress and low tolerance for frustration. Family members don't want to reinforce the sick role; they're more concerned with preventing anxiety from escalating. Clients with borderline personality disorder already maintain intense emotions, and it isn't safe to encourage further expression of them. The family doesn't need to put pressure on the client to change behavior; this approach will only cause inappropriate behavior to escalate.

NP: Planning; CN: Health promotion and maintenance; CNS: Prevention and early detection of disease; CL: Application

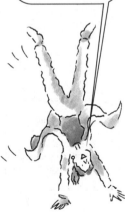

47. In planning care for a client with borderline personality disorder, a nurse must be aware that this client is prone to develop which of the following conditions?

1. Binge eating
2. Memory loss
3. Cult membership
4. Delusional thinking

47. 1. Clients with borderline personality disorder are likely to develop dysfunctional coping and act out in self-destructive ways such as binge eating. They aren't prone to develop memory loss or delusional thinking. Becoming involved in cults may be seen in some clients with antisocial personality disorder.

NP: Planning; CN: Psychosocial integrity; CNS: Coping and adaptation; CL: Analysis

48. Which of the following statements is expected from a client with borderline personality disorder with a history of dysfunctional relationships?

1. "I won't get involved in another relationship."
2. "I'm determined to look for the perfect partner."
3. "I've decided to learn better communication skills."
4. "I'm going to be an equal partner in a relationship."

48. 2. Clients with borderline personality disorder would decide to look for a perfect partner. This characteristic is a result of the dichotomous manner in which these clients view the world. They go from relationship to relationship without taking responsibility for their behavior. It's unlikely that an unsuccessful relationship will cause clients to make a change. They tend to be demanding and impulsive in relationships. There's no thought given to what one wants or needs from a relationship. Because they tend to blame others for problems, it's unlikely they would express a desire to learn communication skills.

NP: Analysis; CN: Psychosocial integrity; CNS: Psychosocial adaptation; CL: Analysis

49. Which of the following nursing interventions is the most appropriate for a client with borderline personality disorder working on developing healthy relationships?

1. Have the client assess current behaviors.
2. Work with the client to develop outgoing behavior.
3. Limit the client's interactions to family members only.
4. Encourage the client to approach others for interactions.

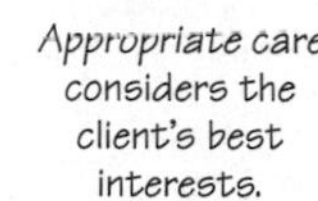

Appropriate care considers the client's best interests.

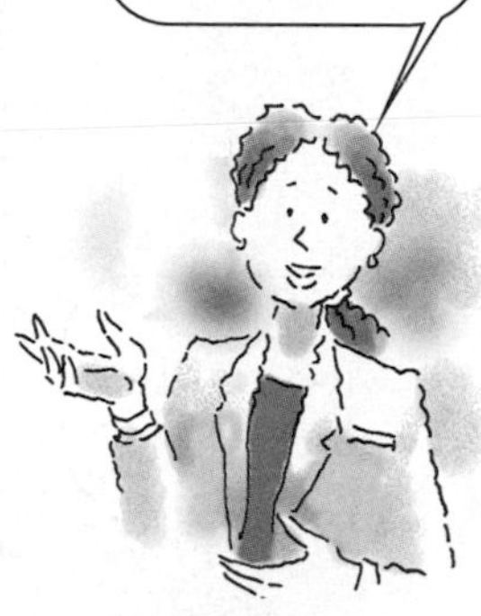

49. 1. Self-assessment of behavior enables the client to look at himself and identify social behaviors that need to be changed. Clients with borderline personality disorder don't tend to have difficulty approaching and interacting with other people. It's unrealistic to have clients with borderline personality disorder limit their interactions to family members only. Clients with borderline personality disorder tend to be demanding and the center of attention. It isn't useful to work on developing outgoing behavior.

NP: Implementation; CN: Psychosocial integrity; CNS: Psychosocial adaptation; CL: Analysis

50. Which of the following defense mechanisms is most likely to be seen in a client with borderline personality disorder?

1. Compensation
2. Displacement
3. Identification
4. Projection

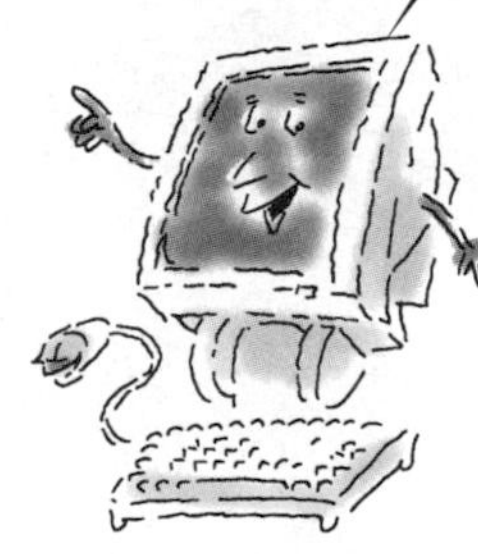

You're waaay into these questions! Keep it up!

50. 4. Clients with borderline personality disorder tend to blame and project their feelings and inadequacies onto others. They don't model themselves after other people or tend to use compensation to handle distress. Clients with borderline personality disorder are impulsive and tend to react immediately. It's unlikely they would displace their feelings onto others.

NP: Assessment; CN: Psychosocial integrity; CNS: Coping and adaptation; CL: Analysis

51. Which of the following conditions is likely to coexist in clients with a diagnosis of borderline personality disorder?

1. Avoidance
2. Delirium
3. Depression
4. Disorientation

51. 3. Chronic feelings of emptiness and sadness predispose a client to depression. About 40% of the clients with borderline personality disorder struggle with depression. Clients with borderline personality disorder don't tend to develop delirium or become disoriented. This is only a possibility if the client becomes intoxicated. Clients with borderline personality disorder tend to disregard boundaries and limits. Avoidance isn't an issue with these clients.

NP: Analysis; CN: Psychosocial integrity; CNS: Coping and adaptation; CL: Comprehension

52. Which of the following nursing interventions has priority for a client with borderline personality disorder?

1. Maintain consistent and realistic limits.
2. Give instructions for meeting basic self-care needs.
3. Engage in daytime activities to stimulate wakefulness.
4. Have the client attend group therapy on a daily basis.

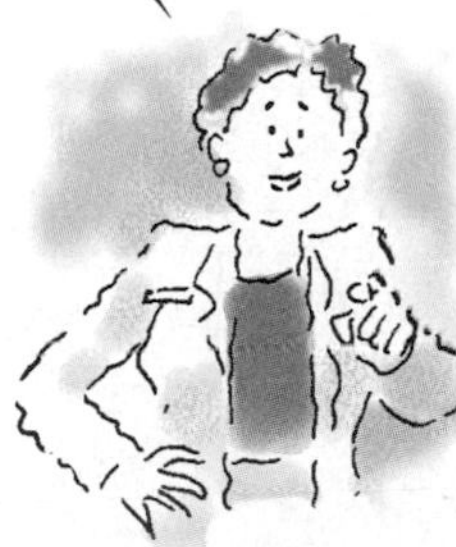

Prioritizing is a crucial part of nursing!

52. 1. Clients with borderline personality disorder who are needy, dependent, and manipulative will benefit greatly from maintaining consistent and realistic limits. They don't tend to have difficulty meeting their self-care needs. They enjoy attending group therapy because they often attempt to use the opportunity to become the center of attention. They don't tend to have sleeping difficulties.

NP: Implementation; CN: Psychosocial integrity; CNS: Psychosocial adaptation; CL: Comprehension

53. Which of the following outcomes indicates individual therapy has been effective for a client with borderline personality disorder?

1. The client accepts that medication isn't a treatment of choice.
2. The client agrees to undergo hypnosis for suppression of memories.
3. The client understands the organic basis for the problematic behavior.
4. The client verbalizes awareness of the consequences for unacceptable behaviors.

53. 4. An indication of effective individual therapy for this client is his expressed awareness of consequences for unacceptable behaviors. Medications can control symptoms. However, monitoring for reckless use or abuse of drugs must be done for the client with borderline personality disorder. Hypnosis isn't a treatment used with a client with borderline personality disorder. There's no organic basis for the development of this disorder.

NP: Evaluation; CN: Psychosocial integrity; CNS: Psychosocial adaptation; CL: Application

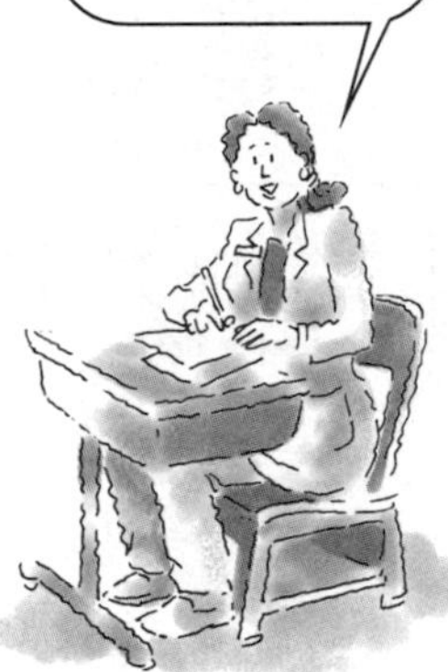

54. Which of the following actions by a client with borderline personality disorder indicates adequate learning about personal behavior?

1. The client talks about intense anger.
2. The client smiles while making demands.
3. The client decides never to engage in conflict.
4. The client stops the family from controlling finances.

54. 1. Learning has occurred when anger is discussed rather than acted out in unhealthy ways. The behavior to change would be the demands placed on others. Smiling while making these demands shows manipulative behavior. Not engaging in conflict is unrealistic. It's important to help this client slowly develop financial responsibility rather than just stopping the family from monitoring the client's overspending.

NP: Evaluation; CN: Psychosocial integrity; CNS: Psychosocial adaptation; CL: Application

55. A nurse is planning care for a client with borderline personality disorder who has been agitated. Which of the following instructions is included for the client and family?

1. Encourage the rebuilding of family relationships.
2. Help the client handle anxiety before it escalates.
3. Have the client participate in a weekly support group.
4. Discuss the client's bad habits that need to be changed.

55. 2. The client needs help handling anxiety because escalating anxiety can trigger self-destructive behaviors in clients with borderline personality disorder. When a client with borderline personality disorder is agitated, it's difficult to communicate, let alone rebuild family relationships. Participation in a weekly support group won't be enough to help the client handle agitation. When a client is agitated, it isn't appropriate to discuss bad habits that need to be changed. This action may further agitate the client.

NP: Planning; CN: Psychosocial integrity; CNS: Psychosocial adaptation; CL: Application

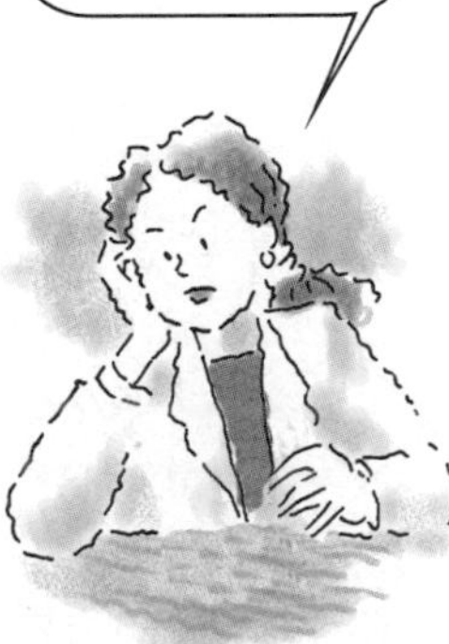

When treatment isn't working, reevaluation may be necessary.

56. A client with a borderline personality disorder isn't making progress on the identified goals. Which of the following client factors should be reevaluated?

1. Memory
2. Motivation
3. Orientation
4. Perception

56. 2. Clients with borderline personality disorders tend to be poorly motivated for treatment. They don't tend to have perception problems such as hallucinations or illusions, problems in orientation, or memory problems.

NP: Evaluation; CN: Psychosocial integrity; CNS: Psychosocial adaptation; CL: Analysis

57. A nurse is assessing a client diagnosed with dependent personality disorder. Which of the following characteristics is a major component of this disorder?

1. Abrasive to others
2. Indifferent to others
3. Manipulative of others
4. Overreliance on others

58. A client with dependent personality disorder is working on goals for self-care. Which of the following short-term goals is most important to the client's everyday activities of daily living?

1. Do all self-care activities independently.
2. Write a daily schedule for each day of the week.
3. Do self-care activities in a minimal amount of time.
4. Determine activities that can be performed without help.

59. Which of the following information must be included for the family of a client diagnosed with dependent personality disorder?

1. Address coping skills.
2. Explore panic attacks.
3. Promote exercise programs.
4. Decrease aggressive outbursts.

60. Which of the following strategies is appropriate for a client with dependent personality disorder?

1. Orient the client to current surroundings.
2. Reassure the client about personal safety.
3. Ask questions to help the client recall problems.
4. Differentiate between positive and negative feedback.

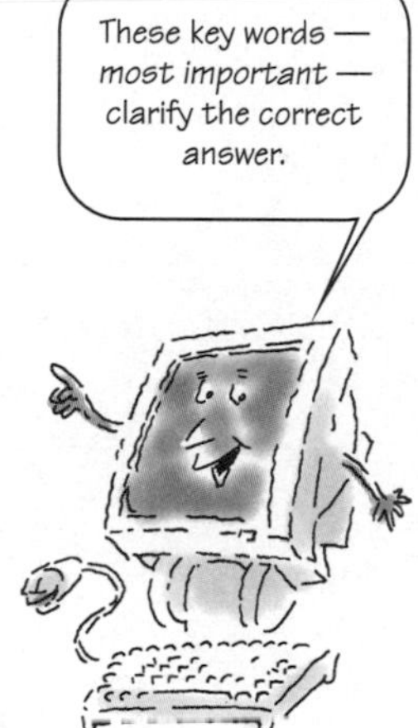

These key words — most important — clarify the correct answer.

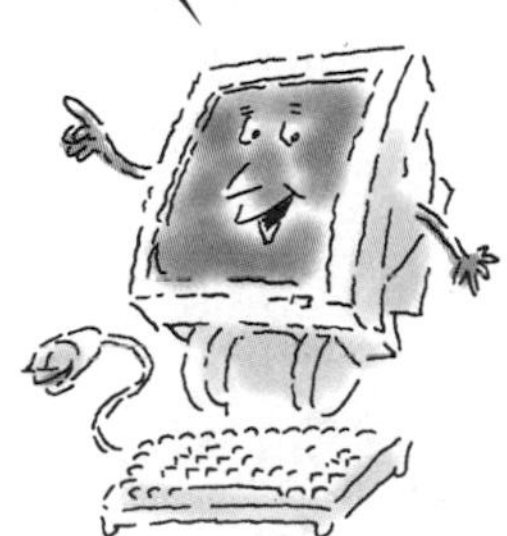

Think carefully. You know the answer to this one.

57. 4. Clients with dependent personality disorder are extremely overreliant on other people; they aren't abrasive or assertive. They're clinging and demanding of others; they don't manipulate. People with dependent personality disorder rely on others and want to be taken care of. They aren't indifferent.

NP: Assessment; CN: Psychosocial integrity; CNS: Coping and adaptation; CL: Knowledge

58. 4. By determining activities that can be performed without assistance, the client can then begin to practice them independently. Writing a daily schedule doesn't help the client focus on what needs to be done to promote self-care. If the nurse only encourages a client to perform self-care activities independently, nothing may change. The amount of time needed to perform self-care activities isn't important. If time pressure is put on the client, there may be more reluctance to perform self-care activities.

NP: Analysis; CN: Psychosocial integrity; CNS: Psychosocial adaptation; CL: Comprehension

59. 1. The family needs information about coping skills to help the client learn to handle stress. Clients with dependent personality disorder don't have aggressive outbursts; they tend to be passive and submit to others. They don't tend to have panic attacks. Exercise is a health promotion activity for all clients. Clients with dependent personality disorder wouldn't need exercise promoted more than other people.

NP: Implementation; CN: Safe, effective care environment; CNS: Management of care; CL: Comprehension

60. 4. Clients with dependent personality disorder tend to view all feedback as criticism; they frequently misinterpret another's remarks. Clients with dependent personality disorder don't need orientation to their surroundings. Memory problems aren't associated with this disorder, so asking questions to stimulate the client's memory isn't necessary. Personal safety isn't an issue because a person with dependent personality disorder typically isn't self-destructive.

NP: Analysis; CN: Psychosocial integrity; CNS: Psychosocial adaptation; CL: Application

61. A client with dependent personality disorder is crying after a family meeting. Which of the following statements by a family member is most likely the cause of upset to this client?
1. "You take advantage of people, especially the people in our family."
2. "You act like you love me one minute but hate me the next minute."
3. "You feel like you deserve everything, whether you work for it or not."
4. "You always agree to everything, but deep down inside you feel differently."

61. 4. The client was confronted by a family member about behavior that doesn't represent the client's true feelings. Clients are afraid they won't be taken care of if they disagree. Clients with a dependent personality disorder don't have a sense of entitlement and don't take advantage of other people, but they subordinate their needs to others. They don't show the defense mechanism of splitting, where a person is valued and then devalued.

NP: Analysis; CN: Psychosocial integrity; CNS: Psychosocial adaptation; CL: Analysis

62. A client with dependent personality disorder is having trouble performing activities of daily living. Which of the following nursing interventions would help facilitate the client's daily activities?
1. Have the client eat three meals a day.
2. Work with the client to establish a budget.
3. Make a chart to document hygiene practices.
4. Discuss how the client can obtain a driver's license.

62. 2. Clients with dependent personality disorder tend to withdraw from adult responsibilities. Managing money through the use of a budget is a first step toward assuming adult responsibilities. Hygiene issues usually aren't a problem for clients with dependent personality disorder. These clients don't tend to have problems with nutritional intake. Clients with a dependent personality disorder don't have any special reasons for not obtaining a driver's license.

NP: Implementation; CN: Psychosocial integrity; CNS: Psychosocial adaptation; CL: Comprehension

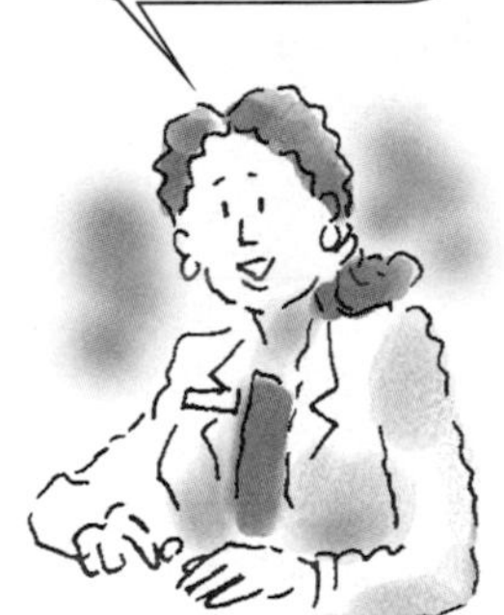

The clients need you to teach them.

63. A client with a dependent personality disorder is taking fluoxetine (Prozac) for depression. Which of the following instructions is included in client teaching?
1. Drink only wine and beer when taking this drug.
2. Add as-needed doses if depression becomes worse.
3. Expect 3 to 4 weeks to go by before effects are seen.
4. Be aware that alterations in usual sleep patterns, especially nightmares, may occur.

63. 3. The client must take the drug for 3 to 4 weeks before therapeutic effects are seen. The nurse must caution the client against the use of alcohol, including wine and beer, when taking fluoxetine. The client is to take the drug as prescribed. Additional doses must not be self-administered. Fluoxetine treats disruptions in sleep and doesn't cause nightmares.

NP: Implementation; CN: Physiological integrity; CNS: Pharmacological and parenteral therapies; CL: Knowledge

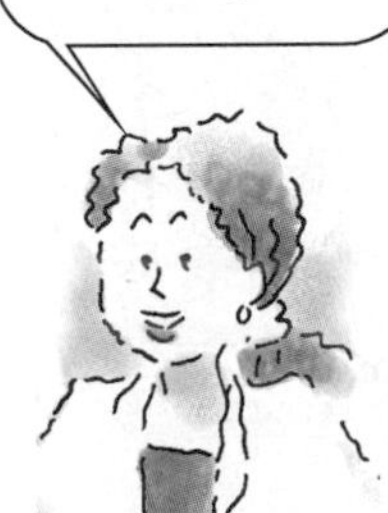

Evaluating the plan is as important as forming it.

64. Which of the following behaviors by a client with dependent personality disorder shows the client has made progress toward the goal of increasing problem-solving skills?
1. The client is courteous.
2. The client asks questions.
3. The client stops acting out.
4. The client controls emotions.

64. 2. The client with dependent personality disorder is passive and tries to please others. By asking questions, the client is beginning to gather information, the first step of decision making. These clients don't tend to have emotional outbursts or to be impolite. They avoid expressing their feelings or acting out for fear of displeasing others.

NP: Evaluation; CN: Psychosocial integrity; CNS: Psychosocial adaptation; CL: Analysis

65. Which of the following information is expected in a history of a client with dependent personality disorder?

1. Lack of relationships
2. Lack of self-confidence
3. Preoccupation with rules
4. Tendency to overvalue self

65. 2. Clients with dependent personality disorder lack self-confidence and have low self-esteem. They tend to undervalue, not overvalue, self. They have unhealthy relationships, allowing others to take over their lives. They aren't preoccupied with rules. They focus on their need to be taken care of by others.
NP: Assessment; CN: Psychosocial integrity; CNS: Coping and adaptation; CL: Knowledge

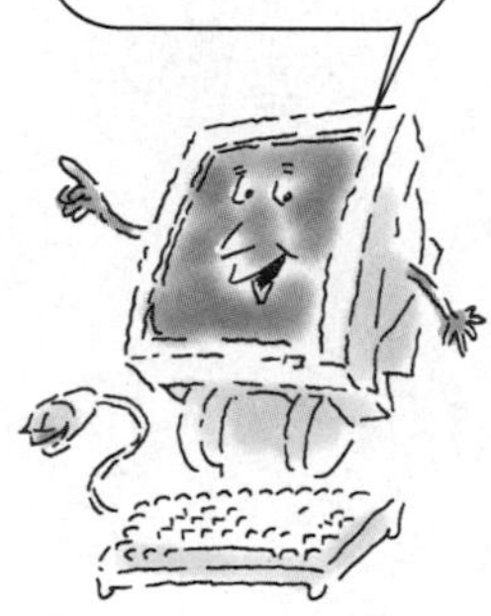

Question 66 asks for short-term goals, not long-term ones. Keep that in mind.

66. Which of the following short-term goals is appropriate for a client with dependent personality disorder experiencing excessive dependency needs?

1. Verbalize self-confidence in own abilities.
2. Decide relationships don't take energy to sustain.
3. Discuss feelings related to frequent mood swings.
4. Stop obsessive thinking that impedes daily social functioning.

66. 1. Individuals with dependent personalities believe they must depend on others to be competent for them. They need to gain more self-confidence in their own abilities. The client must realize that relationships take energy to develop and sustain. Clients with dependent personality disorder usually don't have obsessive thinking or mood swings to interfere with their socialization.
NP: Analysis; CN: Psychosocial integrity; CNS: Psychosocial adaptation; CL: Application

67. A client with dependent personality disorder is thinking about getting a part-time job. Which of the following nursing interventions will help this client when employment is obtained?

1. Help the client develop strategies to control impulses.
2. Explain that there are consequences for inappropriate behaviors.
3. Have the client work to sustain healthy interpersonal relationships.
4. Help the client decrease the use of regression as a defense mechanism.

67. 3. Sustaining healthy relationships will help the client be comfortable with peers in the job setting. Clients with dependent personality disorder don't usually use regression as a defense mechanism. It's common to see denial and introjection used. They don't usually have trouble with impulse control or offensive behavior that would lead to negative consequences.
NP: Implementation; CN: Psychosocial integrity; CNS: Psychosocial adaptation; CL: Analysis

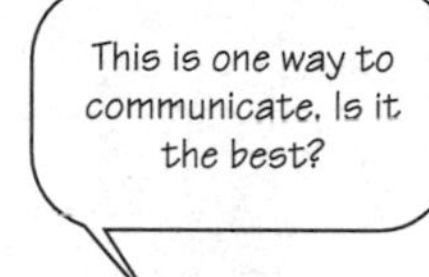

This is one way to communicate. Is it the best?

68. A client with dependent personality disorder has difficulty expressing personal concerns. Which of the following communication techniques is best to teach the client?

1. Questioning
2. Reflection
3. Silence
4. Touch

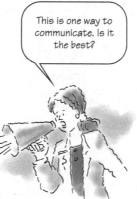

68. 1. Questioning is a way to learn to identify feelings and express self. The use of reflection isn't a communication technique that will help the client express personal feelings and concerns. The use of touch to express feelings and personal concerns must be used very judiciously. Using silence won't help the client identify and discuss personal concerns.
NP: Implementation; CN: Psychosocial integrity; CNS: Psychosocial adaptation; CL: Application

69. A nurse is evaluating the effectiveness of an assertiveness group that a client with dependent personality disorder attended. Which of the following client statements indicates the group had therapeutic value?

1. "I can't seem to do the things other people do."
2. "I wish I could be more organized like other people."
3. "I want to talk about something that's bothering me."
4. "I just don't want people in my family to fight any more."

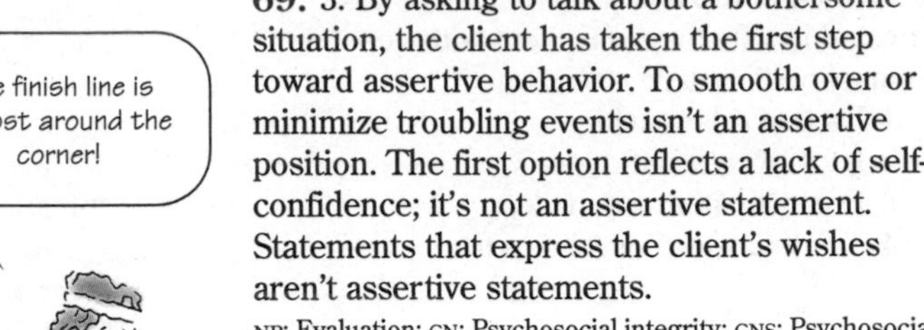

The finish line is almost around the corner!

69. 3. By asking to talk about a bothersome situation, the client has taken the first step toward assertive behavior. To smooth over or minimize troubling events isn't an assertive position. The first option reflects a lack of self-confidence; it's not an assertive statement. Statements that express the client's wishes aren't assertive statements.

NP: Evaluation; CN: Psychosocial integrity; CNS: Psychosocial adaptation; CL: Application

70. After a family visit, a client with dependent personality disorder becomes anxious. Which of the following situations is a possible cause of the anxiety?

1. Sensitivity to criticism
2. Discussion of family rules
3. Being asked personal questions
4. Identification of eccentric behavior

70. 1. Clients with dependent personality disorder are extremely sensitive to criticism and can become very anxious when they feel interpersonal conflict or tension. When they're asked personal questions, they don't necessarily become anxious. When they have discussions about family rules, they try to become submissive and please others rather than become anxious. Clients with dependent personality disorder don't tend to show eccentric behavior that causes them anxiety.

NP: Analysis; CN: Psychosocial integrity; CNS: Coping and adaptation; CL: Application

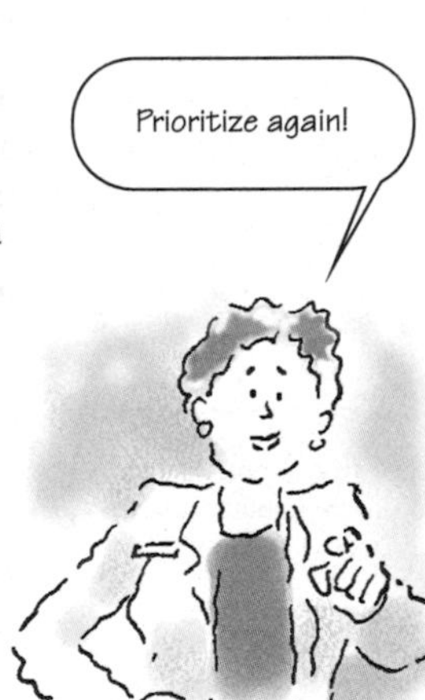

Prioritize again!

71. A client with dependent personality disorder has a history of minor GI problems. Which of the following goals has *priority*?

1. Get a referral to a specialist.
2. Consult with a dietitian regularly.
3. Arrange for a family support meeting.
4. Examine the client's present level of coping skills.

71. 4. Many clients with GI discomfort tend to be anxious and need help developing coping skills. Before a referral is obtained, other factors that could cause GI upset must be addressed. A client with dependent personality disorder usually is overdependent on family members and doesn't tend to need a nurse to advocate for client support. Consulting with a dietitian wouldn't be a priority goal. A consultation would be initiated only after other variables were assessed and a need was identified.

NP: Analysis; CN: Physiological integrity; CNS: Physiological adaptation; CL: Application

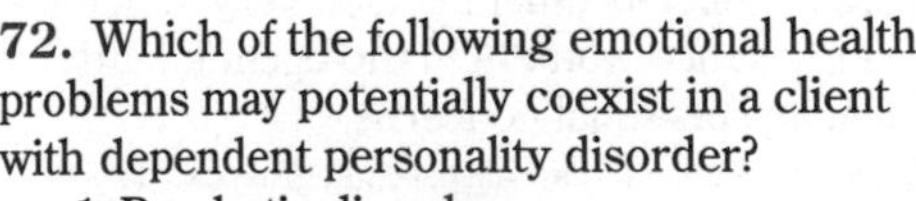

72. Which of the following emotional health problems may potentially coexist in a client with dependent personality disorder?

1. Psychotic disorder
2. Anxiety disorder
3. Alcohol-related disorder
4. Posttraumatic stress disorder

72. 2. Because they've placed their own needs in the hands of others, clients with dependent personalities are extremely vulnerable to anxiety disorder. They don't tend to have coexisting problems of posttraumatic stress disorder, psychotic disorder, or alcohol-related disorder.

NP: Analysis; CN: Psychosocial integrity; CNS: Coping and adaptation; CL: Analysis

73. A nurse notices that a client with dependent personality disorder is depressed. Which of the following factors is assessed as contributing to depression?

1. Unmet needs
2. Sense of smothering
3. Messy, unkempt appearance
4. Difficulty delaying gratification

73. 1. Having many unmet needs is a precursor to depression. Clients with dependent personality disorder don't experience a sense of smothering, a problem seen in clients with panic disorder. Clients with problems delaying gratification tend to have anxiety problems, not problems with depression. Poor hygiene is often a *manifestation, not* a cause, of depression.

NP: Analysis; CN: Psychosocial integrity; CNS: Coping and adaptation; CL: Analysis

Keep in mind the type of personality this client has.

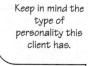

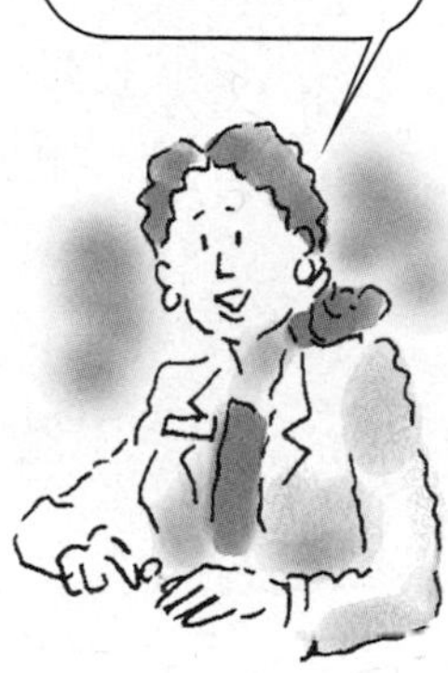

74. A client with dependent personality disorder makes the following statement, "I'll never be able to take care of myself." Which of the following responses is best?

1. "How can you say that? You can function."
2. "Let's talk about what's making you feel so fearful."
3. "I think we need to work on identifying your strengths."
4. "Can we talk about this tomorrow at the family meeting?"

74. 2. The client with dependent personality disorder is afraid of abandonment and being unable to care for himself. Talking about his fears is a useful strategy. The first option is inappropriate because the nurse doesn't recognize the client's feelings. When the client makes a desperate statement, the nurse must respond to the client's feelings, rather than insert her opinion. Working on identifying a client's strengths will add to his feelings of not being strong enough to care for himself. Waiting to talk about his concern until the family meeting minimizes its importance.

NP: Implementation; CN: Psychosocial integrity; CNS: Coping and adaptation; CL: Analysis

75. A client on your unit says the Mafia has a contract out on him. He refuses to leave his semiprivate room and insists on frisking his roommate before allowing him to enter. Which of the following actions should you take first?

1. Transfer the client to a private room.
2. Acknowledge the client's fear when he refuses to leave his room or wants to frisk his roommate.
3. Transfer the roommate to another room.
4. Lock the client out of his room for a while each day so he can see he's safe.

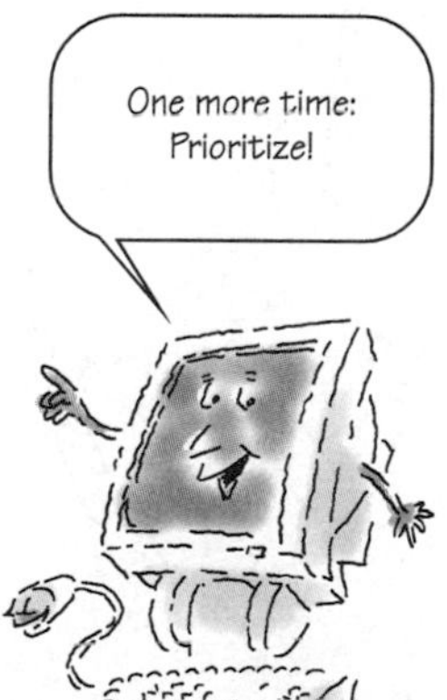

One more time: Prioritize!

75. 2. Acknowledging underlying feelings may help defuse the client's anxiety without promoting his delusional thinking. This, in turn, may help the client distinguish between his emotional state and external reality. Transferring either client to another room would validate the client's delusional thinking. Locking the client out of his room may further escalate the client's anxiety and stimulate aggressive acting-out behavior.

NP: Implementation; CN: Psychosocial integrity; CNS: Coping and adaptation; CL: Application

76. A client with schizotypal personality disorder is sitting in a puddle of urine. She's playing in it, smiling, and softly singing a child's song. Which action would be best?

1. Admonish the client for not using the bathroom.
2. Firmly tell the client that her behavior is unacceptable.
3. Ask the client whether she's ready to get cleaned up now.
4. Help the client to the shower, and change the bedclothes.

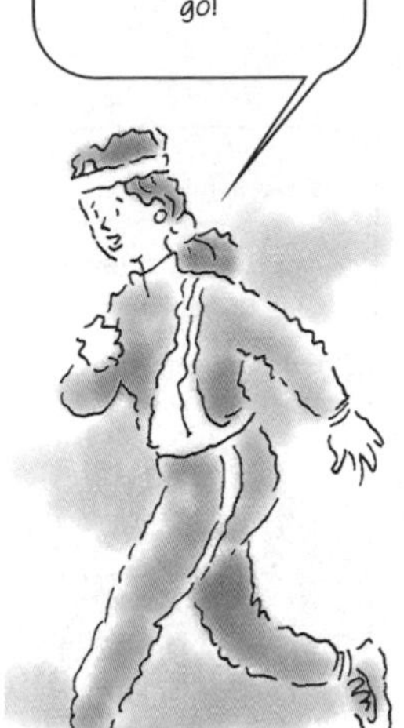

You've passed the 75 mark. Not too much more to go!

76. 4. A client with a schizotypal personality disorder can experience high levels of anxiety and regress to childlike behaviors. This client may require help meeting self-care needs. The client may not respond to the other options or those options may generate more anxiety.

NP: Implementation; CN: Psychosocial integrity; CNS: Coping and adaptation; CL: Application

77. A client with avoidant personality disorder says occupational therapy (OT) is boring and he doesn't want to go. Which action would be best?

1. State firmly that you'll escort him to OT.
2. Arrange with OT for the client to do a project on the unit.
3. Ask the client to talk about why OT is boring.
4. Arrange for the client not to attend OT until he feels better.

77. 1. If given the chance, a client with avoidant personality disorder typically elects to remain immobilized. The nurse should insist that the client participate in OT. Arranging for the client to do a project on the unit validates and reinforces the client's desire to avoid going to OT. Addressing an invalid issue such as the client's perceived boredom avoids the real issue: the client's need for therapy. There's no indication that the client is incapable of participating in OT.

NP: Implementation; CN: Psychosocial integrity; CNS: Coping and adaptation; CL: Application

78. A client with paranoid personality disorder works toward the goal of increasing social interaction. Which behavior indicates that the client is meeting this goal?

1. The client develops and follows a schedule of group activities.
2. The client verbalizes aggressive feelings to the nurse.
3. The client visits the consumer center to use the Internet.
4. The client explores somatic complaints with the staff.

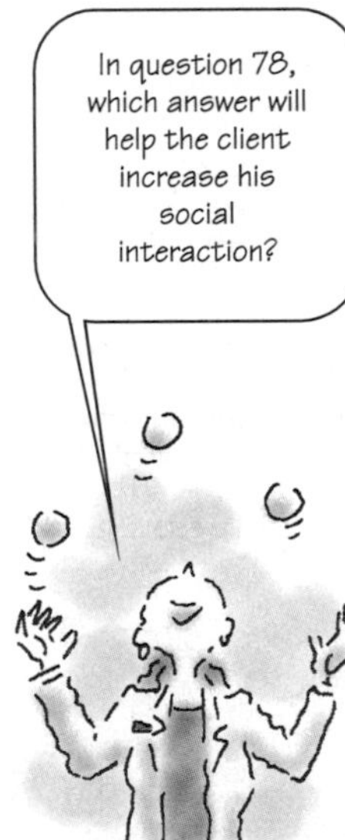

In question 78, which answer will help the client increase his social interaction?

78. 1. By developing and following a schedule of group activities, the client increases opportunities to use social skills and increase interactions with others. Verbalizing aggressive feelings doesn't give the client opportunities to increase social interaction. Using a computer at the consumer center is a solitary activity. Talking to the staff about somatic complaints doesn't provide opportunities for social interaction.

NP: Evaluation; CN: Psychosocial integrity; CNS: Psychosocial adaptation; CL: Application

79. The nurse works with the family of a client diagnosed with schizoid personality disorder, helping them to assist him in making decisions. Which outcome indicates the nurse's interventions have been successful?

1. The family prevents the client from experiencing disappointments.
2. The family encourages the client to talk about specific issues and concerns.
3. The family removes alcohol and unnecessary prescription drugs from the house.
4. The family doesn't let the client obtain secondary gains from illness.

79. 2. A client with schizoid personality disorder typically is vague and has difficulty with self-expression; encouraging the client to talk about specific issues and concerns shows that the nurse's interventions were successful. It's neither realistic nor helpful for the family to protect the client from disappointments. Clients with schizoid personality disorder aren't at high risk for substance abuse and don't seek secondary gains from illness.

NP: Evaluation; CN: Psychosocial integrity; CNS: Psychosocial adaptation; CL: Application

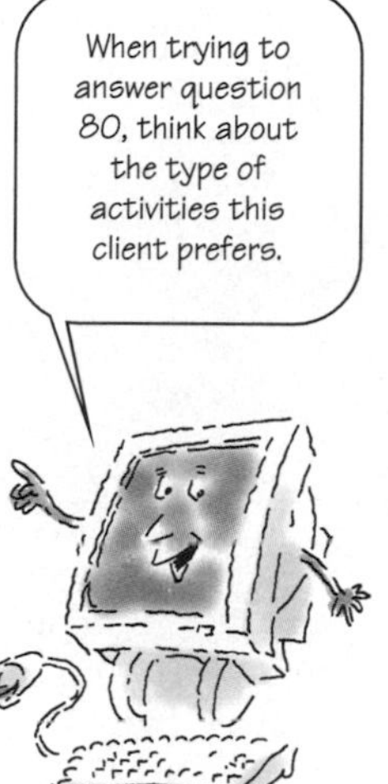

When trying to answer question 80, think about the type of activities this client prefers.

80. A nurse discusses job possibilities with a client with schizoid personality disorder. Which suggestion by the nurse would be helpful?

1. "You could work in a family restaurant part-time on the weekends and holidays."
2. "Maybe your friend could get you that customer service job where you work only in the evenings."
3. "Your idea of applying for the position of filing and organizing records is worth pursuing."
4. "Being an introvert limits the employment opportunities you can pursue."

80. 3. Clients with schizoid personality disorder prefer solitary activities, such as filing, to working with others. Working as a cashier or customer service representative would involve interacting with many people. Not all jobs require extensive interpersonal contact.

NP: Implementation; CN: Psychosocial integrity; CNS: Coping and adaptation; CL: Analysis

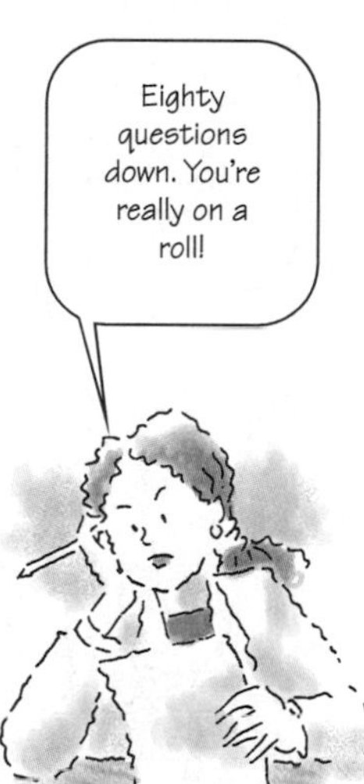

Eighty questions down. You're really on a roll!

81. A client with borderline personality disorder is learning how to verbalize, rather than act on, the desire to hurt herself. Which intervention should the nurse use to help her recognize angry feelings?

1. Explain how pain triggers intense anger and causes the client to act out.
2. Determine how problems with the client's family cause her to act aggressively.
3. Teach the client that being volatile is a normal reaction to unfair events.
4. Have the client work on identifying speech and behavior that accompany anger.

81. 4. Aggressive speech and inappropriate behaviors indicate that the client is angry or upset; these feelings may trigger acting out. Pain rarely triggers intense anger or makes a client act out. Blaming one's family of origin for inappropriate handling of anger isn't helpful. Being volatile isn't a normal reaction to unfair life events. The client needs to express anger in safe and appropriate ways.

NP: Implementation; CN: Psychosocial integrity; CNS: Coping and adaptation; CL: Analysis

82. A client with borderline personality disorder states that she doesn't know how to deal with her impulsive behavior. Which intervention should the nurse implement?

1. Teach the client that impulsive behavior is part of her illness.
2. Explore how depression influences impulsive situations.
3. Select an example of an impulsive situation and explore it.
4. Decrease interactions in which impulsive behavior occurs.

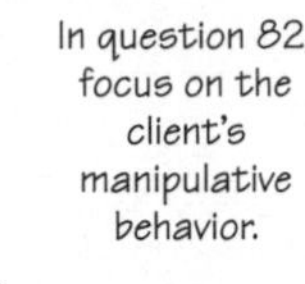

In question 82, focus on the client's manipulative behavior.

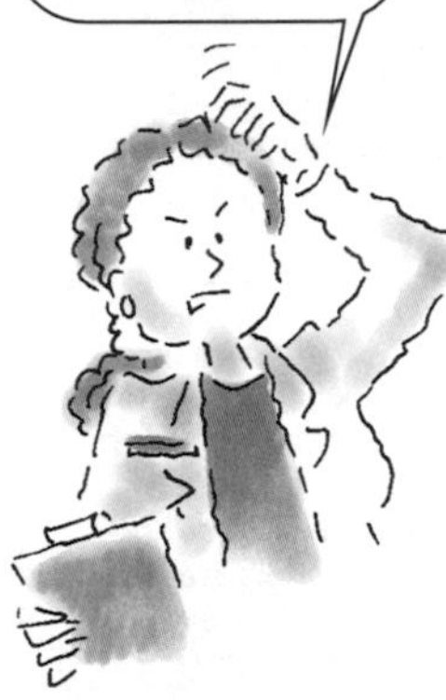

82. 3. By selecting an impulsive situation to explore with the client, the nurse can help her begin to understand the causes and consequences of her behavior and learn how to modify it. Although impulsive behavior is part of borderline personality disorder, the nurse's intervention needs to address ways to handle it. Anxiety, not depression, is strongly related to impulsive behavior. Decreasing social interactions is unrealistic; it's more useful to address the impulsive behavior.

NP: Planning; CN: Psychosocial integrity; CNS: Coping and adaptation; CL: Analysis

83. A client with borderline personality disorder causes conflict between the facility staff and her family. The nurse suspects the client is experiencing which behavior?

1. Disorientation
2. Splitting
3. Grandiosity
4. Hypervigilance

83. 2. Splitting occurs when the client creates situations that alternate between devaluing and idolizing people. This manipulative behavior creates conflict. The client isn't disoriented, being grandiose, or demonstrating hypervigilance in this situation.

NP: Assessment; CN: Psychosocial integrity; CNS: Coping and adaptation; CL: Comprehension

84. A client with borderline personality disorder is in the facility for self-destructive behavior and will attend milieu therapy. Which is the nurse's role in milieu therapy?

1. To provide a structured environment and serve as a model for appropriate behavior
2. To establish a place where the client can verbalize feelings to the nurse
3. To review client skills for the purpose of helping the client obtain employment
4. To encourage the client to do family work to understand the family's rigidity

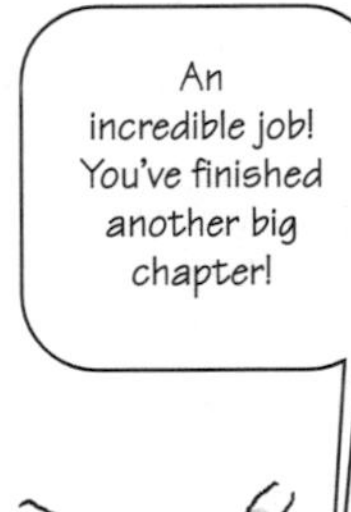

An incredible job! You've finished another big chapter!

84. 1. In milieu therapy, the nurse provides a structured environment and serves as a role model for the mature, responsible behavior expected of the client; this helps the client work on interpersonal problems and decision making. Clients with borderline personality disorder feel inadequate; they experience severe stress and manipulate others to get their needs met. Milieu therapy is a group modality, not a one-to-one modality. The nurse doesn't do family work during milieu therapy.

NP: Implementation; CN: Psychosocial integrity; CNS: Psychosocial adaptation; CL: Comprehension

85. A client in an outpatient clinic is inconsiderate and attention-seeking. Which personality disorder should the nurse suspect?

1. Schizoid
2. Antisocial
3. Histrionic
4. Dependent

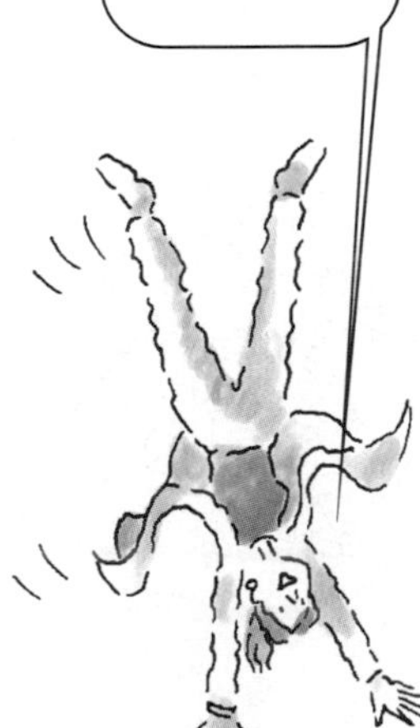

85. 3. A client with histrionic personality disorder is dramatic, inconsiderate, and attention-seeking. A client with schizoid personality disorder is aloof and self-centered. A client with antisocial personality disorder is asocial and aggressive and engages in criminal behavior. A client with dependent personality disorder is submissive and fearful and relies on others.

NP: Assessment; CN: Psychosocial integrity; CNS: Psychosocial adaptation; CL: Knowledge

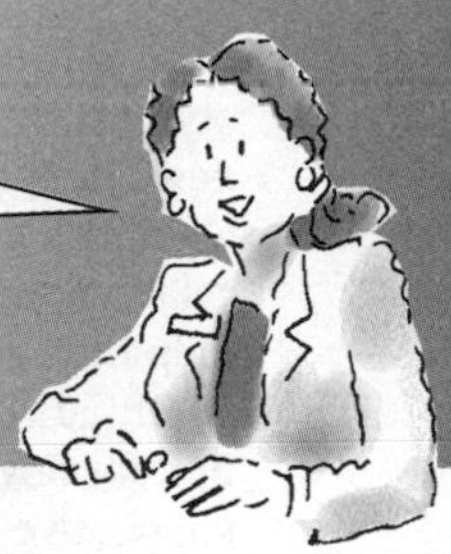
So I'm talking to Queen Elizabeth the other day, and she said you'd do spectacularly well on this chapter. (I'm kidding. What do I look, delusional?) Personally, I think you'll do even better than that. Go for it!

Chapter 17
Schizophrenic & delusional disorders

1. A schizophrenic client tells his primary nurse that he's scheduled to meet the King of Samoa at a special time, making it impossible for the client to leave his room for dinner. Which of the following responses by the nurse is most appropriate?

1. "It's meal time. Let's go so you can eat."
2. "The King of Samoa told me to take you to dinner."
3. "Your physician expects you to follow the unit's schedule."
4. "People who don't eat on this unit aren't being cooperative."

1. 1. A delusional client is so wrapped up in his false beliefs that he tends to disregard activities of daily living, such as nutrition and hydration. He needs clear, concise, firm directions from a caring nurse to meet his needs. The second option belittles and tricks the client, possibly evoking mistrust on the part of the client. The third option evades the issue of meeting his basic needs. The last option is demeaning and doesn't address the delusion.

NP: Implementation; CN: Health promotion and maintenance; CNS: Prevention and early detection of disease; CL: Application

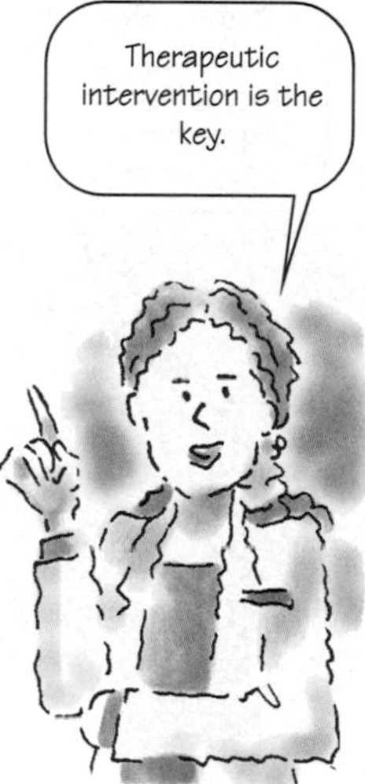
Therapeutic intervention is the key.

2. While looking out the window, a client with schizophrenia remarks, "That school across the street has creatures in it that are waiting for me." Which of the following terms best describes what the creatures represent?

1. Anxiety attack
2. Projection
3. Hallucination
4. Delusion

2. 4. A delusion is a false fixed belief that has no basis in reality. Although anxiety can increase delusional responses, it isn't considered the primary symptom. Projection is the blaming of others in an attempt to justify actions. Hallucinations are perceptual disorders of the five senses and are part of most psychoses. The person sees, tastes, feels, smells, and hears things in the absence of external stimulation.

NP: Analysis; CN: Physiological integrity; CNS: Physiological adaptation; CL: Knowledge

3. A 40-year-old client with a diagnosis of chronic, undifferentiated schizophrenia lives in a rooming house that has a weekly nursing clinic. He scratches while he tells the nurse he feels creatures eating away at his skin. Which of the following interventions should be done first?

1. Talk about his hallucinations and fears.
2. Refer him for anticholinergic adverse reactions.
3. Assess for possible physical problems such as rash.
4. Call his physician to get his medication increased to control his psychosis.

3. 3. Clients with schizophrenia generally have poor visceral recognition because they live so fully in their fantasy world. They need to have an in-depth assessment of physical complaints that may spill over into their delusional symptoms. Talking with the client won't provide an assessment of his itching, and itching isn't an adverse reaction of antipsychotic drugs. Calling the physician to get the client's medication increased doesn't address his physical complaints.

NP: Implementation; CN: Safe, effective care environment; CNS: Safety and infection control; CL: Application

4. A 22-year-old schizophrenic client was admitted to the psychiatric unit during the night. The next morning, he began to misidentify the nurse and call her by his sister's name. Which of the following interventions is best?

1. Assess the client for potential violence.
2. Take the client to his room, where he'll feel safer.
3. Assume the misidentification makes the client feel more comfortable
4. Correct the misidentification, and orient the client to the unit and staff.

4. 4. Misidentification can contribute to anxiety, fear, aggression, and hostility. Orienting a new client to the hospital unit, staff, and other clients, along with establishing a nurse-client relationship, can decrease these feelings and help the client feel in control. Assessing for potential violence is an important nursing function for any psychiatric client, but a perceived supportive environment reduces the risk for violence. Withdrawing to his room, unless interpersonal relationships have become nontherapeutic for him, encourages the client to remain in his fantasy world.

NP: Implementation; CN: Psychosocial integrity; CNS: Coping and adaptation; CL: Application

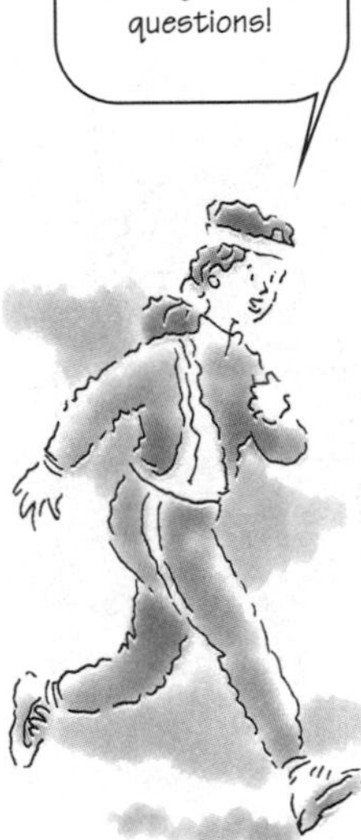

You're really moving through these questions!

5. Which of the following terms describes an effect of isolation?

1. Delusions
2. Hallucinations
3. Lack of volition
4. Waxy flexibility

5. 2. Prolonged isolation can produce sensory deprivation, manifested by hallucinations. A delusion is a false, fixed belief that has no basis in reality. Lack of volition is a symptom associated with type I negative symptoms of schizophrenia. Waxy flexibility is a motor disturbance that's a predominant feature of catatonic schizophrenia.

NP: Analysis; CN: Psychosocial integrity; CNS: Psychosocial adaptation; CL: Application

6. A client diagnosed with schizophrenia several years ago tells the nurse that he feels "very sad." The nurse observes that he's smiling when he says it. Which of the following terms best describes the nurse's observation?

1. Inappropriate affect
2. Extrapyramidal
3. Insight
4. Inappropriate mood

6. 1. Affect refers to behaviors such as facial expression that can be observed when a person is expressing and experiencing feelings. If the client's affect doesn't reflect the emotional content of the statement, the affect is considered inappropriate. Extrapyramidal symptoms are adverse effects of some categories of medication. Insight is a component of the mental status examination and is the ability to perceive oneself realistically and understand if a problem exists. Mood is an extensive and sustained feeling tone.

NP: Analysis; CN: Psychosocial integrity; CNS: Psychosocial adaptation; CL: Comprehension

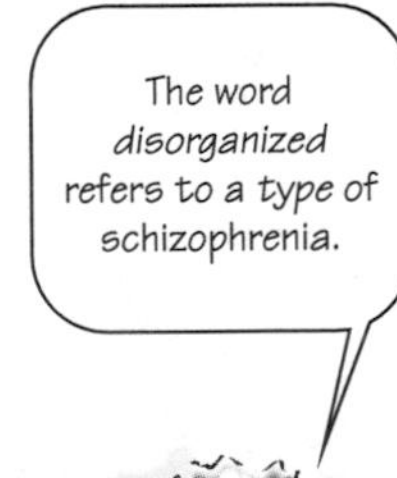

The word disorganized refers to a type of schizophrenia.

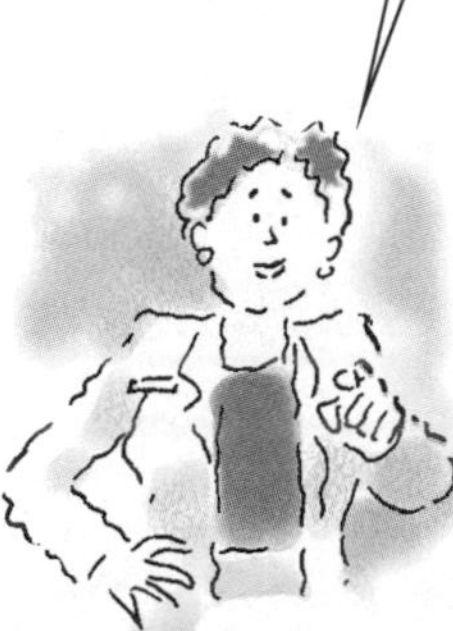

7. Which of the following conditions or characteristics is related to the cluster of symptoms associated with disorganized schizophrenia?

1. Odd beliefs
2. Flat affect
3. Waxy flexibility
4. Systematized delusions

7. 2. Flat affect, the lack of facial or behavioral manifestations of emotion, is related to disorganized schizophrenia. Waxy flexibility occurs in catatonic schizophrenia. Systematized delusions occur most commonly in paranoid residual type schizophrenia, characterized by odd beliefs or unusual perceptions rather than prominent delusions or hallucinations.

NP: Assessment; CN: Psychosocial integrity; CNS: Psychosocial adaptation; CL: Knowledge

8. A client on the psychiatric unit is copying and imitating the movements of his primary nurse. During recovery, he says, "I thought the nurse was my mirror. I felt connected only when I saw my nurse." This behavior is known by which of the following terms?

1. Modeling
2. Echopraxia
3. Ego-syntonicity
4. Ritualism

8. 2. Echopraxia is the copying of another's behaviors and is the result of the loss of ego boundaries. Modeling is the conscious copying of someone's behaviors. Ego-syntonicity refers to behaviors that correspond with the individual's sense of self. Ritualistic behaviors are repetitive and compulsive.

NP: Assessment; CN: Psychosocial integrity; CNS: Coping and adaptation; CL: Application

9. The teenage son of a father with schizophrenia is worried that he might have schizophrenia as well. Which of the following behaviors would be an indication that he should be evaluated for signs of the disorder?

1. Moodiness
2. Preoccupation with his body
3. Spending more time away from home
4. Changes in sleep patterns

9. 4. In conjunction with other signs, changes in sleep patterns are distinctive initial signs of schizophrenia. Other signs include changes in personal care habits and social isolation. Moodiness, preoccupation with the body, and spending more time away from home are normal adolescent behaviors.

NP: Assessment; CN: Health promotion and maintenance; CNS: Prevention and early detection of disease; CL: Application

10. Which of the following symptoms is usually responsive to traditional antipsychotic drugs?

1. Apathy
2. Delusions
3. Social withdrawal
4. Attention impairment

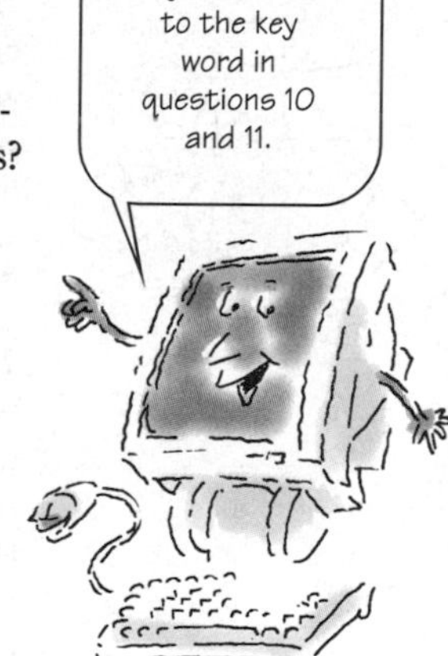
Pay attention to the key word in questions 10 and 11.

10. 2. Positive symptoms, such as delusions, hallucinations, thought disorder, and disorganized speech, respond to traditional antipsychotic drugs. The other options are part of the category of negative symptoms, including affective flattening, restricted thought and speech, apathy, anhedonia, asociality, and attention impairment, and are more responsive to the new atypical antipsychotics, such as clozapine (Clozaril), risperidone (Risperdal), and olanzapine (Zyprexa).

NP: Analysis; CN: Physiological integrity CNS: Pharmacological and parenteral therapies; CL: Comprehension

11. A client was hospitalized after his son filed a petition for involuntary hospitalization for safety reasons. The son seeks out the nurse because his father is angry and refuses to talk with him. He's frustrated and feeling very guilty about his decision. Which of the following responses to this client is the most empathic?

1. "Your father is here because he needs help."
2. "He'll feel differently about you as he gets better."
3. "It sounds like you're feeling guilty about leaving your father here."
4. "This is a stressful time for you, but you'll feel better as he gets well."

11. 3. This response focuses on the son and helps him discuss and deal with his feelings. Unresolved feelings of guilt, shame, isolation, and loss of hope impact on the family's ability to manage the crisis and be supportive to the client. The other options offer premature reassurance and cut off the opportunity for the son to discuss his feelings.

NP: Implementation; CN: Psychosocial integrity; CNS: Coping and adaptation; CL: Application

12. A client followed her antipsychotic medication regimen for a number of years. Her physician treats her urinary tract infection with antibiotic therapy. Which of the following actions are nursing responsibilities?

1. Arrange for possible hospitalization.
2. Have a visiting nurse give the medication.
3. Give instructions on the medication, possible adverse effects, and a return demonstration for teaching effectiveness.
4. Develop a psychoeducational program to address the client's emotional and physical problems arising from physiologic problems.

12. 3. The client has been successful and reliable in carrying out her current medication regimen. The nurse should assume the competency includes self-administration of antibiotics if the instructions are understood. No evidence exists that the client is having a relapse as a result of the infection, so she wouldn't need a psychoeducational program or hospitalization. Having a community nurse give the medication encourages dependency as opposed to self-care.

NP: Implementation; CN: Safe, effective care environment; CNS: Management of care; CL: Application

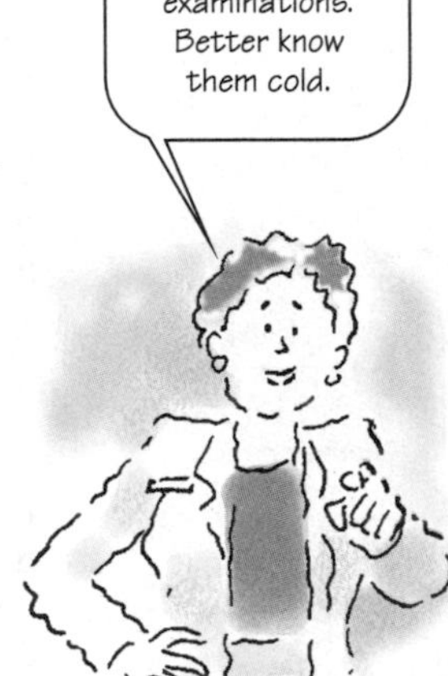

Signs and symptoms are big on NCLEX examinations. Better know them cold.

13. Which of the following signs indicate tardive dyskinesia?

1. Involuntary movements
2. Blurred vision
3. Restlessness
4. Sudden fever

13. 1. Symptoms of tardive dyskinesia include tongue protrusion, lip smacking, chewing, blinking, grimacing, choreiform movements of limbs and trunk, and foot tapping. Blurred vision is a common adverse reaction of antipsychotic drugs and usually disappears after a few weeks of therapy. Restlessness is associated with akathisia. Sudden fever is a symptom of a malignant neurologic disorder.

NP: Analysis; CN: Physiological integrity; CNS: Reduction of risk potential; CL: Application

14. A client approaches a nurse and tells her that he hears a voice telling him that he's evil and deserves to die. Which of the following terms describes the client's perception?

1. Delusion
2. Disorganized speech
3. Hallucination
4. Idea of reference

14. 3. Hallucinations are sensory experiences that are misrepresentations of reality or have no basis in reality. Delusions are beliefs not based in reality. Disorganized speech is characterized by jumping from one topic to the next or using unrelated words. An idea of reference is a belief that an unrelated situation holds special meaning for the client.

NP: Assessment; CN: Psychosocial integrity; CNS: Coping and adaptation; CL: Knowledge

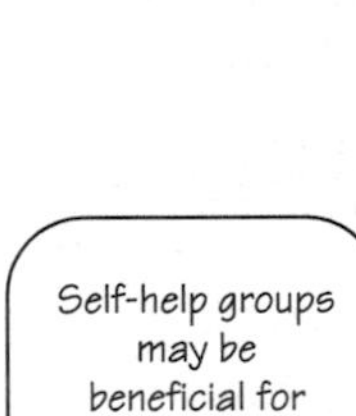

Self-help groups may be beneficial for your client.

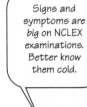

15. A client is referred to a self-help group after discharge from the hospital. Which of the following types of individuals leads these groups?

1. Individuals concerned about coping with mutual concerns
2. Social workers familiar with the problems of the mentally ill
3. Psychiatrists trained to help with stressors in the community
4. Psychiatric nurse specialists able to provide help with monitoring medication

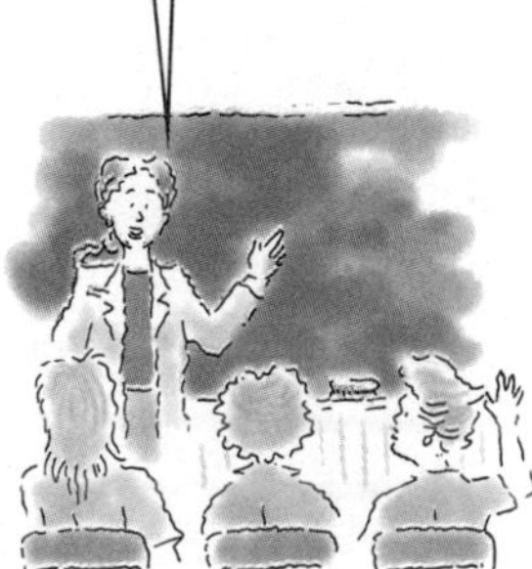

15. 1. Self-help groups are organized and led by consumers of mental health services who come together to share and offer support and advice to each other about a specific problem. These groups aren't led by such professionals as nurses, social workers, and psychiatrists.

NP: Implementation; CN: Psychosocial integrity; CNS: Coping and adaptation; CL: Knowledge

16. Which of the following numbers of members in a therapy group is ideal?
1. 1 to 4
2. 4 to 7
3. 7 to 10
4. 10 to 15

16. 3. The ideal number of members in an inpatient group is 7 to 10. Having fewer than 7 members provides inadequate interaction and material for successful group process. Having more than 10 members doesn't allow for adequate time for individual participation.

NP: Implementation; CN: Psychosocial integrity; CNS: Coping and adaptation; CL: Application

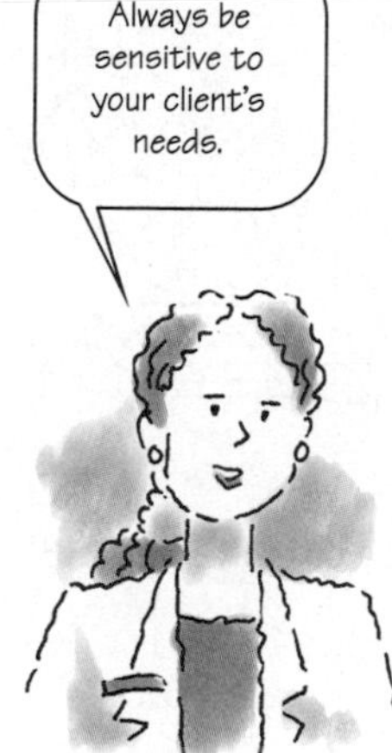

Always be sensitive to your client's needs.

17. A client admitted to an inpatient unit approaches a nursing student saying he descended from a long line of people of a "superrace." Which of the following actions is correct?
1. Smile and walk into the nurse's station.
2. Challenge the client's false belief.
3. Listen for hidden messages in themes of delusion, indicating unmet needs.
4. Introduce yourself, shake hands, and sit down with the client in the day room.

17. 4. The first goal is to establish a relationship with the client, which includes creating psychological space for the creation of trust. The student should sit and make herself available, reflecting concern and interest. Walking into the nurse's station would indicate disinterest and lack of concern about the client's feelings. After establishing a relationship and lessening the client's anxiety, the student can orient the client to reality, listen to his concerns and fears, and try to understand the feelings reflected in the delusions. Delusions are firmly maintained false beliefs, and attempts to dismiss them don't work.

NP: Implementation; CN: Safe, effective care environment; CNS: Management of care; CL: Application

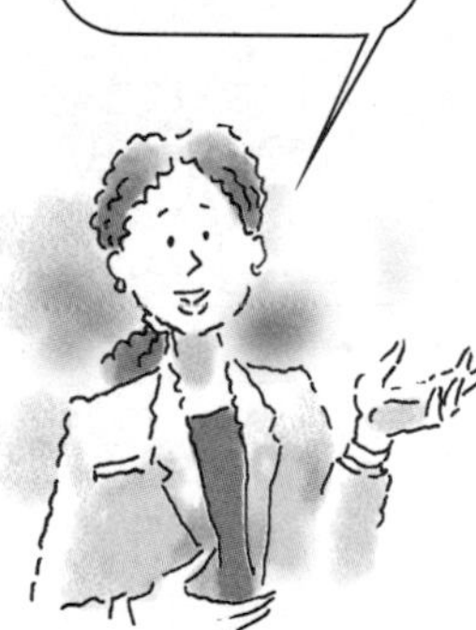

Every nursing diagnosis tells a story that helps all nurses better understand the client.

18. Which of the following nursing diagnoses is most appropriate for a client with acute schizophrenic reaction?
1. Social isolation related to impaired ability to trust
2. Impaired mobility related to fear of hostile impulses
3. Disturbed sleep patterns related to impaired thinking ability
4. Risk for other-directed violence related to perceptual distortions

18. 1. Clients with schizophrenia are mistrustful, which results in withdrawal and social isolation. Mobility isn't a common problem for persons with schizophrenia. Sleep disturbance may be present but isn't the most common symptom. Contrary to popular belief, persons with schizophrenia usually aren't violent.

NP: Analysis; CN: Safe, effective care environment; CNS: Management of care; CL: Analysis

19. A nurse is assisting with morning care when a client suddenly throws off the covers and starts shouting, "My body is changing and disintegrating because I'm not of this world." Which of the following terms best describes this behavior?
1. Depersonalization
2. Ideas of reference
3. Looseness of association
4. Paranoid ideation

19. 1. Depersonalization is a state in which the client feels unreal or believes parts of the body are being distorted. Ideas of reference are beliefs unrelated to situations and hold special meaning for the individual. The term loose associations refers to sentences that have vague connections to each other. Paranoid ideations are beliefs that others intend to harm the client in some way.

NP: Analysis; CN: Psychosocial integrity; CNS: Coping and adaptation; CL: Analysis

20. Many clients with schizophrenia simultaneously have opposing emotions. Which of the following terms describes this phenomenon?

1. Double bind
2. Ambivalence
3. Loose associations
4. Inappropriate affect

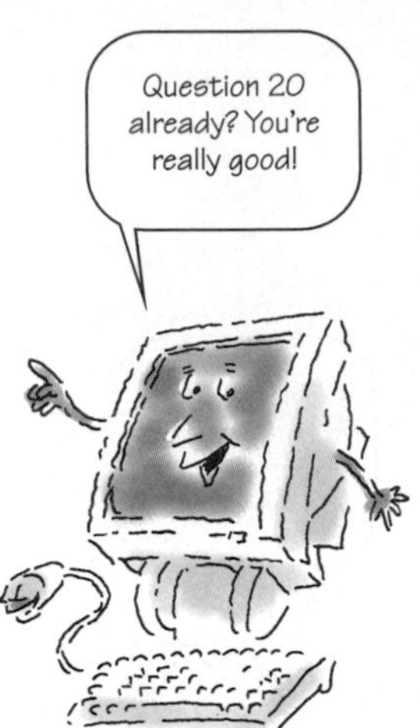

Question 20 already? You're really good!

20. 2. Ambivalence, one of the symptoms associated with schizophrenia, immobilizes the person from acting. A double bind presents two conflicting messages — for example, saying that you trust someone but then not allowing the person into your room. Loose association involves rapid shifts of ideas from one subject to another in an unrelated manner. Inappropriate affect refers to an observable expression of emotions incongruent with the emotion felt.
NP: Assessment; CN: Psychosocial integrity; CNS: Coping and adaptation; CL: Comprehension

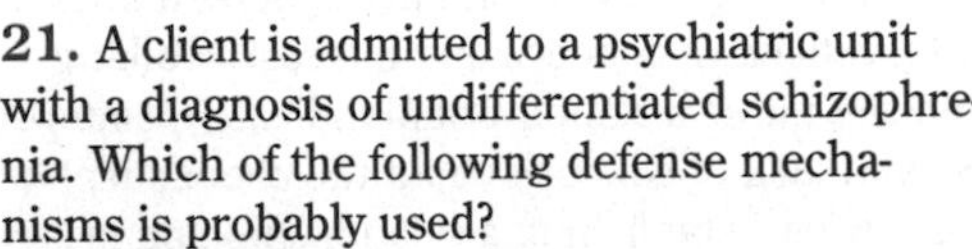

21. A client is admitted to a psychiatric unit with a diagnosis of undifferentiated schizophrenia. Which of the following defense mechanisms is probably used?

1. Projection
2. Rationalization
3. Regression
4. Repression

21. 3. Regression, a return to earlier behavior to reduce anxiety, is the basic defense mechanism in schizophrenia. Projection is a defense mechanism in which one blames others and attempts to justify actions; it's used primarily by people with paranoid schizophrenia and delusional disorder. Rationalization is a defense mechanism used to justify one's actions. Repression is the basic defense mechanism in the neuroses; it's an involuntary exclusion of painful thoughts, feelings, or experiences from awareness.
NP: Analysis; CN: Psychosocial integrity; CNS: Coping and adaptation; CL: Comprehension

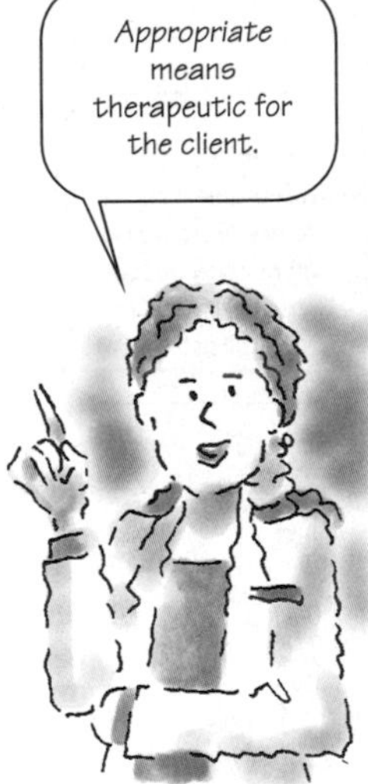

Appropriate means therapeutic for the client.

22. A nurse on a psychiatric unit observes a client in the corner of the room moving his lips as if he were talking to himself. Which of the following actions is the most appropriate?

1. Ask him why he's talking to himself.
2. Leave him alone until he stops talking.
3. Tell him it isn't good for him to talk to himself.
4. Invite him to join in a card game with the nurse.

22. 4. Being with the nurse provides stimulation that competes with the hallucinations. The client doesn't think he's talking to himself, he's responding only to the voices he hears. Being alone keeps the client in his fantasy world. Telling the client that he shouldn't talk to himself fails to understand how real his fantasy world and hallucinations are.
NP: Planning; CN: Psychosocial integrity; CNS: Coping and adaptation; CL: Application

23. A client makes vague statements with no logical connections. He asks whether the nurse understands. Which of the following responses is best?

1. "Why don't we wait until later to talk about it?"
2. "You're not making sense, so I won't talk about this topic."
3. "Yes, I understand the overall sense of the logical connections from the idea."
4. "I want to understand what you're saying, but I'm having difficulty following you."

23. 4. The nurse needs to communicate that she wants to understand without blaming the client for the lack of understanding. Asking the client to wait because he's too confused cuts off an attempt to communicate and asks the client to do what he can't at present. Telling the client that he isn't making sense is judgmental and could impair the therapeutic relationship. Pretending to understand is a violation of trust and can damage the therapeutic relationship.
NP: Implementation; CN: Psychosocial integrity; CNS: Coping and adaptation; CL: Application

24. A client asks a nurse if she hears the voice of the nonexistent man speaking to him. Which of the following responses is best?

1. "No one is in your room except you."
2. "Yes, I hear him, but I won't listen to him."
3. "What has he told you? Is it helpful advice?"
4. "No, I don't hear him, but I know you do. What is he saying?"

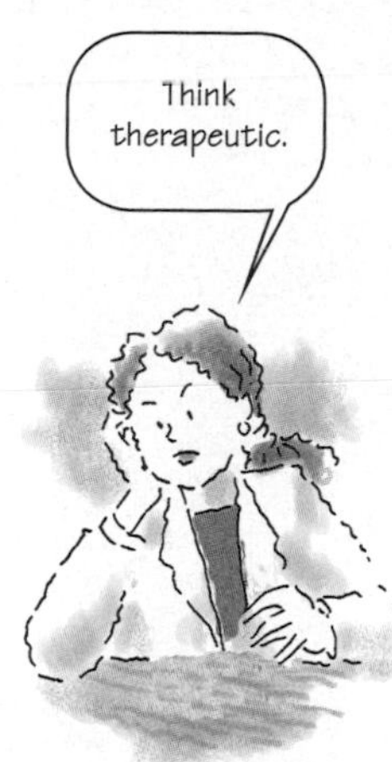
Think therapeutic.

24. 4. This response points out reality and shows concern and support. Attempting to argue the client out of the belief might entrench him more firmly in his belief, making him feel more out of control because of the negative and fearful nature of hallucinations. The other two options violate the trust of the therapeutic relationship.

NP: Implementation; CN: Safe, effective care environment; CNS: Management of care; CL: Application

25. Which of the following instructions is correct for a client taking chlorpromazine (Thorazine)?

1. Reduce the dosage if you feel better.
2. Occasional social drinking isn't harmful.
3. Stop taking the drug immediately if adverse reactions develop.
4. Schedule routine medication checks.

25. 4. Ongoing assessment by a primary health care provider is important to assess for adverse reactions and continued therapeutic effectiveness. The dosage should be changed only after checking with the primary care provider. Alcoholic beverages are contraindicated while taking an antipsychotic drug. Adverse reactions should be reported immediately to determine if the drug should be discontinued.

NP: Implementation; CN: Physiological integrity; CNS: Pharmacological and parenteral therapies; CL: Application

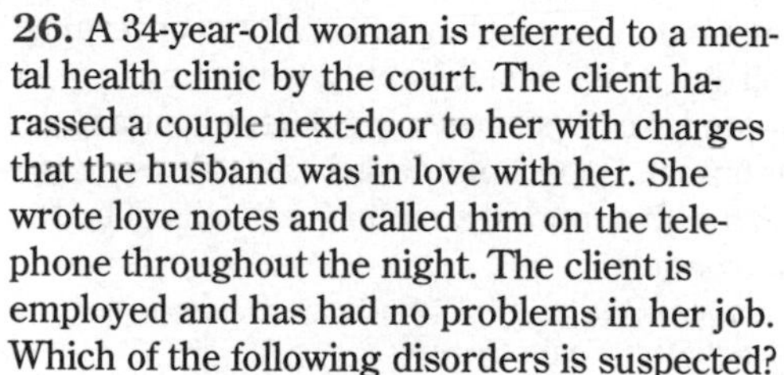

26. A 34-year-old woman is referred to a mental health clinic by the court. The client harassed a couple next-door to her with charges that the husband was in love with her. She wrote love notes and called him on the telephone throughout the night. The client is employed and has had no problems in her job. Which of the following disorders is suspected?

1. Major depression
2. Paranoid schizophrenia
3. Delusional disorder
4. Bipolar affective disorder

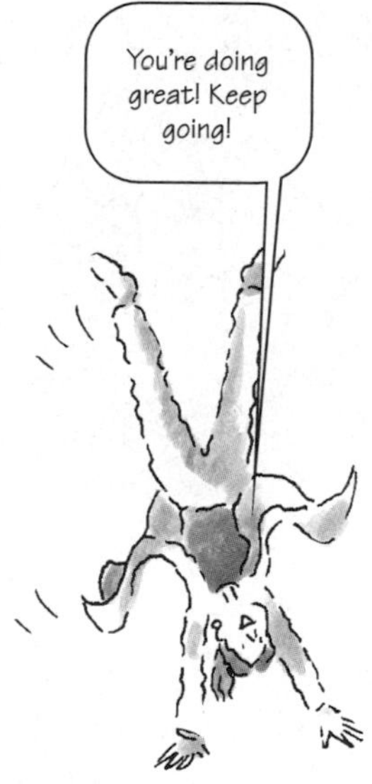
You're doing great! Keep going!

26. 3. The client has a delusional disorder with erotomanic delusions as her primary symptom and believes she's loved intensely by a married person showing no interest in her. No symptoms of major depression exist. The client doesn't believe someone is trying to harm her, the hallmark characteristic of paranoia. Bipolar affective disorder is characterized by cycles of extreme emotional highs (mania) and lows (depression).

NP: Analysis; CN: Psychosocial integrity; CNS: Coping and adaptation; CL: Application

27. A homebound client taking clozapine (Clozaril) tells the nurse he has been feeling tired for 5 days. His temperature is 99.6° F; pulse, 110 beats/minute; and respirations, 20 breaths/minute. Which of the following instructions is correct?

1. Take the medication with milk.
2. Stop the medication at once, and see the physician immediately.
3. Understand that the symptoms will disappear as soon as he gets more rest.
4. Stop the medication gradually, and see the physician next week.

27. 2. He should stop the medication and see his physician immediately because fever can be a sign of agranulocytosis, which is a medical emergency. Taking antipsychotic medication with milk, nicotine, and caffeine will decrease the effectiveness. Rest will have no effect on this client's symptoms. Drowsiness and fatigue usually disappear with continued therapy.

NP: Implementation; CN: Physiological integrity; CNS: Reduction of risk potential; CL: Application

28. A 20-year-old client is admitted to the hospital with a diagnosis of schizophrenia. During the initial assessment, he points to the nurse's stethoscope and says it's a snake. Which of the following terms describes this phenomenon?

1. Abstraction
2. Delusion
3. Hallucination
4. Illusion

28. 4. An illusion is a misinterpretation of an actual sensory stimulation. An abstraction is an idea or concept such as love or a belief that can't be represented by a concrete object. A delusion is a false, fixed belief and an hallucination is a false sensory perception without a stimulus.

NP: Analysis; CN: Psychosocial integrity; CNS: Coping and adaptation; CL: Comprehension

29. When asking a family about the onset of a schizophrenic client's illusions, which of the following periods is the most likely answer?

1. Adolescence
2. Early childhood
3. Late adulthood
4. Late childhood

29. 1. The usual onset of schizophrenia is between adolescence and early adulthood.

NP: Implementation; CN: Psychosocial integrity; CNS: Psychosocial adaptation; CL: Knowledge

It's important to know the correct terminology for making accurate diagnoses.

30. A client can't eat because he believes his bowels have turned against him. Which of the following terms describes this phenomenon?

1. Conversion hysteria
2. Depersonalization
3. Hypochondriasis
4. Somatic delusion

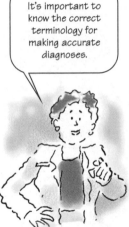

30. 4. A somatic delusion is a fixed, false belief pertaining to the body and body parts. Conversion hysteria is a somatoform disorder in which there are symptoms of some physical illness without any underlying organic cause. Depersonalization is a feeling of unreality concerning self and a loss of self-identity, with things around the person seeming different, strange, or unreal. Hypochondriasis is somatic overconcern with a morbid attention to details of body functioning.

NP: Analysis; CN: Psychosocial integrity; CNS: Coping and adaptation; CL: Comprehension

31. Which of the following actions by the nurse is an appropriate therapeutic intervention for a client experiencing hallucinations?

1. Confine him in his room until he feels better.
2. Provide a competing stimulus that distracts from the hallucinations.
3. Discourage attempts to understand what precipitates his hallucinations.
4. Support perceptual distortions until he gives them up of his own accord.

31. 2. Providing competing stimuli acknowledges the presence of the hallucination and teaches ways to decrease the frequency of hallucinations. The other options support and maintain hallucinations or deny their existence.

NP: Planning; CN: Psychosocial integrity; CNS: Coping and adaptation; CL: Application

32. A client with schizophrenia reports that her hallucinations have decreased in frequency. Which of the following interventions would be appropriate to begin addressing the client's problem with social isolation?
1. Have the client join in a group game.
2. Name the client as the leader of the client support group.
3. Have the client play solitaire.
4. Ask the client to participate in a group sing-along.

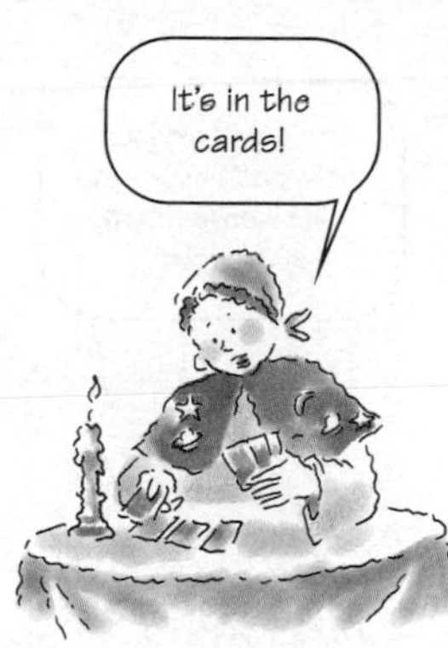

It's in the cards!

32. 4. Having the client participate in a non-competitive group activity that doesn't require individual participation won't present a threat to the client. Games can become competitive and lead to anxiety or hostility. The client probably lacks sufficient social skills to lead a group at this time. Playing solitaire doesn't encourage socialization.
NP: Planning; CN: Psychosocial integrity; CNS: Coping and adaptation; CL: Application

33. A single 24-year-old client is admitted with acute schizophrenic reaction. Which of the following methods is appropriate therapy for this type of schizophrenia?
1. Counseling to produce insight into behavior
2. Biofeedback to reduce agitation associated with schizophrenia
3. Drug therapy to reduce symptoms associated with acute schizophrenia
4. Electroconvulsive therapy to treat the mood component of schizophrenia

33. 3. Drug therapy is usually successful in normalizing behavior and reducing or eliminating hallucinations, delusions, thought disorder, affect flattening, apathy, and asociality. Counseling isn't appropriate at this time. Electroconvulsive therapy might be considered for schizoaffective disorder, which has a mood component, and is a treatment of choice for clinical depression. Biofeedback reduces anxiety and modifies behavioral responses but isn't the major component in the treatment of schizophrenia.
NP: Analysis; CN: Psychosocial integrity; CNS: Coping and adaptation; CL: Comprehension

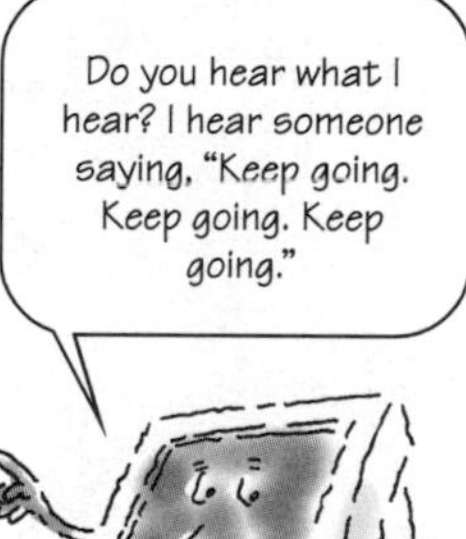

Do you hear what I hear? I hear someone saying, "Keep going. Keep going. Keep going."

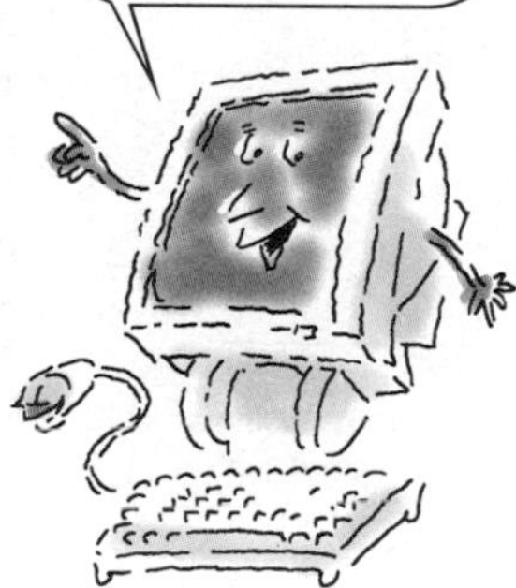

34. A client tells a nurse voices are telling him to do "terrible things." Which of the following actions is part of the initial therapy?
1. Find out what the voices are telling him.
2. Let him go to his room to decrease his anxiety.
3. Begin talking to the client about an unrelated topic.
4. Tell the client the voices aren't real.

34. 1. For safety purposes, the nurse must find out whether the voices are directing the client to harm himself or others. Further assessment can help identify appropriate therapeutic interventions. Isolating a person during this intense sensory confusion often reinforces the psychosis. Changing the topic indicates that the nurse isn't concerned about the client's fears. Dismissing the voices shuts down communication between the client and the nurse.
NP: Implementation; CN: Safe, effective care environment; CNS: Safety and infection control; CL: Application

35. A client is preoccupied with his belief that the CIA has been planning to take him away to save the agency from his influence. These delusions are a defense against which of the following underlying feelings?
1. Aggression
2. Guilt
3. Inferiority
4. Persecution

35. 3. The delusional system contains grandiose ideation that allows the client to feel important rather than inferior. Feelings of aggression will appear as violent or hostile thoughts. Guilt results in beliefs that the person deserves to be punished. Persecution is the fear that others are trying to harm you.
NP: Planning; CN: Psychosocial integrity; CNS: Coping and adaptation; CL: Application

36. A client has started taking haloperidol (Haldol). Which of the following instructions is most appropriate for a client taking haloperidol?

1. You should report feelings of restlessness or agitation at once.
2. Use a sunscreen outdoors on a year-round basis.
3. Be aware you'll feel increased energy taking this drug.
4. This drug will indirectly control essential hypertension.

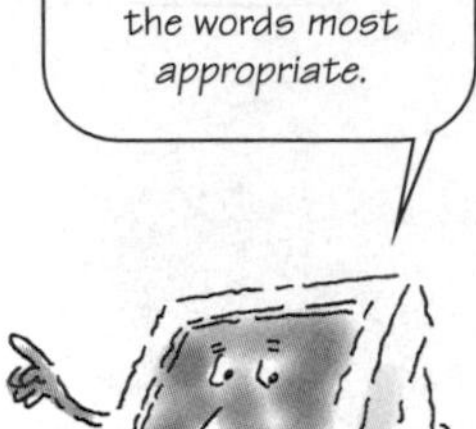

Don't get anxious, now, but check out the words most appropriate.

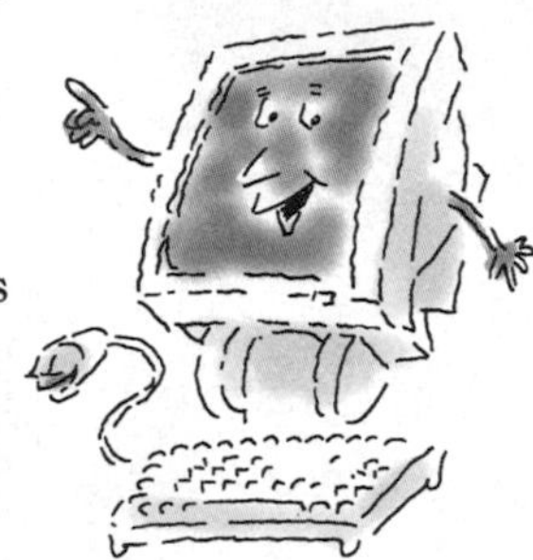

36. 1. Agitation and restlessness are adverse effects of haloperidol and can be treated with anticholinergic drugs. Haloperidol isn't likely to cause photosensitivity or control essential hypertension. Although the client may experience increased concentration and activity, these effects are due to a decrease in symptoms, not the drug itself.

NP: Implementation; CN: Physiological integrity; CNS: Pharmacological and parenteral therapies; CL: Application

37. A 45-year old client experiencing delusions has been admitted to the crisis center. When assessing the content of the delusions, the nurse should look for which of the following aspects of the delusions?

1. Logic
2. Religious beliefs
3. Themes
4. True experiences

37. 3. Understanding the themes inherent in the client's psychotic symptoms may help the nurse learn what stresses trigger the symptoms. A delusion is a false, fixed belief that misrepresents perceptions or experiences and isn't open to rational argument. Assessing for logic, religious beliefs, or true experiences draws the nurse into the delusional thinking and therefore isn't therapeutic.

NP: Assessment; CN: Psychosocial integrity; CNS: Psychosocial adaptation; CL: Analysis

38. Which of the following cluster of symptoms would indicate schizophrenia?

1. Persistent, intrusive thoughts leading to repetitive, ritualistic behaviors
2. Feelings of helplessness and hopelessness
3. Unstable moods and delusions of grandeur
4. Hallucinations or delusions and decreased ability to function in society

38. 4. Schizophrenia is a brain disease characterized by a variety of symptoms, including hallucinations, delusions, and asociality. Clients with obsessive-compulsive disorder experience intrusive thoughts and ritualistic behaviors. Feelings of helplessness and hopelessness are pivotal symptoms of clinical depression. Unstable moods and delusions of grandeur are characteristics of bipolar affective disorder.

NP: Assessment; CN: Psychosocial integrity; CNS: Coping and adaptation; CL: Comprehension

39. Which of the following symptoms indicates that schizophrenia is a thought disorder?

1. Faulty logic
2. Distorted but organized thinking
3. Organized but disruptive thoughts
4. Appropriate perception, but difficulty responding appropriately to people and events

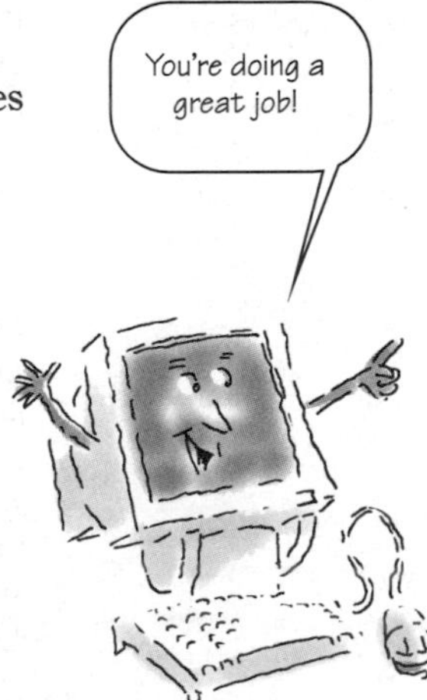

39. 1. Thought disorders are characterized by problems in the form and organization of thinking. They appear as loose associations, word salad, tangentiality, illogicality, circumstantiality, pressure of speech, and poverty of speech that impairs communication. Thinking is disorganized and perceptions are often misinterpreted. The other options are inaccurate characteristics of schizophrenia.

NP: Analysis; CN: Psychosocial integrity; CNS: Psychosocial adaptation; CL: Analysis

40. Which of the following terms describes a marked decrease in the variation or intensity of emotional expression?

1. Anhedonia
2. Depression
3. Flat affect
4. Incongruence

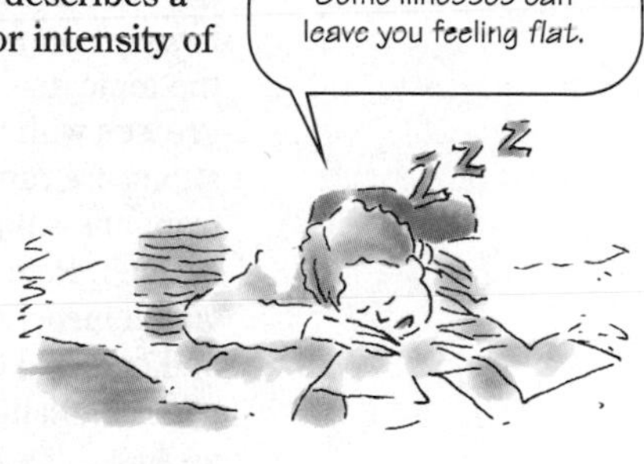

Some illnesses can leave you feeling flat.

40. 3. Flat affect indicates that no expression can be observed while the client is expressing and experiencing feelings and emotions. Anhedonia is decreased ability or inability to express pleasure, joy, intimacy, and closeness. Depression is an extensive and sustained negative feeling. Incongruence is discrepancy between verbal and nonverbal communication.

NP: Assessment; CN: Psychosocial integrity; CNS: Coping and adaptation; CL: Comprehension

41. A client is admitted after being found on a highway, hitting at cars and yelling at motorists. When approached by the nurse, the client shouts, "You're the one who stole my husband from me." Which of the following describes the client's condition?

1. Hallucinatory experience
2. Delusional experience
3. Disorientation to the environment
4. Phobic experience

41. 2. A delusion is a false, fixed belief manufactured without appropriate or sufficient evidence to support it. The client's statements don't represent hallucinations because they aren't perceptual disorders. No information in the question addresses orientation. The client's statements don't represent a phobia because they don't represent an irrational fear.

NP: Assessment; CN: Psychosocial integrity; CNS: Coping and adaptation; CL: Application

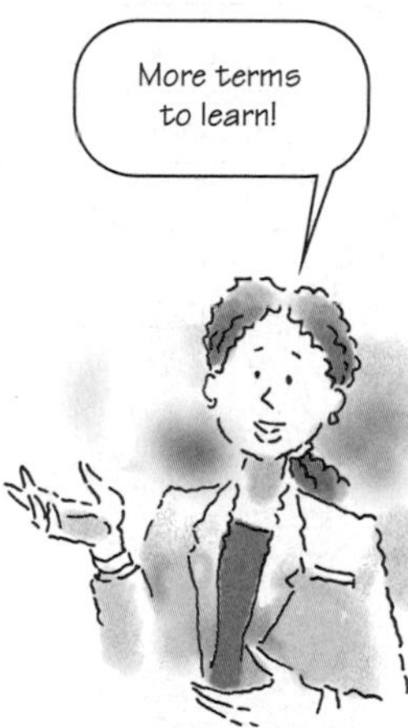

More terms to learn!

42. Which of the following statements describes remission in schizophrenia?

1. The disease is in the prodromal phase.
2. The client no longer has prominent psychotic symptoms.
3. The client is free from all signs of illness and is no longer on medication.
4. The client is free from all signs of illness whether or not he's on medication.

42. 2. Schizophrenia is a chronic disorder with periods of remission and exacerbation. The prodromal phase is the precursor to an exacerbation. Clients aren't usually cured but are treated over time with case management, medication, symptom management skills, social skill training, network support, vocational training, and health promoting practices.

NP: Evaluation; CN: Health promotion and maintenance; CNS: Growth and development through the life span; CL: Comprehension

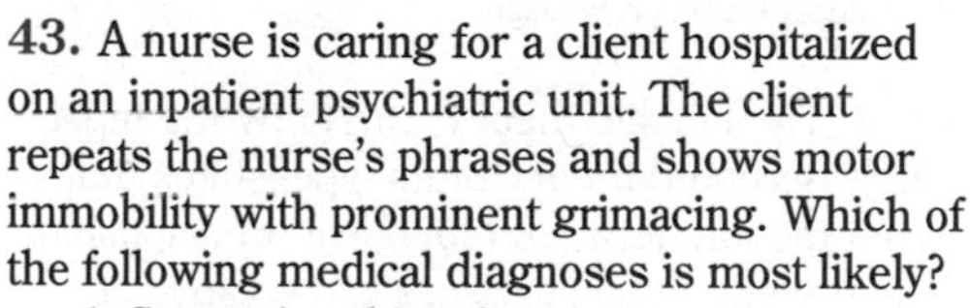

43. A nurse is caring for a client hospitalized on an inpatient psychiatric unit. The client repeats the nurse's phrases and shows motor immobility with prominent grimacing. Which of the following medical diagnoses is most likely?

1. Catatonic schizophrenia
2. Disorganized schizophrenia
3. Residual schizophrenia
4. Undifferentiated schizophrenia

43. 1. Motor immobility, parroting phrases, and grimacing are characteristics of catatonic schizophrenia. Symptoms of disorganized schizophrenia are disorganized speech and behaviors with flat or inappropriate affect. Symptoms of residual schizophrenia include odd beliefs, eccentric behavior, and illogical thinking. Undifferentiated schizophrenia is characterized by delusions or hallucinations and other behaviors common to other types of schizophrenia.

NP: Analysis; CN: Psychosocial integrity; CNS: Coping and adaptation; CL: Comprehension

44. A nurse on an inpatient unit is having a discussion with a client with schizophrenia about his schedule for the day. The client comments that he was highly active at home and then explains the volunteer job he held. Which of the following terms describes the client's thinking?

1. Circumstantiality
2. Loose associations
3. Referential
4. Tangentiality

44. 4. Tangentiality describes thought patterns loosely connected but not directly related to the topic. In circumstantiality, the person digresses with unnecessary details. Loose associations are rapid shifts in the expression of ideas from one subject to another in an unrelated manner. Referential thinking is when an individual incorrectly interprets neutral incidents and external events as having a particular or special meaning for him.

NP: Analysis; CN: Psychosocial integrity; CNS: Coping and adaptation; CL: Application

45. While talking to a client with schizophrenia, a nurse notes the client frequently uses unrecognizable words with no common meaning. Which of the following terms describes this?

1. Echolalia
2. Clang association
3. Neologisms
4. Word salad

45. 3. Neologisms are newly coined words with personal meanings to the client with schizophrenia. Echolalia is parrotlike echoing of spoken words or sounds. Clang association is the linking of words by sound rather than meaning. A word salad is stringing words in sequence that have no connection to one another.

NP: Implementation; CN: Psychosocial integrity; CNS: Psychosocial adaptation; CL: Application

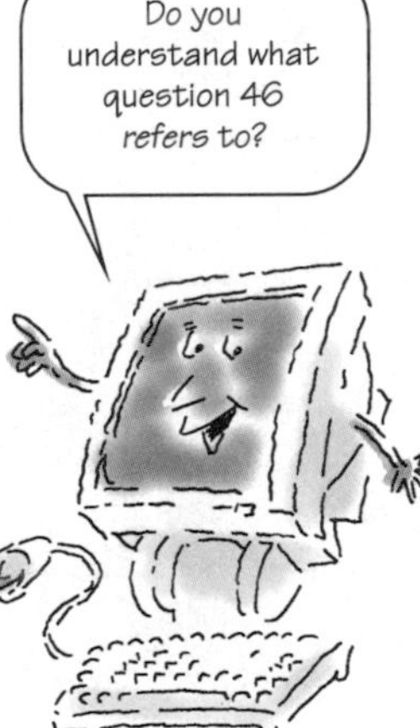

Do you understand what question 46 refers to?

46. While caring for a hospitalized client diagnosed with schizophrenia, a nurse observes the client watching television. The client tells the nurse the television is speaking directly to him. Which of the following terms describes this belief?

1. Autistic thinking
2. Concrete thinking
3. Paranoid thinking
4. Referential thinking

46. 4. Referential, or primary process thinking, is a belief that incidents and events in the environment have special meaning for the client. Autistic thinking is a disturbance in thought due to the intrusion of a private fantasy world, internally stimulated, resulting in abnormal responses to people. Concrete thinking is the literal interpretation of words and symbols. Paranoid thinking is the belief that others are trying to harm you.

NP: Analysis; CN: Psychosocial integrity; CNS: Coping and adaptation; CL: Comprehension

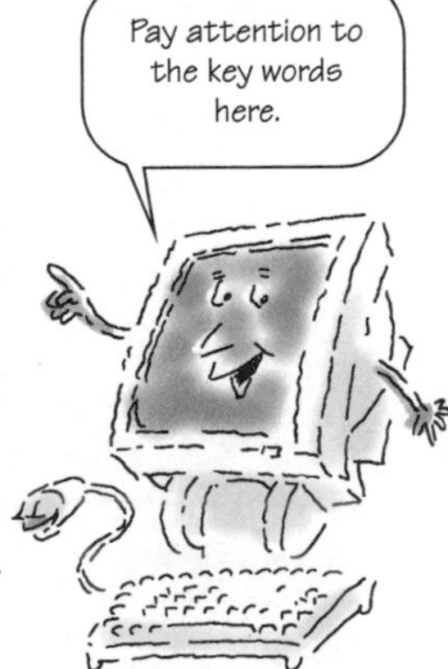

Pay attention to the key words here.

47. A nurse is talking with a family of a client diagnosed with schizophrenia. The mother asks, "What causes this disorder?" Which of the following explanations is the most widely accepted?

1. Prenatal or postpartum central nervous system damage
2. Bacterial infections in the mother during pregnancy or delivery
3. A biological predisposition exacerbated by environmental stressors
4. Lack of bonding and attachment during infancy, which leads to depression in later life

47. 3. The holistic theory, currently the most widely accepted theory of its type, states that an interaction between biological predisposition and environmental stressors is the cause of schizophrenia. The biological explanation states that schizophrenia is caused by a brain disease, a bacterial infection in utero, or early brain damage. The psychoanalytic perspective involves the belief that the mother-infant bond is the source of the schizophrenia.

NP: Implementation; CN: Physiological integrity; CNS: Physiological adaptation; CL: Application

48. Results from current brain research in clients with schizophrenia supports which of the following explanations for clients with enlarged ventricles?

1. Shorter prodromal period for the disease
2. Greater response to treatment for the disease
3. More prominent prodromal period for the disease
4. Lesser amount of cognitive impairment from the disease

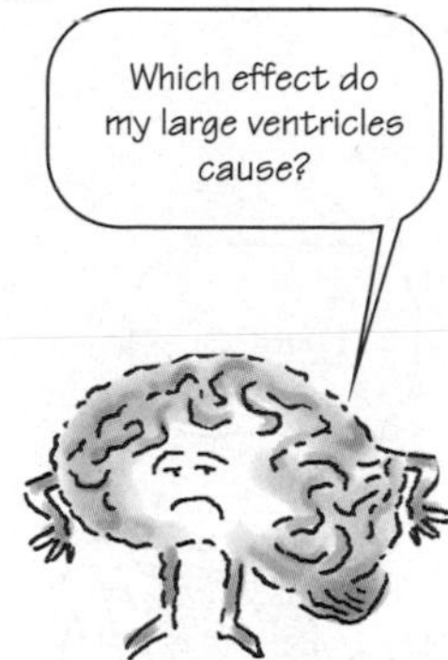

Which effect do my large ventricles cause?

48. 3. Imaging studies of the brain structure of people with schizophrenia suggest there is loss or underdevelopment of brain tissue, manifested by decreased brain volume; larger lateral and third ventricles; atrophy in the frontal lobe, cerebellum, and limbic structures; and increased size of sulci on the surface of the brain. There is a trend for enlarged ventricles to be associated with two indicators of poor prognosis: early age of onset and poor premorbid functioning.

NP: Assessment; CN: Physiological integrity; CNS: Physiological adaptation; CL: Knowledge

49. A client is taking chlorpromazine (Thorazine) for the treatment of schizophrenia. This drug blocks the transmission of which of the following substances?

1. Dopamine
2. Epinephrine
3. Norepinephrine
4. Thyroxine

49. 1. Most antipsychotic agents block the transmission of dopamine to the brain. Other transmitters linked to schizophrenia include serotonin, acetylcholine, and norepinephrine. Epinephrine, norepinephrine, and thyroxine aren't blocked by chlorpromazine.

NP: Implementation; CN: Physiological integrity; CNS: Pharmacological and parenteral therapies; CL: Knowledge

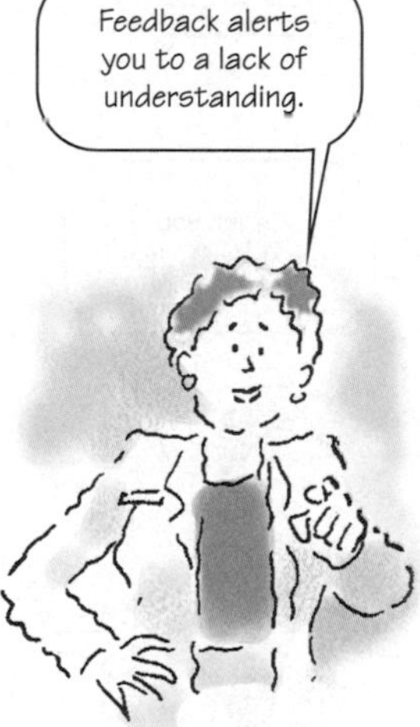

Feedback alerts you to a lack of understanding.

50. In preparation for discharge, a client diagnosed with schizophrenia was taught self-symptom management as part of a relapse prevention program. Which of the following statements indicates the client understands symptom monitoring?

1. "When I hear voices, I become afraid I'll relapse."
2. "My parents aren't involved enough to be aware if I begin to relapse."
3. "My family is more protected from stress if I keep them out of my illness process."
4. "When I'm feeling stressed, I go to a quiet room by myself and do imagery."

50. 4. This statement indicates the client has learned a technique for coping with stress with the use of imagery technique. The other options don't show an understanding of self-symptom monitoring and may result in symptom intensification and possible relapse.

NP: Implementation; CN: Psychosocial integrity; CNS: Coping and adaptation; CL: Application

You'll need to read the key word carefully on this one!

51. A client diagnosed with schizophrenia has been taking haloperidol (Haldol) for 1 week when a nurse observes that the client's eyeball is fixated on the ceiling. Which of the following specific conditions is the client exhibiting?

1. Akathisia
2. Neuroleptic malignant syndrome
3. Oculogyric crisis
4. Tardive dyskinesia

51. 3. An oculogyric crisis involves a fixed positioning of the eyes, typically in an upward gaze. Neuroleptic malignant syndrome causes increased body temperature, muscle rigidity, and altered consciousness. Akathisia is a restlessness that can cause pacing and tapping of the fingers or feet. Stereotyped involuntary movements (tongue protrusion, lip smacking, chewing, blinking, and grimacing) characterize tardive dyskinesia.

NP: Planning; CN: Physiological integrity; CNS: Pharmacological and parenteral therapies; CL: Application

52. A client taking antipsychotic medications shows dystonic reactions, including torticollis and oculogyric crisis. Which of the following medications is given?

1. benztropine (Cogentin)
2. chlordiazepoxide (Librium)
3. diazepam (Valium)
4. fluoxetine (Prozac)

52. 1. Benztropine and trihexyphenidyl are anticholinergic drugs used to counteract the dystonic reactions and adverse reactions of antipsychotic drugs. The antihistamine diphenhydramine is also effective in treating extrapyramidal symptoms. Fluoxetine is an antidepressant, and diazepam and chlordiazepoxide are benzodiazepines.

NP: Implementation; CN: Physiological integrity; CNS: Pharmacological and parenteral therapies; CL: Application

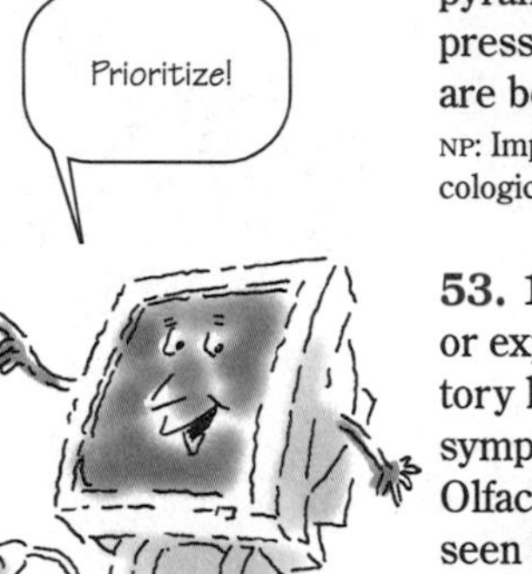
Prioritize!

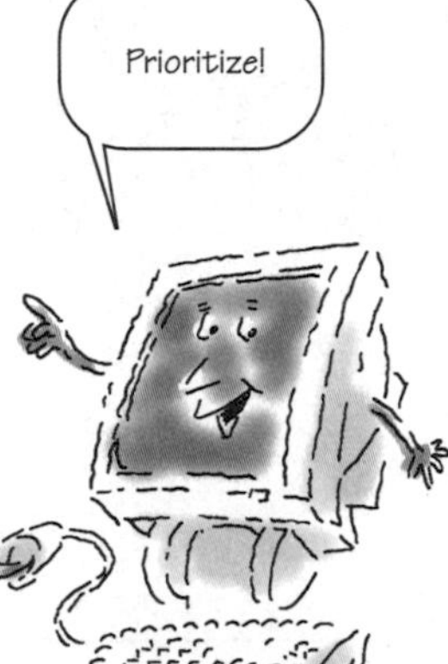

53. A client diagnosed with schizophrenia is having hallucinations. The most common type of hallucination involves which of the following senses?

1. Hearing
2. Smell
3. Touch
4. Vision

53. 1. Hallucinations are sensory impressions or experiences without external stimuli. Auditory hallucinations are the most common symptoms with clients with schizophrenia. Olfactory, tactile, and visual hallucinations are seen in a number of psychiatric disorders, such as substance abuse disorders, delirium, and dementia, but not as often in schizophrenia.

NP: Assessment; CN: Physiological integrity; CNS: Physiological adaptation; CL: Comprehension

54. A 20-year-old client has been diagnosed with schizophrenia. He presently lives by himself, doesn't bathe, doesn't dress himself, and is erratic with eating, drinking, and taking prescribed medications. Which of the following nursing diagnoses for this client has priority?

1. Ineffective role performance related to isolation
2. Activity intolerance related to perceptual distortions
3. Ineffective coping
4. Imbalanced nutrition: Less than body requirements related to symptoms of schizophrenia

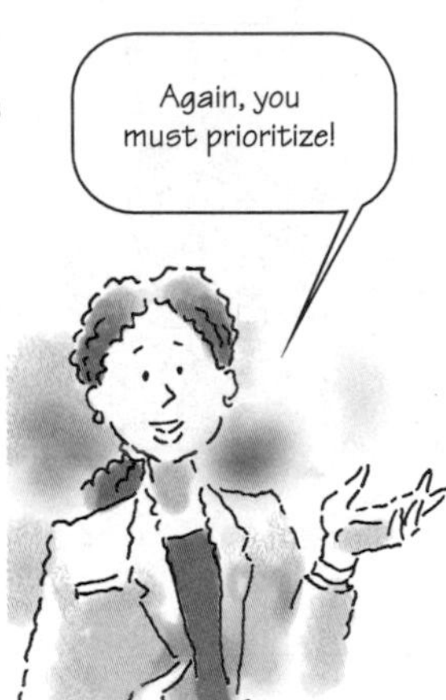
Again, you
must prioritize!

54. 4. The deterioration of the client undergoing a schizophrenic crisis is manifested in multiple self-care deficits. Adequate nutrition in these instances is the primary concern of the nurse. The other problems can be addressed after the client has been stabilized.

NP: Analysis; CN: Safe, effective care environment; CNS: Safety and infection control; CL: Application

55. As a nurse approaches the nursing station, a client with the diagnosis of delusional disorder raises his voice and says, "You're following me. What do you want?" To prevent escalating fear and anger, the nurse takes a nonthreatening posture and makes which of the following responses in a calm voice?

1. "Are you frightened?"
2. "You know I'm not following you."
3. "You'll have to go into seclusion if you continue to threaten me."
4. "I'm sorry if I frightened you. I was returning to the nursing station after going out for lunch."

55. 4. Being clear in communication, remaining calm, and showing concern increases the chance the client will cooperate, lessening potential for violence. The first option tries to identify the client's feelings but doesn't convey warmth and concern. The second option isn't empathic and shows no indication of trying to reach the client at a level beyond content of communication. The third option may increase the client's anxiety, fear, and mistrust when the nurse engages in a power struggle and triggers competitiveness within the client.

NP: Implementation; CN: Psychosocial integrity; CNS: Coping and adaptation; CL: Application

56. Which of the following actions by a client with stable schizophrenia is most important for preventing relapse?

1. Attending group therapy sessions
2. Participating in family support meetings
3. Attending social skills training sessions
4. Consistently taking prescribed medications

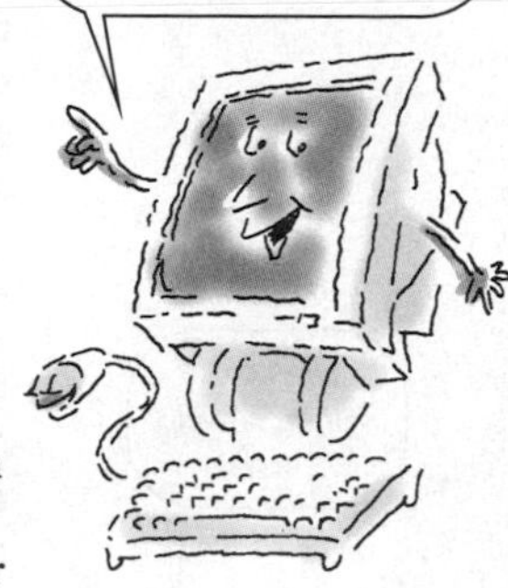

The words *most important* in question 56 indicate the need to prioritize. As a matter of fact, there's lots of prioritizing on this page.

56. 4. Although all of the choices are important for preventing relapse, compliance with the medication regimen is central to the treatment of schizophrenia, a brain disease.

NP: Implementation; CN: Safe, effective care environment; CNS: Management of care; CL: Application

57. A client approaches the nurse and points at the sky, showing her where the men would be coming from to get him. Which of the following responses is most therapeutic?

1. "Why do you think the men are coming here?"
2. "You're safe here, we won't let them harm you."
3. "It seems like the world is pretty scary for you, but you're safe here."
4. "There are no bad men in the sky because no one lives that close to earth."

57. 3. This response acknowledges the client's fears, listens to his feelings, and offers a sense of security as the nurse tries to understand the concerns behind the symbolism. She reflects these concerns to the client, along with reassurance of safety. The first option validates the delusion, not the feelings and fears, and doesn't orient the client to reality. The second option gives false reassurance. Because the nurse isn't sure of the symbolism, she can't make this promise. The last option rejects the client's feelings and doesn't address the client's fears.

NP: Implementation; CN: Safe, effective care environment; CNS: Management of care; CL: Application

58. A client is brought to the crisis response center by his family. During evaluation, he reports being depressed for the last month and complains about voices constantly whispering to him. Which of the following diagnoses is the most likely?

1. Catatonic schizophrenia
2. Disorganized schizophrenia
3. Paranoid schizophrenia
4. Schizoaffective disorder

58. 4. A client with major depressive episode who begins to hear voices and at times thinks someone is after him is most likely schizoaffective. The client who repeats phrases and shows waxy flexibility or stupor with prominent grimaces is most likely catatonic. The client with disorganized speech and behavior and a flat or inappropriate affect most likely has disorganized schizophrenia. The client who expresses thoughts of people spying on him, attributes ulterior motives to others, and has a flat affect is most likely paranoid schizophrenic.

NP: Analysis; CN: Psychosocial integrity; CNS: Coping and adaptation; CL: Analysis

59. Which of the following nursing interventions is most appropriate for use with a client with paranoid schizophrenia?

1. Defend yourself when the client is verbally hostile toward you.
2. Provide a warm approach by touching the client.
3. Explain everything you're doing before you do it.
4. Clarify the content of the client's delusions.

59. 3. Explaining everything you do will prevent misinterpretation of your actions. A nondefensive stance provides an atmosphere in which the client's angry feelings can be explored. Touching the paranoid client should be avoided because it can be interpreted as threatening. The content of delusions should not be the focus of your care because the content is illogical.

NP: Planning; CN: Psychosocial integrity: CNS: Psychosocial adaptation: CL: Analysis

60. During an interview, a nurse expects which of the following conditions or actions from the client with a delusional disorder?

1. Bizarre behavior
2. Agitation
3. Impaired short-term memory
4. Apparently normal functioning

60. 4. The psychosocial functioning of the person with a delusional disorder may be relatively unimpaired. Another common characteristic of the client with a delusional disorder is the apparent normality of his behavior and appearance when his delusional ideas aren't being discussed or acted on. The client with delusional disorder doesn't have such symptoms as concrete thinking, bizarre or agitated behavior, and impaired memory, typical of a client with schizophrenia who functions at a lower level.

NP: Assessment; CN: Psychosocial integrity; CNS: Coping and adaptation; CL: Comprehension

61. A client is admitted to a psychiatric unit for a delusional disorder. He explains to a nurse that he made a contract with God to be the best minister on earth. Now that he has achieved the goal, most of his friends have stopped seeing him out of envy. On mental status examination, there is little impairment in psychosocial functioning. Which of the following conditions is expected?

1. Nonbizarre delusions
2. Fragmentary delusions
3. Regressive behavior
4. Regressive delusions

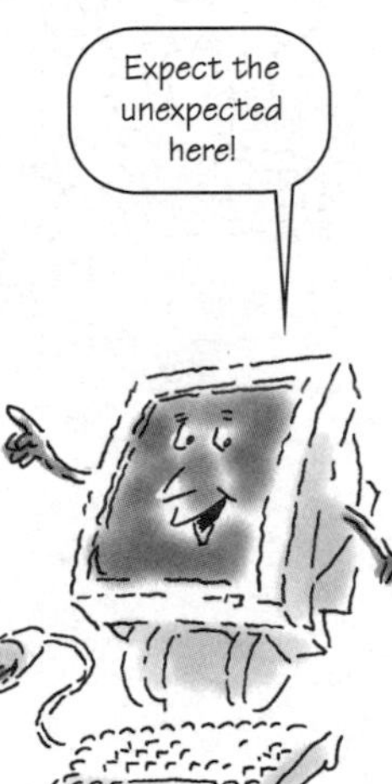
Expect the unexpected here!

61. 1. The essential feature of delusional disorder is the presence of one or more nonbizarre delusions that persist for at least 1 month. The most common delusions by subtypes are erotomanic, grandiose, jealousy, persecutory, and somatic. Bizarre delusions are patently absurd beliefs with absolutely no foundation in reality. Fragmentary delusions are unconnected delusions not organized around a coherent theme. Regressive behaviors revert back to a less mature state and aren't associated with a mental disorder.

NP: Assessment; CN: Psychosocial integrity; CNS: Coping and adaptation; CL: Comprehension

62. Low-potency psychotropic agents are likely to cause which of the following adverse reactions?

1. Akathisia
2. Dystonia
3. Sedation
4. Tardive dyskinesia

62. 3. Low-potency agents usually have a weak affinity for dopamine-2 receptors and cause sedation. Akathisia, dystonia, and tardive dyskinesia are more likely to be caused by high-potency psychotropic agents because more of the drug is needed for therapeutic effects, increasing the likelihood of these extrapyramidal symptoms.

NP: Analysis; CN: Physiological integrity; CNS: Pharmacological and parenteral therapies; CL: Knowledge

63. Thiothixene (Navane) is likely to cause which of the following adverse reactions?

1. Akinesia
2. Hypotension
3. Sedation
4. Weight gain

63. 1. Thiothixene is a high-potency agent with a high affinity for the dopamine-2 receptors, resulting in the increased likelihood of akinesia, a form of extrapyramidal symptoms. Although thiothixene targets other neurotransmitters responsible for hypotension, sedation, and weight gain, their affinity to these receptors is weak and more likely to occur with low-potency psychotropics.

NP: Analysis; CN: Physiological integrity; CNS: Pharmacological and parenteral therapies; CL: Knowledge

64. Inability to carry out daily responsibilities typically occurs during the prodromal phase of schizophrenia. Which of the following may also occur during this phase?

1. Increased energy and motivation
2. Increased social interaction
3. Impaired role functioning and neglect of personal hygiene
4. Heightened work performance

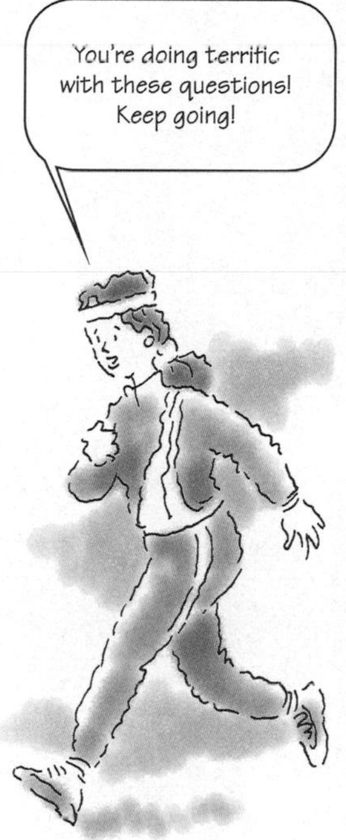

You're doing terrific
with these questions!
Keep going!

64. 3. Prodromal (early) signs and symptoms of schizophrenia can occur 1 month to 1 year before the first psychotic break and represent a clear deterioration in functioning. They may include impaired role functioning and neglect of personal hygiene as well as social withdrawal and depression. Increases in energy and social interaction and heightened work performance don't occur during the prodromal phase.

NP: Assessment; CN: Psychosocial integrity; CNS: Psychosocial adaptation; CL: Application

65. The daughter of a client with schizophrenia states, "I'm afraid I may develop this disease, too." The nurse should teach the client that schizophrenia is linked to which of the following?

1. Sexual abuse
2. A combination of genetic and other factors
3. Both parents having schizophrenia
4. Emotional trauma during childhood

65. 2. Experts believe schizophrenia results from a combination of genetic, environmental, and other factors—such as viruses, birth injuries, and nutritional factors. Schizophrenia incidence is higher among relatives of persons with the disease. It can occur even if both parents don't have schizophrenia. Emotional trauma during childhood hasn't been linked to schizophrenia.

NP: Analysis; CN: Psychosocial integrity; CNS: Psychosocial adaptation; CL: Application

66. A nurse teaches a class of caregivers about the positive and negative behaviors of schizophrenia. Positive behaviors include which of the following?

1. Limited spontaneous speech
2. Inability to initiate and persist in goal-directed activities
3. Misinterpretation of experiences and altered sensory input
4. Extremely brief replies to questions

66. 3. Positive behaviors of schizophrenia include attention-getting behaviors, which can result from misinterpretation of experiences and altered sensing input (such as hallucinations, delusions, and bizarre behavior). Negative behaviors are those that render the client inert and unmotivated, such as lack of spontaneous speech, poverty of thought, apathy, and poor social functioning.

NP: Assessment; CN: Psychosocial integrity; CNS: Psychosocial adaptation; CL: Application

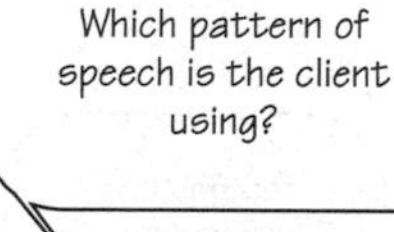

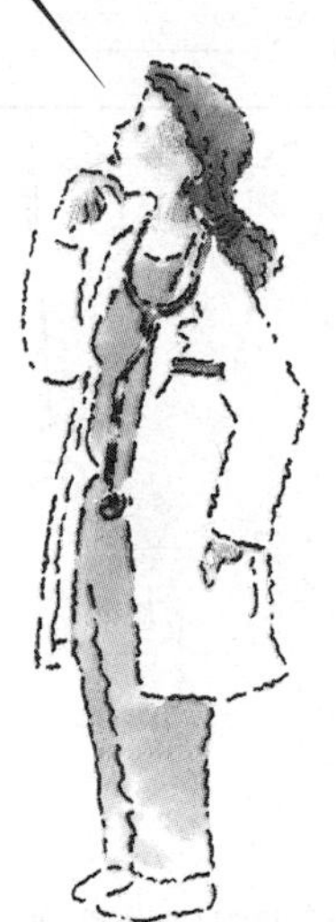

67. The nurse is facilitating a group of schizophrenic clients when one client says, "I like to drive my car, bar, tar, far." This pattern of speech is known as which of the following?

1. Clang association
2. Echolalia
3. Echopraxia
4. Neologisms

67. 1. Linking together words based on their sounds rather than their meanings is called clang association. Echolalia is the involuntary parrotlike repetition of words spoken by others. Echopraxia refers to meaningless imitation of others' motions. Neologisms are new words that a person invents.

NP: Assessment; CN: Psychosocial integrity; CNS: Psychosocial adaptation; CL: Application

68. A schizophrenic client who's receiving antipsychotic medication paces, fidgets, and can't seem to stay still. The nurse recognizes these behaviors as which of the following?

1. Tardive dyskinesia
2. Dystonia
3. Akathisia
4. Akinesia

68. 3. Akathisia is an extrapyramidal adverse effect of some antipsychotic medications, manifested by restlessness and an inability to stay still. Tardive dyskinesia refers to involuntary abnormal movements of the mouth, tongue, face, and jaw. Dystonia refers to difficulty with movement. Akinesia is absence of movement.

NP: Assessment; CN: Physiological integrity; CNS: Pharmacological and parenteral therapies; CL: Analysis

69. Which nursing diagnosis is most appropriate for a client diagnosed with schizophrenia, disorganized type?

1. Self-care deficit
2. Disturbed sleep pattern
3. Impaired verbal communication
4. Social isolation

69. 3. Schizophrenia, disorganized type, is characterized by disorganized speech, disorganized behavior, and inappropriate or flat affect. Self-care deficit, disturbed sleep pattern, and social isolation aren't classic manifestations of this type of schizophrenia.

NP: Analysis; CN: Psychosocial integrity; CNS: Psychosocial adaptation; CL: Analysis

70. A client with paranoid schizophrenia tells the nurse that two people talking in the hall are planning to kidnap and kill him. The client's thought pattern reflects which of the following?

1. Auditory hallucinations
2. Delusions of grandeur
3. Ideas of reference
4. Echolalia

70. 3. A client with ideas of reference mistakenly believes that other people's thoughts, speech, and behaviors refer to the client. Auditory hallucinations are sounds that aren't based in reality. Delusions of grandeur are false beliefs that arise without appropriate external stimuli. Echolalia refers to involuntary repetition of words spoken by others.

NP: Assessment; CN: Psychosocial integrity; CNS: Psychosocial adaptation; CL: Application

71. A client with paranoid schizophrenia states that the nurses are conspiring to kill him. The client perceives the environment as which of the following?

1. Dangerous
2. Supportive
3. Disorganized
4. Bizarre

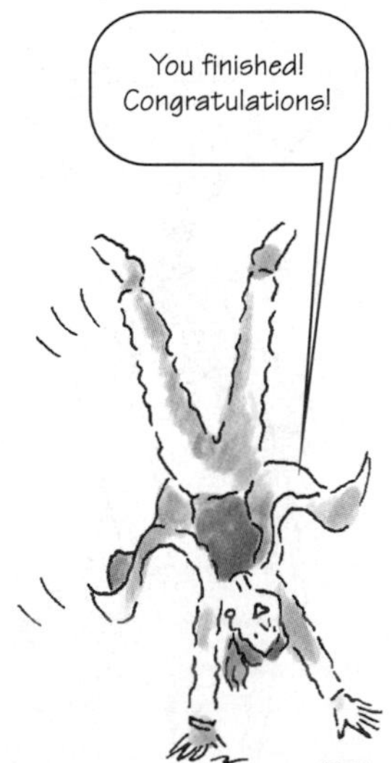
You finished!
Congratulations!

71. 1. This client perceives the environment as dangerous or one in which he is directly threatened. Although a perception that the environment is disorganized or bizarre wouldn't lead the client to believe there's a conspiracy to kill him, it wouldn't foster safety and security. A supportive environment is perceived as nonthreatening and nurturing.

NP: Assessment; CN: Psychosocial integrity; CNS: Psychosocial adaptation; CL: Application

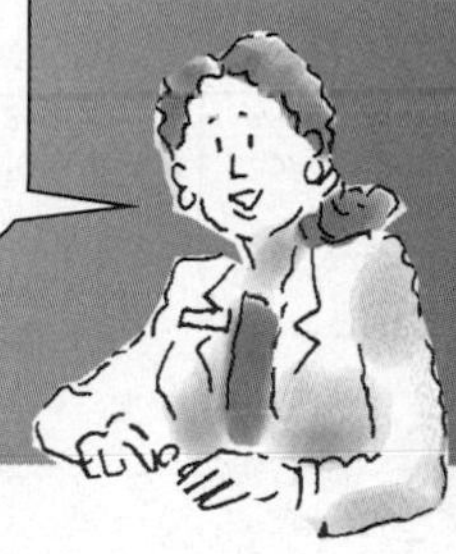

About the only substance of
abuse this chapter doesn't cover
is my personal weakness —
chocolate mousse! Think of me as
you work through this chapter. I'll
be the one with chocolate
smudges on her fingers. Tee-hee!

Chapter 18 Substance abuse disorders

1. Family members of a client who abuses alcohol asks a nurse to help them intervene. Which of the following actions is essential for a successful intervention?

1. All family members must tell the client they're powerless.
2. All family members must describe how the addiction affects them.
3. All family members must come up with their share of financial support.
4. All family members must become caregivers during the detoxification period.

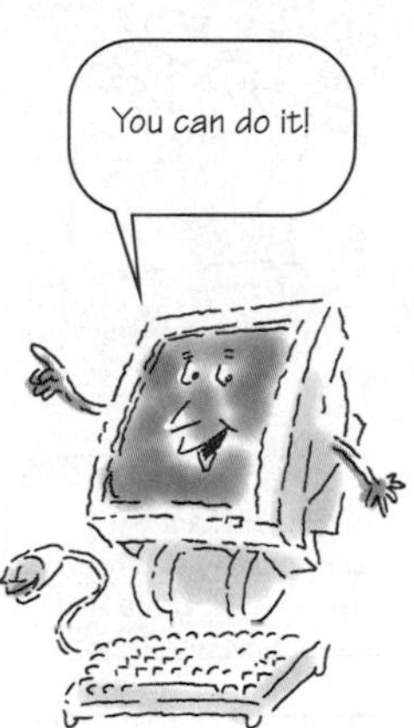

You can do it!

1. 2. After the family is taught about addiction, they must write down examples of how the addiction has affected each of them and use this information during the intervention. It isn't necessary to tell the client the family is powerless. The family is empowered through this intervention experience. In many cases, a third-party payer will help with treatment costs. Doing an intervention doesn't make family members responsible for financial support or providing care and support during the detoxification period.

NP: Implementation; CN: Psychosocial integrity; CNS: Psychosocial adaptation; CL: Analysis

2. A client who abuses alcohol tells a nurse, "I'm sure I can become a social drinker." Which of the following responses is most appropriate?

1. "When do you think you can become a social drinker?"
2. "What makes you think you'll learn to drink normally?"
3. "Does your alcohol use cause major problems in your life?"
4. "How many alcoholic beverages can a social drinker consume?"

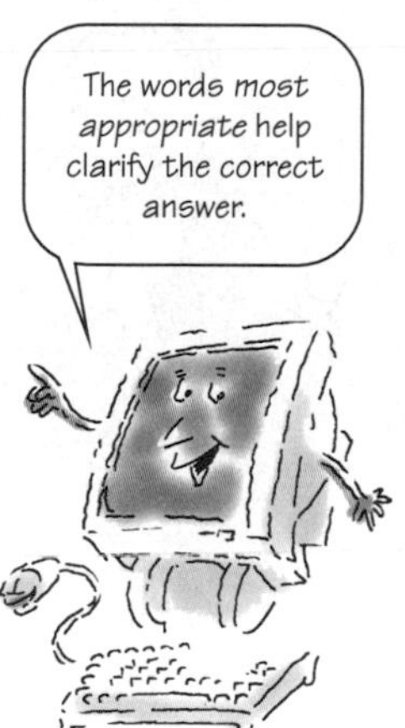

The words *most appropriate* help
clarify the correct
answer.

2. 3. This question may help the client recall the problematic results of using alcohol and the reasons the client began treatment. Asking when he believes he can become a social drinker will only encourage the addicted person to deny the problem and develop an unrealistic, self-defeating goal. Asking how many alcoholic beverages a social drinker can consume and why the client thinks he can drink normally will encourage the addicted person to defend himself and deny the problem.

NP: Implementation; CN: Psychosocial integrity; CNS: Psychosocial adaptation; CL: Application

3. A client asks a nurse not to tell his parents about his alcohol problem. Which of the following responses is most appropriate?

1. "How can you not tell them? Is that being honest?"
2. "Don't you think you'll need to tell them someday?"
3. "Do alcohol problems run in either side of your family?"
4. "What do you think will happen if you tell your parents?"

3. 4. Clients who struggle with addiction problems often believe people will be judgmental, rejecting, and uncaring if they are told that the client is recovering from alcohol abuse. The first option challenges the client and will put him on the defensive. The second option will make the client defensive and construct rationalizations as to why his parents don't need to know. The third option is a good assessment question, but it isn't an appropriate question to ask a client who's afraid to tell others about his addiction.

NP: Implementation; CN: Psychosocial integrity; CNS: Psychosocial adaptation; CL: Analysis

NP: Nursing process CN: Client needs category CNS: Client needs subcategory CL: Cognitive level

4. A nurse assesses a client for signs of alcohol withdrawal. During the period of early withdrawal, which of the following findings are expected?

1. Depression
2. Hyperactivity
3. Insomnia
4. Nausea

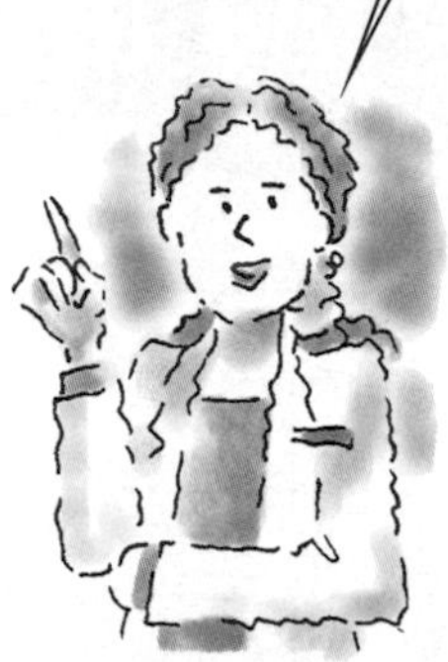

A disease can have many stages, each with its own symptoms.

4. 4. Nausea and, later, vomiting are early signs of alcohol withdrawal. Depression, hyperactivity, and insomnia aren't associated with early alcohol withdrawal.

NP: Assessment; CN: Psychosocial integrity; CNS: Coping and adaptation; CL: Knowledge

5. Which of the following health findings is expected in a client who chronically abuses alcohol?

1. Enlarged liver
2. Nasal irritation
3. Muscle wasting
4. Limb paresthesia

5. 1. A major effect of alcohol on the body is liver impairment, and an enlarged liver is a common physical finding. Nasal irritation is commonly seen with clients who snort cocaine. Muscle wasting and limb paresthesia don't tend to occur with clients who abuse alcohol.

NP: Assessment; CN: Psychosocial integrity; CNS: Coping and adaptation; CL: Knowledge

6. A client with an alcohol problem starts to talk to a nurse about wanting a drink. Which of the following terms best describes what this client is experiencing?

1. Craving
2. Potentiation
3. Recidivism
4. Tolerance

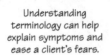

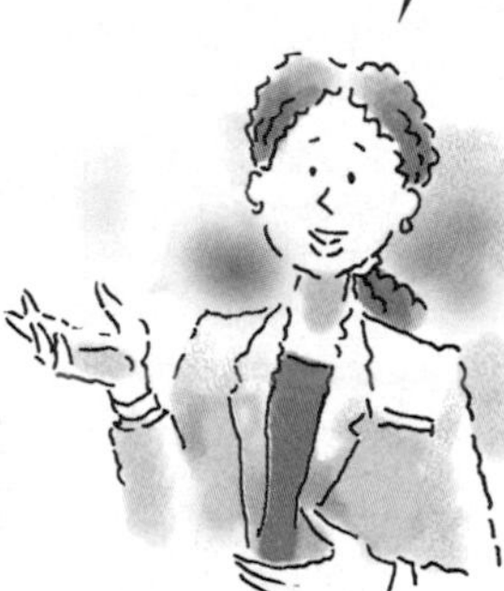

Understanding terminology can help explain symptoms and ease a client's fears.

6. 1. Craving is the strong, overwhelming urge to have the drink. Drug potentiation is the tendency for one drug to increase the activity of another drug. Recidivism is the tendency to relapse. Tolerance occurs when the client needs to drink increasing amounts to achieve the same effects.

NP: Analysis; CN: Psychosocial integrity; CNS: Coping and adaptation; CL: Knowledge

7. A client who abuses alcohol tells a nurse, "Alcohol helps me sleep." Which of the following information about alcohol use and sleep is most accurate?

1. Alcohol doesn't help promote sleep.
2. Continued alcohol use causes insomnia.
3. One glass of alcohol at dinnertime can induce sleep.
4. Sometimes alcohol can make one drowsy enough to fall asleep.

7. 1. Alcohol use may initially promote sleep, but with continued use, it causes insomnia. Evidence shows that alcohol doesn't facilitate sleep. One glass of alcohol at dinnertime won't induce sleep. The last option doesn't give information about how alcohol affects sleep. It makes the client think alcohol use to induce sleep is an appropriate strategy to try.

NP: Assessment; CN: Psychosocial integrity; CNS: Psychosocial adaptation; CL: Analysis

8. A family expresses concern when a family member withdrawing from alcohol is given lorazepam (Ativan). Which of the following information should be given to the family about the medication?

1. The medication promotes a sense of well-being during the client's difficult withdrawal period.
2. The medication is given for a short time to help the client complete the withdrawal process.
3. The medication will help the client forget about the physical sensations that go with alcohol withdrawal.
4. The medication helps in the treatment of coexisting diseases, such as cardiac problems and hypertension.

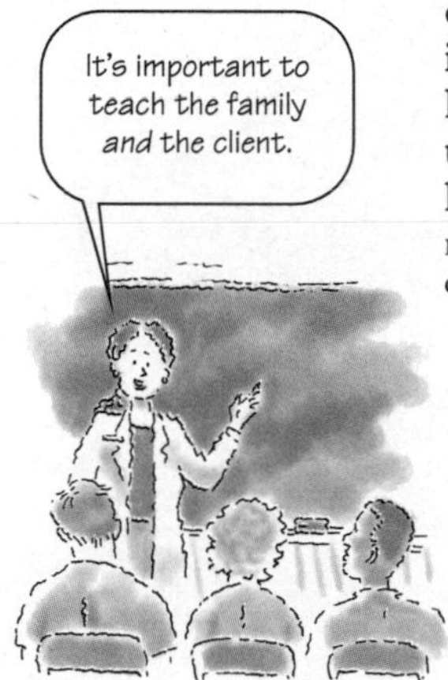
It's important to teach the family and the client.

8. 2. Lorazepam is a short-acting benzodiazepine usually given for 1 week to help the client in alcohol withdrawal. The medication isn't given to help forget the experience; it lessens the symptoms of withdrawal. It isn't used to treat coexisting cardiovascular problems or promote a sense of well-being.

NP: Implementation; CN: Psychosocial integrity; CNS: Psychosocial adaptation; CL: Comprehension

9. A client who abuses alcohol tells a nurse everyone in his family has an alcohol problem and nothing can be done about it. Which of the following responses is the most appropriate?

1. "You're right, it's much harder to become a recovering person."
2. "This is just an excuse for you so you don't have to work on becoming sober."
3. "Sometimes nothing can be done, but you may be the exception in this family."
4. "Alcohol problems can occur in families, but you can decide to take the steps to become and stay sober."

9. 4. This statement challenges the client to become proactive and take the steps necessary to maintain a sober lifestyle. The first option agrees with the client's denial and isn't a useful response. The second option confronts the client and may make him more adamant in defense of this position. The third option agrees with the client's denial and isn't a useful response.

NP: Implementation; CN: Psychosocial integrity; CNS: Psychosocial adaptation; CL: Application

10. Which of the following major cardiovascular problems may occur in a client with chronic alcoholism?

1. Arteriosclerosis
2. Heart failure
3. Heart valve damage
4. Pericarditis

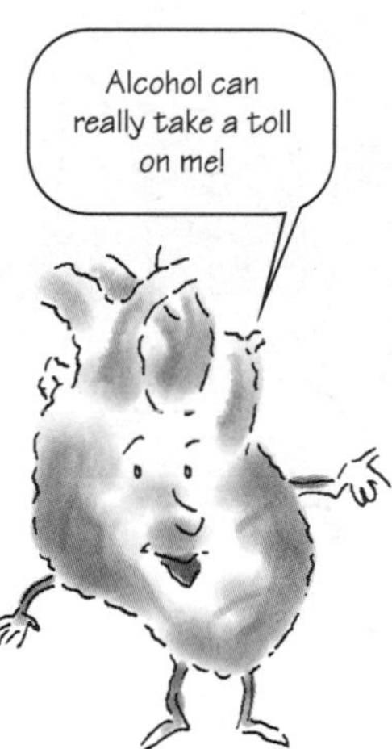
Alcohol can really take a toll on me!

10. 2. Heart failure is a severe cardiac consequence associated with long-term alcohol use. Arteriosclerosis, heart valve damage, and pericarditis aren't medical consequences of alcoholism.

NP: Analysis; CN: Psychosocial integrity; CNS: Coping and adaptation; CL: Knowledge

11. Which of the following assessment findings is commonly associated with the abuse of alcohol in a young, depressed adult woman?

1. Defiant responses
2. Infertility
3. Memory loss
4. Sexual abuse

11. 4. Many women diagnosed with substance abuse problems also have a history of physical or sexual abuse. Alcohol abuse isn't a common finding in a young woman showing defiant behavior or experiencing infertility. Memory loss isn't a common finding in a young woman experiencing alcohol abuse.

NP: Assessment; CN: Psychosocial integrity; CNS: Coping and adaptation; CL: Analysis

12. A nurse determines that a client who abused alcohol has nutritional problems. Which of the following strategies is best for addressing the client's nutritional needs?

1. Encourage the client to eat a diet high in calories.
2. Help the client recognize and follow a balanced diet.
3. Have the client drink liquid protein supplements daily.
4. Have the client monitor the calories consumed each day.

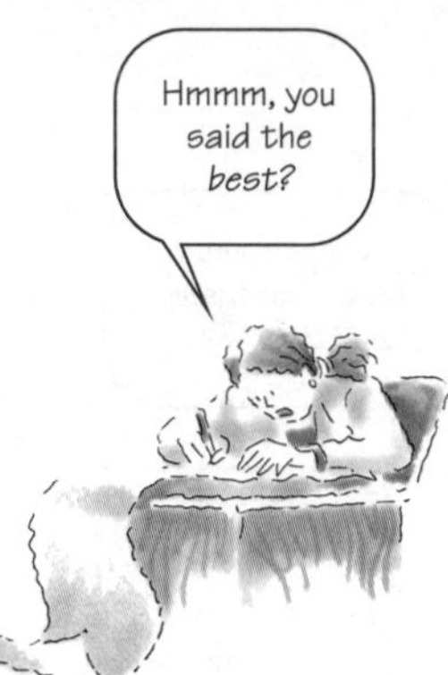

12. 2. Clients who abuse alcohol are often malnourished and need help to follow a balanced diet. Increasing calories may cause the client to just eat empty calories. Having the client monitor calorie intake could be done only after the client recognizes the need to maintain a balanced diet. Calorie counts usually aren't needed in most recovering clients who begin to eat from the basic food groups. The client must be involved in the decision to supplement the daily dietary intake. The nurse can't force the client to drink liquid protein supplements.

NP: Planning; CN: Psychosocial integrity; CNS: Psychosocial adaptation; CL: Comprehension

13. A client with a history of alcohol abuse refuses to take vitamins. Which of the following statements is most appropriate for explaining why vitamins are important?

1. "It's important to take vitamins to stop your craving."
2. "Prolonged use of alcohol can cause vitamin depletion."
3. "For every vitamin you take, you'll help your liver heal."
4. "By taking vitamins, you don't need to worry about your diet."

13. 2. Chronic alcoholism interferes with the metabolism of many vitamins. Vitamin supplements can prevent deficiencies from occurring. Taking vitamins won't stop a person from craving alcohol or help a damaged liver heal. A balanced diet is *essential* in addition to taking multivitamins.

NP: Implementation; CN: Psychosocial integrity; CNS: Psychosocial adaptation; CL: Application

14. Which of the following behaviors in a client who abuses alcohol indicates a knowledge deficit in nutrition?

1. Avoiding foods high in fat
2. Eating only one adequate meal each day
3. Taking vitamin and mineral supplements
4. Eating large portions of foods containing fiber

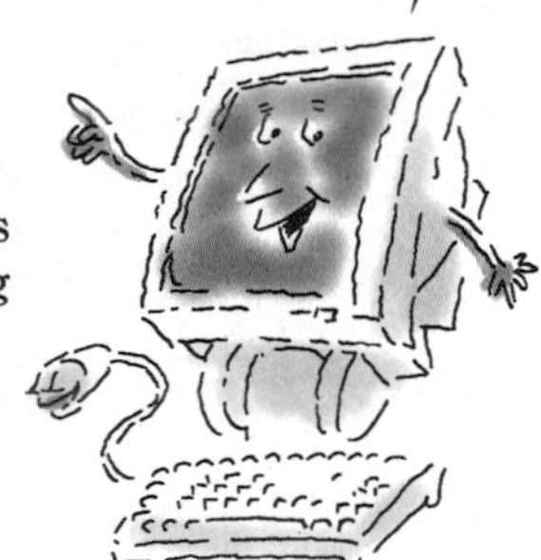

Careful! The word deficit almost makes this a negative question.

14. 2. If the client eats only one adequate meal each day, there will be a deficit of essential nutrients. It's appropriate for the client to take vitamin and mineral supplements to prevent deficiency in these nutrients. Avoiding foods high in fat content and consuming large portions of foods containing fiber indicate the client has good knowledge about nutrition.

NP: Assessment; CN: Psychosocial integrity; CNS: Coping and adaptation; CL: Knowledge

15. A client tells a nurse, "I've been drinking ever since they told me I had learning disabilities." Which of the following rationales does this client's statement indicate?

1. The client is self-medicating.
2. The client has an excuse to drink.
3. The client isn't a productive person.
4. The client will be unable to stop drinking.

15. 1. A client with learning disabilities may experience frustration, depression, or overall feelings of low self-esteem and may self-medicate with alcohol. Many people with learning disabilities don't resort to alcohol but develop other coping skills to handle the disability. People with learning disabilities can be very productive. A person with a learning disability can successfully recover from alcohol addiction.

NP: Analysis; CN: Psychosocial integrity; CNS: Coping and adaptation; CL: Application

16. A nurse is assessing a client who has been actively abusing alcohol for 20 years. Which of the following conditions might be seen during the assessment?

1. Agitated behavior
2. Paranoid thoughts
3. Ritualistic behaviors
4. Cognitive impairment

16. 4. A long-term effect of alcohol is cognitive impairment. Agitated behavior occurs when the client is withdrawing from alcohol, not during active use. Paranoid thoughts and ritualistic behaviors aren't typically seen in a client actively abusing alcohol.

NP: Assessment; CN: Psychosocial integrity; CNS: Coping and adaptation; CL: Comprehension

17. A nurse has a meeting with a family of a recovering client. The client tells a family member, "You made it easy for me to use alcohol. You always made excuses for my behavior." Which of the following important issues should the family be encouraged to address?

1. Giving up enabling behaviors
2. Managing the client's self-care
3. Dealing with negative behaviors
4. Evaluating the home environment

17. 1. Enabling the behaviors of family members allows the client to continue the addiction by rationalizing, denying, or otherwise excusing the problem. Managing the client's self-care isn't an issue that needs to be addressed based on the client's statement. Dealing with negative behaviors and evaluating the home environment don't address the client's statement about the family's enabling behavior.

NP: Implementation; CN: Psychosocial integrity; CNS: Psychosocial adaptation; CL: Comprehension

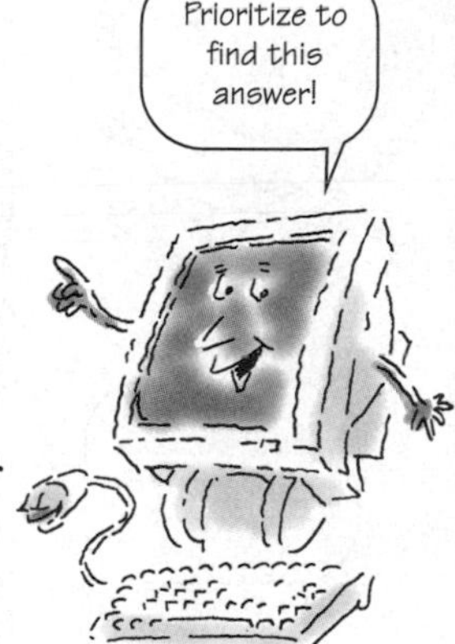

Prioritize to find this answer!

18. Which of the following short-term goals should be a priority for a client with a knowledge deficit about the effects of alcohol on the body?

1. Test blood chemistries daily.
2. Verbalize the results of substance use.
3. Talk to a pharmacist about the substance.
4. Attend a weekly aerobic exercise program.

18. 2. It's important for the client to talk about the health consequences of the continued use of alcohol. Testing blood chemistries daily gives the client minimal knowledge about the effects of alcohol on the body and isn't the most useful information in a teaching plan. A pharmacist isn't the appropriate health care professional to educate the client about the effects of alcohol use on the body. Although exercise is an important goal of self-care, it doesn't address the client's knowledge deficit about the effects of alcohol on the body.

NP: Analysis; CN: Psychosocial integrity; CNS: Psychosocial adaptation; CL: Application

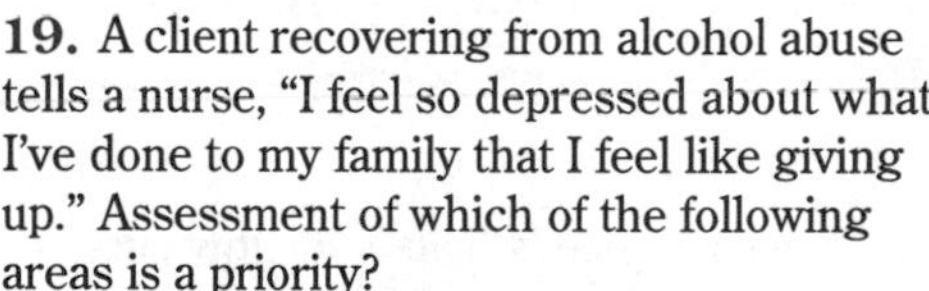

19. A client recovering from alcohol abuse tells a nurse, "I feel so depressed about what I've done to my family that I feel like giving up." Assessment of which of the following areas is a priority?

1. Family support
2. A plan for self-harm
3. A sponsor for the client
4. Other ambivalent feelings

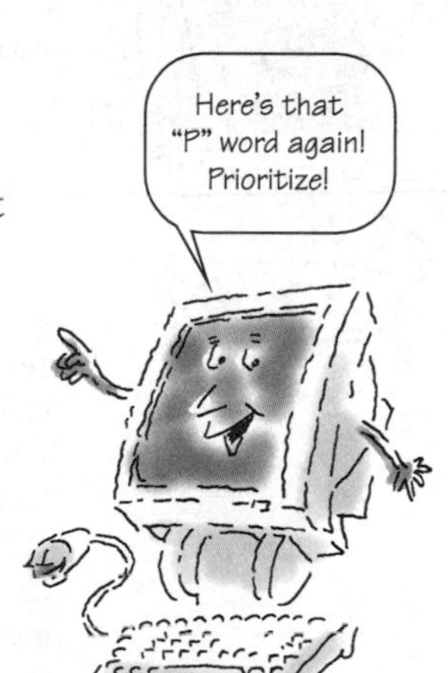

Here's that "P" word again! Prioritize!

19. 2. When a client talks about giving up, the nurse must explore the potential for suicidal behavior. Although questioning the client about family support, the availability of a sponsor, or ambivalent feelings are important, the priority action is to assess for suicide.

NP: Analysis; CN: Psychosocial integrity; CNS: Psychosocial adaptation; CL: Application

20. A client withdrawing from alcohol says he's worried about periodic hallucinations. Which of the following interventions is best for this client's problem?

1. Point out that the sensation doesn't exist.
2. Allow the client to talk about the experience.
3. Encourage the client to wash the body areas well.
4. Determine if the client has a cognitive impairment.

20. 2. The client needs to talk about the periodic hallucinations to prevent them from becoming triggers to acting out behaviors and possible self-injury. The client's experience of sensory-perceptual alterations must be acknowledged; therefore, denying that the client's hallucinations exist isn't a helpful strategy. Determining if the client has a cognitive impairment and encouraging the client to wash the body areas well don't address the problem of periodic hallucinations.

NP: Implementation; CN: Psychosocial integrity; CNS: Psychosocial adaptation; CL: Application

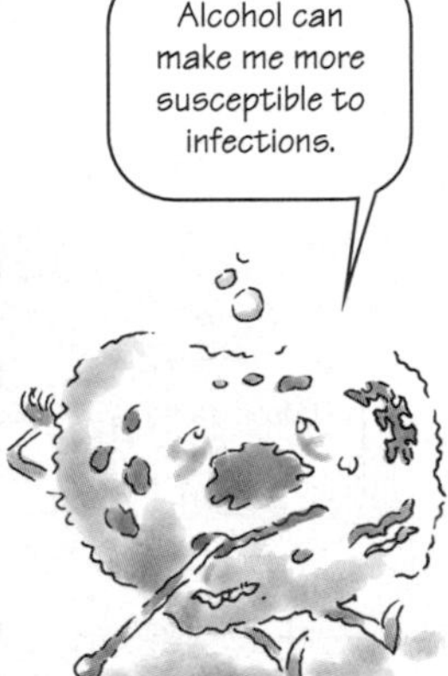

Alcohol can make me more susceptible to infections.

21. A client who has been drinking alcohol for 30 years asks a nurse if permanent damage has occurred to the immune system. Which of the following responses is the best?

1. "There is often less resistance to infections."
2. "Sometimes the body's metabolism will increase."
3. "Put your energies into maintaining sobriety for now."
4. "Drinking puts you at high risk for disease later in life."

21. 1. Chronic alcohol use depresses the immune system and causes increased susceptibility to infections. A nutritionally well-balanced diet that includes foods high in protein and B vitamins will help develop a strong immune system. The potential damage to the immune system doesn't increase the body's metabolism. Drinking alcohol may put the client at risk for immune system problems at any time in life. The third option negates the client's concern and isn't an appropriate or caring response.

NP: Implementation; CN: Psychosocial integrity; CNS: Psychosocial adaptation; CL: Analysis

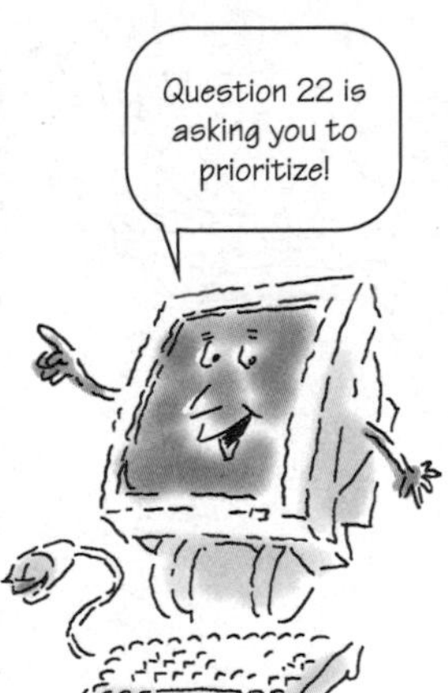

Question 22 is asking you to prioritize!

22. A client experiencing alcohol withdrawal is upset about going through detoxification. Which of the following goals is a priority?

1. The client will commit to a drug-free lifestyle.
2. The client will work with the nurse to remain safe.
3. The client will drink plenty of fluids on a daily basis.
4. The client will make a personal inventory of strengths.

22. 2. The priority goal is for client safety. Although drinking enough fluids, identifying personal strengths, and committing to a drug-free lifestyle are important goals, the nurse's first priority must be to promote client safety.

NP: Planning; CN: Psychosocial integrity; CNS: Psychosocial adaptation; CL: Comprehension

23. A client recovering from alcohol abuse needs to develop effective coping skills to handle daily stressors. Which of the following interventions is most useful to the client?

1. Determine the client's level of verbal skills.
2. Help the client avoid areas that cause conflict.
3. Discuss examples of successful coping behavior.
4. Teach the client to accept uncomfortable situations.

23. 3. The client needs help to identify successful coping behavior and develop ways to incorporate that behavior into daily functioning. There are many skills for coping with stress, and determining the client's level of verbal skills may not be important. Encouraging the client to avoid conflict prevents him from learning skills to handle daily stressors.

NP: Implementation; CN: Psychosocial integrity; CNS: Psychosocial adaptation; CL: Analysis

24. A client is struggling with alcohol dependence. Which of the following communication strategies would be most effective?

1. Speak briefly and directly.
2. Avoid blaming or preaching to the client.
3. Confront feelings and examples of perfectionism.
4. Determine if nonverbal communication will be more effective.

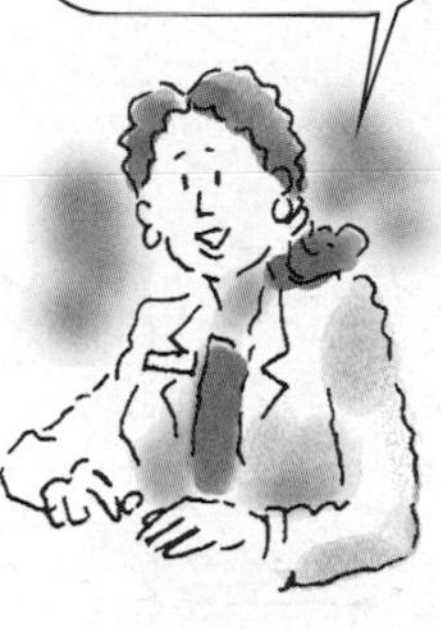
Effective communication helps in all areas of recovery.

24. 2. Blaming or preaching to the client causes negativity and prevents the client from hearing what the nurse has to say. Speaking briefly to the client may not allow time for adequate communication. Perfectionism doesn't tend to be an issue. Determining if nonverbal communication will be more effective is better suited for a client with cognitive impairment.

NP: Implementation; CN: Psychosocial integrity; CNS: Psychosocial adaptation; CL: Analysis

25. A nurse is working with a client on recognizing the relationship between alcohol abuse and interpersonal problems. Which of the following interventions has priority?

1. Help the client identify personal strengths.
2. Help the client decrease compulsive behaviors.
3. Examine the client's use of defense mechanisms.
4. Have the client work with peers who can serve as role models.

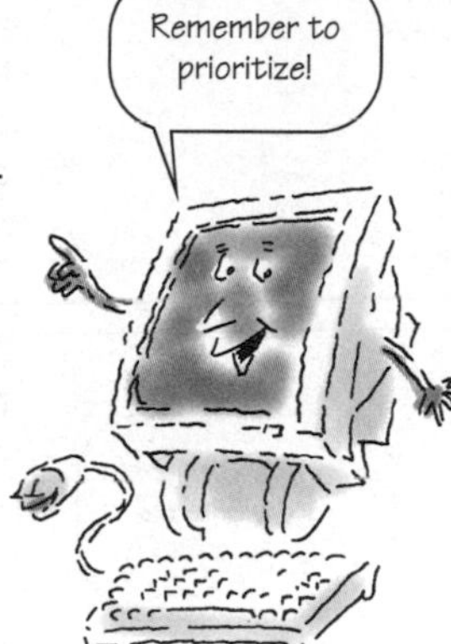
Remember to prioritize!

25. 3. Defense mechanisms can impede the development of healthy relationships and cause the client pain. After identifying barriers to relationship problems, it would be appropriate to identify or clarify personal strengths. Compulsive behavior doesn't tend to be a problem for alcoholic clients who struggle with interpersonal problems. Working with peers who are role models would be useful after the client recognizes and gains some insight into the problems. It isn't the priority intervention.

NP: Implementation; CN: Psychosocial integrity; CNS: Psychosocial adaptation; CL: Analysis

26. A client recovering from alcohol addiction has limited coping skills. Which of the following characteristics would indicate relationship problems?

1. The client is prone to panic attacks.
2. The client doesn't pay attention to details.
3. The client has poor problem-solving skills.
4. The client ignores the need to relax and rest.

26. 3. To have satisfying relationships, a person must be able to communicate and problem solve. Relationship problems don't predispose people to panic attacks more than other psychosocial stressors. Paying attention to details isn't a major concern when addressing the client's relationship difficulties. Although ignoring the need for rest and relaxation is unhealthy, it shouldn't pose a major relationship problem.

NP: Analysis; CN: Psychosocial integrity; CNS: Coping and adaptation; CL: Analysis

27. A nurse suggests to a client struggling with alcohol addiction that keeping a journal may be helpful. Which of the following reasons best explains this?

1. The client can identify stressors and responses to them.
2. The client will be better able to understand the diagnosis.
3. The client can help others by reading the journal to them.
4. The client will develop an emergency plan for use in a crisis.

27. 1. Keeping a journal enables the client to identify problems and patterns of coping. From this information, the difficulties the client faces can be addressed. A journal isn't necessarily kept to promote better understanding of the client's illness, but it helps the client understand himself better. Journals aren't read to other people unless the client wants to share a particular part. Journals aren't typically used for identifying an emergency plan for use in a crisis.

NP: Planning; CN: Psychosocial integrity; CNS: Coping and adaptation; CL: Application

28. Which of the following information is most important to use in a teaching plan for a client who abused alcohol?

1. Personal needs
2. Illness exacerbation
3. Cognitive distortions
4. Communication skills

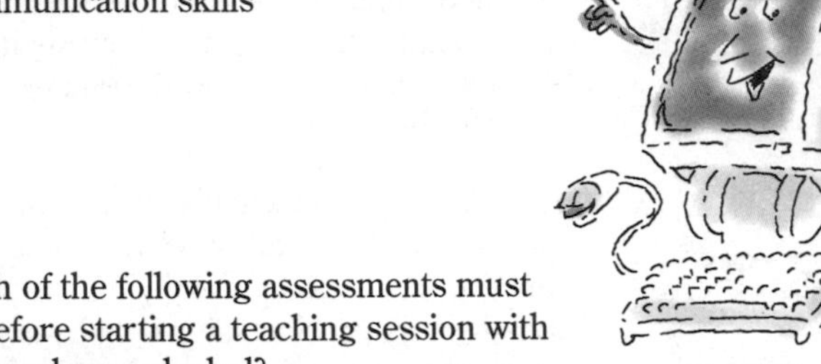
Prioritize!

28. 4. Addicted clients often have difficulty communicating their needs in an appropriate way. Learning appropriate communication skills is a major goal of treatment. Next, behavior that focuses on the self and meeting personal needs will be addressed. The identification of cognitive distortions would be difficult if the client has poor communication skills. Teaching about illness exacerbation isn't a skill, but it is essential for relaying information about relapse.
NP: Planning; CN: Psychosocial integrity; CNS: Psychosocial adaptation; CL: Analysis

29. Which of the following assessments must be done before starting a teaching session with a client who abuses alcohol?

1. Sleep patterns
2. Decision making
3. Note-taking skills
4. Readiness to learn

29. 4. It's important to know if the client's current situation helps or hinders the potential to learn. Decision making and sleep patterns aren't factors that must be assessed before teaching about addiction. Note-taking skills aren't a factor in determining whether the client will be receptive to teaching.
NP: Assessment; CN: Psychosocial integrity; CNS: Coping and adaptation; CL: Knowledge

30. A nurse is developing strategies to prevent relapse with a client who abuses alcohol. Which of the following client interventions is important?

1. Avoid taking over-the-counter medications.
2. Limit monthly contact with the family of origin.
3. Refrain from becoming involved in group activities.
4. Avoid people, places, and activities from the former lifestyle.

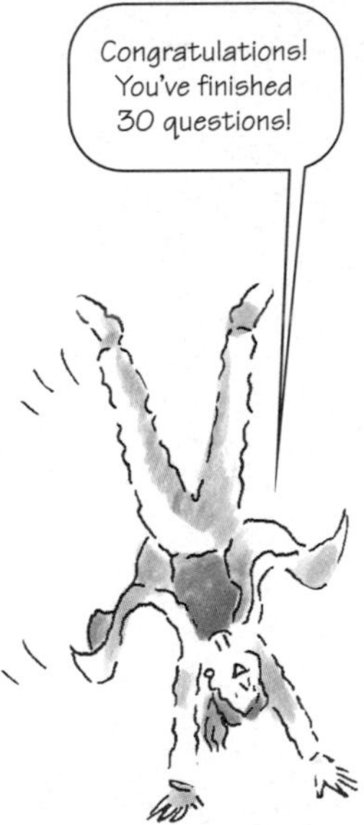
Congratulations!
You've finished
30 questions!

30. 4. Changing the client's old habits is essential for sustaining a sober lifestyle. Certain over-the-counter medications that don't contain alcohol will probably need to be used by the client at certain times. It's unrealistic to have the client abstain from all such medications. Contact with the client's family of origin may not be a trigger to relapse, so limiting contact wouldn't be useful. Refraining from group activities isn't a good strategy to prevent relapse. Going to Alcoholics Anonymous and other support groups will help prevent relapse.
NP: Implementation; CN: Psychosocial integrity; CNS: Psychosocial adaptation; CL: Analysis

31. A client recovering from alcohol abuse tells the nurse, "I get nothing out of Alcoholics Anonymous (AA) meetings." Which of the following responses is most appropriate?

1. "What were you told about going to AA meetings?"
2. "What do you want to get out of the AA meetings?"
3. "When do you think you'll stop going to the meetings?"
4. "Do you think you can control what happens in a meeting?"

31. 2. This response puts some of the responsibility for staying sober on the client and encourages the client to take a more active role. Asking what the client was told about AA meetings opens up a discussion that allows the client to continue to discuss disappointments rather than taking a proactive stand to support the value of AA meetings. The third option condones the client's desire to stop going to the meetings. The fourth option changes the issue from being responsible for staying sober to focusing on what the client can't control.
NP: Implementation; CN: Psychosocial integrity; CNS: Psychosocial adaptation; CL: Analysis

32. A client asks a nurse, "Why does it matter if I talk to my peers in group therapy?" Which of the following responses is most appropriate?
1. "Group therapy lets you see what you're doing wrong in your life."
2. "Group therapy acts as a defense against your disorganized behavior."
3. "Group therapy provides a way to ask for support as well as to support others."
4. "In group therapy, you can vent your frustrations and others will listen."

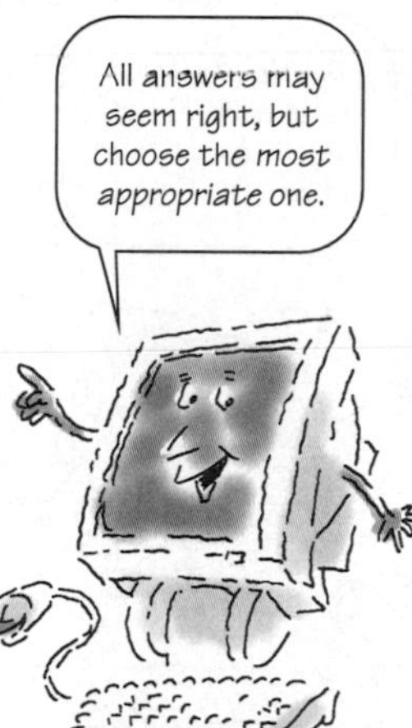

All answers may seem right, but choose the most appropriate one.

32. 3. The best response addresses how group therapy provides opportunities to communicate, learn, and give and get support. Group members will give a client feedback, not just point out what a client is doing wrong. Group therapy isn't a defense against disorganized behavior. People can express all kinds of feelings and discuss a variety of topics in group therapy. Interactions are goal oriented and not just vehicles to vent one's frustrations.

NP: Implementation; CN: Psychosocial integrity; CNS: Psychosocial adaptation; CL: Application

33. A family meeting is held with a client who abuses alcohol. While listening to the family, which of the following unhealthy communication patterns might be identified?
1. Use of descriptive jargon
2. Disapproval of behaviors
3. Avoidance of conflicting issues
4. Unlimited expression of nonverbal communication

33. 3. The interaction pattern of a family with a member who abuses alcohol often revolves around denying the problem, avoiding conflict, or rationalizing the addiction. Health care providers are more likely to use jargon. The family might have problems setting limits and expressing disapproval of the client's behavior. Nonverbal communication often gives the nurse insight into family dynamics.

NP: Analysis; CN: Psychosocial integrity; CNS: Psychosocial adaptation; CL: Analysis

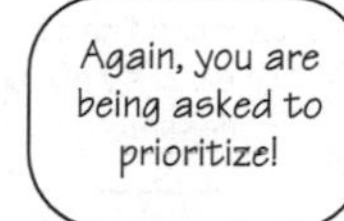

Again, you are being asked to prioritize!

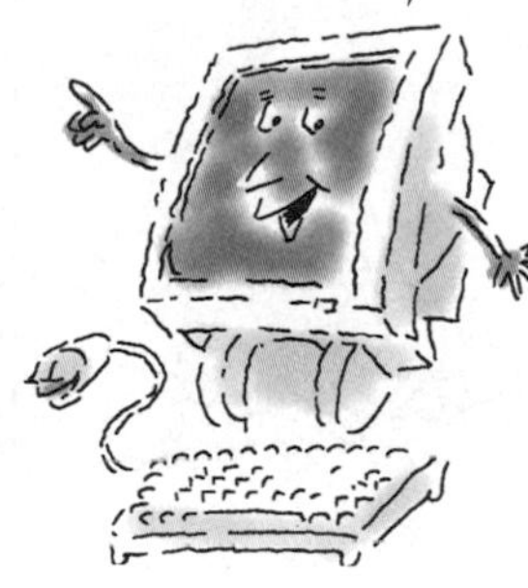

34. A client addicted to alcohol begins individual therapy with a nurse. Which of the following interventions should be a priority?
1. Learn to express feelings.
2. Establish new roles in the family.
3. Determine strategies for socializing.
4. Decrease preoccupation with physical health.

34. 1. The client must address issues, learn ways to cope effectively with life stressors, and express his needs appropriately. After the client establishes sobriety, the possibility of taking on new roles can become a reality. Determining strategies for socializing isn't the priority intervention for an addicted client. Usually, these clients need to change former socializing habits. Clients addicted to alcohol don't tend to be preoccupied with physical health problems.

NP: Implementation; CN: Psychosocial integrity; CNS: Psychosocial adaptation; CL: Comprehension

35. A client recovering from alcohol addiction asks a nurse how to talk to his children about the impact of his addiction on them. Which of the following responses is most appropriate?
1. "Try to limit references to the addiction, and focus on the present."
2. "Talk about all the hardships you've had in working to remain sober."
3. "Tell them you're sorry, and emphasize that you're doing so much better now."
4. "Talk to them by acknowledging the difficulties and pain your drinking caused."

35. 4. Part of the healing process for the family is to acknowledge the pain, embarrassment, and overall difficulties the client's drinking problem caused family members. The first option facilitates the client's ability to deny the problem. The second prevents the client from acknowledging the difficulties the children endured. The third leads the client to believe only a simple apology is needed. The addiction must be addressed and the children's pain acknowledged.

NP: Implementation; CN: Psychosocial integrity; CNS: Psychosocial adaptation; CL: Comprehension

36. A client with a diagnosis of alcohol dependency is being discharged from the hospital. Which of the following major goals will the client address in outpatient therapy?

1. Find a way to drink socially.
2. Allow self to grieve recent losses.
3. Work to bring others into treatment.
4. Develop relapse prevention strategies.

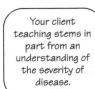

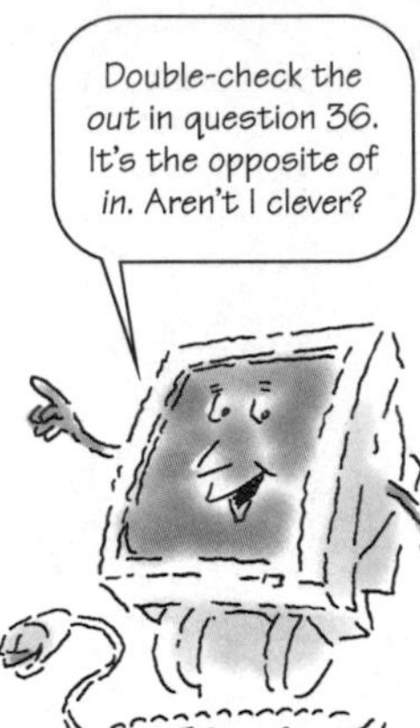

Double-check the out in question 36. It's the opposite of in. Aren't I clever?

36. 4. The primary goal for a client in outpatient treatment is to focus on strategies that prevent relapse. Finding ways to drink socially and working to bring others into treatment aren't goals of outpatient therapy. Allowing self to grieve the losses the addiction caused is a part of the early work of inpatient therapy and may be continued in outpatient therapy.

NP: Analysis; CN: Psychosocial integrity; CNS: Coping and adaptation; CL: Knowledge

37. A client addicted to alcohol tells a nurse, "Making friends used to be hard for me." Which of the following statements by the client indicates that client teaching about relationships was successful?

1. "I've set limits on my behaviors toward others."
2. "I've decided I need to be judgmental of others."
3. "I won't become intimately involved with others."
4. "I can't bear to see myself hurt again in a relationship."

37. 1. When the client can set personal limits and maintain boundaries, the ability to have successful interpersonal relationships can occur. Being judgmental is contraindicated if a client wants to have successful relationships. Setting arbitrary limits on relationships indicates the client needs to learn more interpersonal relationship skills. The universal truth about relationships is that they bring both joy and pain. The last statement indicates a need to learn more about relationships.

NP: Evaluation; CN: Psychosocial integrity; CNS: Psychosocial adaptation; CL: Application

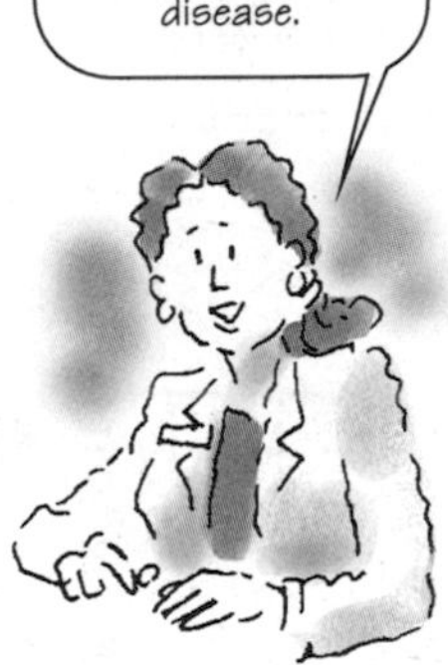

Your client teaching stems in part from an understanding of the severity of disease.

38. A client who abused alcohol for more than 20 years is diagnosed with cirrhosis of the liver. Which of the following statements by the client shows that teaching has been effective?

1. "If I decide to stop drinking, I won't kill myself."
2. "If I watch my blood pressure, I should be okay."
3. "If I take vitamins, I can undo some liver damage."
4. "If I use nutritional supplements, I won't have problems."

38. 1. This statement reflects the client's perception of the severity of the condition and the life-threatening complications that can result from continued use of alcohol. Aggressive treatment is required, not merely watching one's blood pressure. At this point in the illness, there is little likelihood that liver damage from cirrhosis can be altered. The fourth option denies the severity of the problem and negates the life-threatening complications common with a diagnosis of cirrhosis.

NP: Evaluation; CN: Psychosocial integrity; CNS: Psychosocial adaptation; CL: Comprehension

39. A client tells a nurse, "I'm not going to have problems from smoking marijuana." Which of the following responses is most accurate?

1. "Evidence shows it can cause major health problems."
2. "Marijuana can cause reproductive problems later in life."
3. "Smoking marijuana isn't as dangerous as smoking cigarettes."
4. "Some people have minor or no reactions to smoking marijuana."

39. 2. Marijuana causes cardiac, respiratory, immune, and reproductive health problems. Most people who smoke marijuana don't have major health problems. All people who smoke marijuana have symptoms of intoxication. The residues from marijuana are more toxic than those from cigarettes.

NP: Implementation; CN: Psychosocial integrity; CNS: Psychosocial adaptation; CL: Comprehension

40. During an assessment of a client with a history of polysubstance abuse, which of the following information should be obtained after the names of the drugs?
1. Age at last use
2. Route of administration
3. How the drug was obtained
4. The place the drug was used

41. A client says, "I started using cocaine as a recreational drug, but now I can't seem to control the use." That statement identifies which of the following drug behaviors?
1. Toxic dose
2. Dual diagnosis
3. Cross-tolerance
4. Compulsive use

42. A client says he used amphetamines to be productive at work. Which of the following symptoms commonly occurs when the drug is abruptly discontinued?
1. Severe anxiety
2. Increased yawning
3. Altered perceptions
4. Amotivational syndrome

43. The use of which of the following drugs since early adolescence could lead to bone marrow depression?
1. Amphetamines
2. Cocaine
3. Inhalants
4. Marijuana

44. Which of the following reasons best explains why it's important to monitor behavior in a client who has stopped using phencyclidine (PCP)?
1. Fatigue can cause feelings of being overwhelmed.
2. Agitation and mood swings can occur during withdrawal.
3. Bizarre behavior can be a precursor to a psychotic episode.
4. Memory loss and forgetfulness can cause unsafe conditions.

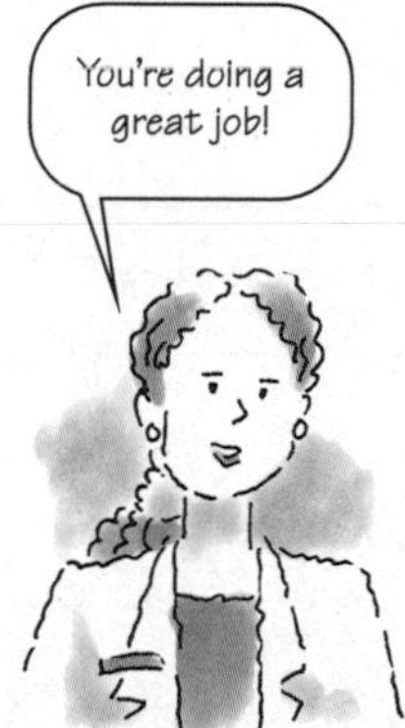
You're doing a great job!

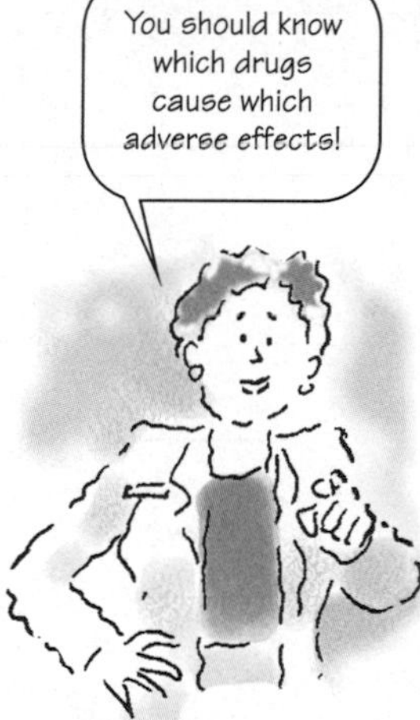
You should know which drugs cause which adverse effects!

40. 2. The route of administration gives information about the effects of the drug and what immediate treatment is necessary. How the drug was obtained, place it was used, and age at last use aren't essential information for treatment.

NP: Analysis; CN: Psychosocial integrity; CNS: Coping and adaptation; CL: Knowledge

41. 4. Compulsive drug use involves taking a substance for a period of time significantly longer than intended. A toxic dose is the amount of a drug that causes a poisonous effect. Dual diagnosis is the coexistence of a drug problem and a mental health problem. Cross-tolerance occurs when the effects of a drug are decreased and the client takes larger amounts to achieve the desired drug effect.

NP: Analysis; CN: Psychosocial integrity; CNS: Coping and adaptation; CL: Comprehension

42. 1. When amphetamines are abruptly discontinued, the client may experience severe anxiety or agitation. Increased yawning is a symptom of opioid withdrawal. Altered perceptions occur when a client is withdrawing from hallucinogens. Amotivational syndrome is seen with clients using marijuana.

NP: Analysis; CN: Psychosocial integrity; CNS: Coping and adaptation; CL: Application

43. 3. Inhalants cause severe bone marrow depression. Marijuana, cocaine, and amphetamines don't cause bone marrow depression.

NP: Analysis; CN: Psychosocial integrity; CNS: Psychosocial adaptation; CL: Knowledge

44. 3. Bizarre behavior and speech are associated with PCP withdrawal and can indicate psychosis. Fatigue isn't necessarily a problem when a client stops using PCP. Agitation, mood swings, memory loss, and forgetfulness don't tend to occur when a client has stopped using PCP.

NP: Analysis; CN: Psychosocial integrity; CNS: Psychosocial adaptation; CL: Analysis

45. A client is seeking help to stop using amphetamines. Which of the following assessment data indicates the client is experiencing withdrawal?

1. Disturbed sleep
2. Increased yawning
3. Psychomotor agitation
4. Inability to concentrate

46. Which of the following conditions can occur in a client who has just used cocaine?

1. Increased heart rate
2. Elevated temperature
3. Increased neck distention
4. Decreased respiratory rate

47. Which of the following information is most important in teaching a client who abuses prescription drugs?

1. Herbal substitutes are safer to use.
2. Medication should be used only for the reason prescribed.
3. The client should consult a physician before using a drug.
4. Consider if family members influence the client to use drugs.

48. The family of an adolescent who smokes marijuana asks a nurse if the use of marijuana leads to abuse of other drugs. Which of the following responses is best?

1. "Use of marijuana is a stage your child will go through."
2. "Many people use marijuana and don't use other street drugs."
3. "Use of marijuana can lead to abuse of more potent substances."
4. "It's difficult to answer that question as I don't know your child."

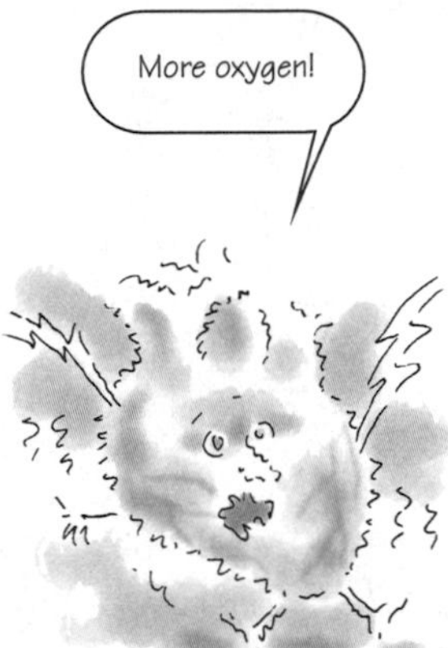
More oxygen!

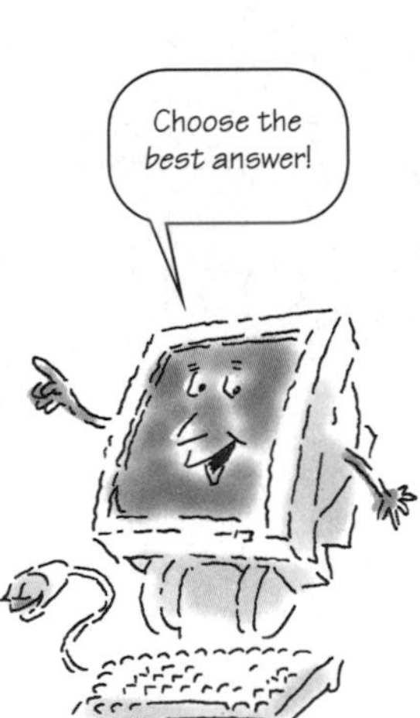
Choose the best answer!

45. 1. It's common for a person withdrawing from amphetamines to experience disturbed sleep and unpleasant dreams. Increased yawning is seen with clients withdrawing from opioids. Psychomotor agitation is seen in cocaine withdrawal, and the inability to concentrate is seen in caffeine withdrawal.

NP: Assessment; CN: Psychosocial integrity; CNS: Coping and adaptation; CL: Knowledge

46. 1. An increase in heart rate is common because cocaine increases the heart's demand for oxygen. Cocaine doesn't decrease the client's respiratory rate, increase body temperature, or cause increased neck distention.

NP: Analysis; CN: Psychosocial integrity; CNS: Coping and adaptation; CL: Application

47. 2. People often take prescribed drugs for reasons other than those intended, primarily to self-medicate or experience a sense of euphoria. The safety and efficacy of most herbal remedies hasn't been established. Sometimes over-the-counter medications are necessary for minor problems. There may be a family history of substance abuse, but it isn't a priority when planning nursing care.

NP: Planning; CN: Psychosocial integrity; CNS: Psychosocial adaptation; CL: Application

48. 3. Marijuana is considered a "gateway drug" because it tends to lead to the abuse of more potent drugs. People who use marijuana tend to use or at least experiment with more potent substances. Marijuana isn't a part of a developmental stage that adolescents go through. It isn't important that the nurse knows the child.

NP: Implementation; CN: Psychosocial integrity; CNS: Psychosocial adaptation; CL: Application

49. A pregnant client is thinking about stopping cocaine use. Which of the following statements by the client indicates effective teaching about pregnancy and drug use?

1. "Right after birth, I'll give the baby up for adoption."
2. "I'll help the baby get through the withdrawal period."
3. "I don't want the baby to have withdrawal symptoms."
4. "It's scary to think the baby may have Down syndrome."

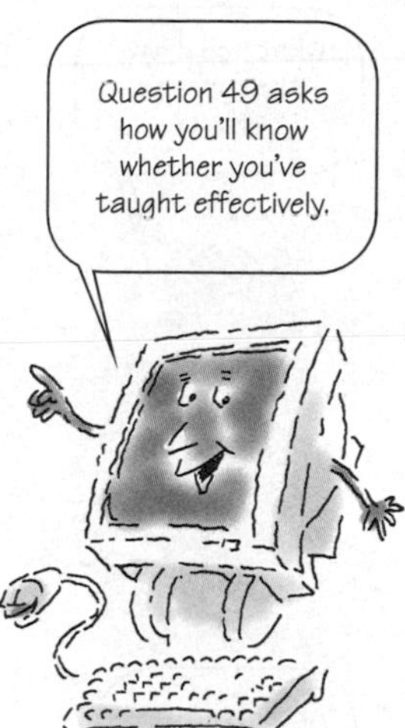

Question 49 asks how you'll know whether you've taught effectively.

49. 3. Neonates born to mothers addicted to cocaine have withdrawal symptoms at birth. If the client says she'll give the baby up for adoption after birth or help the baby get through the withdrawal period, the teaching was ineffective because the mother doesn't see the impact of her drug use on the child. Use of cocaine during pregnancy doesn't contribute to the baby having Down syndrome.

NP: Evaluation; CN: Psychosocial integrity; CNS: Psychosocial adaptation; CL: Analysis

50. A client with a history of cocaine abuse returns from a pass to an inpatient drug and alcohol facility showing behavior changes. Which of the following tests shows the presence of cocaine in the body?

1. Antibody screen
2. Glucose screen
3. Hepatic screen
4. Urine screen

50. 4. A urine toxicology screen would show the presence of cocaine in the body. Glucose, hepatic, or antibody screening wouldn't show the presence of cocaine in the body.

NP: Analysis; CN: Psychosocial integrity; CNS: Psychosocial adaptation; CL: Knowledge

51. A client says, "I didn't mean to keep taking the drug. I just had a lot of difficulty sleeping." Which of the following drug classifications is the client most at risk for abusing?

1. Amphetamines
2. Barbiturates
3. Cannabis
4. Opioids

51. 2. Barbiturates are frequently prescribed to relieve insomnia, and a client can easily become addicted. Amphetamines are stimulants and aren't used to promote sleep. Cannabis isn't used to promote sleep. Opioids are prescribed for pain, not sleep disorders.

NP: Analysis; CN: Psychosocial integrity; CNS: Coping and adaptation; CL: Knowledge

52. Which of the following interventions is most important in planning care for a client recovering from cocaine use?

1. Skin care
2. Suicide precautions
3. Frequent orientation
4. Nutrition consultation

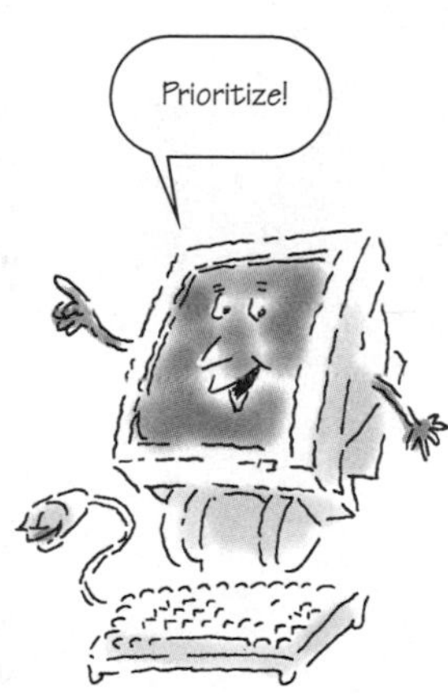

52. 2. Clients recovering from cocaine use are prone to "postcoke depression" and have a likelihood of becoming suicidal if they can't take the drug. Frequent orientation and skin care are routine nursing interventions but aren't the most immediate considerations for this client. Nutrition consultation isn't the most pressing intervention for this client.

NP: Planning; CN: Psychosocial integrity; CNS: Psychosocial adaptation; CL: Comprehension

53. Which of the following clinical conditions is frequently seen with substance abuse clients who repeatedly use cocaine?

1. Panic attacks
2. Bipolar cycling
3. Attention deficits
4. Expressive aphasia

53. 2. Clients who frequently use cocaine will experience the rapid cycling effect of excitement and then severe depression. They don't tend to experience panic attacks, expressive aphasia, or attention deficits.

NP: Assessment; CN: Psychosocial integrity; CNS: Coping and adaptation; CL: Analysis

54. A client who uses cocaine finally admits other drugs were also abused to equalize the effect of cocaine. Which of the following substances might be included in the client's pattern of polysubstance abuse?

1. Alcohol
2. Amphetamines
3. Caffeine
4. Phencyclidine

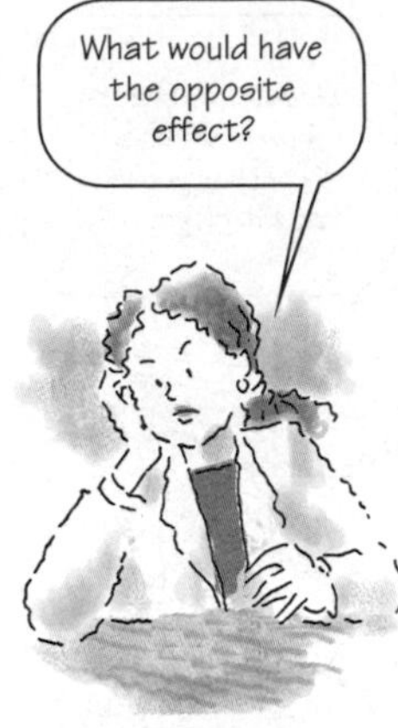
What would have
the opposite
effect?

54. 1. A cocaine addict will often use alcohol to decrease or equalize the stimulating effects of cocaine. Caffeine, phencyclidine, and amphetamines aren't used to equalize the stimulating effects of cocaine.

NP: Analysis; CN: Psychosocial integrity; CNS: Coping and adaptation; CL: Application

55. A group of teenagers tell the school nurse they used cocaine because they were bored. Which of the following short-term goals is the most important for the nurse to immediately initiate?

1. Prepare a drug lecture.
2. Restrict school privileges.
3. Establish an activity schedule.
4. Report the incident to their parents.

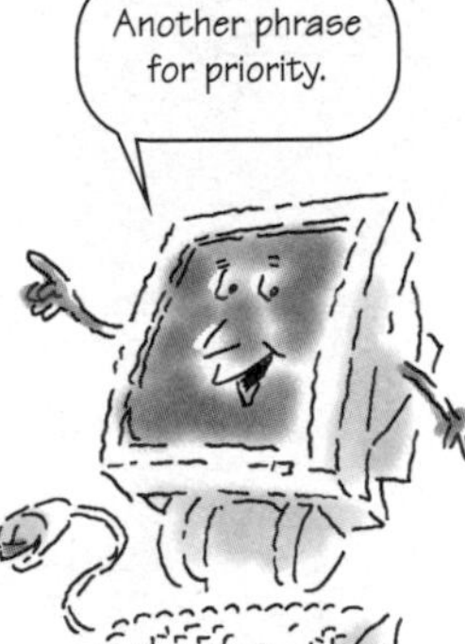
Another phrase
for priority.

55. 3. Having an activity schedule enables the adolescents to focus, become involved in constructive activities, and make better choices about what to do with their free time. Preparing a drug lecture or restricting school privileges won't be seen as useful by the adolescents and may inadvertently contribute to their inappropriate behavior. As the nurse works with the adolescents, it would be more effective to have the children talk to their parents about their drug use.

NP: Planning; CN: Psychosocial integrity; CNS: Psychosocial adaptation; CL: Comprehension

56. Which of the following statements by a client indicates teaching about cocaine use has been effective?

1. "I wasn't using cocaine to feel better about myself."
2. "I started using cocaine more and more until I couldn't stop."
3. "I'm not addicted to cocaine because I don't use it every day."
4. "I'm not going to be a chronic user, I only use it on holidays."

56. 2. This statement reflects the trajectory or common pattern of cocaine use and indicates successful teaching. The first option reflects the client's denial. People gravitate to the drug and continue its use because it gives them a sense of well-being, competency, and power. Cocaine abusers tend to be binge users and can be drug-free for days or weeks between use, but they still have a drug problem. The fourth option indicates the client is in denial about the drug's potential to become a habit. Effective teaching didn't occur.

NP: Evaluation; CN: Psychosocial integrity; CNS: Psychosocial adaptation; CL: Analysis

57. A client who formerly used lysergic acid diethylamide (LSD) is seeking counseling. Which of the following characteristics or conditions in the mental health history would be seen in this client?

1. Lack of trust
2. Panic attacks
3. Recurrent depression
4. Loss of ego boundaries

57. 2. Clients who used LSD often have a history of panic attacks or psychotic behavior. This is often referred to as a "bad trip." Loss of ego boundaries, recurrent depression, and lack of trust don't tend to be problems for this type of client.

NP: Assessment; CN: Psychosocial integrity; CNS: Coping and adaptation; CL: Analysis

58. Which of the following psychiatric or medical emergencies is most likely to occur when a client is using phencyclidine (PCP)?

1. Cardiac arrest
2. Seizure disorder
3. Violent behavior
4. Delirium reaction

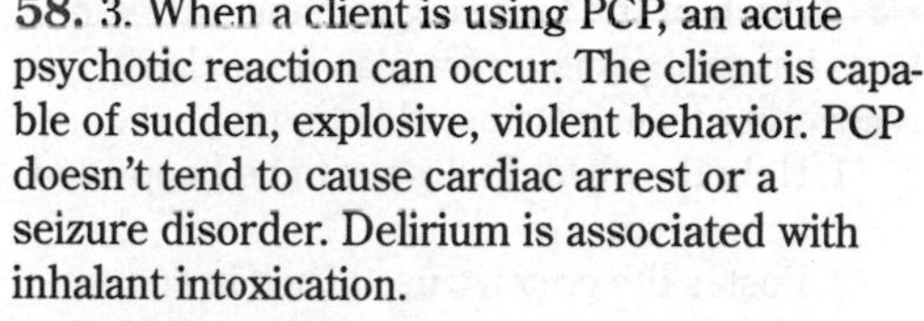

58. 3. When a client is using PCP, an acute psychotic reaction can occur. The client is capable of sudden, explosive, violent behavior. PCP doesn't tend to cause cardiac arrest or a seizure disorder. Delirium is associated with inhalant intoxication.

NP: Analysis; CN: Psychosocial integrity; CNS: Psychosocial adaptation; CL: Knowledge

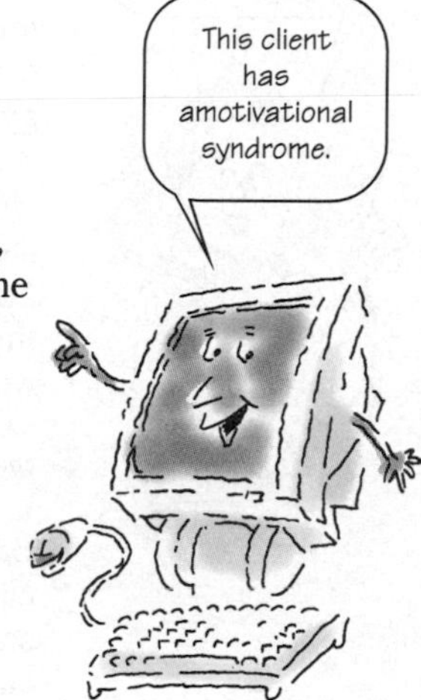
This client has amotivational syndrome.

59. A client who smoked marijuana daily for 10 years tells a nurse, "I don't have any goals, and I just don't know what to do." Which of the following communication techniques is the most useful when talking to this client?

1. Focus the interaction.
2. Use nonverbal methods.
3. Use reflection techniques.
4. Ask open-ended questions.

59. 1. A client with amotivational syndrome from chronic use of marijuana tends to talk in tangents and needs the nurse to focus the conversation. Nonverbal communication or reflection techniques wouldn't be useful as this client must focus and learn to identify and accomplish goals. Using only open-ended questions won't allow the client to focus and establish specific goals.

NP: Implementation; CN: Psychosocial integrity; CNS: Psychosocial adaptation; CL: Comprehension

60. A nurse is assessing a client who uses heroin to determine if there are physical health problems. Which of the following medical consequences of heroin use frequently occurs?

1. Hepatitis
2. Peptic ulcers
3. Hypertension
4. Chronic pharyngitis

60. 1. Hepatitis is the most frequent medical complication of heroin abuse. Peptic ulcers are more likely to be a complication of caffeine use, hypertension is a complication of amphetamine use, and chronic pharyngitis is a complication of marijuana use.

NP: Assessment; CN: Psychosocial integrity; CNS: Coping and adaptation; CL: Application

61. The family of a client withdrawing from heroin asks a nurse why the client is receiving naltrexone (ReVia). Which of the following responses is correct?

1. To help reverse withdrawal symptoms
2. To keep the client sedated during withdrawal
3. To take the place of detoxification with methadone
4. To decrease the client's memory of the withdrawal experience

61. 1. Naltrexone is an opioid antagonist and helps reverse the symptoms of opioid withdrawal. Keeping the client sedated during withdrawal isn't the reason for giving this drug. The drug doesn't decrease the client's memory of the withdrawal experience and isn't used in place of detoxification with methadone.

NP: Implementation; CN: Psychosocial integrity; CNS: Psychosocial adaptation; CL: Application

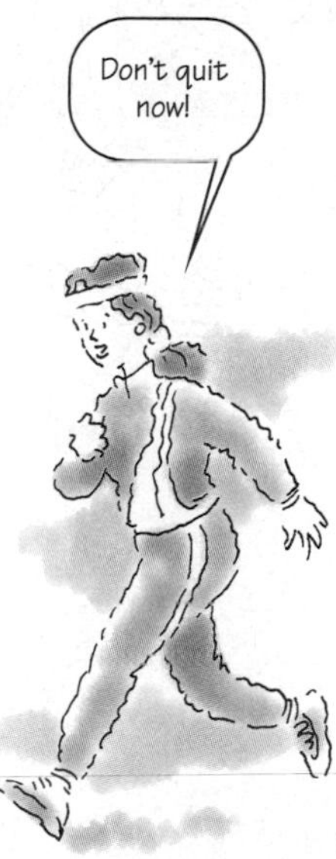
Don't quit now!

62. Which of the following nursing interventions has priority in a care plan for a client recovering from cocaine addiction?

1. Help the client find ways to be happy and competent.
2. Foster the creative use of self in community activities.
3. Teach the client to handle stresses in the work setting.
4. Help the client acknowledge the current level of dependency.

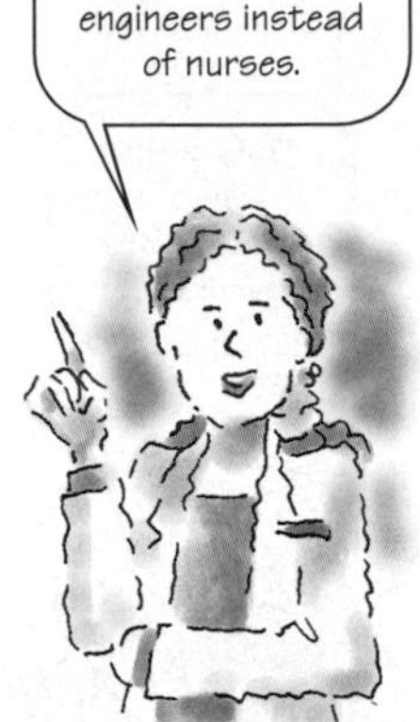
Maybe we should
be called priority
engineers instead
of nurses.

62. 1. The major component of a treatment program for a client with cocaine addiction is to have the client feel happy and competent. Cocaine addiction is difficult to treat because the drug actions reinforce its use. There are often perceived positive effects. Clients often credit the drug with giving them creative energy instead of looking within themselves. The second option may inadvertently reinforce the client's drug use. The third option is appropriate but isn't the most immediate nursing action. Examining the client's level of dependency isn't the immediate choice as the client needs to work on remaining drug free.

NP: Planning; CN: Psychosocial integrity; CNS: Psychosocial adaptation; CL: Application

63. A client tells a nurse, "I've been clean from drugs for the past 5 years, but my life really hasn't changed." Which of the following concepts should be explored with this client?

1. Further education
2. Conflict resolution
3. Career development
4. Personal development

63. 4. True recovery involves changing the client's distorted thinking and working on personal and emotional development. Before the client pursues further education, career development, or conflict resolution skills, it's imperative the client devotes energy to emotional and personal development.

NP: Planning; CN: Psychosocial integrity; CNS: Psychosocial adaptation; CL: Analysis

64. A client discusses how drug addiction has made life unmanageable. Which of the following information does the client need to start coping with the drug problem?

1. How peers have committed to sobriety
2. How to accomplish family of origin work
3. The addiction process and tools for recovery
4. How environmental stimuli serve as drug triggers

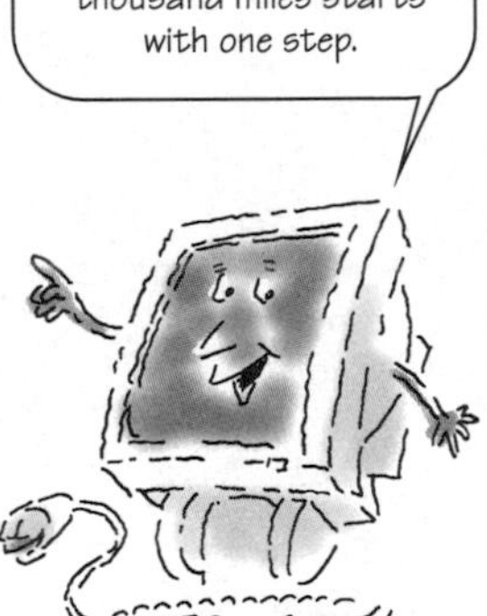
A journey of a
thousand miles starts
with one step.

64. 3. When the client admits life has become unmanageable, the best strategy is to teach about the addiction, how to obtain support, and how to develop new coping skills. Information about how peers committed to sobriety would be shared with the client as the treatment process begins. Identification of how environmental stimuli serve as drug triggers would be a later part of the treatment process and family of origin work. Initially, the client must commit to sobriety and learn skills for recovery.

NP: Planning; CN: Psychosocial integrity; CNS: Psychosocial adaptation; CL: Analysis

65. Which of the following physical health findings is expected during an assessment of a client with a history of cocaine abuse?

1. Glossitis
2. Pharyngitis
3. Bilateral ear infections
4. Perforated nasal septum

65. 4. When cocaine is snorted frequently, the client often develops a perforated nasal septum. Bilateral ear infections, pharyngitis, and glossitis aren't common physical findings for a client with a history of cocaine abuse.

NP: Assessment; CN: Psychosocial integrity; CNS: Coping and adaptation; CL: Knowledge

66. A client recovering from cocaine abuse is participating in group therapy. Which of the following statements by the client indicates the client has benefited from the group?

1. "I think the laws about drug possession are too strict in this country."
2. "I'll be more careful about talking about my drug use to my children."
3. "I finally realize the short high from cocaine isn't worth the depression."
4. "I can't understand how I could get all these problems that we talked about in group."

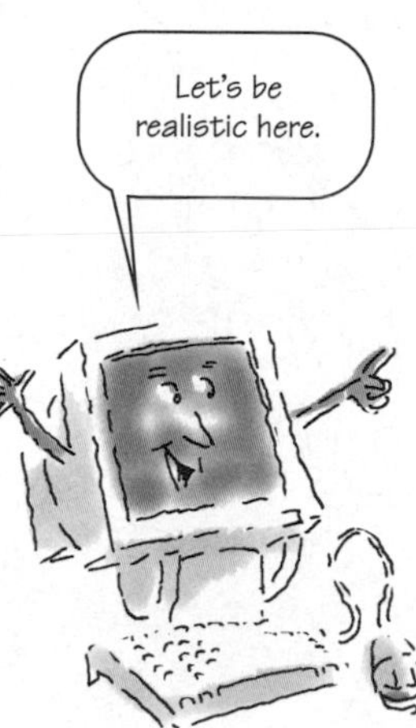
Let's be realistic here.

66. 3. This is a realistic appraisal of a client's experience with cocaine and how harmful the experience is. The first option indicates the client was distracting self from personal issues and isn't working on goals in the group setting. Talking about drugs to children must be reinforced with nonverbal behavior, and not talking about drugs may give children the wrong message about drug use. The fourth option indicates the client is in denial about the consequences of cocaine use.

NP: Evaluation; CN: Psychosocial integrity; CNS: Psychosocial adaptation; CL: Analysis

67. A family expresses concern that a member who stopped using amphetamines 3 months ago is acting paranoid. Which of the following explanations is the best?

1. A person gets symptoms of paranoia with polysubstance abuse.
2. When a person uses amphetamines, paranoid tendencies may continue for months.
3. Sometimes family dynamics and a high suspicion of continued drug use make a person paranoid.
4. Amphetamine abusers may have severe anxiety and paranoid thinking.

67. 2. After a client uses amphetamines, there may be long-term effects that exist for months after use. Two common effects are paranoia and ideas of reference. Even with polysubstance abuse, the paranoia comes from the chronic use of amphetamines. The third option blames the family when the paranoia comes from the drug use. Severe anxiety isn't typically manifested in paranoid thinking.

NP: Implementation; CN: Psychosocial integrity; CNS: Psychosocial adaptation; CL: Analysis

68. A nurse is trying to determine if a client who abuses heroin has any drug-related legal problems. Which of the following assessment questions is the best to ask the client?

1. When did your spouse become aware of your use of heroin?
2. Do you have a probation officer that you report to periodically?
3. Have you experienced any legal violations while being intoxicated?
4. Do you have a history of frequent visits with the employee assistance program manager?

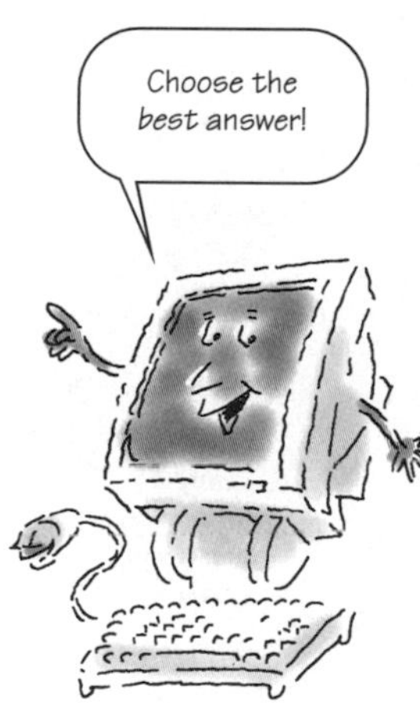
Choose the best answer!

68. 3. This question focuses on obtaining direct information about drug-related legal problems. When a spouse becomes aware of a partner's substance abuse, the first action isn't necessarily to institute legal action. Even if the client reports to a probation officer, the offense isn't necessarily a drug-related problem. Asking if the client has a history of frequent visits with the employee assistance program manager isn't useful. It assumes any visit to the employee assistance program manager is related to drug issues.

NP: Assessment; CN: Psychosocial integrity; CNS: Coping and adaptation; CL: Analysis

69. Which of the following areas requires thorough assessment before the nurse can determine if a client who stopped using heroin will have severe withdrawal symptoms?

1. Ego strength
2. Liver function
3. Seizure history
4. Kidney function

69. 2. Liver function status is an important variable that can be used to indicate the severity of a client's drug withdrawal. Ego strength, seizure history, and kidney function aren't variables that can be used to predict the severity of withdrawal symptoms.

NP: Assessment; CN: Psychosocial integrity; CNS: Coping and adaptation; CL: Comprehension

70. A client who uses cocaine denies that drug use is a problem. Which of the following intervention strategies would be best to confront the client's denial?

1. State ways to cope with stress.
2. Repeat the drug facts as needed.
3. Identify the client's ambivalence.
4. Use open-ended, factual questions.

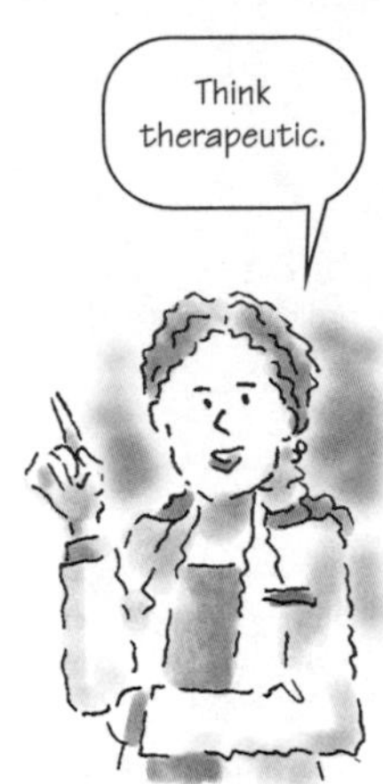
Think therapeutic.

70. 4. The use of open-ended, factual questions will help the client acknowledge that a drug problem is present. Stating ways to cope with stress and identifying the client's ambivalence won't be effective for breaking through a client's denial. Repeating drug facts won't be effective, as the client will perceive it as preaching or nagging.

NP: Implementation; CN: Psychosocial integrity; CNS: Psychosocial adaptation; CL: Application

71. A nurse is working with parents of an adolescent client who abuses inhalants. Which of the following information about consequences is best to include in a teaching plan?

1. Consequences must be enforceable.
2. Everything can become a consequence.
3. When setting consequences, be verbally forceful.
4. Consequences are seldom needed with adolescents.

71. 1. Consequences must be specific and enforceable. Sometimes parents are prone to make consequences that are too difficult to enforce or that actually become a punishment for the parents. Everything can't be made into a consequence. Being verbally forceful isn't appropriate because the consequence can occur in a civil tone of voice. A consequence can be used with every person regardless of developmental stage.

NP: Planning; CN: Psychosocial integrity; CNS: Psychosocial adaptation; CL: Analysis

72. Which of the following conditions may be present when a client addicted to cocaine becomes pessimistic about treatment?

1. Depression
2. Estrangement
3. Fatigue
4. Impulsiveness

72. 1. Clients withdrawing from drugs such as cocaine frequently experience depression. It's common for drug-addicted clients to experience fatigue without becoming pessimistic. Being impulsive or having feelings of estrangement aren't necessarily related to a client becoming pessimistic about treatment.

NP: Assessment; CN: Psychosocial integrity; CNS: Coping and adaptation; CL: Knowledge

73. A nurse is working with a client addicted to cocaine who is in denial. Which of the following approaches is most useful for dealing with the client's denial?

1. Ask whether the client sees the drug use as a problem.
2. Focus on the pain the client is having during withdrawal.
3. Reinforce the connection between drug use and harmful results.
4. Help the client recognize reality by pointing out withdrawal symptoms.

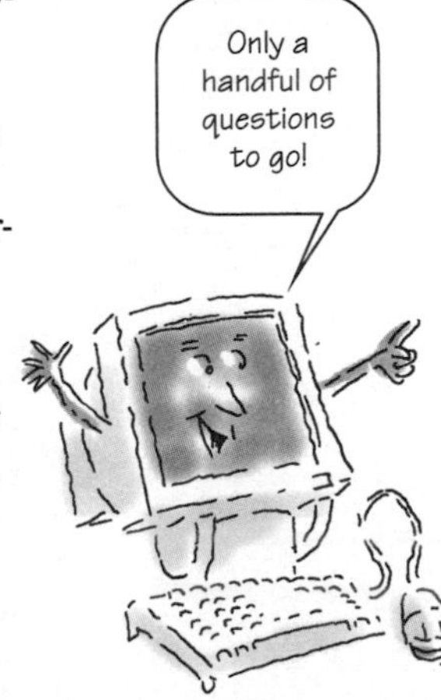
Only a handful of questions to go!

73. 3. To deal with the client's denial, the nurse must confront the drug use and point out the results of the behavior. Asking if the client sees the drug use as a problem will only reinforce the client's denial and provide a forum to intellectualize the problem or provide excuses for it. Pain isn't associated with withdrawal from cocaine. Pointing out withdrawal symptoms may not be the most effective strategy as the client often downplays the significance of the problem.

NP: Implementation; CN: Psychosocial integrity; CNS: Psychosocial adaptation; CL: Analysis

24. A 14-year-old client is admitted to an inpatient adolescent unit. The treatment team believes she has dissociative identity disorder (DID). Based on this information, which of the following interventions should the nurse anticipate using?

1. Request a social work consultation.
2. Institute elopement precautions.
3. Confront the parents about the staff's suspicion of child abuse.
4. Prevent the client from interacting with other clients on the unit.

25. When asked about behaviors of a client with dissociative identity disorder (DID), family members might include which of the following observations?

1. Statements by the client that he feels "like a robot"
2. A desire to sleep for long periods
3. Unpredictable and sometimes bizarre changes in behavior
4. A need to continually verbalize feelings about the abuse he suffered as a child

26. A client with dissociative identity disorder (DID) is admitted to an inpatient psychiatric unit. A nurse-manager asked all staff to attend a meeting. Which of the following reasons for the meeting is the most likely?

1. To review the restraint protocol with the staff
2. To inform the staff that no one should refuse to work with the client
3. To warn the staff that this client may be difficult and challenging to work with
4. To allow staff members to discuss concerns about working with a client with DID

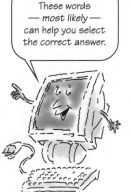

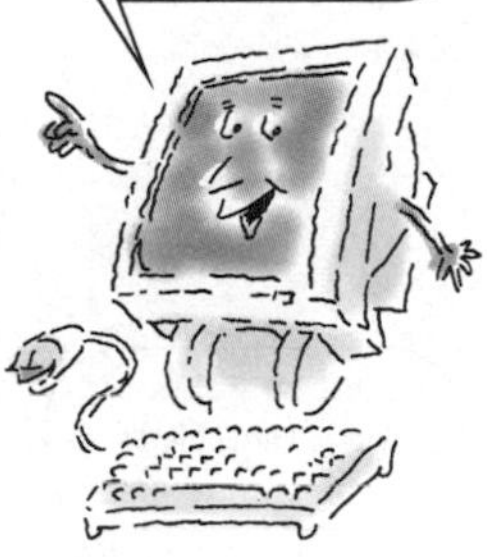

These words
— most likely —
can help you select
the correct answer.

27. A 26-year-old man is reported missing after being the victim of a violent crime. Two months later, a family member finds him working in a city 100 miles from his home. The man doesn't recognize the family member or recall being the victim of a crime. He most likely has which of the following conditions?

1. Depersonalization disorder
2. Dissociative amnesia
3. Dissociative fugue
4. Dissociative identity disorder

24. 1. In many cases, clients with DID have been subjected to child abuse. The social worker is the appropriate person to investigate the child's home setting. The client isn't at any more risk for elopement than the other adolescent clients. Until there has been an investigation into the client's home setting, confrontation wouldn't be appropriate or therapeutic. Clients with DID are always encouraged to interact with other clients on the unit.

NP: Planning; CN: Safe, effective care environment; CNS: Management of care; CL: Application

25. 3. Changes in behavior are one of the cardinal findings of DID. This occurs as the alter personalities take control. Feeling like a robot is more likely to occur in depersonalization disorder. The desire to sleep for long periods is more descriptive of depression. Often, the client with DID isn't aware of the occurrence of child abuse.

NP: Assessment; CN: Psychosocial integrity; CNS: Psychosocial adaptation; CL: Knowledge

26. 4. Allowing all staff members to meet together may prevent the staff from splitting into groups of those who believe the validity of this diagnosis and those who don't. Unless this client shows behaviors harmful to himself or others, restraints aren't needed. Telling the staff no one should refuse to work with the client or this client will probably be very difficult and challenging sets a very negative tone as staff plan and provide care for the client.

NP: Planning; CN: Safe, effective care environment; CNS: Management of care; CL: Application

27. 3. Dissociative fugue is sudden flight after a traumatic event. During the episode, the person may assume a new identity and not recognize people from his past. Depersonalization disorder is the sudden loss of the sense of one's own reality. Dissociative amnesia doesn't involve flight from work or home. Dissociative identity disorder is the coexistence of two or more personalities in one person.

NP: Assessment; CN: Psychosocial integrity; CNS: Psychosocial adaptation; CL: Knowledge

28. Which of the following nursing interventions is most appropriate for a client who has just had an episode of dissociative fugue?

1. Let the client verbalize the fear and anxiety he feels.
2. Encourage the client to share his experiences during the episode.
3. Have the client sign a contract stating he won't leave the premises again.
4. Tell the client he won't resolve his problems by running away from them.

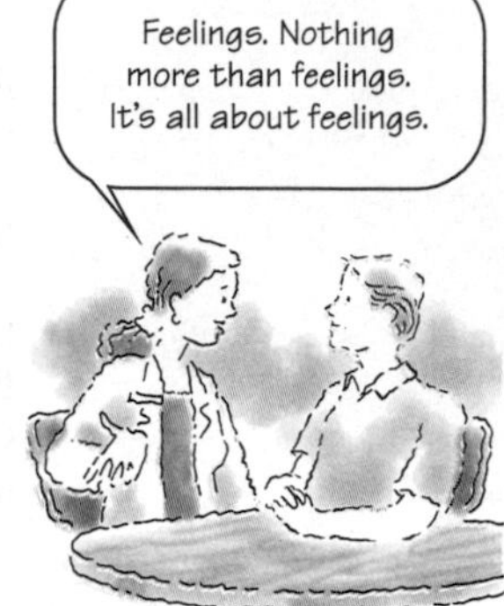

Feelings. Nothing more than feelings. It's all about feelings.

28. 1. An episode of dissociative fugue can be a very frightening experience. The client rarely remembers the events during the episode. Signing a contract would have little effect because a dissociative fugue episode isn't something the client consciously wanted to do. Because the client isn't conscious of "running away," this response isn't helpful.

NP: Implementation; CN: Health promotion and maintenance; CNS: Growth and development through the life span; CL: Analysis

29. Which of the following statements is correct about dissociative disorders?

1. They occur as a result of incest.
2. They occur as a result of substance abuse.
3. They occur in more than 40% of all people.
4. They occur as result of the brain trying to protect the person from severe stress.

29. 4. This answer best describes the cause of a dissociative disorder. Incest is only one of many reasons dissociative disorders occur. Typically, substance abuse isn't a cause (but may be an effect) of a dissociative disorder. Dissociative disorders are actually very rare.

NP: Assessment; CN: Psychosocial integrity; CNS: Psychosocial adaptation; CL: Knowledge

30. Which of the following nursing interventions would be most appropriate when working with a client who had a recent episode of dissociative fugue?

1. Place the client on elopement precautions.
2. Help the client identify resources to deal with stressful situations.
3. Allow the client to share his experiences about the dissociative fugue episode.
4. Confront the client about his running away from problems instead of dealing with them.

30. 2. Dissociative fugue is precipitated by stressful situations. Helping the client identify resources could prevent recurrences. Once the dissociative fugue episode is over, the client returns to normal functioning; he wouldn't be an elopement risk. The client often has amnesia about the events during the dissociative fugue episode, which limits his ability to share the experience. The client doesn't realize that he's running away from his problems.

NP: Implementation; CN: Psychosocial integrity; CNS: Psychosocial adaptation; CL: Analysis

31. A 32-year-old client lost her home in a flood last month. When questioned about her feelings about the loss, she doesn't remember being in a flood or owning a home. This client most likely has which of the following disorders?

1. Depersonalization disorder
2. Dissociative amnesia
3. Dissociative fugue
4. Dissociative identity disorder

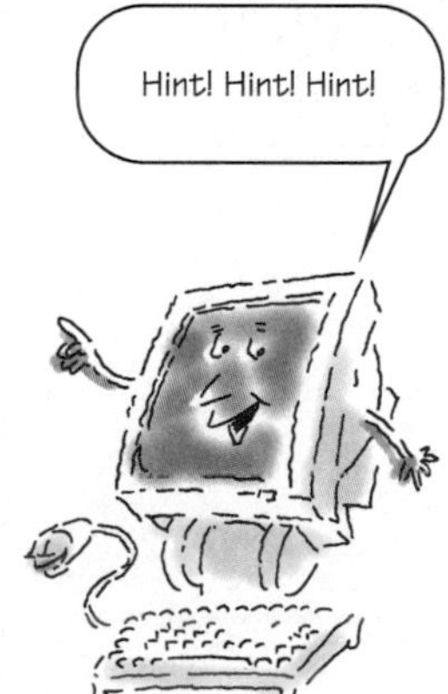

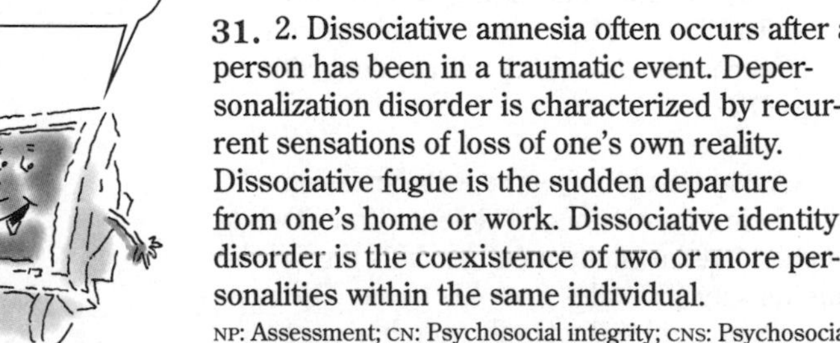

31. 2. Dissociative amnesia often occurs after a person has been in a traumatic event. Depersonalization disorder is characterized by recurrent sensations of loss of one's own reality. Dissociative fugue is the sudden departure from one's home or work. Dissociative identity disorder is the coexistence of two or more personalities within the same individual.

NP: Assessment; CN: Psychosocial integrity; CNS: Psychosocial adaptation; CL: Knowledge

32. Dissociative amnesia is most likely to occur as a result of which of the following circumstances?

1. Binge drinking
2. A hostage situation
3. A closed-head injury
4. A fight with a family member

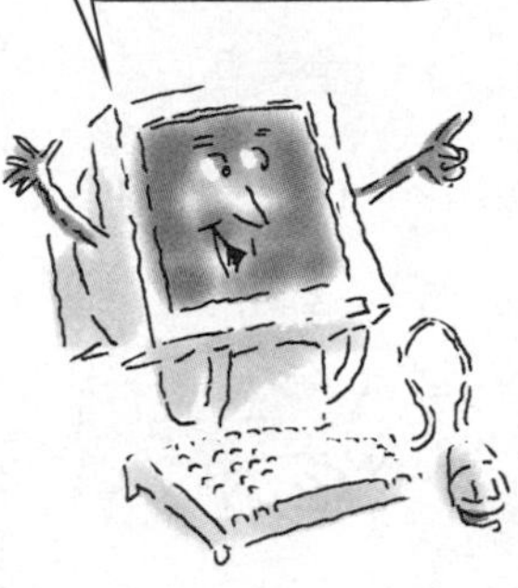

Perhaps all of these circumstances can cause dissociative amnesia, but which is most likely?

32. 2. Dissociative amnesia typically occurs after the person has experienced a very stressful, traumatic situation. Binge drinking doesn't cause dissociative amnesia. A closed-head injury could result in physiologic but not dissociative amnesia. Having a fight with a family member typically wouldn't be stressful enough to cause dissociative amnesia.

NP: Assessment; CN: Psychosocial integrity; CNS: Coping and adaptation; CL: Knowledge

33. A client was the driver in an auto accident in which a 3-year-old boy was killed. The client now has dissociative amnesia. He verbalizes understanding of his treatment plan when he makes which of the following statements?

1. "I won't drive a car again for at least a year."
2. "I'll take my Ativan anytime I feel upset about this situation."
3. "I'll visit the child's grave as soon as I'm released from the hospital."
4. "I'll attend my hypnotic therapy sessions prescribed by my psychiatrist."

33. 4. Hypnosis can be beneficial to this client because it allows repressed feelings and memories to surface. The client may be ready to drive again, and circumstances may dictate that he drives again before a year has passed. The client needs to learn other coping mechanisms besides taking a highly addictive drug such as lorazepam (Ativan). Visiting the child's grave on release from the hospital may be too traumatic and encourage continuation of the amnesia.

NP: Evaluation; CN: Psychosocial integrity; CNS: Coping and adaptation; CL: Application

34. A client with dissociative amnesia shows understanding of her condition when she makes which of the following statements?

1. "I'll probably never be able to regain my memories of the fire."
2. "I have problems with my memory due to my abuse of tranquilizers."
3. "If I concentrate hard enough, I'll be able to bring up memories of the car accident."
4. "To protect my mental well-being, my brain has temporarily hidden my memories of the rape from me."

34. 4. One of the cardinal features of dissociative amnesia is that the person has loss of memory of a traumatic event. With therapy and time, the person will probably be able to recall the traumatic event. This type of amnesia isn't related to substance abuse. With this disorder, the loss of memory is a protective function performed by the brain and isn't within the person's conscious control.

NP: Evaluation; CN: Psychosocial integrity; CNS: Coping and adaptation; CL: Analysis

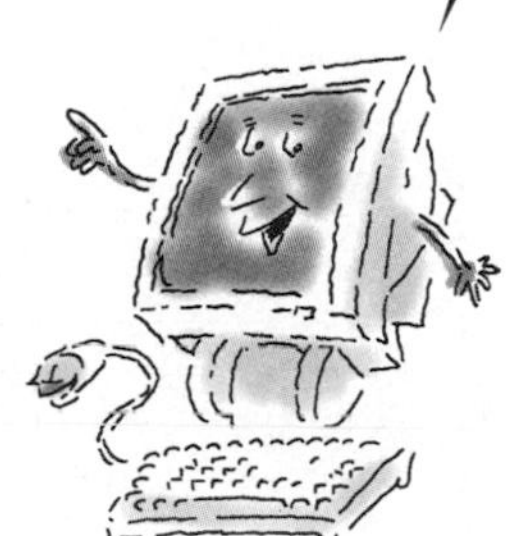

Gotta love those words, most appropriate. They're hints to the answer.

35. Which of the following interventions is most appropriate in the treatment of a client admitted for a diagnostic workup for possible dissociative amnesia?

1. Restrain the client if he attempts to wander off the unit.
2. Question the client every hour about orientation to time, place, and person.
3. Provide teaching on computed tomography scans and other imaging tests.
4. Encourage the client not to dwell on the traumatic event that lead to his memory loss.

35. 3. Clients with a type of memory problem commonly have a diagnostic workup to rule out any physical cause. Clients with dissociative amnesia typically don't have a problem with wandering. Frequent attempts to assess the client's orientation level could easily make the client more distressed and agitated. In many cases, the client doesn't have memories of the traumatic events before amnesia.

NP: Planning; CN: Health promotion and maintenance; CNS: Growth and development through the life span; CL: Application

36. A client with dissociative amnesia indicates understanding about the use of amobarbital (Amytal) in her treatment when she makes which of the following statements?

1. "This medication helps me sleep."
2. "This medication helps me control my anxiety."
3. "I must take this drug once a day after discharge if the drug is to be therapeutically beneficial."
4. "I'm given this medication during therapy sessions to increase my ability to remember forgotten events."

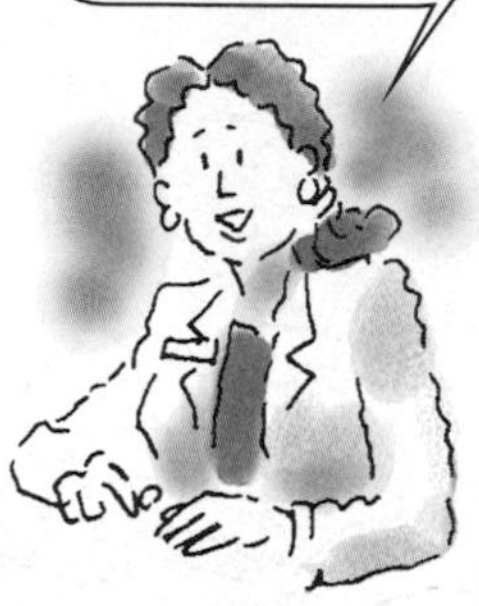

Which of these statements can you almost hear one of your brightest clients saying?

36. 4. This drug is given to the client with dissociative amnesia to help her remember forgotten events. It isn't prescribed as a sleep aid or antianxiety agent. Because the drug is given during therapy to recall forgotten events, there would be no therapeutic benefit to taking this drug at home.

NP: Evaluation; CN: Psychosocial integrity; CNS: Coping and adaptation; CL: Analysis

37. A client with dissociative amnesia says, "You must think I'm really stupid because I have no recollection of the accident." Which of the following responses would be most appropriate?

1. "Why would I think you're stupid?"
2. "Have I acted like I think you're stupid?"
3. "What kind of grades did you get in school?"
4. "As a protective measure, the brain sometimes doesn't let us remember traumatic events."

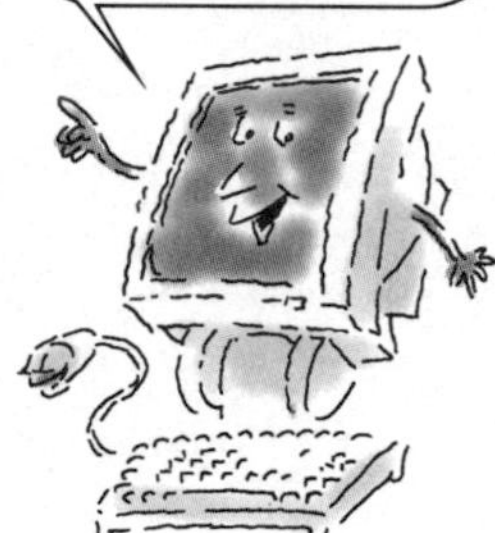

Question 37 cries out for the most appropriate response.

37. 4. This provides a simple explanation for the client. The use of "why" can put someone on the defensive. The second choice takes the focus off the client. The third choice changes the topic.

NP: Implementation; CN: Psychosocial integrity; CNS: Psychosocial adaptation; CL: Application

38. Which of the following nursing interventions is important in caring for the client with a dissociative disorder?

1. Encourage the client to participate in unit activities and meetings.
2. Question the client about the events triggering the dissociative disorder.
3. Allow the client to remain in his room anytime he's experiencing feelings of dissociation.
4. Encourage the client to form friendships with other clients in his therapy groups to decrease his feelings of isolation.

38. 1. Attending unit activities and meetings helps decrease the client's sense of isolation. Often, the client can't recall the events that triggered the dissociative disorder, so questioning him would not be helpful. The client would need to be isolated from others only if he's unable to interact appropriately. A client with a dissociative disorder has typically had few healthy relationships. Forming friendships with others in therapy could be setting the client up to continue in unhealthy relationships.

NP: Implementation; CN: Safe, effective care environment; CNS: Management of care; CL: Application

39. Which of the following characteristics applies to depersonalization disorder?
1. Disorientation to time, place, and person
2. Sensation of detachment from body or mind
3. Unexpected and sudden travel to another location
4. A feeling that one's environment will never change

39. 2. In depersonalization disorder, the person feels detached from his body and mental processes. The person is usually oriented to time, place, and person. Unexpected and sudden travel to another location is one of the characteristics of dissociative fugue. Clients with depersonalization disorder often feel the outside world has changed.

NP: Assessment; CN: Psychosocial integrity; CNS: Psychosocial adaptation; CL: Comprehension

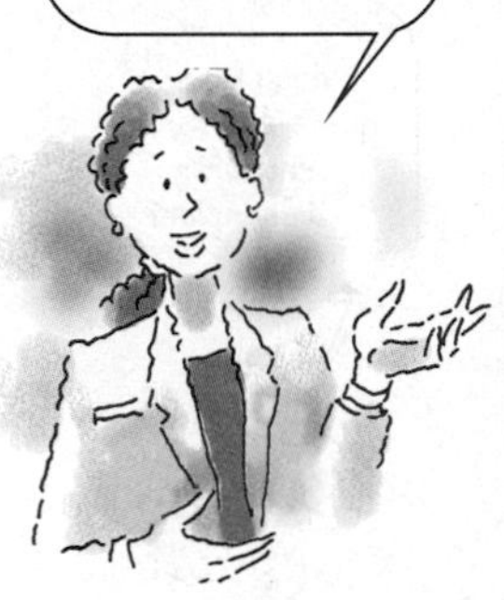

How can you tell when your client understands your instructions?

40. A client with depersonalization disorder verbalizes understanding of the ways to decrease his symptoms when he makes which of the following statements?
1. "I'll avoid any stressful situation."
2. "Meditation will help control my symptoms."
3. "I'll need to practice relaxation exercises regularly."
4. "I may need to remain on antipsychotic medication for the rest of my life."

40. 3. Relaxation can lead to a decrease in maladaptive responses. Although stress can be a predisposing factor in depersonalization disorder, it's impossible to avoid all stressful situations. Meditation is the voluntary induction of the sensation of depersonalization. This isn't a psychotic disorder, so antipsychotic medication wouldn't be therapeutic or beneficial.

NP: Evaluation; CN: Psychosocial integrity; CNS: Coping and adaptation; CL: Analysis

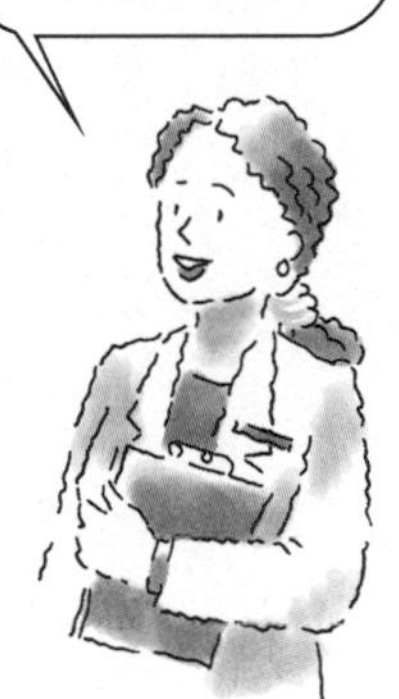

Making the right nursing diagnosis is critical for effective nursing care.

41. A client with depersonalization disorder spends much of her day in a dreamlike state during which she ignores personal care needs. Which of the following nursing diagnoses is most appropriate for this client?
1. Disturbed thought processes related to organic brain damage
2. Impaired memory related to frequently being in a dreamlike state
3. Dressing or grooming self-care deficit related to perceptual impairment
4. Deficient knowledge related to performance or personal care needs due to lack of information

41. 3. Because of time spent in a dreamlike state, many clients with depersonalization disorder ignore self-care needs. There's no known organic brain damage with this disorder. Memory impairment is more of a problem with other dissociative disorders, such as dissociative identity disorder and dissociative amnesia. The dreamlike state can lead to problems meeting personal care needs, not a knowledge deficit.

NP: Planning; CN: Safe, effective care environment; CNS: Safety and infection control; CL: Application

42. A client reports frequently feeling that he's floating above his body. During these times, he says he's aware of who he is and where he's located. The client is describing which of the following types of dissociative disorder?
1. Depersonalization disorder
2. Dissociative amnesia
3. Dissociative identity disorder
4. Dissociative fugue

42. 1. One of the cardinal symptoms of depersonalization disorder is feeling detached from one's body or mental processes. During the feelings of detachment, the person doesn't become disoriented. Dissociative amnesia is defined as one or more episodes of being unable to recall important information. Dissociative identity disorder is the existence of two or more personalities that take control of the person's behavior. In a dissociative fugue, the person has no memory of his life before the flight.

NP: Assessment; CN: Psychosocial integrity; CNS: Psychosocial adaptation; CL: Knowledge

43. In which of the following settings does treatment for clients with depersonalization disorder typically occur?
1. Inpatient psychiatric hospital
2. Community mental health clinic
3. Family practice physician's office
4. Support group for clients with depersonalization disorder

43. 2. Most clients with depersonalization disorder can be treated successfully on an outpatient basis. These clients only need to be hospitalized if they become suicidal or have severe depression or anxiety. Because no organic basis for the disorder usually exists, these clients aren't treated in a family practice physician's office. Because the disorder is rare, few support groups are composed only of clients with this disorder.
NP: Assessment; CN: Psychosocial integrity; CNS: Psychosocial adaptation; CL: Knowledge

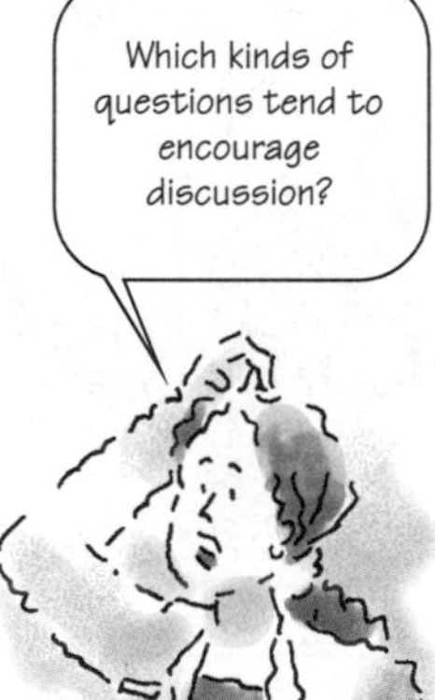

Which kinds of questions tend to encourage discussion?

44. A client with depersonalization disorder tells the nurse, "I feel like such a freak when I have an out-of-body experience." Which of the following responses would be most appropriate?
1. "How often do you have these feelings?"
2. "I don't understand what you mean by a freak."
3. "Tell me more about these out-of-body experiences."
4. "How does your husband feel about you having these experiences?"

44. 3. This open-ended response allows the client to focus and expand on this topic. Asking how often the experiences occur is a closed-ended question that doesn't encourage discussion of the experience. The second option could cause the client to focus too narrowly on only one aspect of the topic. Asking how the client's husband feels makes it appear that the nurse wants to change the topic.
NP: Implementation; CN: Psychosocial integrity; CNS: Psychosocial adaptation; CL: Analysis

45. Which of the following characteristics best applies to dissociative disorders?
1. A group of disorders with the common symptom of hallucinations
2. A group of disorders with a rapid disruption of the client's memory
3. A group of disorders with impairment of memory or identity due to the development of organic changes in the brain
4. A group of disorders with impairment of memory or identity due to an unconscious attempt to protect the person from emotional pain or traumatic experiences

45. 4. A group of disorders in which there is impairment of memory or identity due to an unconscious attempt to protect the client from emotional pain or traumatic experiences describes dissociative disorders. Hallucinations are associated with schizophrenic disorders. The onset of dissociative disorders may be gradual, sudden, or chronic. There's no known organic cause for dissociative disorders.
NP: Assessment; CN: Psychosocial integrity; CNS: Psychosocial adaptation; CL: Knowledge

46. A client with depersonalization disorder tells the nurse, "I feel like my arm isn't attached to my body." Which of the following responses would be most appropriate?
1. "Do you know where you are?"
2. "What makes you feel that way?"
3. "Don't worry because I can see your arm is attached to your body."
4. "This disorder causes people to feel that body parts may be unattached to the rest of the body."

46. 4. Reinforcing that what the client feels is an expected result of the disease process would be most appropriate. Asking if the client knows where he is changes the topic. Asking why he feels that way could put the client on the defensive. Stating that his arm is attached to his body belittles the client's feelings.
NP: Implementation; CN: Psychosocial integrity; CNS: Psychosocial adaptation; CL: Comprehension

47. A client with a dissociative disorder suddenly wanders away from the facility. When the nurse finds him, he can't recall what happened. The nurse identifies this behavior as which of the following?

1. Repression
2. Depersonalization
3. Derealization
4. Dissociative fugue

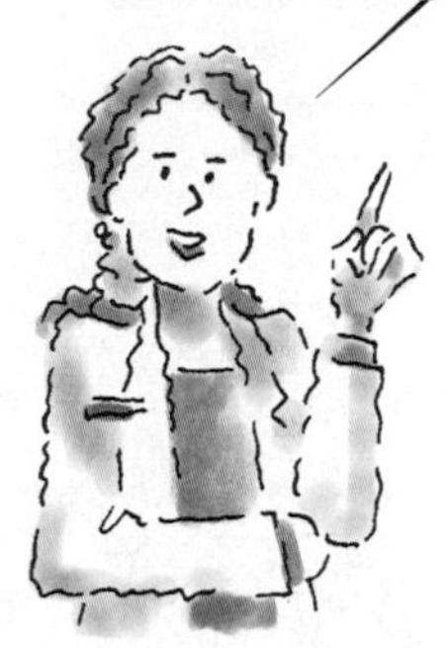

Which behavior is the client exhibiting in question 47?

47. 4. Dissociative fugue is characterized by suddenly wandering away from one's usual place, accompanied by amnesia for all or part of the past. Repression is a defense mechanism in which thoughts and feelings are kept from consciousness. Depersonalization is a feeling of detachment or separation from one's self. Derealization is a feeling that the external world is unreal.

NP: Assessment; CN: Psychosocial integrity; CNS: Psychosocial adaptation; CL: Application

48. The nurse conducts an admission assessment on a client diagnosed with dissociative identity disorder. Which sign or symptom supports this diagnosis?

1. A sense of being in a dream
2. Inability to remember a particular event
3. Having two or more personalities
4. Ritualistic behavior

48. 3. Dissociative identity disorder is characterized by having two or more distinct personalities, often in conflict with one another. A sense of being in a dream is common in depersonalization disorders. Selective amnesia refers to an inability to recall certain events that occurred during a specified period and is more common in traumatic stress disorders. Ritualistic behavior is seen in obsessive-compulsive disorders.

NP: Assessment; CN: Psychosocial integrity; CNS: Psychosocial adaptation; CL: Application

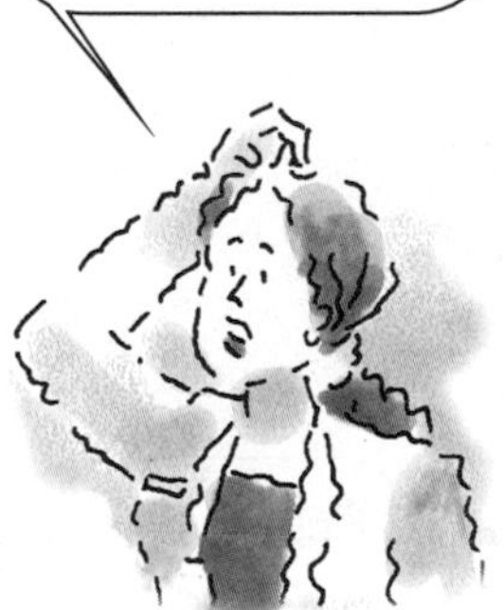

49. A client with a dissociative disorder can't recall any experiences. This symptom suggests which type of amnesia?

1. Localized amnesia
2. Generalized amnesia
3. Selective amnesia
4. Continuous amnesia

49. 2. Generalized amnesia refers to the inability to recall a whole lifetime of experiences. Localized amnesia is amnesia for a brief period (usually hours) after an upsetting event. Selective amnesia is amnesia for some but not all events. In continuous amnesia, the person forgets successive events as they occur.

NP: Assessment; CN: Psychosocial integrity; CNS: Psychosocial adaptation; CL: Knowledge

50. Which statement about dissociative disorder is true?

1. It can result from drug use.
2. It's a protective defense mechanism used to cope with anxiety.
3. It's caused by gradual memory loss.
4. It arises from a desire to avoid adult responsibilities.

50. 2. Dissociative disorder reflects dissociation—a defense mechanism used to prevent anxiety regarding traumatic events. Dissociative disorder doesn't result from drug use, doesn't involve gradual memory loss, and isn't linked to a desire to avoid adult responsibilities.

NP: Assessment; CN: Psychosocial integrity; CNS: Psychosocial adaptation; CL: Application

51. A client with a dissociative identity disorder experiences amnesia. Which nursing diagnosis is most appropriate?
1. Powerlessness
2. Ineffective coping
3. Disturbed sensory perception
4. Risk for self-directed violence

51. 2. Amnesia may result from an inability to cope with anxiety. Powerlessness, disturbed sensory perception, and risk for self-directed violence aren't appropriate in this situation.
NP: Analysis; CN: Psychosocial integrity; CNS: Psychosocial adaptation; CL: Analysis

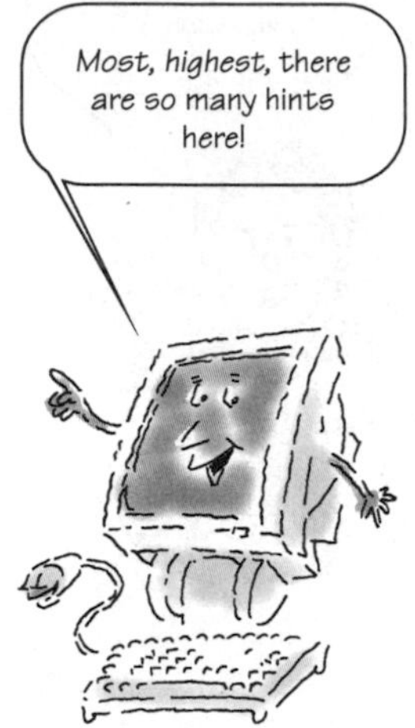

Most, highest, there are so many hints here!

52. After taking a potentially lethal drug overdose, a client tells the nurse that his alter "did it." Which nursing diagnosis takes highest priority?
1. Posttrauma syndrome
2. Anxiety
3. Risk for self-directed violence
4. Disturbed personal identity

52. 3. Taking a potentially lethal drug overdose indicates that the client poses a danger to himself. Because the alter may act again, the risk for self-directed violence persists. The other nursing diagnoses either aren't relevant or take lower priority.
NP: Assessment; CN: Psychosocial integrity; CNS: Psychosocial adaptation; CL: Analysis

53. A 42-year-old client with dissociative identity disorder confides to the nurse that he thinks he caused his brother to become ill during an earlier period in his life. Dissociative identity disorder is linked to which of the following?
1. Genetic predisposition
2. Severe childhood trauma
3. Developmental delays
4. Lack of learning

53. 2. Many studies indicate that dissociative identity disorder is a coping mechanism related to severe childhood trauma; developing one or more alternate personalities (common in dissociative identity disorders) helps the child cope with pain and fear stemming from the traumatic event. The disorder hasn't been linked to genetic predisposition, developmental delays, or lack of learning.
NP: Analysis; CN: Psychosocial integrity; CNS: Psychosocial adaptation; CL: Application

54. A client with dissociative identity disorder experiences frequent periods of memory loss. Which nursing intervention can help the client deal with the memory loss?
1. Orienting the client to time, place, person, and situation
2. Explaining to the client the circumstances surrounding the memory loss
3. Assessing for cues that the client is ready to discuss the memory loss
4. Telling the client not to worry because the memory loss has no physiologic base

54. 3. Memory loss serves as a protective mechanism for many clients with dissociative identity disorder; the nurse should wait until the client is ready to discuss the problem, as shown by certain cues. Orienting the client may force the client out of the protective mechanism of the memory loss (which the client may not be ready for and can result in further harm). Explaining the circumstances surrounding the memory loss and telling the client not to worry aren't therapeutic interventions.
NP: Analysis; CN: Psychosocial integrity; CNS: Psychosocial adaptation; CL: Application

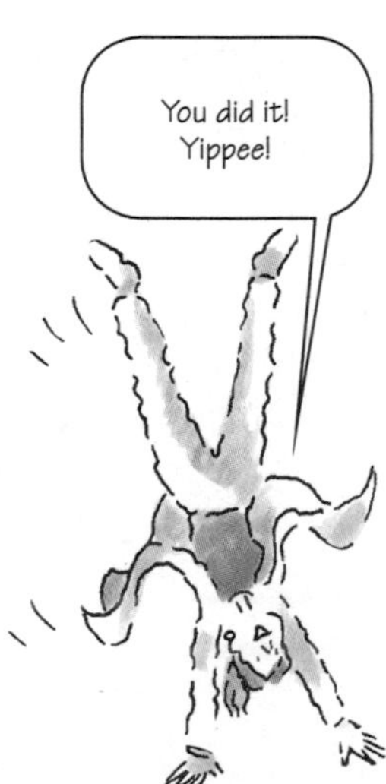

You did it!
Yippee!

NP: Nursing process CN: Client needs category CNS: Client needs subcategory CL: Cognitive level

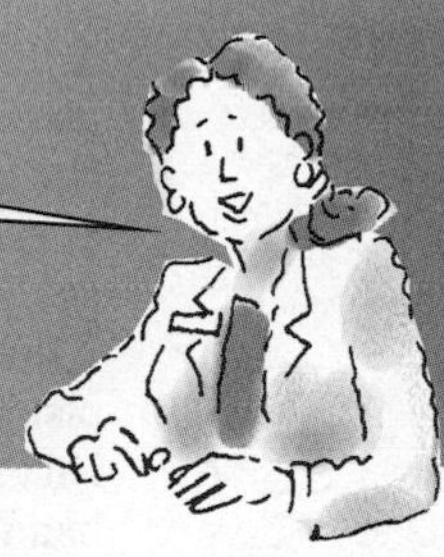

This chapter will test your knowledge of disorders of a highly sensitive nature. Remain professional at all times, and you'll do great. Good luck!

Chapter 20 Sexual & gender identity disorders

1. A male client has undergone surgery for the repair of an abdominal aortic aneurysm. Which of the following responses is most appropriate to the client's wife when she asks if her husband will be impotent?

1. "Don't worry, he will be all right."
2. "He has other problems to worry about."
3. "We will cross that bridge when we come to it."
4. "There is a chance of impotence after repair of an abdominal aortic aneurysm."

2. Which of the following discharge instructions would be most accurate to provide to a female client who has suffered a spinal cord injury at the C4 level?

1. After a spinal cord injury, women usually remain fertile; therefore, you may consider contraception if you don't want to become pregnant.
2. After a spinal cord injury, women usually are unable to conceive a child.
3. Sexual intercourse shouldn't be different for you.
4. After a spinal cord injury, menstruation usually stops.

3. Which of the following permanent complications might the nurse expect to see in a client who has just undergone a perineal prostatectomy?

1. Bleeding
2. Erectile dysfunction
3. Infection
4. Pneumonia

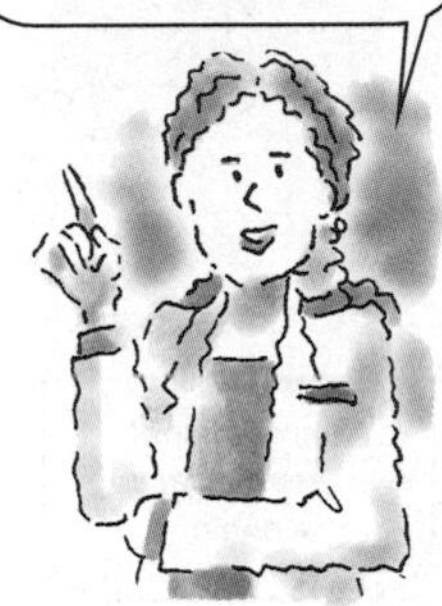

Therapeutic communication involves demonstrating sensitivity to your client's and his family's concerns.

1. 4. Impotence and retrograde ejaculation are sexual dysfunctions commonly experienced by male clients after abdominal aortic aneurysm. Telling a family member that the client will be all right is offering false assurance. Telling the client's wife to "cross that bridge when we come to it" ignores her concerns and isn't therapeutic. Stating that he has other problems isn't therapeutic and doesn't address the wife's concern.

NP: Application; CN: Psychosocial integrity; CNS: Coping and adaptation; CL: Application

2. 1. After a spinal cord injury, women remain fertile and can conceive and deliver a child. If a woman doesn't want to become pregnant, she *must* use contraception. Menstruation isn't affected by a spinal cord injury, but sexual functioning may be different.

NP: Implementation; CN: Physiological integrity; CNS: Physiological adaptation; CL: Application

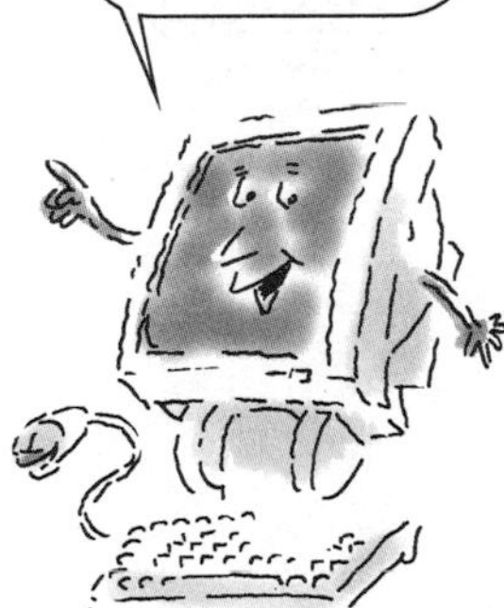

Note the word *permanent* in question 3 before you answer.

3. 2. After a perineal prostatectomy, a major complication is erectile dysfunction. As with any surgery, the client also is at risk for bleeding, pneumonia, and infection, but these aren't permanent conditions.

NP: Assessment; CN: Physiological integrity; CNS: Reduction of risk potential; CL: Comprehension

4. A client with chronic obstructive pulmonary disease (COPD) tells the nurse, "I no longer have enough energy to make love to my husband." Which of the following nursing interventions would be most appropriate?

1. Refer the couple to a sex therapist.
2. Advise the woman to seek a gynecologic consult.
3. Suggest methods and measures that facilitate sexual activity.
4. Tell the client, "If you talk this over with your husband, he'll understand."

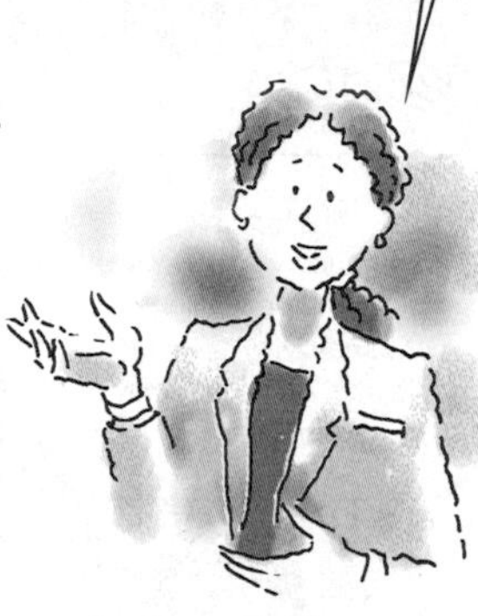

In question 4, you've got to choose the most appropriate answer, not just a possible one.

4. 3. Sexual dysfunction in COPD clients is the direct result of dyspnea and reduced energy levels. Measures to reduce physical exertion, enhance oxygenation, and accommodate decreased energy levels may aid sexual activity. If the problem persists, a consult with a therapist might be necessary. A gynecologic consult isn't necessary. Discussing this with her husband may not resolve the problem.

NP: Implementation; CN: Physiological integrity; CNS: Reduction of risk potential; CL: Application

5. A client with an ileostomy tells the nurse he can't have an erection. Which of the following pertinent information should the nurse know?

1. The client will never regain functioning.
2. The client needs an abdominal X-ray.
3. The client has no problem with self-control.
4. Impotence is uncommon following an ileostomy.

5. 4. Sexual dysfunction is uncommon after an ileostomy. Psychological causes of impotence should be explored. An abdominal X-ray isn't indicated for sexual dysfunction. An ileostomy can change a person's self-control, making sexual functioning difficult.

NP: Analysis; CN: Psychosocial integrity; CNS: Psychosocial adaptation; CL: Analysis

6. A recently divorced 40-year-old male who has undergone radiation therapy for testicular cancer tells the nurse he is unable to achieve an erection. Which of the following nursing diagnoses is most appropriate?

1. Ineffective coping related to radiation therapy
2. Sexual dysfunction related to the effects of radiation therapy
3. Disturbed body image related to the effects of radiation therapy
4. Imbalanced nutrition: Less than body requirements related to radiation therapy

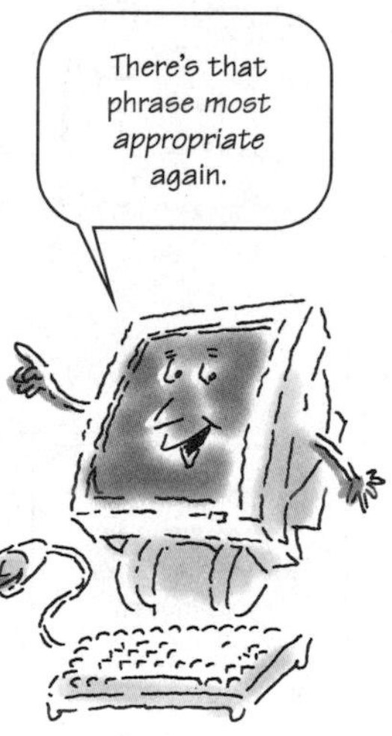

There's that phrase most appropriate again.

6. 2. Radiation or chemotherapy may cause sexual dysfunction. Libido may only be temporarily affected, and the client should be provided with emotional support. The client may experience alopecia or skin changes as well as weight loss, but the client isn't verbalizing concern in this area. The client hasn't verbalized fear or concern related to the cancer. Nutrition hasn't been mentioned.

NP: Analysis; CN: Psychosocial integrity; CNS: Coping and adaptation; CL: Analysis

7. Which of the following actions should the nurse include in the teaching plan of a newly married female client with a cervical spinal cord injury who doesn't wish to become pregnant at this time?

1. Provide the client with brochures on sexual practice.
2. Provide the client's husband with material on vasectomy.
3. Instruct the client on the rhythm method of contraception.
4. Instruct the client's husband on inserting a diaphragm with contraceptive jelly.

7. 4. Because the client experienced a cervical spinal cord injury, she won't be able to insert any form of contraception protection; therefore, it's vital to provide her husband with instruction on insertion of a diaphragm. Providing the couple with literature on sexual practice doesn't address the client's concerns. During this time of crisis, the couple doesn't wish to have children, but they may reconsider, so providing information on vasectomy isn't appropriate. The rhythm method isn't the most effective way to prevent pregnancy.

NP: Implementation; CN: Psychosocial integrity; CNS: Coping and adaptation; CL: Application

8. A client tells the nurse she is having her menstrual period every 2 weeks and it lasts for 1 week. Which of the following conditions is best defined by this menstrual pattern?

1. Amenorrhea
2. Dyspareunia
3. Menorrhagia
4. Metrorrhagia

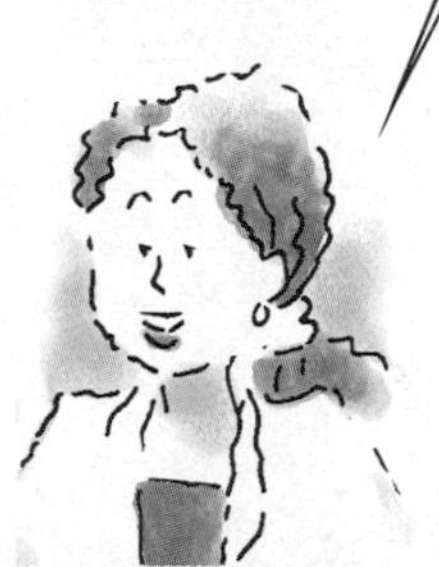

What's the difference between menorrhagia and metrorrhagia? You've got to know to answer question 8.

8. 3. Menorrhagia is an excessive menstrual period. Amenorrhea is lack of menstruation. Dyspareunia is painful intercourse. Metrorrhagia is uterine bleeding from another cause other than menstruation.

NP: Assessment; CN: Physiological integrity; CNS: Reduction of risk potential; CL: Knowledge

9. Which of the following aspects might be a major stressor for a couple being treated for infertility?

1. Examinations
2. Giving specimens
3. Scheduling intercourse
4. Finding out which partner is infertile

9. 3. The major cause of stress in infertile couples is planning sexual intercourse to correlate to fertility cycles. The inconvenience and discomfort of producing specimens and receiving examinations isn't a major stressor. Most couples undergoing fertility treatment understand that one partner is usually infertile.

NP: Implementation; CN: Health promotion and maintenance; CNS: Growth and development through the life span; CL: Application

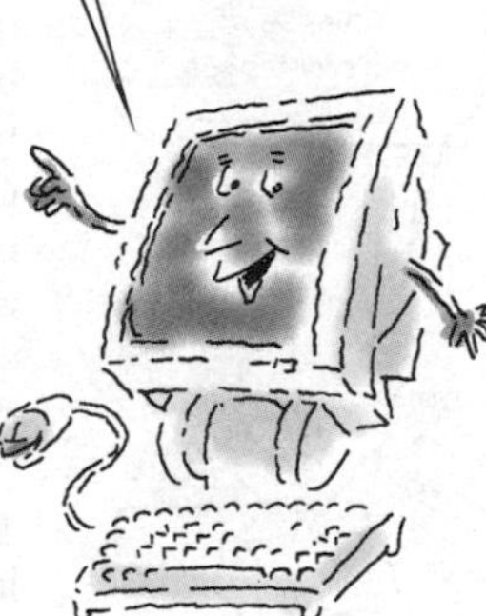

10 out of 56 done! Keep going!

10. A 38-year-old woman must undergo a hysterectomy for uterine cancer. The nurse planning her care should include which of the following actions to meet the woman's body image changes?

1. Ask her if she is having pain.
2. Refer her to a psychotherapist.
3. Don't discuss the subject with her.
4. Encourage her to verbalize her feelings.

10. 4. Encourage the client to verbalize her feelings because loss of one's reproductive organs may bring on feelings of loss of sexuality. Referring her to a psychotherapist may be premature; the client should be given time to work through her feelings. Avoidance of the subject isn't a therapeutic nursing intervention. Pain is a concern after surgery, but it has no bearing on body image.

NP: Implementation; CN: Psychosocial integrity; CNS: Coping and adaptation; CL: Application

11. A 50-year-old male who had a myocardial infarction 8 weeks ago tells a nurse, "My wife wants to make love, but I don't think I can. I'm worried that it might kill me." Which of the following responses from the nurse would be most appropriate?

1. "Tell me about your feelings."
2. "Let's increase your rehabilitation schedule."
3. "Let me call the primary health care provider for you."
4. "Tell your wife when you're able you'll make love."

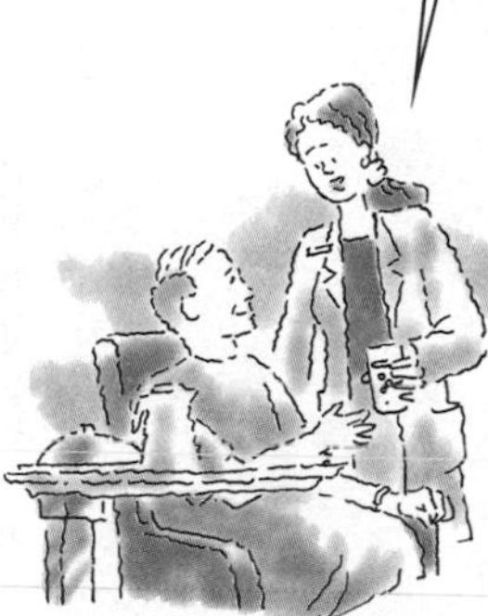

Let's put together a plan of care that serves both your needs.

11. 1. The nurse should address the client's concerns. Asking the client to verbalize his feelings will permit the nurse to gain insight into the problem. Telling the wife that eventually the client will make love may place strain on the marriage. Calling the primary health care provider before a complete assessment is made is inappropriate. The rehabilitation schedule shouldn't be increased until the nurse assesses the situation and is sure no harm will come to the client.

NP: Implementation; CN: Psychosocial integrity; CNS: Coping and adaptation; CL: Application

12. A 55-year-old female client who's in cardiac rehabilitation tells a nurse that she's unable to make love to her husband because she often feels fatigued and has a sense of doom. Which of the following nursing interventions is most appropriate?

1. Instruct her not to have intercourse until she is ready.
2. Instruct her to take a nitroglycerin tablet prior to intercourse.
3. Encourage her to learn additional methods to use for sexual intercourse.
4. Encourage her to verbalize her feelings while you perform a physical examination on her.

12. 4. Because the client has a complaint of fatigue, she should be examined and her feelings should be explored. Instructing her not to have intercourse doesn't address her concerns. She shouldn't take nitroglycerin before intercourse until her fatigue is evaluated. Before recommending alternative methods for intercourse, the client should be assessed physically and psychologically.

NP: Implementation; CN: Psychosocial integrity; CNS: Coping and adaptation; CL: Application

13. A 33-year-old female tells the nurse she has never had an orgasm. She tells the nurse that her partner is upset that he is unable to meet her needs. Which of the following nursing interventions is most appropriate?

1. Ask the client if she desires intercourse.
2. Assess the couple's perception of the problem.
3. Tell the client that most women don't reach orgasm.
4. Refer the client to a therapist because she has sexual aversion disorder.

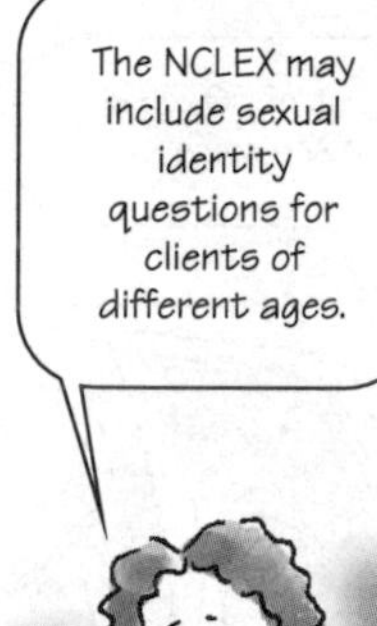

The NCLEX may include sexual identity questions for clients of different ages.

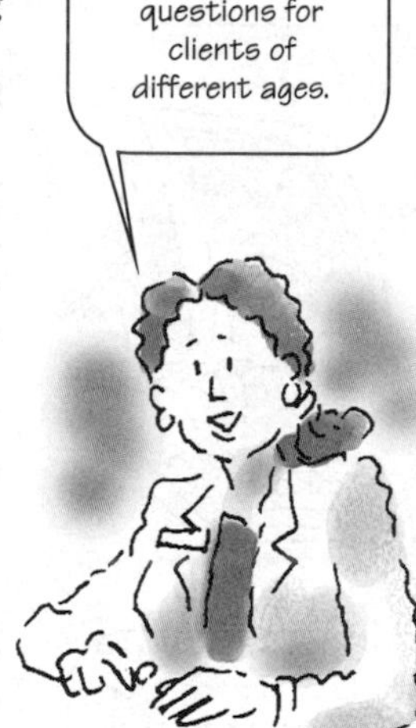

13. 2. Assessing the couple's perception of the problem will define the problem and assist the couple and the nurse in understanding it. A nurse can't make a medical diagnosis such as sexual aversion disorder. Most individuals can be taught to reach orgasm if there is no underlying medical condition. When assessing the client, the nurse should be professional and matter of fact and shouldn't make the client feel inadequate or defensive.

NP: Planning; CN: Psychosocial integrity; CNS: Coping and adaptation; CL: Application

14. Which of the following complications is most likely the cause for a 35-year-old male client who complains to the nurse that he has an orgasm too quickly?

1. Fear of intimacy
2. Premature ejaculation
3. Sexual aversion disorder
4. Hypoactive sexual desire disorder

14. 2. Premature ejaculation is defined as having an orgasm with ejaculation after minimal stimulation, often leaving the male feeling inadequate for not fulfilling his partner's desires. Sexual aversion disorder is the avoidance of sexual activity. Hypoactive sexual desire disorder is a decline in the drive for sexual activity. Fear doesn't cause premature ejaculation.

NP: Assessment; CN: Psychosocial integrity; CNS: Coping and adaptation; CL: Comprehension

15. A 50-year-old male who is taking antihypertensive medication tells the office nurse who's monitoring his blood pressure that he can't have sexual intercourse with his wife anymore. Which of the following problems is most likely the cause?

1. His advancing age
2. His blood pressure
3. His stressful lifestyle
4. His blood pressure medication

15. 4. Antihypertensive medication may cause impotence in men. Men are usually able to have an erection throughout their life. Blood pressure itself doesn't cause impotence but its treatment does. Stress may cause erectile dysfunction, but there's no evidence that the client is under stress.

NP: Assessment; CN: Psychosocial integrity; CNS: Coping and adaptation; CL: Knowledge

16. Research performed on sexual disorders has shown that victims of sexual abuse have a tendency to experience which of the following results?
1. Have higher hormonal levels
2. Remain celibate throughout life
3. Become sex offenders themselves
4. Have normal sexual experiences throughout life

16. 3. Children who have been sexually abused have a predisposition for becoming a sex offender. Research doesn't show that victims of sexual abuse have higher hormonal levels. They probably won't have normal sexual experiences throughout life without intense therapy. Research also shows that victims of sexual abuse are at risk for paraphiliac disorders.
NP: Implementation; CN: Psychosocial integrity; CNS: Psychosocial adaptation; CL: Analysis

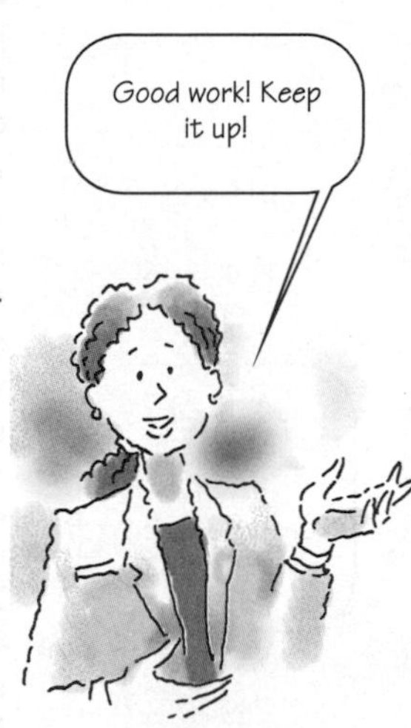

Good work! Keep it up!

17. Which of the following interventions is important for a client who engages in sexual acts with animals (zoophilia)?
1. Place the client in the seclusion room.
2. Assess triggers that stimulate the behaviors.
3. Have the primary health care provider order antidepressant medication.
4. Counsel the client not to discuss his sexual behaviors with anyone.

17. 2. Assessing the triggers that stimulate inappropriate sexual behavior helps to prevent recurrence. The seclusion room should be used only to ensure the safety of the client and staff. Antidepressants aren't indicated for sexual disorders; hormonal therapy is the usual drug treatment. Clinical support and group therapy are used to teach sexually acceptable behavior.
NP: Implementation; CN: Psychosocial integrity; CNS: Psychosocial adaptation; CL: Analysis

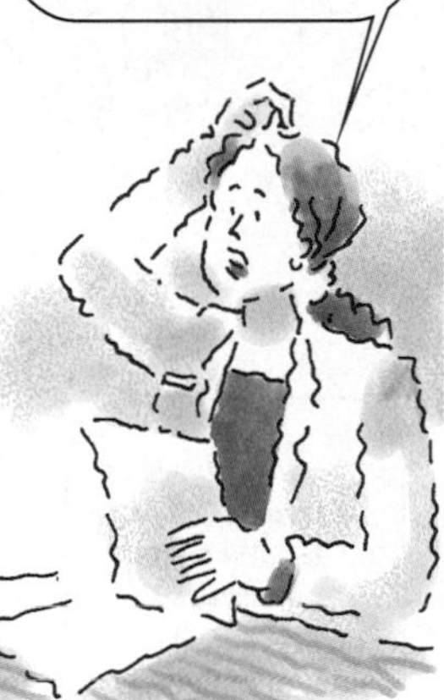

Sometimes, the nurse must assess her own feelings about a client before planning care.

18. A 25-year-old male client convicted of raping a female college student has completed his parole and has been attending a sex offenders group for 5 years. The client no longer wishes to participate in the group. Which of the following actions should the nurse take?
1. Insist that the client remain in therapy.
2. Perform a self-evaluation, and assess the discomfort level.
3. Call the parole board, and tell them of the client's decision.
4. Call the client's family, and tell them of his decision and progress.

18. 2. If the client has successfully completed therapy, then the nurse must evaluate her own value system. Calling the parole board may be an inappropriate decision, especially if the client has met all of his requirements. A nurse can't release confidential information to the client's family without his permission and consent. Insisting that the client remain in therapy may not prove to be successful, as he must be motivated to undergo therapy.
NP: Planning; CN: Psychosocial integrity; CNS: Psychosocial adaptation; CL: Analysis

19. A 32-year-old client who engages in voyeurism has come to the hospital for treatment so his family and friends don't find out. The nurse planning care for this client should include which of the following interventions?
1. Encourage the client to inform his family and friends so that he isn't living a lie
2. Suggest individual therapy to discuss socially unacceptable behavior
3. Develop the care plan without input from the client
4. Evaluate the client's defense mechanism

19. 2. Discussing inappropriate sexual behavior with the client increases compliance with treatment and decreases the risk of relapse. Informing family and friends isn't an initial intervention; disclosure to family and friends is usually delayed until the client acknowledges his behavior. All care planning should involve the client. An initial evaluation should focus on the antecedents to the inappropriate behavior.
NP: Planning; CN: Psychosocial integrity; CNS: Psychosocial adaptation; CL: Application

20. A client is admitted to the psychiatric unit for paraphiliac coercive disorder: rape. Which of the following assessment questions will provide the nurse with insight toward this client's cognitive distortion?

1. "Tell me what you're feeling."
2. "Do you have any lifestyle problems?"
3. "What brings you to the hospital for treatment?"
4. "Do you believe you're here for a sexual disorder?"

20. 4. If a client had a cognitive disorder, then the client would be using denial as a defense mechanism and would deny having a sexual disorder. Asking why the client is at the hospital will tell the nurse if the client has insight into his illness. Asking about lifestyle problems will provide the nurse with information related to problems with relationships. Asking what a client is feeling is important, but it doesn't provide information on the use of defense mechanisms.

NP: Assessment; CN: Psychosocial integrity; CNS: Coping and adaptation; CL: Application

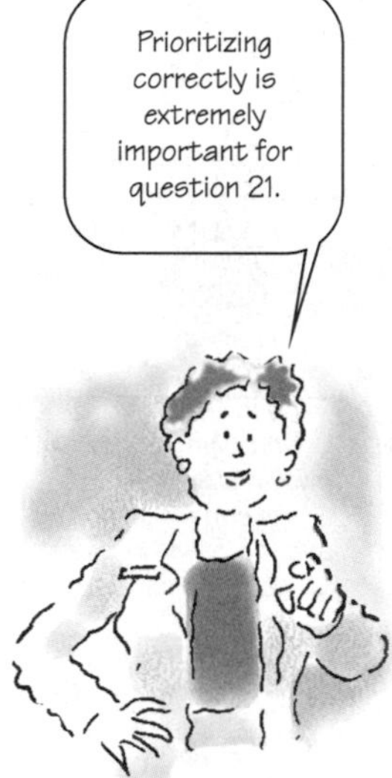

Prioritizing correctly is extremely important for question 21.

21. A 38-year-old woman was returning home from the store late one evening and was sexually assaulted. When she's brought to the emergency department, she's crying. Which of the following concerns for this client should be the nurse's first priority?

1. Filing a police report
2. Calling the client's family
3. Encouraging the client to enroll in a self-defense class
4. Remaining with the client and assisting her through the crisis

21. 4. Sexual assault is treated as a medical emergency, and the client requires constant attention and assistance during the crisis. Filing a police report wouldn't take precedence over a medical emergency. Comforting the client by contacting family should be carried out after the client's injuries are treated. Encouraging the client to enroll in a self-defense class isn't appropriate during crisis.

NP: Implementation; CN: Psychosocial integrity; CNS: Psychosocial adaptation; CL: Application

22. A client is admitted to the psychiatric unit as part of his probation period for exhibitionism and fetishism. The client seems to be adjusting well, but several clients report that their undergarments are missing. Which of the following actions would be most appropriate?

1. Notify the primary health care provider.
2. Search the client's room.
3. Call a community meeting, and let the clients settle the matter.
4. Privately assess whether the client is engaging in sexual activities on the unit.

22. 4. Meeting with the client privately establishes trust. This client needs to be assessed for what triggers might be present to prompt this behavior. Searching the client's room without discussion is a violation of a trusting milieu. It isn't therapeutic to encourage the unit to confront one member of the community. Notification of the primary health care provider shouldn't be done without assessment of the client.

NP: Implementation; CN: Psychosocial integrity; CNS: Psychosocial adaptation; CL: Application

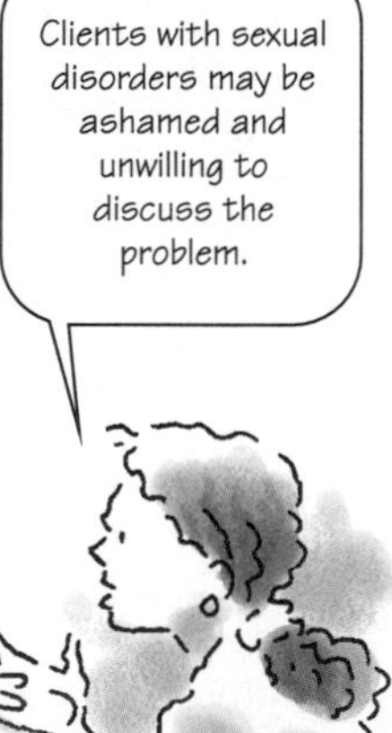

Clients with sexual disorders may be ashamed and unwilling to discuss the problem.

23. A client is admitted to the hospital for scatophilia and tells the nurse that he doesn't want to talk to her about his sexual behaviors. Which of the following responses from the nurse is most appropriate?

1. "I need to ask you the questions on the database."
2. "It's your right not to answer my questions."
3. "OK, I'll just write 'no comment.'"
4. "I know this must be difficult for you."

23. 4. Stating "I know this must be difficult for you" acknowledges the client's feelings and opens communications. Insisting that the form needs to be completed doesn't open up communications or acknowledge the client's feelings. Clients have rights, but data collection is necessary so that help with the problem can be offered. Writing "no comment" alone would be inappropriate.

NP: Implementation; CN: Psychosocial integrity; CNS: Psychosocial adaptation; CL: Application

24. Which of the following therapies may be used with a client who admits to frottage?

1. Electroconvulsive therapy
2. Relaxation therapy
3. Administration of psychotropic agents
4. Positive reinforcement and group therapy

24. 4. Frottage involves rubbing against someone in a public place. Positive reinforcement and group therapy are used to assist a client with frottage to develop new sexual response patterns. Electroconvulsive therapy and relaxation therapy aren't indicated for this condition. Psychotropic medications are used for dangerous and compulsive practices and aren't indicated for this condition.

NP: Planning; CN: Psychosocial integrity; CNS: Psychosocial adaptation; CL: Analysis

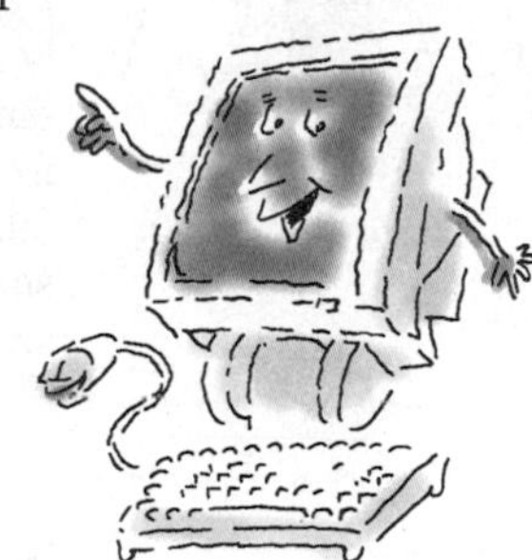
Keep going; you're doing great!

25. When treating a client admitted to the psychiatric unit for transvestic fetishism, the nurse should develop a care plan based on which of the following diagnoses?

1. Ineffective health maintenance
2. Ineffective sexuality patterns
3. Dysfunctional grieving
4. Self-care deficit

25. 2. Ineffective sexuality patterns would be appropriate because transvestic fetishism refers to intense sexual arousal with cross-dressing. Ineffective health maintenance is an appropriate diagnosis for someone experiencing a health problem. Self-care deficit is a diagnosis for the inability to meet self-care needs. Dysfunctional grieving refers to the inability to recover from a loss. The client hasn't exhibited any problems with health, self-care, or loss.

NP: Planning; CN: Psychosocial integrity; CNS: Coping and adaptation; CL: Application

26. When working with a client with a paraphiliac disorder, which of the following goals is appropriate for the client?

1. To attend all meetings on the unit
2. To use triggers to initiate sexual behaviors
3. To inform his employer of the reason for hospitalization
4. To verbalize appropriate methods to meet sexual needs upon discharge

26. 4. Upon discharge, the client should verbalize an alternative appropriate method to meet his sexual needs and effective strategies to prevent relapse. It isn't imperative that the client attend all meetings on the unit, but it's important that the client attend the prescribed group sessions. The client may wish to discuss the disorder with his spouse but not necessarily his employer. A client with a paraphiliac disorder should recognize triggers that initiate inappropriate sexual behaviors and learn ways to direct his impulses.

NP: Planning; CN: Psychosocial integrity; CNS: Psychosocial adaptation; CL: Analysis

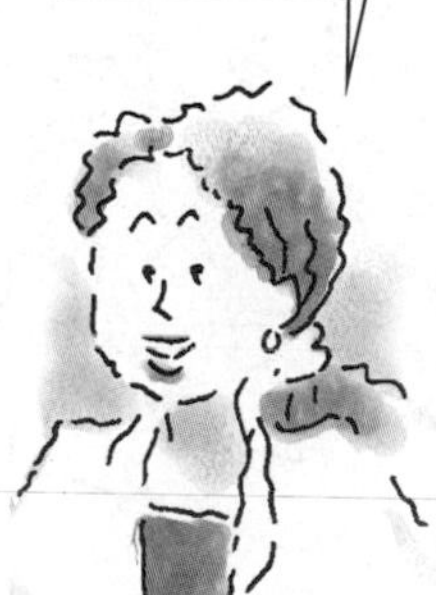
Effective care may involve managing interactions between clients.

27. A client admitted to the hospital with a diagnosis of pedophilia tells his roommate about his problems. His roommate runs down the hall yelling at the nurse, "I don't want to be in here with a child molester." Which of the following responses from the nurse is most appropriate?

1. "Stop acting out."
2. "Calm down, and go back to your room."
3. "Your roommate isn't a child molester."
4. "I can see you're upset. Sit down and we'll talk."

27. 4. Acknowledging that the client is upset and sitting down and talking with him will allow the client to verbalize his feelings. If a client were agitated or anxious over his roommate, it wouldn't be therapeutic or safe to keep those clients together without intervention. Stating that the pedophile isn't a child molester doesn't acknowledge the client's feelings. Telling the client to stop acting out isn't a therapeutic response.

NP: Implementation; CN: Psychosocial integrity; CNS: Psychosocial adaptation; CL: Application

28. When assigning rooms for clients, the nurse should *not* place which of the following clients with a client who has a diagnosis of sexual sadism?

1. A client with a diagnosis of sexual masochism
2. A client with a diagnosis of voyeurism
3. A client who's an exhibitionist
4. A client who's a homosexual

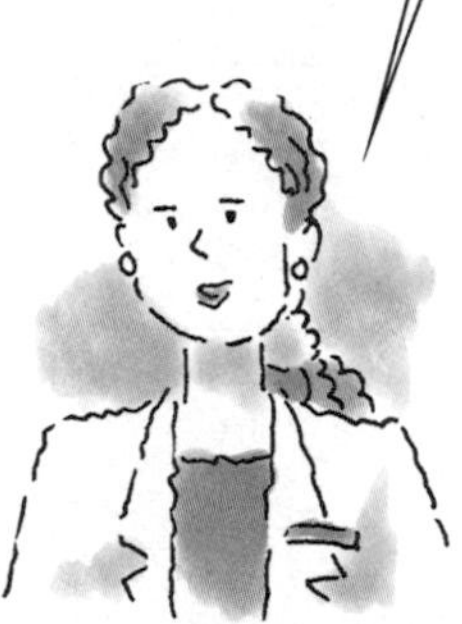

Be aware of the compatibility of the clients you select as roommates.

28. 1. A client who's admitted with a diagnosis of sexual masochism is aroused through suffering and, therefore, shouldn't be placed with a client who's diagnosed with sexual sadism, who's aroused by inflicted pain. An exhibitionist is aroused through the exposure of one's genitals to an unsuspecting person. A homosexual enjoys relationships with someone of the same sex. A voyeur is aroused by secretly observing someone who's naked or engaged in sexual activity.

NP: Planning; CN: Safe, effective care environment; CNS: Management of care; CL: Application

29. The nurse is obtaining a health history from a client when he states he has been diagnosed with voyeurism. The nurse knows which of the following actions is characteristic of a voyeur?

1. Observing others while they disrobe
2. Wearing clothing of the opposite sex
3. Rubbing against a nonconsenting person
4. Using rubber sheeting for sexual arousal

29. 1. Voyeurism is sexual arousal from secretly observing someone who is disrobing. Rubbing against someone who is nonconsenting is frottage. Using objects for sexual arousal is fetishism. Transvestic fetishism describes someone who enjoys cross-dressing.

NP: Assessment; CN: Psychosocial integrity; CNS: Psychosocial adaptation; CL: Comprehension

30. Which of the following characteristics best describes the client with scatophilia?

1. The client uses the telephone for sexual arousal.
2. The client uses the Internet for sexual gratification.
3. The client is aroused through contact with children.
4. The client is aroused by rubbing against a nonconsenting person.

30. 1. Telephone scatophilia is a paraphilia in which a person derives sexual arousal by engaging in lewd conversations on the telephone. As of present, there are no *DSM-IV* criteria for sexual gratification through the Internet. Pedophiles engage in fondling or sexual activities with children under 13 years of age. Frottage is rubbing against a nonconsenting person for sexual arousal.

NP: Assessment; CN: Psychosocial integrity; CNS: Psychosocial adaptation; CL: Comprehension

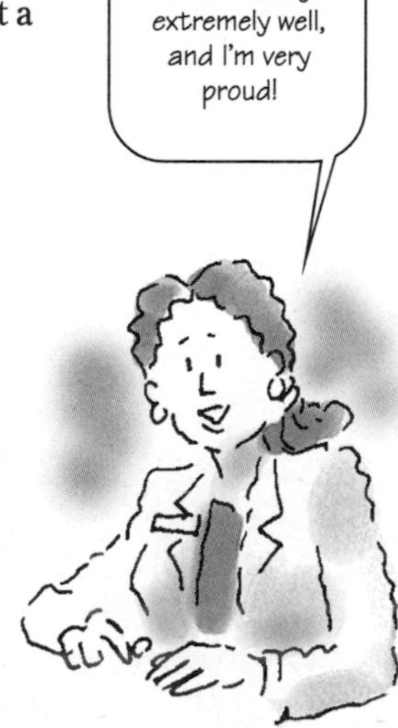

You're doing extremely well, and I'm very proud!

31. Which of the following factors is the biological cause of paraphilias?

1. Hormonal levels
2. Hereditary factors
3. Environmental factors
4. History of sexual abuse

31. 1. Hormonal levels are biologically based factors. Heredity, a history of sexual abuse, and environmental factors are all non-biological factors in the development of paraphilias.

NP: Assessment; CN: Psychosocial integrity; CNS: Psychosocial adaptation; CL: Comprehension

32. Which of the following definitions best describes necrophilia?

1. Obscene phone calling
2. Sexual activity with animals
3. Sexual activity with corpses
4. Sexual arousal by contact with urine

32. 3. The definition of necrophilia is sexual activity with corpses. Scatophilia is sexual arousal through obscene telephone calling. Zoophilia is sexual activity with animals. Sexual arousal by contact with urine is known as urophilia.

NP: Implementation; CN: Psychosocial integrity; CNS: Coping and adaptation; CL: Comprehension

33. A nurse lecturing on paraphilias informs her audience that recidivism is high for paraphilias. Which of the following definitions best describes recidivism?

1. Insight into treatment
2. Aggressive sexual assault
3. Behaviors associated with sexual deviation
4. Continued inappropriate behavior after treatment

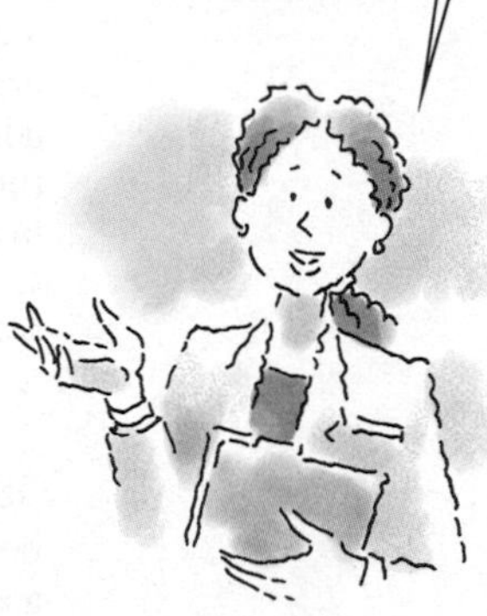

The NCLEX often tests your ability to educate accurately.

33. 4. Recidivism is defined as continuing in an unacceptable behavior after completing treatment to correct that behavior. Sexually deviant behaviors are known as paraphilias. High level of insight isn't connected with any specific disorder. Aggressive sexual assault is a type of paraphilia.

NP: Assessment; CN: Psychosocial integrity; CNS: Coping and adaptation; CL: Analysis

34. Which of the following nursing diagnoses is most appropriate for a client with sexual masochism?

1. Risk for self-mutilation
2. Ineffective role performance
3. Ineffective coping
4. Risk for other-directed violence

34. 1. A person with sexual masochism is sexually aroused by being the receiver of pain and, therefore, may injure himself. There is no evidence that this client isn't coping. A person diagnosed with transvestic fetishism may have ineffective role performance. A sexual sadist would be a danger to others.

NP: Planning; CN: Psychosocial integrity; CNS: Psychosocial adaptation; CL: Analysis

35. Which of the following statements made by a client with paraphilia indicates a potential for relapse?

1. "I am going to outpatient therapy."
2. "I am going to try to attend all therapy sessions."
3. "I don't need this, and I can't imagine why the judge sent me here."
4. "The physician wants me to take leuprolide acetate (Lupron). I think that will help."

35. 3. A lack of insight to the problem may indicate a potential for relapse. Attending all therapy sessions and outpatient therapy demonstrates compliance with the treatment plan. Lupron is an anti-androgenic that lowers testosterone levels and decreases the libido.

NP: Evaluation; CN: Psychosocial integrity; CNS: Psychosocial adaptation; CL: Analysis

36. The nurse knows that gender is part of one's identity. Which of the following events signifies when gender is first ascribed?

1. A baby is born.
2. A child attends school.
3. A child receives sex-specific toys.
4. A child receives sex-specific clothing.

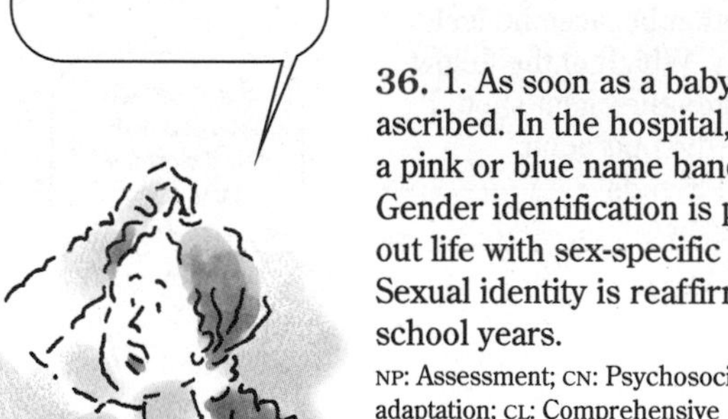

So, when do gender differences start?

36. 1. As soon as a baby is born, gender is ascribed. In the hospital, a baby is given either a pink or blue name band, card, or blanket. Gender identification is perpetuated throughout life with sex-specific clothing and toys. Sexual identity is reaffirmed throughout the school years.

NP: Assessment; CN: Psychosocial integrity; CNS: Coping and adaptation; CL: Comprehensive

37. A mother brings her 14-year-old son to the psychiatric crisis room. The client's mother states, "He's always dressing in female clothing. There must be something wrong with him." Which of the following responses from the nurse would be most appropriate?

1. "Your son will be evaluated shortly."
2. "I'll tell your son that this isn't appropriate."
3. "I know you're upset. Would you like to talk?"
4. "I wouldn't want my son to dress in girl's clothing."

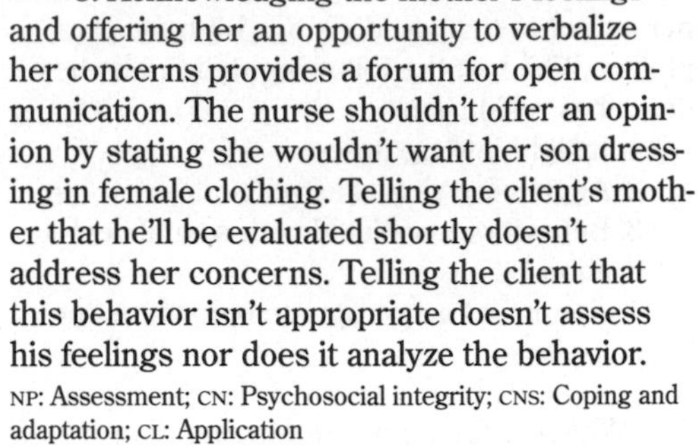

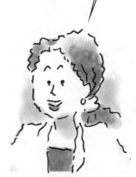

37. 3. Acknowledging the mother's feelings and offering her an opportunity to verbalize her concerns provides a forum for open communication. The nurse shouldn't offer an opinion by stating she wouldn't want her son dressing in female clothing. Telling the client's mother that he'll be evaluated shortly doesn't address her concerns. Telling the client that this behavior isn't appropriate doesn't assess his feelings nor does it analyze the behavior.

NP: Assessment; CN: Psychosocial integrity; CNS: Coping and adaptation; CL: Application

38. A 17-year-old female who enjoys playing ball with "the boys" and is most comfortable in jeans tells her mother she doesn't want to go to the prom if she has to wear a frilly dress. Her mother asks, "What should I do with my daughter?" Which of the following responses from the nurse would be most appropriate?

1. Tell the client's mother, "She'll grow out of it."
2. Offer to speak to the client about her dressing habits.
3. Ask the client's mother to talk about her fears for her daughter.
4. Tell the client's mother to make her go to the prom but not wear a dress.

38. 3. Asking the client's mother to verbalize her fears will permit the nurse to accurately assess the mother's distress. The client's mother may be upset over the boyish behavior or the fact that her daughter doesn't wish to go to the prom. The nurse shouldn't speak to the client about her boyish ways as this implies a value judgment on the part of the nurse. Forcing her to go to the prom isn't therapeutic, and doesn't address the mother's fears. Telling the client's mother that her daughter will grow out of it may be offering the mother false reassurance.

NP: Assessment; CN: Psychosocial integrity; CNS: Coping and adaptation; CL: Application

39. A 39-year-old male wishes to undergo a sex-reassignment operation because he feels trapped in his male body. Which of the following actions is the next step the client should take if he wants to have the operation?

1. Tell his family and friends
2. Attend psychotherapy
3. Visit transsexual bars
4. See a surgeon

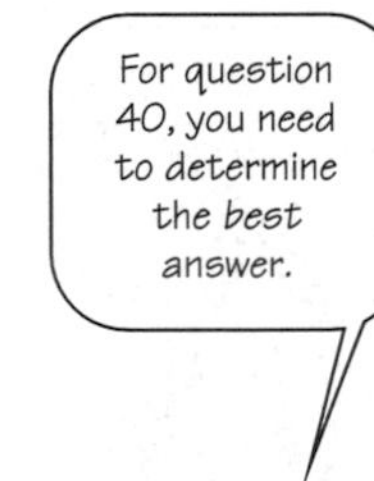

For question 40, you need to determine the best answer.

39. 2. Before having a sex-reassignment operation, the client should have several years of psychotherapy. The family, as well as friends, should be told of the client's plans. Seeing a surgeon isn't usually done on a regular basis until after the completion of psychotherapy. Visiting transsexual bars has no bearing on having a sex-reassignment operation.

NP: Assessment; CN: Psychosocial integrity; CNS: Psychosocial adaptation; CL: Analysis

40. Which of the following reasons best explains the rationale for estrogen therapy for a male client who wishes to undergo sexual reassignment surgery?

1. To develop breasts
2. To cause menstruation
3. To assist with cross-dressing
4. To develop body hair and lack of menstruation

40. 1. A male who receives long-term estrogen therapy will develop female secondary sexual characteristics such as breasts. Androgens would be taken by a female to develop body hair and stop menstruation. A male on estrogen won't menstruate as he doesn't have a uterus. Estrogen has no bearing on cross-dressing.

NP: Implementation; CN: Psychosocial integrity; CNS: Psychosocial adaptation; CL: Analysis

41. The nurse is caring for several clients with gender identity disorders. The nurse understands that which of the following clients is most at risk for anxiety related to transsexualism?

1. Elderly
2. Adolescent
3. Young adult
4. Prepubescent child

42. What is the gender identity disorder that results in the person believing he or she is really the opposite sex?

1. Exhibitionism
2. Homosexuality
3. Transsexualism
4. Transvestitism

43. A transsexual client wishes to have a sexual reassignment operation and tells the nurse he's ready to begin hormonal therapy. Which of the following facts about the client must be true before estrogen therapy is administered?

1. He has cross-dressed and lived as the opposite sex for several years.
2. He has decided against undergoing the operation.
3. He has decided he needs more psychotherapy.
4. He has been functioning sexually as a female.

44. According to Erikson, an adolescent who is suffering from gender identity disorder is unable to progress through which of the following developmental tasks?

1. Initiative versus guilt
2. Intimacy versus isolation
3. Industry versus inferiority
4. Identity versus role confusion

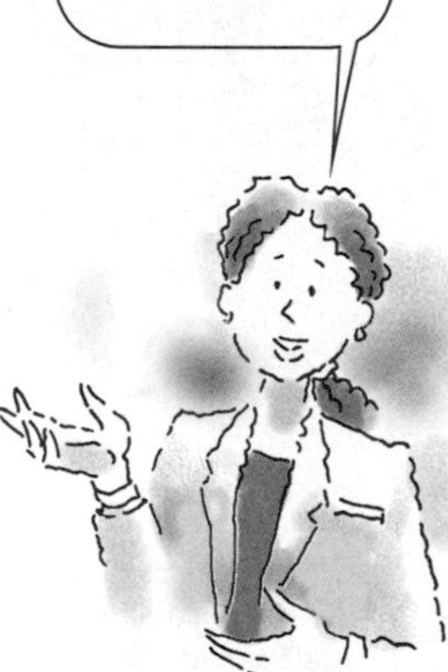

For question 43, you need to determine the proper order of events for this client.

41. 2. Adolescents who are transsexuals are usually very distraught over the changes occurring within their body. Children, young adults, and elderly persons aren't experiencing rapidly developing secondary sexual characteristics in their bodies; therefore, they aren't at high risk for anxiety.

NP: Implementation; CN: Psychosocial integrity; CNS: Coping and adaptation; CL: Analysis

42. 3. Transsexuals believe they're really of the opposite sex. A homosexual enjoys sexual relations with a person of the same sexual orientation. A transvestite enjoys cross-dressing. An exhibitionist is someone who's sexually aroused by displaying one's genitals in a public place.

NP: Analysis; CN: Psychosocial integrity; CNS: Coping and adaptation; CL: Application

43. 1. Before a sexual reassignment operation, the client should live as the opposite sex after undergoing several years of psychotherapy. A client wishing to take hormonal therapy is in the final step before receiving the operation. A male doesn't have female reproductive organs, so he couldn't have been functioning sexually as a female. Psychotherapy is an ongoing modality for someone requesting a sexual reassignment operation.

NP: Implementation; CN: Psychosocial integrity; CNS: Psychosocial adaptation; CL: Analysis

44. 4. According to developmentalist Erik Erikson, adolescence is a time when role identity is found as a result of independence and sexual maturity; role confusion would result from the inability to integrate all experiences. Initiative versus guilt is when a child begins to conceptualize and interpersonalize relationships. Industry versus inferiority is when a child incorporates and acquires social skills. Intimacy versus isolation is a stage in which the adult meets other adults and establishes relationships.

NP: Assessment; CN: Health promotion and maintenance; CNS: Growth and development through the life span; CL: Analysis

45. A 35-year-old male who has been married for 10 years arrives at the psychiatric clinic stating, "I can't live this lie any more. I wish I were a woman. I don't want my wife. I need a man." Which of the following initial actions would be most appropriate from the nurse?

1. Call the primary health care provider.
2. Encourage the client to speak to his wife.
3. Have the client admitted.
4. Sit down with the client, and talk about his feelings.

45. 4. Sitting down with the client and exploring his feelings will allow the nurse to assess him. The primary health care provider shouldn't be notified until an assessment is made. An assessment of the client should be made *before* admitting the client to the unit. He shouldn't speak to his wife until he has processed his feelings.

NP: Implementation; CN: Psychosocial integrity; CNS: Psychosocial adaptation; CL: Application

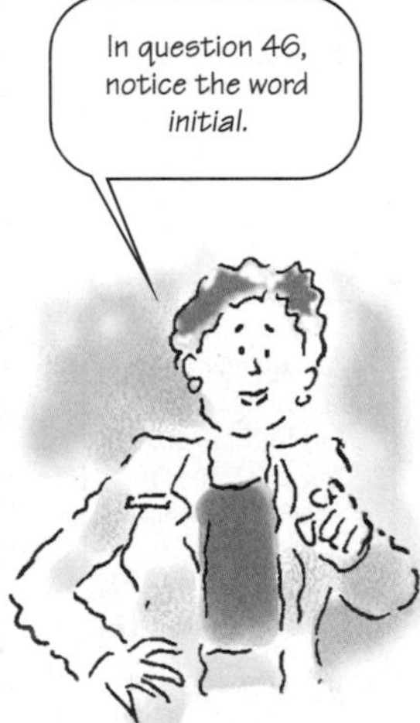

In question 46, notice the word *initial.*

46. A 14-year-old female client admits to having transsexual feelings and states, "I would rather die than live in this body." Which of the following initial actions would be most appropriate for the nurse to take?

1. Explain to her that she is too young to have these feelings.
2. Call her parents, and let them know about her feelings.
3. Encourage her to verbalize her feelings.
4. Ask her if she plans to kill herself.

46. 4. Whenever a client verbalizes feelings of preferring death to life, the nurse should always make sure that the client doesn't have a plan. Transsexual tendencies usually arise during the adolescent years, so it is appropriate for the client to have these feelings. Calling her parents wouldn't be a priority until after a psychological safety assessment is completed. Encouraging her to verbalize her feelings isn't an initial action for the nurse.

NP: Assessment; CN: Psychosocial integrity; CNS: Psychosocial adaptation; CL: Application

47. A female client enjoys wearing men's clothing. Her sister tells the nurse that the client wishes a sexual reassignment operation. The client tells the nurse she just wants to be left alone. Which of the following initial nursing interventions is most appropriate?

1. Allow the client to deal with her sister.
2. Encourage the client to verbalize her feelings.
3. Tell the client's sister to mind her own business.
4. Encourage the client to continue doing what is comfortable for her.

47. 2. The client needs to verbalize her feelings regarding wearing male attire as well as her desire to be left alone. It's inappropriate for a nurse to tell a family member to mind her own business. The client shouldn't be encouraged to do whatever makes her comfortable until she is assessed.

NP: Assessment; CN: Psychosocial integrity; CNS: Coping and adaptation; CL: Application

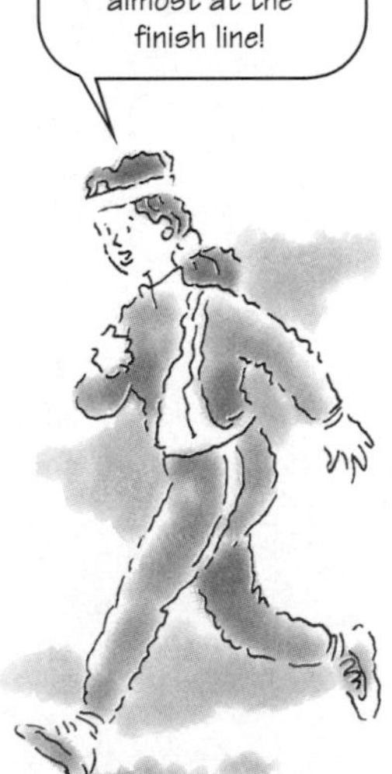

Keep going! You're almost at the finish line!

48. A mother is concerned about her son and says he's 10 years old and has been playing with dolls since he was 2. Which of the following initial strategies should be included in his care plan?

1. Providing counseling for his mother
2. Instructing the mother to throw away the dolls
3. Instructing the mother on play that's age-appropriate
4. Exploring with the child his feelings related to the dolls

48. 4. It's important to assess the child's feelings as well as to explore his preference for dolls rather than sports. There's no evidence of age-inappropriate play. Until proper assessment is made, it's inappropriate to remove the dolls. The mother may need to be instructed on methods to cope with his behaviors but only after the child is permitted to verbalize.

NP: Planning; CN: Psychosocial integrity; CNS: Psychosocial adaptation; CL: Application

NP: Nursing process CN: Client needs category CNS: Client needs subcategory CL: Cognitive level

49. A newly graduated nurse expresses concern to the nurse-manager about working with clients who want to discuss sexual problems. Which response by the nurse-manager is appropriate?

1. "If you find sexual dysfunction an interesting subject, you're qualified to provide counseling to that client."
2. "You can refer those types of questions to other health care professionals."
3. "If you've graduated from nursing school and passed the NCLEX, you qualify as a sex counselor."
4. "Any nurse should be able to give basic information about sexual health and to screen for sexual dysfunction."

49. 4. Basic nursing education provides a knowledge base sufficient to assess for sexual dysfunction and to perform sexual health teaching. Sex therapists have additional training and education.

NP: Analysis; CN: Psychosocial integrity; CNS: Coping and adaptation; CL: Application

50. A 57-year-old hypertensive male client expresses concern about his sexual functioning. Which question is most helpful in obtaining further assessment data?

1. Medication history
2. Sexual practices
3. Medical conditions
4. Family history

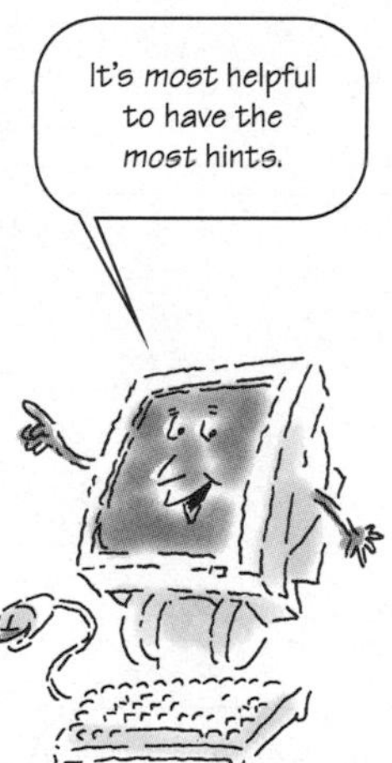

It's most helpful
to have the
most hints.

50. 1. Many antihypertensive medications can affect sexual functioning; the nurse must assess if the client is taking other medications that may also alter sexual functioning. Sexual practices are part of the nursing assessment, as are other medical conditions and family history. However, obtaining a thorough medication history and reviewing effects on the client may help alleviate misconceptions and easily identify the source of the problem.

NP: Assessment; CN: Physiological integrity; CNS: Pharmacological and parenteral therapies; CL: Application

51. A male client brings a list of his prescribed medications to the clinic. During the initial assessment, he tells the nurse that he has been experiencing delayed ejaculation. Which drug class is associated with this problem?

1. Anticoagulants
2. Antibiotics
3. Antihypertensives
4. Steroids

51. 3. Antihypertensive agents can cause or contribute to sexual dysfunction. Anticoagulants, antibiotics, and steroids have no known effect on sexual function.

NP: Assessment; CN: Physiological integrity; CNS: Pharmacological and parenteral therapies; CL: Knowledge

52. After a myocardial infarction (MI), a client tells the nurse he's afraid he'll have another heart attack if he attempts sexual intercourse. Which nursing diagnosis is most appropriate?

1. Deficient knowledge related to sexual dysfunction
2. Disturbed body image related to lifestyle changes
3. Sexual dysfunction related to disturbances in self-esteem
4. Disturbed body image related to effects of treatment

52. 1. After an MI, many clients fear that engaging in sex will trigger another MI. The nurse should teach the client about when he can safely resume sexual activity and which positions to use during intercourse to conserve energy. The client's fears result from lack of knowledge, not disturbances in self-esteem or body image.

NP: Assessment; CN: Psychosocial integrity; CNS: Psychosocial adaptation; CL: Application

53. A 42-year-old woman complains of painful intercourse. Which nursing diagnosis is <u>most</u> useful in planning this client's care?

1. Ineffective coping
2. Disturbed body image
3. Ineffective sexuality patterns
4. Sexual dysfunction

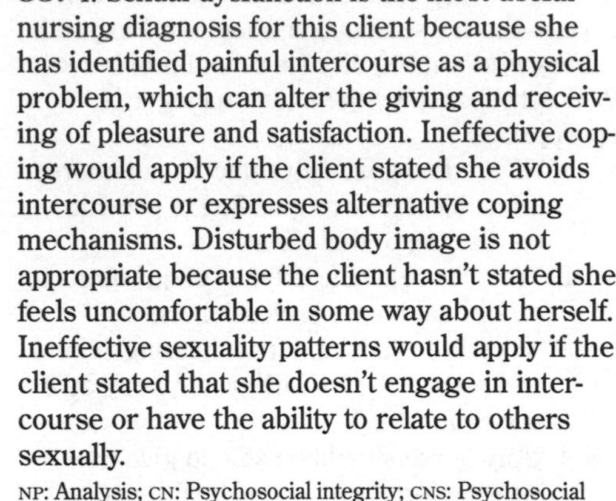

53. 4. Sexual dysfunction is the most useful nursing diagnosis for this client because she has identified painful intercourse as a physical problem, which can alter the giving and receiving of pleasure and satisfaction. Ineffective coping would apply if the client stated she avoids intercourse or expresses alternative coping mechanisms. Disturbed body image is not appropriate because the client hasn't stated she feels uncomfortable in some way about herself. Ineffective sexuality patterns would apply if the client stated that she doesn't engage in intercourse or have the ability to relate to others sexually.

NP: Analysis; CN: Psychosocial integrity; CNS: Psychosocial adaptation; CL: Application

54. A 46-year-old female client is diagnosed with a problem in sexual functioning. When planning her care, which nursing action takes <u>highest priority</u>?

1. Assessing the client's sexual functioning
2. Assessing the client's role in her sexual relationship
3. Determining the nurse's own beliefs and feelings about this issue
4. Interviewing the client's sexual partner

54. 3. The nurse must first identify her own beliefs and feelings about the issue and remain nonjudgmental. The other actions may be relevant but take lower priority.

NP: Analysis; CN: Psychosocial integrity; CNS: Psychosocial adaptation; CL: Application

55. Which of the following disorders would the nurse expect to encounter <u>most</u> often when working in a sexual dysfunction treatment clinic?

1. Sexual aversion disorder
2. Dyspareunia
3. Decreased sexual desire
4. Vaginismus

55. 3. Decreased sexual desire is the most common problem seen in sexual dysfunction treatment clinics. Sexual aversion, dyspareunia, and vaginismus are encountered less commonly.

NP: Assessment; CN: Physiological integrity; CNS: Physiological adaptation; CL: Knowledge

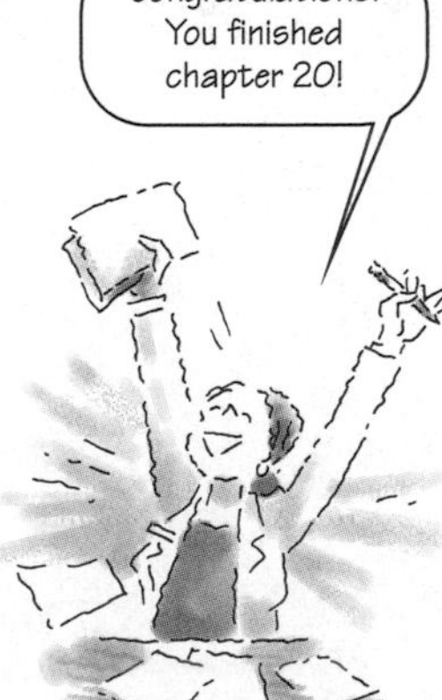
Congratulations! You finished chapter 20!

56. A client in a psychiatric unit has been identified as a peeping Tom. What's the medical term for the client's disorder?

1. Voyeurism
2. Gender identity disorder
3. Pedophilia
4. Fetishism

56. 1. A "peeping Tom" has a disorder called voyeurism and is sexually excited by sexual fantasies, urges, or behaviors involving observing an unknowing and nonconsenting person (usually unclothed or engaged in sex). Gender identity disorder is characterized by a feeling of being trapped in a body of the wrong gender. Pedophilia is characterized by sexual fantasies, urges, or behaviors involving sexual activity with a prepubescent child. Fetishism refers to sexual fantasies, urges, or behaviors involving the use of nonhuman objects to produce or enhance sexual arousal with or without a partner.

NP: Assessment; CN: Psychosocial integrity; CNS: Psychosocial adaptation; CL: Knowledge

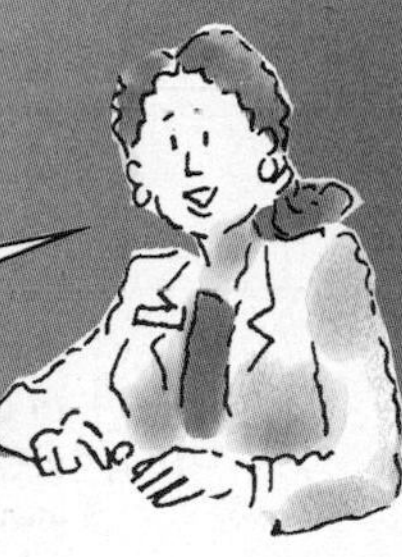

New information about eating disorders is released almost continuously. For the latest about disorders of critical importance for young people, check the Internet site of the National Eating Disorders Association at www.nationaleatingdisorders.org/.

Chapter 21 Eating disorders

1. A parent with a daughter with bulimia nervosa asks a nurse, "How can my child have an eating disorder when she isn't underweight?" Which of the following responses is best?

1. "A person with bulimia nervosa can maintain a normal weight."
2. "It's hard to face this type of problem in a person you love."
3. "At first there is no weight loss; it comes later in the disease."
4. "This is a serious problem even though there is no weight loss."

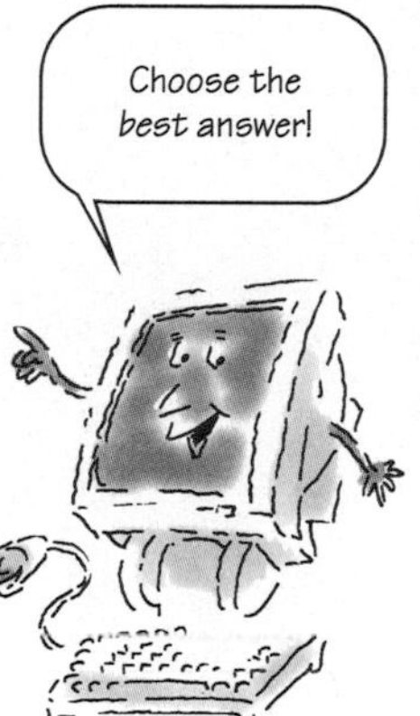

2. A nurse is assessing an adolescent girl recently diagnosed with an eating disorder and symptoms of bulimia nervosa. Which of the following findings is expected based on laboratory test results?

1. Hypocalcemia
2. Hypoglycemia
3. Hypokalemia
4. Hypophosphatemia

3. Which of the following statements about the binge-purge cycle that occurs with bulimia nervosa is correct?

1. There are emotional triggers connected to bingeing.
2. Over time, people often grow out of bingeing behaviors.
3. Bingeing isn't the problem; purging is the issue to address.
4. When a person gets too hungry, there's a tendency to binge.

Help your client understand her behavior.

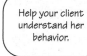

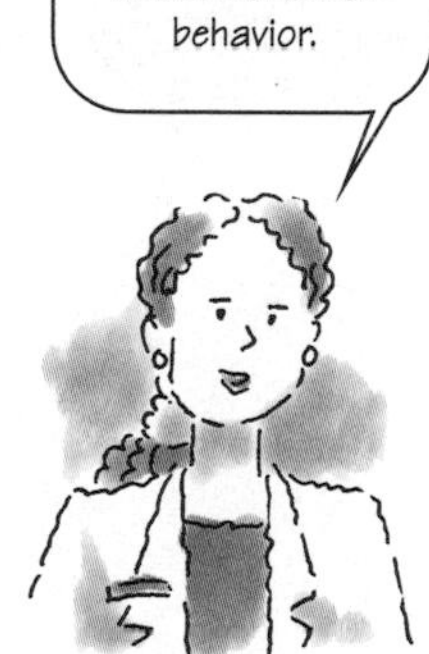

1. 1. A client with bulimia nervosa may be of normal weight, overweight, or underweight. Weight loss isn't a clinical criterion for bulimia nervosa. The second option doesn't address the need for information about the relationship between weight change and bulimia nervosa. The third option is incorrect because there may be little or no weight loss. The fourth option doesn't address the issue of weight change in a client with bulimia nervosa.

NP: Implementation; CN: Psychosocial integrity; CNS: Psychosocial adaptation; CL: Knowledge

2. 3. Clients who are newly diagnosed with bulimia nervosa will have hypokalemia, or decreased potassium levels, due to purging behaviors. Hypocalcemia and hypophosphatemia don't tend to occur in these clients until they have experienced the disorder for a longer period of time. Hypoglycemia doesn't tend to occur in these clients.

NP: Assessment; CN: Psychosocial integrity; CNS: Coping and adaptation; CL: Knowledge

3. 1. It's important for the client to understand the emotional triggers to bingeing, such as disappointment, depression, and anxiety. People don't outgrow eating behaviors. This leads a person to believe binge eating is a normal part of growth and development when it definitely isn't. The third option negates the seriousness of bingeing and leads the client to believe only vomiting is a problem, not overeating. Physiologic hunger doesn't predispose a client to binge behaviors.

NP: Implementation; CN: Physiological integrity; CNS: Reduction of risk potential; CL: Comprehension

4. A client with bulimia nervosa tells a nurse she has periods of depression. Which of the following areas is assessed to determine if the depression has affected her daily functioning?

1. Chronic fatigue
2. Paranoid thinking
3. Verbal manipulation
4. Threatening behaviors

4. 1. Chronic fatigue is highly symptomatic of depression and interferes with a client's routine activities of daily living. Clients with an eating disorder who have periods of depression don't necessarily show paranoid thinking, threatening behaviors, or engage in verbal manipulation of others.

NP: Assessment; CN: Psychosocial integrity; CNS: Coping and adaptation; CL: Comprehension

5. A client with a diagnosis of bulimia nervosa is working on relationship issues. Which of the following nursing interventions is the most important?

1. Have the client work on developing social skills.
2. Focus on how relationships cause bulimic behavior.
3. Help the client identify feelings about relationships.
4. Discuss how to prevent getting overinvolved in relationships.

5. 3. The client needs to address personal feelings, especially uncomfortable ones because they may trigger bingeing behavior. Social skills are important to a client's well-being, but they aren't typically a major problem for the client with bulimia nervosa. Relationships ***don't cause*** bulimic behaviors. It's the inability to handle stress or conflict that arises from interactions that causes the client to be distressed. The client isn't necessarily overinvolved in relationships; the issue may be the lack of satisfying relationships in the person's life.

NP: Implementation; CN: Psychosocial integrity; CNS: Psychosocial adaptation; CL: Application

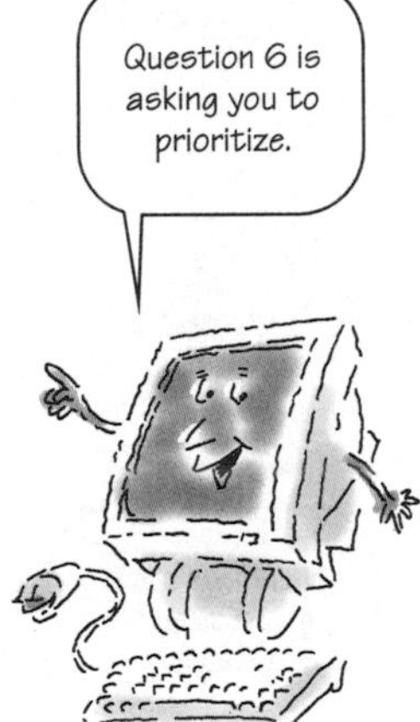
Question 6 is
asking you to
prioritize.

6. A young woman with bulimia nervosa wants to lessen her feelings of powerlessness. Which of the following short-term goals is most important initially?

1. Learn problem-solving skills.
2. Decrease symptoms of anxiety.
3. Perform self-care activities daily.
4. Verbalize how to set limits with others.

6. 1. If the client can learn effective problem-solving skills, she'll gain a sense of control and power over her life. Anxiety is commonly caused by feelings of powerlessness. Verbalizing how to set limits and protect self from the intrusive behavior of others is a necessary life skill, but problem-solving skills take priority. Performing daily self-care activities won't reduce one's sense of powerlessness.

NP: Analysis; CN: Psychosocial integrity; CNS: Psychosocial adaptation; CL: Comprehension

7. A client with bulimia nervosa tells a nurse her parents don't know about her eating disorder. Which of the following goals is appropriate for this client and her family?

1. Decrease the chaos in the family unit.
2. Learn effective communication skills.
3. Spend time together in social situations.
4. Discuss the client's need to be responsible.

7. 2. A major goal for the client and her family is to learn to communicate directly and honestly. To change the chaotic environment, the family must first learn to communicate effectively. Families with a member who has an eating disorder are often enmeshed and don't need to spend more time together. Before discussing the client's level of responsibility, the family needs to establish effective ways to communicate with each other.

NP: Analysis; CN: Psychosocial integrity; CNS: Psychosocial adaptation; CL: Comprehension

8. When discussing self-esteem with a client with bulimia nervosa, which of the following areas is the most important?
1. Personal fears
2. Family strengths
3. Negative thinking
4. Environmental stimuli

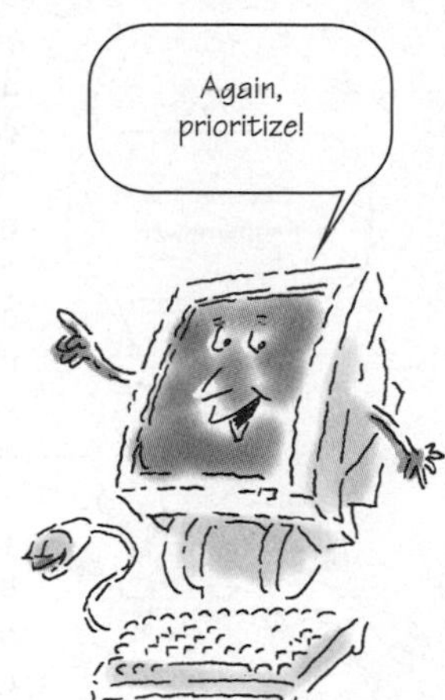
Again, prioritize!

8. 3. Clients with bulimia nervosa need to work on identifying and changing their negative thinking and distortion of reality. Personal fears are related to negative thinking. Exploring family strengths isn't a priority; it's more appropriate to explore the client's strengths. Environmental stimuli don't cause bulimic behaviors.

NP: Planning; CN: Psychosocial integrity; CNS: Psychosocial adaptation; CL: Application

9. Which of the following complications of bulimia nervosa is life-threatening?
1. Amenorrhea
2. Bradycardia
3. Electrolyte imbalance
4. Yellow skin

9. 3. Electrolyte imbalance can be a life-threatening complication of bulimia nervosa due to purging behaviors. Amenorrhea, bradycardia, and yellow skin are complications of bulimia nervosa that don't tend to be life-threatening.

NP: Assessment; CN: Psychosocial integrity; CNS: Coping and adaptation; CL: Knowledge

10. A nurse is talking to a client with bulimia nervosa about the complications of laxative abuse. Which of the following complications should be included?
1. Loss of taste
2. Swollen glands
3. Dental problems
4. Malabsorption of nutrients

10. 4. A serious complication of laxative abuse is malabsorption of nutrients, such as proteins, fats, and calcium. Laxative abuse doesn't tend to affect the client's sense of taste. Swollen glands and dental problems are complications associated with purging.

NP: Implementation; CN: Psychosocial integrity; CNS: Psychosocial adaptation; CL: Knowledge

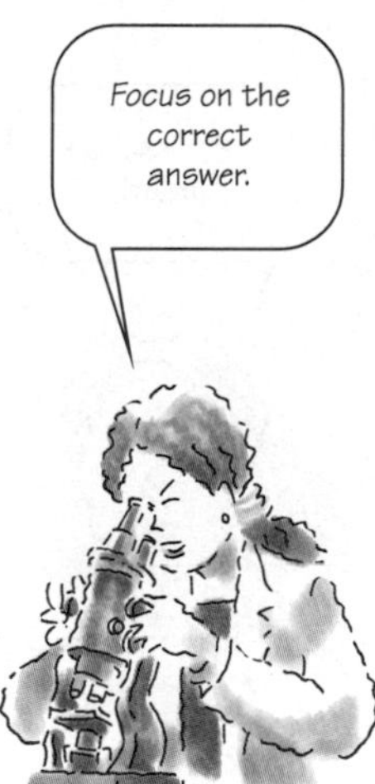
Focus on the correct answer.

11. A client with bulimia nervosa tells a nurse she and her parents don't agree on anything. Which of the following methods is best to address this problem when the family comes for a family meeting?
1. Focus on conflict resolution skills.
2. Establish an internal locus of control.
3. Construct a three-generation genogram.
4. Discuss age-specific developmental problems.

11. 1. To decrease conflict and promote family harmony, the nurse would teach the family conflict resolution skills. Establishing a plan to promote internal control or constructing a three-generation genogram won't help the family solve conflicts. Discussion of age-specific developmental problems won't promote conflict resolution or promote family harmony.

NP: Planning; CN: Psychosocial integrity; CNS: Psychosocial adaptation; CL: Comprehension

12. A client is talking to a nurse about her binge-purge cycle. Which of the following questions should the nurse ask about the cycle?
1. "Do you know how to stop the binge-purge cycle?"
2. "Does the binge-purge cycle help you lose weight?"
3. "Can the binge-purge cycle take away your anxiety?"
4. "How often do you go through the binge-purge cycle?"

12. 4. This is an important question because there's often a range of frequencies, such as from a once-a-week pattern to multiple times per day. Asking the client if she knows how to stop the binge-purge cycle isn't appropriate as it will generate feelings of self-blame and shame. It's common for clients to experience daily fluctuations in weight (some report variations of up to 10 lb). The binge-purge cycle doesn't decrease anxiety; it tends to generate overall negative feelings about self.

NP: Assessment; CN: Psychosocial integrity; CNS: Coping and adaptation; CL: Application

13. A nurse is assessing a client with bulimia nervosa for possible substance abuse. Which of the following questions is best to obtain information about this possible problem?

1. "Have you ever used diet pills?"
2. "Where would you go to buy drugs?"
3. "At what age did you start drinking?"
4. "Do your peers ever offer you drugs?"

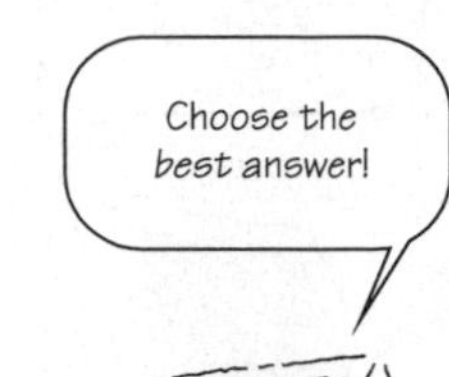
Choose the best answer!

13. 1. Some clients with bulimia nervosa have a history of or actively use amphetamines to control weight. The use of alcohol and street drugs is also common. The second and fourth questions could be answered by the client without revealing drug use. The age the client started drinking may not show current substance use.

NP: Assessment; CN: Psychosocial integrity; CNS: Coping and adaptation; CL: Comprehension

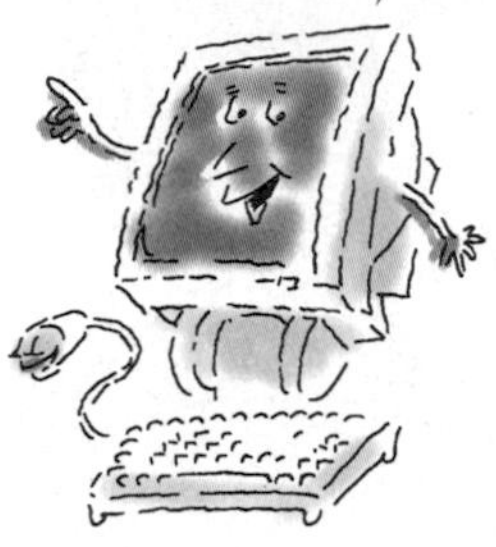

14. A client with bulimia nervosa is discussing her abnormal eating behaviors. Which of the following statements by the client indicates she's beginning to understand this eating disorder?

1. "When my loneliness gets to me, I start to binge."
2. "I know that when my life gets better I'll eat right."
3. "I know I waste food and waste my money on food."
4. "After my parents divorce, I'll talk about bingeing and purging."

14. 1. Binge eating is a way to handle the uncomfortable feelings of frustration, loneliness, anger, and fear. The second option indicates the client is experiencing denial of the eating disorder. The third option addresses the client's guilt feelings; it doesn't reflect knowledge of her eating disorder. The fourth option shows the client isn't ready to discuss her eating disorder.

NP: Analysis; CN: Psychosocial integrity; CNS: Psychosocial adaptation; CL: Analysis

15. A nurse is assessing a client to determine the distress experienced after binge eating. Which of the following symptoms are typical after bingeing?

1. Ageusia
2. Headache
3. Pain
4. Sore throat

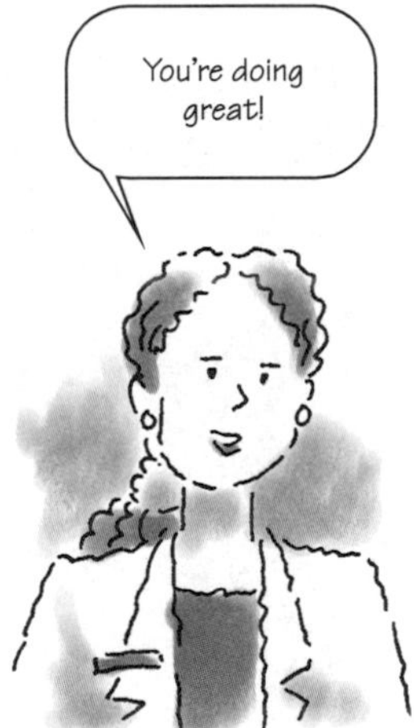
You're doing great!

15. 3. After a binge episode, the client commonly has abdominal distention and stomach pain. A sore throat is associated with vomiting. Ageusia (loss of taste) or headache aren't associated with binge eating.

NP: Assessment; CN: Physiological integrity; CNS: Physiological adaptation; CL: Knowledge

16. A mother of a client with bulimia nervosa asks a nurse if bulimia nervosa will stop her daughter from menstruating. Which of the following responses is best?

1. "All women with anorexia nervosa or bulimia nervosa will have amenorrhea."
2. "When your daughter is bingeing and purging, she won't have normal periods."
3. "The eating disorder must be ongoing for your daughter's menstrual cycle to change."
4. "Women with bulimia nervosa may have a normal or abnormal menstrual cycle, depending on the severity of the problem."

16. 4. Women with bulimia nervosa may have a normal or abnormal menstrual cycle, depending on the severity of the eating disorder. Not all women with eating disorders have amenorrhea. The eating disorder can disrupt the menstrual cycle at any point in the illness.

NP: Implementation; CN: Psychosocial integrity; CNS: Psychosocial adaptation; CL: Analysis

17. Which of the following difficulties are frequently found in families with a member who has bulimia nervosa?

1. Mental illness
2. Multiple losses
3. Chronic anxiety
4. Substance abuse

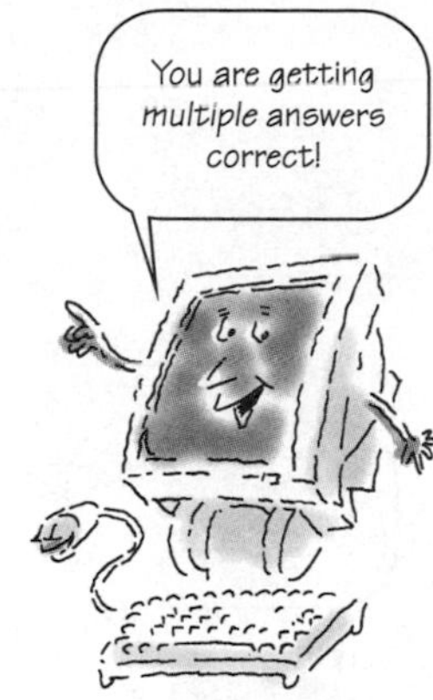
You are getting multiple answers correct!

17. 2. Families with a member who has bulimia nervosa often struggle with multiple losses. Mental illness, chronic anxiety, or substance abuse doesn't tend to be a theme in the family background of the client with bulimia nervosa.
NP: Assessment; CN: Psychosocial integrity; CNS: Coping and adaptation; CL: Analysis

18. A client with bulimia nervosa tells a nurse her major problem is eating too much food in a short period of time and then vomiting. Which of the following short-term goals is the most important?

1. Help the client understand every person has a satiety level.
2. Encourage the client to verbalize fears and concerns about food.
3. Determine the amount of food the client will eat without purging.
4. Obtain a therapy appointment to look at the emotional causes of bulimia nervosa.

18. 3. The client must meet her nutritional needs to prevent further complications, so she must identify the amount of food she can eat without purging as her first short-term goal. Binge eaters can't recognize their satiety level or their feelings of fullness. Obtaining knowledge or verbalizing her fears and feelings about food are *not* priority goals for this client. After meeting immediate physiological needs, therapy is an important part of dealing with this disorder.
NP: Planning; CN: Physiological integrity; CNS: Reduction of risk potential; CL: Application

19. Which of the following statements indicates a client with bulimia nervosa is making progress in interrupting the binge-purge cycle?

1. "I called my friend the last two times I got upset."
2. "I know I'll have this problem with eating forever."
3. "I started asking my mother or sister to watch me eat each meal."
4. "I can have my boyfriend bring me home from parties if I want to purge."

19. 1. A sign of progress is when the client begins to verbalize feelings and interact with people instead of going to food for comfort. The second option indicates the client needs more information on how to handle the disorder. Having another person watch the client eat isn't a helpful strategy as the client will depend on others to help control food intake. The last option indicates the client is in denial about the severity of the problem.
NP: Evaluation; CN: Psychosocial integrity; CNS: Psychosocial adaptation; CL: Application

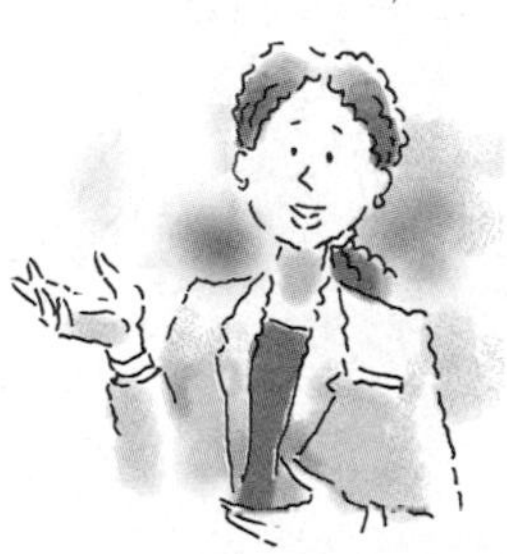
These key words mean prioritize.

20. A client with bulimia nervosa asks a nurse, "How can I ask for help from my family?" Which of the following responses is the most appropriate?

1. "When you ask for help, make sure you really need it."
2. "Have you ever asked for help before?"
3. "Ask family members to spend time with you at mealtime."
4. "Think about how you can handle this situation without help."

20. 2. Determine whether the client has ever been successful in asking for help. Previous experiences affect the client's ability to ask for help now. The client needs to ask for help anytime without analyzing the level of need. Having other people around at mealtime isn't the only way to ask for help. Developing a support system is imperative for this client.
NP: Implementation; CN: Psychosocial integrity; CNS: Psychosocial adaptation; CL: Analysis

21. A client with bulimia nervosa tells a nurse that she doesn't eat during the day, but after 5:00 p.m., she begins to binge and vomit. Which of the following interventions would be the most useful to this client?

1. Help the client stop eating the foods on which she binges.
2. Discuss the effects of fasting on the client's pattern of eating.
3. Encourage the client to become involved in food preparation.
4. Teach the client to eat earlier in the day and decrease intake at night.

21. 2. If a person fasts for most of the day, it's common to become extremely hungry, overeat by bingeing, and then feel the need to purge. Restricting food intake can actually trigger the binge-purge cycle. In treatment, the client is taught to identify foods that trigger eating, discuss the feelings associated with these foods, and work to eat them in normal amounts. Involvement in food preparation won't promote changes in the client's behaviors. The last option doesn't address how fasting can trigger the binge-purge cycle.

NP: Implementation; CN: Psychosocial integrity; CNS: Psychosocial adaptation; CL: Application

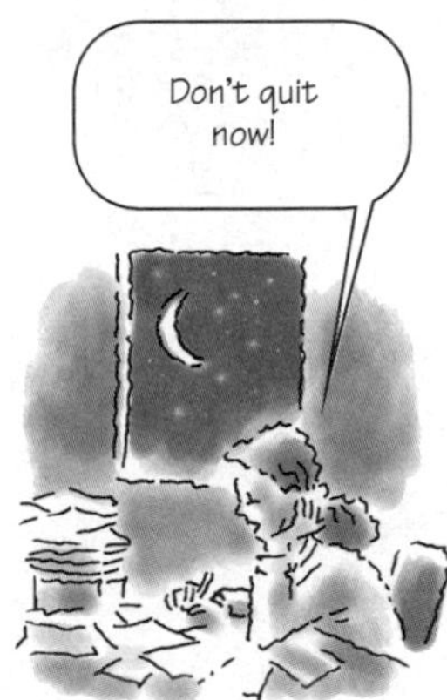

22. A client with bulimia nervosa tells a nurse she was doing well until last week, when she had a fight with her father. Which of the following nursing interventions would help most?

1. Examine the relationship between feelings and eating.
2. Discuss the importance of therapy for the entire family.
3. Encourage the client to avoid certain family members.
4. Identify daily stressors and learn stress management skills.

22. 1. The client needs to understand her feelings and develop healthy coping skills to handle unpleasant situations. Family therapy may be indicated but shouldn't be an immediate intervention. Avoidance isn't a useful coping strategy; eventually the underlying issues need to be explored. All clients can benefit from stress management skills, but for this client, care must focus on the relationship between feelings and eating behaviors.

NP: Implementation; CN: Psychosocial integrity; CNS: Psychosocial adaptation; CL: Application

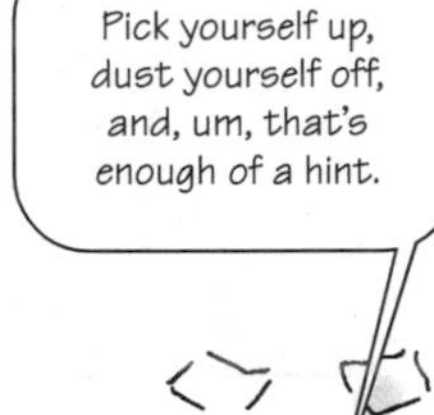

Pick yourself up, dust yourself off, and, um, that's enough of a hint.

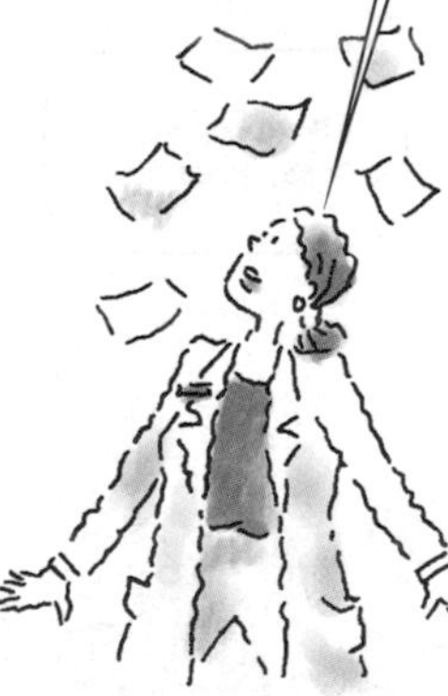

23. Which of the following statements from a bulimic client shows that she understands the concept of relapse?

1. "If I can't maintain control over things, I'll have problems."
2. "If I have problems, then that says I haven't learned much."
3. "If this illness becomes chronic, I won't be able to handle it."
4. "If I have problems, I can start over again and not feel hopeless."

23. 4. This statement indicates that the client knows a relapse is just a slip, and positive gains made from treatment haven't been lost. Negative self-statements can lead to relapse. Control issues relate to powerlessness, which contribute to relapse.

NP: Evaluation; CN: Psychosocial integrity; CNS: Psychosocial adaptation; CL: Comprehension

24. Which of the following areas in the client or family history is important to explore for an adolescent with bulimia nervosa?

1. Lack of social skills
2. Depression in relatives
3. Neurologic conditions
4. Chronic fatigue syndrome

24. 2. There's a high rate of depression in the relatives of a client with bulimia nervosa. Clients with bulimia nervosa often show appropriate social skills and frequently hide their eating disorder from others. There's no evidence to suggest a relationship between bulimia nervosa and neurologic conditions or to associate chronic fatigue syndrome with bulimia nervosa.

NP: Assessment; CN: Psychosocial integrity; CNS: Coping and adaptation; CL: Knowledge

25. Which of the following medical conditions is commonly found in clients with bulimia nervosa?

1. Allergies
2. Cancer
3. Diabetes
4. Hepatitis A

25. 3. Diabetes, heart disease, and hypertension are medical complications frequently seen in clients with bulimia nervosa. Allergies, cancer, and hepatitis A are *not* medical complications commonly associated with bulimia nervosa.

NP: Analysis; CN: Health promotion and maintenance; CNS: Prevention and early detection of disease; CL: Application

26. A client with anorexia nervosa attended psychoeducational sessions on principles of adequate nutrition. Which of the following statements by the client indicates the teaching was effective?

1. "I eat while I'm doing things to distract myself."
2. "I eat all my food at night right before I go to bed."
3. "I eat small amounts of food slowly at every meal."
4. "I eat only when I'm with my family and trying to be social."

26. 3. Slowly eating small amounts of food facilitates adequate digestion and prevents distention. Healthy eating is best accomplished when a person isn't doing other things while eating. Eating right before bedtime isn't a healthy eating habit. If a client eats only when the family is present or when trying to be social, eating is tied to social or emotional cues rather than nutritional needs.

NP: Evaluation; CN: Psychosocial integrity; CNS: Psychosocial adaptation; CL: Comprehension

All options may be good, but choose the *best* one.

27. A client with anorexia nervosa tells a nurse, "I'll never have the slender body I want." Which of the following interventions is best to handle this problem?

1. Call a family meeting to get help from the parents.
2. Help the client work on developing a realistic body image.
3. Make an appointment to see the dietitian on a weekly basis.
4. Develop an exercise program the client can do twice a week.

27. 2. With anorexia nervosa, the client pursues thinness and has a distorted view of self. A family meeting may not help the client develop a more realistic view of the body. Although meeting with a dietitian might be helpful, it isn't a priority. Clients with anorexia nervosa typically exercise excessively.

NP: Implementation; CN: Psychosocial integrity; CNS: Psychosocial adaptation; CL: Application

28. A client with anorexia nervosa tells a nurse, "My parents never hug me or say I've done anything right." Which of the following interventions is the best to use with this family?

1. Teach the family principles of assertive behavior.
2. Discuss the difficulties the family has in social situations.
3. Help the family convey a positive attitude toward the client.
4. Explore the family's ability to express affection appropriately.

28. 4. There's often a lack of affection and warmth in families who have a member with an eating disorder. Although assertiveness is an important skill, the family member needs to realize assertiveness isn't always rewarded. Difficulties in social situations are important to address, but the intervention must focus on how to express positive feelings and affection. A positive attitude helps a person become better able to handle the pressures of life, but it may not change the family's display of affection.

NP: Implementation; CN: Psychosocial integrity; CNS: Psychosocial adaptation; CL: Application

29. Which of the following communication strategies is best to use with a client with anorexia nervosa who is having problems with peer relationships?

1. Use concrete language and maintain a focus on reality.
2. Direct the client to talk about what is causing the anxiety.
3. Teach the client to communicate feelings and express self appropriately.
4. Confront the client about being depressed and self-absorbed.

29. 3. Clients with anorexia nervosa often communicate on a superficial level and avoid expressing feelings. Identifying feelings and learning to express them are initial steps in decreasing isolation. Clients with anorexia nervosa are usually able to discuss abstract and concrete issues. Discussions shouldn't be limited to the client's feelings of anxiety. Confrontation usually isn't an effective communication strategy as it may cause the client to withdraw and become more depressed.

NP: Implementation; CN: Psychosocial integrity; CNS: Psychosocial adaptation; CL: Application

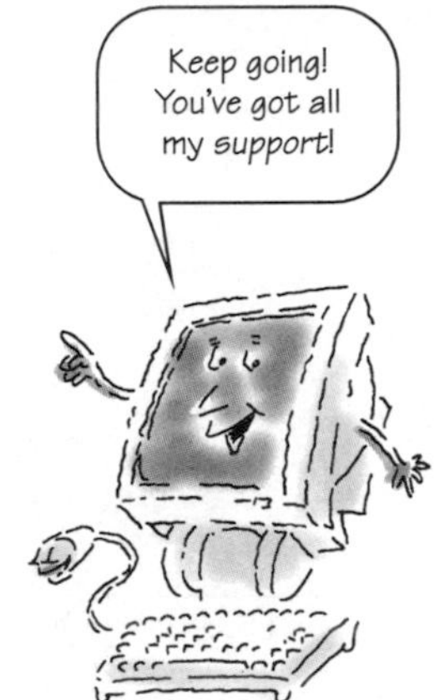

Keep going! You've got all my support!

30. A nurse is working with a family who has a member with anorexia nervosa. Which of the following actions is essential to teach this family?

1. How to be supportive
2. How to encourage grieving
3. How to set limits on behavior
4. How to monitor social interactions

30. 1. The most important intervention to teach the family is how to be there for the client and express their support. These clients need to be encouraged to handle all feelings, not just grief. The client often needs to be encouraged to express negative feelings appropriately, especially anger. Setting limits may prevent important dialogue from occurring. Social interactions are usually limited because the client is withdrawn and self-absorbed. The client needs to develop peer relationships.

NP: Implementation; CN: Psychosocial integrity; CNS: Psychosocial adaptation; CL: Comprehension

31. A nurse is talking to a family of a client with anorexia nervosa. Which of the following family behaviors is most likely to be seen during the family's interaction?

1. Sibling rivalry
2. Rage reactions
3. Parental disagreement
4. Excessive independence

31. 3. In many families with a member with anorexia nervosa, there is marital conflict and parental disagreement. Sibling rivalry is a common occurrence and not specific to a family with a member with anorexia nervosa. Emotions are overcontrolled and there's difficulty appropriately expressing negative feelings. In these families, the members tend to be enmeshed and dependent on each other. The family with an anorexic member is often one that looks good to the outside observer.

NP: Assessment; CN: Psychosocial integrity; CNS: Coping and adaptation; CL: Comprehension

32. A nurse is working with a client with anorexia nervosa who has skin problems in her extremities. Which of the following short-term goals is the most important for the client?

1. Do daily range of motion exercises.
2. Eat some fatty foods daily.
3. Check neurologic reflexes.
4. Promote adequate circulation.

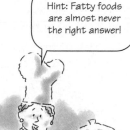

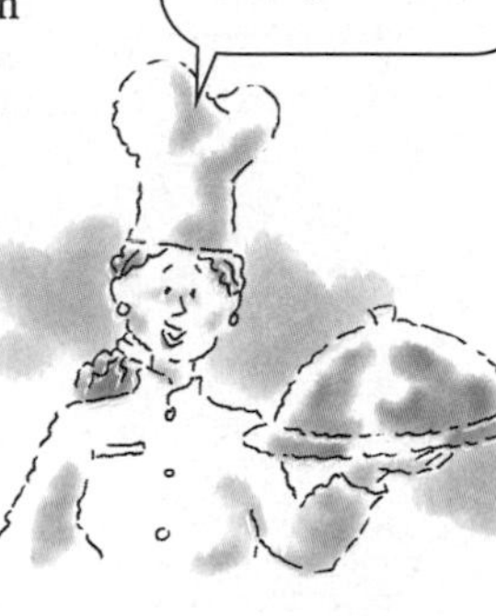

Hint: Fatty foods are almost never the right answer!

32. 4. Circulation changes will cause extremities to be cold, numb, and have dry and flaky skin. Exercise may help prevent contractures and muscle atrophy, but it may have only a limited secondary effect on promoting circulation. Intake of fatty foods won't have an impact on the client's skin problems. Checking neurologic reflexes won't necessarily assist with handling skin problems.

NP: Planning; CN: Psychosocial integrity; CNS: Psychosocial adaptation; CL: Knowledge

33. A woman with anorexia nervosa is discharged from the hospital after gaining 12 lb. Which of the following statements indicates the client still has a lack of knowledge about her condition?

1. "I plan to eat six small meals a day."
2. "I feel this is scary, and I need to write in my journal about it."
3. "I have to diet because I've gained 12 pounds."
4. "I'll need to attend therapy for support to stay healthy."

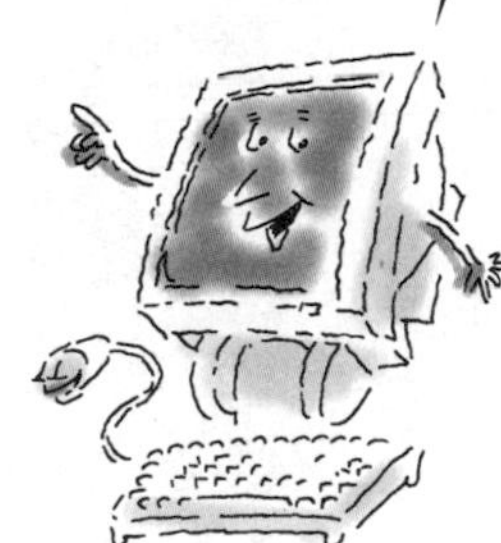

Careful! Here's one of those cleverly disguised further teaching questions.

33. 3. The client is still relying on a mental image of herself as being fat. Eating small meals each day is a realistic plan for meeting nutritional needs without feeling bloated. Feeling insecure when leaving a controlled environment is a common response to discharge. Planning to attend therapy after discharge shows an understanding of the need for continued therapy.

NP: Evaluation; CN: Psychosocial integrity; CNS: Psychosocial adaptation; CL: Analysis

34. A client with anorexia nervosa tells a nurse she always feels fat. Which of the following interventions is the best for this client?

1. Talk about how important the client is.
2. Encourage her to look at herself in a mirror.
3. Address the dynamics of the disorder.
4. Talk about how she's different from her peers.

34. 3. The client can benefit from understanding the underlying dynamics of the eating disorder. The client with anorexia nervosa has low self-esteem and won't believe the positive statements. Although the client may look at herself in the mirror, in her mind she'll still see herself as fat. Pointing out differences will only diminish her already low self-esteem.

NP: Implementation; CN: Psychosocial integrity; CNS: Psychosocial adaptation; CL: Application

35. The grandparents of a client with anorexia nervosa want to support the client, but aren't sure what they should do. Which of the following interventions is best?

1. Promote positive expressions of affection.
2. Encourage behaviors that enhance socialization.
3. Discuss how eating disorders create powerlessness.
4. Discuss the meaning of hunger and body sensations.

35. 1. Clients with eating disorders need emotional support and expressions of affection from family members. It wouldn't be an appropriate strategy to have the grandparents promote socialization. Although clients with eating disorders feel powerless, it's better to have the grandparents focus on something positive. Talking about hunger and other sensations won't give the grandparents useful strategies.

NP: Implementation; CN: Psychosocial integrity; CNS: Psychosocial adaptation; CL: Application

36. A nurse is analyzing the need for health teaching in a client with anorexia nervosa who lives in a chaotic family situation. Which of the following questions is most important for the nurse to ask the client?

1. "How many months have your periods been irregular?"
2. "How often do you think about food in a 24-hour period?"
3. "What were the circumstances before your eating disorder?"
4. "How much and what kinds of exercise do you engage in every day?"

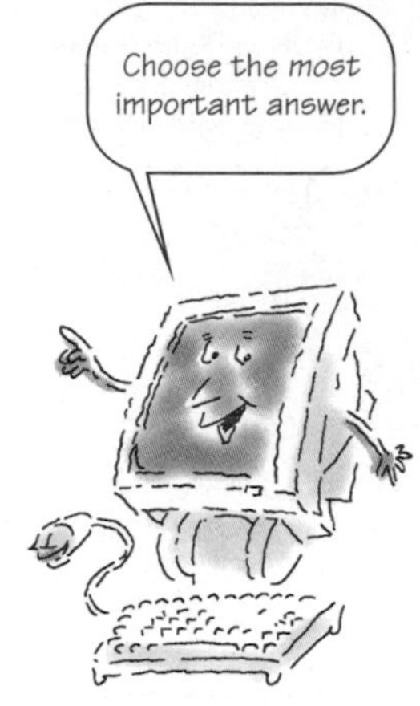

Choose the most important answer.

36. 3. This question lets the nurse get information about the family and background situations that influenced the client's needs and distorted eating. The other options deal with menstrual history, exercise patterns, and food obsessions. Although they're relevant, they don't provide information.

NP: Analysis; CN: Psychosocial integrity; CNS: Psychosocial adaptation; CL: Comprehension

37. An adolescent client with anorexia nervosa tells a nurse about her outstanding academic achievements and her thoughts about suicide. Which of the following factors must the nurse consider when making a care plan for this client?

1. Self-esteem
2. Physical illnesses
3. Paranoid delusions
4. Relationship avoidance

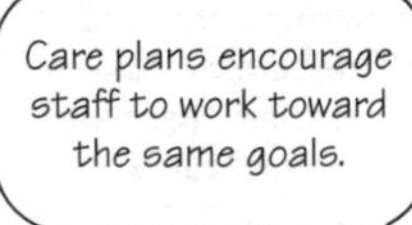

Care plans encourage staff to work toward the same goals.

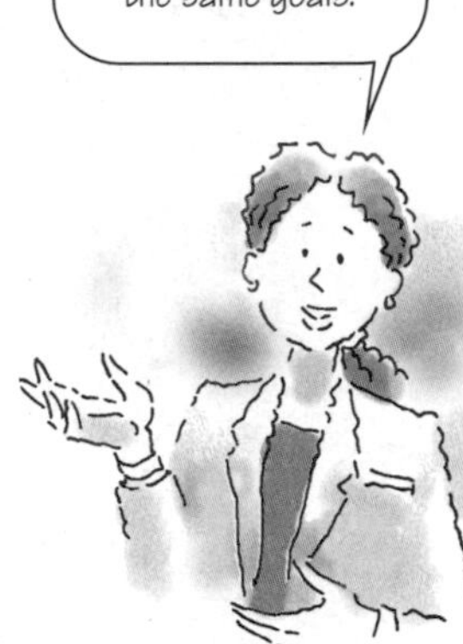

37. 1. The client lacks self-esteem, which contributes to her level of depression and feelings of personal ineffectiveness, which in turn may lead to suicidal thoughts. Physical illnesses are common with clients with anorexia nervosa, but they don't relate to this situation. Paranoid delusions refer to false ideas that others want to harm you. No evidence exists that this client is socially isolated.

NP: Planning; CN: Psychosocial integrity; CNS: Psychosocial adaptation; CL: Analysis

38. In making a care plan for a family with a member who has anorexia nervosa, which of the following information should be included?

1. Coping mechanisms used in the past
2. Concerns about changes in lifestyle and daily activities
3. Rejection of feedback from family and significant others
4. Appropriate eating habits and social behaviors centering on eating

38. 1. Examination of positive and negative coping mechanisms used by the family allows the nurse to build a care plan specific to the family's strengths and weaknesses. The way the family copes with concerns is more important than the concerns themselves. Feedback from the family and significant others is vital when building a care plan. Eating habits and behaviors are symptoms of the way people cope with problems.

NP: Planning; CN: Psychosocial integrity; CNS: Psychosocial adaptation; CL: Application

39. Which of the following goals is best to help a client with anorexia nervosa recognize self-distortions?

1. Identify the client's misperceptions of self.
2. Acknowledge immature and childlike behaviors.
3. Determine the consequences of a faulty support system.
4. Recognize the age-appropriate tasks to be accomplished.

39. 1. Questioning the client's misperceptions and distortions will create doubt about how the client views himself. Acknowledging immature behaviors or determining the consequences of a faulty support system won't promote client recognition of self-distortions. Recognizing the age-appropriate tasks to be accomplished by the client won't help the client recognize distortions.

NP: Implementation; CN: Psychosocial integrity; CNS: Psychosocial adaptation; CL: Analysis

40. Parents of a client with anorexia nervosa ask about the risk factors for this disorder. Which of the following definitions is the most accurate?

1. Inability to be still and emotional lability
2. High level of anxiety and disorganized behavior
3. Low self-esteem and problems with family relationships
4. Lack of life experiences and no opportunities to learn skills

40. 3. There are several risk factors for eating disorders, including low self-esteem, history of depression, substance abuse, and dysfunctional family relationships. Restlessness and emotional lability are symptoms of manic depressive illness. Anxiety and disorganized behavior could be signs of a psychotic disorder. A lack of life experiences and an absence of opportunities to learn life skills may be a result of anorexia.

NP: Assessment; CN: Psychosocial integrity; CNS: Psychosocial adaptation; CL: Knowledge

41. A client with anorexia nervosa has started taking fluoxetine hydrochloride (Prozac). Which of the following adverse reactions complicates the treatment of this eating disorder?

1. Drowsiness
2. Dry mouth
3. Light-headedness
4. Nausea

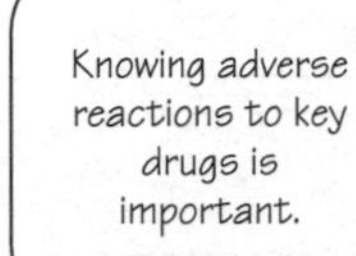

Knowing adverse reactions to key drugs is important.

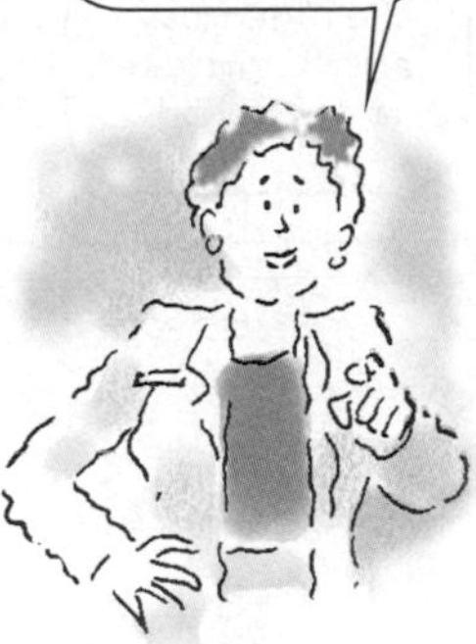

41. 4. Nausea is an adverse reaction to the drug that compounds the eating disorder problem, and the client must be closely monitored. Although the adverse reactions of drowsiness, dry mouth, or light-headedness may occur, they aren't likely to interfere with treatment.

NP: Analysis; CN: Physiological integrity; CNS: Pharmacological and parenteral therapies; CL: Knowledge

42. A client with anorexia nervosa is worried about rectal bleeding. Which of the following questions should be asked to obtain more information about this problem?

1. "How often do you use laxatives?"
2. "How many days ago did you stop vomiting?"
3. "Are you eating anything that causes irritation?"
4. "Do you have bleeding before or after exercise?"

42. 1. Excessive use of laxatives will cause GI irritation and rectal bleeding. If the client stopped vomiting but is still using laxatives, rectal bleeding can occur. Clients who are anorexic eat very little, and what they eat won't cause rectal bleeding. Exercise doesn't cause rectal bleeding.

NP: Assessment; CN: Health promotion and maintenance; CNS: Prevention and early detection of disease; CL: Application

43. A client with anorexia nervosa tells a nurse she has developed hair on most of her body. Which of the following conditions may be associated with this condition?

1. Anemia
2. Osteoporosis
3. Dehydration
4. Electrolyte imbalance

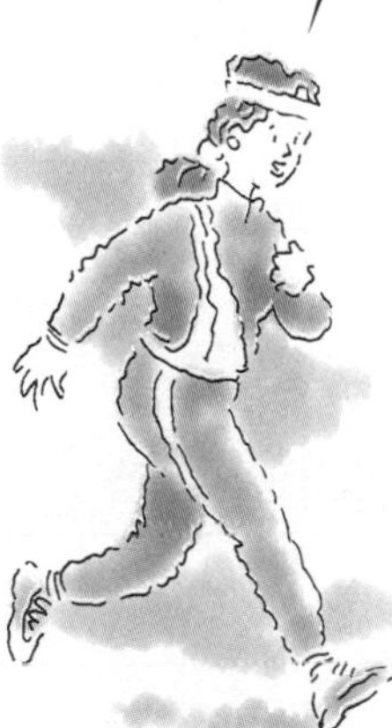

You're heading down the home stretch! Keep going!

43. 3. When a client with anorexia nervosa has fine hair all over her body (lanugo), the nurse would perform a more extensive assessment of the skin. Lanugo indicates dehydration due to starvation. Anemia is associated with hematologic complications. Osteoporosis is associated with the musculoskeletal system. Electrolyte imbalance is associated with body metabolism.

NP: Assessment; CN: Health promotion and maintenance; CNS: Prevention and early detection of disease; CL: Knowledge

44. A client with anorexia nervosa is talking to a nurse about her group therapy. Which of the following statements shows the group experience has helped the client?

1. "I feel I'm different and I don't need a lot of friends."
2. "I'll tell my parents it's not just me who has problems."
3. "I can see how to do things better and become the best."
4. "I think I have some unrealistic expectations of myself."

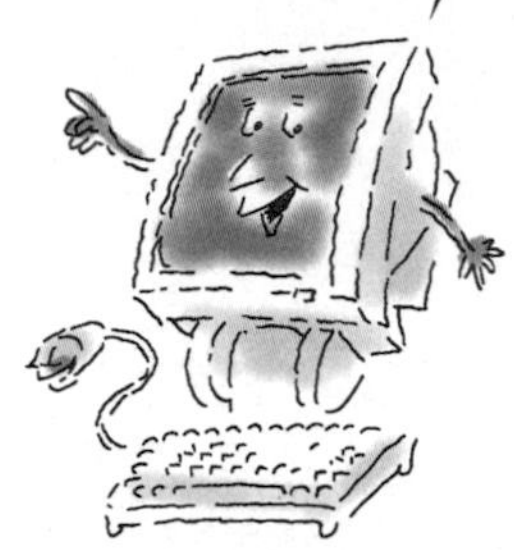

Question 44 is looking for something that proved helpful.

44. 4. A goal of group therapy is to provide methods to assess whether personal expectations are unrealistic. Other goals are to learn to handle problems; not to blame parents or others; decrease perfectionist tendencies; and decrease isolation and learn to have healthy peer relationships.

NP: Evaluation; CN: Psychosocial integrity; CNS: Psychosocial adaptation; CL: Application

45. A nurse and her client who has anorexia nervosa are working on the goal of developing social relationships. Which of the following actions by the client is an indication the client is meeting her goal?

1. The client talks about the value of peer relationships.
2. The client decides to talk to her parents about her friends.
3. The client expresses the need to establish trust relationships.
4. The client attends an activity without prompting from others.

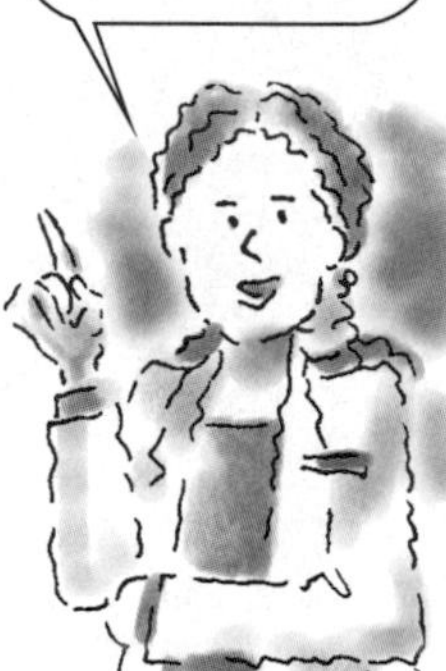

The client must agree to the goal or it won't work.

45. 4. When a client with anorexia nervosa attends an activity without prompting from others, it's a positive sign the client is working toward developing social relationships. Talking about the value of relationships is also beneficial but is only the first step in establishing them. Talking to parents about friends is a start but doesn't necessarily indicate that the client can establish relationships. Expressing the need to establish trust relationships is a first step, but an indication of success would be actually initiating such a relationship.

NP: Evaluation; CN: Psychosocial integrity; CNS: Psychosocial adaptation; CL: Application

46. What initial action should the nurse take when a young woman with anorexia nervosa says, "I'll try to eat something"?

1. Provide a small portion of a healthy food.
2. Weigh the client before and after eating.
3. Ask the client what she thinks she can eat.
4. Suggest the client drink something before eating.

46. 1. Small amounts of food won't overwhelm the client when given at frequent intervals. They also won't overtax the GI and cardiac systems. Weighing the client before and after meals is a useless, stress-provoking action. Asking the client questions may provoke anxiety. It's better to give the client food when she asks. Drinking something before eating isn't necessary; the fluid may prevent the client from being able to eat a sufficient amount of the food.

NP: Implementation; CN: Physiological integrity; CNS: Reduction of risk potential; CL: Application

47. A client with anorexia nervosa tells a nurse, "I feel so awful and inadequate." Which of the following responses is best?

1. "You're being too hard on yourself."
2. "Someday you'll feel better about things."
3. "Tell me something you like about yourself."
4. "Maybe relaxing by yourself will help you feel better."

47. 3. This statement redirects the client to talk about positive aspects of self. The other options minimize her feelings or don't address the client's concerns or encourage the client to change her self-image.

NP: Implementation; CN: Psychosocial integrity; CNS: Psychosocial adaptation; CL: Application

48. Which of the following physiologic complications of anorexia nervosa can quickly become life-threatening?
1. Cardiac arrhythmias
2. Decreased blood pressure
3. Decreased metabolic rate
4. Altered thyroid functioning

48. 1. With starvation, the heart muscle becomes irritable and less efficient, causing sudden, severe arrhythmias and, possibly, death. None of the other options tend to be life-threatening.
NP: Analysis; CN: Health promotion and maintenance; CNS: Prevention and early detection of disease; CL: Knowledge

49. An adolescent client with anorexia nervosa starts outpatient treatment. Which client statement indicates that she has a basic understanding of her eating disorder?
1. "I'm not worried because no one ever dies from anorexia."
2. "I still feel fat even though I'm told that I'm not."
3. "My old school friends aren't important to me anymore."
4. "I don't feel right unless I do an intense workout every day."

49. 2. A client with anorexia nervosa shows a basic understanding of the disorder if she can talk about feeling fat even though she's actually underweight, or if she expresses an intense fear of gaining weight. Anorexia nervosa has a mortality of approximately 10% to 15%. People with eating disorders tend to isolate themselves from friends and family members because of their intense focus on food, weight, and exercise. A client with anorexia nervosa may exercise compulsively to prevent weight gain; this behavior indicates continuing presence of the eating disorder.
NP: Analysis; CN: Psychosocial integrity; CNS: Coping and adaptation; CL: Analysis

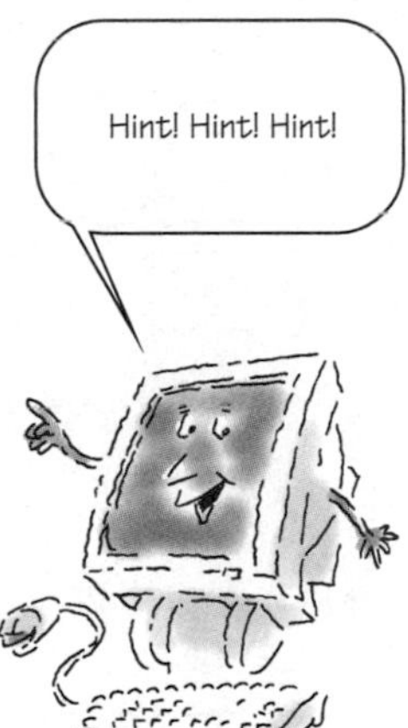

50. Which question is most useful in assessing the self-esteem of a client with anorexia nervosa?
1. "How would you describe yourself to others?"
2. "What activities do you enjoy doing with your friends?"
3. "Do you play any sports at school or in your community?"
4. "How do you decide how to spend your free time?"

50. 1. Clients with anorexia nervosa tend to have low self-esteem even if they're high achievers in school, activities, and sports; asking for a self-description can uncover the client's distorted body image and low self-esteem. Questions about activities with friends, involvement in sports, or how the client decides to spend her free time don't necessarily elicit information about self-esteem.
NP: Assessment; CN: Psychosocial integrity; CNS: Coping and adaptation; CL: Analysis

51. Which psychosocial finding should the nurse expect when assessing a client with anorexia nervosa?
1. Avoidant behavior
2. Antisocial behavior
3. Introverted behavior
4. Hypervigilant behavior

51. 3. Clients with anorexia nervosa typically demonstrate introverted behavior. Clients with bulimia, not anorexia nervosa, tend to show avoidant and dependent behaviors. Clients with eating disorders don't necessarily demonstrate antisocial behavior. Hypervigilant behavior is common in clients with posttraumatic stress disorder, not eating disorders.
NP: Assessment; CN: Psychosocial integrity; CNS: Coping and adaptation; CL: Analysis

52. The nurse notes severe hypocalcemia in a client with anorexia nervosa. Which history finding supports a diagnosis of osteoporosis?

1. Eating a vegetarian diet
2. Drinking well water
3. Going scuba diving
4. Smoking cigarettes

52. 4. Hypocalcemia and cigarette smoking increase the risk for osteoporosis. Eating a vegetarian diet, drinking well water, and going scuba diving don't predispose the client to osteoporosis.

NP: Analysis; CN: Physiological integrity; CNS: Reduction of risk potential; CL: Analysis

53. A client with anorexia nervosa is receiving care from her family after successfully completing the refeeding stage of treatment. Which nursing intervention takes priority at this time?

1. Providing a strong support system and opportunities to do reality testing
2. Teaching the family stress-reduction skills to help promote family harmony
3. Promoting anticipatory grieving over the loss each family member is experiencing
4. Assisting the family to work on the issues of autonomy and separation

53. 4. When a client with anorexia nervosa successfully completes the refeeding stage of treatment, the family must work on separation and individuation of the client and on decreasing family rigidity and overprotectiveness. Although the client needs a strong support system, developing a sense of self is more important at this time; also, reality testing isn't a typical problem in clients with eating disorders. All families can benefit from learning stress-reduction skills; however, at this time, these skills take lower priority than developing client independence. Anticipatory grieving isn't particularly relevant for family members of a client with an eating disorder.

NP: Analysis; CN: Psychosocial integrity; CNS: Coping and adaptation; CL: Application

54. A client with bulimia nervosa has a history of severe GI problems caused by excessive purging. Based on this finding, the nurse must stay alert for which physiologic problem?

1. Renal calculi
2. Esophageal tears
3. Focal seizures
4. Muscle atrophy

54. 2. A bulimic client with severe GI problems from excessive purging is at increased risk for esophageal tears and irritation or esophagitis. Although clients with eating disorders may develop renal calculi, this client is at greater risk for developing esophageal tears. Focal seizures and muscle atrophy aren't related to severe GI problems.

NP: Planning; CN: Physiological integrity; CNS: Reduction of risk potential; CL: Analysis

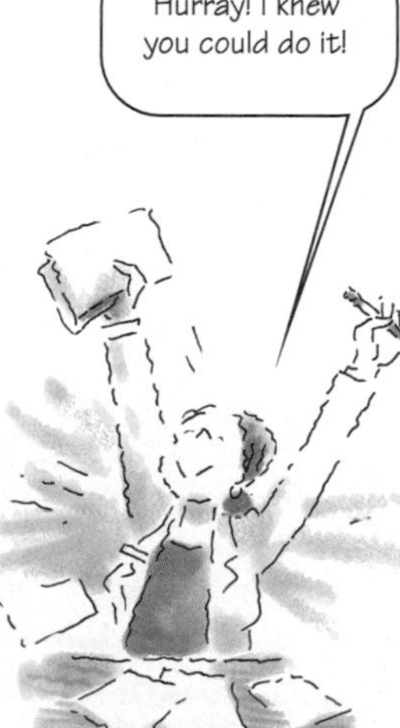
Hurray! I knew you could do it!

55. A client with bulimia nervosa struggles to talk about how her eating behavior relates to her emotions. Which nursing intervention is most important?

1. Having the client verbalize her thoughts about her recent situational crises
2. Instructing the client to keep a daily journal to evaluate how she acts on her feelings of hunger
3. Using group therapy to assist the client in learning how others identify their feelings
4. Examining the client's coping skills and teaching her to trust herself as well as others

55. 2. By keeping a daily journal, the client can examine her eating behaviors and her responses to her feelings of hunger. The client may be unable to verbalize her thoughts and perceptions about recent situational crises. She needs to identify her own feelings rather than others'. Although she needs to practice coping skills and learn how to trust herself, these goals are less important than understanding the link between her feelings and her dysfunctional eating behavior.

NP: Planning; CN: Psychosocial integrity; CNS: Coping and adaptation; CL: Analysis

Part IV Maternal-neonatal care

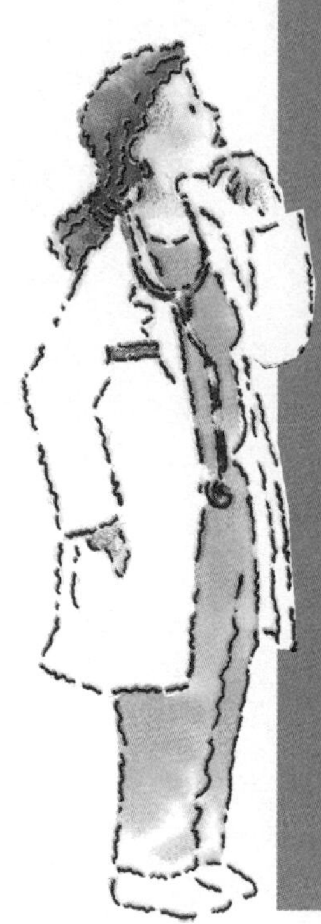

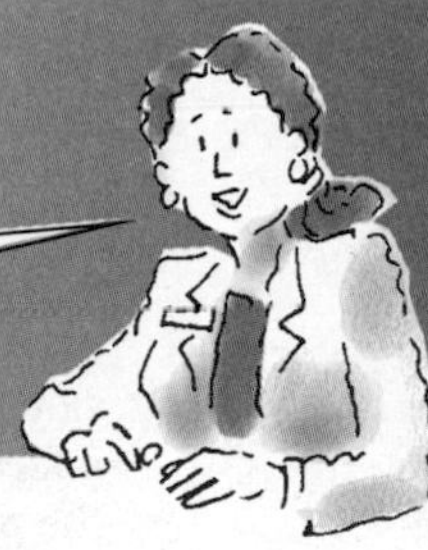

Looking for information
about antepartum care
before tackling this chapter?
Visit **www.obgyn.net/**, an
independent Internet site
dedicated to obstetric and
gynecologic health problems.

Chapter 22
Antepartum care

1. Usually individual twins will grow appropriately and at the same rate as singletons until how many weeks' gestation?

1. 16 to 18 weeks
2. 18 to 22 weeks
3. 30 to 32 weeks
4. 38 to 40 weeks

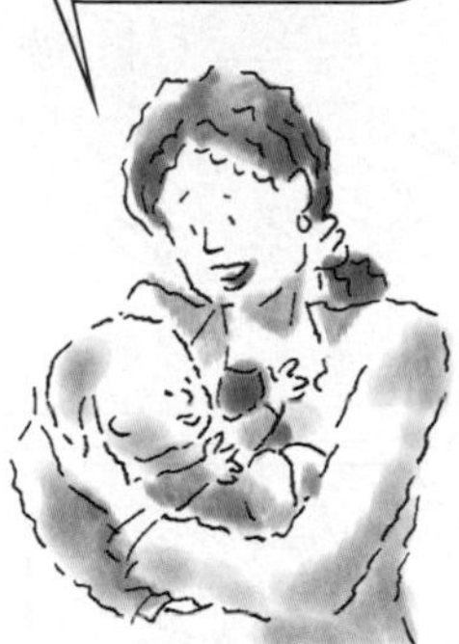

Think back to your

for the answer to

1. 3. Individual twins usually grow at the same rate as singletons until 30 to 32 weeks' gestation, then twins don't gain weight as rapidly as singletons of the same gestational age. The placenta can no longer keep pace with the nutritional requirements of both fetuses after 32 weeks, so there's some growth retardation in twins if they remain *in utero* at 38 to 40 weeks.

NP: Analysis; CN: Health promotion and maintenance; CNS: Growth and development through the life span; CL: Knowledge

2. Which of the following classifications applies to monozygotic twins for whom the cleavage of the fertilized ovum occurs more than 13 days after fertilization?

1. Conjoined twins
2. Diamniotic dichorionic twins
3. Diamniotic monochorionic twins
4. Monoamniotic monochorionic twins

2. 1. The type of placenta that develops in monozygotic twins depends on the time at which cleavage of the ovum occurs. Cleavage in conjoined twins occurs more than 13 days after fertilization. Cleavage that occurs less than 3 days after fertilization results in diamniotic dichorionic twins. Cleavage that occurs between days 3 and 8 results in diamniotic monochorionic twins. Cleavage that occurs between days 8 and 13 results in monoamniotic monochorionic twins.

NP: Analysis; CN: Health promotion and maintenance; CNS: Growth and development through the life span; CL: Knowledge

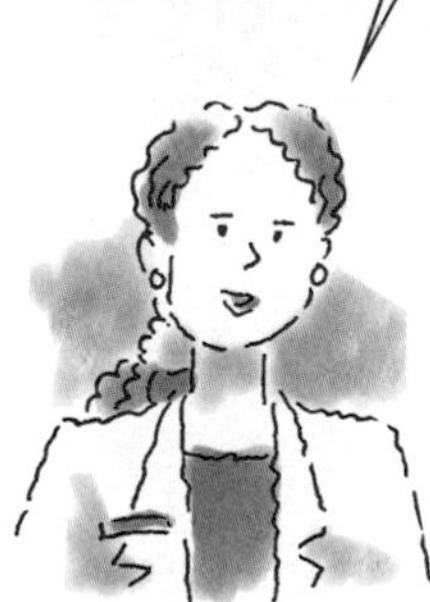

3 asks about the

3. In twin-to-twin transfusion syndrome, the arterial circulation of one twin is in communication with the venous circulation of the other twin. One fetus is considered the "donor" twin and one becomes the "recipient" twin. Assessment of the recipient twin would most likely show which of the following conditions?

1. Anemia
2. Oligohydramnios
3. Polycythemia
4. Small fetus

3. 3. The recipient twin in twin-twin transfusion syndrome is transfused by the other twin. The recipient twin then becomes polycythemic and often has heart failure due to circulatory overload. The donor twin becomes anemic. The recipient twin has polyhydramnios, not oligohydramnios. The recipient twin is usually large, whereas the donor twin is often small.

NP: Analysis; CN: Physiological integrity; CNS: Physiological adaptation; CL: Analysis

4. A pregnant client who reports painless vaginal bleeding at 28 weeks' gestation is diagnosed with placenta previa. The placental edge reaches the internal os. This type of placenta previa is known as which of the following types?

1. Low-lying placenta previa
2. Marginal placenta previa
3. Partial placenta previa
4. Total placenta previa

4. 2. A marginal placenta previa is characterized by implantation of the placenta in the margin of the cervical os, not covering the os. A low-lying placenta is implanted in the lower uterine segment but doesn't reach the cervical os. A partial placenta previa is the partial occlusion of the cervical os by the placenta. The internal cervical os is completely covered by the placenta in a total placenta previa.

NP: Analysis; CN: Physiological integrity; CNS: Physiological adaptation; CL: Analysis

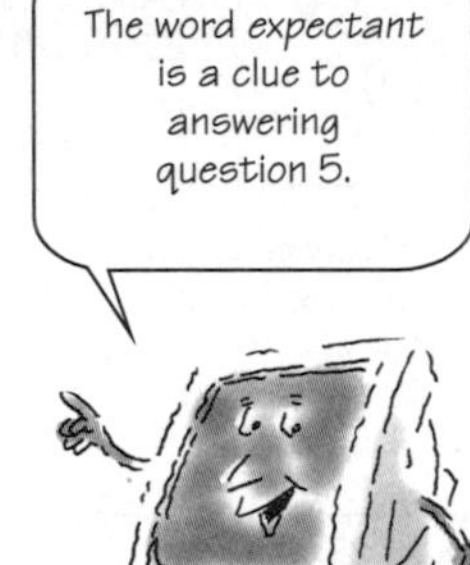
The word *expectant* is a clue to answering question 5.

5. Expectant management of the client with a placenta previa includes which of the following procedures or treatments?

1. Stat culture and sensitivity
2. Antenatal steroids after 34 weeks' gestation
3. Ultrasound examination every 2 to 3 weeks
4. Scheduled delivery of the fetus before fetal maturity in a hemodynamically stable mother

5. 3. Fetal surveillance through ultrasound examination every 2 to 3 weeks is indicated to evaluate fetal growth, amnionic fluid, and placental location in clients with placenta previa being expectantly managed. A stat culture and sensitivity would be done for severe bleeding or maternal or fetal distress and isn't part of expectant management. Antenatal steroids may be given to clients between 26 and 32 weeks' gestation to enhance fetal lung maturity. In a hemodynamically stable mother, delivery of the fetus should be delayed until fetal lung maturity is attained.

NP: Assessment; CN: Physiological integrity; CNS: Reduction of risk potential; CL: Knowledge

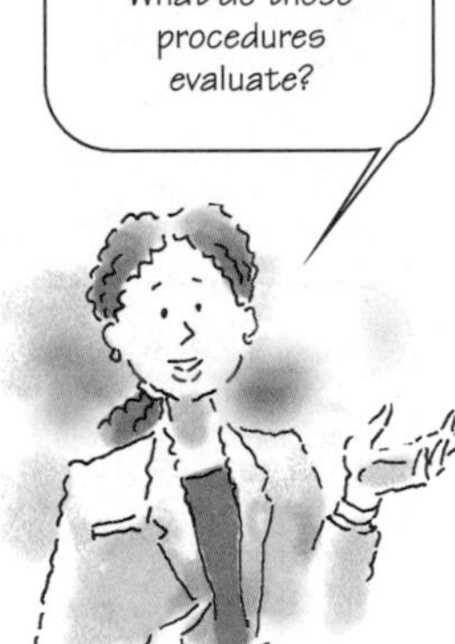
What do these procedures evaluate?

6. A client with painless vaginal bleeding has just been diagnosed as having a placenta previa. Which of the following procedures is usually performed to diagnose placenta previa?

1. Amniocentesis
2. Digital or speculum examination
3. External fetal monitoring
4. Ultrasound

6. 4. Once the mother and fetus are stabilized, ultrasound evaluation of the placenta should be done to determine the cause of the bleeding. Amniocentesis is contraindicated in placenta previa. A digital or speculum examination shouldn't be done as this may lead to severe bleeding or hemorrhage. External fetal monitoring won't detect a placenta previa, although it will detect fetal distress, which may result from blood loss or placental separation.

NP: Implementation; CN: Physiological integrity; CNS: Reduction of risk potential; CL: Knowledge

7. Clients with placenta previa are at increased risk for the placenta to form an abnormally firm attachment to the uterine wall, known as placenta accreta. Which of the following statements best describes this abnormal attachment?

1. The placenta invades the myometrium.
2. The placenta covers the cervical os.
3. The placenta penetrates the myometrium.
4. The placenta attaches to the myometrium.

7. 4. Placenta accreta is the abnormal attachment of the placenta to the myometrium of the uterus. When the placenta invades the myometrium, it's called placenta increta. When the placenta covers the cervical os, it's called placenta previa. Placenta percreta occurs when the villi of the placenta penetrate the myometrium to the serosa level.

NP: Assessment; CN: Health promotion and maintenance; CNS: Growth and development through the life span; CL: Knowledge

8. Which of the following symptoms occurs with a hydatidiform mole?

1. Heavy, bright red bleeding every 21 days
2. Fetal cardiac motion after 6 weeks' gestation
3. Benign tumors found in the smooth muscle of the uterus
4. "Snowstorm" pattern on ultrasound with no fetus or gestational sac

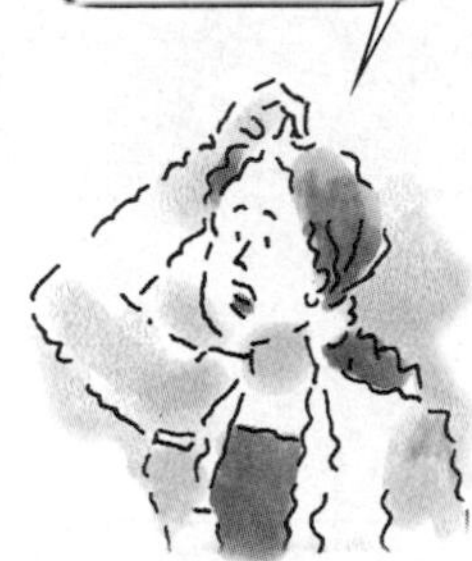

Sometimes it's hard to keep your symptoms straight, isn't it?

8. 4. Ultrasound is the technique of choice in diagnosing a hydatidiform mole. The chorionic villi of a molar pregnancy resemble a snowstorm pattern on ultrasound. Bleeding with a hydatidiform mole is often dark brown and may occur erratically for weeks or months. There's no cardiac activity because there's no fetus. Benign tumors found in the smooth muscle of the uterus are leiomyomas or fibroids.

NP: Analysis; CN: Physiological integrity; CNS: Reduction of risk potential; CL: Analysis

9. A 21-year-old client has just been diagnosed with having a hydatidiform mole. Which of the following factors is considered a risk factor for developing a hydatidiform mole?

1. Age in 20s or 30s
2. High socioeconomic status
3. Primigravida
4. Prior molar gestation

9. 4. A previous molar gestation increases a woman's risk for developing a subsequent molar gestation by 4 to 5 times. Adolescents and women ages 40 years and older are at increased risk for molar pregnancies. Multigravidas, especially women with a prior pregnancy loss, and women with lower socioeconomic status are at an increased risk for this problem.

NP: Analysis; CN: Physiological integrity; CNS: Physiological adaptation; CL: Analysis

10. A 21-year-old client arrives at the emergency department with complaints of cramping abdominal pain and mild vaginal bleeding. Pelvic examination shows a left adnexal mass that is tender when palpated. Culdocentesis shows blood in the cul-de-sac. This client probably has which of the following conditions?

1. Abruptio placentae
2. Ectopic pregnancy
3. Hydatidiform mole
4. Pelvic inflammatory disease

10. 2. Most ectopic pregnancies don't appear as obvious life-threatening medical emergencies. Ectopic pregnancies must be considered in any sexually active woman of childbearing age who complains of menstrual irregularity, cramping abdominal pain, and mild vaginal bleeding. Pelvic inflammatory disease, abruptio placentae, and hydatidiform moles won't show blood in the cul-de-sac.

NP: Analysis; CN: Physiological integrity; CNS: Reduction of risk potential; CL: Analysis

11. A client, 34 weeks' pregnant, arrives at the emergency department with severe abdominal pain, uterine tenderness, and an increased uterine tone. The client denies vaginal bleeding. The external fetal monitor shows fetal distress with severe, variable decelerations. The client most likely has which of the following conditions?

1. Abruptio placentae
2. Ectopic pregnancy
3. Molar pregnancy
4. Placenta previa

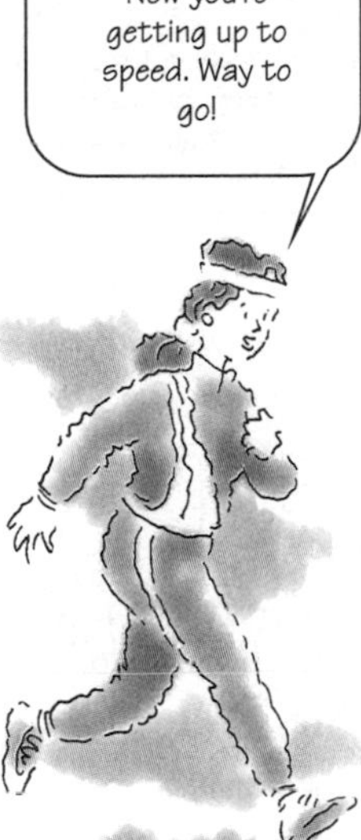

Now you're getting up to speed. Way to go!

11. 1. A client with severe abruptio placentae will often have severe abdominal pain. The uterus will have increased tone with little to no return to resting tone between contractions. The fetus will start to show signs of distress, with decelerations in the heart rate or even fetal death with a large placental separation. A molar pregnancy generally would be detected before 34 weeks' gestation. Placenta previa usually involve painless vaginal bleeding without uterine contractions. An ectopic pregnancy, which usually occurs in the fallopian tubes, would rupture well before 34 weeks.

NP: Analysis; CN: Physiological integrity; CNS: Reduction of risk potential; CL: Analysis

12. Before the placenta functions, the corpus luteum is the primary source for synthesis of which of the following hormones?
1. Cortisol and thyroxine
2. Estrogen and progesterone
3. Luteinizing hormone (LH) and follicle-stimulating hormone (FSH)
4. Thyroxine (T_4) and triiodothyronine (T_3)

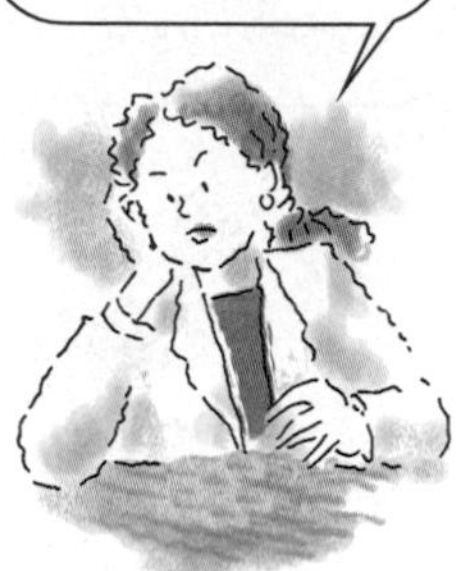

So many hormones to learn; so little time!

12. 2. The corpus luteum produces progesterone and estrogen for the first 8 to 10 weeks of pregnancy until the placenta takes over this function. The high levels of estrogen and progesterone cause suppression of LH and FSH. T_4 and T_3 are produced in the thyroid. Cortisol is produced in the adrenal gland.

NP: Analysis; CN: Health promotion and maintenance; CNS: Growth and development through the life span; CL: Knowledge

13. Which of the following changes in respiratory functioning during pregnancy is considered normal?
1. Increased tidal volume
2. Increased expiratory volume
3. Decreased inspiratory capacity
4. Decreased oxygen consumption

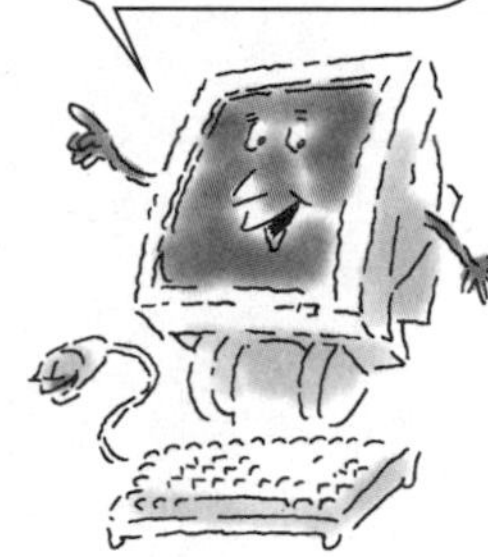

Be careful with question 13. It asks what's *normal* during pregnancy.

13. 1. A pregnant client breathes deeper, which increases the tidal volume of gas moved in and out of the respiratory tract with each breath. The expiratory volume and residual volume decrease as the pregnancy progresses. The inspiratory capacity increases during pregnancy. The increased oxygen consumption in the pregnant client is 15% to 20% greater than in the nonpregnant state.

NP: Assessment; CN: Health promotion and maintenance; CNS: Growth and development through the life span; CL: Knowledge

14. Which of the following terms applies to the tiny, blanched, slightly raised end arterioles found on the face, neck, arms, and chest during pregnancy?
1. Epulis
2. Linea nigra
3. Striae gravidarum
4. Telangiectasias

14. 4. The dilated arterioles that occur during pregnancy are due to the elevated level of circulating estrogen. An epulis is a red raised nodule on the gums that may develop at the end of the first trimester and continue to grow as the pregnancy progresses. The linea nigra is a pigmented line extending from the symphysis pubis to the top of the fundus during pregnancy. Striae gravidarum, or stretch marks, are slightly depressed streaks that commonly occur over the abdomen, breast, and thighs during the second half of pregnancy.

NP: Assessment; CN: Health promotion and maintenance; CNS: Growth and development through the life span; CL: Knowledge

15. Which of the following statements is true about dizygotic twins?
1. They occur most frequently in Asian women.
2. There's a decreased risk with increased parity.
3. There's an increased risk with increased maternal age.
4. There's no increased risk with the use of fertility drugs.

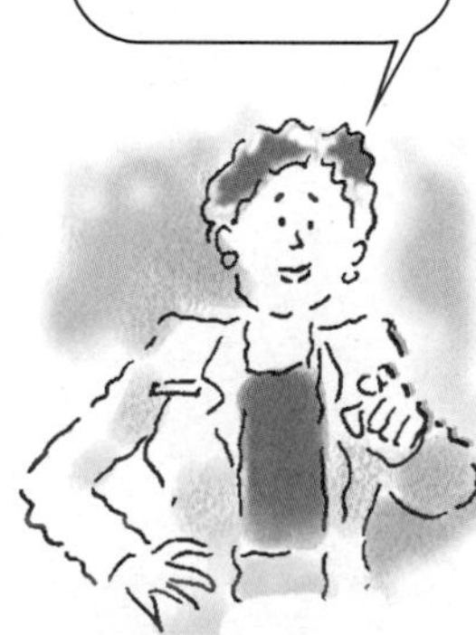

Watch out for these true-false kinds of questions. Read carefully!

15. 3. Dizygotic twinning is influenced by race (most frequent in Black women and least frequent in Asian women), age (increased risk with increased maternal age), parity (increased risk with increased parity), and fertility drugs (increased risk with the use of fertility drugs, especially ovulation-inducing drugs). The incidence of monozygotic twins isn't affected by race, age, parity, heredity, or fertility medications.

NP: Analysis; CN: Health promotion and maintenance; CNS: Growth and development through the life span; CL: Knowledge

NP: Nursing process CN: Client needs category CNS: Client needs subcategory CL: Cognitive level

16. Which of the following conditions is common in pregnant clients in the second trimester of pregnancy?

1. Mastitis
2. Metabolic alkalosis
3. Physiologic anemia
4. Respiratory acidosis

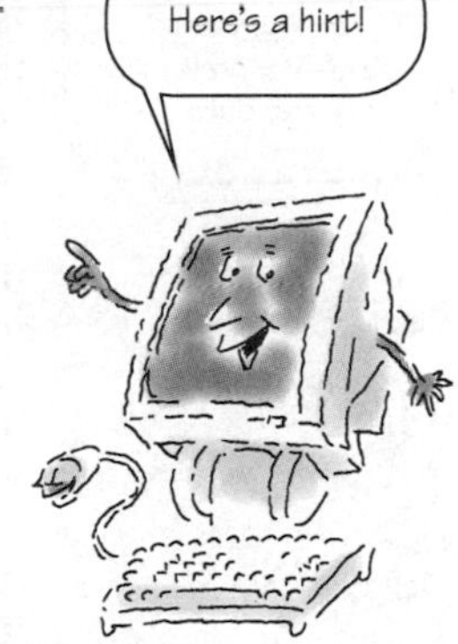

Here's a hint!

16. 3. Hemoglobin and hematocrit values decrease during pregnancy as the increase in plasma volume exceeds the increase in red blood cell production. Alterations in acid-base balance during pregnancy result in a state of respiratory alkalosis, compensated by mild metabolic acidosis. Mastitis is an infection in the breast characterized by a swollen tender breast and flulike symptoms. This condition is most frequently seen in breast-feeding clients.

NP: Analysis; CN: Health promotion and maintenance; CNS: Growth and development through the life span; CL: Knowledge

17. A 21-year-old client, 6 weeks' pregnant, is diagnosed with hyperemesis gravidarum. This excessive vomiting during pregnancy will often result in which of the following conditions?

1. Bowel perforation
2. Electrolyte imbalance
3. Miscarriage
4. Pregnancy-induced hypertension

17. 2. Excessive vomiting in clients with hyperemesis gravidarum often causes weight loss and fluid, electrolyte, and acid-base imbalances. Pregnancy-induced hypertension and bowel perforation aren't related to hyperemesis. The effects of hyperemesis on the fetus depend on the severity of the disorder. Clients with severe hyperemesis may have a low-birth-weight infant, but the disorder generally isn't life-threatening to the fetus.

NP: Analysis; CN: Physiological integrity; CNS: Reduction of risk potential; CL: Analysis

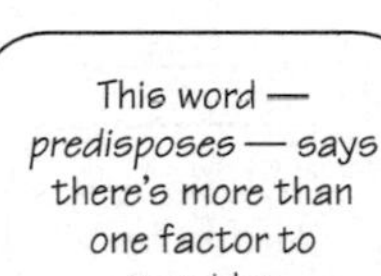

This word — predisposes — says there's more than one factor to consider.

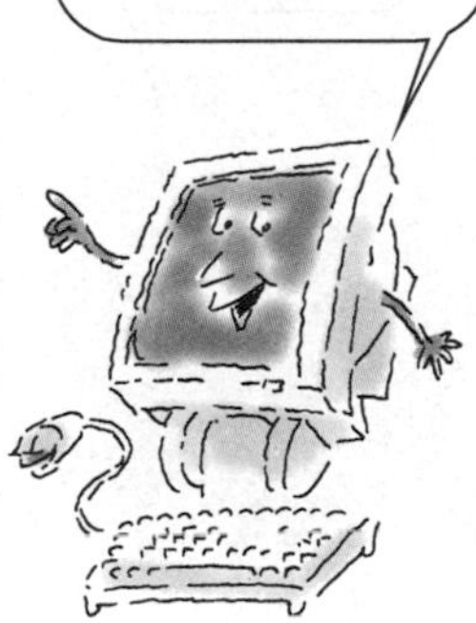

18. A client is being admitted to the antepartum unit for hypovolemia secondary to hyperemesis gravidarum. Which of the following factors predisposes a client to the development of this condition?

1. Trophoblastic disease
2. Maternal age older than 35 years
3. Malnourished or underweight clients
4. Low levels of human chorionic gonadotrophin (HCG)

18. 1. Trophoblastic disease is associated with hyperemesis gravidarum. Obesity and maternal age younger than 20 years are risk factors for developing hyperemesis gravidarum. High levels of estrogen and HCG have been associated with hyperemesis.

NP: Analysis; CN: Physiological integrity; CNS: Reduction of risk potential; CL: Knowledge

19. Clients with gestational diabetes are usually managed by which of the following therapies?

1. Diet
2. Long-acting insulin
3. Oral hypoglycemic drugs
4. Oral hypoglycemic drugs and insulin

19. 1. Clients with gestational diabetes are usually managed by diet alone to control their glucose intolerance. Oral hypoglycemic drugs are contraindicated in pregnancy. Long-acting insulin usually isn't needed for blood glucose control in the client with gestational diabetes.

NP: Analysis; CN: Health promotion and maintenance; CNS: Growth and development through the life span; CL: Knowledge

20. Magnesium sulfate is given to pregnant clients with preeclampsia to prevent which of the following conditions?

1. Hemorrhage
2. Hypertension
3. Hypomagnesemia
4. Seizures

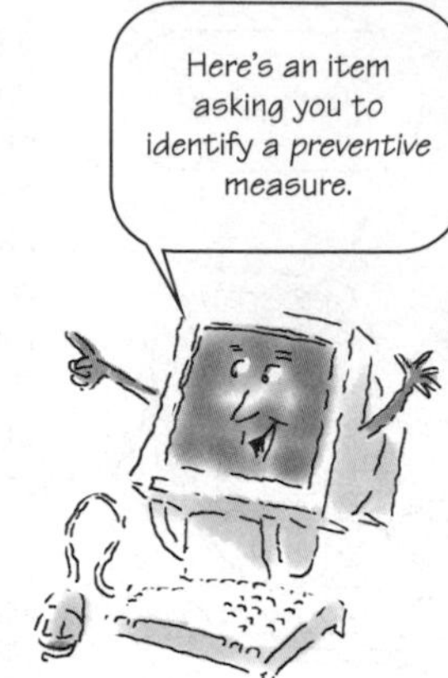

Here's an item asking you to identify a preventive measure.

20. 4. The anticonvulsant mechanism of magnesium is believed to depress seizure foci in the brain and peripheral neuromuscular blockade. Hypomagnesemia isn't a complication of preeclampsia. Antihypertensive drugs other than magnesium are preferred for sustained hypertension. Magnesium doesn't help prevent hemorrhage in preeclamptic clients.

NP: Implementation; CN: Physiological integrity; CNS: Pharmacological and parenteral therapies; CL: Analysis

21. A pregnant client has a negative contraction stress test (CST). Which of the following statements describes negative CST results?

1. Persistent late decelerations in fetal heartbeat occurred, with at least three contractions in a 10-minute window.
2. Accelerations of fetal heartbeat occurred, with at least 15 beats/minute, lasting 15 to 30 seconds in a 20-minute period.
3. Accelerations of fetal heartbeat were absent or didn't increase by 15 beats/minute for 15 to 30 seconds in a 20-minute period.
4. There was good fetal heart rate variability and no decelerations from contraction in a 10-minute period in which there were three contractions.

21. 4. A CST measures the fetal response to uterine contractions. A client must have three contractions in a 10-minute period. A negative CST shows good fetal heart rate variability with no decelerations from uterine contractions. No accelerations in the heartbeat of at least 15 beats/minute for 15 to 30 seconds in a 20-minute period indicates a nonreactive nonstress test (NST). Reactive NSTs have accelerations in the fetal heartbeat of at least 15 beats/minute lasting 15 to 30 seconds in a 20-minute period. Persistent late decelerations with contractions is a positive CST.

NP: Analysis; CN: Health promotion and maintenance; CNS: Growth and development through the life span; CL: Analysis

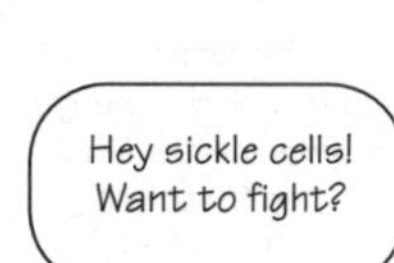

Hey sickle cells! Want to fight?

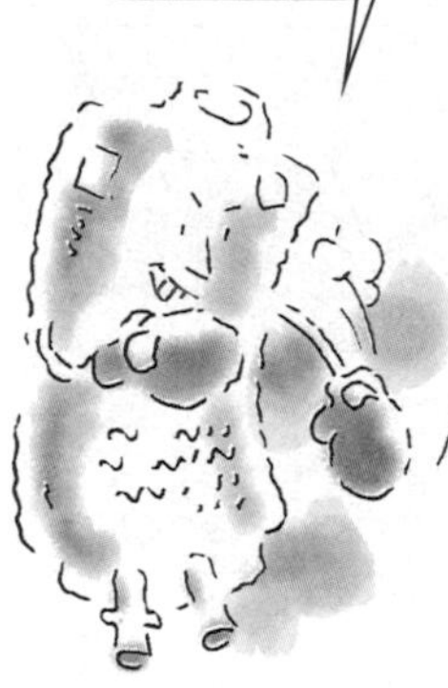

22. A pregnant client with sickle cell anemia is at an increased risk for having a sickle cell crisis during pregnancy. Aggressive management of a sickle cell crisis includes which of the following measures?

1. Antihypertensive agents
2. Diuretic agents
3. I.V. fluids
4. Acetaminophen (Tylenol) for pain

22. 3. A sickle cell crisis during pregnancy is usually managed by exchange transfusion, oxygen, and I.V. fluids. The client usually needs a stronger analgesic than acetaminophen to control the pain of a crisis. Antihypertensive drugs usually aren't necessary. Diuretics wouldn't be used unless fluid overload resulted.

NP: Planning; CN: Physiological integrity; CNS: Reduction of risk potential; CL: Analysis

23. Which of the following cardiac conditions is normal during pregnancy?

1. Cardiac tamponade
2. Heart failure
3. Endocarditis
4. Systolic murmur

23. 4. Systolic murmurs are heard in up to 90% of pregnant clients, and the murmur disappears soon after the delivery. Cardiac tamponade, which causes effusion of fluid into the pericardial sac, isn't normal during pregnancy. Despite the increases in intravascular volume and work load of the heart associated with pregnancy, heart failure isn't normal in pregnancy. Endocarditis is most often associated with I.V. drug use and isn't a normal finding in pregnancy.

NP: Assessment; CN: Health promotion and maintenance; CNS: Growth and development through the life span; CL: Knowledge

NP: Nursing process CN: Client needs category CNS: Client needs subcategory CL: Cognitive level

24. In a complete hydatidiform mole, which of the following karyotypes is typically found?

1. 46XX
2. 69XXY
3. 69XXX
4. 69XYY

24. 1. A complete hydatidiform mole results from the fertilization of an egg in which the nucleus is lost or inactivated. This causes the nucleus of the sperm (23X) to duplicate itself (46XX). 69XXY, 69XXX, and 69XYY are karyotypes of partial moles that result from two sperm fertilizing an apparently normal ovum.

NP: Analysis; CN: Health promotion and maintenance; CNS: Growth and development through the life span; CL: Knowledge

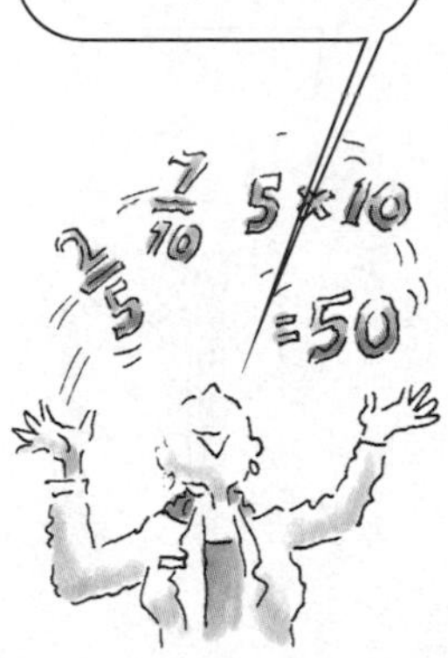

Keep those numbers and letters straight, now.

25. Magnesium sulfate is given to clients with pregnancy-induced hypertension to prevent seizure activity. Which of the following magnesium levels is therapeutic for clients with preeclampsia?

1. 4 to 7 mEq/L
2. 8 to 10 mEq/L
3. 10 to 12 mEq/L
4. Greater than 15 mEq/L

25. 1. The therapeutic level of magnesium for clients with pregnancy-induced hypertension is 4 to 7 mEq/L. A serum level of 8 to 10 mEq/L may cause the absence of reflexes in the client. Serum levels of 10 to 12 mEq/L may cause respiratory depression, and a serum level of magnesium greater than 15 mEq/L may result in respiratory paralysis.

NP: Assessment; CN: Physiological integrity; CNS: Pharmacological and parenteral therapies; CL: Knowledge

26. A client is receiving I.V. magnesium sulfate for severe preeclampsia. Which of the following adverse effects is associated with magnesium sulfate?

1. Anemia
2. Decreased urine output
3. Hyperreflexia
4. Increased respiratory rate

26. 2. Decreased urine output may occur in clients receiving I.V. magnesium and should be monitored closely to keep urine output at greater than 30 ml/hour, because magnesium is excreted through the kidneys and can easily accumulate to toxic levels. Anemia isn't associated with magnesium therapy. The client should be monitored for respiratory depression and paralysis when serum magnesium levels reach approximately 15 mEq/L. Magnesium infusions may cause depression of deep tendon reflexes or hyporeflexia.

NP: Analysis; CN: Physiological integrity; CNS: Pharmacological and parenteral therapies; CL: Analysis

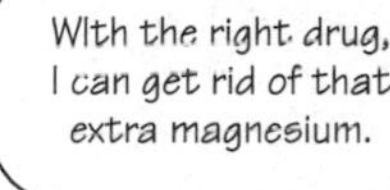

With the right drug, I can get rid of that extra magnesium.

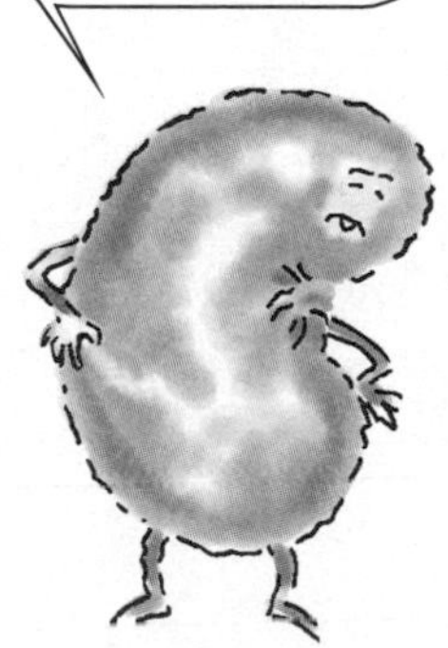

27. The antagonist for magnesium sulfate should be readily available to any client receiving I.V. magnesium. Which of the following drugs is the antidote for magnesium toxicity?

1. Calcium gluconate (Kalcinate)
2. Hydralazine (Apresoline)
3. Naloxone (Narcan)
4. Rh_0(D) immune globulin (RhoGAM)

27. 1. Calcium gluconate is the antidote for magnesium toxicity. Ten milliliters of 10% calcium gluconate is given I.V. push over 3 to 5 minutes. Hydralazine is given for sustained elevated blood pressures in preeclamptic clients. Rh_0(D) immune globulin is given to women with Rh-negative blood to prevent antibody formation from Rh-positive conceptions. Naloxone is used to correct narcotic toxicity.

NP: Analysis; CN: Physiological integrity; CNS: Reduction of risk potential; CL: Analysis

28. A pregnant client is screened for tuberculosis during her first prenatal visit. An intradermal injection of purified protein derivative (PPD) of the tuberculin bacilli is given. The client is considered to have a positive test for which of the following results?

1. An indurated wheal under 10 mm in diameter appears in 6 to 12 hours.
2. An indurated wheal over 10 mm in diameter appears in 48 to 72 hours.
3. A flat circumcised area under 10 mm in diameter appears in 6 to 12 hours.
4. A flat circumcised area over 10 mm in diameter appears in 48 to 72 hours.

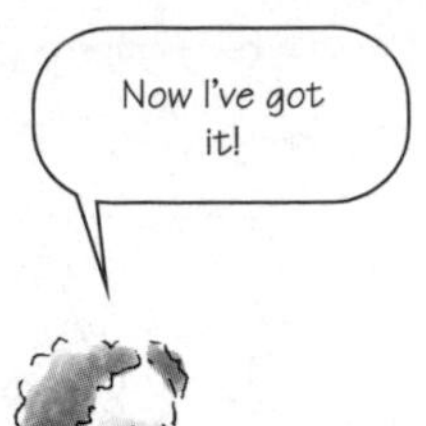

Now I've got it!

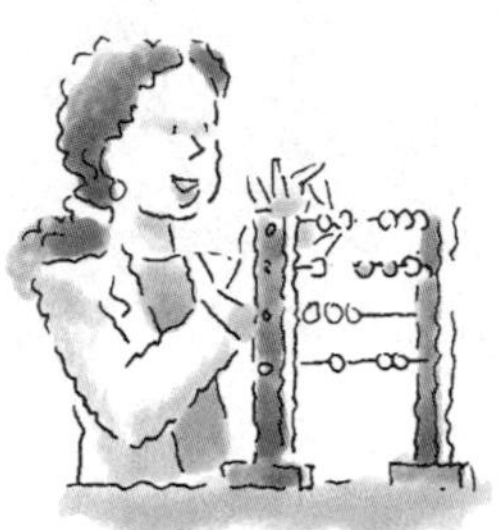

28. 2. A positive PPD result would be an indurated wheal over 10 mm in diameter that appears in 48 to 72 hours. The area must be a raised wheal, not a flat circumcised area to be considered positive.

NP: Assessment; CN: Health promotion and maintenance; CNS: Prevention and early detection of disease; CL: Knowledge

29. A 23-year-old client who is 27 weeks' pregnant arrives at her physician's office with complaints of fever, nausea, vomiting, malaise, unilateral flank pain, and costovertebral angle tenderness. Which of the following diagnoses is the most likely?

1. Asymptomatic bacteriuria
2. Bacterial vaginosis
3. Pyelonephritis
4. Urinary tract infection (UTI)

29. 3. The symptoms indicate acute pyelonephritis, a serious condition in a pregnant client. UTI symptoms include dysuria, urgency, frequency, and suprapubic tenderness. Asymptomatic bacteriuria doesn't cause symptoms. Bacterial vaginosis causes milky white vaginal discharge but no systemic symptoms.

NP: Analysis; CN: Physiological integrity; CNS: Reduction of risk potential; CL: Analysis

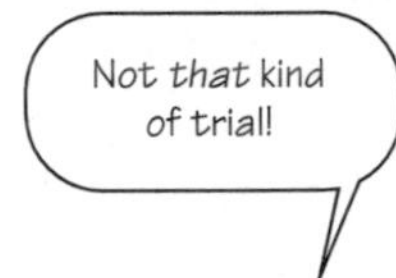

Not that kind of trial!

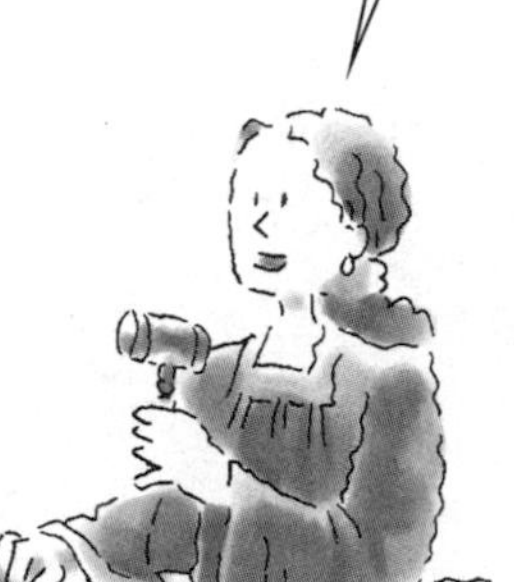

30. Clients with which of the following conditions would be appropriate for a trial of labor after a prior cesarean delivery?

1. Complete placenta previa
2. Invasive cervical cancer
3. Premature rupture of membranes
4. Prior classical cesarean delivery

30. 3. Clients with premature rupture of membranes are permitted a trial of labor after a previous cesarean delivery. A client with invasive cervical cancer should be scheduled for a cesarean delivery. Clients with placenta previa or a prior classical cesarean delivery shouldn't be given a trial of labor due to the risk of uterine rupture or severe bleeding.

NP: Analysis; CN: Physiological integrity; CNS: Physiological adaptation; CL: Analysis

31. Rh isoimmunization in a pregnant client develops during which of the following conditions?

1. Rh-positive maternal blood crosses into fetal blood, stimulating fetal antibodies.
2. Rh-positive fetal blood crosses into maternal blood, stimulating maternal antibodies.
3. Rh-negative fetal blood crosses into maternal blood, stimulating maternal antibodies.
4. Rh-negative maternal blood crosses into fetal blood, stimulating fetal antibodies.

31. 2. Rh isoimmunization occurs when Rh-positive fetal blood cells cross into the maternal circulation and stimulate maternal antibody production. In subsequent pregnancies with Rh-positive fetuses, maternal antibodies may cross back into the fetal circulation and destroy the fetal blood cells.

NP: Analysis; CN: Physiological integrity; CNS: Reduction of risk potential; CL: Knowledge

32. Which of the following doses of Rh_o(D) immune globulin (RhoGAM) is appropriate for a pregnant client at 28 weeks' gestation?

1. 50 mcg in a sensitized client
2. 50 mcg in an unsensitized client
3. 300 mcg in a sensitized client
4. 300 mcg in an unsensitized client

32. 4. An Rh-negative unsensitized woman should be given 300 mcg of RhoGAM at 28 weeks' after an indirect Coombs test is done to verify that sensitization hasn't occurred. For a first-trimester abortion or ectopic pregnancy, 50 mcg of RhoGAM is given.

NP: Analysis; CN: Health promotion and maintenance; CNS: Growth and development through the life span; CL: Analysis

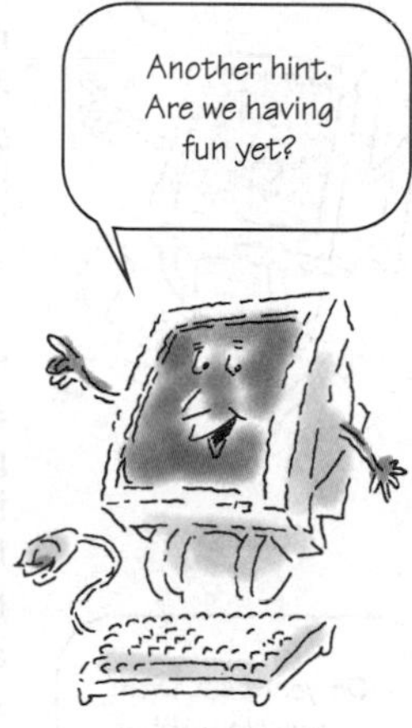
Another hint.
Are we having
fun yet?

33. A client hospitalized for premature labor tells the nurse she's having occasional contractions. Which of the following nursing interventions would be the most appropriate?

1. Teach the client the possible complications of premature birth.
2. Tell the client to walk to see if she can get rid of the contractions.
3. Encourage her to empty her bladder and drink plenty of fluids, and give I.V. fluids.
4. Notify anesthesia for immediate epidural placement to relieve the pain associated with contractions.

33. 3. An empty bladder and adequate hydration may help decrease or stop labor contractions. Walking may encourage contractions to become stronger. Teaching the potential complications is likely to increase the client's anxiety rather than help her relax. It would be inappropriate to call anesthesia and have an epidural placed because further assessment of contractions is necessary.

NP: Planning; CN: Physiological integrity; CNS: Reduction of risk potential; CL: Application

34. The phrase *gravida 4, para 2* indicates which of the following prenatal histories?

1. A client has been pregnant four times and had two miscarriages.
2. A client has been pregnant four times and had two live-born children.
3. A client has been pregnant four times and had two cesarean deliveries.
4. A client has been pregnant four times and had two spontaneous abortions.

34. 2. *Gravida* refers to the number of times a client has been pregnant; *para* refers to the number of viable children born. Therefore, the client who is *gravida 4, para 2* has been pregnant four times and had two live-born children.

NP: Assessment; CN: Health promotion and maintenance; CNS: Growth and development through the life span; CL: Knowledge

35. Which of the following factors would contribute to a high-risk pregnancy?

1. Blood type O positive
2. First pregnancy at age 33 years
3. History of allergy to honey bee pollen
4. History of insulin-dependent diabetes mellitus

35. 4. A woman with a history of diabetes has an increased risk for perinatal complications, including hypertension, preeclampsia, and neonatal hypoglycemia. The age of 33 years without other risk factors doesn't increase risk, nor does type O positive blood or environmental allergens.

NP: Assessment; CN: Health promotion and maintenance; CNS: Prevention and early detection of disease; CL: Comprehension

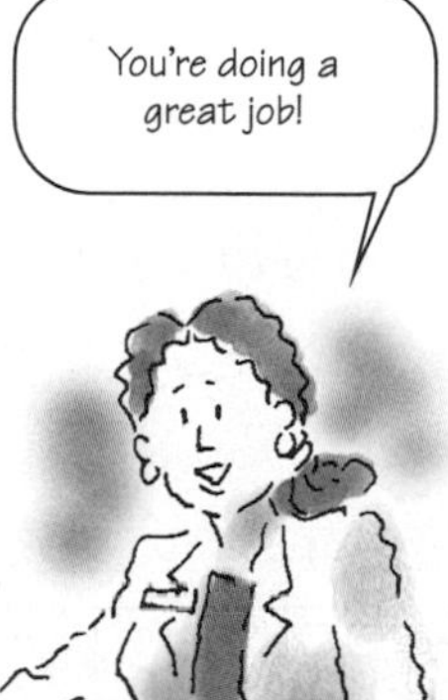
You're doing a
great job!

36. Which of the following complications can be potentially life-threatening and can occur in a client receiving a tocolytic agent?

1. Diabetic ketoacidosis
2. Hyperemesis gravidarum
3. Pulmonary edema
4. Sickle cell anemia

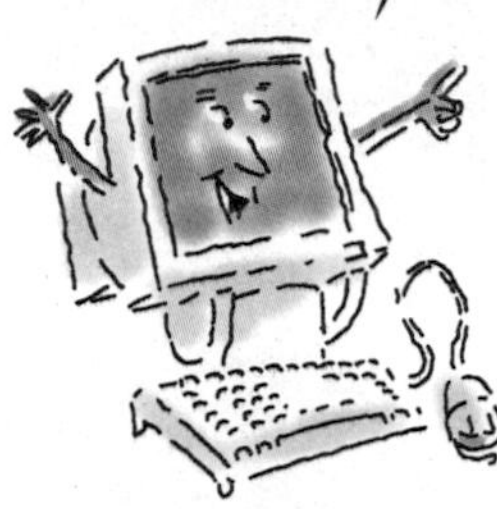

The answer to question 36 has to be correct in two ways.

36. 3. Tocolytics are used to stop labor contractions. The most common adverse effect associated with the use of these drugs is pulmonary edema. Clients who don't have diabetes don't need to be observed for diabetic ketoacidosis. Hyperemesis gravidarum doesn't result from tocolytic use. Sickle cell anemia is an inherited genetic condition and doesn't develop spontaneously.

NP: Assessment; CN: Physiological integrity; CNS: Pharmacological and parenteral therapies; CL: Knowledge

37. Which of the following hormones would be administered for the stimulation of uterine contractions?

1. Estrogen
2. Fetal cortisol
3. Oxytocin
4. Progesterone

37. 3. Oxytocin is the hormone responsible for stimulating uterine contractions. Pitocin, the synthetic form, may be given to clients who are past their due date. Progesterone has a relaxing effect on the uterus. Fetal cortisol is believed to slow the production of progesterone by the placenta. Although estrogen has a role in uterine contractions, it isn't given in a synthetic form to help uterine contractility.

NP: Planning; CN: Physiological integrity; CNS: Pharmacological and parenteral therapies; CL: Knowledge

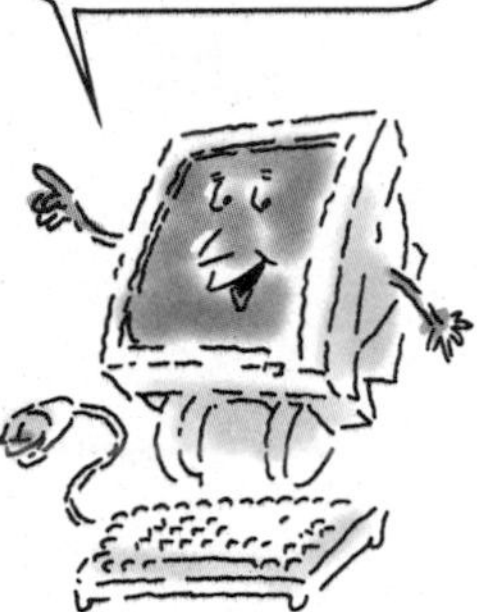

Do your best with question 38! (Best, get it? It's a clue!)

38. Which of the following answers best describes the stage of pregnancy in which maternal and fetal blood are exchanged?

1. Conception
2. 9 weeks' gestation, when the fetal heart is well developed
3. 32 to 34 weeks' gestation (third trimester)
4. Maternal and fetal blood are never exchanged

38. 4. Only nutrients and waste products are transferred across the placenta. Blood exchange never occurs. Complications and some medical procedures can cause an exchange to occur accidentally.

NP: Analysis; CN: Physiological integrity; CNS: Physiological adaptation; CL: Comprehension

39. Which of the following rationales best explains why a pregnant client should lie on her left side when resting or sleeping in the later stages of pregnancy?

1. To facilitate digestion
2. To facilitate bladder emptying
3. To prevent compression of the vena cava
4. To avoid the development of fetal anomalies

39. 3. The weight of the pregnant uterus is sufficiently heavy to compress the vena cava, which could impair blood flow to the uterus, possibly decreasing oxygen to the fetus. The side-lying position hasn't been shown to prevent fetal anomalies, nor does it facilitate bladder emptying or digestion.

NP: Planning; CN: Physiological integrity; CNS: Reduction of risk potential; CL: Analysis

40. A pregnant client is concerned about lack of fetal movement. What instructions would the nurse give that might offer reassurance?

1. Start taking two prenatal vitamins.
2. Take a warm bath to facilitate fetal movement.
3. Eat foods that contain a high sugar content to enhance fetal movement.
4. Lie down once a day and count the number of fetal movements for 15 to 30 minutes.

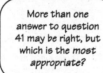

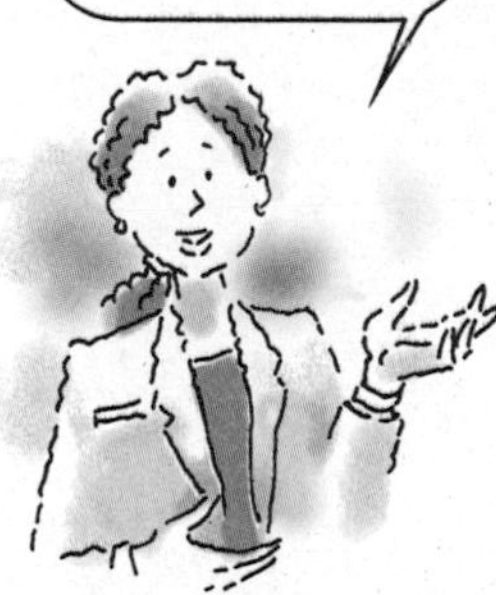

Client teaching is an important role for the nurse.

40. 4. Having the client lie down once during the day will allow her to concentrate on detecting fetal movement, which can be reassuring. Additionally, when the mother is up and actively walking around, it tends to be soothing to the fetus, resulting in sleep promotion. Lying down will make it easier for the client to detect movement. Eating additional sugary foods isn't recommended as some pregnant clients are more susceptible to cavities. Taking a warm bath is again likely to be soothing to the fetus. There's also a risk for hyperthermia if the water is too warm or the client is immersed too long. Instructing her to take additional prenatal vitamins isn't recommended as vitamins can be toxic.

NP: Planning; CN: Psychosocial integrity; CNS: Coping and adaptation; CL: Application

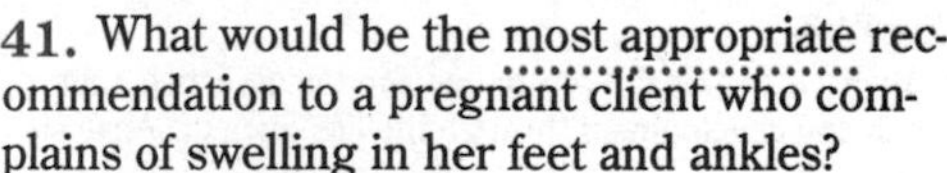

41. What would be the most appropriate recommendation to a pregnant client who complains of swelling in her feet and ankles?

1. Limit fluid intake.
2. Buy walking shoes.
3. Sit and elevate the feet twice daily.
4. Start taking a diuretic as needed daily.

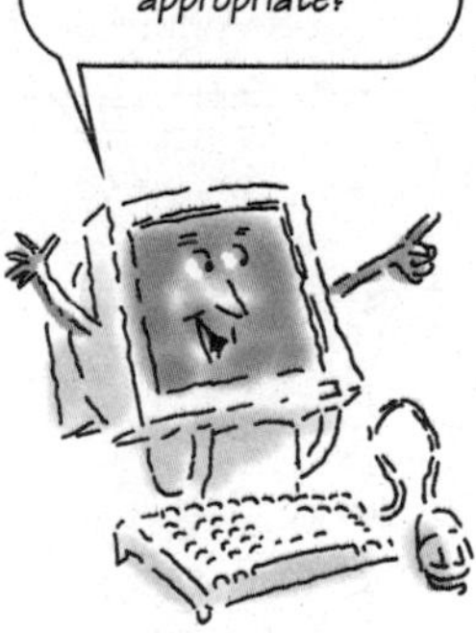

More than one answer to question 41 may be right, but which is the most appropriate?

41. 3. Sitting down and putting up her feet at least once daily will promote venous return and therefore decrease edema. Buying walking shoes won't necessarily decrease edema. Limiting fluid intake isn't recommended unless there are additional medical complications such as heart failure. Diuretics aren't recommended during pregnancy because it's important to maintain an adequate circulatory volume.

NP: Planning; CN: Physiological integrity; CNS: Basic care and comfort; CL: Application

42. Which of the following interventions would the nurse recommend to a client having severe heartburn during her pregnancy?

1. Eat several small meals daily.
2. Eat crackers on waking every a.m.
3. Drink a preparation of salt and vinegar.
4. Drink orange juice frequently during the day.

42. 1. Eating small frequent meals will place less pressure on the esophageal sphincter, reducing the likelihood of the regurgitation of stomach contents into the lower esophagus. None of the other suggestions have been shown to decrease heartburn.

NP: Planning; CN: Physiological integrity; CNS: Basic care and comfort; CL: Application

43. Which of the following maternal complications is associated with obesity in pregnancy?

1. Mastitis
2. Placenta previa
3. Preeclampsia
4. Rh isoimmunization

43. 3. The incidence of preeclampsia in obese clients is about seven times more than that in pregnant nonobese clients. Placenta previa, mastitis, and Rh isoimmunization aren't associated with increased incidence in obese pregnant clients.

NP: Analysis; CN: Physiological integrity; CNS: Reduction of risk potential; CL: Analysis

44. Because uteroplacental circulation is compromised in clients with preeclampsia, a nonstress test (NST) is performed to detect which of the following conditions?

1. Anemia
2. Fetal well-being
3. Intrauterine growth retardation (IUGR)
4. Oligohydramnios

45. A client is 33 weeks' pregnant and has had diabetes since she was 21. When checking her fasting blood sugar level, which of the following values would indicate the client's disease was controlled?

1. 45 mg/dl
2. 85 mg/dl
3. 120 mg/dl
4. 136 mg/dl

46. Which of the following techniques is best to monitor the fetus of a client with diabetes in her third trimester?

1. Ultrasound examination weekly
2. Nonstress test (NST) twice weekly
3. Daily contraction stress test (CST) at 32 weeks' gestation
4. Monitoring of fetal activity by client weekly

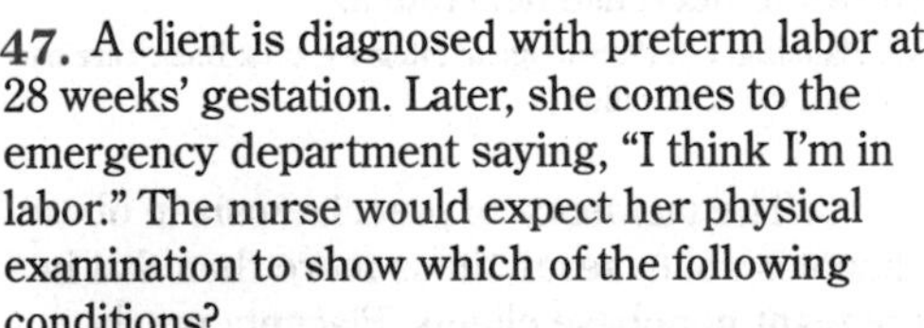

47. A client is diagnosed with preterm labor at 28 weeks' gestation. Later, she comes to the emergency department saying, "I think I'm in labor." The nurse would expect her physical examination to show which of the following conditions?

1. Painful contractions with no cervical dilation
2. Regular uterine contractions with cervical dilation
3. Irregular uterine contraction with no cervical dilation
4. Irregular uterine contractions with cervical effacement

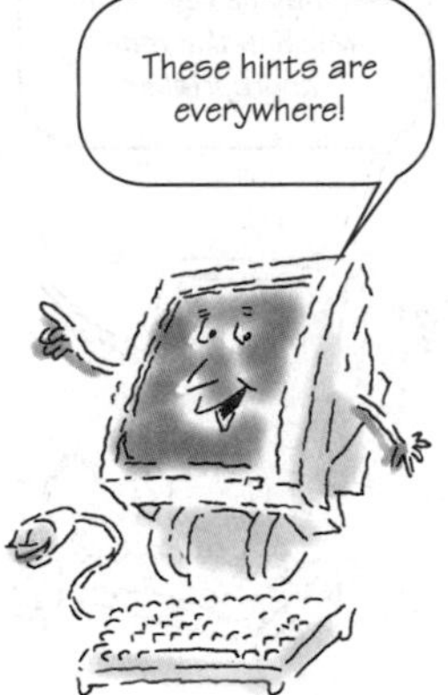
These hints are everywhere!

44. 2. An NST is based on the theory that a healthy fetus will have transient fetal heart rate accelerations with fetal movement. A fetus with compromised uteroplacental circulation usually won't have these accelerations, which indicate a nonreactive NST. Serial ultrasounds will detect IUGR and oligohydramnios in a fetus. An NST can't detect anemia in a fetus.

NP: Analysis; CN: Health promotion and maintenance; CNS: Growth and development through the life span; CL: Analysis

45. 2. Recommended fasting blood sugar levels in pregnant clients with diabetes are 60 to 90 mg/dl. A fasting blood sugar level of 45 mg/dl is low and may result in symptoms of hypoglycemia. A blood sugar level below 120 mg/dl is recommended for 1-hour postprandial values. A blood sugar level above 136 mg/dl in a pregnant client indicates hyperglycemia.

NP: Analysis; CN: Health promotion and maintenance; CNS: Growth and development through the life span; CL: Analysis

46. 2. Of the techniques listed, the NST is the preferred antepartum heart rate screening test for pregnant clients with diabetes. NSTs should be done at least twice weekly, starting at 32 weeks' gestation, as fetal deaths in clients with diabetes have been noted within 1 week of a reactive NST. Ultrasounds should be done every 4 to 6 weeks to monitor fetal growth. CST wouldn't be initiated at 32 weeks' gestation. Maternal fetal activity monitoring should be done daily.

NP: Planning; CN: Physiological integrity; CNS: Reduction of risk potential; CL: Knowledge

47. 2. Regular uterine contractions (every 10 minutes or more) along with cervical dilation change before 36 weeks is considered preterm labor. No cervical change with uterine contractions isn't considered preterm labor.

NP: Analysis; CN: Health promotion and maintenance; CNS: Growth and development through the life span; CL: Knowledge

NP: Nursing process CN: Client needs category CNS: Client needs subcategory CL: Cognitive level

48. Which of the following conditions is the most common cause of anemia in pregnancy?

1. Alpha thalassemia
2. Beta thalassemia
3. Iron deficiency anemia
4. Sickle cell anemia

48. 3. Iron deficiency anemia accounts for approximately 95% of anemia in pregnancy. Sickle cell anemia is an inherited chronic disease that results from abnormal hemoglobin synthesis. Thalassemias are the most common genetic disorders of the blood. These anemias cause a reduction or absence of the alpha or beta hemoglobin chain.

NP: Analysis; CN: Health promotion and maintenance; CNS: Growth and development through the life span; CL: Knowledge

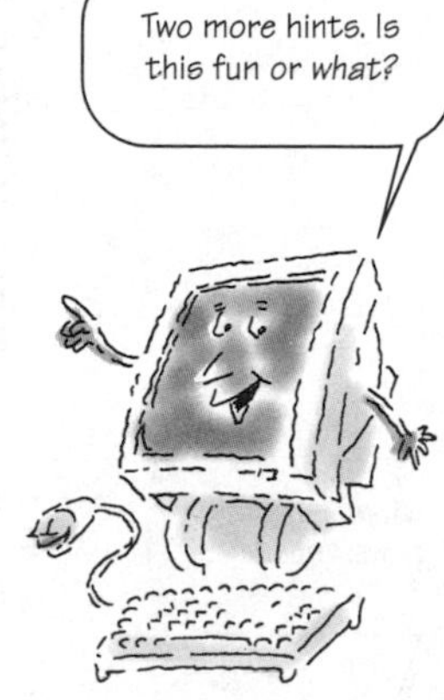

Two more hints. Is this fun or what?

49. Which of the following tests should be ordered to confirm a diagnosis of beta thalassemia?

1. Complete blood count (CBC)
2. Hemoglobin A_{1c}
3. Hemoglobin electrophoresis
4. Iron level

49. 3. Diagnosis of the specific type of thalassemia is achieved by hemoglobin electrophoresis. This test detects high levels of hemoglobin A_2 or F. The CBC includes white blood cell, hemoglobin, hematocrit, and platelet values. Hemoglobin A_{1c} values show the client's blood sugar levels over the past 120 days. A direct iron level can't be tested. Iron status is indirectly assessed through hemoglobin, hematocrit, mean corpuscular volume, and other such values. A client history and diet record can also help determine iron intake.

NP: Analysis; CN: Physiological integrity; CNS: Reduction of risk potential; CL: Knowledge

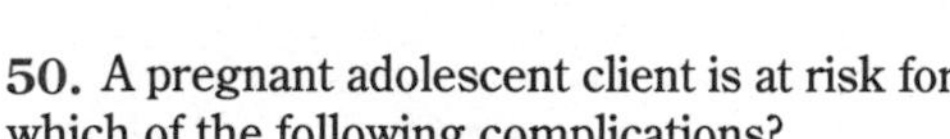

50. A pregnant adolescent client is at risk for which of the following complications?

1. Gestational diabetes
2. Low-birth-weight infant
3. Macrosomic infant
4. Placenta previa

50. 2. Adolescent clients are at risk for delivering low-birth-weight neonates, not macrosomic neonates. Nutritional counseling should be included as part of prenatal care for adolescent clients. Adolescents aren't at increased risk for developing gestational diabetes or placenta previa.

NP: Analysis; CN: Health promotion and maintenance; CNS: Growth and development through the life span; CL: Knowledge

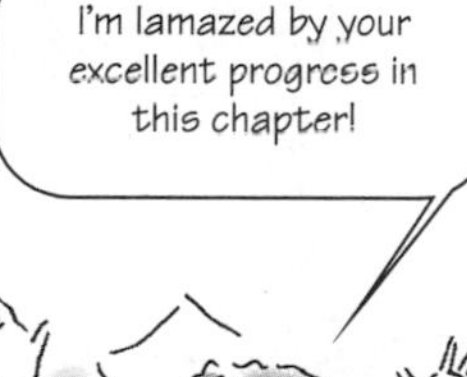

I'm lamazed by your excellent progress in this chapter!

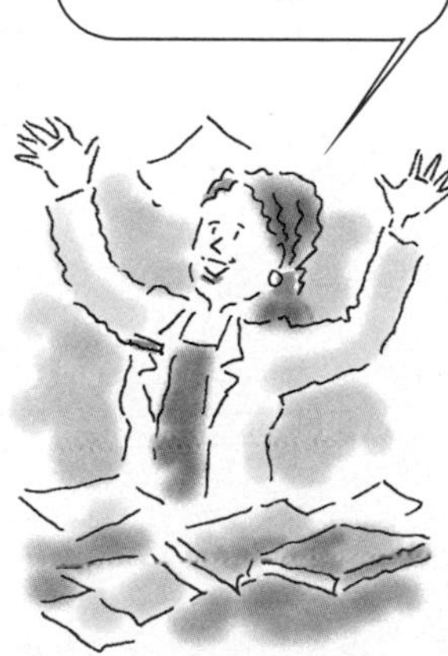

51. Which of the following methods of pain control incorporates effleurage as a technique to displace pain?

1. Bradley method
2. Hydrotherapy
3. Lamaze method
4. Nubain method

51. 3. The Lamaze method incorporates effleurage, or light abdominal massage, to reduce pain during labor. With the Bradley method, the client reduces pain through abdominal breathing, ambulation, and using an internal focus point as a disassociation technique. Hydrotherapy is the use of water during labor, including showers and tubs. Nubain, a narcotic analgesic, is commonly used during labor.

NP: Assessment; CN: Physiological integrity; CNS: Physiological adaptation; CL: Knowledge

52. Which drug would the nurse choose to utilize as an antagonist for magnesium sulfate?

1. Oxytocin (Pitocin)
2. Terbutaline (Brethaire)
3. Calcium gluconate (Kalcinate)
4. Naloxone (Narcan)

52. 3. Calcium gluconate should be kept at the bedside while a client is receiving a magnesium infusion. If magnesium toxicity occurs, calcium gluconate is administered as an antidote. Oxytocin is the synthetic form of the naturally occurring pituitary hormone used to initiate or augment uterine contractions. Terbutaline is a beta$_2$-adrenergic agonist that may be used to relax the smooth muscle of the uterus, especially for preterm labor and uterine hyperstimulation. Naloxone is an opiate antagonist administered to reverse the respiratory depression that may follow administration of opiates.

NP: Implementation; CN: Physiological integrity; CNS: Reduction of risk potential; CL: Analysis

53. The nurse receives an order to start an infusion for a client who's hemorrhaging due to a placenta previa. What supplies will be needed?

1. Y tubing, normal saline solution, and a 20G catheter
2. Y tubing, lactated Ringer's solution, and an 18G catheter
3. Y tubing, normal saline solution, and an 18G catheter
4. Y tubing, lactated Ringer's solution, and a 20G catheter

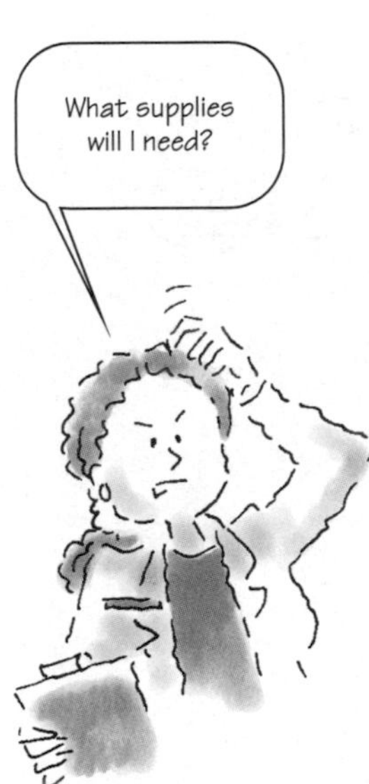
What supplies will I need?

53. 3. Blood transfusions require Y tubing, normal saline solution to mix with the blood product, and an 18G catheter to avoid lysing (breaking) the red blood cells. A 20G catheter lumen isn't large enough for a blood transfusion. Lactated Ringer's solution isn't the I.V. solution of choice with a blood transfusion.

NP: Implementation; CN: Physiological integrity; CNS: Pharmacological and parenteral therapies; CL: Comprehension

54. During the last 6 weeks of gestation, which of the following tests is not used to determine fetal well-being?

1. Biophysical profile
2. Nonstress test
3. Maternal blood count
4. Fetal movement count

54. 3. Maternal blood count evaluates maternal, not fetal, well-being. The biophysical profile uses ultrasound to evaluate fetal body movements, fetal breathing movements, fetal muscle tone, reactive fetal cardiac rate, and amniotic fluid volume. The nonstress test evaluates the fetal heart rate for accelerations during fetal movement. Fetal movement counts are used during the last trimester to obtain a rough index of fetal health; the number of fetal movements are counted at different times throughout the day and then charted to detect any change in overall activity over a number of days.

NP: Analysis; CN: Physiological integrity; CNS: Reduction of risk potential; CL: Knowledge

55. The GTPAL system is used to document a client's previous pregnancies. Which phrase does GTPAL stand for?

1. Total neonates, Preterm neonates, Anacephalic neonates, and Live births
2. Total neonates, Problem pregnancies, Abortions, and Live births
3. Term neonates, Preterm neonates, Anacephalic neonates, and Live births
4. Term neonates, Preterm neonates, Abortions, and Living children

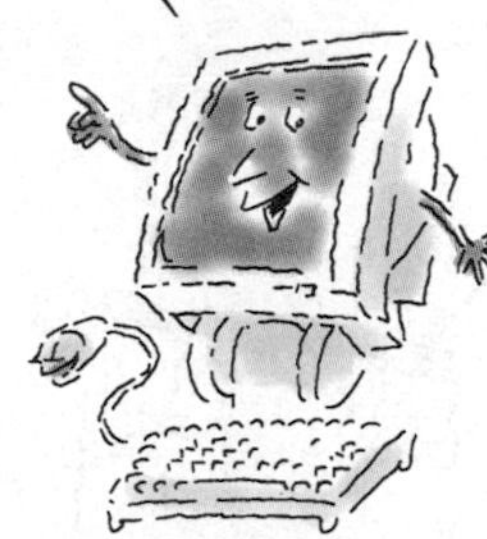

You've got to really think about this question.

55. 4. In GTPAL, G stands for gravida; T denotes the number of term neonates born after 37 weeks' gestation; P, the number of preterm neonates born before 37 weeks' gestation; A, the number of pregnancies ending with spontaneous or therapeutic abortion; and L, the number of children currently living.

NP: Assessment; CN: Health promotion and maintenance; CNS: Growth and development through the life span; CL: Knowledge

56. Gravida refers to which of the following descriptions?

1. A serious pregnancy
2. Number of times a female has been pregnant
3. Number of children a female has delivered
4. Number of term pregnancies a female has had

56. 2. Gravida refers to the number of times a female has been pregnant, regardless of pregnancy outcome or the number of neonates delivered.

NP: Assessment; CN: Health promotion and maintenance; CNS: Growth and development through the life span; CL: Knowledge

57. A 32-year-old woman is 15 weeks' pregnant when admitted to the labor unit. According to the GTPAL system, she is a G5 P1212. Which description does this indicate?

1. Total of 5 pregnancies, 1 full-term pregnancy, 2 problem pregnancies, 1 spontaneous abortion, and 2 live births
2. Total of 5 children, 1 full-term pregnancy, 2 preterm pregnancies, 1 abortion, 2 live births
3. Total of 5 pregnancies, 1 full-term pregnancy, 2 preterm pregnancies, 1 abortion, 2 living children
4. Total of 5 pregnancies, 1 full-term pregnancy, 2 problem pregnancies, 1 abortion, 2 living children

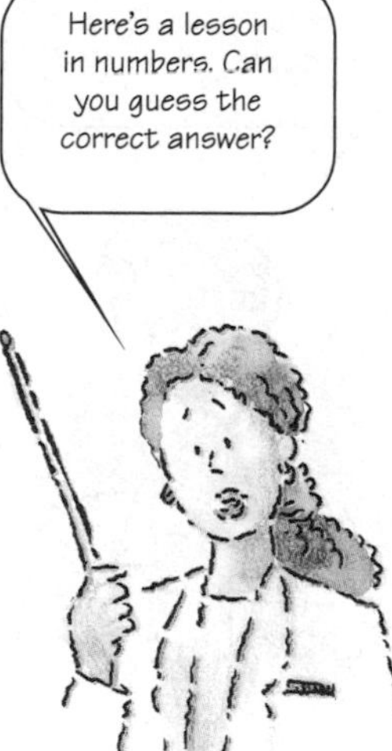

Here's a lesson in numbers. Can you guess the correct answer?

57. 3. T indicates the number of term neonates born at 37 weeks' gestation or after; P, the number of preterm neonates born before 37 weeks' gestation; A, the number of pregnancies ending with spontaneous or therapeutic abortion; and L, the number of children currently living. In this case, the client has been pregnant five times (including the current pregnancy); has had one pregnancy of at least 37 weeks' gestation, two preterm pregnancies, and one abortion; and has two living children.

NP: Assessment; CN: Health promotion and maintenance; CNS: Growth and development through the life span; CL: Knowledge

58. Which of the following conditions poses the greatest risk to a 32-year-old woman who is 15 weeks' pregnant and has a history of hypertension?

1. Abruptio placentae
2. Preterm labor
3. Spontaneous abortion
4. Anemia

58. 1. A history of hypertension predisposes the client for developing abruptio placentae. She isn't at risk for developing preterm labor, spontaneous abortion, or anemia.

NP: Analysis; CN: Physiological integrity; CNS: Reduction of risk potential; CL: Analysis

59. A 32-year-old woman has her first prenatal visit at 15 weeks' gestation. Which finding during this visit is abnormal?

1. Fundal height of 18 cm
2. Blood pressure of 124/72 mm Hg
3. Urine negative for protein
4. Weight of 144 lb (65.3 kg)

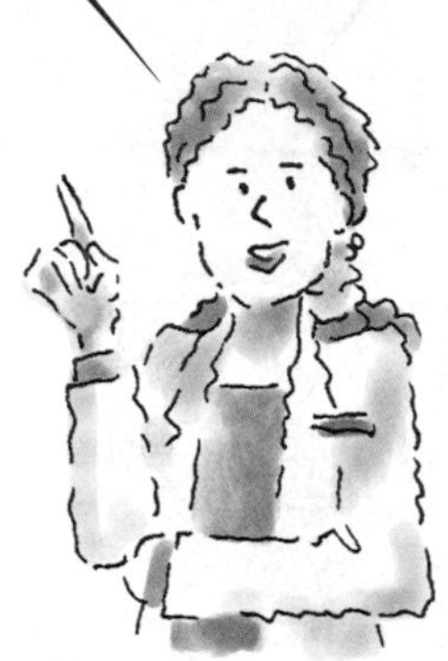

Question 59 is asking for an abnormal finding.

59. 1. Fundal height (in centimeters) should equal the number of weeks' gestation. This client should have a fundal height of 15 to 16 cm. The blood pressure, urine, and weight findings are within normal limits for the information given.

NP: Assessment; CN: Physiological integrity; CNS: Reduction of risk potential; CL: Analysis

60. A 25-year-old primiparous client arrives for her first prenatal visit at 10 weeks' gestation. She seems nervous and has many questions. Which action should the nurse take first?

1. Assess the client's concerns while taking a comprehensive history.
2. Ask the client to undress to prepare for the physical examination.
3. Reassure the client that all her questions will be answered during the visit.
4. Tell the client there's nothing to worry about; the physician will take care of her.

60. 3. Providing initial reassurance helps set the client's mind at ease. Assessing the client's concerns while taking a history would be appropriate only if the client wrote down her questions in advance. Asking her to disrobe immediately may make the client even more nervous. She should be treated as an intelligent partner in her care rather than be told that the physician will take care of everything.

NP: Implementation; CN: Psychosocial integrity; CNS: Coping and adaptation; CL: Application

61. Accompanied by her father, a primiparous 15-year-old client arrives for her first prenatal visit at 30 weeks' gestation. Her father refuses to leave the room, stating that the girl is shy and he will answer the questions for her. Which aspect of this situation should be of most concern to the nurse?

1. The possibility of preterm labor with an adolescent pregnancy
2. Lack of prenatal care until this visit
3. Possible child abuse or domestic violence
4. Difficulties of an overprotective parent in dealing with his daughter

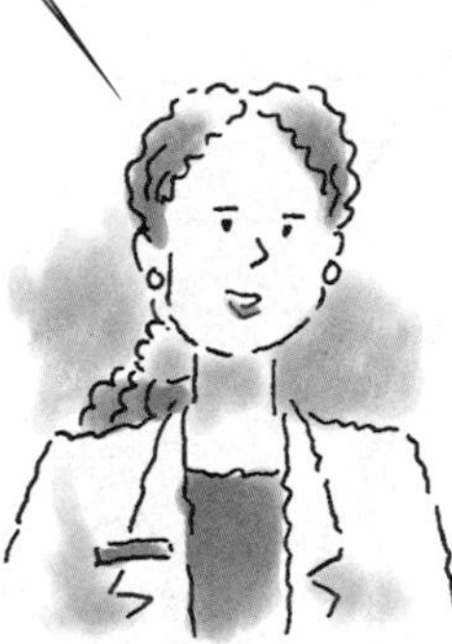

Question 61 poses a serious situation. What should the nurse be most concerned about?

61. 3. Generally, a father would be somewhat uncomfortable staying in a room while his pregnant daughter is examined. If he insists on staying during the history and physical examination, the nurse should gently but firmly ask him to wait in another room. If the nurse suspects possible child abuse or domestic violence, the father may not want the girl to be alone with the nurse, fearing that she might reveal the abuse or violence. (Typically, a victim of domestic violence says nothing if the perpetrator is in the room with her.) The possibility of preterm labor and lack of prenatal care should be considered — but they aren't the primary concerns in this situation. An overprotective parent can be supported and taught how to let go of a child as time goes by; a social work referral may be warranted.

NP: Assessment; CN: Psychosocial integrity; CNS: Psychosocial adaptation; CL: Knowledge

62. Which statement describes the best way for the nurse to determine if a pregnant client is the victim of domestic abuse or violence?

1. Interview the client with her partner in the room.
2. Interview the client with the physician present.
3. Interview the client alone in a nonjudgmental way.
4. Interview the client in a nonjudgmental way, with the partner present.

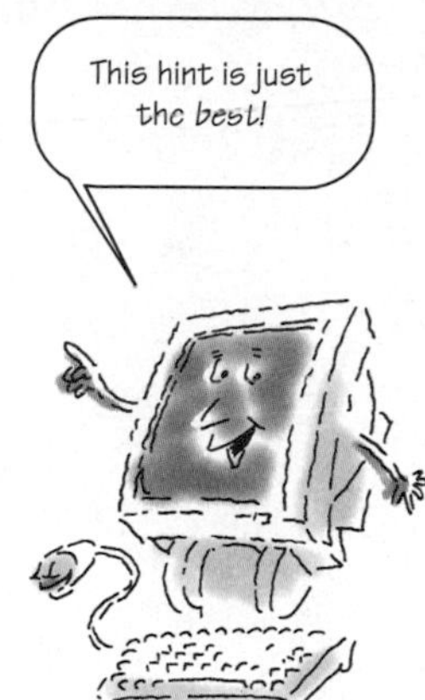

This hint is just
the best!

62. 3. To help the client feel protected and develop enough trust in the nurse to share her "secret," the nurse should interview her alone in a nonjudgmental way. If the partner is present, the client is likely to clam up for fear of retaliation the next time they're alone together.
NP: Assessment; CN: Psychosocial integrity; CNS: Psychosocial adaptation; CL: Knowledge

63. Pregnancy causes multiple body changes that are normal but can cause discomfort. Which change does not normally occur during the first trimester?

1. Hemorrhoids
2. Increased vaginal discharge
3. Breast tenderness
4. Fatigue

63. 1. Hemorrhoids generally occur during the second and third trimesters as blood stagnates in the lower extremities, resulting from pressure on the pelvic veins and inferior vena cava from the enlarged uterus. Increased vaginal discharge, breast tenderness, and fatigue are typical discomforts of the first trimester.
NP: Assessment; CN: Health promotion and maintenance; CNS: Growth and development through the life span; CL: Knowledge

64. During the second and third trimesters, common pregnancy discomforts may increase in number and severity. Which discomforts are normal during this time?

1. Ankle edema, hemorrhoids, nausea and vomiting, and shortness of breath
2. Ankle edema, shortness of breath, leg cramps, and increased vaginal discharge
3. Leg cramps, Braxton Hicks contractions, and nausea and vomiting
4. Leg cramps, ankle edema, and shortness of breath

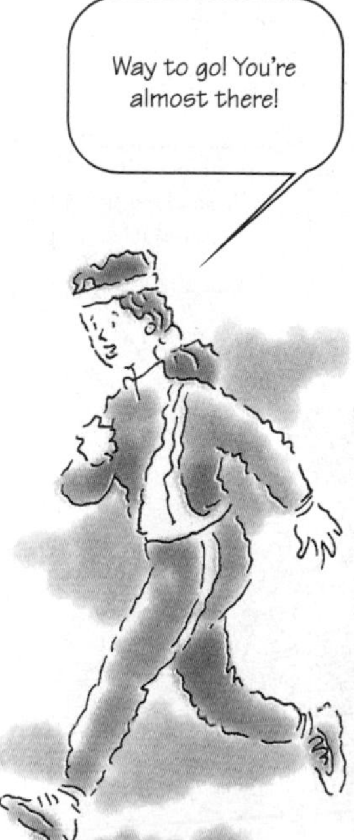

Way to go! You're
almost there!

64. 4. Leg cramps, ankle edema, and shortness of breath are normal during the second and third trimesters. The nurse should teach the client how to relieve minor discomforts and what to report if the discomfort becomes unbearable. Nausea and vomiting should subside by the end of the first trimester; if they don't, the nurse should suspect an undiagnosed problem, such as hyperemesis gravidarum or emotional factors that may be exacerbating the nausea and vomiting. Increased vaginal discharge generally occurs during the first trimester and decreases at the end of this period. A yellow, curdlike, or malodorous discharge suggests an abnormal vaginal infection, which should be reported to the physician.
NP: Assessment; CN: Health promotion and maintenance; CNS: Growth and development through the life span; CL: Knowledge

65. Which of the following conditions isn't diagnosed by abdominal ultrasound during the prenatal period?

1. Fetal presentation
2. Fetal heart activity
3. Maternal diabetes
4. Amniotic fluid volume

65. 3. Abdominal ultrasound evaluates fetal presentation, fetal heart activity, and amniotic fluid volume. Although it may show increased amniotic fluid, thus helping to diagnose maternal diabetes, it isn't used for that purpose.
NP: Analysis; CN: Physiological integrity; CNS: Reduction of risk potential; CL: Analysis

66. A glucose tolerance test is generally performed if the client has an abnormal result in the 1-hour glucose-screening test. Which condition does the glucose tolerance test diagnose?

1. Type 1 diabetes mellitus
2. Gestational diabetes
3. Diabetic neuropathy
4. Fetal diabetes

66. 2. The glucose tolerance test diagnoses gestational diabetes—a type of diabetes that occurs during pregnancy. The client with this disorder is typically prescribed a special diet and, after delivery, has no further problems unless she becomes pregnant again. Type 1 diabetes mellitus generally is diagnosed in preadolescents. Diabetic neuropathy may occur in clients with long-standing diabetes. Fetal diabetes can't be diagnosed because the maternal pancreas regulates fetal glucose levels.

NP: Analysis; CN: Health promotion and maintenance; CNS: Prevention and early detection of disease; CL: Knowledge

67. Which of the following problems doesn't typically result from uncontrolled gestational diabetes?

1. Maternal hyperglycemia
2. Fetal demise
3. Insufficient amniotic fluid
4. Maternal hypertension

67. 3. Excess, not insufficient, amniotic fluid may occur in a pregnant client with gestational diabetes. Maternal hyperglycemia or hypertension and fetal demise are possible consequences of uncontrolled gestational diabetes.

NP: Analysis; CN: Health promotion and maintenance; CNS: Prevention and early detection of disease; CL: Knowledge

68. When measuring fundal height in a primiparous client during her 24-week checkup, which measurement should the nurse expect?

1. 30 cm
2. 20 cm
3. 24 cm
4. 16 cm

68. 3. Fundal height measurement correlates directly to the number of weeks of gestation. At 24 weeks' gestation, the desired measurement from the symphysis pubis to the fundus is 24 cm. The other measurements correlate to the corresponding weeks of gestation.

NP: Assessment; CN: Health promotion and maintenance; CNS: Growth and development through the life span; CL: Knowledge

69. During her first prenatal visit, a client at 20 weeks' gestation has a fundal measurement of 24 cm. Which is the most likely reason for this abnormal finding?

1. Gestational diabetes
2. Multiple gestation
3. Inaccurate date of last menstrual period
4. A large fetus

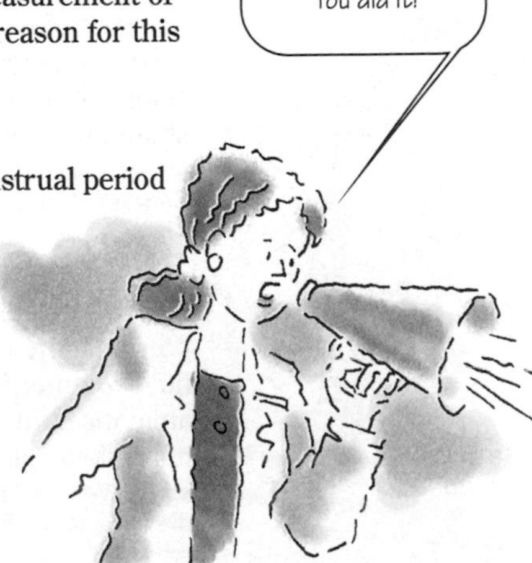

69. 3. Generally, a fundal height that's inconsistent with weeks of gestation results from inaccurate menses dates. Gestational diabetes generally leads to a larger fundal height later than week 20. Although multiple gestation generally causes increased fundal height after 16 weeks' gestation, this is a less likely explanation for the abnormal fundal height. A fetus that's large for gestational age is usually diagnosed during the third trimester.

NP: Analysis; CN: Health promotion and maintenance; CNS: Prevention and early detection of disease; CL: Analysis

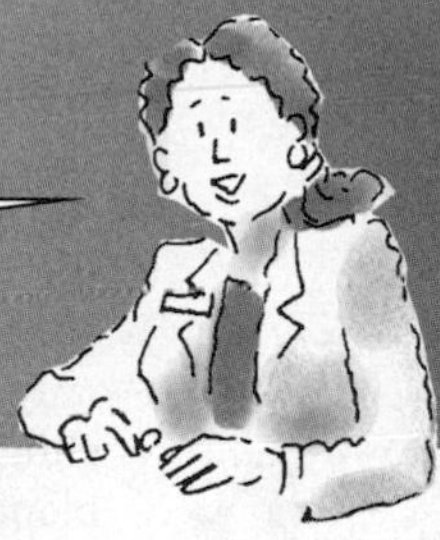

The prepartum and postpartum periods are important to know about. However, the intrapartum period — that's where the action is! This chapter covers the intrapartum period, perhaps the most critical of the three.

Chapter 23
Intrapartum care

1. A woman with a term, uncomplicated pregnancy comes into the labor-and-delivery unit in early labor saying that she thinks her water has broken. Which of the following actions by the nurse would be most appropriate?

1. Prepare the woman for delivery.
2. Note the color, amount, and odor of the fluid.
3. Immediately contact the physician.
4. Collect a sample of the fluid for microbial analysis.

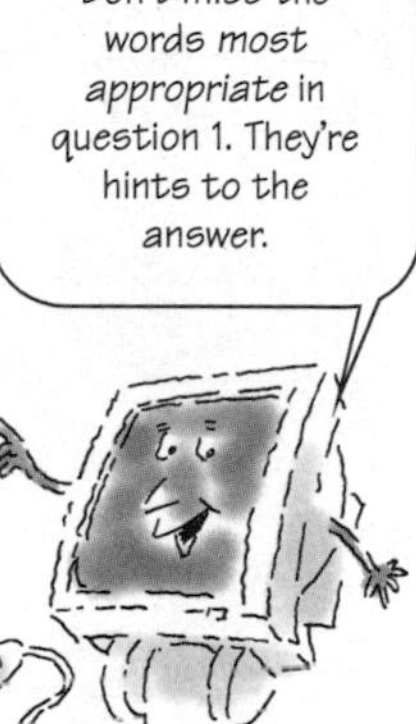

Don't miss the words *most appropriate* in question 1. They're hints to the answer.

1. 2. Noting the color, amount, and odor of the fluid, as well as the time of the rupture, will help guide the nurse in her next action. There's no need to call the client's physician immediately or prepare the client for delivery if the fluid is clear and delivery isn't imminent. Rupture of membranes isn't unusual in the early stages of labor. Fluid collection for microbial analysis isn't routine if there's no concern for infection (maternal fever).

NP: Assessment; CN: Physiological integrity; CNS: Reduction of risk potential; CL: Application

2. A woman who's 36 weeks pregnant comes into the labor-and-delivery unit with mild contractions. Which of the following complications should the nurse watch for when the client informs her that she has placenta previa?

1. Sudden rupture of membranes
2. Vaginal bleeding
3. Emesis
4. Fever

2. 2. Contractions may disrupt the microvascular network in the placenta of a client with placenta previa and result in bleeding. If the separation of the placenta occurs at the margin of the placenta, the blood will escape vaginally. Sudden rupture of the membranes isn't related to placenta previa. Fever would indicate an infectious process, and emesis isn't related to placenta previa.

NP: Assessment; CN: Physiological integrity; CNS: Reduction of risk potential; CL: Application

3. A client's labor doesn't progress. After ruling out cephalopelvic disproportion, the physician orders I.V. administration of 1,000 ml normal saline solution with oxytocin (Pitocin) 10 U to run at 2 milliunits/minute. Two milliunits/minute is equivalent to how many ml/minute?

1. 0.002
2. 0.02
3. 0.2
4. 2.0

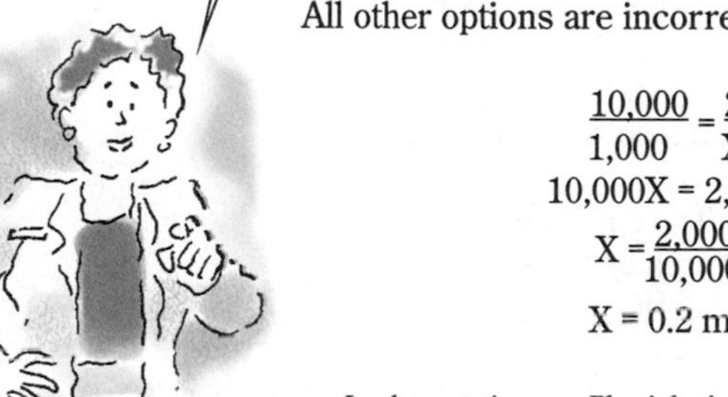

That's three down, 67 to go. Keep at it!

3. 3. The answer is found by setting up a ratio and following through with the calculations, shown below. Each unit of oxytocin contains 1,000 milliunits. Therefore, 1,000 ml of I.V. fluid contains 10,000 milliunits (10 units) of Pitocin. All other options are incorrect.

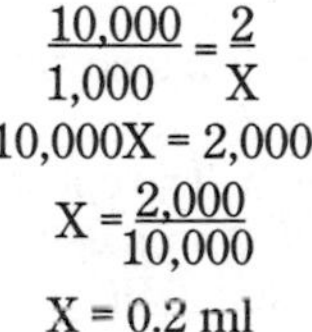

$$\frac{10{,}000}{1{,}000} = \frac{2}{X}$$

$$10{,}000X = 2{,}000$$

$$X = \frac{2{,}000}{10{,}000}$$

$$X = 0.2 \text{ ml}$$

NP: Implementation; CN: Physiological integrity; CNS: Pharmacological and parenteral therapies; CL: Analysis

4. A client in labor has been receiving oxytocin (Pitocin) to aid her progress. The nurse caring for her notes that a contraction has remained strong for 60 seconds. Which of the following actions should the nurse take first?

1. Stop the oxytocin infusion.
2. Notify the physician.
3. Monitor fetal heart tones as usual.
4. Turn the client on her left side.

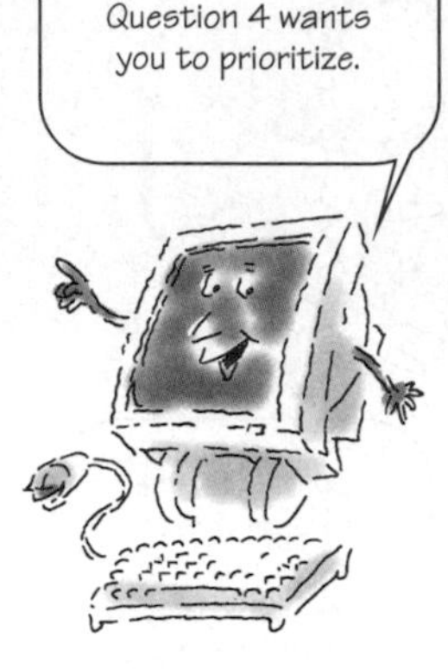
Question 4 wants you to prioritize.

4. 1. Oxytocin stimulates contractions and should be stopped. A contraction that remains strong for 60 seconds with no sign of easing off signals approaching tetany and could lead to uterine rupture. The nurse should monitor the fetal heart tones and notify the physician but only after stopping the oxytocin. The client should be turned on her left side to increase blood flow to the fetus, which can be decreased with tetany. This decreased blood flow can potentially compromise the fetus.

NP: Implementation; CN: Physiological integrity; CNS: Reduction of risk potential; CL: Knowledge

5. A client at term arrives in the labor unit experiencing contractions every 4 minutes. After a brief assessment, she's admitted and an electric fetal monitor is applied. Which of the following observations would alert the nurse to an increased potential for fetal distress?

1. Total weight gain of 30 lb (13.6 kg)
2. Maternal age of 32 years
3. Blood pressure of 146/90 mm Hg
4. Treatment for syphilis at 15 weeks' gestation

5. 3. A blood pressure of 146/90 mm Hg may indicate pregnancy-induced hypertension (PIH). Over time, PIH reduces blood flow to the placenta and can cause intrauterine growth retardation and other problems that make the fetus less able to tolerate the stress of labor. A weight gain of 30 lb is within expected parameters for a healthy pregnancy. A woman over age 30 doesn't have a greater risk of complications if her general condition is healthy before pregnancy. Syphilis that has been treated doesn't pose an additional risk.

NP: Assessment; CN: Physiological integrity; CNS: Reduction of risk potential; CL: Application

6. Which of the following observations indicates fetal distress?

1. Fetal scalp pH of 7.14
2. Fetal heart rate of 144 beats/minute
3. Acceleration of fetal heart rate with contractions
4. Presence of long-term variability

6. 1. A scalp pH below 7.25 indicates acidosis and fetal hypoxia. A fetal heart rate of 144 beats/minute, acceleration of the fetal heart rate with contractions, and long-term variability are normal responses of a healthy fetus to labor.

NP: Assessment; CN: Safe, effective care environment; CNS: Management of care; CL: Comprehension

7. During labor a client's amniotic membranes rupture. Meconium is present in the amniotic fluid. Meconium in amniotic fluid is a normal finding in which of the following situations?

1. Preterm labor
2. Cephalopelvic disproportion
3. Prolonged latent phase
4. Breech presentation

7. 4. Meconium in a breech presentation may be caused by compression of the fetus's intestinal tract during descent. Meconium in the amniotic fluid in preterm labor, cephalopelvic disproportion, or a prolonged latent phase would indicate fetal distress caused by a brief period of hypoxia.

NP: Assessment; CN: Physiological integrity; CNS: Reduction of risk potential; CL: Comprehension

8. A client at 42 weeks' gestation is 3 cm dilated, 30% effaced, with membranes intact and the fetus at +2 station. Fetal heart rate (FHR) is 140 to 150 beats/minute. After 2 hours, the nurse notes on the external fetal monitor that, for the past 10 minutes, the FHR ranged from 160 to 190 beats/minute. The client states that her baby has been extremely active. Uterine contractions are strong, occurring every 3 to 4 minutes and lasting 40 to 60 seconds. Which of the following findings would indicate fetal hypoxia?

1. Abnormally long uterine contractions
2. Abnormally strong uterine intensity
3. Excessively frequent contractions, with rapid fetal movement
4. Excessive fetal activity and fetal tachycardia

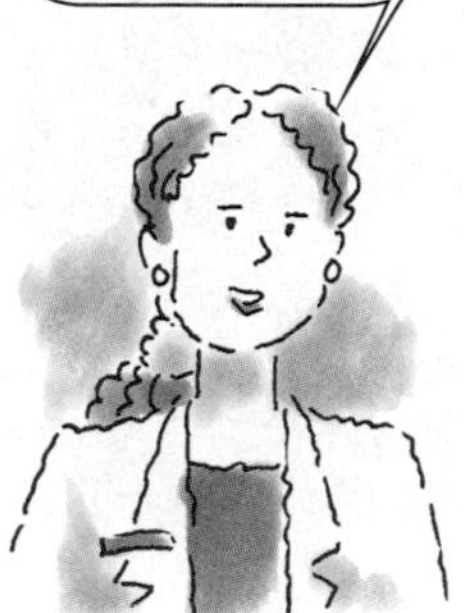

Remember that every piece of information provided may not be necessary to answer the question.

8. 4. Fetal tachycardia and excessive fetal activity are the first signs of fetal hypoxia. The duration of uterine contractions is within normal limits. Uterine intensity can be mild to strong and still be within normal limits. The frequency of contractions is within the normal limits for the active phase of labor.

NP: Evaluation; CN: Physiological integrity; CNS: Reduction of risk potential; CL: Analysis

9. A client at 33 weeks' gestation and leaking amniotic fluid is placed on an external fetal monitor. The monitor indicates uterine irritability, and contractions are occurring every 4 to 6 minutes. The physician orders terbutaline (Brethine). Which of the following teaching statements is appropriate for this client?

1. "This medicine will make you breathe better."
2. "You may feel a fluttering or tight sensation in your chest."
3. "This will dry your mouth and make you feel thirsty."
4. "You'll need to replace the potassium lost by this drug."

9. 2. A fluttering or tight sensation in the chest is a common adverse reaction to terbutaline. Terbutaline relieves bronchospasm, but the client is receiving it to reduce uterine motility. Mouth dryness and thirst occur with the inhaled form of terbutaline but are unlikely with the subcutaneous form. Hypokalemia is a potential adverse reaction following large doses of terbutaline but not at doses of 0.25 mg.

NP: Implementation; CN: Health promotion and maintenance; CNS: Prevention and early detection of disease; CL: Application

10. A 17-year-old primigravida with severe pregnancy-induced hypertension (PIH) has been receiving magnesium sulfate I.V. for 3 hours. The latest assessment reveals deep tendon reflexes (DTR) of +1, blood pressure of 150/100 mm Hg, a pulse of 92 beats/minute, a respiratory rate of 10 breaths/minute, and urine output of 20 ml/hour. Which of the following actions would be most appropriate?

1. Continue monitoring per standards of care.
2. Stop the magnesium sulfate infusion.
3. Increase the infusion rate by 5 gtt/minute.
4. Decrease the infusion rate by 5 gtt/minute.

10. 2. Magnesium sulfate should be withheld if the client's respiratory rate or urine output falls or if reflexes are diminished or absent, all of which are true for this client. The client also shows other signs of impending toxicity, such as flushing and feeling warm. Inaction won't resolve the client's suppressed DTRs and low respiratory rate and urine output. The client is already showing central nervous system depression because of excessive magnesium sulfate, so increasing the infusion rate is inappropriate. Impending toxicity indicates that the infusion should be stopped rather than just slowed down.

NP: Implementation; CN: Physiological integrity; CNS: Pharmacological and parenteral therapies; CL: Application

11. During a vaginal examination of a client in labor, the nurse palpates the fetus's larger, diamond-shaped fontanelle toward the anterior portion of the client's pelvis. Which of the following statements best describes this situation?

1. The client can expect a brief and intense labor, with potential for lacerations.
2. The client is at risk for uterine rupture and needs constant monitoring.
3. The client may need interventions to ease back pain and change the fetal position.
4. The fetus will be delivered using forceps or a vacuum extractor.

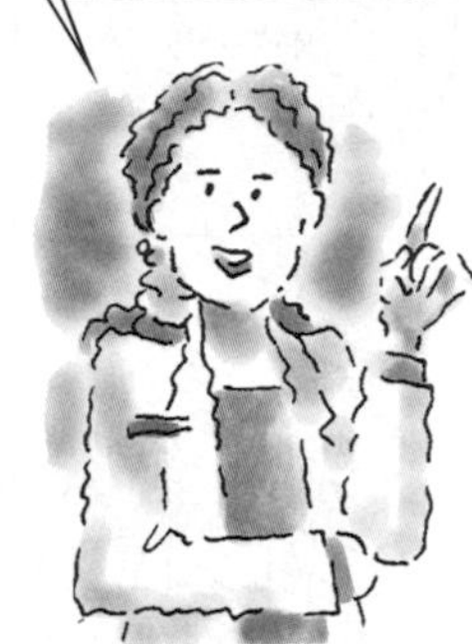

Be careful of the words will be in option 4. They indicate an absolute, a near rarity in health care.

11. 3. The fetal position is occiput posterior, a position that commonly produces intense back pain during labor. Most of the time, the fetus rotates during labor to occiput anterior position. Positioning the client on her side can facilitate this rotation. An occiput posterior position would most likely result in prolonged labor. Occiput posterior alone doesn't create a risk of uterine rupture. The fetus would be delivered with forceps or vacuum extractor only if its presenting part doesn't rotate and descend spontaneously.

NP: Planning; CN: Safe, effective care environment; CNS: Management of care; CL: Analysis

12. The cervix of a 26-year-old primigravida in labor is 5 cm dilated and 75% effaced, and the fetus is at 0 station. The physician prescribes an epidural regional block. Into which of the following positions should the nurse place the client when the epidural is administered?

1. Lithotomy
2. Supine
3. Prone
4. Lateral

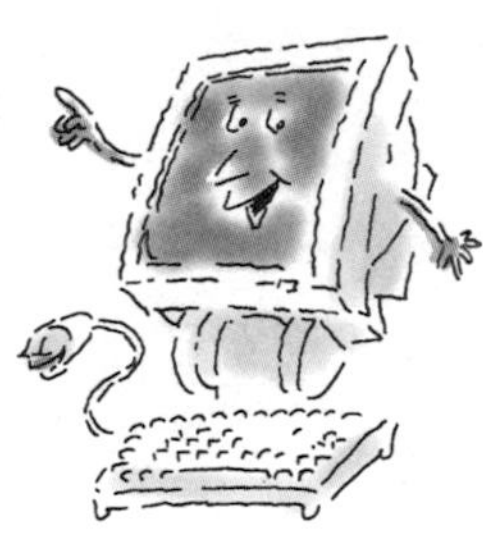

I can tell you love to face a challenge! (Tee-hee!)

12. 4. The client should be placed on her left side or sitting upright, with her shoulders parallel and legs slightly flexed. Her back shouldn't be flexed because this position increases the possibility that the dura may be punctured and the anesthetic will accidentally be given as spinal, not epidural, anesthesia. None of the other positions allows proper access to the epidural space.

NP: Implementation; CN: Safe, effective care management; CNS: Safety and infection control; CL: Application

13. Which of the following terms is used to describe the thinning and shortening of the cervix that occurs just before and during labor?

1. Ballottement
2. Dilation
3. Effacement
4. Multiparous

13. 3. Effacement is cervical shortening and thinning while dilation is widening of the cervix; both facilitate opening the cervix in preparation for delivery. Ballottement is the ability of another individual to move the fetus by externally manipulating the maternal abdomen. A ballotable fetus hasn't yet engaged in the maternal pelvis. Multiparous refers to a woman who has had previous live births.

NP: Assessment; CN: Physiological integrity; CNS: Physiological adaptation; CL: Comprehension

14. Which of the following fetal positions is most favorable for birth?

1. Vertex presentation
2. Transverse lie
3. Frank breech presentation
4. Posterior position of the fetal head

14. 1. Vertex presentation (flexion of the fetal head) is the optimal presentation for passage through the birth canal. Transverse lie is an unacceptable fetal position for vaginal birth and requires a cesarean birth delivery. Frank breech presentation, in which the buttocks present first, can be a difficult vaginal delivery. Posterior positioning of the fetal head can make it difficult for the fetal head to pass under the maternal symphysis pubis bone.

NP: Analysis; CN: Physiological integrity; CNS: Reduction of risk potential; CL: Analysis

15. Which of the following stages of labor is the one in which birth occurs?
1. First stage of labor
2. Second stage of labor
3. Third stage of labor
4. Fourth stage of labor

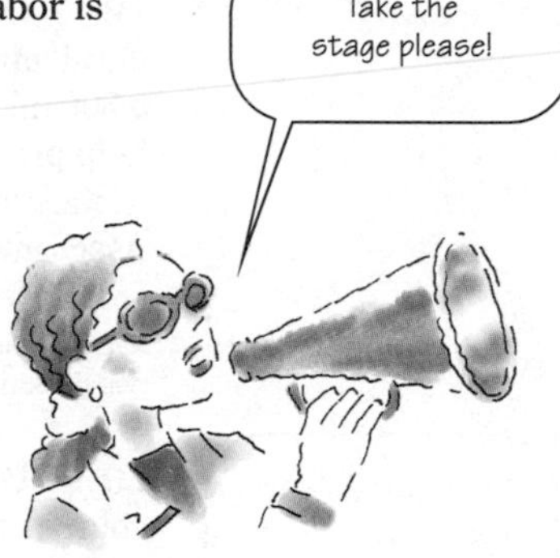
Take the stage please!

15. 2. The second stage of labor begins with complete dilation (10 cm) and ends with the expulsion of the fetus. The first stage of labor is the stage of dilation, which is divided into three distinct phases: latent, active, and transition. The third stage of labor begins with the birth of the infant and ends with the expulsion of the placenta. The fourth stage of labor is the first 4 hours after placental expulsion, in which the client's body begins the recovery process.

NP: Planning; CN: Physiological integrity; CNS: Basic care and comfort; CL: Knowledge

16. Which of the following laboratory results would be critical for a client admitted to the labor-and-delivery unit?
1. Blood type
2. Calcium
3. Iron
4. Oxygen saturation

16. 1. Blood type would be a critical value to have because the risk of blood loss is always a potential complication during the labor-and-delivery process. Approximately 40% of a woman's cardiac output is delivered to the uterus, therefore, blood loss can occur quite rapidly in the event of uncontrolled bleeding. Calcium and iron aren't critical values and oxygen saturation isn't a laboratory value.

NP: Planning; CN: Physiological integrity; CNS: Reduction of risk potential; CL: Analysis

17. Which of the following fetal heart rates would be expected in the fetus of a laboring woman who is full-term?
1. 80 to 100 beats/minute
2. 100 to 120 beats/minute
3. 120 to 160 beats/minute
4. 160 to 180 beats/minute

17. 3. A rate of 120 to 160 beats/minute in the fetal heart is appropriate for filling the heart with blood and pumping it out to the system. Faster or slower rates don't accomplish perfusion adequately and could indicate fetal compromise.

NP: Assessment; CN: Health promotion and maintenance; CNS: Growth and development through the life span; CL: Knowledge

18. A laboring client has external electronic fetal monitoring in place. Which of the following assessment data can be determined by examining the fetal heart rate strip produced by the external electronic fetal monitor?
1. Gender of the fetus
2. Fetal position
3. Labor progress
4. Oxygenation

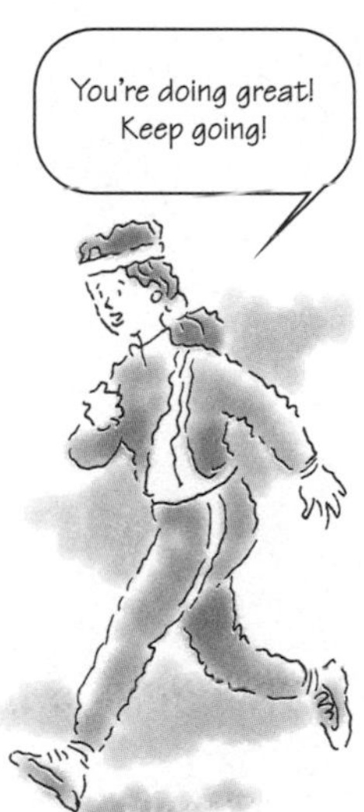
You're doing great! Keep going!

18. 4. Oxygenation of the fetus may be indirectly assessed through fetal monitoring by closely examining the fetal heart rate strip. Accelerations in the fetal heart rate strip indicate good oxygenation, while decelerations in the fetal heart rate sometimes indicate poor fetal oxygenation. The fetal heart rate strip can't determine the gender of the fetus or assess fetal position. Labor progress can be directly assessed only through cervical examination.

NP: Analysis; CN: Physiological integrity; CNS: Reduction of risk potential; CL: Comprehension

19. Which of the following nursing actions is required before a client in labor receives an epidural?

1. Give a fluid bolus of 500 ml.
2. Check for maternal pupil dilation.
3. Assess maternal reflexes.
4. Assess maternal gait.

19. 1. One of the major adverse effects of epidural administration is hypotension. Therefore, a 500-ml fluid bolus is usually administered to help prevent hypotension in the client who wishes to receive an epidural for pain relief. Assessments of maternal reflexes, pupil response, and gait aren't necessary.

NP: Analysis; CN: Physiological integrity; CNS: Reduction of risk potential; CL: Analysis

20. Which of the following complications is possible with an episiotomy?

1. Blood loss
2. Uterine disfigurement
3. Prolonged dyspareunia
4. Hormonal fluctuation postpartum

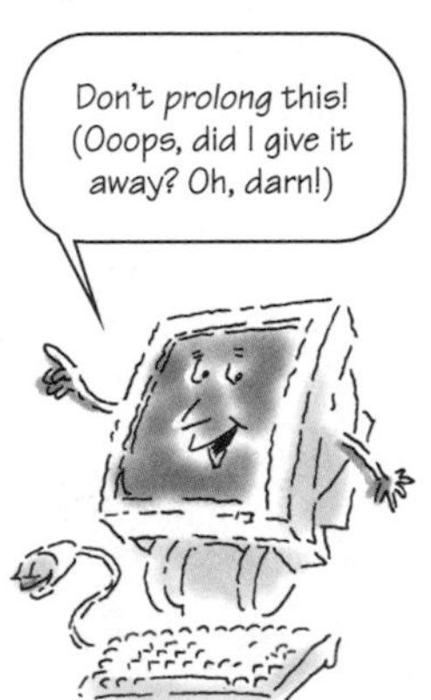

Don't prolong this! (Ooops, did I give it away? Oh, darn!)

20. 3. Prolonged dyspareunia (painful intercourse) may result when complications such as infection interfere with wound healing. Minimal blood loss occurs when an episiotomy is performed. The uterus isn't affected by episiotomy because it's the perineum that is cut to accommodate the fetus. Hormonal fluctuations that occur during the postpartum period aren't the result of an episiotomy.

NP: Planning; CN: Physiological integrity; CNS: Basic care and comfort; CL: Analysis

21. A client in early labor states that she has a thick, yellow discharge from both of her breasts. Which of the following actions by the nurse would be most appropriate?

1. Tell her that her milk is starting to come in because she's in labor.
2. Complete a thorough breast examination, and document the results in the chart.
3. Perform a culture on the discharge, and inform the client that she might have mastitis.
4. Inform the client that the discharge is colostrum, normally present after the 4th month of pregnancy.

21. 4. After the 4th month, colostrum may be expressed. The breasts normally produce colostrum for the first few days after delivery. Milk production begins 1 to 3 days postpartum. A clinical breast examination isn't usually indicated in the intrapartum setting. Although a culture may be indicated, it requires advanced assessment as well as a medical order.

NP: Implementation; CN: Health promotion and maintenance; CNS: Growth and development through the life span; CL: Knowledge

22. While performing an admission nursing assessment of a client in early labor, the nurse observes a brown, raised lesion resembling a mole, 2″ (5 cm) below the left breast. Which of the following observations by the nurse would be most appropriate?

1. That looks like a mole and is clinically insignificant.
2. That looks like seborrhea keratosis and is a precancerous lesion.
3. That's a supernumerary nipple, a common finding.
4. That's a skin tag and is clinically insignificant.

22. 3. Supernumerary nipples are common in men and women and are usually located 2″ to 2½″ (5 to 6 cm) below the breast near the midline. A supernumerary nipple resembles a mole, although closer inspection will reveal a small nipple and areola and is clinically insignificant. A mole (nevus) may be macular or papular, tan to brown in color, and usually has smooth borders. Keratosis lesions are raised, thickened areas of pigmentation that look scaly and warty. They don't become cancerous. Skin tags (acrochordons) are overgrowths of normal skin that form a stalk and are polyplike.

NP: Assessment; CN: Health promotion and maintenance; CNS: Growth and development through the life span; CL: Analysis

23. A client in early labor is concerned about the pinkish "stretch marks" on her abdomen. Which of the following observations by the nurse shows an accurate understanding of the marks on the client's abdomen?

1. Striae are common in pregnancy and will fade away completely after the uterus contracts to its prepregnant state.
2. Striae are common in pregnancy, will fade after delivery, but don't disappear.
3. Striae are common in pregnancy and will fade away after application of an emollient cream.
4. This is a sign of a separation of the rectus muscle and will require further assessment by the physician.

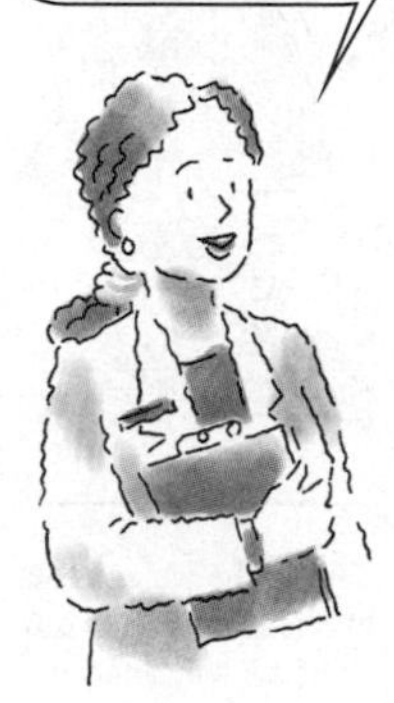
Stretch marks
are yet another
reminder of the
joy of giving birth!

23. 2. Striae are wavy, depressed streaks that may occur over the abdomen, breasts, or thighs as pregnancy progresses. They fade with time to a silvery color but won't disappear. Creams may soften the skin but won't remove the striae. Separation of the rectus muscle, diastasis, is a condition of pregnancy whereby the abdominal wall has difficulty stretching enough to accommodate the growing fetus, causing the muscle to separate.

NP: Implementation; CN: Health promotion and maintenance; CNS: Growth and development through the life span; CL: Knowledge

24. Which of the following positions increases cardiac output and stroke volume of a client in labor?

1. Supine
2. Sitting
3. Side-lying
4. Semi-Fowler's

24. 3. In the side-lying position, cardiac output increases, stroke volume increases, and the pulse rate decreases. In the supine position, the blood pressure can drop severely, due to the pressure of the fetus and enlarged uterus on the vena cava, resulting in supine hypotensive or vena caval syndrome. Neither the sitting nor semi-Fowler's position increase cardiac output or stroke volume.

NP: Assessment; CN: Health promotion and maintenance; CNS: Prevention and early detection of disease; CL: Application

25. Which of the following ranges is considered severe bradycardia for a full-term fetus?

1. Fewer than 70 beats/minute.
2. 70 to 100 beats/minute.
3. 120 to 160 beats/minute.
4. 160 to 200 beats/minute.

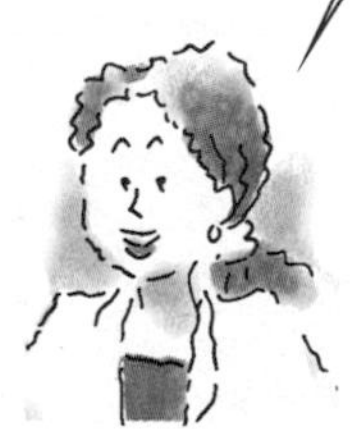
Think of the range
of possibilities in
question 25.

25. 1. A fetal heart rate (FHR) below 70 beats/minute is considered severe bradycardia and is associated with rapidly occurring fetal acidosis. Normal FHR for a full-term fetus is 120 to 160 beats/minute. FHR from 70 to 100 beats/minute is considered moderate fetal bradycardia. Fetal tachycardia, an FHR above 160 beats/minute can result from early fetal hypoxia, maternal fever, parasympathetic drugs, beta sympathomimetic drugs, amnionitis, maternal hyperthyroidism, or fetal anemia.

NP: Assessment; CN: Health promotion and maintenance; CNS: Growth and development through the life span; CL: Knowledge

26. Which of the following Leopold's maneuvers assesses the descent of the presenting part into the pelvis?

1. First
2. Second
3. Third
4. Fourth

26. 4. The fourth maneuver assesses the descent of the presenting part into the pelvis. The first maneuver determines the shape, size, consistency, and mobility of the form that is found. The second maneuver determines the location of the fetal back and fetal extremities. The third maneuver reveals what part is presenting above the pelvic inlet.

NP: Assessment; CN: Health promotion and maintenance; CNS: Growth and development through the life span; CL: Knowledge

27. A client who's 35 weeks pregnant arrives at a labor-and-delivery unit leaking clear fluid from her vagina. Which of the following interventions would be most appropriate?

1. Perform a vaginal examination.
2. Obtain a catheterized urine specimen.
3. Encourage the client to ambulate.
4. Obtain a sterile speculum sample of the fluid.

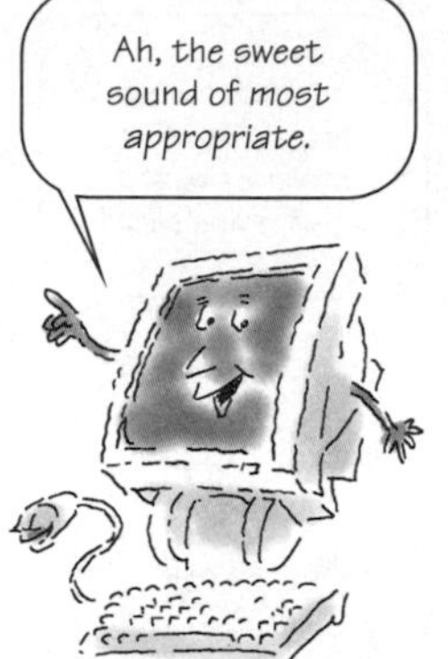

Ah, the sweet sound of most appropriate.

27. 4. A sterile speculum examination is performed to identify ruptured membranes. Confirmation is done with nitrazine paper and a positive ferning test. With premature rupture of membranes in a client under 37 weeks' gestation, vaginal examinations are contraindicated to reduce the incidence of infection. Clean catch urine specimens would be appropriate to rule out infection but not a catheterized specimen. The client should ambulate only after a thorough nursing assessment and examination to determine the safety of walking for the client and fetus.

NP: Implementation; CN: Physiological integrity; CNS: Reduction of risk potential; CL: Application

28. Which of the following descriptions best fits Braxton Hicks contractions?

1. Contractions beginning irregularly, becoming regular and predictable
2. Contractions causing cervical effacement and dilation
3. Contractions felt initially in the lower back and radiating to the abdomen in a wavelike motion
4. Contractions that begin and remain irregular

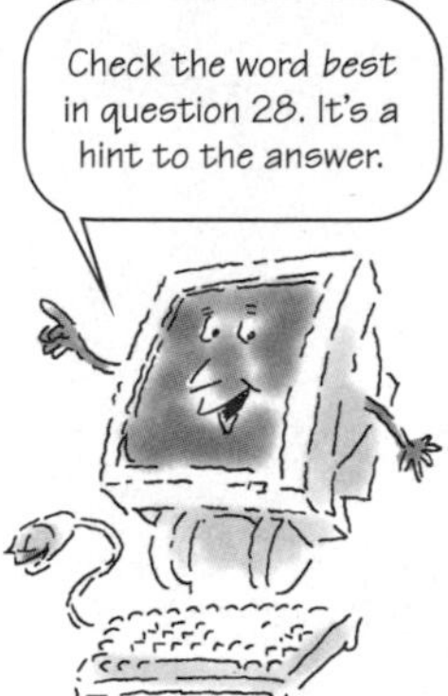

Check the word best in question 28. It's a hint to the answer.

28. 4. Braxton Hicks contractions begin and remain irregular. They're felt in the abdomen and remain confined to the abdomen and groin. They commonly disappear with ambulation and don't dilate the cervix. True contractions begin irregularly but become regular and predictable, causing cervical effacement and dilation. True contractions are felt initially in the lower back and radiate to the abdomen in a wavelike motion.

NP: Assessment; CN: Physiological integrity; CNS: Physiological adaptation; CL: Knowledge

29. Which of the following descriptions best fits the term effacement?

1. Enlargement of the cervical canal
2. Expulsion of the mucus plug
3. Shortening and thinning of the cervical canal
4. Downward movement of the fetal head

29. 3. With effacement, the cervical canal shortens and thins due to longitudinal traction from the contracting uterine fundus. Dilation is the enlargement of the cervical os from 1 to 10 cm. Expulsion of the cervical mucus plug followed by a seepage of cervical capillary blood is called "show." Descent is a mechanism of labor whereby the presenting part of the fetus descends into the pelvic inlet.

NP: Assessment; CN: Health promotion and maintenance; CNS: Growth and development through the life span; CL: Knowledge

30. A laboring client is in the first stage of labor and has progressed from 4 to 7 cm in cervical dilation. In which of the following phases of the first stage does cervical dilation occur most rapidly?

1. Preparatory phase
2. Latent phase
3. Active phase
4. Transition phase

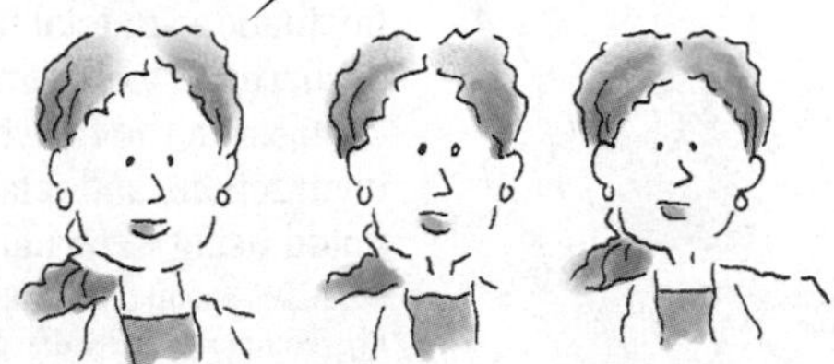

Which phase is the correct answer here?

30. 3. Cervical dilation occurs more rapidly during the active phase than any of the previous phases. The active phase is characterized by cervical dilation that progresses from 4 to 7 cm. The preparatory, or latent, phase begins with the onset of regular uterine contractions and ends when rapid cervical dilation begins. Transition is defined as cervical dilation beginning at 8 cm and lasting until 10 cm or complete dilation.

NP: Assessment; CN: Health promotion and maintenance; CNS: Growth and development through the life span; CL: Comprehension

31. During which of the following stages of labor does crowning take place?

1. First
2. Second
3. Third
4. Fourth

31. 2. The second stage of labor begins at full cervical dilation (10 cm) and ends when the infant is born. Crowning is present during this stage as the fetal head, pushed against the perineum, causes the vaginal introitus to open, allowing the fetal scalp to be visible. The first stage begins with true labor contractions and ends with complete cervical dilation. The third stage is from the time the infant is born until the delivery of the placenta. The fourth stage is the first 1 to 4 hours following delivery of the placenta.

NP: Assessment; CN: Health promotion and maintenance; CNS: Growth and development through the life span; CL: Comprehension

32. The nurse suspects that the laboring client may have been physically abused by her male partner. Which of the following interventions by the nurse would be most appropriate?

1. Confront the male partner.
2. Question the woman in front of her partner.
3. Contact hospital security.
4. Collaborate with the physician to make a referral to social services.

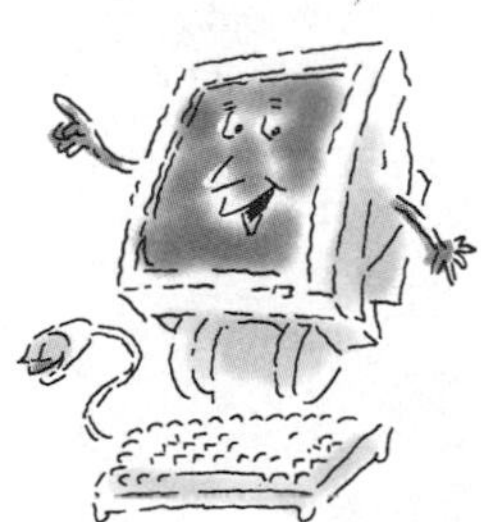

Did you notice the words most appropriate in question 32? Another hint!

32. 4. Collaborating with the physician to make a referral to social services will aid the client by creating a plan and providing support. Additionally, by law, the nurse or nursing supervisor must report the suspected abuse to the police and follow up with a written report. Although confrontation can be used therapeutically, this action will most likely provoke anger in the suspected abuser. Questioning the woman in front of her partner doesn't allow her the privacy required to address this issue and may place her in greater danger. If the woman isn't in imminent danger, there's no need to call hospital security.

NP: Implementation; CN: Physiological integrity; CNS: Reduction of risk potential; CL: Analysis

33. Which of the following assessments requires internal fetal monitoring?

1. Fetal heart rate (FHR)
2. Long-term variability (LTV)
3. Short-term variability (STV)
4. Periodic changes in the heart rate

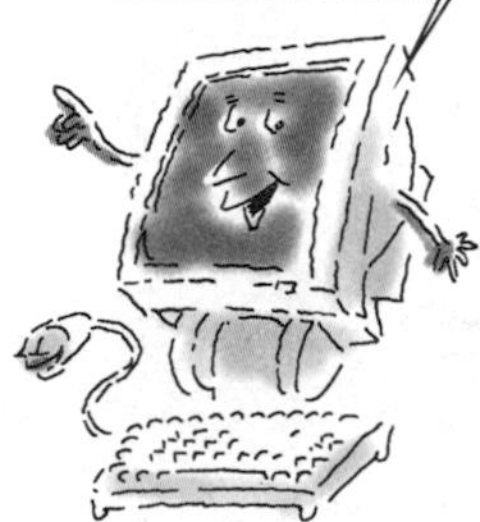

Be careful. One or more options might be applicable here, but only one will be required.

33. 3. STV can be assessed only by using internal fetal monitoring and a pressure-sensing catheter that's placed inside the uterine cavity. FHR may be determined using external or internal fetal monitoring. LTV is observed with external and internal fetal monitoring and shows the fluctuations in fetal heart rate of 6 to 10 beats occurring 3 to 10 times per minute. Periodic changes in the heart rate occur in response to contractions and fetal movement and may be noted using external or internal fetal monitoring.

NP: Assessment; CN: Health promotion and maintenance; CNS: Prevention and early detection of disease; CL: Knowledge

34. The nurse has just admitted a client in the labor-and-delivery unit who has been diagnosed by her physician as having diabetes mellitus. Which of the following measures would be most appropriate for this situation?

1. Ask the client about her most recent blood glucose levels.
2. Prepare oral hypoglycemic medications for administration during labor.
3. Notify the neonatal intensive care unit that you'll be admitting a client with diabetes.
4. Prepare the client for cesarean delivery.

34. 1. As part of the history, asking about the client's most recent blood glucose levels will indicate how well her diabetes has been controlled. Oral hypoglycemic drugs are never used during pregnancy because they cross the placental barrier, stimulate fetal insulin production, and are potentially teratogenic. Plans to admit the infant to the neonatal intensive care unit are premature. Cesarean delivery is no longer the preferred delivery for clients with diabetes. Vaginal birth is preferred and presents a lower risk to the mother and fetus.

NP: Assessment; CN: Physiological integrity; CNS: Reduction of risk potential; CL: Application

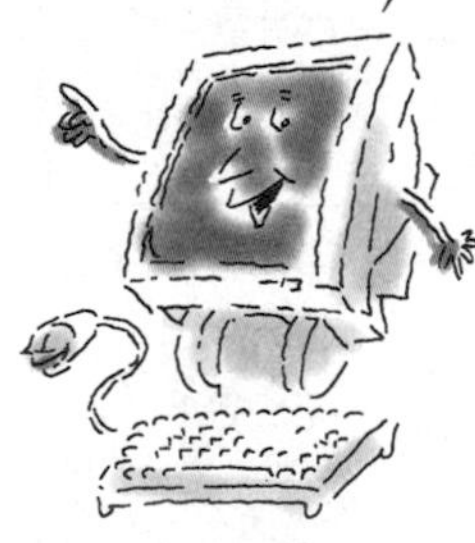

Watch out for question 35; it's a negative stem.

35. A client is admitted to the labor-and-delivery unit with a known anencephalic fetus. Which of the following measures would not be appropriate for the nurse to perform?

1. Assess fetal heart tones.
2. Notify the physician of her admission.
3. Monitor uterine contractions.
4. Provide privacy.

35. 1. Fetal heart tones are rarely assessed in a client with an anencephalic fetus; most fetuses won't survive due to lack of cerebral function. Notifying the physician and monitoring uterine contractions are both appropriate because many of these clients experience difficult labor. Providing privacy is an appropriate therapeutic intervention because the client and family will grieve their loss.

NP: Implementation; CN: Physiological integrity; CNS: Reduction of risk potential; CL: Comprehension

36. A 30-year-old multiparous client admitted to the labor-and-delivery unit hasn't received prenatal care for this pregnancy. Which of the following data is most relevant to the nursing assessment?

1. Date of last menstrual period (LMP)
2. Family history of sexually transmitted diseases (STDs)
3. Name of insurance provider
4. Number of siblings

36. 1. The date of the LMP is essential to estimate the date of delivery. The nursing history would also include subjective information, such as personal (but not necessarily family) history of STDs, gravidity, and parity. Although beneficial to the hospital for financial reimbursement, the insurance provider has no bearing on the nursing history. Likewise, the number of siblings isn't pertinent to the assessment.

NP: Assessment; CN: Health promotion and maintenance; CNS: Prevention and early detection of disease; CL: Analysis

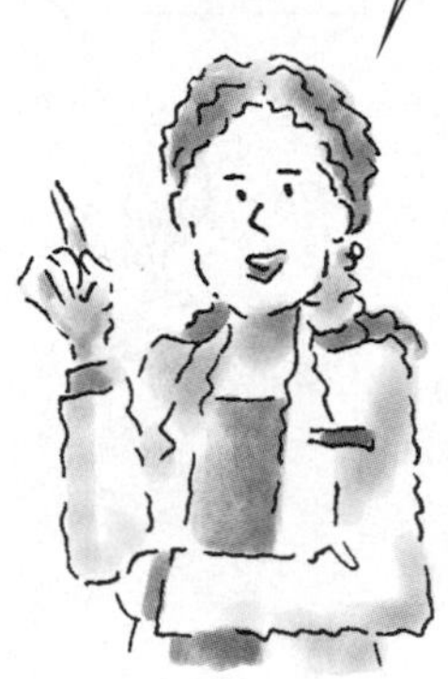
Careful! Another negative question here!

37. Which of the following symptoms isn't usually observed in laboring clients with pregnancy-induced hypertension (PIH)?

1. Elevated blood pressure
2. Polyuria
3. Facial and hand edema
4. Epigastric discomfort

37. 2. Renal plasma flow and glomerular filtration are decreased in PIH, so increasing oliguria indicates a worsening condition. Blood pressure increases as a result of increased peripheral resistance. Facial and hand edema is due to protein loss, sodium retention, and a lowered glomerular filtration rate, moving fluid from intravascular to extravascular spaces. Epigastric discomfort may be due to abdominal edema or pancreatic or hepatic ischemia.
NP: Assessment; CN: Health promotion and maintenance; CNS: Prevention and early detection of disease; CL: Application

38. While performing a vaginal examination, the nurse feels pulsating tissue against her fingertips. What would be the most appropriate nursing intervention?

1. Leave the client, and call the physician.
2. Put the client in a semi-Fowler's position.
3. Ask the client to push with the next contraction.
4. Leave the fingers in place, and press the nurse call light.

38. 4. When the umbilical cord precedes the fetal presenting part, it's known as a prolapsed cord. Leaving the fingers in place and calling for assistance is the safest intervention for the fetus, as you'll need to keep the fetus off the cord to reduce cord compression. The nursing staff will contact the physician, and the client will probably need a cesarean delivery because of the risk of fetal demise with the fetus pressing against the cord during delivery. Placing the client in the semi-Fowler's position would increase the pressure of the fetus on the umbilical cord. Asking the client to push with the next contraction would be contraindicated, as it would also force the presenting part against the cord, causing severe bradycardia and possible fetal demise.
NP: Evaluation; CN: Physiological integrity; CNS: Reduction of risk potential; CL: Application

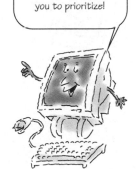

Item 39 is asking you to prioritize!

39. A client is admitted to the labor-and-delivery unit in labor, with blood flowing down her legs. Which of the following nursing interventions would be most appropriate?

1. Place an indwelling catheter.
2. Assess fetal heart tones.
3. Perform a vaginal examination.
4. Prepare the client for cesarean delivery.

39. 2. Assessing fetal heart tones would be the first step because it's necessary to establish fetal well-being due to a possible placenta previa or abruptio placentae. Although an indwelling catheter may be placed, it isn't an early intervention. Performing a vaginal examination would be contraindicated because any agitation of the cervix with a previa can result in hemorrhage and death for the mother or fetus. Preparing the client for a cesarean delivery may not be indicated. A sonogram will need to be performed to determine the cause of bleeding. If the diagnosis is a partial placenta previa, the client may still be able to deliver vaginally.
NP: Implementation; CN: Physiological integrity; CNS: Reduction of risk potential; CL: Comprehension

40. A client in labor is receiving magnesium sulfate to treat pregnancy-induced hypertension. How should this drug be administered?

1. As a loading dose of 4 g in normal saline solution, followed by a continuous infusion of 1 to 2 g/hour
2. As a loading dose of 2 g in normal saline solution, followed by a continuous infusion of 2 g/hour
3. As a loading dose of 4 g in dextrose 5% in water (D_5W), followed by a continuous infusion of 1 to 2 g/hour
4. As a loading dose of 4 grams in D_5W, followed by a continuous infusion of 4 g/hour

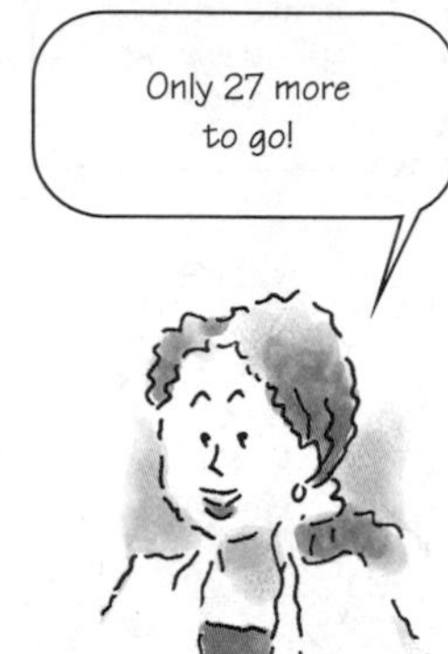

Only 27 more to go!

40. 3. A loading dose of magnesium sulfate should be given as a 4-g bolus, followed by a continuous infusion of 1 to 2 g/hour in D_5W for maintenance. Magnesium sulfate shouldn't be administered in normal saline solution.

NP: Implementation; CN: Physiological integrity; CNS: Pharmacological and parenteral therapies; CL: Application

41. A multiparous client who has been in labor for 2 hours states that she feels the urge to move her bowels. How should the nurse respond?

1. Let the client get up to use the toilet.
2. Allow the client to use a bedpan.
3. Perform a pelvic examination.
4. Check the fetal heart rate.

41. 3. A complaint of rectal pressure usually indicates a low presenting fetal part, signaling imminent delivery. The nurse should perform a pelvic examination to assess the dilation of the cervix and station of the presenting fetal part. Don't let the client use the toilet or a bedpan before she's examined because she could deliver on the toilet or in the bedpan. Checking the fetal heart rate is important but comes after the nurse evaluates the client's complaint.

NP: Implementation; CN: Health promotion and maintenance; CNS: Prevention and early detection of disease; CL: Application

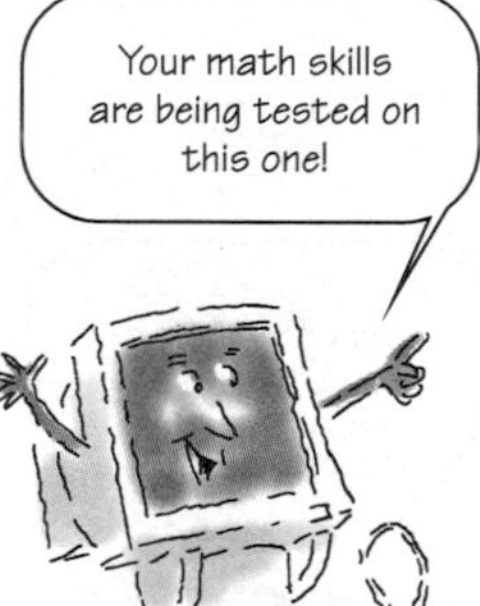

Your math skills are being tested on this one!

42. The physician has ordered an I.V. of 5% dextrose in lactated Ringer's solution at 125 ml/hr. The I.V. tubing delivers 10 drops per ml. How many drops per minute should fall into the drip chamber?

1. 10 to 11
2. 12 to 13
3. 20 to 21
4. 22 to 24

42. 3. Multiply the number of milliliters to be infused (125) by the drop factor (10); $125 \times 10 = 1{,}250$. Then divide the answer by the number of minutes to run the infusion (60); $1{,}250 \div 60 = 20.83$, or 20 to 21 gtt/minute.

NP: Evaluation; CN: Physiological integrity; CNS: Pharmacological and parenteral therapies; CL: Knowledge

43. Which type of contractions signal true labor?

1. Contractions that achieve cervical dilation
2. Contractions that are felt abdominally
3. Contractions that may be irregular
4. Contractions that may disappear with ambulation

43. 1. True labor is indicated by contractions that achieve cervical dilation. Contractions that are felt abdominally, occur irregularly, or disappear with ambulation usually indicate false labor.

NP: Assessment; CN: Health promotion and maintenance; CNS: Growth and development through the life span; CL: Comprehension

44. Which of the following drugs is preferred for treating pregnancy-induced hypertension (PIH)?

1. Terbutaline (Brethaire)
2. Oxytocin (Pitocin)
3. Magnesium sulfate
4. Calcium gluconate (Kalcinate)

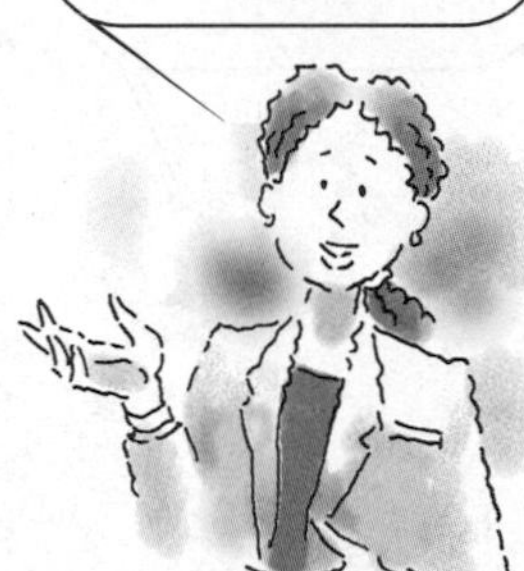

What's the preferred drug for treating PIH?

44. 3. Magnesium sulfate is the drug of choice to treat PIH because it reduces edema by causing a shift from the extracellular spaces into the intestines. It also depresses the central nervous system, which decreases the incidence of seizures. Terbutaline is a smooth-muscle relaxant that relaxes the uterus. Oxytocin is the synthetic form of the pituitary hormone used to stimulate uterine contractions. Calcium gluconate is the antagonist for magnesium toxicity.

NP: Planning; CN: Physiological integrity; CNS: Pharmacological and parenteral therapies; CL: Knowledge

45. Which of the following characteristics best describes variable decelerations?

1. Predictable
2. Indicators of fetal well-being
3. Indicative of cord compression
4. Periodic decreases in fetal heart rate resulting from pressure on the fetal head

45. 3. Variable decelerations are common in labor when the membranes are ruptured, which decrease to protect the cord, as the fetus descends the birth canal. Variable decelerations are unpredictable. Atypical variable decelerations suggest of fetal hypoxia. Decreases in fetal heart rate are due to decreased protection on the cord, not the fetal head. *Early* decelerations are related to pressure on the fetal head.

NP: Assessment; CN: Physiological integrity; CNS: Physiological adaptation; CL: Knowledge

46. Which of the following characteristics best describes early decelerations?

1. Reassuring, beginning at the onset of the contraction and ending with the end of the contraction
2. Decelerations initiated 30 to 40 seconds after the onset of the contraction
3. Decreased blood flow to the fetus due to uteroplacental insufficiency
4. Loss of variability with fetal hypoxia

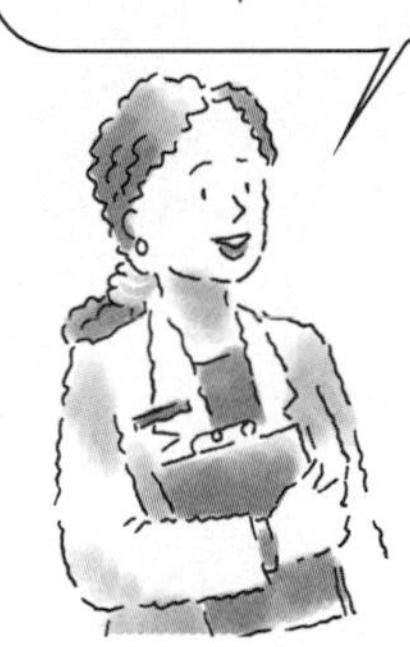

In question 46, remembering when these decelerations occur is important!

46. 1. Early decelerations are reassuring and are due to pressure on the fetal head as it progresses down the birth canal. They have a uniform waveform that resembles an inverted mirror of the corresponding contraction. They begin at the onset of the contraction and end with the end of the contraction. Decelerations initiated 30 to 40 seconds after the onset of the contraction are termed late decelerations and are due to uteroplacental insufficiency from decreased blood flow during uterine contractions. Early decelerations aren't associated with loss of variability or fetal hypoxia.

NP: Assessment; CN: Physiological integrity; CNS: Physiological adaptation; CL: Knowledge

47. Which characteristic best describes spontaneous (periodic) accelerations?

1. Occur with contractions
2. Reflect the shape of contractions
3. Associated with decelerations
4. Indicate fetal well-being and aren't associated with contractions

47. 4. Spontaneous accelerations are symmetrical, uniform increases in fetal heart rate. They indicate fetal well-being, represent an intact central nervous system response to fetal movement or stimulation, and aren't associated with contractions. Uniform accelerations are symmetric, occur with contractions, and reflect the shape of the contraction. Decelerations are periodic decreases in fetal heart rate from the baseline heart rate.

NP: Assessment; CN: Physiological integrity; CNS: Physiological adaptation; CL: Knowledge

48. The first day of a client's last menstrual period (LMP) was October 10. Using Nägele's rule, what is the estimated date of delivery?

1. July 10
2. July 17
3. August 10
4. August 17

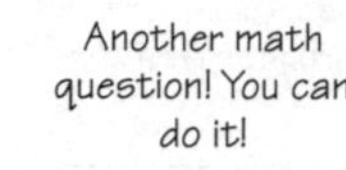
Another math
question! You can
do it!

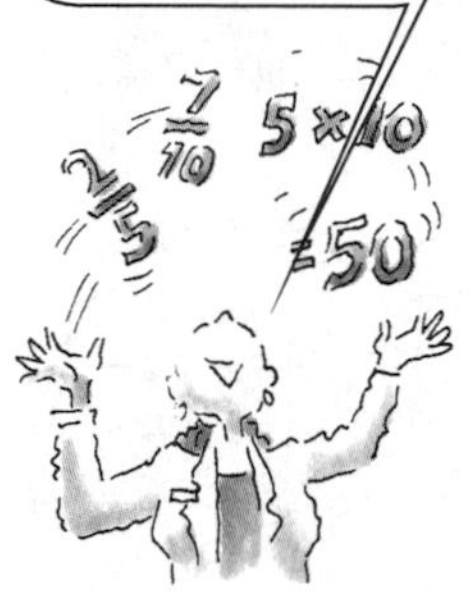

48. 2. After determining the first day of the LMP, the nurse would subtract 3 months and add 7 days. If the client's LMP was October 10, subtracting 3 months is July 10, and adding 7 days brings the date to July 17.
NP: Assessment; CN: Health promotion and maintenance; CNS: Growth and development through the life span; CL: Analysis

49. At 1 minute of life, a neonate is crying vigorously, has a heart rate of 98, is active with normal reflexes, and has a pink body and blue extremities. Which of the following Apgar scores would be correct for this neonate?

1. 6
2. 7
3. 8
4. 9

49. 3. Heart rate, respiratory effort, muscle tone, reflex irritability, and color are used to assess the Apgar score. Each of the signs is assigned a score of 0, 1, or 2. The highest possible score is 10. This neonate lost 1 point for a slower-than-normal heart rate and 1 point for its acrocyanosis, a common finding in which the trunk is pink but the extremities are bluish.
NP: Assessment; CN: Physiological integrity; CNS: Reduction of risk potential; CL: Analysis

50. A client at 30 weeks' gestation enters the labor-and-delivery unit with ruptured membranes. Which of the following drugs is administered from the 24th to 32nd week of pregnancy to promote fetal lung maturity?

1. Betamethasone (Celestone)
2. Magnesium sulfate
3. Oxytocin (Pitocin)
4. Terbutaline (Brethaire)

50. 1. Betamethasone is a glucocorticoid that induces pulmonary maturation in the fetus and decreases respiratory distress syndrome in preterm infants when administered prior to delivery. Magnesium sulfate is also a beta-adrenergic used for tocolysis. Oxytocin is the synthetic form of the pituitary hormone used to stimulate uterine contractions. Terbutaline is a beta-adrenergic used to relax the smooth muscle of the uterus, especially for preterm labor and uterine hyperstimulation.
NP: Planning; CN: Physiological integrity; CNS: Reduction of risk potential; CL: Knowledge

51. Immediately after delivery, the nurse observes that the neonate is wimpering and grimaces when touched. His fingers and toes are bluish, and his heart rate is 130 beats/minute. Which step should the nurse take next?

1. Tell the physician that the neonate appears abnormal.
2. Assign an Apgar score of 8.
3. Assign an Apgar score of 10.
4. Call the pediatrician to diagnose the neonate's problem.

51. 2. The nurse should assign an Apgar score of 8. Of a maximum possible score of 10, the nurse deducts 1 point for acrocyanosis and 1 point for a less-than-robust cry. This 1-minute Apgar score is within normal limits, so it isn't necessary to call the physician or pediatrician.
NP: Implementation; CN: Physiological integrity; CNS: Basic care and comfort; CL: Comprehension

52. A pregnant client has a total hemoglobin level of 9 g/dl. Which risk is greatest during the intrapartum period?
1. Small-for-gestational-age neonate
2. Fetal distress
3. Excessive postpartum bleeding
4. Shortness of breath

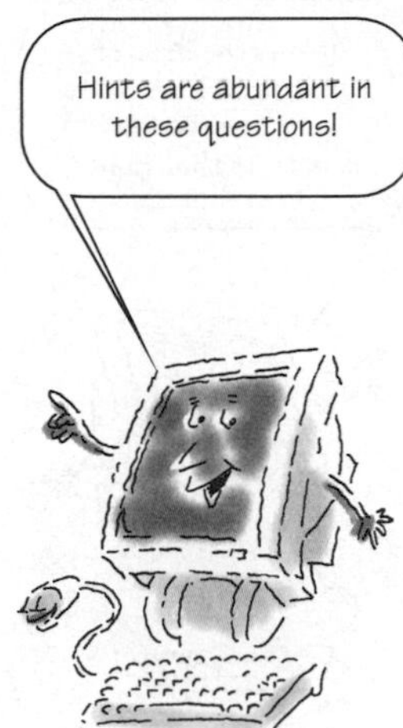
Hints are abundant in these questions!

52. 2. Fetal distress is common in women with anemia than in the general nonanemic population. Shortness of breath occurs more commonly antepartally; the risk for developing shortness of breath doesn't increase during the intrapartum period. A small-for-gestational-age neonate and excessive postpartum bleeding are diagnosed after the intrapartum period.
NP: Analysis; CN: Health promotion and maintenance; CNS: Prevention and early detection of disease; CL: Comprehension

53. Which is the most common and popular method for assessing fetal status throughout labor?
1. Fetal heart rate auscultation using a stethoscope
2. Fetal heart rate auscultation and recording using electronic fetal monitoring
3. Asking the client how she feels and whether the fetus is moving
4. Doing pelvic examinations to check the location of the fetal presenting part

53. 2. The most common and popular method for fetal assessment throughout labor is electronic monitoring, which records the fetal heart rate and maternal contractions and shows how the fetus reacts to the stress of contractions. Although fetal heart rate auscultation can be done with a stethoscope, it's less common because it requires advanced skills. Asking the client how she feels and whether the fetus is moving are important but don't provide specifics about fetal well-being. A pelvic examination reveals cervical dilation and fetal station but doesn't reveal fetal well-being.
NP: Assessment; CN: Health promotion and maintenance; CNS: Prevention and early detection of disease; CL: Analysis

54. Labor is a series of events affected by the coordination of five essential factors. One of these is the passenger (fetus). Which are the other four factors?
1. Contractions, passageway, placental position and function, pattern of care
2. Contractions, maternal response, placental position, psychological response
3. Passageway, contractions, placental position and function, psychological response
4. Passageway, placental position and function, paternal response, psychological response

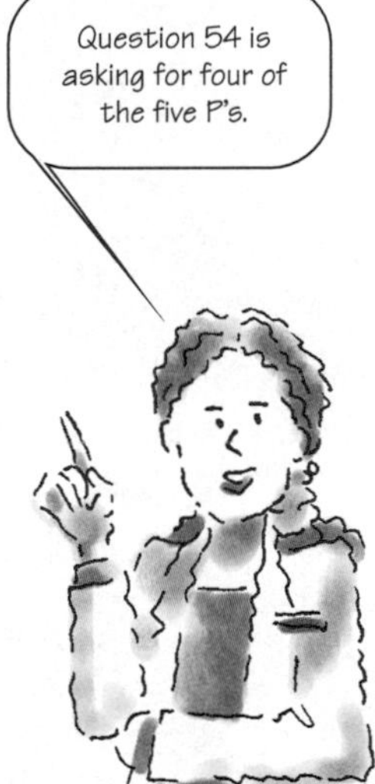
Question 54 is asking for four of the five P's.

54. 3. The five essential factors (sometimes called the five P's) are passenger (fetus), passageway (pelvis), powers (contractions), placental position and function, and psychological response of the mother. These factors must work in concert for labor to progress smoothly.
NP: Assessment; CN: Health promotion and maintenance; CNS: Growth and development through the life span; CL: Comprehension

55. Fetal presentation refers to which of the following descriptions?
1. Fetal body part that enters the maternal pelvis first
2. Relationship of the presenting part to the maternal pelvis
3. Relationship of the long axis of the fetus to the long axis of the mother
4. A classification according to the fetal part

55. 1. Presentation is the fetal body part that enters the pelvis first; it's classified by the presenting part; the three main presentations are cephalic, breech, and shoulder. The relationship of the presenting fetal part to the maternal pelvis refers to fetal position. The relationship of the long axis of the fetus to the long axis of the mother refers to fetal lie; the three possible lies are longitudinal, transverse, and oblique.
NP: Assessment; CN: Physiological integrity; CNS: Physiological adaptation; CL: Knowledge

56. Fetal lie is the relationship of the long axis of the fetus to the long axis of the mother. Which fetal lie is the most common and best suited for vaginal delivery?
1. Transverse
2. Longitudinal
3. Oblique
4. Compound

56. 2. A longitudinal lie is the only lie that can result in a vaginal birth. Generally, an oblique lie converts to a longitudinal lie, enabling vaginal delivery. Transverse and compound lies are incompatible with a vaginal birth and necessitate cesarean delivery.
NP: Analysis; CN: Physiological integrity; CNS: Physiological adaptation; CL: Knowledge

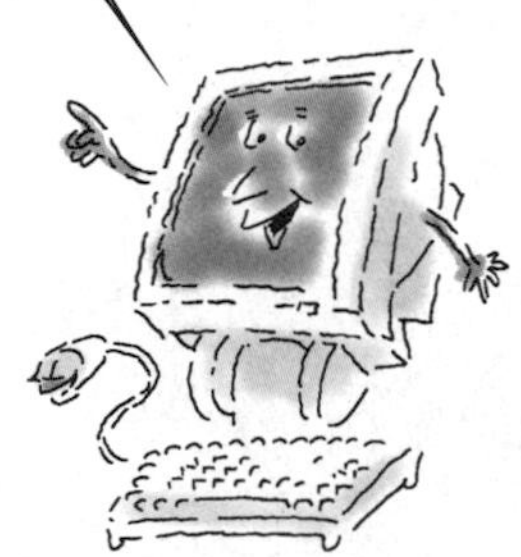

It was the best of times, it was the most of times. Wait a minute, is that right?

57. Which component must the nurse evaluate when assessing labor contractions?
1. Pelvic type, duration, and frequency
2. Contraction type and frequency, and pelvic type
3. Contraction duration, frequency, and intensity
4. Contraction type, duration, and intensity

57. 3. The three components of a contraction that the nurse must evaluate are the duration, frequency, and intensity of each contraction. Pelvic type has no bearing on contractions.
NP: Assessment; CN: Safe, effective care environment; CNS: Management of care; CL: Comprehension

58. A client in labor is using the Lamaze method of prepared childbirth. Her cervix is dilated 5 cm, with contractions occurring 2 to 3 minutes apart. The nurse should instruct the client to breathe at which level?
1. Level 1
2. Level 2
3. Level 3
4. Level 4

58. 2. Level 2 breathing techniques are useful when cervical dilation is between 4 and 6 cm. Level 1 breathing techniques are useful for early contractions; level 3, for the transition stage of labor; and level 4, for the transition stage of labor.
NP: Implementation; CN: Safe, effective care environment; CNS: Management of care; CL: Application

59. A client has received dinoprostone (Prostin E2) for cervical ripening. The nurse should assess her for which adverse drug effect?
1. Vomiting
2. Euphoria
3. Uterine inversion
4. Constipation

59. 1. Headache, nausea and vomiting, chills, fever, and hypertension are adverse effects of dinoprostone. Euphoria and uterine inversion are rare adverse effects of this drug. Diarrhea, not constipation, is a possible adverse effect.
NP: Assessment; CN: Health promotion and maintenance; CNS: Prevention and early detection of disease; CL: Analysis

60. The first stage of labor is divided into the latent and active states. Each is characterized by which of the following events?
1. Progressive cervical dilation and fetal descent
2. Progressive maternal anxiety
3. Progressive fetal descent
4. Progressive cervical dilation

60. 1. Progressive cervical dilation and effacement and fetal descent characterize the first stage of labor. Progressive maternal anxiety may occur but doesn't characterize this stage.
NP: Analysis; CN: Health promotion and maintenance; CNS: Growth and development through the life span; CL: Comprehension

61. At 39 weeks' gestation, a primiparous client arrives at the labor and delivery unit complaining of lower back pain that started 6 hours ago. A pelvic examination reveals that her cervix is dilated 3 cm and 75% effaced. Which explanation is most likely for what's happening?

1. The client is complaining of a common discomfort of pregnancy.
2. The client is in active labor.
3. The client is in the latent phase of labor.
4. The client has a urinary tract infection (UTI).

61. 3. The latent phase of labor is characterized by lower back pain, abdominal cramping, and cervical dilation of 3 to 4 cm. A UTI doesn't present as a backache. Pyelonephritis may present with flank pain, among other symptoms. Active labor is the active progression of labor from 3 or 4 cm to 10 cm, or complete dilation.

NP: Analysis; CN: Physiological integrity; CNS: Physiological adaptation; CL: Knowledge

62. Labor length is determined by multiple factors, including the number of previous labors. In primiparous clients, labor lasts an average of 13 to 15 hours. Which is the average length of labor for multiparous clients?

1. 6 to 7 hours
2. 8 to 9 hours
3. 10 to 11 hours
4. 12 to 15 hours

62. 2. The average length of labor for multiparous clients is 8 to 9 hours. Of course, labor may be shorter or longer for the individual client, depending on circumstances.

NP: Assessment; CN: Physiological integrity; CNS: Physiological adaptation; CL: Knowledge

63. A client is admitted to the labor-and-delivery suite at 36 weeks' gestation. She has a history of cesarean delivery and complains of severe abdominal pain that started less than 1 hour earlier. When the nurse palpates tetanic contractions, the client again complains of severe pain. After the client vomits, she states that the pain is better and then passes out. Which is the probable cause of her signs and symptoms?

1. Hysteria compounded by influenza
2. Placental abruption
3. Uterine rupture
4. Dysfunctional labor

63. 3. Uterine rupture is a medical emergency that may occur before or during labor. Signs and symptoms typically include abdominal pain that may ease after uterine rupture, vomiting, vaginal bleeding, hypovolemic shock, and fetal distress. With influenza, a person usually doesn't feel better or pass out after vomiting. With placental abruption, the client typically complains of vaginal bleeding and constant abdominal pain. Dysfunctional labor doesn't cause such dramatic symptoms.

NP Analysis; CN: Health promotion and maintenance; CNS: Prevention and early detection of disease; CL: Comprehension

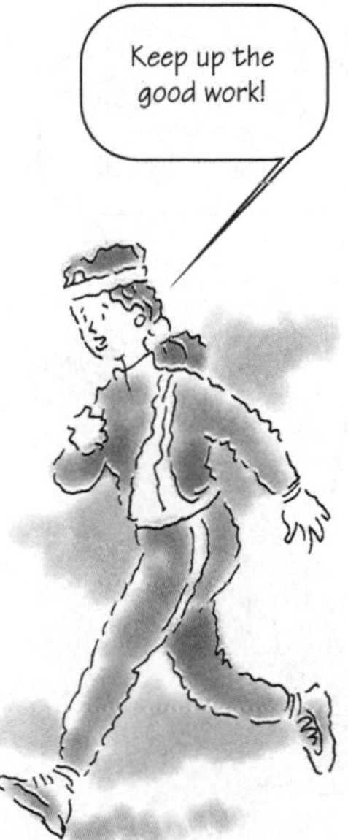

64. Which is the classic sign of premature rupture of the amniotic membranes (PROM)?

1. Contractions with leakage of clear fluid from the vagina
2. Contractions alone
3. Leakage of clear fluid from the vagina
4. Decreased fetal movement

64. 3. In PROM, the amniotic sac ruptures before the onset of contractions. General treatment guidelines include minimizing vaginal examinations, watching for signs and symptoms of labor, and monitoring the mother and fetus for potential infection. Occasionally, PROM causes a decrease in fetal movement, but this isn't a classic sign.

NP: Assessment; CN: Health promotion and maintenance; CNS: Prevention and early detection of disease; CL: Knowledge

65. Which phrase refers to the degree of flexion that the fetus assumes or the relationship of the fetal parts to one another?

1. Fetal attitude
2. Fetal position
3. Fetal lie
4. Fetal presentation

65. 1. Fetal attitude refers to the degree of flexion that the fetus assumes or the relationship of the fetal parts to one another. Fetal position is the relationship of the presenting part to the specific quadrant of the woman's pelvis. Fetal lie refers to the relationship of the long axis of the fetal body to the long axis of the mother's body. Fetal presentation is the fetal body part that will deliver first.

NP: Analysis; CN: Physiological integrity; CNS: Physiological adaptation; CL: Comprehension

66. Pregnancy-induced hypertension (PIH) may be diagnosed initially when the client is in labor. Besides elevated blood pressure, which are classic signs of PIH?

1. Proteinuria and generalized neuralgia
2. Edema and generalized neuralgia
3. Headache and edema
4. Proteinuria and edema

66. 4. The three classic signs of PIH are high blood pressure, proteinuria, and edema, which may affect the face, hands, and lower extremities. Neuralgia isn't a symptom of PIH. Headache may occur but isn't a classic sign.

NP: Assessment; CN: Health promotion and maintenance; CNS: Prevention and early detection of disease; CL: Knowledge

67. As the fetus passes through the birth canal, it makes various positional changes, called cardinal movements of labor. Which is the first cardinal movement?

1. Descent
2. Flexion
3. Extension
4. Internal rotation

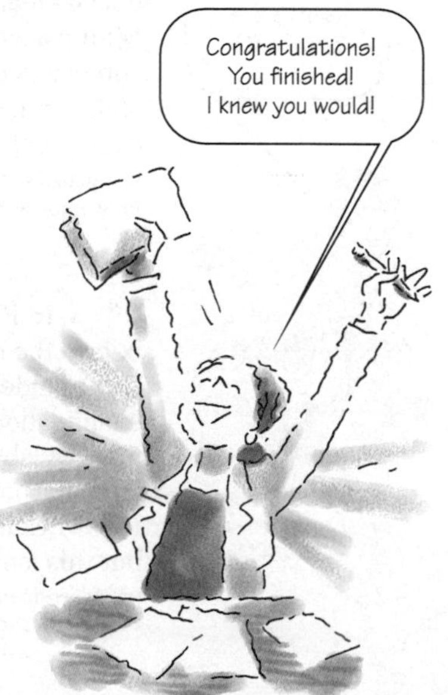
Congratulations!
You finished!
I knew you would!

67. 1. Descent, the first cardinal movement, is the downward movement of the fetal presenting part. Flexion, the second cardinal movement, occurs as pressure from the pelvic floor causes the fetal head to bend forward into the chest. Internal rotation, the third cardinal movement, puts the fetal shoulders into the optimal position to enter the inlet or puts the widest diameter of the shoulders inline with the inlet's widest diameter. Extension, the fourth cardinal movement, occurs as the occiput is delivered, the back of the neck stops beneath the pelvic arch, the head extends, and the foremost parts of the face and chin are delivered.

NP: Assessment; CN: Physiological integrity; CNS: Physiological adaptation; CL: Knowledge

NP: Nursing process CN: Client needs category CNS: Client needs subcategory CL: Cognitive level

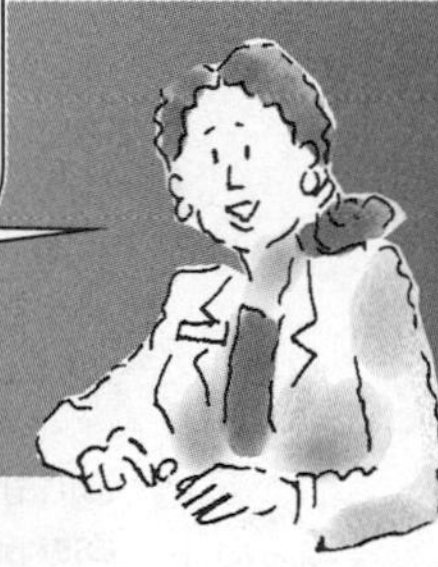

Before taking off through this chapter, why not spend a few minutes browsing the birthing stories at www.birthstories.com/. It'll get you in just the right mood to tackle care of the postpartum patient. Enjoy!

Chapter 24 Postpartum care

1. When completing the morning postpartum assessment, the nurse notices the client's perineal pad is completely saturated with lochia rubra. Which of the following actions should be the nurse's first response?

1. Vigorously massage the fundus.
2. Immediately call the primary care provider.
3. Have the charge nurse review the assessment.
4. Ask the client when she last changed her perineal pad.

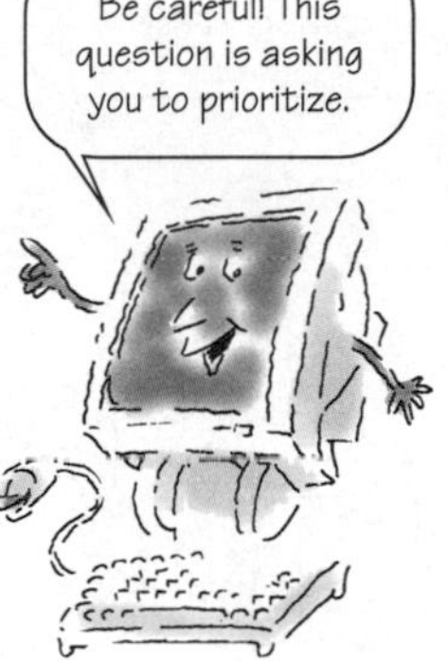

Be careful! This question is asking you to prioritize.

1. 4. If the morning assessment is done relatively early, it's possible that the client hasn't yet been to the bathroom, in which case her perineal pad may have been in place all night. Secondly, her lochia may have pooled during the night, resulting in a heavy flow in the morning. Vigorous massage of the fundus isn't recommended for heavy bleeding or hemorrhage. The nurse wouldn't want to call the primary care provider unnecessarily. If the nurse were uncertain, it would be appropriate to have another qualified individual check the client but only after a complete assessment of the client's status.

NP: Analysis; CN: Physiological integrity; CNS: Physiological adaptation; CL: Analysis

2. Which of the following factors might result in a decreased supply of breast milk in a postpartum mother?

1. Supplemental feedings with formula
2. Maternal diet high in vitamin C
3. An alcoholic drink
4. Frequent feedings

2. 1. Routine formula supplementation may interfere with establishing an adequate milk volume because decreased stimulation to the mother's nipples affects hormonal levels and milk production. Vitamin C levels haven't been shown to influence milk volume. One drink containing alcohol generally tends to relax the mother, facilitating letdown. Excessive consumption of alcohol may block letdown of milk to the infant, though supply isn't necessarily affected. Frequent feedings are likely to increase milk production.

NP: Analysis; CN: Physiological integrity; CNS: Physiological adaptation; CL: Application

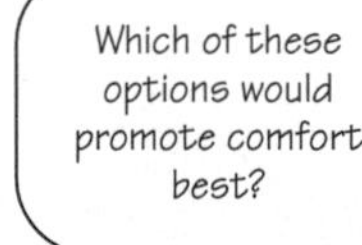

Which of these options would promote comfort best?

3. Which of the following interventions would be helpful to a breast-feeding mother who is experiencing engorged breasts?

1. Applying ice
2. Applying a breast binder
3. Teaching how to express her breasts in a warm shower
4. Administering bromocriptine (Parlodel)

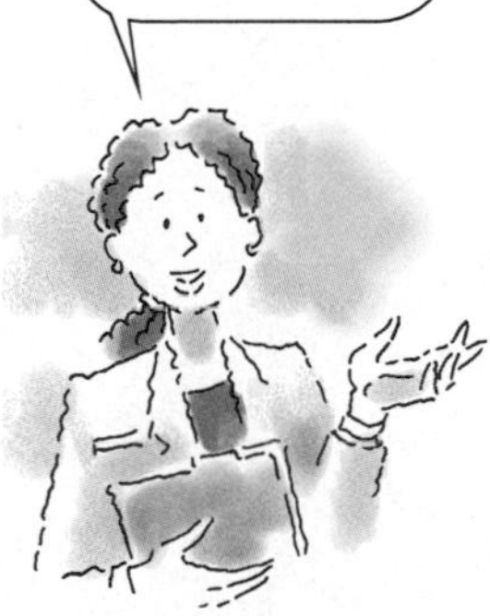

3. 3. Teaching the client how to express her breasts in a warm shower aids with letdown and will give temporary relief. Ice can promote comfort by decreasing blood flow (vasoconstriction), numbing, and discouraging further letdown of milk; however, this is followed by a rebound reaction of more letting down once the ice is removed. Breast binders aren't effective in relieving the discomforts of engorgement. Bromocriptine is no longer indicated for lactation suppression.

NP: Implementation; CN: Physiological integrity; CNS: Basic care and comfort; CL: Application

4. Which of the following assessments should be performed routinely in the postpartum client?

1. Antibody screen
2. Babinski's reflex
3. Homans' sign
4. Patellar reflex

4. 3. Homans' sign, or pain on dorsiflexion of the foot, may indicate deep vein thrombosis (DVT). Postpartum women are at increased risk of DVT because of changes in clotting mechanisms to control bleeding at delivery. An antibody screen wouldn't be classified as an assessment technique. Both Babinski's reflex and the patellar reflex need not be routinely assessed in the postpartum woman.

NP: Planning; CN: Health promotion and maintenance; CNS: Prevention and early detection of disease; CL: Analysis

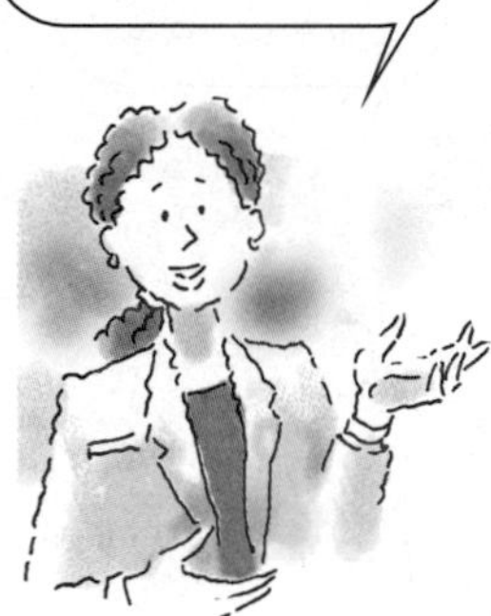

If you know what Kegel exercises are, you should get question 5 correct easily.

5. Which of the following reasons explains why Kegel exercises are advantageous to women after they deliver a child?

1. They assist with lochia removal.
2. They promote the return of normal bowel function.
3. They promote blood flow, allowing for healing and strengthening the musculature.
4. They assist the woman in burning calories for rapid postpartum weight loss.

5. 3. Exercising the pubococcygeal muscle increases blood flow to the area. The increased blood flow brings oxygen and other nutrients to the perineal area to aid in healing. Additionally, these exercises help to strengthen the musculature, thereby decreasing the risk of future complications, such as incontinence and uterine prolapse. Performing Kegel exercises may assist with lochia removal but that isn't their main purpose. Bowel function isn't influenced by Kegel exercises. Kegel exercises don't expend sufficient energy to burn many calories.

NP: Analysis; CN: Health promotion and maintenance; CNS: Prevention and early detection of disease; CL: Analysis

6. When the nurse is performing a psychosocial assessment on a postpartum client, the nurse is aware that what percentage of women experience "postpartum blues"?

1. 20 to 25%
2. 50 to 80%
3. 30 to 45%
4. 95 to 100%

6. 2. The "postpartum blues" are a transient mood alteration that arise within the first 3 postpartum weeks and are typically self-limiting, occurring in 50 to 80% of clients. A more severe mood alteration occurs in approximately 20% of clients. These changes occur within a few days after delivery and may last for a few days to a year or more. The most severe condition, a major depressive episode occurs in approximately 0.1% of clients and in many cases requires hospitalization for psychiatric care.

NP: Planning; CN: Psychosocial integrity; CNS: Coping and adaptation; CL: Knowledge

7. Which of the following practices would the nurse recommend to a client who has had a cesarean delivery?

1. Frequent douching after she's discharged
2. Coughing and deep-breathing exercises
3. Sit-ups at 2 weeks postoperatively
4. Side-rolling exercises

7. 2. As for any postoperative client, coughing and deep-breathing exercises should be taught to keep the alveoli open and prevent infection. Frequent douching isn't recommended for any group of women and is contraindicated in women who have just given birth. Sit-ups at 2 weeks postpartum could potentially damage the healing of the incision. Side-rolling exercises aren't an accepted medical practice.

NP: Implementation; CN: Physiological integrity; CNS: Reduction of risk potential; CL: Application

8. Which of the following reasons explains why a client might express disappointment after having a cesarean delivery instead of a vaginal delivery?

1. Cesarean deliveries cost more.
2. Depression is more common after a cesarean delivery.
3. The client is usually more fatigued after cesarean delivery.
4. The client may feel a loss for not having experienced a "normal" birth.

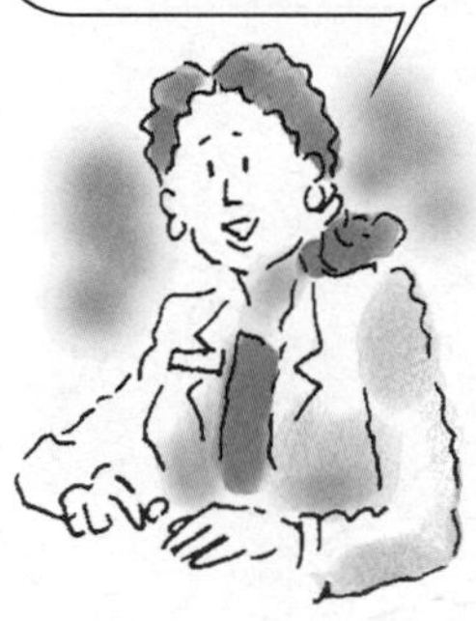

Remember to be sensitive to your postpartum client's needs.

8. 4. Clients occasionally feel a loss after a cesarean delivery. They may feel they're inadequate because they couldn't deliver their infant vaginally. The cost of cesarean delivery doesn't generally apply because the woman isn't directly responsible for payment. No conclusive studies support the theory that depression is more common after cesarean delivery when compared to vaginal delivery. Although clients are usually more fatigued after a cesarean delivery, fatigue hasn't been shown to cause feelings of disappointment over the method of delivery.

NP: Analysis; CN: Psychosocial integrity; CNS: Coping and adaptation; CL: Analysis

9. Which of the following findings is normal during the postpartum period of a client who has experienced a vaginal birth?

1. Redness or swelling in the calves
2. A palpable uterine fundus beyond 6 weeks postpartum
3. Vaginal dryness after the lochial flow has ended
4. Dark red lochia for approximately 6 weeks after the birth

9. 3. Vaginal dryness is a normal finding during the postpartum period due to hormonal changes. Redness or swelling in the calves may indicate thrombophlebitis. The fundus shouldn't be palpable beyond 6 weeks. Dark red lochia (indicating fresh bleeding) should only last 2 to 3 days postpartum.

NP: Assessment; CN: Physiological integrity; CNS: Physiological adaptation; CL: Knowledge

10. On completing a fundal assessment, the nurse notes the fundus is situated on the client's left abdomen. Which of the following actions is appropriate?

1. Ask the client to empty her bladder.
2. Straight catheterize the client immediately.
3. Call the client's primary health care provider for direction.
4. Straight catheterize the client for half of her urine volume.

10. 1. A full bladder may displace the uterine fundus to the left or right side of the abdomen. A straight catheterization is unnecessarily invasive if the woman can urinate on her own. Nursing interventions should be completed before notifying the primary health care provider in a nonemergency situation.

NP: Assessment; CN: Physiological integrity; CNS: Physiological adaptation; CL: Application

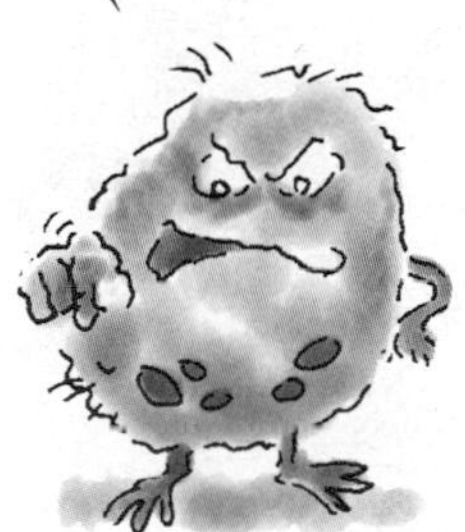

Bacteria can strike when you least expect us!

11. The nurse should inform the client with mastitis that the disorder is most commonly caused by which of the following organisms?

1. *Escherichia coli*
2. Group A beta-hemolytic streptococci (GBS)
3. *Staphylococcus aureus*
4. *Streptococcus pyogenes*

11. 3. The most common cause of mastitis is *S. aureus*, transmitted from the baby's mouth. Mastitis isn't harmful to the baby. *E. coli*, GBS, and *S. pyogenes* aren't associated with mastitis. GBS infection *is* associated with neonatal sepsis and death.

NP: Analysis; CN: Health promotion and maintenance; CNS: Growth and development through the life span; CL: Knowledge

12. A client had a spontaneous vaginal delivery after 18 hours of labor. Her excessive vaginal bleeding has now become a postpartum hemorrhage. Immediate nursing care of this client should include which of the following interventions?
1. Avoiding massaging the uterus
2. Monitoring vital signs every hour
3. Placing the client in Trendelenburg's position
4. Elevating the head of the bed to increase blood flow

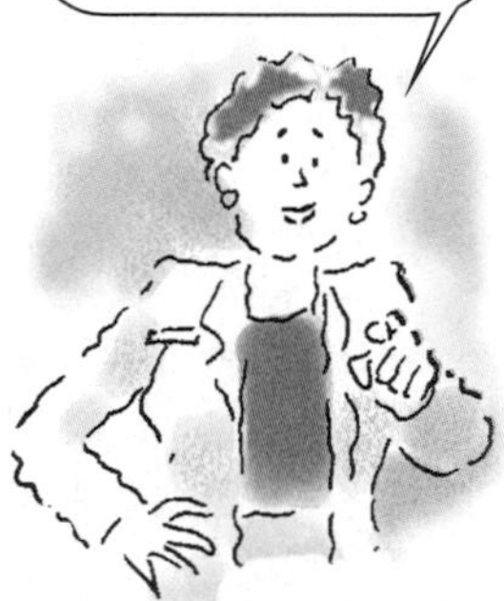

Be careful. One word may change a seemingly correct answer into a wrong one.

12. 3. The client should be placed in Trendelenburg's position to prevent or control hypovolemic shock. The uterus should be palpated to determine if it's contracting and should be massaged if it's boggy or not contracting. Vital signs should be monitored continuously, or at least every 10 to 15 minutes, until the client's condition stabilizes. The head of the bed shouldn't be elevated because this will further lower the blood pressure.

NP: Implementation; CN: Physiological integrity; CNS: Physiological adaptation; CL: Analysis

13. Which of the following complications should the nurse assess for in a client with type 1 diabetes mellitus whose delivery was complicated by polyhydramnios and macrosomia?
1. Postpartum mastitis
2. Increased insulin needs
3. Postpartum hemorrhage
4. Pregnancy-induced hypertension (PIH)

13. 3. The client is at risk for a postpartum hemorrhage from the overdistention of the uterus because of the extra amniotic fluid and the large baby. The uterus may not be able to contract as well as it would normally. The diabetic mother usually has decreased insulin needs for the first few days postpartum. Neither polyhydramnios nor macrosomia would increase the client's risk of PIH or mastitis.

NP: Assessment; CN: Physiological integrity; CNS: Reduction of risk potential; CL: Knowledge

14. Infections in mothers with diabetes tend to be more severe and can quickly lead to which of the following complications?
1. Anemia
2. Ketoacidosis
3. Respiratory acidosis
4. Respiratory alkalosis

14. 2. Women with diabetes who become pregnant tend to become sicker and develop illnesses quicker than pregnant woman without diabetes. Severe infections in diabetes can lead to diabetic ketoacidosis. Anemia, respiratory acidosis, and respiratory alkalosis aren't generally associated with infections in mothers with diabetes.

NP: Analysis; CN: Health promotion and maintenance; CNS: Growth and development through the life span; CL: Knowledge

Is it getting chilly in here or is it just me? (Hey, that's a hint!)

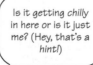

15. Which of the following statements regarding mastitis is correct?
1. The most common pathogen is group A beta-hemolytic streptococci.
2. A breast abscess is a common complication of mastitis.
3. Mastitis usually develops in both breasts of a breast-feeding woman.
4. Symptoms include fever, chills, malaise, and localized breast tenderness.

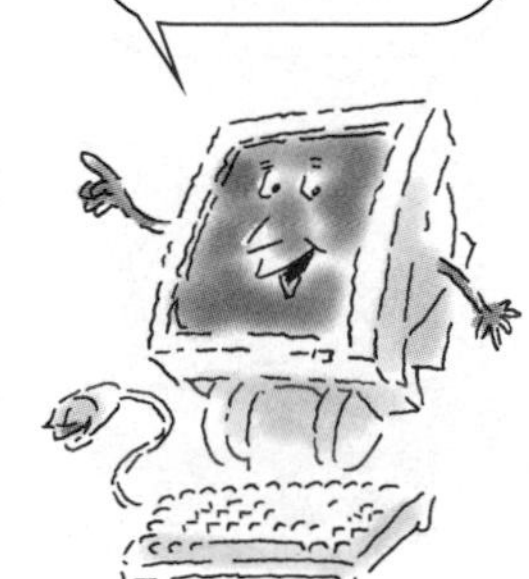

15. 4. Mastitis is an infection of the breast characterized by flulike symptoms, along with redness and tenderness in the breast. The most common causative agent is *Staphylococcus aureus*. Breast abscess is rarely a complication of mastitis if the woman continues to empty the affected breast. Mastitis usually occurs in one breast, not bilaterally.

NP: Analysis; CN: Physiological integrity; CNS: Physiological adaptation; CL: Knowledge

16. Which of the following measurements best describes delayed postpartum hemorrhage?
1. Blood loss in excess of 300 ml, occurring 24 hours to 6 weeks after delivery
2. Blood loss in excess of 500 ml, occurring 24 hours to 6 weeks after delivery
3. Blood loss in excess of 800 ml, occurring 24 hours to 6 weeks after delivery
4. Blood loss in excess of 1,000 ml, occurring 24 hours to 6 weeks after delivery

16. 2. Postpartum hemorrhage involves blood loss in excess of 500 ml. Most delayed postpartum hemorrhages occur between the fourth and ninth days postpartum. The most frequent causes of a delayed postpartum hemorrhage include retained placental fragments, intrauterine infection, and fibroids.

NP: Analysis; CN: Physiological integrity; CNS: Reduction of risk potential; CL: Knowledge

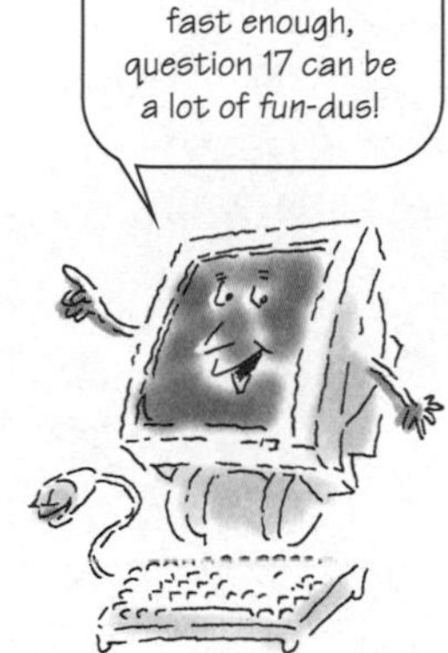

If you catch on fast enough, question 17 can be a lot of fun-dus!

17. Which of the following assessments of the mother should be made in the immediate postpartum period (first 2 hours)?
1. Blood glucose level
2. Electrocardiogram (ECG)
3. Height of fundus
4. Stool test for occult blood

17. 3. A complete physical assessment should be performed every 15 minutes for the first 1 to 2 hours postpartum, including assessment of the fundus, lochia, perineum, blood pressure, pulse, and bladder function. A blood glucose level needs to be obtained only if the woman has risk factors for an unstable blood glucose level or if she has symptoms of an altered blood glucose level. An ECG would be necessary only if the woman is at risk for cardiac difficulty. A stool test for occult blood generally wouldn't be valid during the immediate postpartum period; it's difficult to sort out lochial bleeding from rectal bleeding.

NP: Assessment; CN: Health promotion and maintenance; CNS: Growth and development through the life span; CL: Knowledge

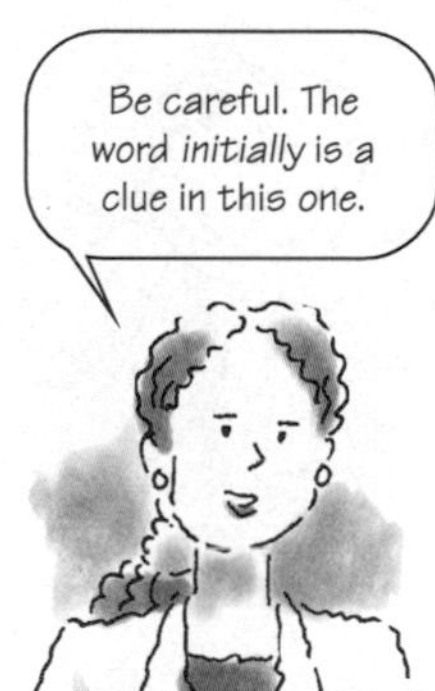

Be careful. The word *initially* is a clue in this one.

18. In performing an assessment of a postpartum client 2 hours after delivery, the nurse notices heavy bleeding with large clots. Which of the following responses is most appropriate initially?
1. Massaging the fundus firmly
2. Performing bimanual compressions
3. Administering ergonovine (Ergotrate)
4. Notifying the primary health care provider

18. 1. Initial management of excessive postpartum bleeding is firm massage of the fundus along with a rapid infusion of oxytocin or lactated Ringer's solution. Ergotrate should be used only if the bleeding doesn't respond to massage and oxytocin. Bimanual compression is performed by a primary health care provider. The primary health care provider should be notified if the client doesn't respond to fundal massage, but other measures can be taken in the meantime.

NP: Implementation; CN: Physiological integrity; CNS: Physiological adaptation; CL: Analysis

19. The nurse is about to give a class B diabetic (age of onset greater than 20 years, duration less than 10 years) her insulin before breakfast on her first day postpartum. Which of the following answers best describes insulin requirements immediately postpartum?
1. Lower than during her pregnancy
2. Higher than during her pregnancy
3. Lower than before she became pregnant
4. Higher than before she became pregnant

19. 3. Postpartum insulin requirements are usually significantly lower than prepregnancy requirements. Occasionally, clients may require little to no insulin during the first 24 to 48 hours postpartum.

NP: Analysis; CN: Physiological integrity; CNS: Reduction of risk potential; CL: Knowledge

20. Which of the following findings would be expected when assessing the postpartum client?

1. Fundus 1 cm above the umbilicus 1 hour postpartum
2. Fundus 1 cm above the umbilicus on postpartum day 3
3. Fundus palpable in the abdomen at 2 weeks postpartum
4. Fundus slightly to right; 2 cm above umbilicus on postpartum day 2

20. 1. Within the first 12 hours postpartum, the fundus usually is approximately 1 cm above the umbilicus. The fundus should be below the umbilicus by postpartum day 3. The fundus shouldn't be palpated in the abdomen after day 10. A uterus that isn't midline or is above the umbilicus on postpartum day 3 might be caused by a full, distended bladder or a uterine infection.

NP: Assessment; CN: Health promotion and maintenance; CNS: Growth and development through the life span ; CL: Knowledge

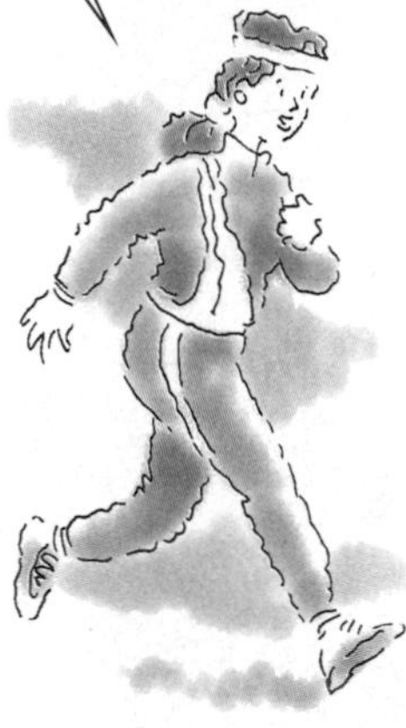

You're hustling! Keep up the good work!

21. A client is complaining of painful contractions, or afterpains, on postpartum day 2. Which of the following conditions could increase the severity of afterpains?

1. Bottle-feeding
2. Diabetes
3. Multiple gestation
4. Primiparity

21. 3. Multiple gestation, breast-feeding, multiparity, and conditions that cause overdistention of the uterus will increase the intensity of afterpains. Bottle-feeding and diabetes aren't directly associated with increasing severity of afterpains, unless the client has delivered a macrosomic infant.

NP: Analysis; CN: Health promotion and maintenance; CNS: Growth and development through the life span; CL: Knowledge

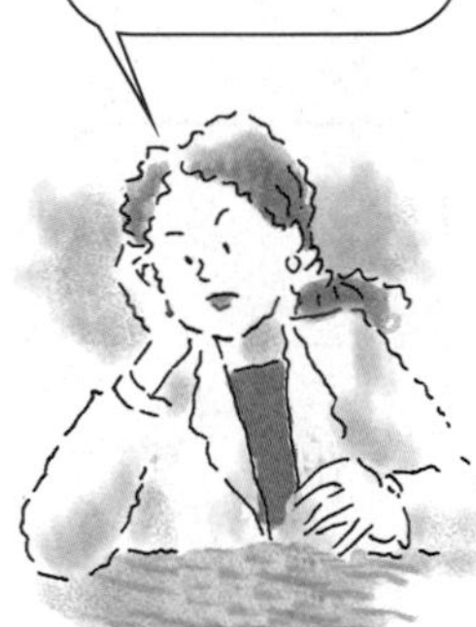

This item is asking you to distinguish between heavy and excessive bleeding.

22. When giving a postpartum client self-care instructions, the nurse instructs her to report heavy or excessive bleeding. Which of the following would indicate heavy bleeding?

1. Saturating a pad in 15 minutes
2. Saturating a pad in 1 hour
3. Saturating a pad in 4 to 6 hours
4. Saturating a pad in 8 hours

22. 2. Bleeding is considered heavy when a woman saturates a sanitary pad in 1 hour. Excessive bleeding occurs when a postpartum client saturates a pad in 15 minutes. Moderate bleeding occurs when the bleeding saturates less than 6″ (15 cm) of a pad in 1 hour.

NP: Assessment; CN: Health promotion and maintenance; CNS: Growth and development through the life span; CL: Knowledge

23. On which of the following postpartum days can the client expect lochia serosa (old blood, serum, leukocytes, and tissue debris)?

1. Days 3 and 4 postpartum
2. Days 3 to 10 postpartum
3. Days 10 to 14 postpartum
4. Days 14 to 42 postpartum

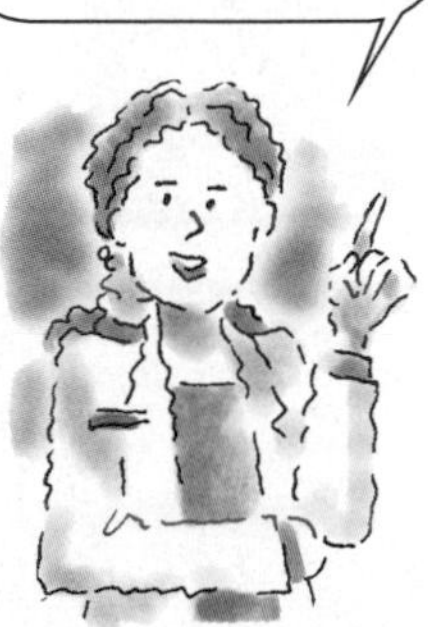

Before you answer, make sure you know which type of lochia this item is asking for.

23. 2. On the third and fourth postpartum days, the lochia becomes a pale pink or brown and contains old blood, serum, leukocytes, and tissue debris. This type of lochia usually lasts until postpartum day 10. Lochia rubra usually last for the first 3 to 4 days postpartum and consists of blood, decidua, and trophoblastic debris. Lochia alba, which contains leukocytes, decidua, epithelial cells, mucus, and bacteria, may continue for 2 to 6 weeks postpartum.

NP: Analysis; CN: Health promotion and maintenance; CNS: Growth and development through the life span; CL: Knowledge

24. A client and her neonate have a blood incompatibility, and the neonate has had a positive direct Coombs' test. Which of the following nursing interventions is appropriate?

1. Because the woman has been sensitized, give Rh_0(D) immune globulin (RhoGAM).
2. Because the woman hasn't been sensitized, give RhoGAM.
3. Because the woman has been sensitized, don't give RhoGAM.
4. Because the woman hasn't been sensitized, don't give RhoGAM.

24. 3. A positive Coombs' test means that the Rh-negative woman is now producing antibodies to the Rh-positive blood of the neonate. RhoGAM shouldn't be given to a sensitized client because it won't be able to prevent antibody formation.

NP: Analysis; CN: Physiological integrity; CNS: Reduction of risk potential; CL: Analysis

25. Which of the following definitions best describes a puerperal infection?

1. An infection in the uterus of a postpartum woman
2. An infection in the bladder of a postpartum woman
3. An infection in the perineum of a postpartum woman
4. An infection in the genital tract of a postpartum woman

25. 4. A puerperal infection is an infection of the genital tract, after delivery through the first 6 weeks postpartum. Endometritis is an infection of the mucous membrane or endometrium of the uterus. Cystitis is an infection of the bladder. Infection of the perineum or episiotomy site usually results in localized pain, low-grade fever, and redness and swelling at the wound edges.

NP: Analysis; CN: Physiological integrity; CNS: Reduction of risk potential; CL: Knowledge

Don't pass on this question. It's important! (Now *that's* a subtle hint!)

26. Which of the following behaviors characterizes the postpartum mother in the taking-in phase?

1. Passive and dependent
2. Striving for independence and autonomy
3. Curious and interested in care of the baby
4. Exhibiting maximum readiness for new learning

26. 1. During the taking-in phase, which usually lasts 2 to 3 days, the mother is passive and dependent and expresses her own needs rather than the neonate's needs. The taking-hold phase usually lasts from days 3 to 10 postpartum. During this stage, the mother strives for independence and autonomy; she also becomes curious and interested in the care of the baby and is most ready to learn.

NP: Assessment; CN: Psychosocial integrity; CNS: Coping and adaptation; CL: Knowledge

27. Which of the following verbalizations should be cause for concern to the nurse treating a postpartum client within a few days of delivery?

1. The client is nervous about taking the baby home.
2. The client feels empty since she delivered the baby.
3. The client would like to watch the nurse give the baby her first bath.
4. The client would like the nurse to take her baby to the nursery so she can sleep.

27. 2. A mother experiencing postpartum blues may say she feels empty now that the infant is no longer in her uterus. She may also verbalize that she feels unprotected now. Many first-time mothers are nervous about caring for their neonates by themselves after discharge. New mothers may want a demonstration before doing a task themselves. A client may want to get some uninterrupted sleep so she may ask that the baby be taken to the nursery.

NP: Assessment; CN: Psychosocial integrity; CNS: Psychosocial adaptation; CL: Knowledge

28. Which of the following complications may be indicated by continuous seepage of blood from the vagina of a postpartum client, when palpation of the uterus reveals a firm uterus 1 cm below the umbilicus?

1. Retained placental fragments
2. Urinary tract infection (UTI)
3. Cervical laceration
4. Uterine atony

28. 3. Continuous seepage of blood may be due to cervical or vaginal lacerations if the uterus is firm and contracting. Retained placental fragments and uterine atony may cause subinvolution of the uterus, making it soft, boggy, and larger than expected. UTI won't cause vaginal bleeding, although hematuria may be present.

NP: Assessment; CN: Physiological integrity; CNS: Reduction of risk potential; CL: Knowledge

29. Discharge teaching of the postpartum client who is receiving anticoagulant therapy for a deep venous thrombophlebitis includes which of the following instructions?

1. Avoid iron replacement therapy.
2. Avoid over-the-counter salicylates.
3. Wear girdles and knee-high stockings when possible.
4. Shortness of breath is a common adverse effect of the medication.

29. 2. Discharge teaching should include informing the client to avoid salicylates, which may potentiate the effects of anticoagulant therapy. Iron won't affect anticoagulation therapy. Restrictive clothing should be avoided to prevent the recurrence of thrombophlebitis. Shortness of breath should be reported immediately because it may be a symptom of pulmonary embolism.

NP: Planning; CN: Physiological integrity; CNS: Reduction of risk potential; CL: Knowledge

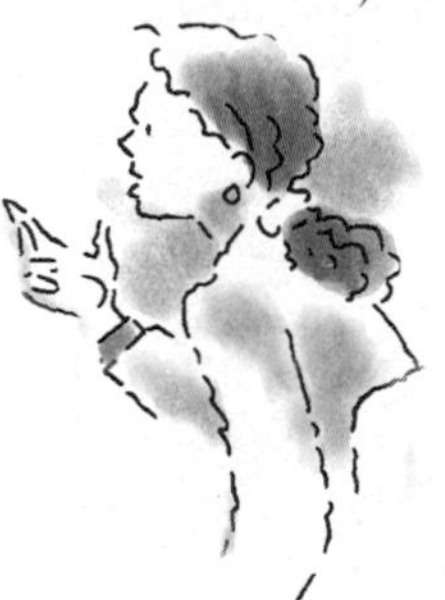

Another 30 down! Keep at it!

30. TORCH is an acronym for maternal infections associated with an increase in congenital malformations and disorders. Which of the following disorders does the *H* represent?

1. Hemophilia
2. Hepatitis B virus
3. Herpes simplex virus
4. Human immunodeficiency virus

30. 3. TORCH represents the following maternal infections: **T**oxoplasmosis; **O**thers, such as gonorrhea, syphilis, varicella, hepatitis, and human immunodeficiency virus; **R**ubella; **C**ytomegalovirus; and **H**erpes simplex virus. Hemophilia is a clotting disorder in which factors VII and X are deficient.

NP: Analysis; CN: Physiological integrity; CNS: Reduction of risk potential; CL: Knowledge

31. Which of the following signs of grieving is dysfunctional in a client 3 days after a perinatal loss?

1. Lack of appetite
2. Denial of the death
3. Blaming herself
4. Frequent crying spells

31. 2. Denial of the perinatal loss is dysfunctional grieving in the client. Lack of appetite, blaming oneself, and frequent crying spells are part of a normal grieving process.

NP: Assessment; CN: Psychosocial integrity; CNS: Psychosocial adaptation; CL: Knowledge

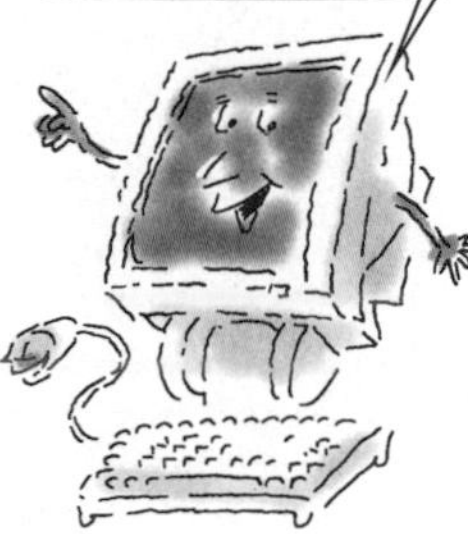

Use of the word *dysfunctional* in this item almost makes it a negative question.

32. Which of the following conditions in a postpartum client may cause fever not caused by infection?

1. Breast engorgement
2. Endometritis
3. Mastitis
4. Uterine involution

32. 1. Breast engorgement and dehydration are noninfectious causes of postpartum fevers. Mastitis and endometritis are both postpartum infections. Involution of the uterus won't cause temperature elevations.

NP: Analysis; CN: Health promotion and maintenance; CNS: Growth and development through the life span; CL: Knowledge

33. An RH-positive client delivers a 6 lb, 10 oz neonate vaginally after 17 hours of labor. Which of the following conditions puts this client at risk for infection?

1. Length of labor
2. Maternal Rh status
3. Method of delivery
4. Size of the baby

33. 1. A prolonged length of labor places the mother at increased risk for developing an infection. The average size of the baby, vaginal delivery, and Rh status of the client don't place the mother at increased risk.

NP: Analysis; CN: Physiological integrity; CNS: Physiological adaptation; CL: Analysis

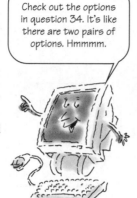

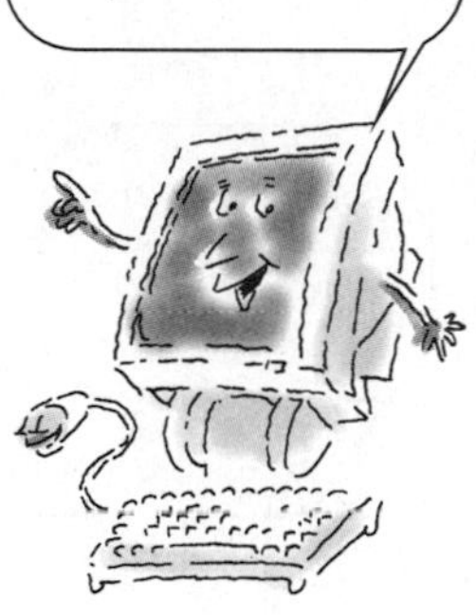

Check out the options in question 34. It's like there are two pairs of options. Hmmmm.

34. Which of the management strategies should be implemented regarding breast-feeding after cesarean delivery?

1. Delay breast-feeding until 24 hours after delivery.
2. Breast-feed frequently during the day and every 4 to 6 hours at night.
3. Use the cradle hold position to avoid incisional discomfort.
4. Use the football hold position to avoid incisional discomfort.

34. 4. When breast-feeding after a cesarean delivery, the client should be encouraged to use the football hold to avoid incisional discomfort. Breast-feeding should be initiated as soon after birth as possible. The mother should be encouraged to breast-feed her infant every 2 to 4 hours throughout the night as well as during the day to increase the milk supply.

NP: Analysis; CN: Physiological integrity; CNS: Basic care and comfort; CL: Analysis

35. What type of milk is present in the breasts 7 to 10 days postpartum?

1. Colostrum
2. Hind milk
3. Mature milk
4. Transitional milk

35. 4. Transitional milk comes after colostrum and usually lasts until 2 weeks postpartum. Colostrum is a thin yellow fluid released by the breasts before and up to 2 weeks postpartum. Hind milk, which satisfies the infant's hunger and promotes weight gain, arrives approximately 10 minutes after each feeding starts. Mature milk is white and thinner than transitional milk and is present after 2 weeks postpartum.

NP: Analysis; CN: Health promotion and maintenance; CNS: Growth and development through the life span; CL: Knowledge

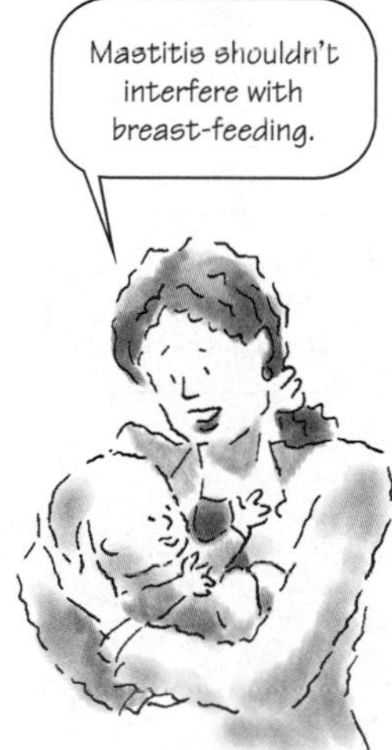

36. Which of the following recommendations should be given to a client with mastitis who is concerned about breast-feeding her neonate?

1. She should stop breast-feeding until completing the antibiotic.
2. She should supplement feeding with formula until the infection resolves.
3. She shouldn't use analgesics because they aren't compatible with breast-feeding.
4. She should continue to breast-feed; mastitis won't infect the infant.

36. 4. The client with mastitis should be encouraged to continue breast-feeding while taking antibiotics for the infection. No supplemental feedings are necessary because breast-feeding doesn't need to be altered and actually encourages resolution of the infection. Analgesics are safe and should be administered as needed.

NP: Analysis; CN: Health promotion and maintenance; CNS: Growth and development through the life span; CL: Analysis

37. Which of the following terms is used to describe maladaptation to the stress and conflicts of the postpartum period, characterized by disabling feelings of inadequacy and an inability to cope?
1. Postpartum blues
2. Postpartum depression
3. Postpartum neurosis
4. Postpartum psychosis

37. 2. Postpartum depression occurs in approximately 10% to 15% of all postpartum women. This depression is characterized by disabling feelings of inadequacy and an inability to cope that can last up to 3 years. The client is often tearful and despondent. The client with postpartum blues experiences crying and sadness, generally between 3 to 5 days postpartum, but this condition resolves itself quickly. Postpartum neurosis includes neurotic behavior during the initial 6 weeks after birth. Postpartum psychosis includes hallucinations, delusions, and phobias.

NP: Analysis; CN: Psychosocial integrity; CNS: Psychosocial adaptation; CL: Knowledge

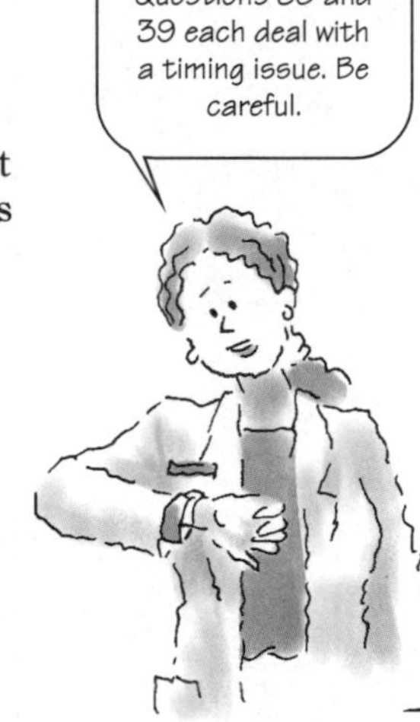

Questions 38 and 39 each deal with a timing issue. Be careful.

38. In which of the following time periods is it most likely for a client who has delivered twins to experience late postpartum hemorrhage?
1. 24 to 48 hours after delivery
2. 24 hours to 6 weeks after delivery
3. 6 weeks to 3 months after delivery
4. 6 weeks to 6 months after delivery

38. 2. Late or secondary postpartum hemorrhages occur more than 24 hours but less than 6 weeks postpartum. Early or primary postpartum hemorrhages occur within 24 hours of delivery.

NP: Analysis; CN: Physiological integrity; CNS: Reduction of risk potential; CL: Knowledge

39. Which of the following complications is most likely responsible for a delayed postpartum hemorrhage?
1. Cervical laceration
2. Clotting deficiency
3. Perineal laceration
4. Uterine subinvolution

39. 4. Late postpartum bleeding is often the result of subinvolution of the uterus. Retained products of conception or infection often cause subinvolution. Cervical or perineal lacerations can cause an immediate postpartum hemorrhage. A client with a clotting deficiency may also have an immediate postpartum hemorrhage, if the deficiency isn't corrected at the time of delivery.

NP: Analysis; CN: Physiological integrity; CNS: Physiological adaptation; CL: Knowledge

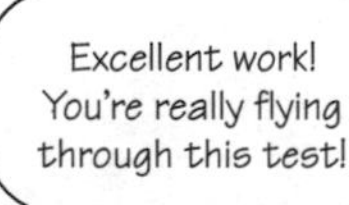

Excellent work! You're really flying through this test!

40. A client needs to void 3 hours after a vaginal delivery. Which of the following risk factors necessitates assisting her out of bed?
1. Chest pain
2. Breast engorgement
3. Orthostatic hypotension
4. Separation of episiotomy incision

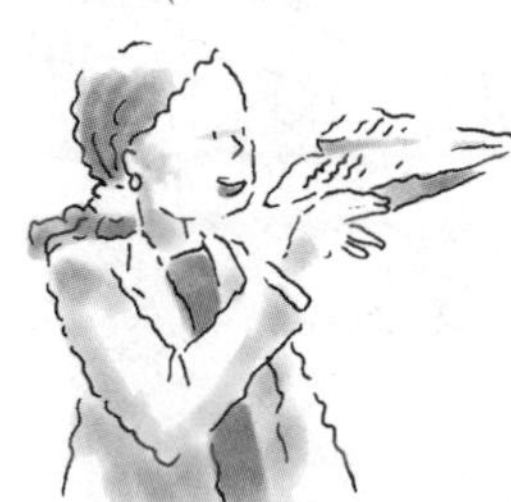

40. 3. The rapid decrease in intra-abdominal pressure occurring after birth causes splanchnic engorgement. The client is at risk for orthostatic hypotension when standing due to the blood pooling in this area. Breast engorgement is caused by vascular congestion in the breast before true lactation. The client shouldn't experience separation of the episiotomy incision or chest pain when standing.

NP: Implementation; CN: Health promotion and maintenance; CNS: Growth and development through the life span; CL: Knowledge

41. Before giving a postpartum client the rubella vaccine, which of the following facts should the nurse include in client teaching?

1. The vaccine is safe in clients with egg allergies.
2. Breast-feeding isn't compatible with the vaccine.
3. Transient arthralgia and rash are uncommon adverse effects.
4. The client should avoid getting pregnant for 3 months after the vaccination because the vaccine has teratogenic effects.

41. 4. The client must understand that she must not become pregnant for 2 to 3 months after the vaccination because of its potential teratogenic effects. The rubella vaccine is made from duck eggs so an allergic reaction may occur in clients with egg allergies. The virus isn't transmitted into the breast milk, so clients may continue to breast-feed after vaccination. Transient arthralgia and rash are common adverse effects of the vaccine.

NP: Planning; CN: Health promotion and maintenance; CNS: Growth and development through the life span; CL: Knowledge

42. Which of the following medications is most commonly used to treat preeclampsia during the prenatal and postpartum periods?

1. Diazepam (Valium)
2. Hydralazine (Apresoline)
3. Magnesium sulfate
4. Nifedipine (Procardia)

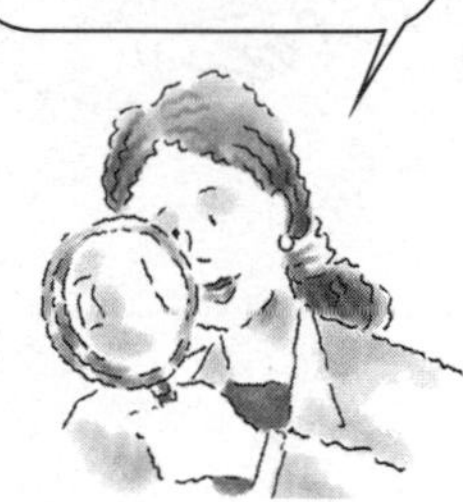

Don't lose your focus. Pay attention to the words most commonly in this item.

42. 3. Magnesium sulfate is commonly used in the treatment of preeclampsia to prevent seizures. It also produces a smooth muscle depression effect, which can lower blood pressure. Diazepam may also be given for seizure activity. Nifedipine and hydralazine are used for severely hypertensive preeclamptic women.

NP: Implementation; CN: Physiological integrity; CNS: Pharmacological and parenteral therapies; CL: Knowledge

43. Which of the following complications is associated with magnesium sulfate therapy?

1. Hypotension
2. Postpartum depression
3. Postpartum hemorrhage
4. Uterine infection

43. 3. Because magnesium sulfate produces a smooth muscle depressive effect, the uterus should be assessed for uterine atony, which would increase the risk of postpartum hemorrhage. Uterine infection and postpartum depression aren't associated with magnesium sulfate therapy. Magnesium sulfate is considered more of an anticonvulsant than an antihypertensive.

NP: Evaluation; CN: Physiological integrity; CNS: Pharmacological and parenteral therapies; CL: Comprehension

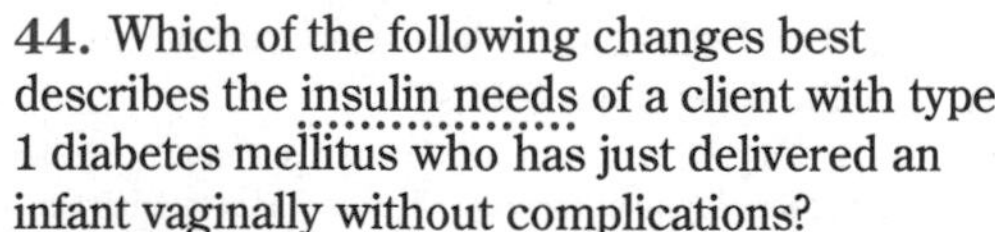

44. Which of the following changes best describes the insulin needs of a client with type 1 diabetes mellitus who has just delivered an infant vaginally without complications?

1. Increase
2. Decrease
3. Remain the same as before pregnancy
4. Remain the same as during pregnancy

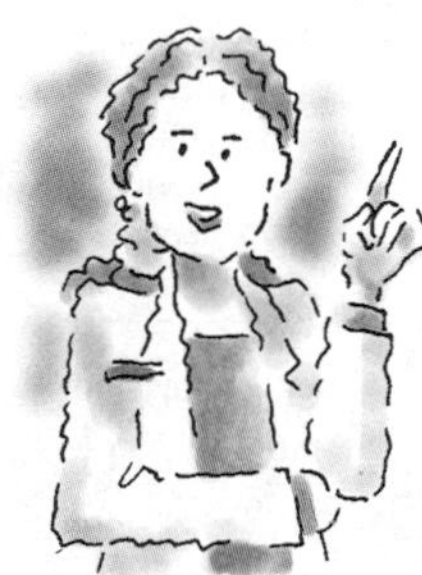

To answer question 44, think about how insulin works in the body. Take it one step at a time.

44. 2. The placenta produces the hormone human placental lactogen, an insulin antagonist. After birth, the placenta, the major source of insulin resistance, is gone. Insulin needs decrease and women with type 1 diabetes may need only one-half to two-thirds of the prenatal insulin dose during the first few postpartum days. Blood glucose levels should be monitored and insulin dosages adjusted as needed. The client should be encouraged to maintain appropriate dietary schedules, even if their infants are feeding on demand.

NP: Evaluation; CN: Physiological integrity; CNS: Physiological adaptation; CL: Comprehension

45. Which of the following responses is most appropriate for a mother with diabetes who wants to breast-feed but is concerned about the effects of breast-feeding on her health?

1. Mothers with diabetes who breast-feed have a hard time controlling their insulin needs.
2. Mothers with diabetes shouldn't breast-feed because of potential complications.
3. Mothers with diabetes shouldn't breast-feed; insulin requirements are doubled.
4. Mothers with diabetes may breast-feed; insulin requirements may decrease from breast-feeding.

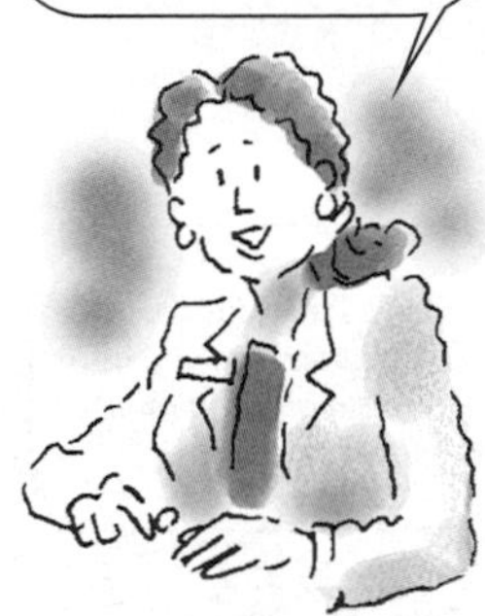

To breast-feed or not to breast-feed, that is the question for mothers today.

45. 4. Breast-feeding has an antidiabetogenic effect. Insulin needs are decreased because carbohydrates are used in milk production. Breast-feeding mothers are at a higher risk of hypoglycemia in the first postpartum days after birth because the glucose levels are lower. Mothers with diabetes should be encouraged to breast-feed.

NP: Implementation; CN: Physiological integrity; CNS: Pharmacological and parenteral therapies; CL: Comprehension

46. A multiparous client vaginally delivered an infant at 38 weeks without complications. She has three other children at home, two of whom were full-term and one a preterm. Which of the following classifications would accurately describe this client?

1. Gravida 3 Para 4104
2. Gravida 3 Para 3113
3. Gravida 4 Para 2103
4. Gravida 4 Para 3104

46. 4. Gravida is the number of times a woman has been pregnant. Parity is the number of pregnancies that have reached viability (whether the fetus was born alive or was stillborn). The *T* is term births; the *P* is preterm births; the *A* is abortions; and the *L* is living children. This client is a gravida 4 (counting this pregnancy and delivery of a full-term infant). In her obstetrical history, she delivered two other full-term infants and one preterm infant; therefore, she is P3104.

NP: Assessment; CN: Health promotion and maintenance; CNS: Growth and development through the life span; CL: Knowledge

47. Which of the following factors puts a multiparous client on her first postpartum day at risk for developing hemorrhage?

1. Hemoglobin level of 12 g/dl
2. Uterine atony
3. Thrombophlebitis
4. Moderate amount of lochia rubra

47. 2. Multiparous women often experience a loss of uterine tone due to frequent distentions of the uterus from past pregnancies. As a result, this client is also at higher risk for hemorrhage. Thrombophlebitis doesn't increase the risk of hemorrhage during the postpartal period. The hemoglobin level and lochia flow are within acceptable limits.

NP: Assessment; CN: Health promotion and maintenance; CNS: Growth and development through the life span; CL: Analysis

48. On the first postpartum night, a client requests that her baby be sent back to the nursery so she can get some sleep. The client is most likely in which of the following phases?

1. Depression phase
2. Letting-go phase
3. Taking-hold phase
4. Taking-in phase

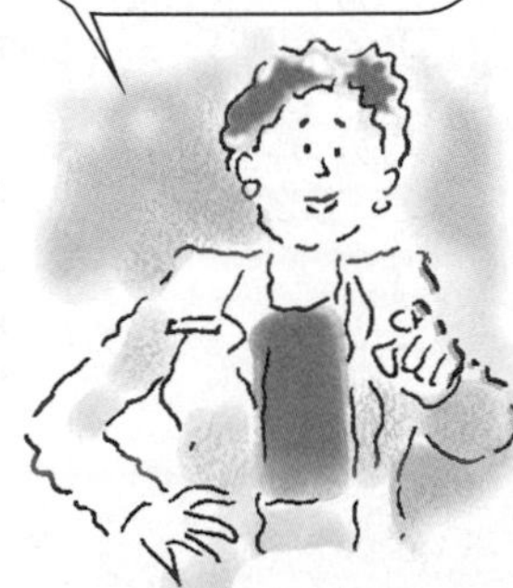

Remember, when you're dealing with a postpartum patient, you've got two patients to think about.

48. 4. The taking-in phase occurs in the first 24 hours after birth. The mother is concerned with her own needs and requires support from staff and relatives. The taking-hold phase occurs when the mother is ready to take responsibility for her care as well as her infant's care. The letting-go phase begins several weeks later, when the mother incorporates the new infant into the family unit. The depression phase isn't an appropriate answer.

NP: Assessment; CN: Health promotion and maintenance; CNS: Growth and development through the life span; CL: Analysis

49. Four clients each gave birth 12 hours ago. Which one would most likely suffer complications after birth?

1. Gravida 2 Para 2002, cesarean birth, incisional site intact, hemoglobin level 9.8 g/dl
2. Gravida 2 Para 1011, cesarean birth, incisional site intact, pulse 84 beats/minute
3. Gravida 1 Para 1001, vaginal delivery, midline episiotomy, temperature 99.8° F (37.7° C)
4. Gravida 1 Para 1001, vaginal delivery, ruptured membranes 10 hours before delivery

49. 1. Women who are anemic in pregnancy (defined as a hemoglobin < 10 g/dl) may experience more complications, such as poor wound healing and inability to tolerate activity. The vital signs in answers 2 and 3 are within normal limits. Dehydration can cause a slightly elevated temperature. Women whose membranes are ruptured more than 24 hours before birth are more prone to developing chorioamnionitis.

NP: Planning; CN: Health promotion and maintenance; CNS: Growth and development through the life span; CL: Analysis

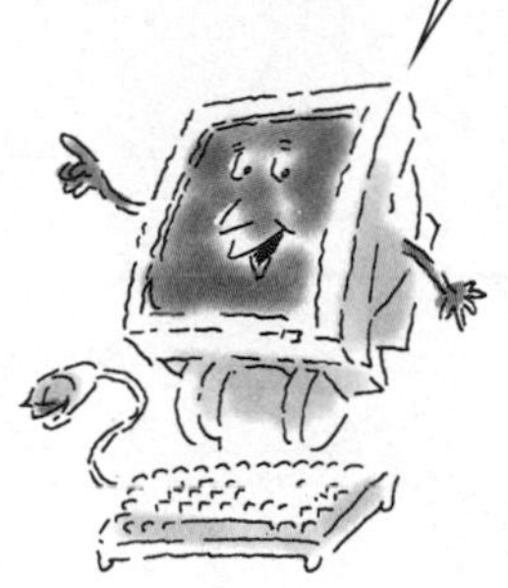

I've got two words for you: *most commonly*. Need I say more?

50. Which of the following groups of symptoms is most commonly associated with preeclampsia?

1. Edema, hyporeflexia, and glycosuria
2. Hypotension, hyporeflexia, and proteinuria
3. Hypertension, hyperreflexia, and proteinuria
4. Hyperglycemia, hyperreflexia, and glycosuria

50. 3. The hallmark signs and symptoms of preeclampsia include hypertension, hyperreflexia, and proteinuria. Preeclampsia is classified as mild or severe, according to signs and symptoms. The other choices are incorrect.

NP: Assessment; CN: Physiological integrity; CNS: Reduction of risk potential; CL: Knowledge

51. A client has delivered twins. Which of the following intervention would be most important for the nurse to perform?

1. Assess fundal tone and lochia flow.
2. Apply a cold pack to the perineal area.
3. Administer analgesics, as ordered.
4. Encourage voiding by offering the bedpan.

51. 1. Women who deliver twins are at a higher risk for postpartum hemorrhage due to overdistention of the uterus, which causes uterine atony. Assessing fundal tone and lochia flow helps to determine risks for hemorrhage. Applying cold packs to the perineum, administering analgesics as ordered, and offering the bedpan are all significant nursing interventions but not as important as preventing postpartum hemorrhage.

NP: Implementation; CN: Health promotion and maintenance; CNS: Growth and development through the life span; CL: Comprehension

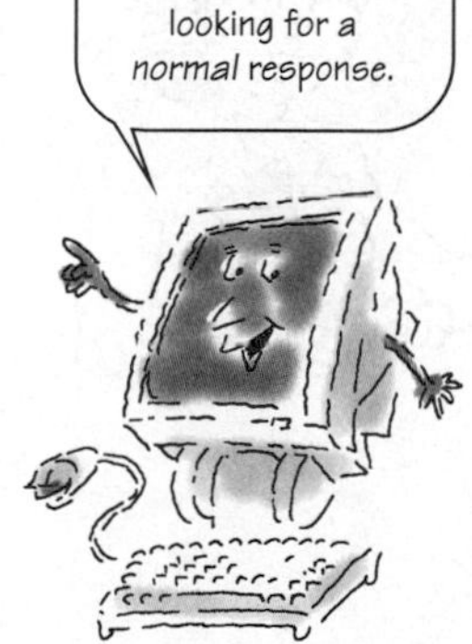

Watch it! Question 52 is looking for a *normal response*.

52. Which of the following physiological responses is considered normal in the early postpartum period?

1. Urinary urgency and dysuria
2. Rapid diuresis
3. Decrease in blood pressure
4. Increased motility of the GI system

52. 2. In the early postpartum period, there's an increase in the glomerular filtration rate and a drop in progesterone levels, which result in rapid diuresis. There should be no urinary urgency, though a woman may feel anxious about voiding. There's minimal change in blood pressure following childbirth, and a residual decrease in GI motility.

NP: Assessment; CN: Physiological integrity; CNS: Physiological adaptation; CL: Knowledge

53. During the third postpartum day, which of the following observations about the client would the nurse be most likely to make?

1. The client appears interested in learning more about neonatal care.
2. The client talks a lot about her birth experience.
3. The client sleeps whenever the neonate isn't present.
4. The client requests help in choosing a name for the neonate.

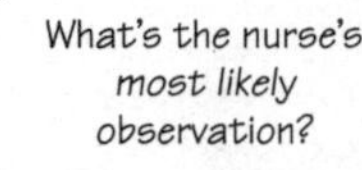

What's the nurse's most likely observation?

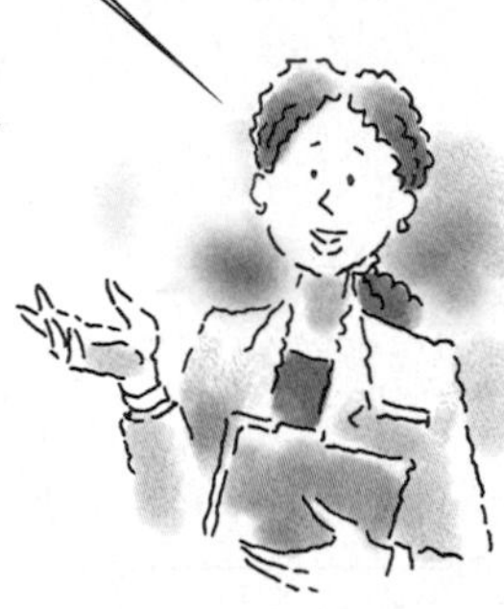

53. 1. The third to tenth days of postpartum care are the "taking-hold" phase, in which the new mother strives for independence and is eager for her neonate. The other options describe the phase in which the mother relives her birth experience.

NP: Evaluation; CN: Health promotion and maintenance; CNS: Growth and development through the life span; CL: Analysis

54. Which of the following circumstances is most likely to cause uterine atony and lead to postpartum hemorrhage?

1. Hypertension
2. Cervical and vaginal tears
3. Urine retention
4. Endometritis

54. 3. Urine retention causes a distended bladder to displace the uterus above the umbilicus and to the side, which prevents the uterus from contracting. The uterus needs to remain contracted if bleeding is to stay within normal limits. Cervical and vaginal tears can cause postpartum hemorrhage but are less common occurrences in the postpartal period. Endometritis and maternal hypertension don't cause postpartum hemorrhage.

NP: Implementation; CN: Health promotion and maintenance; CNS: Growth and development through the life span; CL: Knowledge

55. Which type of lochia should the nurse expect to find in a client 2 days postpartum?

1. Foul-smelling
2. Lochia serosa
3. Lochia alba
4. Lochia rubra

55. 4. Lochia rubra lasts about 4 days. Then comes lochia serosa, which extends through the 7th day, and then lochia alba, which occurs during the 2nd and 3rd postpartal weeks. Foul-smelling lochia is a sign of infection.

NP: Implementation; CN: Health promotion and maintenance; CNS: Growth and development through the life span; CL: Knowledge

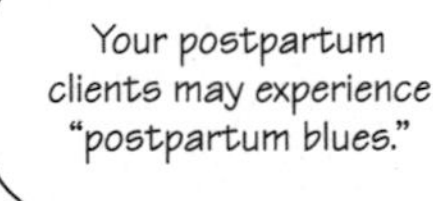

Your postpartum clients may experience "postpartum blues."

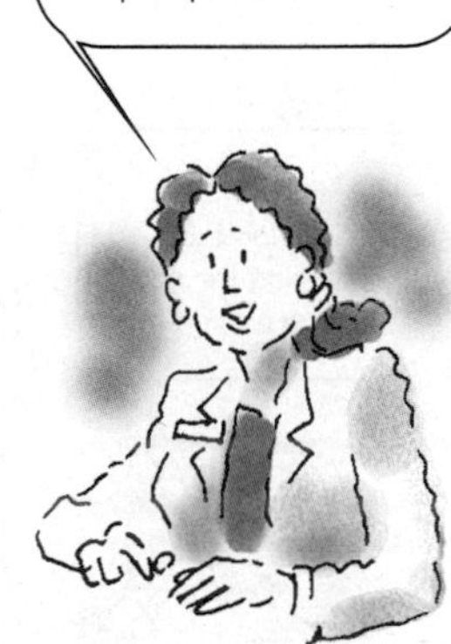

56. Which percentage of postpartum clients experiences "postpartum blues"?

1. 20% to 25%
2. 50% to 80%
3. 30% to 45%
4. 100%

56. 2. "Postpartum blues" — a transient mood alteration that arises during the first 3 weeks postpartum and is typically self-limiting — affects 50% to 80% of postpartum clients. A more severe mood alteration, seen in approximately 20% of clients, involves changes that occur within a few days after delivery and may last for a few days to more than 1 year.

NP: Assessment; CN: Psychosocial integrity; CNS: Psychosocial adaptation; CL: Application

57. When performing a comprehensive fundal check during a postpartum assessment, the nurse evaluates which fundal state?

1. Fundal consistency, location, and height
2. Fundal consistency and height
3. Fundal location and potential fundal distention
4. Fundal location and height

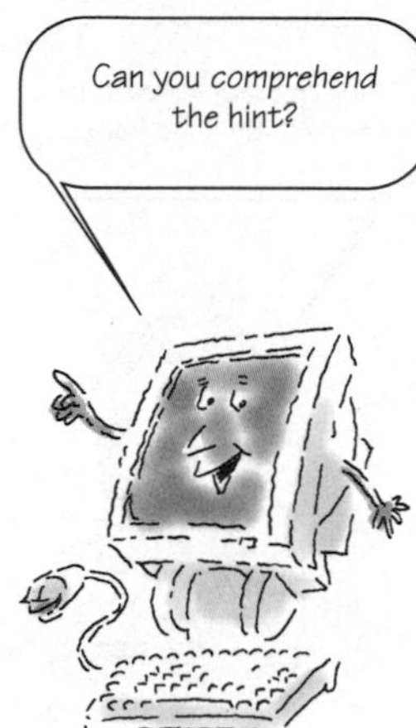

Can you comprehend the hint?

57. 1. A comprehensive fundal check includes evaluation of fundal consistency, height, and location. Normal results are a firm fundus that's at the correct height for the postpartum day and located in the center of the pelvis. Options 2, 3, and 4 don't reflect a comprehensive fundal check because they're missing valuable components.

NP: Assessment; CN: Physiological integrity; CNS: Physiological adaptation; CL: Analysis

58. During the postpartum period, which situation does a firm fundus indicate?

1. A firm tumor at the top of the uterus
2. Contraction of the uterus
3. Continuing labor contractions
4. Bladder distention

58. 2. A firm postpartum fundus means that the uterus has contracted and is constricting blood vessels, thereby decreasing lochial flow. A uterine tumor doesn't necessarily cause a firm fundus. The client wouldn't experience labor contractions during the postpartum period. Bladder distention restricts the uterus from contracting downward, resulting in a soft, boggy uterus and increased vaginal bleeding.

NP: Assessment; CN: Physiological integrity; CNS: Physiological adaptation; CL: Knowledge

59. To encourage uterine involution in a primigravid client on the first postpartum day, the nurse should instruct her to assume which position?

1. Prone
2. Knee-to-chest
3. Supine
4. Side-lying

59. 1. A prone position (lying on the abdomen) supports the abdominal muscles and aids uterine involution. To avoid air embolism, a postpartum client shouldn't assume a knee-to-chest position until at least the third postpartum week. The supine and side-lying positions don't promote involution.

NP: Implementation; CN: Health promotion and maintenance; CNS: Reduction of risk potential; CL: Comprehension

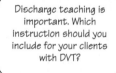

60. A postpartum client is receiving anticoagulant therapy for deep vein thrombophlebitis. Discharge teaching should include which instruction?

1. Avoid iron replacement therapy.
2. Wear a girdle and knee-high stockings whenever possible.
3. Avoid over-the-counter salicylates.
4. Be aware that shortness of breath is a common adverse effect of anticoagulants.

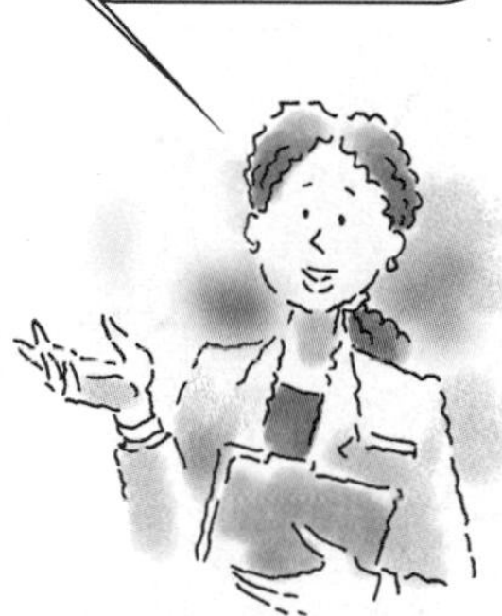

Discharge teaching is important. Which instruction should you include for your clients with DVT?

60. 3. Discharge teaching should include an instruction to avoid salicylates, which may magnify the effects of anticoagulant therapy. Iron doesn't affect anticoagulant therapy. The client should avoid restrictive clothing to prevent recurrence of thrombophlebitis. She should report shortness of breath immediately because it may indicate pulmonary embolus.

NP: Implementation; CN: Health promotion and maintenance; CNS: Reduction of risk potential; CL: Comprehension

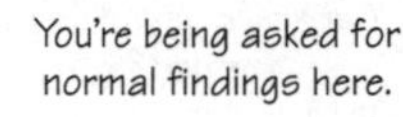

You're being asked for normal findings here.

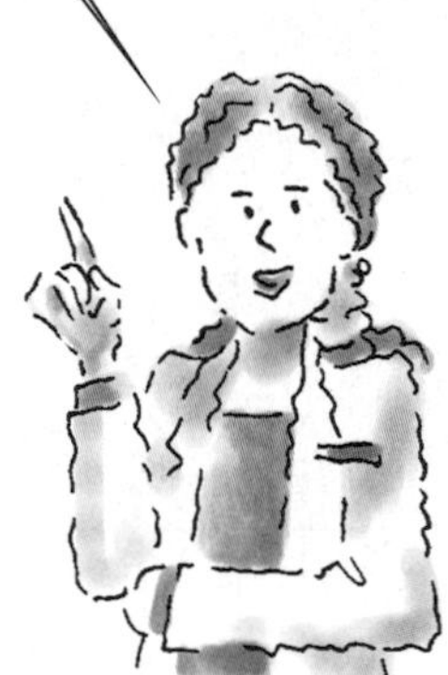

61. For a breast-feeding client on the fourth postpartum day, which breast examination findings are normal?
1. Symmetrical breast shape and size
2. Engorged breasts with inflamed, radiating areas that are sore to the touch
3. Slightly tender, cracked nipples; slightly firm, nontender breasts; transitional milk
4. Tender, intact nipples; firm, nontender breasts; transitional milk

61. 4. Tender, intact nipples; firm, nontender breasts; and transitional milk are normal in a breast-feeding client on the fourth postpartum day. Engorged, inflamed breasts signal mastitis. Tender, cracked nipples aren't a normal finding; they require intervention and client teaching to help the nipples heal and help the client avoid the problem in the future.

NP: Assessment; CN: Physiological integrity; CNS: Physiological adaptation; CL: Comprehension

62. How many additional calories should a breast-feeding primiparous client consume to ensure high-quality breast milk?
1. 500 calories/day
2. 300 calories/day
3. 400 calories/day
4. 1,000 calories/day

62. 1. A breast-feeding client should consume an additional 500 calories/day to ensure that she produces high-quality breast milk. An additional 300 or 400 calories are insufficient for breast-feeding. An additional 1,000 calories a day aren't necessary to ensure high quality breast milk and may lead to an increase in the client's weight.

NP: Planning; CN: Health promotion and maintenance; CNS: Growth and development through the life span; CL: Knowledge

63. The nurse is teaching a breast-feeding primiparous client how to prevent sore nipples. Which client statement indicates the need for further instruction?
1. "I should breast-feed for only 3 to 4 minutes at a time until my milk flow is established."
2. "I should position the baby properly during feedings."
3. "I should pull the baby gently away from my nipple after the feeding."
4. "I should prevent the baby from feeding after my breast has been emptied."

63. 1. In some cases, it takes 7 minutes for the letdown reflex to cause milk to fill the breast. The other answers indicate that the client understands the nurse's instructions.

NP: Evaluation; CN: Physiological integrity; CNS: Reduction of risk potential; CL: Application

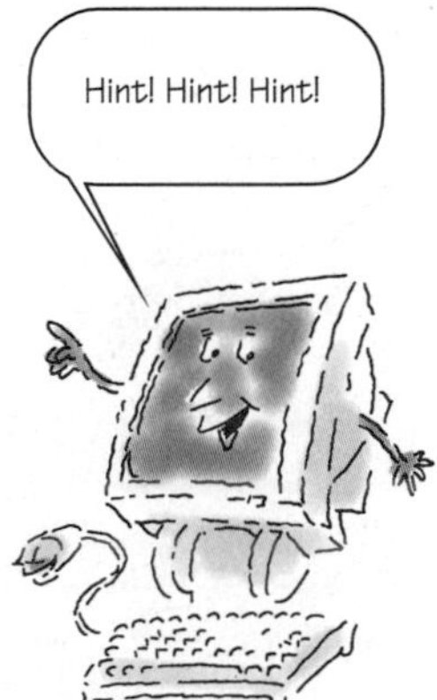

64. Which of the following statements best describes lochia rubra?
1. It contains a mixture of mucus, tissue debris, and blood.
2. It contains placental fragments and blood.
3. It contains mucus, placental fragments, and blood.
4. It contains tissue debris and blood.

64. 1. Lochia rubra contains a mixture of mucus, tissue debris, and blood. Normal lochia rubra contains no placental fragments.

NP: Assessment; CN: Physiological integrity; CNS: Physiological adaptation; CL: Knowledge

65. On the second postpartum day, a client complains that she's urinating more often than when she was pregnant. Which is the primary cause of increased urinary output after delivery?

1. Postpartum diuresis
2. Postpartum renal malfunctioning
3. Increased postpartum fluid intake
4. Postpartum breast-feeding

65. 1. Postpartum diuresis occurs as the body starts to reduce the extracellular fluid volume that increased during pregnancy. Renal plasma flow and glomerular filtration rate also increase slightly until approximately 1 week postpartum. Renal malfunctioning is more likely to decrease urinary output—not increase it. Increased postpartum fluid intake and breast-feeding aren't major causes of postpartum diuresis.

NP: Analysis; CN: Physiological integrity; CNS: Physiological adaptation; CL: Knowledge

66. Lochia alba follows lochia serosa and usually lasts from the first to third week postpartum. Which of the following statements best describes lochia alba?

1. It's creamy white to brown and may have a stale odor.
2. It's creamy white to brown, contains decidual cells, and may have a stale odor.
3. It's brown to red, contains tissue fragments, and may have an odor.
4. It's brown to red and contains decidual cells and leukocytes.

66. 2. Lochia alba is creamy white to brown, contains decidual cells, and may have a stale odor. It also contains leukocytes. Lochia alba shouldn't contain tissue fragments or have a foul odor.

NP: Assessment; CN: Physiological integrity; CNS: Physiological adaptation; CL: Comprehension

67. What's the most common major complication of retained placental fragments?

1. Puerperal infection
2. Postpartum depression
3. Postpartum hemorrhage
4. Postpartum subinvolution

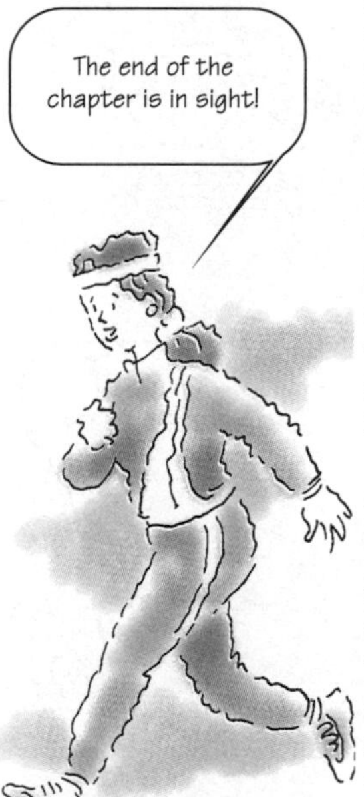

The end of the chapter is in sight!

67. 3. Retained placental fragments, which prevent the uterus from contracting properly, increase postpartum blood loss. This loss may be dramatic and lead to postpartum hemorrhage of 500 ml of blood or more. Although retained placental fragments may also lead to uterine subinvolution or infection, these are less common complications. Postpartum depression is a psychiatric disorder not related to retained placental fragments.

NP: Assessment; CN: Health promotion and maintenance; CNS: Prevention and early detection of disease; CL: Comprehension

68. Postpartum involution refers to which of the following descriptions?

1. Normal postpartum psychiatric developmental stages of the mother
2. Normal postpartum coping stages of the mother
3. Normal postpartum uterine contractions that force the uterus to shrink
4. Abnormal postpartum uterine activity

68. 3. Uterine involution is the normal contraction of the uterus during the immediate and prolonged postpartum periods, during which the uterine walls shrink rapidly and lochial contents are evacuated. Involution isn't a psychiatric developmental or coping stage.

NP: Assessment; CN: Physiological integrity; CNS: Physiological adaptation; CL: Knowledge

69. Which of the following descriptions refers to a puerperal infection?

1. Infection of the neonate's umbilicus
2. Infection of the breast-feeding mother's nipples
3. Infection of the maternal genital tract postpartally
4. Infection of the maternal blood

69. 3. A puerperal infection is an infection of the maternal genital tract after delivery. Generally, it results from invasion by bacteria, such as group A beta-hemolytic streptococci, staphylococcus, coliform, and other organisms. Labor and delivery may reduce a woman's resistance to infection by bacteria usually found in the body. A puerperal infection isn't related to infection of the neonate's umbilicus or to a maternal nipple or blood infection.

NP: Analysis; CN: Physiological integrity; CNS: Physiological adaptation; CL: Comprehension

70. Uterine involution begins immediately after delivery and continues until the uterus is as close to its prepregnant size as possible. Immediately after delivery, the uterine fundus should be at which level?

1. Above the symphysis pubis
2. At the umbilicus
3. Midway between the symphysis pubis and umbilicus
4. Two or three fingerbreadths above the umbilicus

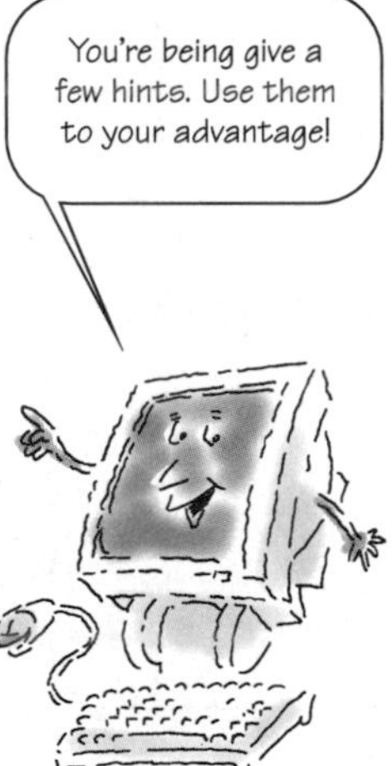

You're being give a few hints. Use them to your advantage!

70. 2. Immediately postpartum, the uterine fundus should be at the level of the umbilicus. Thereafter, the fundus generally is 1 fingerbreadth below the umbilicus for each postpartum day—until day 9 or 10, when it's just above the symphysis pubis. For example, in a client who's 3 days postpartum, the fundus should be located approximately 3 fingerbreadths below the umbilicus.

NP: Assessment; CN: Physiological integrity; CNS: Physiological adaptation; CL: Comprehension

71. On the tenth postpartum day, a primiparous client is admitted to the hospital with a diagnosis of femoral thrombophlebitis. Her treatment plan includes bed rest, analgesic therapy, and subcutaneous heparin administration. During assessment, which action takes highest priority?

1. Measurement of the pulse rate
2. Evaluation of lochial flow
3. Measurement of blood pressure
4. Evaluation of breast-feeding status

71. 2. Because heparin's anticoagulant effects may contribute to postpartum hemorrhage, evaluating the amount of lochial flow takes highest priority. Although the nurse should assess vital signs frequently, pulse rate and blood pressure evaluation aren't priorities at this time. A breast-feeding client can continue to take heparin; evaluation of her breast-feeding status isn't relevant.

NP: Assessment; CN: Safe, effective care management; CNS: Management of care; CL: Knowledge

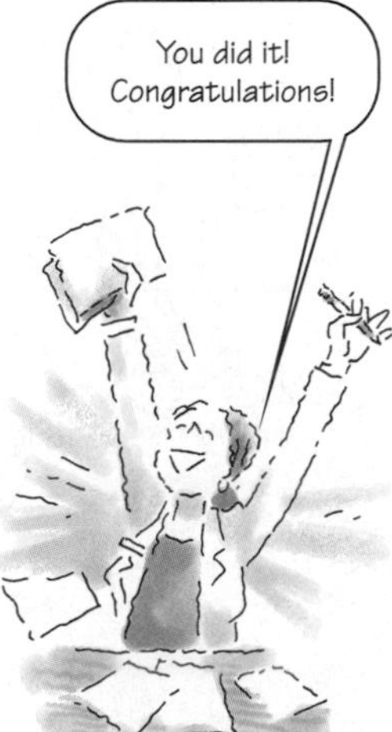

You did it! Congratulations!

72. A multiparous client with pelvic thrombophlebitis is being treated with bed rest and anticoagulant therapy. The nurse should call for assistance immediately if the client experiences which sign or symptom?

1. Pain in the pelvic area
2. Increased blood pressure
3. Urine retention
4. Sudden, sharp chest pain

72. 4. Sudden, sharp chest pain and difficulty breathing indicate pulmonary embolism—a medical emergency that may result from thrombophlebitis. Pain in the pelvic area may be associated with pelvic thrombophlebitis but doesn't require immediate assistance. Increased blood pressure and urine retention aren't associated with pulmonary embolism or anticoagulant therapy.

NP: Implementation; CN: Physiological integrity; CNS: Reduction of risk potential; CL: Application

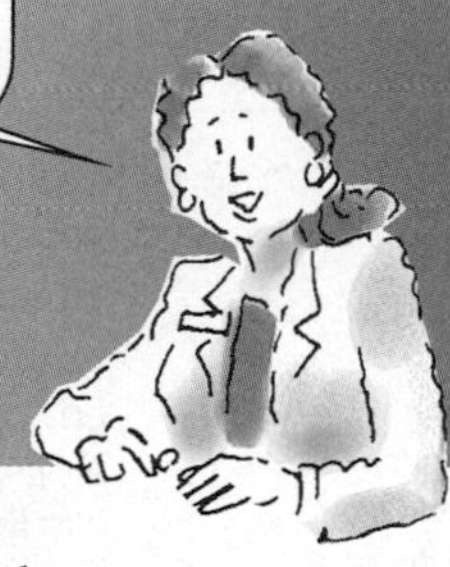

Neonates depend on you for everything. Let's show 'em you've got what it takes for neonatal care!

Chapter 25 Neonatal care

1. A client has given birth to a preterm male neonate. The client tells the nurse that she still wants to breast-feed her neonate. The nurse should explain to the mother that:

1. Breast milk contains antibodies that help protect her neonate.
2. Commercial formula will provide better nutrition for the neonate.
3. Breast-feeding can be started when the neonate is ready for discharge.
4. The neonate will be less likely to develop an infection on commercial formula.

1. 1. Studies have proven that breast milk provides preterm neonates with better protection from infection, such as necrotizing enterocolitis, because of the antibodies contained in breast milk. Commercial formula doesn't provide any better nutrition than breast milk. Breast milk feedings can be started as soon as the neonate is stable, and the neonate is more likely to develop infections when fed formula rather than breast milk.

NP: Planning; CN: Health promotion and maintenance; CNS: Reduction of risk potential; CL: Application

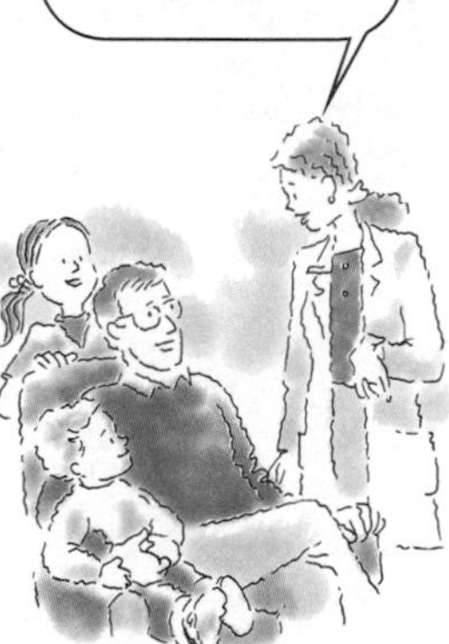

Your baby is being given a drug to help him breathe better.

2. Which action best explains the main role of surfactant in the neonate?

1. Assists with ciliary body maturation in the upper airways
2. Helps maintain a rhythmic breathing pattern
3. Promotes clearing mucus from the respiratory tract
4. Helps the lungs remain expanded after the initiation of breathing

2. 4. Surfactant works by reducing surface tension in the lung. Surfactant allows the lung to remain slightly expanded, decreasing the amount of work required for inspiration. Surfactant hasn't been shown to influence ciliary body maturation, clear the respiratory tract, or regulate the neonate's breathing pattern.

NP: Assessment; CN: Health promotion and maintenance; CNS: Growth and development through the life span; CL: Knowledge

3. While assessing a 2-hour-old neonate, the nurse observes the neonate to have acrocyanosis. Which of the following nursing actions should be performed initially?

1. Activate the code blue or emergency system.
2. Do nothing because acrocyanosis is normal in the neonate.
3. Immediately take the neonate's temperature according to hospital policy.
4. Notify the physician of the need for a cardiac consult.

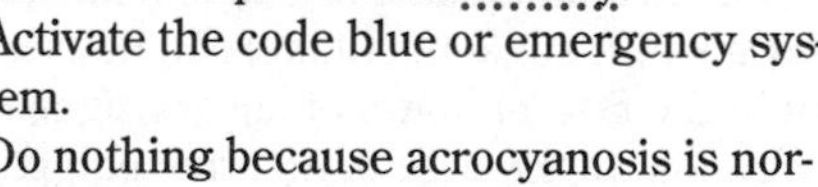

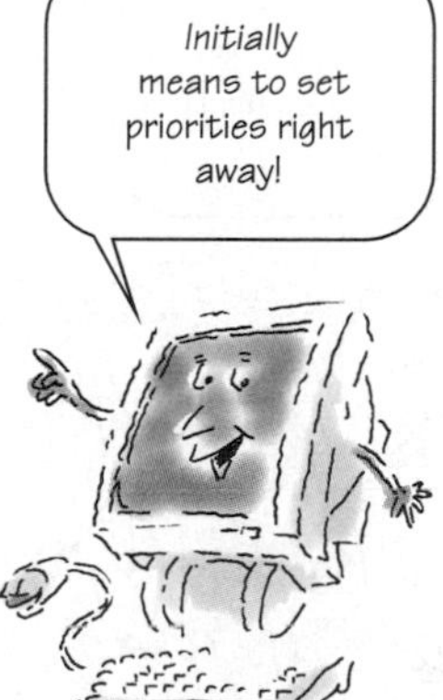

Initially means to set priorities right away!

3. 2. Acrocyanosis, or bluish discoloration of the hands and feet in the neonate (also called peripheral cyanosis), is a normal finding and shouldn't last more than 24 hours after birth. The other choices are inappropriate.

NP: Assessment; CN: Physiological integrity; CNS: Physiological adaptation; CL: Application

4. When teaching parents of a neonate the proper position for the neonate's sleep, the nurse stresses the importance of placing the neonate on his back to reduce the risk of which of the following?

1. Aspiration
2. Sudden infant death syndrome (SIDS)
3. Suffocation
4. Gastroesophageal reflux (GER)

4. 2. Supine positioning is recommended to reduce the risk of SIDS in infancy. The risk of aspiration is slightly increased with the supine position. Suffocation would be less likely with an infant supine than prone and the position for GER requires the head of the bed to be elevated.

NP: Implementation; CN: Health promotion and maintenance; CNS: Reduction of risk potential; CL: Application

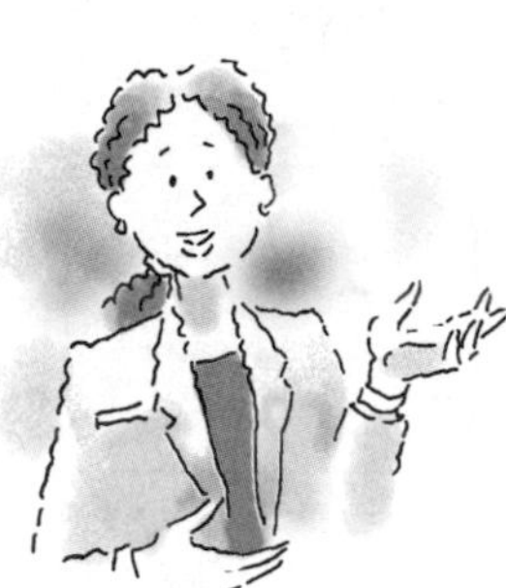

Knowing the risk factors can help guide your assessment.

5. The nurse is aware that a neonate of a mother with diabetes is at risk for which complication?

1. Anemia
2. Hypoglycemia
3. Nitrogen loss
4. Thrombosis

5. 2. Neonates of mothers with diabetes are at risk for hypoglycemia due to increased insulin levels. During gestation, an increased amount of glucose is transferred to the fetus through the placenta. The neonate's liver can't initially adjust to the changing glucose levels after birth. This may result in an overabundance of insulin in the neonate, resulting in hypoglycemia. Neonates of mothers with diabetes aren't at increased risk for anemia, nitrogen loss, or thrombosis.

NP: Analysis; CN: Physiological integrity; CNS: Reduction of risk potential; CL: Knowledge

6. Which complication is common in neonates who receive prolonged mechanical ventilation at birth?

1. Bronchopulmonary dysplasia
2. Esophageal atresia
3. Hydrocephalus
4. Renal failure

6. 1. Bronchopulmonary dysplasia commonly results from the high pressures that must sometimes be used to maintain adequate oxygenation. Esophageal atresia, a structural defect in which the esophagus and trachea communicate with each other, doesn't relate to mechanical ventilation. Hydrocephalus and renal failure don't typically occur in these clients.

NP: Analysis; CN: Physiological integrity; CNS: Reduction of risk potential; CL: Analysis

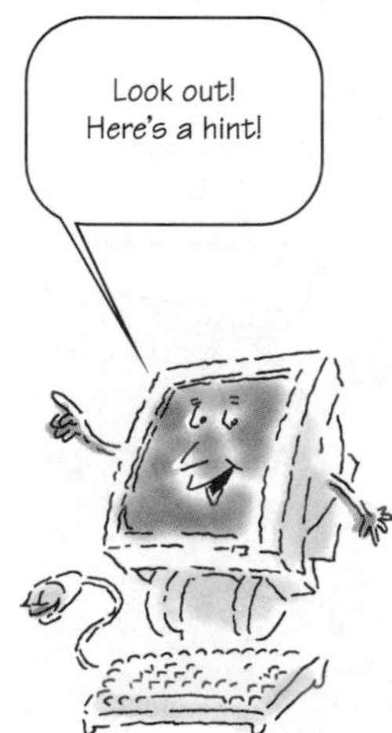

Look out!
Here's a hint!

7. When performing neonatal assessment, which is the best indication of adequate hydration?

1. Soft, smooth skin
2. A sunken fontanel
3. Frequent spitting up
4. No urine output in the first 24 hours of life

7. 1. Soft, smooth skin is a sign of adequate hydration. A sunken fontanel and no urine output in the first 24 hours of life are signs of poor hydration. In the case of no urine output, kidney dysfunction would also be a concern. Frequent spitting up is normal in neonates. Excessive spitting up, however, may result in poor hydration.

NP: Assessment; CN: Physiological integrity; CNS: Physiological adaptation; CL: Analysis

8. When performing a neurologic assessment, which sign is considered a normal finding in a neonate?

1. Doll eyes
2. "Sunset" eyes
3. Positive Babinski's sign
4. Pupils that don't react to light

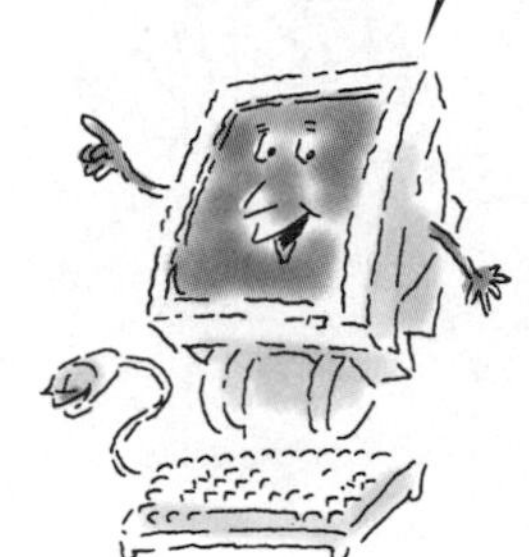

Question 8 asks what's normal. It could just as easily ask what's abnormal. Always double-check this kind of term.

8. 3. A positive Babinski's sign is present in infants until approximately age 1. A positive Babinski's reflex is normal in neonates but abnormal in adults. The appearance of "sunset" eyes, in which the sclera is visible above the iris, results from cranial nerve palsies and may indicate increased intracranial pressure. Doll eyes is also a neurologic response but it's noted in adults. A neonate's pupils normally react to light as in an adult.

NP: Analysis; CN: Physiologic integrity; CNS: Basic care and comfort; CL: Analysis

9. At what gestational age is a conceptus considered viable (able to live outside the womb)?

1. 9 weeks
2. 14 weeks
3. 24 weeks
4. 30 weeks

9. 3. At approximately 23 to 24 weeks' gestation, the lungs are developed enough to sometimes maintain extrauterine life. The lungs are the most immature system during the gestational period. Medical care for premature labor begins much earlier (aggressively at 21 weeks' gestation).

NP: Assessment; CN: Health promotion and maintenance; CNS: Growth and development through the life span; CL: Knowledge

10. A client's mother asks the nurse why her newborn grandson is getting an injection of vitamin K. Which best explains why this drug is given to neonates?

1. Vitamin K assists with coagulation.
2. Vitamin K assists the gut to mature.
3. Vitamin K initiates the immunization process.
4. Vitamin K protects the brain from excess fluid production.

10. 1. Vitamin K, deficient in the neonate, is needed to activate clotting factors II, VII, IX, and X. In the event of trauma, the neonate would be at risk for excessive bleeding. Vitamin K doesn't assist the gut to mature, but the gut produces vitamin K once maturity is achieved. Vitamin K doesn't influence fluid production in the brain or the immunization process.

NP: Planning; CN: Physiological integrity; CNS: Reduction of risk potential; CL: Application

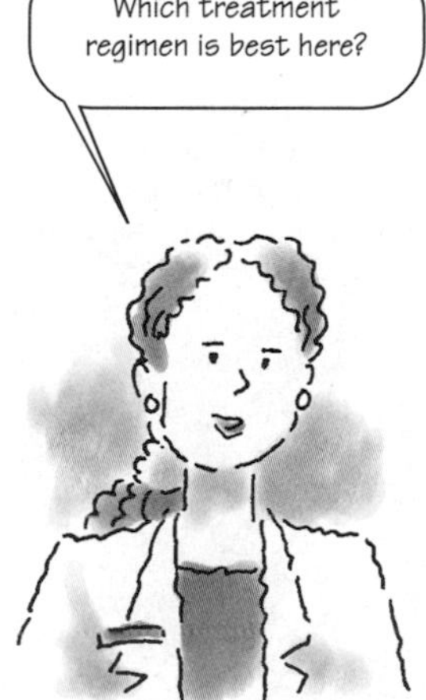

Which treatment regimen is best here?

11. Neonates born to women infected with hepatitis B should undergo which treatment regimen?

1. Hepatitis B vaccine at birth and 1 month
2. Hepatitis B immune globulin at birth; no hepatitis B vaccine
3. Hepatitis B immune globulin within 48 hours of birth and hepatitis B vaccine at 1 month
4. Hepatitis B immune globulin within 12 hours of birth and hepatitis B vaccine at birth, 1 month, and 6 months

11. 4. Hepatitis B immune globulin should be given as soon as possible after birth but within 12 hours. Neonates should also receive hepatitis B vaccine at regularly scheduled intervals. This sequence of care has been determined as superior to the others provided.

NP: Planning; CN: Health promotion and maintenance; CNS: Prevention and early detection of disease; CL: Knowledge

12. When a neonate is delivered with meconium staining in the amnionic fluid, which sequence of events will most effectively decrease the risk of meconium aspiration?

1. Deliver the thorax, then suction the nose.
2. Clamp the umbilical cord, then suction the neonate's mouth.
3. Deliver the head, then suction the mouth and then the nose.
4. Deliver the thorax, then suction the nose and then the mouth.

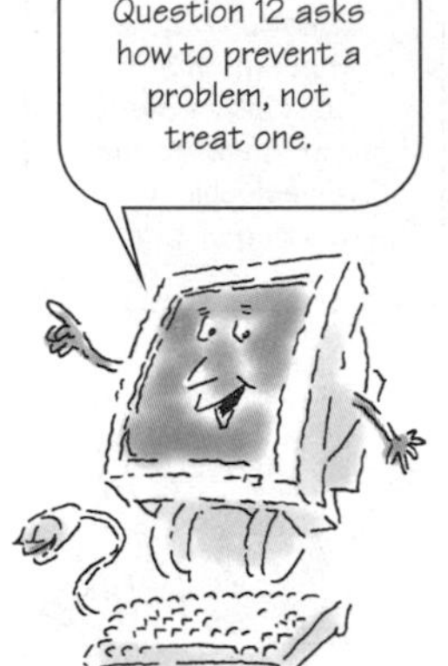

Question 12 asks how to prevent a problem, not treat one.

12. 3. To minimize the risk of aspiration of meconium after delivery, the neonate's mouth, then nose, should be suctioned after delivery of the head. This suctioning shouldn't be delayed until after delivery of the thorax because the neonate will take its first breath with meconium in its mouth.

NP: Implementation; CN: Physiological integrity; CN: Reduction of risk potential; CL: Analysis

13. Erythromycin ointment is administered to the neonate's eyes shortly after birth to prevent which disorder?

1. Cataracts
2. Diabetic retinopathy
3. Ophthalmia neonatorum
4. Strabismus

13. 3. Eye prophylaxis is administered to the neonate immediately or soon after birth to prevent ophthalmia neonatorum. Strabismus is neuromuscular incoordination of the eye alignment. Cataracts are opacity of the lens of the eye associated with children with congenital rubella, galactosemia, and cortisone therapy. Diabetic retinopathy occurs in clients with diabetes when the retina bleeds into the vitreous causing scarring, after which neovascularization occurs.

NP: Planning; CN: Health promotion and maintenance; CNS: Prevention and early detection of disease; CL: Knowledge

14. A client with group AB blood whose husband has group O blood has just given birth. The major sign of ABO blood incompatibility in the neonate is which complication or test result?

1. Negative Coombs' test
2. Bleeding from nose or ear
3. Jaundice after the first 24 hours of life
4. Jaundice within the first 24 hours of life

14. 4. The neonate with an ABO blood incompatibility with its mother will have jaundice within the first 24 hours of life. The neonate would have a positive Coombs' test result. Jaundice after the first 24 hours of life is physiologic jaundice. Bleeding from the nose and ear should be investigated for possible causes but probably isn't related to ABO incompatibility.

NP: Analysis; CN: Health promotion and maintenance; CNS: Growth and development through the life span; CL: Knowledge

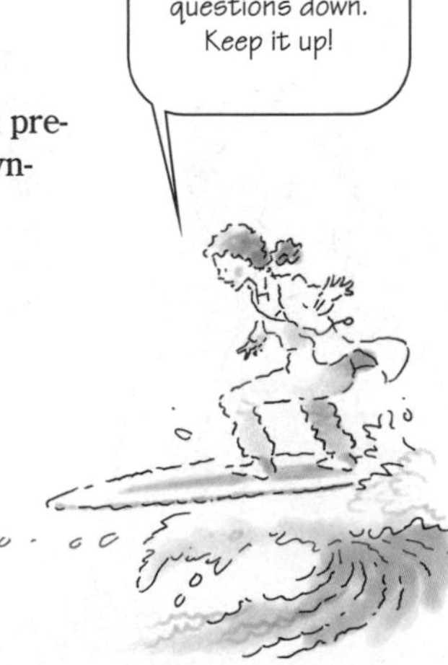

That's 15 questions down. Keep it up!

15. Which circumstance of delivery would predispose a neonate to respiratory distress syndrome (RDS)?

1. Premature birth
2. Vaginal delivery
3. First born of twins
4. Postdate pregnancy

15. 1. Prematurity is the single most important risk factor for developing RDS. The second born of twins and neonates born by cesarean delivery are also at increased risk for RDS. Surfactant deficiency, which frequently results in RDS, isn't a problem for postdate neonates.

NP: Analysis; CN: Health promotion and maintenance; CNS: Growth and development through the life span; CL: Analysis

16. Two days after circumcision, the nurse notes a yellow-white exudate around the head of the neonate's penis. What would be the most appropriate nursing intervention?
1. Leave the area alone as this is a normal finding.
2. Report the findings to the physician and document it.
3. Take the neonate's temperature because an infection is suspected.
4. Try to remove the exudate with a warm washcloth.

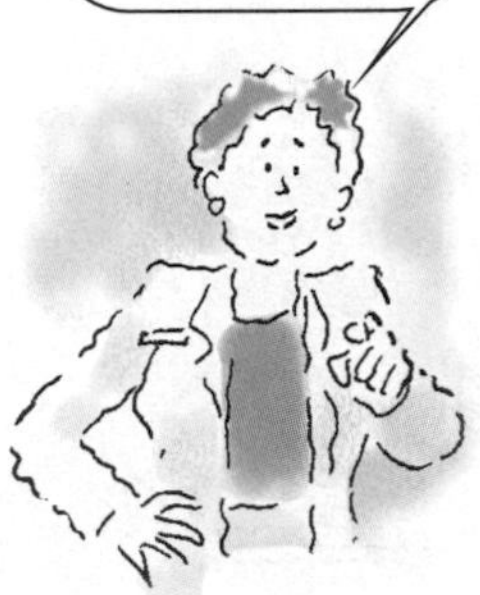

The color of an exudate helps determine its cause.

16. 1. The yellow-white exudate is part of the granulation process and a normal finding for a healing penis after circumcision. Therefore, notifying the physician isn't necessary. There's no indication of an infection that would necessitate taking the neonate's temperature. The exudate shouldn't be removed.

NP: Implementation; CN: Health promotion and maintenance; CNS: Growth and development through the life span; CL: Analysis

17. A client has just given birth at 42 weeks' gestation. When assessing the neonate, which physical finding is expected?
1. A sleepy, lethargic baby
2. Lanugo covering the body
3. Desquamation of the epidermis
4. Vernix caseosa covering the body

17. 3. Postdate fetuses lose the vernix caseosa, and the epidermis may become desquamated. These neonates are usually very alert. Lanugo is missing in the postdate neonate.

NP: Assessment; CN: Health promotion and maintenance; CNS: Growth and development through the life span; CL: Knowledge

18. The small-for-gestation neonate is at increased risk during the transitional period for which complication?
1. Anemia probably due to chronic fetal hypoxia
2. Hyperthermia due to decreased glycogen stores
3. Hyperglycemia due to decreased glycogen stores
4. Polycythemia probably due to chronic fetal hypoxia

18. 4. The small-for-gestation neonate is at risk for developing polycythemia during the transitional period in an attempt to decrease hypoxia. The neonates are also at increased risk for developing hypoglycemia and hypothermia due to decreased glycogen stores.

NP: Analysis; CN: Health promotion and maintenance; CNS: Growth and development through the life span; CL: Analysis

19. Which finding might be seen in a neonate suspected of having an infection?
1. Flushed cheeks
2. Increased temperature
3. Decreased temperature
4. Increased activity level

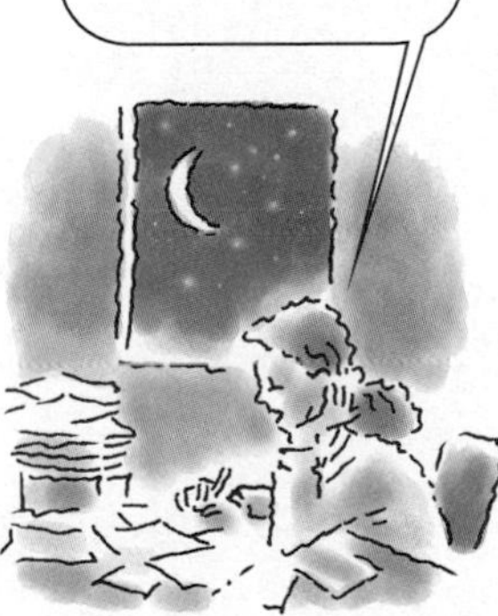

The test-taking expertise you're gaining from answering these questions will be well worth the effort you're putting in. Keep at it!

19. 3. Temperature instability, especially when it results in a low temperature in the neonate, may be a sign of infection. The neonate's color often changes with an infection process but generally becomes ashen or mottled. The neonate with an infection will usually show a decrease in activity level or lethargy.

NP: Assessment; CN: Health promotion and maintenance; CNS: Growth and development through the life span; CL: Analysis

20. Which symptom would indicate the neonate was adapting appropriately to extrauterine life without difficulty?

1. Nasal flaring
2. Light audible grunting
3. Respiratory rate 40 to 60 breaths/minute
4. Respiratory rate 60 to 80 breaths/minute

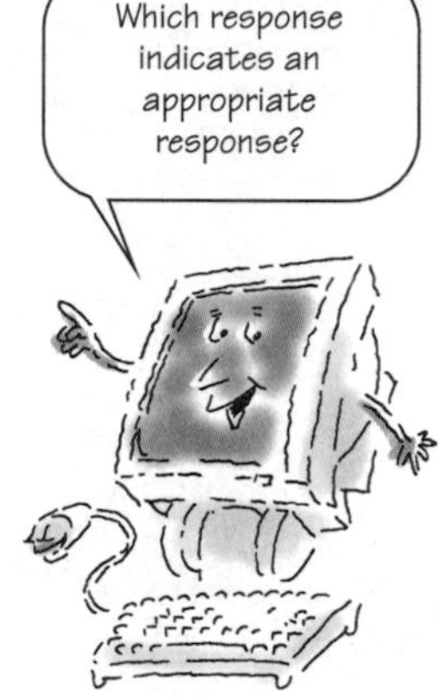
Which response indicates an appropriate response?

20. 3. A respiratory rate 40 to 60 breaths/minute is normal for a neonate during the transitional period. Nasal flaring, respiratory rate more than 60 breaths/minute, and audible grunting are signs of respiratory distress.

NP: Assessment; CN: Health maintenance and promotion; CNS: Growth and development through the life span; CL: Knowledge

21. After reviewing the client's maternal history of magnesium sulfate during labor, which condition would the nurse anticipate as a potential problem in the neonate?

1. Hypoglycemia
2. Jitteriness
3. Respiratory depression
4. Tachycardia

21. 3. Magnesium sulfate crosses the placenta and adverse neonatal effects are respiratory depression, hypotonia, and bradycardia. The serum blood sugar isn't affected by magnesium sulfate. The neonate would be floppy, not jittery.

NP: Analysis; CN: Physiological integrity; CNS: Pharmacological and parenteral therapies; CL: Analysis

22. Which intervention is helpful for the neonate experiencing drug withdrawal?

1. Place the isolette in a quiet area of the nursery.
2. Withhold all medication to improve the liver's metabolization of drugs.
3. Dress the neonate in loose clothing so he won't feel restricted.
4. Place the isolette near the nurses' station for frequent contact with health care workers.

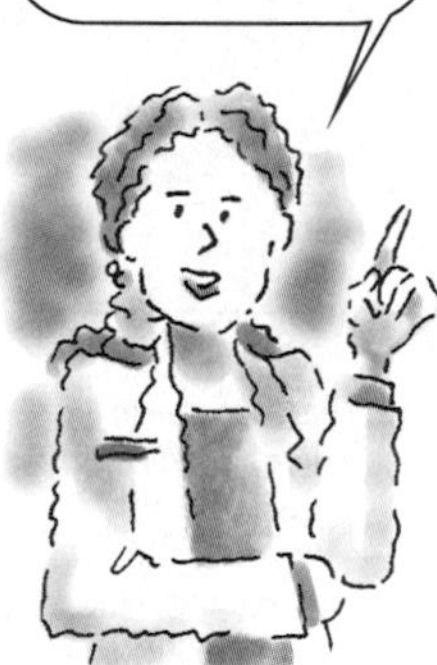
Some neonates need special interventions.

22. 1. Neonates experiencing drug withdrawal often have sleep disturbance. The neonate should be moved to a quiet area of the nursery to minimize environmental stimuli. The neonate should be swaddled to prevent him from flailing and stimulating himself. Medications, such as phenobarbital and paregoric, should be given as needed.

NP: Implementation; CN: Psychosocial integrity; CNS: Psychosocial adaptation; CL: Analysis

23. Neonates of mothers with diabetes are at risk for which complication following birth?

1. Atelectasis
2. Microcephaly
3. Pneumothorax
4. Macrosomia

23. 4. Neonates of mothers with diabetes are at increased risk for macrosomia (excessive fetal growth) as a result of the combination of the increased supply of maternal glucose and an increase in fetal insulin. Along with macrosomia, neonates of diabetic mothers are at risk for respiratory distress syndrome, hypoglycemia, hypocalcemia, hyperbilirubinemia, and congenital anomalies. They aren't at greater risk for atelectasis or pneumothorax. Microcephaly is usually the result of cytomegalovirus or rubella virus infection.

NP: Analysis; CN: Health promotion and maintenance; CNS: Growth and development through the life span; CL: Knowledge

24. Neonates are given which medication to prevent hemorrhagic disease of the neonate?

1. Vitamin K
2. Heparin
3. Iron
4. Warfarin

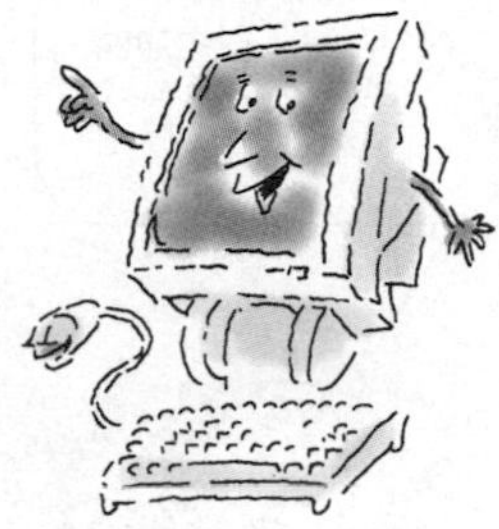

Which measure is
preventive, rather
than curative or

24. 1. Neonates have coagulation deficiencies because of a lack of vitamin K in the intestines, which helps the liver synthesize clotting factors II, VII, IX, and X. Heparin and warfarin are given as anticoagulant therapy, not to prevent hemorrhagic disease in the neonate. Iron is stored in the fetal liver; hemoglobin binds to iron and carries oxygen.

NP: Implementation; CN: Health promotion and maintenance; CNS: Growth and development through the life span; CL: Knowledge

25. During the transition period, a neonate can lose heat in many different ways. A neonate who isn't completely dried immediately after birth or a bath loses heat through which of the following methods?

1. Conduction
2. Convection
3. Evaporation
4. Radiation

25. 3. Evaporation is the loss of heat that occurs when a liquid is converted to a vapor. In the neonate, heat loss by evaporation occurs as a result of vaporization of moisture from the skin. Convection is the flow of heat from the body surface to cooler air. Conduction is the loss of heat from the body surface to cooler surfaces in direct contact. Radiation is the loss of heat to a cooler surface that isn't in direct contact with the neonate.

NP: Implementation; CN: Health promotion and maintenance; CNS: Growth and development through the life span; CL: Knowledge

26. By keeping the nursery temperature warm and wrapping the neonate in blankets, the nurse is preventing which type of heat loss?

1. Conduction
2. Convection
3. Evaporation
4. Radiation

26. 2. Convection heat loss is the flow of heat from the body surface to cooler air. Evaporation is the loss of heat that occurs when a liquid is converted to a vapor. Conduction is the loss of heat from the body surface to cooler surfaces in direct contact. Radiation is the loss of heat from the body surface to cooler solid surfaces not in direct contact but in relative proximity.

NP: Implementation; CN: Health promotion and maintenance; CNS: Growth and development through the life span; CL: Knowledge

27. Which statement is the best explanation for physiologic hyperbilirubinemia?

1. The neonate usually also has a medical problem.
2. In term neonates, it usually appears after 24 hours.
3. It's caused by elevated conjugated bilirubin levels.
4. It's usually progressive from the neonate's feet to his head.

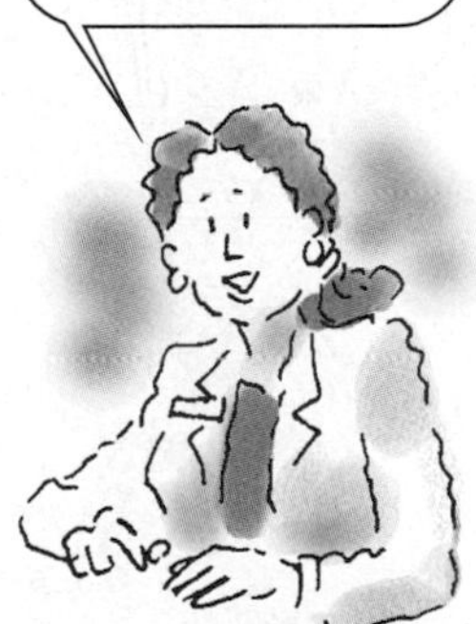

Be careful with this
prefix. Hyper is
almost identical to
hypo but its
meaning, of course,
is vastly different.

27. 2. Physiologic jaundice in term neonates first appears after 24 hours. Jaundice usually appears in a cephalocaudal progression from head to feet. Neonates are otherwise healthy and have no medical problems. Hyperbilirubinemia is caused almost exclusively from unconjugated bilirubin.

NP: Analysis; CN: Physiological integrity; CNS: Reduction of risk potential; CL: Knowledge

28. A neonate has been diagnosed with caput succedaneum. Which statement is correct about caput succedaneum?

1. It usually resolves in 3 to 6 weeks.
2. It doesn't cross the cranial suture line.
3. It's a collection of blood between the skull and periosteum.
4. It involves swelling of the tissue over the presenting part of the fetal head.

28. 4. Caput succedaneum is the swelling of tissue over the presenting part of the fetal scalp due to sustained pressure. This boggy edematous swelling is present at birth, crosses the suture line, and most commonly occurs in the occipital area. A cephalhematoma is a collection of blood between the skull and periosteum that doesn't cross cranial suture lines and resolves in 3 to 6 weeks. Caput succedaneum resolves within 3 to 4 days.

NP: Analysis; CN: Physiological integrity; CNS: Reduction of risk potential; CL: Knowledge

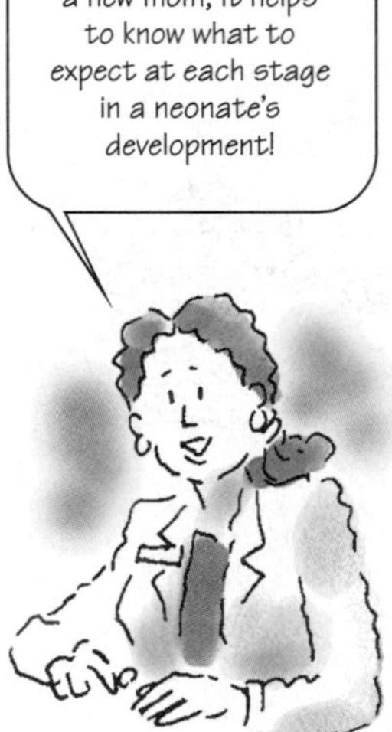

When you're teaching a new mom, it helps to know what to expect at each stage in a neonate's development!

29. The nurse is teaching a postpartum client about the normal stooling pattern of a neonate. Which color and consistency best describes the typical appearance of meconium?

1. Soft, pale yellow
2. Hard, pale brown
3. Sticky green, black
4. Loose, golden yellow

29. 3. Meconium collects in the GI tract during gestation and is initially sterile. Meconium is greenish black because of occult blood and is viscous. The stools of breast-fed neonates are loose golden yellow after the transition to extrauterine life. The stools of formula-fed babies are typically soft and pale yellow after feeding is well established.

NP: Assessment; CN: Health promotion and maintenance; CNS: Growth and development through the life span; CL: Knowledge

30. A 3-day-old neonate needs phototherapy for hyperbilirubinemia. Nursery care of a neonate receiving phototherapy would include which nursing intervention?

1. Tube feedings
2. Feeding the neonate under phototherapy lights
3. Mask over the eyes to prevent retinal damage
4. Temperature monitored every 6 hours during phototherapy

30. 3. The neonate's eyes must be covered with eye patches to prevent damage. The mouth of the neonate doesn't need to be covered during phototherapy. The neonate can be removed from the lights and held for feeding. The neonate's temperature should be monitored at least every 2 to 4 hours due to the risk of hyperthermia with phototherapy.

NP: Analysis; CN: Physiological integrity; CNS: Physiological adaptation; CL: Analysis

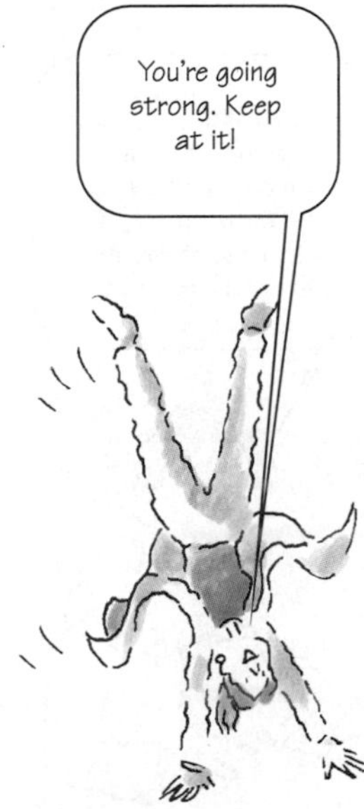

You're going strong. Keep at it!

31. Which of the following neonates would be most likely to develop hyperbilirubinemia?

1. Blacks
2. Neonate of Rh-positive mother
3. Neonate with ABO incompatibility
4. Neonate with Apgar scores 9 and 10 at 1 and 5 minutes

31. 3. The mother's blood type, which is different from the neonate's, has an impact on the neonate's bilirubin level due to the antigen-antibody reaction. Black neonates tend to have lower mean levels of bilirubin. Chinese, Japanese, Korean, and Greek neonates tend to have higher incidences of hyperbilirubinemia. Neonates of Rh-negative, not Rh-positive, mothers tend to have hyperbilirubinemia. Low Apgar scores may indicate a risk for hyperbilirubinemia.

NP: Analysis; CN: Physiological integrity; CNS: Physiological adaptation; CL: Knowledge

32. Gram-positive cocci are responsible for causing 15% to 25% of the major neonatal infections. Which is an example of a gram-positive bacteria?

1. *Escherichia coli*
2. Group B streptococci
3. *Klebsiella* species
4. *Pseudomonas aeruginosa*

32. 2. Group B streptococci are gram-positive cocci that the neonate is exposed to if these bacteria are colonized in the vaginal tract. *Escherichia coli, Pseudomonas aeruginosa,* and *Klebsiella* species are gram-negative rods that produce 78% to 85% of the bacterial infection in neonates.

NP: Analysis; CN: Physiological integrity; CNS: Physiological adaptation; CL: Knowledge

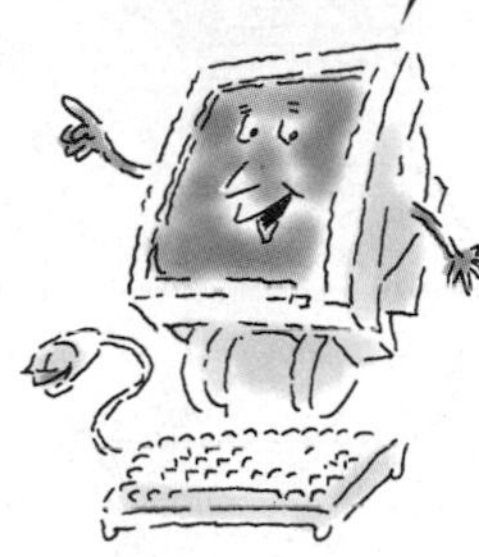

Here's an important clue to the correct answer: most common.

33. The most common neonatal sepsis and meningitis infections seen within 24 hours after birth are caused by which organism?

1. *Candida albicans*
2. *Chlamydia trachomatis*
3. *Escherichia coli*
4. Group B beta-hemolytic streptococci

33. 4. Transmission of group B beta-hemolytic streptococci to the fetus results in respiratory distress that can rapidly lead to septic shock. *E. coli* is the second most common cause. *C. trachomatis* infection causes neonatal conjunctivitis and pneumonia. Candidiasis may be acquired from the birth canal.

NP: Analysis; CN: Physiological integrity; CNS: Physiological adaptation; CL: Knowledge

34. The nurse understands that eythromycin ointment is applied to a neonate's eyes immediately after birth for what purpose?

1. To eliminate the incidence of viral infections
2. To prevent chlamydia infections
3. To prevent syphilis infection of the eyes
4. To reduce the incidence of group B streptococcal conjunctivitis

34. 2. Both chlamydia and gonorrhea are common causes of neonatal conjunctival infections, and erthromycin effectively treats these infections. Viral infections aren't treated with antibiotics, and syphilis and group B streptococcal infections are treated with other antibiotics.

NP: Analysis; CN: Physiological integrity; CNS: Pharmacological and parenteral therapies; CL: Comprehension

35. When attempting to interact with a neonate experiencing drug withdrawal, which behavior would indicate that the neonate is willing to interact?

1. Gaze aversion
2. Hiccups
3. Quiet alert state
4. Yawning

35. 3. When caring for a neonate experiencing drug withdrawal, the nurse needs to be alert for distress signals from the neonate. Stimuli should be introduced one at a time when the neonate is in a quiet alert state. Gaze aversion, yawning, sneezing, hiccups, and body arching are distress signals that the neonate can't handle stimuli at that time.

NP: Assessment; CN: Psychosocial integrity; CNS: Psychosocial adaptation; CL: Knowledge

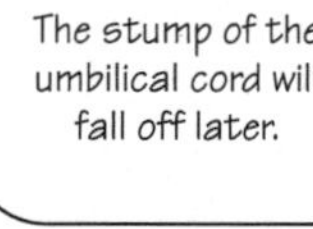

The stump of the umbilical cord will fall off later.

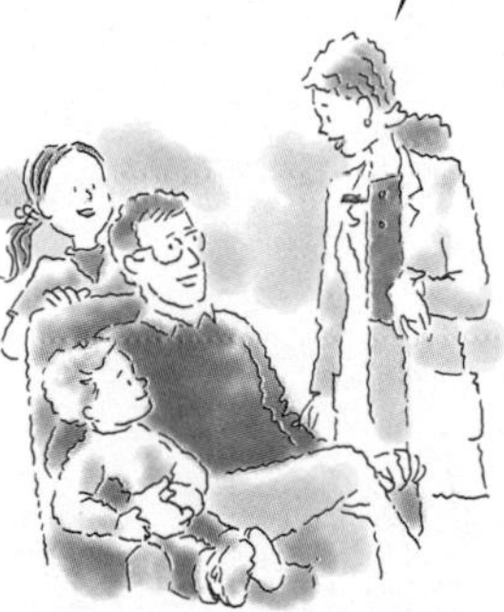

36. When teaching umbilical cord care to a new mother, the nurse would include which information?

1. Apply peroxide to the cord with each diaper change.
2. Cover the cord with petroleum jelly after bathing.
3. Keep the cord dry and open to air.
4. Wash the cord with soap and water each day during a tub bath.

36. 3. Keeping the cord dry and open to air helps reduce infection and hastens drying. Infants aren't given tub baths but are sponged off until the cord falls off. Petroleum jelly prevents the cord from drying and encourages infection. Peroxide could be painful and isn't recommended.

NP: Application; CN: Physiological integrity; CNS: Physiological adaptation; CL: Application

37. When caring for an infant of a mother with diabetes, which physiological finding is most indicative of a hypoglycemic episode?

1. Hyperalert state
2. Jitteriness
3. Positive Babinski reflex
4. Serum glucose level of 60 mg/dl

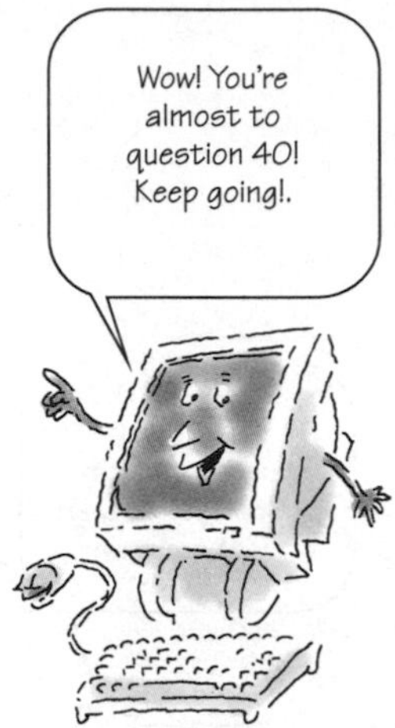
Wow! You're
almost to
question 40!
Keep going!.

37. 2. Hypoglycemia in a neonate is expressed as jitteriness, lethargy, diaphoresis, and a serum glucose level below 40 mg/dl. A hyperalert state in a neonate is more suggestive of neurological irritability and has no correlation to blood glucose levels. Neither does a positive Babinski reflex, which is a normal finding in neonates. A serum glucose level of 60 mg/dl is a normal level.

NP: Analysis; CN: Physiological integrity; CNS: Physiological adaptation; CL: Analysis

38. A mother of a term neonate asks what the thick, white, cheesy coating is on his skin. Which correctly describes this finding?

1. Lanugo
2. Milia
3. Nevus flammeus
4. Vernix

38. 4. Vernix is a white, cheesy material present on the neonate's skin at birth. Lanugo is the fine body hair on a neonate at birth. Milia are small white papules on the skin. Nevus flammeus is a reddish discoloration of an area of skin.

NP: Assessment; CN: Health promotion and maintenance; CNS: Growth and development through the life span; CL: Knowledge

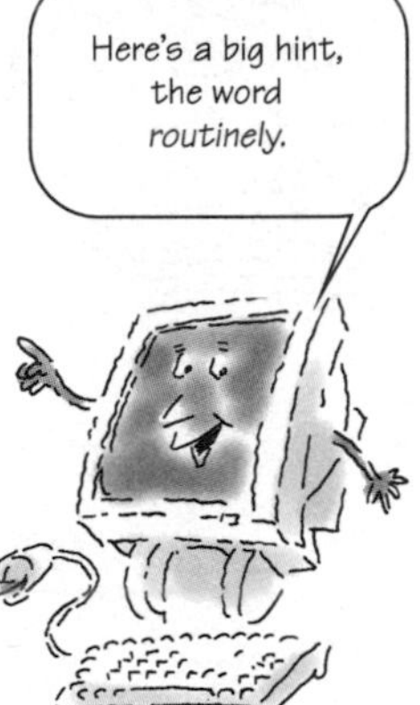
Here's a big hint,
the word
routinely.

39. Which drug is routinely given to the neonate within 1 hour of birth?

1. Erythromycin ophthalmic ointment
2. Gentamycin
3. Nystatin
4. Vitamin A

39. 1. Erythromycin ophthalmic ointment is given for prophylactic treatment of ophthalmic neonatorum. Vitamin K, not vitamin A, is given. Gentamycin is an antibiotic used in the treatment of an infection of the neonate. Nystatin is used for treatment of neonate thrush.

NP: Evaluation; CN: Physiological integrity; CNS: Pharmacological and parenteral therapies; CL: Analysis

40. Which condition or treatment best ensures lung maturity in a neonate?

1. Meconium in the amniotic fluid
2. Glucocorticoid treatment just before delivery
3. Lecithin to sphingomyelin ratio more than 2:1
4. Absence of phosphatidylglycerol in amniotic fluid

40. 3. Lecithin and sphingomyelin are phospholipids that help compose surfactant in the lungs; lecithin peaks at 36 weeks, and sphingomyelin concentrations remain stable. The presence of phosphatidylglycerol indicates lung maturity. Glucocorticoids must be given at least 48 hours before delivery. Meconium is released due to fetal stress before delivery, but it's chronic fetal stress that matures lungs.

NP: Analysis; CN: Physiological integrity; CNS: Physiological adaptation; CL: Knowledge

41. Which assessment finding would be the most unlikely risk factor for respiratory distress syndrome (RDS)?

1. Second born of twins
2. Neonate born at 34 weeks
3. Neonate of a diabetic mother
4. Chronic maternal hypertension

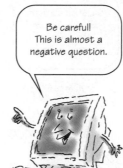

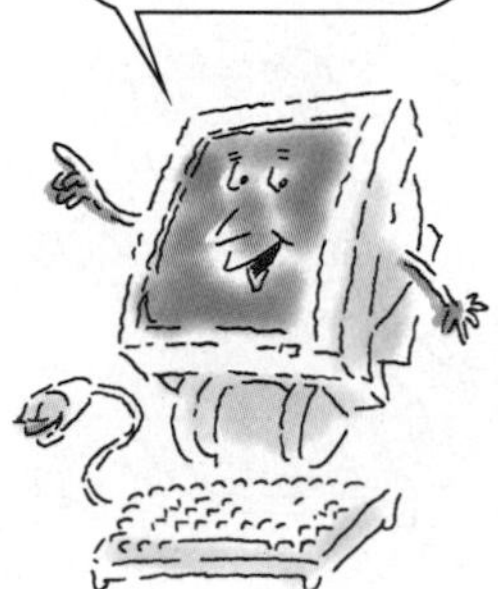
Be careful!
This is almost a
negative question.

41. 4. Chronic maternal hypertension is an unlikely factor because chronic fetal stress tends to increase lung maturity. Premature neonates younger than 35 weeks are associated with RDS. Even with a mature lecithin to sphingomyelin ratio, neonates of mothers with diabetes may still develop respiratory distress. Second born of twins may be prone to greater risk of asphyxia.

NP: Analysis; CN: Physiological integrity; CNS: Physiological adaptation; CL: Analysis

42. A nurse is performing an assessment on a neonate. Which of the following findings is considered common in the healthy neonate?

1. Simian crease
2. Conjunctival hemorrhages
3. Cystic hygroma
4. Bulging fontanelle

42. 2. Conjunctival hemorrhages are commonly seen in neonates secondary to the cranial pressure applied during the birth process. Bulging fontanelles are a sign of intracranial pressure. Simian creases are present in 40% of the neonates with trisomy 21. Cystic hygroma is a neck mass that can affect the airway.

NP: Assessment; CN: Health promotion and maintenance; CNS: Growth and development through the life span; CL: Analysis

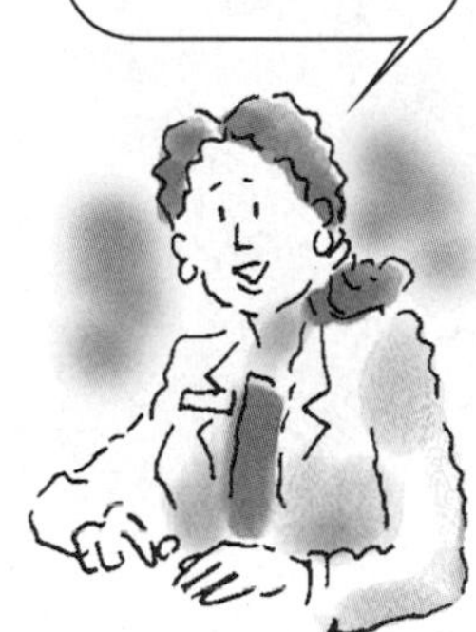
Only one of these
actions is a
priority right after
birth. Which one?

43. When performing nursing care for a neonate after a birth, which intervention has the highest nursing priority?

1. Obtain a Dextrostix.
2. Give the initial bath.
3. Give the vitamin K injection.
4. Cover the neonate's head with a cap.

43. 4. Covering the neonate's head with a cap helps prevent cold stress due to excessive evaporative heat loss from a neonate's wet head. Initial baths aren't given until the neonate's temperature is stable. Dextrostix, appropriate for neonates with risk factors, are obtained at 30 minutes to 1 hour of age. Vitamin K can be given within 4 hours after birth.

NP: Evaluation; CN: Health promotion and maintenance; CNS: Growth and development through the life span; CL: Analysis

44. When assessing a neonate's skin, the nurse observes small white papules surrounded by erythematous dermatitis. This finding is characteristic of which condition?

1. Cutis marmorata
2. Epstein's pearls
3. Erythema toxicum
4. Mongolian spots

44. 3. Erythema toxicum has lesions that come and go on the face, trunk, and limbs. They're small white or yellow papules or vesicles with erythematous dermatitis. Cutis marmorata is bluish mottling of the skin. Mongolian spots are large macules or patches that are gray or blue green. Epstein's pearls, found in the mouth, are similar to facial milia.

NP: Assessment; CN: Health promotion and maintenance; CNS: Growth and development through the life span; CL: Knowledge

45. Which nursing consideration is most important when giving a neonate his initial bath?

1. Give a tub bath.
2. Use water and mild soap.
3. Give it right after delivery.
4. Use hexachlorophene soap.

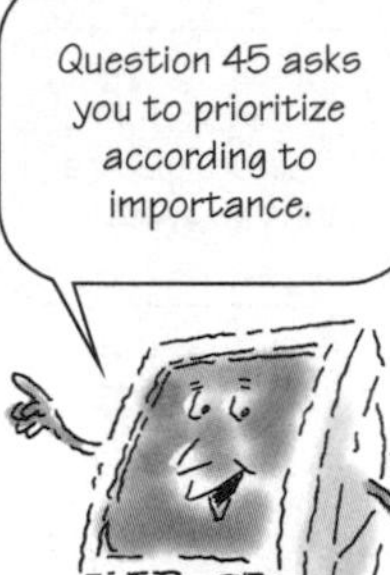
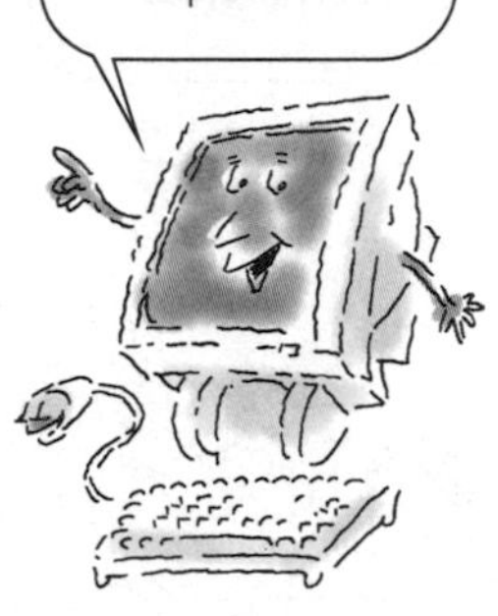

Question 45 asks you to prioritize according to importance.

45. 2. Use only water and mild soap on a neonate to prevent drying out the skin. The initial bath is given when the neonate's temperature is stable. Hexachlorophene soaps should be avoided; they're neurotoxic and may be absorbed through a neonate's skin. Tub baths are delayed until the umbilical cord falls off.

NP: Planning; CN: Health promotion and maintenance; CNS: Growth and development through the life span; CL: Analysis

46. The Centers for Disease Control and Prevention (CDC) recommends the hepatitis B vaccine be administered to which neonates?

1. All neonates
2. Exposed neonates only
3. Neonates showing symptoms
4. Neonates of mothers with human immunodeficiency virus

46. 1. The CDC recommends hepatitis B vaccine be given to all neonates, including those born to hepatitis B surface antigen–negative mothers.

NP: Evaluation; CN: Health promotion and maintenance; CNS: Prevention and early detection of disease; CL: Knowledge

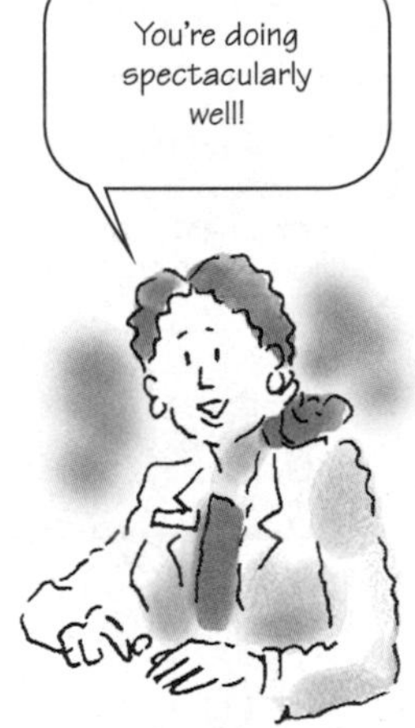
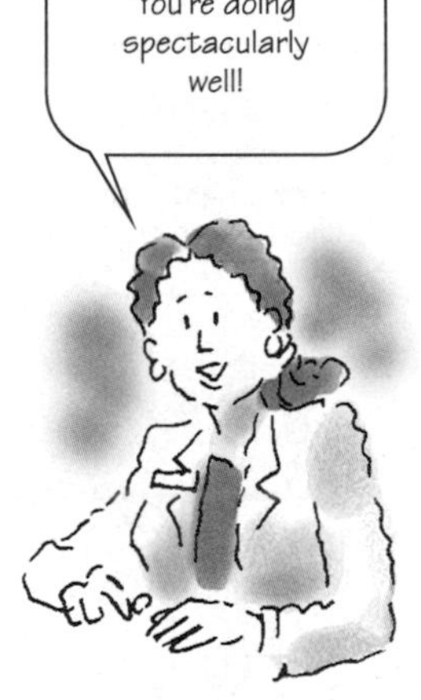

You're doing spectacularly well!

47. A male neonate has just been circumcised. Which nursing intervention is part of the initial care of a circumcised neonate?

1. Apply alcohol to the site.
2. Change the diaper as needed.
3. Keep the neonate in the supine position.
4. Apply petroleum gauze to the site for 24 hours.

47. 4. Petroleum gauze is applied to the site for the first 24 hours to prevent the skin edges from sticking to the diaper. Neonates are initially kept in the prone position. Diapers are changed more frequently to inspect the site. Alcohol is contraindicated for circumcision care.

NP: Implementation; CN: Health promotion and maintenance; CNS: Growth and development through the life span; CL: Application

48. When performing an assessment on a neonate, which assessment finding is most suggestive of hypothermia?

1. Bradycardia
2. Hyperglycemia
3. Metabolic alkalosis
4. Shivering

48. 1. Hypothermic neonates become bradycardic proportional to the degree of core temperature. Hypoglycemia is seen in hypothermic neonates. Shivering is rarely observed in neonates. Metabolic acidosis, not alkalosis, is seen due to slowed respirations.

NP: Assessment; CN: Health promotion and maintenance; CNS: Growth and development through the life span; CL: Analysis

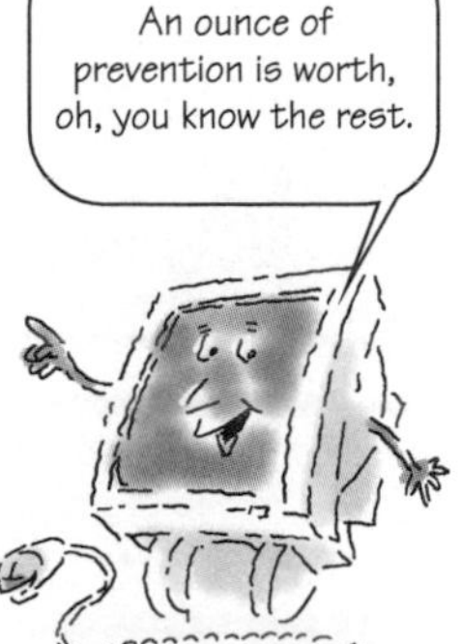

An ounce of prevention is worth, oh, you know the rest.

49. Which nursing intervention helps prevent evaporative heat loss in the neonate immediately after birth?

1. Administering warm oxygen
2. Controlling the drafts in the room
3. Immediately drying the neonate
4. Placing the neonate on a warm, dry towel

49. 3. Immediately drying the neonate decreases evaporative heat loss from his moist body from birth. Placing the neonate on a warm, dry towel decreases conductive losses. Controlling the drafts in the room and administering warmed oxygen help reduce convective loss.

NP: Implementation; CN: Health promotion and maintenance; CNS: Growth and development through the life span; CL: Analysis

50. Which assessment finding in a neonate would indicate a metabolic response to cold stress?
1. Arrhythmias
2. Hypoglycemia
3. Increase in liver function
4. Increase in blood pressure

50. 2. Hypoglycemia occurs as the consumption of glucose increases with the increase in metabolic rate. Arrhythmias and increases in blood pressure occur due to cardiorespiratory manifestations. Liver function declines in cold stress.

NP: Analysis; CN: Health promotion and maintenance; CNS: Growth and development through the life span; CL: Knowledge

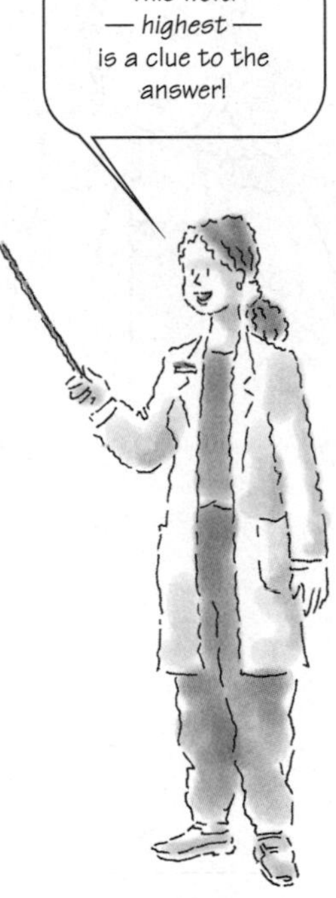

This word

is a clue to the

51. Which would be the highest priority in regulating the temperature of a neonate?
1. Supply extra heat sources to the neonate.
2. Keep the ambient room temperature less than 100° F (37.8° C).
3. Minimize the energy needed for the neonate to produce heat.
4. Block radiant, convective, conductive, and evaporative losses.

51. 4. Prevention of heat loss is always the first goal in thermoregulation to avoid hypothermia. The second goal is to minimize the energy necessary for neonates to produce heat. Adding extra heat sources is a means of correcting hypothermia. The ambient room temperature should be kept at approximately 100° F.

NP: Planning; CN: Health promotion and maintenance; CNS: Growth and development through the life span; CL: Application

52. When maintaining thermoregulation, which neonatal characteristics negatively affect the establishment of a thermal neutral zone?
1. Flexed posture
2. Blood vessels that aren't close to the skin
3. Decreased subcutaneous fat and thin epidermis
4. Increased subcutaneous fat and thick epidermis

52. 3. Decreased subcutaneous fat and a thin epidermis affect the establishment of a thermal neutral zone. The more insulated a neonate is, the greater the ability to cope with lower environmental temperatures. Blood vessels in neonates are close to the skin, so circulating blood is influenced by temperature changes. The flexed posture decreases the surface area exposed and decreases heat loss.

NP: Assessment; CN: Health promotion and maintenance; CNS: Growth and development through the life span; CL: Knowledge

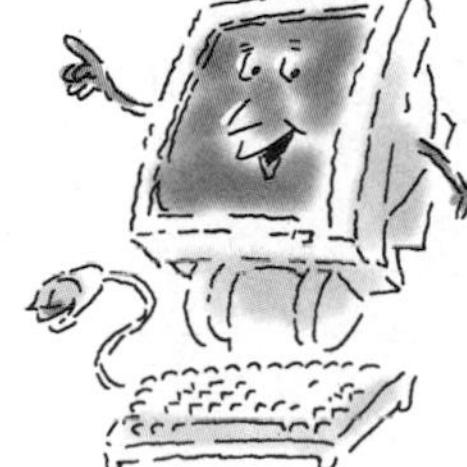

Did you remember
to double-check
that puzzling
prefix? Excellent!

53. Which clinical finding is most suggestive of physiologic hyperbilirubinemia in a neonate?
1. Clinical jaundice before 36 hours of age
2. Clinical jaundice lasting beyond 14 days
3. Bilirubin levels of 12 mg/dl by 3 days of life
4. Serum bilirubin level increasing by more than 5 mg/dl/day

53. 3. Increased bilirubin levels in the liver usually cause bilirubin levels of 12 mg/dl by the 3rd day of life. This is from the impaired conjugation and excretion of bilirubin and difficulty clearing bilirubin from plasma. The other answers suggest nonphysiologic jaundice.

NP: Assessment; CN: Health promotion and maintenance; CNS: Growth and development through the life span; CL: Analysis

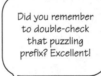

54. What's the desired effect of phenobarbital used in neonates with hyperbilirubinemia?

1. To sedate the neonate during treatment
2. To decrease the conjugation of bilirubin
3. To increase the concentration of ligandin
4. To convert unconjugated bilirubin into water-soluble bilirubin

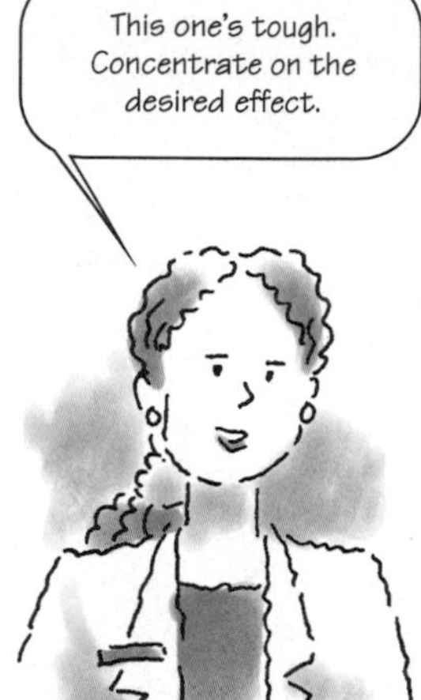

This one's tough. Concentrate on the desired effect.

54. 3. Phenobarbital increases the concentration of ligandin, which transports bilirubin for conjugation. Phenobarbital isn't used in this circumstance for its sedative purposes. Phenobarbital doesn't directly convert bilirubin, but it helps in the process. Phenobarbital helps increase the conjugation of bilirubin.

NP: Evaluation; CN: Physiological integrity; CNS: Pharmacological and parenteral therapies; CL: Analysis

55. A neonate undergoing phototherapy treatment needs to be monitored for which adverse effect?

1. Hyperglycemia
2. Increased insensible water loss
3. Severe decrease in platelet count
4. Increased GI transit time

55. 2. Increased insensible water loss is due to absorbed photon energy from the lights. GI transit time may decrease with use of phototherapy. Hyperglycemia isn't a characteristic effect of phototherapy treatment. There may be a mild decrease in platelet count.

NP: Assessment; CN: Health promotion and maintenance; CNS: Growth and development through the life span; CL: Analysis

56. Which assessment finding might be seen in a neonate suspected of having breast-milk jaundice?

1. History of being a poor feeder
2. Decreased bilirubin level around day 3 of life
3. Clinical jaundice evident after 24 hours
4. Interruption of breast-feeding, resulting in decreased bilirubin levels between 24 and 72 hours

56. 4. The exact cause of breast-milk jaundice is unknown. If bilirubin levels don't decrease after 3 days, human milk is eliminated as a cause. These babies are typically good eaters with good weight gain. Bilirubin levels increase, rather than decrease, at day 3. Jaundice in the first 24 hours of life is characteristic of hemolytic disease.

NP: Assessment; CN: Health promotion and maintenance; CNS: Growth and development through the life span; CL: Analysis

57. Which sign is the earliest indication of respiratory distress syndrome in a neonate?

1. Bilateral crackles
2. Pale gray color
3. Tachypnea more than 60 breaths/minute
4. Poor capillary filling time (3 to 4 seconds)

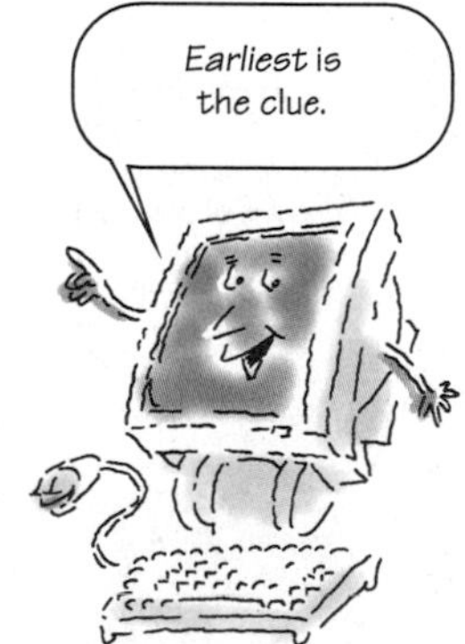

Earliest is the clue.

57. 3. Tachypnea and expiratory grunting occur early in respiratory distress syndrome to help improve oxygenation. Poor capillary filling time, a later manifestation, occurs if signs and symptoms aren't treated. Crackles occur as the respiratory distress progressively worsens. A pale gray skin color obscures earlier cyanosis as respiratory distress symptoms persist and worsen.

NP: Assessment; CN: Health promotion and maintenance; CNS: Growth and development through the life span; CL: Analysis

58. Which of the following disorders is a nonrespiratory cause of respiratory distress?

1. Choanal atresia
2. Meconium aspiration
3. Pulmonary hemorrhage
4. Retained lung fluid syndrome

58. 1. Choanal atresia is caused by protrusion of bone or membrane into nasal passages, causing blockage or narrowing. Meconium aspiration is meconium aspirated into the lungs during birth. Retained lung fluid syndrome is caused by a delay in removing excessive amounts of lung fluid. Pulmonary hemorrhage is bleeding into the alveoli.

NP: Evaluation; CN: Health promotion and maintenance; CNS: Growth and development through the life span; CL: Knowledge

59. A neonate is admitted to the neonatal intensive care unit with persistent pulmonary hypertension. Which pulmonary vasodilator is the drug of choice for this disorder?

1. Dobutamine (Dobutrex)
2. Isoproterenol (Isuprel)
3. Prostaglandin E_2
4. Tolazoline (Priscoline)

59. 4. Tolazoline dilates pulmonary arteries and decreases pulmonary vascular resistance. Isoproterenol dilates pulmonary arteries but doesn't decrease pulmonary vascular resistance. Dobutamine is a vasopressor, not a vasodilator. Prostaglandin E_2 is an oxytocic substance used to induce abortion and doesn't affect pulmonary vasodilation.

NP: Evaluation; CN: Physiological integrity; CNS: Pharmacological and parenteral therapies; CL: Analysis

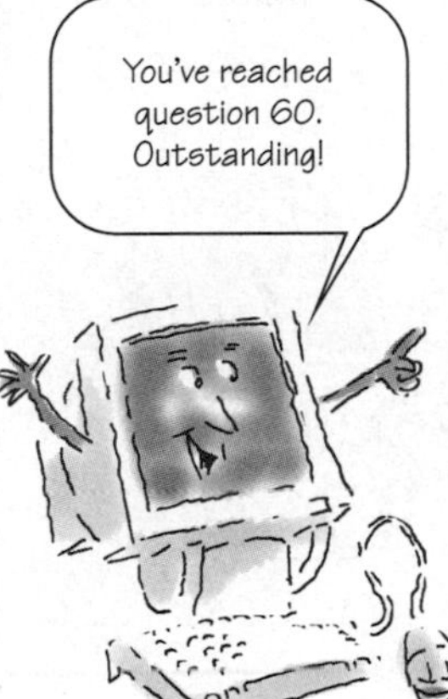

You've reached question 60. Outstanding!

60. Which neonatal respiratory disorder is usually mild and runs a self-limited course?

1. Pneumonia
2. Meconium aspiration syndrome
3. Transient tachypnea of neonate
4. Persistent pulmonary hypertension

60. 3. Transient tachypnea has an invariably favorable outcome after several hours to several days. The outcome of pneumonia depends on the causative agent involved and may have complications. Meconium aspiration, depending on severity, may have long-term adverse effects. In persistent pulmonary hypertension, the mortality rate is more than 50%.

NP: Assessment; CN: Physiological integrity; CNS: Physiological adaptation; CL: Analysis

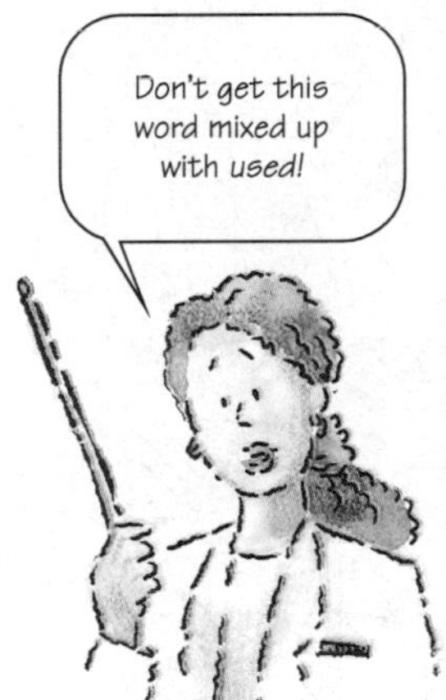

Don't get this word mixed up with used!

61. Which procedure should be avoided in a neonate born with diaphragmatic hernia?

1. Chest X-ray
2. Mask ventilation
3. Placement of orogastric tube
4. Immediate endotracheal intubation

61. 2. Mask ventilation should be avoided to prevent air from being introduced into the GI tract by this technique. An emergency chest X-ray will help in diagnosing this defect. An orogastric tube is needed to decompress the bowel and stomach within the chest. Intubation is needed to ventilate the neonate due to the defect.

NP: Implementation; CN: Physiological integrity; CNS: Physiological adaptation; CL: Application

62. Which immunoglobulin (Ig) provides immunity against bacterial and viral pathogens through passive immunity?

1. IgA
2. IgE
3. IgG
4. IgM

62. 3. IgG is a major Ig of serum and interstitial fluid that crosses the placenta. IgE has a major role in allergic reactions. IgM and IgA don't cross the placenta.

NP: Analysis; CN: Health promotion and maintenance; CNS: Growth and development through the life span; CL: Knowledge

63. Which cranio-facial change is most characteristic in a neonate with fetal alcohol syndrome (FAS)?

1. Macrocephaly
2. Microophthalmia
3. Wide palpebral fissures
4. Well-developed philtrum

63. 2. Distinctive facial dysmorphology of children with FAS most commonly involves the eyes (microophthalmia). Microcephaly is generally seen, as are a poorly developed philtrum and short palpebral fissures.

NP: Assessment; CN: Physiological integrity; CNS: Physiological adaptation; CL: Knowledge

64. A 36-week neonate born weighing 1,800 g has microcephaly and microphthalmia. Based on these findings, which risk factor might be expected in the maternal history?

1. Use of alcohol
2. Use of marijuana
3. Gestational diabetes
4. Positive group B streptococci

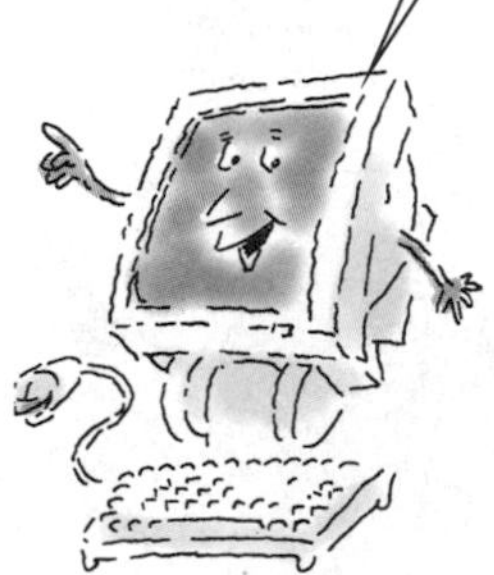

Read closely. Question 64 asks about maternal history, not the neonate's current condition.

64. 1. The most common sign of the effects of alcohol on fetal development is retarded growth in weight, length, and head circumference. Gestational diabetes usually produces large-for-gestational-age neonates. Intrauterine growth retardation isn't characteristic of marijuana use. Positive group B streptococcus isn't a relevant risk factor.

NP: Analysis; CN: Health promotion and maintenance; CNS: Growth and development through the life span; CL: Analysis

65. Which neonatal behavior is most commonly associated with fetal alcohol syndrome (FAS)?

1. Hypoactivity
2. High birth weight
3. Poor wake and sleep patterns
4. High threshold of stimulation

65. 3. Altered sleep patterns are caused by disturbances in the central nervous system from alcohol exposure in utero. Hyperactivity is a characteristic deficit generally noted. Low birth weight is a physical defect seen in neonates with FAS. Neonates with FAS generally have a low threshold for stimulation.

NP: Assessment; CN: Physiological integrity; CNS: Physiological adaptation; CL: Knowledge

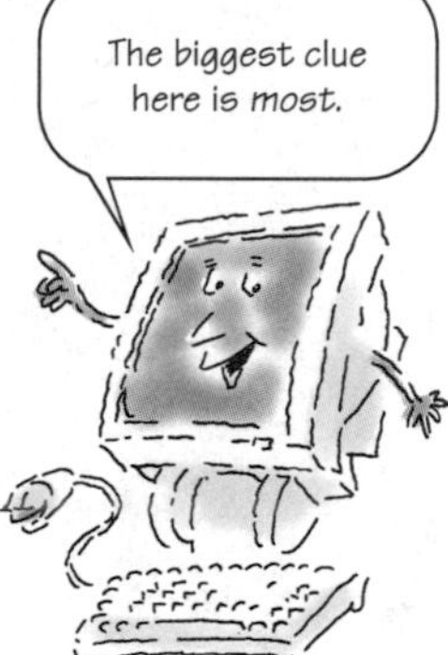

The biggest clue here is most.

66. Which GI disorder is most suggestive of cystic fibrosis?

1. Duodenal obstruction
2. Jejunal atresia
3. Malrotation
4. Meconium ileus

66. 4. Meconium ileus is a luminal obstruction of the distal small intestine by abnormal meconium seen in neonates with cystic fibrosis. Duodenal obstruction, malrotation, and jejunal atresia aren't characteristic findings in neonates with cystic fibrosis.

NP: Analysis; CN: Physiological integrity; CNS: Physiological adaptation; CL: Knowledge

67. Which orthopedic disorder of the neonate results in multiple fractures and skeletal deformities?

1. Klippel-Feil syndrome
2. Osteogenesis imperfecta
3. Congenital hip dislocation
4. Arthrogryposis multiplex congenita

Keep reading carefully and you'll do well.

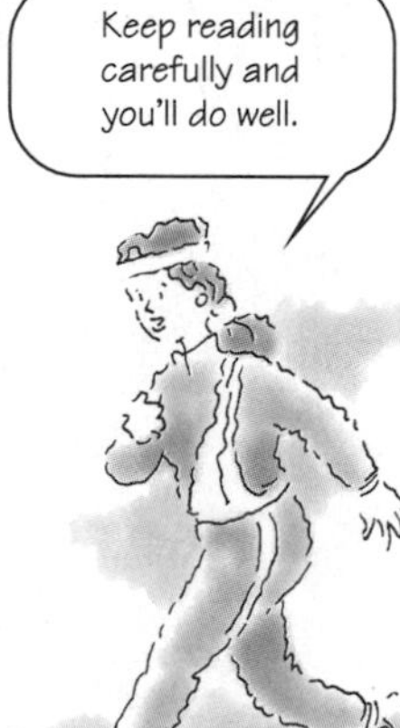

67. 2. Osteogenesis imperfecta is a connective tissue disorder with the primary defect involving the collagen structure. Arthrogryposis multiplex congenita involves multiple, congenitally rigid joints. Congenital hip dislocation is dislocation of the hip joints. Klippel-Feil syndrome involves defective segmentation of cervical vertebrae.

NP: Analysis; CN: Physiological integrity; CNS: Physiological adaptation; CL: Knowledge

68. A neonate has an imperforate anus, tracheoesophageal fistula, and a single umbilical artery. A nurse suspects that the neonate might have which congenital disorder?

1. Beckwith-Wiedemann syndrome
2. Trisomy 13
3. Turner's syndrome
4. VATER association

68. 4. VATER association clinically presents with three or more defects, including the three mentioned. Trisomy 13 and Turner's syndrome are chromosomal aberrations that aren't typically seen with the other defects. These defects aren't associated with Beckwith-Wiedemann syndrome.

NP: Analysis; CN: Physiological integrity; CNS: Physiological adaptation; CL: Analysis

69. An initial assessment of a female neonate shows pink-streaked vaginal discharge. Which factor is the probable cause?

1. Cystitis
2. Birth trauma
3. Neonatal candidiasis
4. Withdrawal of maternal hormones

69. 4. Withdrawal of maternal estrogen can produce pseudomenstruation. Cystitis or a urinary tract infection in a neonate would show generalized signs of sepsis. Birth trauma may cause surface abrasions but not vaginal discharge. Neonates with candidal infections usually have oral lesions (thrush) or monilial diaper rash.

NP: Assessment; CN: Health promotion and maintenance; CNS: Prevention and early detection of disease; CL: Knowledge

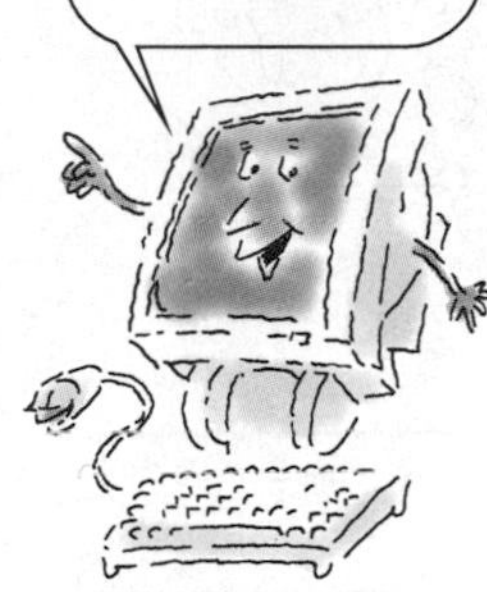

70. When assessing for congenital anomalies in a neonate, which symptom is seen first with tracheoesophageal atresia?

1. Torticollis
2. Nasal stuffiness
3. Oligohydramnios
4. Excessive oral secretions

70. 4. Accumulated secretions are copious because the neonate can't swallow. Torticollis would only be present if there was a defect of muscle or bone. Nasal stuffiness is very common in neonates and doesn't indicate esophageal abnormalities. Atresia will produce polyhydramnios because the fetus can't swallow the amniotic fluid.

NP: Analysis; CN: Physiological integrity; CNS: Physiological adaptation; CL: Analysis

71. The neonate is vulnerable to heat loss because of which anatomic characteristic?

1. Immature liver
2. Immature brain
3. Large skin surface area to body weight ratio
4. More brown fat (adipose tissue) than an adult

71. 3. The neonate has proportionally more surface area through which heat can dissipate. The liver isn't involved in thermoregulation. Brown fat is used to produce body heat and doesn't predispose the neonate to heat loss. The part of the brain that regulates temperature is mature at birth.

NP: Assessment; CN: Physiological integrity; CNS: Reduction of risk potential; CL: Knowledge

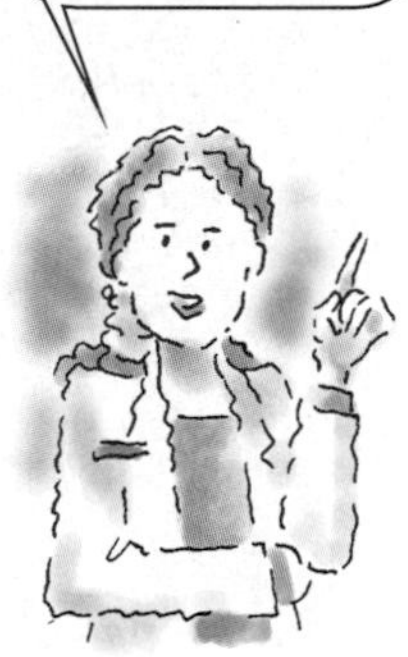

You're doing quite
nicely and will be
done before you
realize it.

72. Maintaining thermoregulation in the neonate is an important nursing intervention because cold stress in the neonate can lead to which condition?

1. Anemia
2. Hyperglycemia
3. Metabolic alkalosis
4. Increased oxygen consumption

72. 4. The neonate's metabolic rate increases as a result of cold stress, which leads to an increased oxygen requirement. Cold stress doesn't increase erythrocyte destruction. Cold stress leads to anaerobic glycolysis, which results in metabolic acidosis. The increased metabolic rate leads to the use of glycogen stores and produces hypoglycemia.

NP: Analysis; CN: Physiological integrity; CNS: Reduction of risk potential; CL: Analysis

73. Which initial nursing intervention best addresses the needs of a term neonate with adequate respiratory and heart rates but who has central cyanosis?

1. Provide tactile stimulation.
2. Give supplemental free-flow oxygen.
3. Assist ventilation with bag and mask.
4. Intubate and suction the lower airway.

73. 2. Room air is currently insufficient, seen by the central cyanosis. Tactile stimulation is only needed if the neonate is apneic or gasping. Intubation is only indicated in special circumstances, such as prematurity or a diaphragmatic hernia. Bag and mask ventilation is only indicated if the heart rate is less than 100 beats/minute.

NP: Implementation; CN: Health promotion and maintenance; CNS: Growth and development through the life span; CL: Application

74. A woman delivers a 3,250-g neonate at 42 weeks' gestation. Which physical finding is expected during an examination of this neonate?

1. Abundant lanugo
2. Absence of sole creases
3. Breast bud of 1 to 2 mm in diameter
4. Leathery, cracked, and wrinkled skin

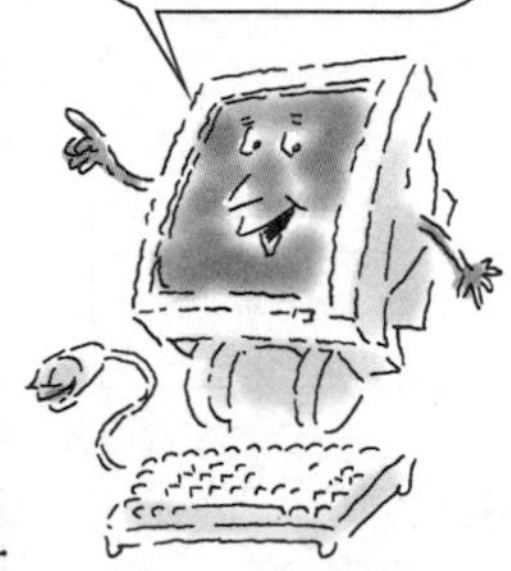

Question 74 asks about an *expected* finding, not necessarily an abnormal one.

74. 4. Neonatal skin thickens with maturity and is often peeling by postterm. Lanugo disappears as pregnancy progresses, with very little remaining on the postterm neonate. As sole creases increase in number and depth with gestational age, a postterm neonate would have deep sole creases. A postterm neonate would have a well-developed breast bud of 5 to 10 mm in diameter.

NP: Assessment; CN: Health promotion and maintenance; CNS: Prevention and early detection of disease; CL: Knowledge

75. While performing an initial assessment on a term neonate with an Asian mother, a bluish marking is observed across the neonate's lower back. What is the significance of this finding?

1. It's probably a sign of birth trauma.
2. It's probably a telangiectatic hemangioma.
3. It's probably a typical marking in dark-skinned races.
4. It probably indicates that hyperbilirubinemia may follow.

75. 3. This is a Mongolian spot, commonly found over the lumbosacral area in neonates of Black, Asian, Latin American, or Native American origin. The coloration is due to the deposition of melanocytes, not erythrocytes, and, without other findings, isn't a bruise. A Mongolian spot is a deep dermal infiltration of melanocytes, so there would be no breakdown of erythrocytes to cause hyperbilirubinemia. A telangiectatic hemangioma is a salmon-pink coloration found at the nape of the neck, eyelids, and forehead.

NP: Assessment; CN: Health promotion and maintenance; CNS: Prevention and early detection of disease; CL: Knowledge

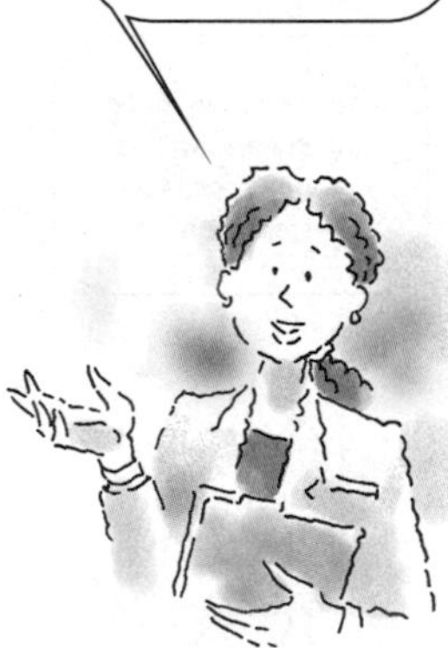

How should the nurse respond to the student?

76. A nurse in the neonate nursery is serving as preceptor for a student nurse. The student asks the nurse why the neonate's head is cone-shaped. Which response is accurate?

1. "It results from caput succendum. The difficult labor caused bruising and swelling of the neonate's head."
2. "It results from molding. Overriding of the cranial sutures allows the neonate's head to pass though the birth canal."
3. "It results from cephalohematoma. Some blood has collected between the skull bone and periosteum."
4. "It results from hydrocephalus. Either too much cerebrospinal fluid is being formed or too little is being absorbed."

76. 2. Molding refers to overlapping of the cranial sutures, which causes the neonate's head to appear cone-shaped. Caput succendum, cephalohematoma, and hydrocephalus don't result in a cone-shaped head. Caput succendum is an area of localized swelling and bruising over a presenting part. Cephalohematoma is a collection of blood between the skull bone and periosteum. Hydrocephalus is an increase in the size of the entire head as a result of increased cerebrospinal fluid volume.

NP: Assessment; CN: Growth and development through the life span; CNS: Prevention and early detection of disease; CL: Analysis

77. A neonate receiving formula feedings is discharged from the neonate nursery. Twenty-four hours later, the mother calls the hospital, stating that the neonate is vomiting most of his feedings. Which statement by the mother indicates that she needs further discharge instructions?

1. "Every time I feed him, he spits up about a teaspoonful of formula onto his bib."
2. "I'm using prepared formula, and he takes ½ oz to 1 oz every 3 to 4 hours."
3. "I feed him every time he cries. Sometimes he eats 4 oz at a time every couple of hours."
4. "I burp him after each ½ oz of formula."

77. 3. Feeding the neonate every time he cries results in overfeeding. A neonate's crying doesn't always signal hunger; sometimes it means his diaper is wet, he needs to suck, or he wants to be held. For the first few days, the neonate's normal stomach capacity is 15 ml, so he should be fed every 3 to 4 hours. All neonates spit up a small amount because of an immature cardiac sphincter. A neonate who's spitting up should be burped after every ounce of formula or less.

NP: Evaluation; CN: Physiologic integrity; CNS: Basic care and comfort; CL: Application

78. A healthy term neonate born by cesarean delivery was admitted to the transitional nursery 30 minutes ago and placed under a radiant warmer. The neonate has an axillary temperature of 99.5° F (37.5° C), a respiratory rate of 80 breaths/minute, and a heelstick glucose value of 60 mg/dl. Which action should the nurse take?

1. Wrap the neonate warmly and place her in an open crib.
2. Administer an oral glucose feeding of dextrose 10% in water.
3. Increase the temperature setting on the radiant warmer.
4. Obtain an order for I.V. fluid administration.

78. 4. Assessment findings indicate that the neonate is in respiratory distress — most likely from transient tachypnea, which is common after cesarean delivery. The normal respiratory rate is 30 to 60 breaths/minute; a neonate with a rate of 80 breaths/minute shouldn't be fed but should receive I.V. fluids until the respiratory rate returns to normal. To allow close observation for worsening respiratory distress, the neonate should be kept unclothed in the radiant warmer. Temperature is in the normal range; raising the warmer's temperature setting would cause overheating and worsen the neonate's respiratory distress.

NP: Implementation; CN: Physiologic integrity; CNS: Basic care and comfort; CL: Application

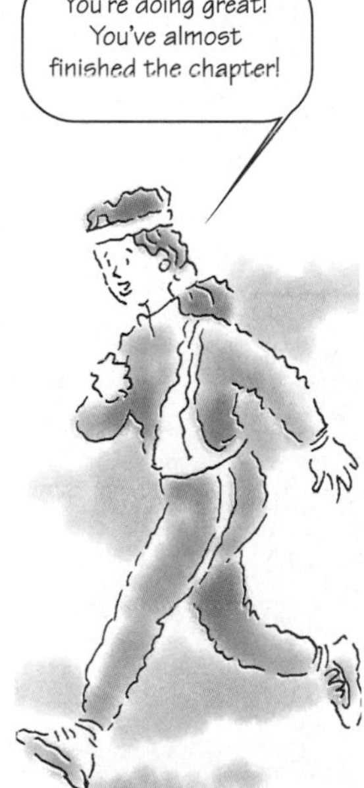

You're doing great!
You've almost
finished the chapter!

79. A home health nurse assesses a neonate who is 48 hours old and was discharged from the hospital 24 hours ago. Which assessment finding indicates a potential problem?

1. The neonate cries but no tears appear.
2. Small papules appear all over the neonate's skin.
3. The neonate doesn't turn his head in the direction that his cheek is stroked.
4. The neonate produces a greenish, tarry stool.

79. 3. A normal, healthy neonate turns in the direction that the cheek is stroked. Failure to do so may indicate a neurologic problem, which the nurse should report to the physician. A neonate's lacrimal glands are immature, resulting in tearless crying for up to 2 months. Erythema toxicum neonatorum causes a transient maculopapular rash—a normal finding in all neonates. Greenish, tarry stools at 48 hours are normal and indicate that the neonate is eliminating formula or breast milk instead of meconium.

NP: Assessment; CN: Health promotion and maintenance; CNS: Growth and development through the life span; CL: Application

80. One minute after birth, a neonate has a heart rate of 60 beats/minute. Five minutes after birth, his heart rate is 80 beats/minute. Which Apgar heart rate score should he receive?

1. 0
2. 1
3. 2
4. 3

80. 2. In Apgar scoring, the heart rate gets a normal score of 2 if it's greater than 100 beats/minute, 1 if it's less than 100, and 0 if there's no heart rate. At 1 and 5 minutes, Apgar scoring is the same. The other answers are either too high or low.

NP: Assessment; CN: Physiologic Integrity; CNS: Physiologic adaptation; CL: Comprehension

81. When assessing a male neonate, the nurse notices that the urinary meatus is located on the ventral surface of the penis. How should the nurse document this finding?

1. As the normal location for the urinary meatus
2. As epispadias
3. As hypospadias
4. As cryptorchidism

81. 3. In hypospadias, the urinary meatus is located on the ventral surface of the penis. The neonate with this finding shouldn't be circumcised in case the foreskin is needed to help reposition the meatus to its normal location (the end of the penis). In epispadias, the urinary meatus is located on the dorsal surface. Cryptorchidism refers to an undescended testicle.

NP: Assessment; CN: Health promotion and maintenance; CNS: Growth and development through the life span; CL: Application.

82. A postpartum client asks the nurse, "Why does my baby have those red areas on his eyelids?" Which response is appropriate?

1. "They're called milia. They're clogged oil glands, which are normal in a neonate."
2. "They're called telangiectasia or stork bites. They usually disappear within 1 year."
3. "We'll watch them closely. They could indicate a bleeding disorder."
4. "They're nothing to worry about. The physician will order topical cream to help them go away."

82. 2. Telangiectasia refers to the flat, reddened, vascular areas commonly found on a neonate's eyelids. Calling them stork bites and telling the mother that they'll disappear within 1 year is reassuring. Milia are found primarily on the nose and result from clogged sebaceous glands. Telling the mother that the red areas will be watched closely and could indicate a bleeding disorder would cause her needless concern. There's no treatment for telangiectasia; the condition fades over time.

NP: Implementation; CN: Health promotion and maintenance; CNS: Growth and development through the life span; CL: Application

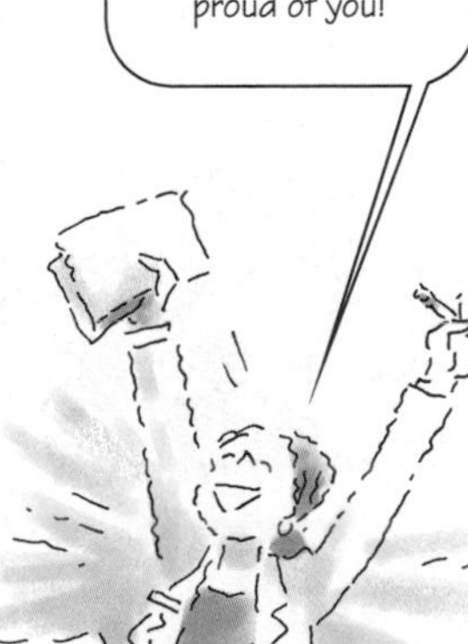

Success! We're super-de-dooper proud of you!

Part V Care of the child

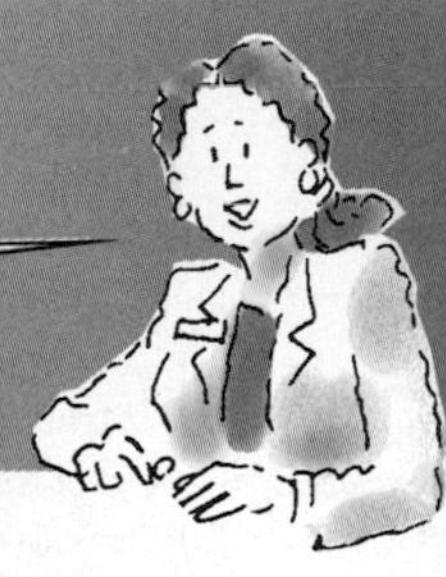

Chapter 27 Cardiovascular disorders

1. A nurse is performing a cardiac assessment on a 2-year-old. The first heart sound (S_1) can best be heard at which of the following locations?

1. Third or fourth intercostal space
2. The apex with the stethoscope bell
3. Second intercostal space, midclavicular line
4. Fifth intercostal space, left midclavicular line

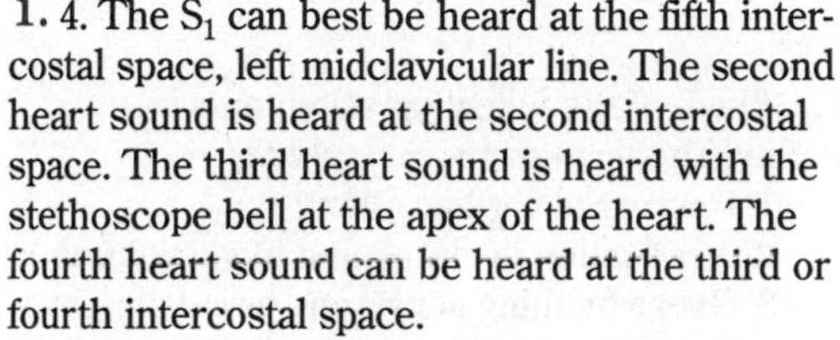

1. 4. The S_1 can best be heard at the fifth intercostal space, left midclavicular line. The second heart sound is heard at the second intercostal space. The third heart sound is heard with the stethoscope bell at the apex of the heart. The fourth heart sound can be heard at the third or fourth intercostal space.

NP: Assessment; CN: Health promotion and maintenance; CNS: Prevention and early detection of disease; CL: Knowledge

2. When auscultating the heart, which of the following characteristics or statements best describes the first heart sound (S_1)?

1. Heard late in diastole
2. Heard early in diastole
3. Closure of the mitral and tricuspid valves
4. Closure of the aortic and pulmonic valves

2. 3. The S_1 occurs during systole with closure of the mitral and tricuspid valves. The second heart sound occurs during diastole with closure of the aortic and pulmonic valves. The third heart sound is heard early in diastole. The fourth heart sound is heard late in diastole.

NP: Assessment; CN: Health promotion and maintenance; CNS: Prevention and early detection of disease; CL: Knowledge

3. Which of the following characteristics best describes a grade 1 heart murmur?

1. Equal to the heart sounds
2. Softer than the heart sounds
3. Can be heard with the naked ear
4. Associated with a precordial thrill

3. 2. A grade 1 heart murmur is commonly difficult to hear and softer than the heart sounds. A grade 2 murmur is usually equal to the heart sounds. A grade 4 murmur is associated with a precordial thrill. A thrill is a palpable manifestation associated with a loud murmur. A grade 6 murmur can be heard with the naked ear or with the stethoscope off the chest.

NP: Assessment; CN: Health promotion and maintenance; CNS: Prevention and early detection of disease; CL: Knowledge

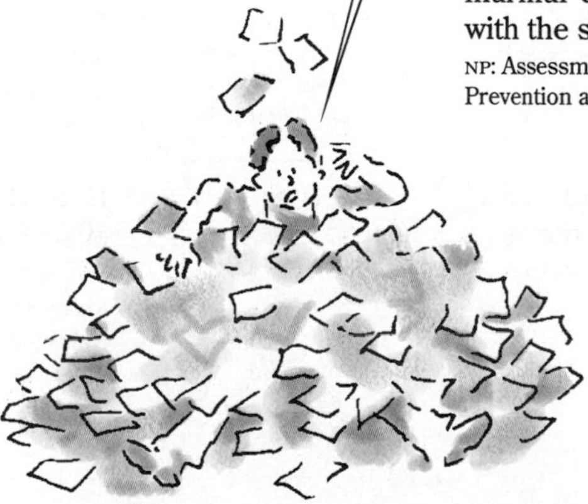

You might have a lot of questions ahead of you, but I know you can do it!

NP: Nursing process CN: Client needs category CNS: Client needs subcategory CL: Cognitive level

4. Which of the following phrases best defines the term *stroke volume?*

1. Volume of blood returning to the heart
2. Ability of the cardiac muscle to act as an efficient pump
3. Resistance the ventricles pump against when ejecting blood
4. Amount of blood ejected by the heart in any one contraction

4. 4. Stroke volume is the amount of blood ejected by the heart in any one contraction. It's influenced by preload, afterload, and contractility. Preload is the amount of blood returning to the heart. Afterload is the resistance the ventricles pump against when ejecting blood. Contractility is the ability of the cardiac muscle to act as an efficient pump.

NP: Evaluation; CN: Physiological integrity; CNS: Physiological adaptation; CL: Knowledge

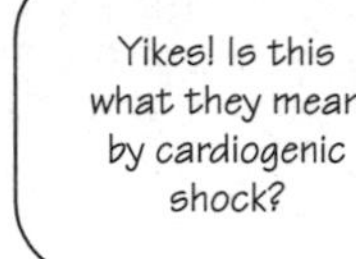

Yikes! Is this what they mean by cardiogenic shock?

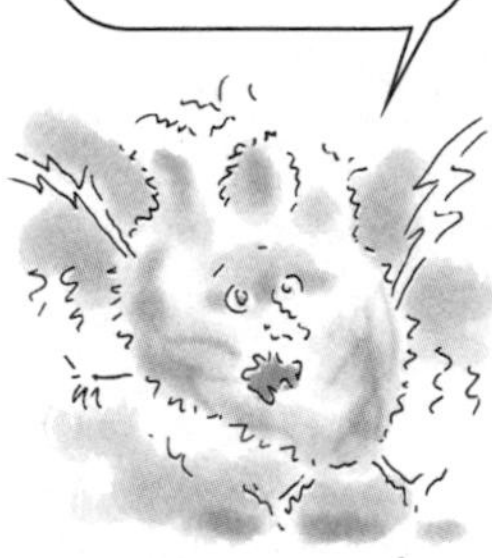

5. Which of the following statements best defines the term *cardiogenic shock?*

1. Decreased cardiac output
2. A reduction in circulating blood volume
3. Overwhelming sepsis and circulating bacterial toxins
4. Inflow or outflow obstruction of the main bloodstream

5. 1. Cardiogenic shock occurs when cardiac output is decreased and tissue oxygen needs aren't adequately met. Hypovolemic shock describes a reduction in circulating blood volume. Septic shock describes overwhelming sepsis and circulating bacterial toxins. Obstructive shock is seen with an inflow or outflow obstruction of the main bloodstream.

NP: Evaluation; CN: Physiological integrity; CNS: Physiological adaptation; CL: Knowledge

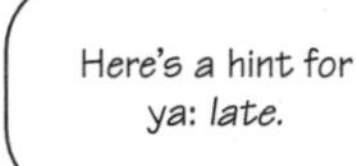

Here's a hint for ya: late.

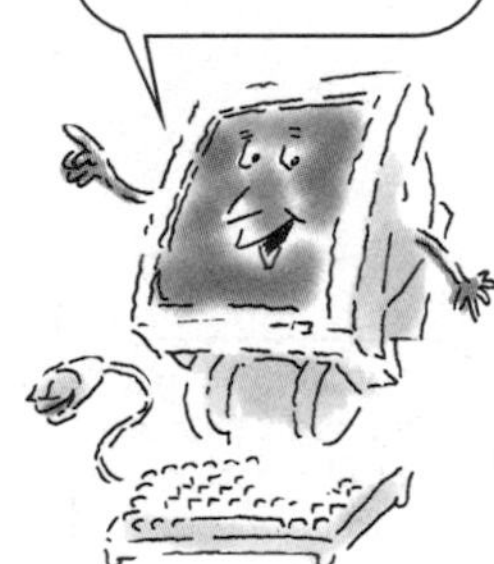

6. Which of the following signs is considered a late sign of shock in children?

1. Tachycardia
2. Hypotension
3. Delayed capillary refill
4. Pale, cool, mottled skin

6. 2. Hypotension is considered a late sign of shock in children. This represents a decompensated state and impending cardiopulmonary arrest. Tachycardia; pale, cool, mottled skin; and delayed capillary refill are earlier indicators of shock that may show compensation.

NP: Assessment; CN: Physiological integrity; CNS: Physiological adaptation; CL: Analysis

7. Which of the following factors indicating a cardiac defect might be found when assessing a 1-month-old infant?

1. Weight gain
2. Hyperactivity
3. Poor nutritional intake
4. Pink mucous membranes

7. 3. Children with heart defects tend to have poor nutritional intake and weight loss, indicating poor cardiac output, heart failure, or hypoxemia. Pink, moist mucous membranes are normal. Gray, pale, or mottled skin may indicate hypoxia or poor cardiac output. The child appears lethargic or tired because of the heart failure or hypoxia.

NP: Assessment; CN: Health promotion and maintenance; CNS: Prevention and early detection of disease; CL: Analysis

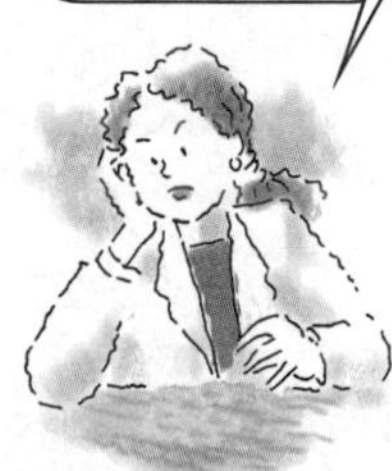

Yes, this is a math question. Stay cool, and you'll do great!

8. A 2-year-old child is showing signs of shock. A 10-ml/kg bolus of normal saline solution is ordered. The child weighs 20 kg. How many milliliters should be administered?

1. 20 ml
2. 100 ml
3. 200 ml
4. 2,000 ml

8. 3. The correct formula for this calculation is 10 ml/kg × 20 kg. The correct answer is 200 ml. The other options are incorrect.

NP: Evaluation; CN: Physiological integrity; CNS: Pharmacological and parenteral therapies; CL: Analysis

9. Which of the following arrhythmias is commonly found in neonates and infants?

1. Atrial fibrillation
2. Bradyarrhythmias
3. Premature atrial contractions
4. Premature ventricular contractions

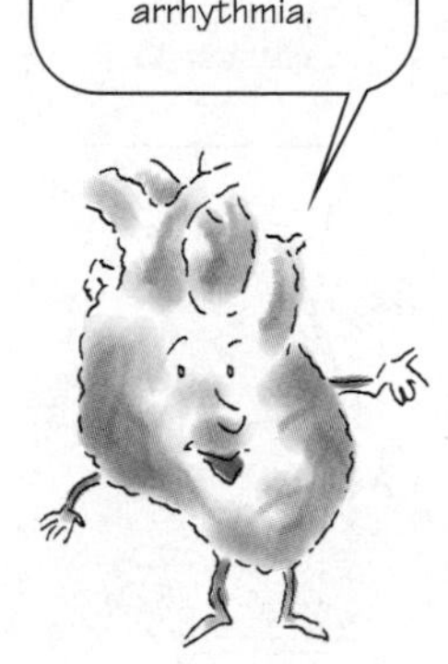

Pick an arrhythmia, any correct arrhythmia.

9. 3. Premature atrial contractions are common in fetuses, neonates, and children. They occur from increased automaticity of an atrial cell anywhere except the sinoatrial node. Premature ventricular contractions are more common in adolescents. Bradyarrhythmias are usually congenital, surgically acquired, or caused by infection. Atrial fibrillation is an uncommon arrhythmia in children occurring from a disorganized state of electrical activity in the atria.

NP: Evaluation; CN: Physiological integrity; CNS: Physiological adaptation; CL: Knowledge

10. Which part of an electrocardiogram reflects ventricular depolarization and contraction?

1. P wave
2. PR interval
3. QRS complex
4. T wave

10. 3. The QRS complex reflects ventricular depolarization and contraction. The P wave represents atrial depolarization and contraction. The PR interval represents the time it takes an impulse to trace from the atrioventricular node to the bundle of His. The T wave represents repolarization of the ventricles.

NP: Analysis; CN: Physiological integrity; CNS: Physiological adaptation; CL: Knowledge

11. Which of the following evaluations of cardiovascular status is noninvasive?

1. Echocardiogram
2. Cardiac enzyme levels
3. Cardiac catheterization
4. Transesophageal pacing

11. 1. An echocardiogram is a noninvasive procedure to visualize the anatomy of the heart. Blood testing determines cardiac enzyme levels. Transesophageal pacing requires a probe to be placed in the esophagus for high-frequency ultrasound. Cardiac catheterization involves passing a catheter into the chambers of the heart for direct visualization of the heart and great vessels.

NP: Evaluation; CN: Physiological integrity; CNS: Physiological adaptation; CL: Analysis

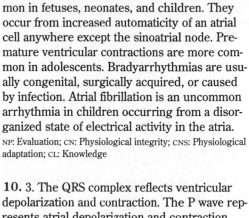

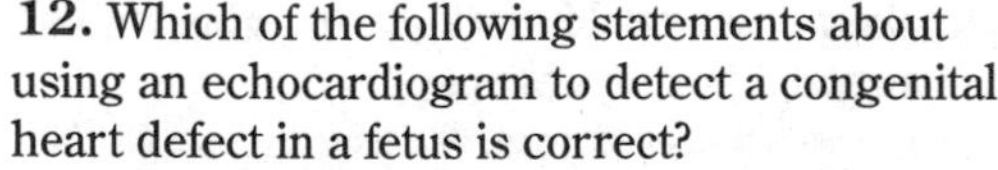

12. Which of the following statements about using an echocardiogram to detect a congenital heart defect in a fetus is correct?

1. A level 1 ultrasound is required to detect this condition.
2. A level 2 ultrasound is required to detect this condition.
3. The mother having the test is generally considered at low risk for problems.
4. Ultrasound can't detect the condition until the 24th week of gestation.

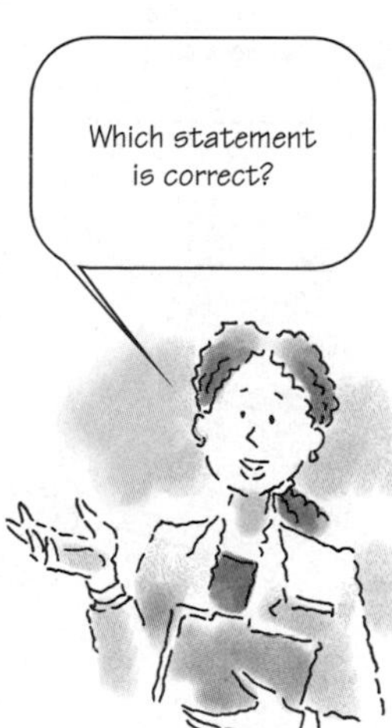

Which statement is correct?

12. 2. A level 2 ultrasound is required to detect a congenital heart defect. Level 1 ultrasounds are routine and aren't able to detect a defect. The mother is usually considered high risk when there's congenital heart disease in the family, maternal diabetes, maternal drug abuse, and other factors. Detection of a congenital heart defect can be made as early as 16 to 18 weeks.

NP: Planning; CN: Health promotion and maintenance; CNS: Prevention and early detection of disease; CL: Analysis

13. Before a cardiac catheterization, which of the following interventions is most appropriate for a child and his parents?

1. Supplying a map of the hospital
2. Limiting visitors to parents only
3. Offering a guided tour of the hospital and catheterization laboratory
4. Explaining that the child can't eat or drink for 1 to 2 days postoperatively

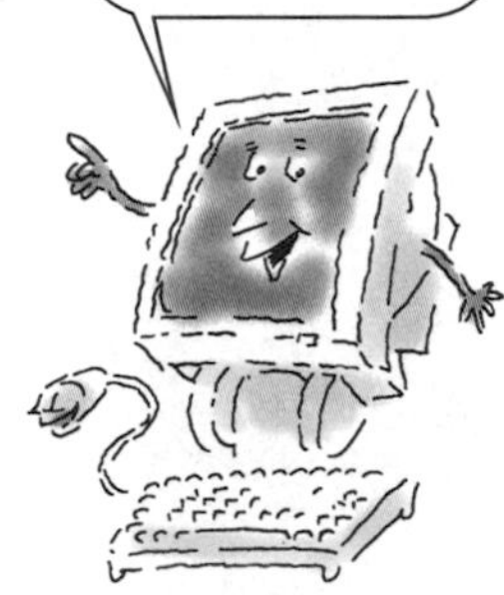

13. 3. A guided tour will help minimize fears and allay anxieties for the child and parents. It gives the opportunity for questions and teaching. A map of the hospital is helpful, but a tour provides the family with more information. The child will be able to start clear liquids and advance as tolerated after the procedure is completed and the child is fully awake. Visitors should include all significant others and siblings as part of the preoperative teaching.
NP: Planning; CN: Physiological integrity; CNS: Physiological adaptation; CL: Analysis

14. Which of the following statements about cardiac catheterization is correct?

1. It's a noninvasive procedure.
2. General anesthesia is required.
3. High-frequency sound waves produce an image of the heart in motion.
4. It provides visualization of the heart and great vessels with radiopaque dye.

14. 4. Cardiac catheterization provides visualization of the heart and great vessels. High-frequency sound waves describe ultrasound and echocardiography. Conscious sedation is usually given before cardiac catheterization. General anesthesia may be used for more complex catheterizations or procedures that place the child at greater risk. It's an invasive procedure in which a thin catheter is passed into the chambers of the heart through a peripheral vein or artery.
NP: Planning; CN: Physiological integrity; CNS: Physiological adaptation; CL: Knowledge

15. Which of the following nursing interventions is most appropriate when caring for a child in the immediate postcatheterization phase?

1. Elevate the head of the bed 45 degrees.
2. Encourage the child to remain flat.
3. Assess vital signs every 2 to 4 hours.
4. Replace a bloody groin dressing with a new dressing.

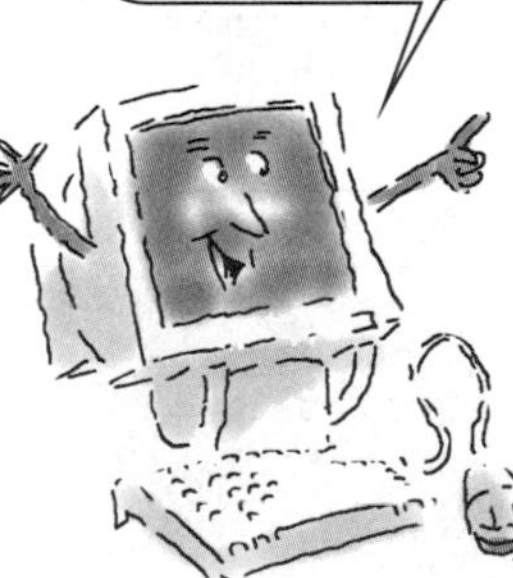

You've already answered 15 questions! See how time flies when you're taking a test?

15. 2. During recovery, the child should remain flat in bed, keeping the punctured leg straight for the prescribed time. The child should avoid raising the head, sitting, straining the abdomen, or coughing. Vital signs are taken every 15 minutes until the child is awake and stable, then every half hour, then hourly as ordered. If bleeding occurs at the insertion site, the nurse should mark the margins with a pen and monitor for changes.
NP: Implementation; CN: Physiological integrity; CNS: Physiological adaptation; CL: Analysis

16. Which of the following home care instructions is included for a child postcatheterization?

1. Encourage fluids and regular diet.
2. Encourage physical activities.
3. The child can routinely bathe after returning home.
4. The child may return to school the next day.

16. 1. A regular diet and increased fluids are encouraged postcatheterization. Increased fluids may flush the injected dyes out of the system. Prolonged bathing can be resumed in 3 days. A sponge bath is encouraged until then. The child may return to school 3 days after discharge. Normal activities may be resumed, but strenuous physical activities or sports should be avoided for about 3 days.
NP: Planning; CN: Physiological integrity; CNS: Physiological adaptation; CL: Analysis

17. A 2-year-old child is being monitored after cardiac surgery. Which of the following signs represents a decrease in cardiac output?

1. Hypertension
2. Increased urine output
3. Weak peripheral pulses
4. Capillary refill less than 2 seconds

18. A 3-year-old child is experiencing distress after having cardiac surgery. Which of the following signs indicates cardiac tamponade?

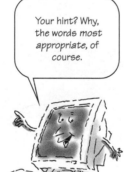

1. Hypertension
2. Muffled heart sounds
3. Widened pulse pressures
4. Increased chest tube drainage

19. A nurse is monitoring fluid and electrolyte balance in a child after cardiac surgery requiring cardiopulmonary bypass. Which of the following findings is expected?

1. Increased urine output
2. Increased sodium level
3. Decreased sodium level
4. Increased potassium level

20. A nurse is teaching wound care to parents after cardiac surgery. Which of the following statements is most appropriate?

1. Lotions and powders are acceptable.
2. Your child can take a complete bath tomorrow.
3. Tingling, itching, and numbness are normal sensations at the wound site.
4. If the sterile adhesive strips over the incision fall off, call the physician.

21. Parents ask a nurse about their 8-year-old son's activity level after cardiac surgery. Which of the following responses would be best?

1. There are no exercise limitations.
2. The child may resume school in 3 days.
3. Encourage a balance of rest and exercise.
4. Climbing and contact sports are restricted for 1 week.

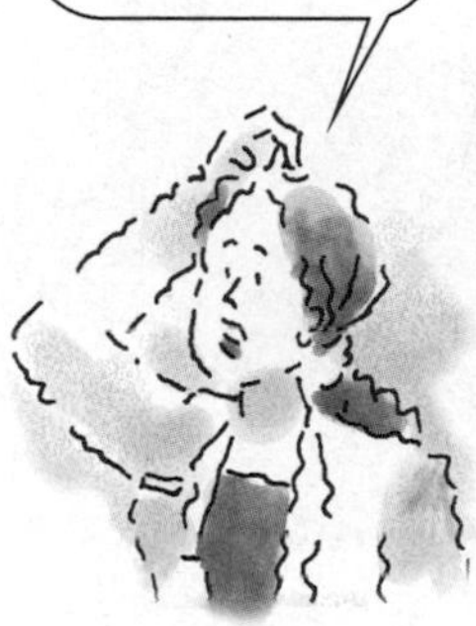

All of these signs may appear, but only one indicates cardiac tamponade. Which one?

Your hint? Why, the words most appropriate, of course.

17. 3. Signs of decreased cardiac output include weak peripheral pulses, low urine output, delayed capillary refill, hypotension, and cool extremities.

NP: Assessment; CN: Physiological integrity; CNS: Physiological adaptation; CL: Analysis

18. 2. Symptoms of cardiac tamponade include muffled heart sounds, hypotension, sudden cessation of chest tube drainage, and a narrowing pulse pressure. Cardiac tamponade occurs when a large volume of fluid interferes with ventricular filling and pumping and collects in the pericardial sac, decreasing cardiac output.

NP: Assessment; CN: Physiological integrity; CNS: Physiological adaptation; CL: Analysis

19. 2. In response to surgery and cardiopulmonary bypass, the body secretes aldosterone and antidiuretic hormone. This in turn increases sodium levels, decreases potassium levels, increases water retention, and decreases urine output.

NP: Assessment; CN: Physiological integrity; CNS: Physiological adaptation; CL: Analysis

20. 3. As the area heals, tingling, itching, and numbness are normal sensations and will eventually go away. A complete bath should be delayed for the first week. Lotions and powders should be avoided during the first 2 weeks after surgery. Steri-Strips may loosen or fall off on their own. This is a common and normal occurrence.

NP: Evaluation; CN: Physiological integrity; CNS: Physiological adaptation; CL: Analysis

21. 3. Activity should be increased gradually each day, allowing for a sensible balance of rest and exercise. School and large crowds should be avoided for at least 2 weeks to prevent exposure to people with active infections. Sports and contact activities should be restricted for about 6 weeks, giving the sternum enough time to heal.

NP: Evaluation; CN: Physiological integrity; CNS: Physiological adaptation; CL: Analysis

22. Which of the following home care instructions is most appropriate for a child after cardiac surgery?

1. Don't stop giving the child the prescribed drugs until the physician says so.
2. Maintain a sodium-restricted diet.
3. Routine dental care can be resumed.
4. Immunizations are delayed indefinitely.

22. 1. Drugs, such as digoxin and furosemide, shouldn't be stopped abruptly. Immunizations are delayed at least 6 weeks after surgery. Routine dental care is usually delayed 6 months after surgery. There are no diet restrictions and the child may resume his regular diet.

NP: Evaluation; CN: Physiological integrity; CNS: Physiological adaptation; CL: Analysis

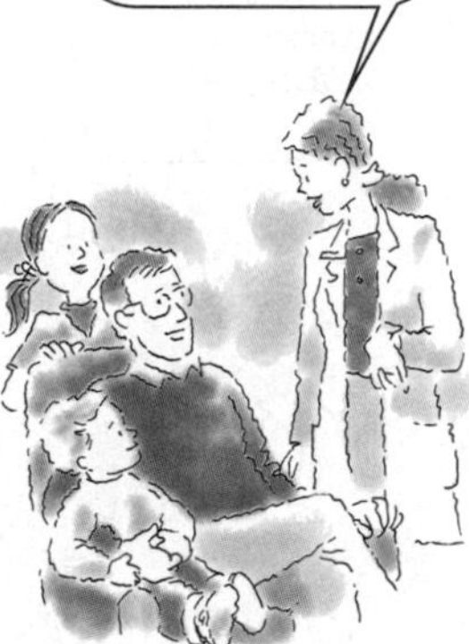

OK, let's talk about what you need to know when you take Timmy home from the hospital.

23. A 4-year-old client with a chest tube is placed on water seal. Which of the following statements is correct?

1. The water level rises with inhalation.
2. Bubbling is seen in the suction chamber.
3. Bubbling is seen in the water seal chamber.
4. Water seal is obtained by clamping the tube.

23. 1. The water seal chamber is functioning appropriately when the water level rises in the chamber with inhalation and falls with expiration. This shows that negative pressure required in the lung is being maintained. Bubbling in the water seal chamber generally indicates the presence of an air leak. Bubbling in the suction chamber should only be seen when suction is being used. The chest tube should never be clamped; a tension pneumothorax may occur. Water seal is activated when the suction is disconnected.

NP: Analysis; CN: Physiological integrity; CNS: Physiological adaptation; CL: Application

24. Which of the following interventions is most appropriate when a chest tube falls out or becomes dislodged?

1. Place a dry gauze dressing over the insertion site.
2. Place a petroleum gauze dressing over the insertion site.
3. Wipe the tube with alcohol and reinsert it.
4. Call the physician immediately.

24. 2. Petroleum gauze should be placed over the site immediately to prevent a pneumothorax. The physician should be notified after this step. The tube is only reinserted by a physician using a sterile thoracotomy tray. A dry gauze dressing will allow air to escape, leading to a pneumothorax.

NP: Analysis; CN: Physiological integrity; CNS: Physiological adaptation; CL: Application

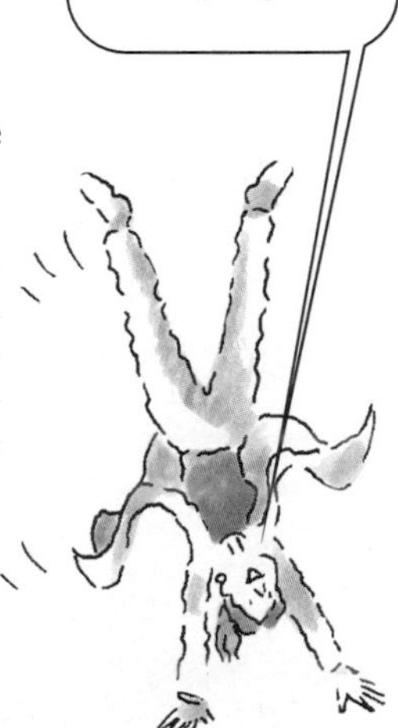

Question 25 is a milestone. Way to go!

25. When assessing a child with heart failure, which of the following findings would the nurse expect to find?

1. Bradycardia
2. Weight gain
3. Gallop murmur
4. Strong, bounding pulses

25. 3. When the heart stretches beyond efficiency, an extra heart sound or S_3 gallop murmur may be audible. This is related to excessive preload and ventricular dilation. Tachycardia occurs as a compensatory mechanism to the decrease in cardiac output. It also attempts to increase the force and rate of myocardial contraction and increase oxygen consumption of the heart. Pulses are usually weak and thready. Children with heart failure tend to have difficulty feeding and tire easily. They're commonly diagnosed as failure to thrive and are in the lower percentiles of their growth charts for weight.

NP: Assessment; CN: Physiological integrity; CNS: Physiological adaptation; CL: Analysis

26. Which of the following symptoms is seen with pulmonary venous congestion or left-sided heart failure?

1. Weight gain
2. Peripheral edema
3. Neck vein distention
4. Tachypnea and dyspnea

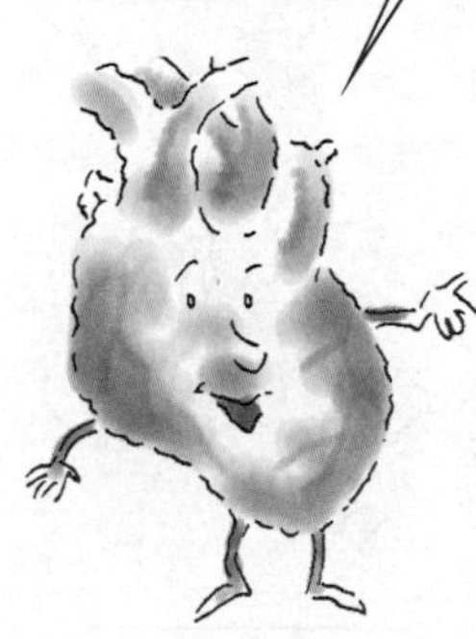

What happens when my left side isn't working properly?

26. 4. Respiratory symptoms, such as tachypnea and dyspnea, are seen due to pulmonary congestion. Peripheral edema, neck vein distention, and weight gain are seen with systemic venous congestion or right-sided heart failure. Fluid accumulates in the interstitial spaces due to blood pooling in the venous circulation.

NP: Assessment; CN: Physiological integrity; CNS: Physiological adaptation; CL: Knowledge

27. Which of the following interventions is most appropriate when caring for an infant with heart failure?

1. Limit fluid intake.
2. Avoid using infant seats.
3. Cluster nursing activities.
4. Place the infant prone or supine.

27. 3. Energy expenditures need to be limited to reduce metabolic and oxygen needs. Nursing care should be clustered, followed by long periods of undisturbed rest. Infants should be placed in the semi-Fowler or upright position. Infant seats help maintain an upright position. This facilitates lung expansion, provides less restrictive movement of the diaphragm, relieves pressure from abdominal organs, and decreases pulmonary congestion. Fluid may be restricted in older children, but infants' nutritional requirements depend on fluid needs.

NP: Analysis; CN: Physiological integrity; CNS: Physiological adaptation; CL: Analysis

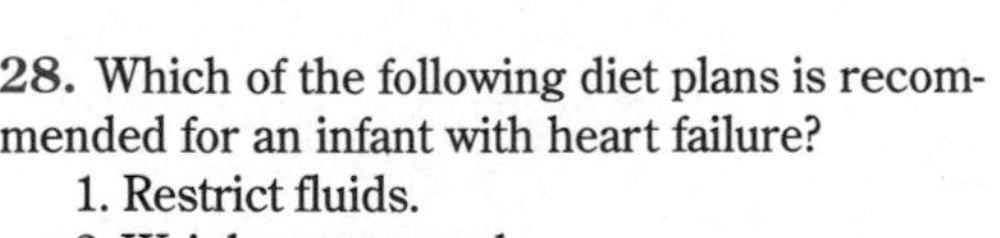

28. Which of the following diet plans is recommended for an infant with heart failure?

1. Restrict fluids.
2. Weigh once a week.
3. Use low-sodium formula.
4. Increase caloric content per ounce.

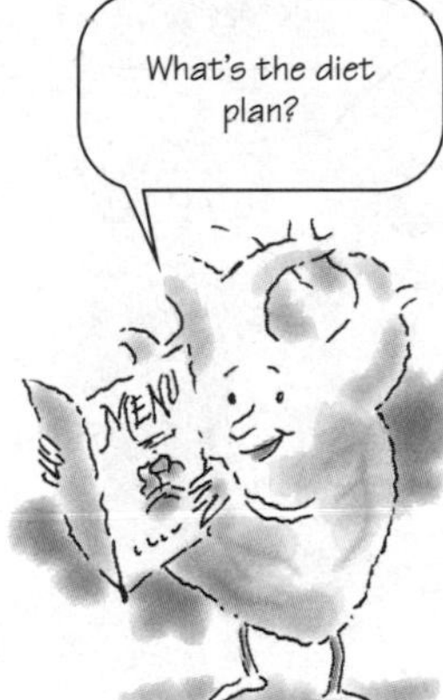

What's the diet plan?
MENU

28. 4. Formulas with increased caloric content are given to meet the greater caloric requirements from the overworked heart and labored breathing. Daily weights at the same time of the day on the same scale before feedings are recommended to follow trends in nutritional stability and diuresis. Fluid restriction and low-sodium formulas aren't recommended. An infant's nutritional needs depend on fluid. Low-sodium formulas may cause hyponatremia.

NP: Implementation; CN: Physiological integrity; CNS: Physiological adaptation; CL: Application

29. Which of the following statements is true about giving oxygen to a client with heart failure?

1. Oxygen is usually given only if the client has concurrent illness.
2. Oxygen is given at high levels only.
3. Oxygen is a pulmonary bed constrictor.
4. Oxygen decreases the work of breathing.

29. 1. Because oxygen is a pulmonary bed dilator, it typically worsens heart failure, which is also referred to as pulmonary overcirculation in children. So, unless there's concurrent illness such as pneumonia, oxygen usually worsens heart failure and increases the work of breathing. Oxygen is usually administered at low levels with humidification.

NP: Implementation; CN: Physiological integrity; CNS: Physiological adaptation; CL: Analysis

30. A teenage client with heart failure is prescribed digoxin. To which of the following classifications does this drug belong?

1. Angiotensin-converting enzyme (ACE) inhibitor
2. Cardiac glycoside
3. Diuretic
4. Vasodilator

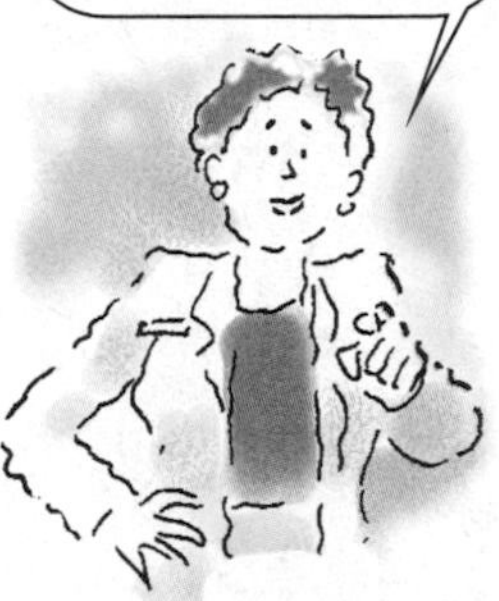

Knowing the classification of a drug can help you remember its actions.

30. 2. Digoxin is a cardiac glycoside. It decreases the workload of the heart and improves myocardial function. Diuretics help remove excess fluid. Vasodilators enhance cardiac output by decreasing afterload. ACE inhibitors cause vasodilation and increase sodium excretion.

NP: Evaluation; CN: Physiological integrity; CNS: Pharmacological and parenteral therapies; CL: Knowledge

31. Which of the following toxic adverse reactions can be seen in a child taking digoxin?

1. Weight gain
2. Tachycardia
3. Nausea and vomiting
4. Seizures

31. 3. Digoxin toxicity in infants and children may present with nausea, vomiting, anorexia, or a slow, irregular apical heart rate. Weight gain, tachycardia, or seizures wouldn't be seen in digoxin toxicity.

NP: Evaluation; CN: Physiological integrity; CNS: Pharmacological and parenteral therapies; CL: Analysis

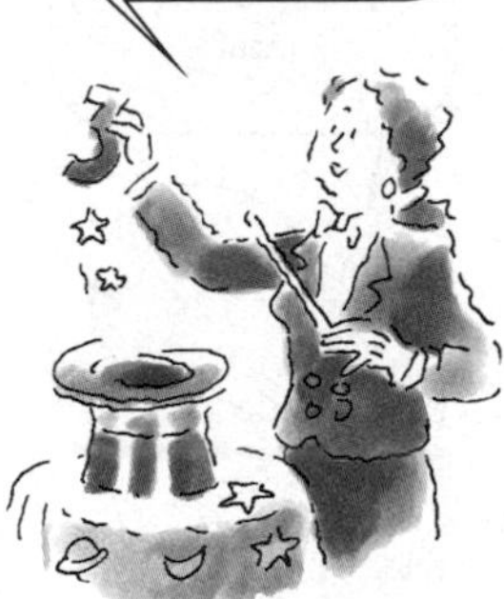

How are you figuring that dosage?

32. An 11-month-old infant with heart failure weighs 10 kg. Digoxin is prescribed as 10 mcg/kg/day in divided doses every 12 hours. How much is given per dose?

1. 10 mcg
2. 50 mcg
3. 100 mcg
4. 500 mcg

32. 2. 10 kg × 10 mcg/kg/day = 100 mcg/day divided by 2 doses = 50 mcg/dose

NP: Evaluation; CN: Physiological integrity; CNS: Pharmacological and parenteral therapies; CL: Analysis

33. A client with heart failure is given captopril (Capoten), an angiotensin-converting enzyme (ACE) inhibitor. Which of the following actions occurs with this type of drug?

1. Vasoconstriction
2. Increased sodium excretion
3. Decreased sodium excretion
4. Increased vascular resistance

33. 2. ACE inhibitors block the conversion of angiotensin I to angiotensin II in the kidney. This causes decreased aldosterone, vasodilation, and increased sodium excretion. As a vasodilator, it also acts to reduce vascular resistance by the manipulation of afterload.

NP: Evaluation; CN: Physiological integrity; CNS: Pharmacological and parenteral therapies; CL: Knowledge

34. Which of the following statements about patent ductus arteriosus is correct?

1. Heart failure is uncommon.
2. The ductus normally closes completely by age 6 weeks.
3. An open ductus arteriosus causes decreased blood flow to the lungs.
4. It represents a cyanotic defect with decreased pulmonary blood flow.

34. 2. At birth, oxygenated blood normally causes the ductus to constrict, and the vessel closes completely by age 6 weeks. This defect is considered an acyanotic defect with increased pulmonary blood flow. The open ductus arteriosus can cause an excessive blood flow to the lungs because of the high pressure in the aorta. Heart failure is common in premature infants with a patent ductus arteriosus.

NP: Assessment; CN: Physiological integrity; CNS: Physiological adaptation; CL: Knowledge

35. Which of the following interventions or drugs is recommended initially for preterm neonates to close a patent ductus arteriosus?
1. Indomethacin
2. Prostaglandin E_1
3. Surgical ligation
4. Cardiac catheterization

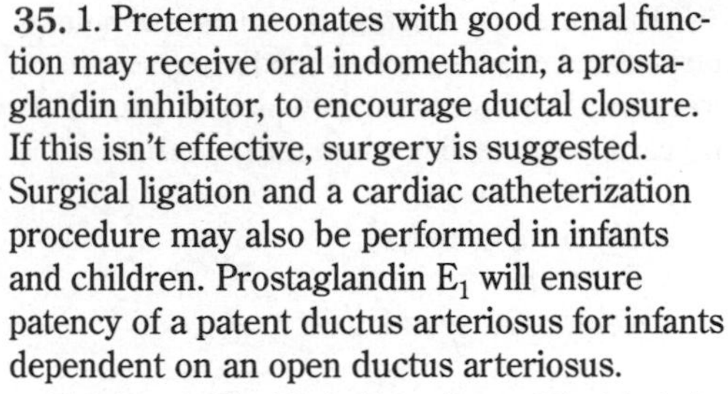

35. 1. Preterm neonates with good renal function may receive oral indomethacin, a prostaglandin inhibitor, to encourage ductal closure. If this isn't effective, surgery is suggested. Surgical ligation and a cardiac catheterization procedure may also be performed in infants and children. Prostaglandin E_1 will ensure patency of a patent ductus arteriosus for infants dependent on an open ductus arteriosus.
NP: Planning; CN: Physiological integrity; CNS: Physiological adaptation; CL: Analysis

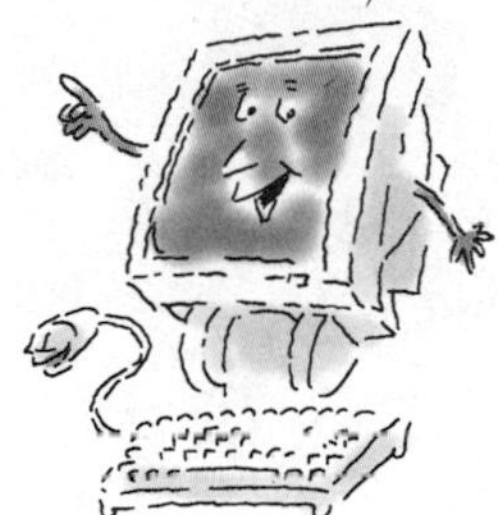

Question 36 asks which finding you *expect*, not necessarily one that may or may not occur.

36. Which of the following findings is expected in a child with patent ductus arteriosus?
1. Weak peripheral pulses
2. Machine-like murmur
3. Narrowed pulse pressure
4. Right ventricular hypertrophy

36. 2. The continuous, turbulent flow of blood from the aorta through the patent ductus arteriosus to the pulmonary artery produces a machine-like murmur. There's a widened pulse pressure and bounding peripheral pulses from the runoff of blood from the aorta to the pulmonary artery. Left ventricular hypertrophy created from the left to right shunting of blood can be seen on X-ray.
NP: Assessment; CN: Physiological integrity; CNS: Physiological adaptation; CL: Knowledge

37. Which of the following cardiovascular disorders is considered acyanotic?
1. Patent ductus arteriosus
2. Tetralogy of Fallot
3. Tricuspid atresia
4. Truncus arteriosus

37. 1. A patent ductus arteriosus represents an acyanotic heart defect with increased pulmonary blood flow. Tricuspid atresia and tetralogy of Fallot are cyanotic defects with decreased pulmonary blood flow. Truncus arteriosus is a cyanotic defect with increased pulmonary blood flow.
NP: Assessment; CN: Physiological integrity; CNS: Physiological adaptation; CL: Knowledge

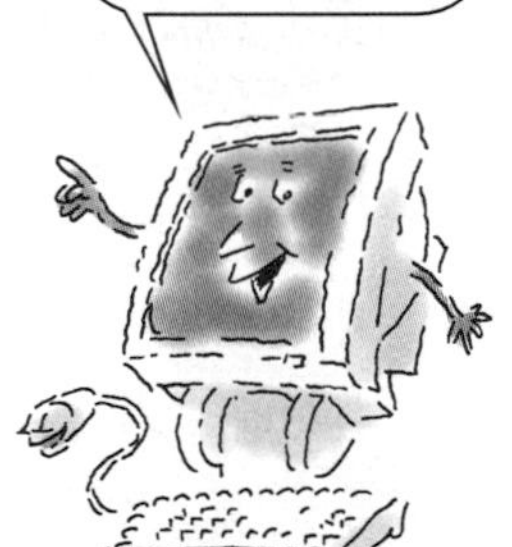

Don't be fooled; this word asks what is NOT expected. Be wary of questions phrased as a negative.

38. Which of the following findings is not expected during an assessment of a child with an acyanotic heart defect?
1. Poor weight gain
2. Bradycardia
3. Hepatomegaly
4. Increased respiratory rate

38. 2. The increase in blood flow to the lungs may cause tachycardia (not bradycardia) and increased respiratory rates to compensate. Hepatomegaly may result from blood backing up into the liver due to the difficulty of entering the right side of the heart. Poor growth and development may be seen due to the increased energy required for breathing.
NP: Assessment; CN: Physiological integrity; CNS: Physiological adaptation; CL: Analysis

39. Eisenmenger's complex consists of pulmonary vascular resistance exceeding systemic pressure. This can occur in which of the following cardiac anomalies when untreated?

1. Aortic stenosis
2. Atrial septal defect
3. Pulmonary stenosis
4. Ventricular septal defect

39. 4. In moderate to large untreated ventricular septal defects, the constant excess flow will increase pulmonary vascular resistance. As time progresses, pressures in the right ventricle and left ventricle may change, causing higher pressures on the right side. A right-to-left shunt results, and pulmonary hypertension occurs.

NP: Assessment; CN: Physiological integrity; CNS: Physiological adaptation; CL: Knowledge

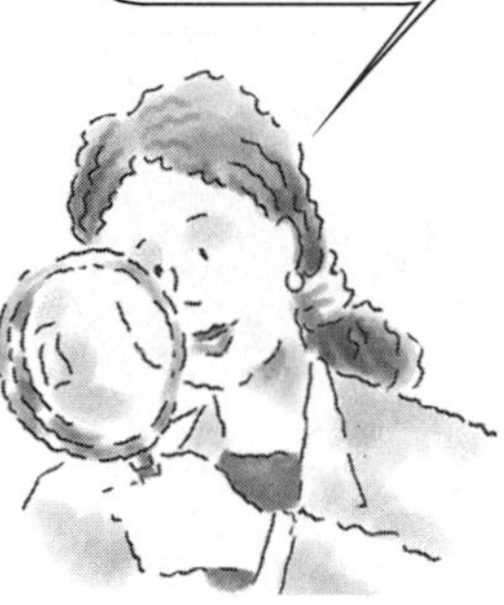

You can see these signs without a magnifying glass!

40. Which of the following signs may be seen in a child with ventricular septal defect?

1. Cyanosis of the nailbeds
2. Above average height on growth chart
3. Above average weight gain on growth chart
4. Pink nailbeds with capillary refill less than 2 seconds

40. 1. Cyanotic nailbeds can be seen when pulmonary resistance increases and causes the left to right shunt to reverse and shunt right to left. This shift leads to signs of heart failure and cyanosis. Children with the defect usually present with symptoms of heart failure, poor growth and development, and failure to thrive.

NP: Assessment; CN: Physiological integrity; CNS: Physiological adaptation; CL: Analysis

41. Which of the following conditions best describes ventricular septal defect?

1. Narrowing of the aortic arch
2. Failure of a septum to develop completely between the atria
3. Narrowing of the valves at the entrance of the pulmonary artery
4. Failure of a septum to develop completely between the ventricles

41. 4. Failure of a septum to develop between the ventricles results in a left-to-right shunt, which is noted as a ventricular septal defect. When the septum fails to develop between the atria, it's considered an atrial septal defect. The narrowing of the aortic arch describes coarctation of the aorta. Narrowing of the valves at the pulmonary artery describes pulmonic stenosis.

NP: Assessment; CN: Physiological integrity; CNS: Physiological adaptation; CL: Knowledge

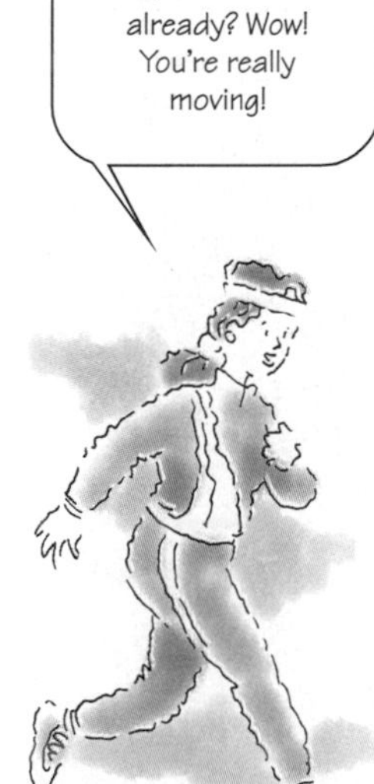

Question 42 already? Wow! You're really moving!

42. Which of the following curative surgical interventions is recommended for a child with ventricular septal defect?

1. Surgery with pulmonary artery banding
2. Defect repair through cardiac catheterization
3. Surgery with purse-string suture or Dacron patch repair
4. Surgery when severe pulmonary hypertension is noted

42. 3. Surgery is recommended for children ages 1 to 4. A median sternotomy incision is placed with the heart on cardiopulmonary bypass. For small defects, a stitch closure is performed. For larger defects, a patch is sewn. Cardiac catheterization repairs have been performed for selective cases but aren't approved for general care. Surgery with pulmonary artery banding is only a palliative procedure for children too small or too ill but in heart failure. Severe pulmonary hypertension would lead to an inoperable condition. If repaired, the excess blood flow to the lungs by patching the defect may be fatal.

NP: Planning; CN: Physiological integrity; CNS: Physiological adaptation; CL: Application

43. A client with a ventricular septal repair is receiving dopamine (Intropin) postoperatively. Which of the following responses is expected?

1. Decreased heart rate
2. Decreased urine output
3. Increased cardiac output
4. Decreased cardiac contractility

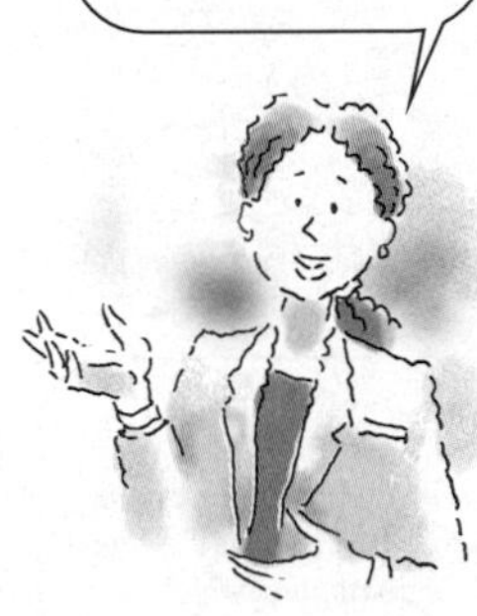

You know more about drugs than you realize!

43. 3. Dopamine stimulates $beta_1$ and $beta_2$ receptors. It's a selective cardiac stimulant that will increase cardiac output, heart rate, and cardiac contractility. Urine output increases in response to dilation of the blood vessels to the mesentery and kidneys.

NP: Evaluation; CN: Physiological integrity; CNS: Pharmacological and parenteral therapies; CL: Knowledge

44. Which of the following descriptions is correct for a complete endocardial cushion defect?

1. Absent tricuspid valve
2. Opening or hole in the atrial septum
3. Opening or hole in the ventricular septum
4. Involves the mitral valve, tricuspid valve, atrial septum, and ventricular septum

44. 4. A complete endocardial cushion defect develops early in fetal life because of inappropriate fusion of the endocardial cushions. It involves the mitral valve, tricuspid valve, atrial septum, and ventricular septum. An opening in the atria is considered an atrial septal defect. An opening in the ventricles is considered a ventricular septal defect. An absent tricuspid valve is considered tricuspid atresia.

NP: Evaluation; CN: Health promotion and maintenance; CNS: Growth and development through the life span; CL: Knowledge

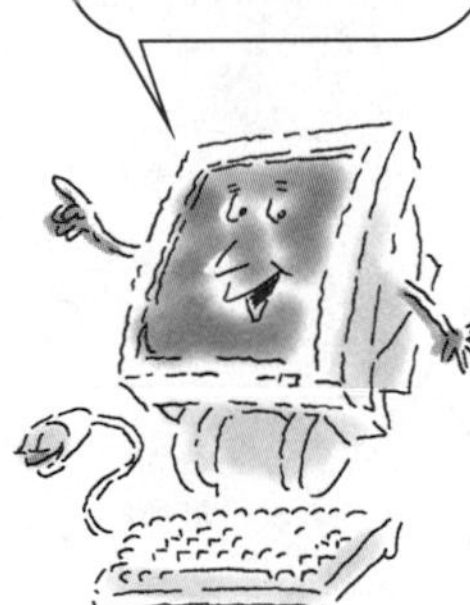

The words most often hint at the answer.

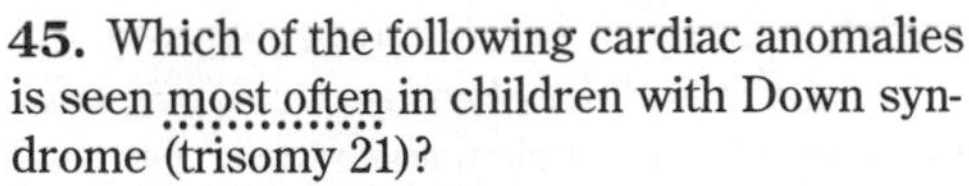

45. Which of the following cardiac anomalies is seen most often in children with Down syndrome (trisomy 21)?

1. Atrial septal defect
2. Pulmonic stenosis
3. Ventricular septal defect
4. Endocardial cushion defect

45. 4. Endocardial cushion defects are seen most in children with Down syndrome. Ventricular septal defects are the most common of the cardiac anomalies. Atrial septal defects account for about 10% of all cardiac anomalies. Pulmonic stenosis is responsible for about 8% of all cardiac anomalies.

NP: Evaluation; CN: Health promotion and maintenance; CNS: Prevention and early detection of disease; CL: Knowledge

46. Which of the following classifications best describes an atrioventricular canal defect or endocardial cushion defect?

1. Cyanotic with increased pulmonary blood flow
2. Cyanotic with decreased pulmonary blood flow
3. Acyanotic with increased pulmonary blood flow
4. Acyanotic with obstructive flow from the ventricles

46. 3. Endocardial cushion defects shunt left to right, which depicts an acyanotic defect with increased pulmonary blood flow. An example of an acyanotic defect with obstructive flow from the ventricles is aortic stenosis. Examples of cyanotic defects include tricuspid atresia and truncus arteriosus.

NP: Evaluation; CN: Health promotion and maintenance; CNS: Prevention and early detection of disease; CL: Knowledge

47. Which of the following cardiac anomalies produces a left-to-right shunt?
1. Atrial septal defect
2. Pulmonic stenosis
3. Tetralogy of Fallot
4. Total anomalous pulmonary venous return

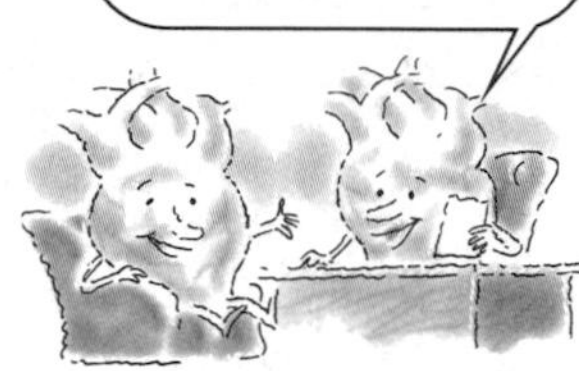

My shunt is left to right. How about yours?

47. 1. Atrial septal defects shunt from left to right because pressures are greater on the left side of the heart. Pulmonic stenosis, tetralogy of Fallot, and total anomalous pulmonary venous return will show a right-to-left shunting of blood.

NP: Evaluation; CN: Health promotion and maintenance; CNS: Prevention and early detection of disease; CL: Analysis

48. A child with an atrial septal repair is entering postoperative day 3. Which of the following interventions would be most appropriate?
1. Give the child nothing by mouth.
2. Maintain strict bed rest.
3. Take vital signs every 8 hours.
4. Administer an analgesic as needed.

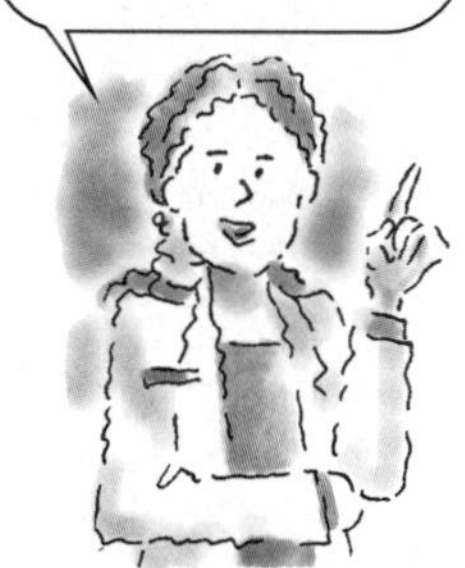

All of these interventions may be appropriate at some point, but which is *most appropriate* for this situation?

48. 4. Pain management is always a priority and should be given on an as needed basis. By day 3, the child should be advancing to a regular diet. Vital signs should be performed routinely every 2 to 4 hours. Activity should include activity as able in the step-down unit, with coughing and deep breathing exercises.

NP: Planning; CN: Physiological integrity; CNS: Physiological adaptation; CL: Application

49. A 3-year-old child is on postoperative day 5 for an atrial septal repair. Which of the following nursing diagnoses would be most appropriate?
1. Activity intolerance
2. Chronic pain
3. Social isolation
4. Excess fluid volume, potential

49. 4. Diuretics may still be used as needed at this point. By day 5, the child's activity level will be normal, and there will be little to no pain. The child isn't isolated from anyone and can usually attend the playroom on day 3 or 4.

NP: Evaluation; CN: Physiological integrity; CNS: Physiological adaptation; CL: Analysis

50. Which of the following conditions best describes coarctation of the aorta?
1. Absent tricuspid valve
2. Narrowing in the area of the aortic valve
3. Localized constriction or narrowing of the aortic wall
4. Narrowing at some location along the right ventricular outflow tract

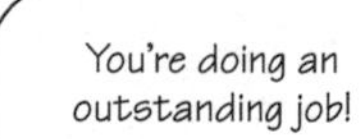

You're doing an outstanding job!

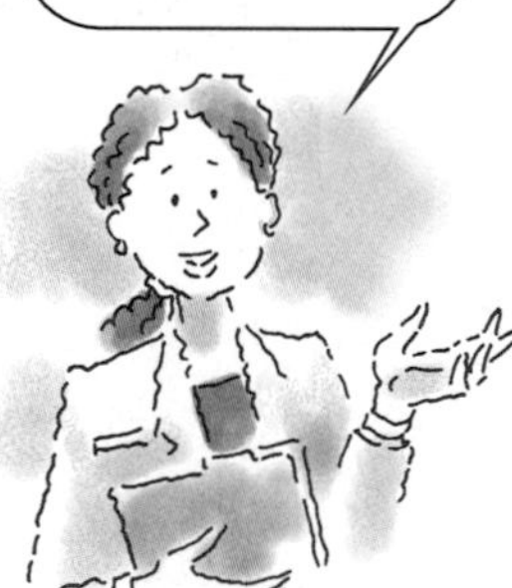

50. 3. Coarctation of the aorta consists of a localized constriction or narrowing of the aortic wall. Aortic stenosis is a narrowing in the area of the aortic valve. Tricuspid atresia is characterized by an absent tricuspid valve. Pulmonic stenosis consists of a narrowing along the right ventricular outflow tract.

NP: Evaluation; CN: Health promotion and maintenance; CNS: Prevention and early detection of disease; CL: Knowledge

51. A client is diagnosed with coarctation of the aorta. Which of the following findings would the nurse expect during an assessment?
1. Normal blood pressure
2. Increased blood pressure in the upper extremities
3. Decreased blood pressure in the upper extremities
4. Decreased or absent pulses in the upper extremities

51. 2. As blood is pumped from the left ventricle to the aorta, some blood flows to the head and upper extremities while the rest meets obstruction and jets through the constricted area. Pressures and pulses are greater in the upper extremities. Decreased or absent pulses are found in the lower extremities.

NP: Assessment; CN: Physiological integrity; CNS: Physiological adaptation; CL: Analysis

52. Which of the following procedures is recommended to treat coarctation of the aorta?

1. Drug therapy
2. Balloon angioplasty
3. Surgery without cardiopulmonary bypass
4. Surgery with cardiopulmonary bypass

52. 3. Balloon angioplasty is reserved for recoarctation of the aorta or for clients initially diagnosed when older than age 1. Surgery is usually performed without cardiopulmonary bypass. Drugs won't help this type of defect.
NP: Planning; CN: Physiological integrity; CNS: Physiological adaptation; CL: Knowledge

53. Which of the following factors is an important part of assessment for a child with a possible cardiac anomaly?

1. Heart rate
2. Temperature
3. Blood pressure
4. Blood pressure in four extremities

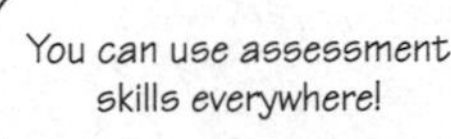

You can use assessment skills everywhere!

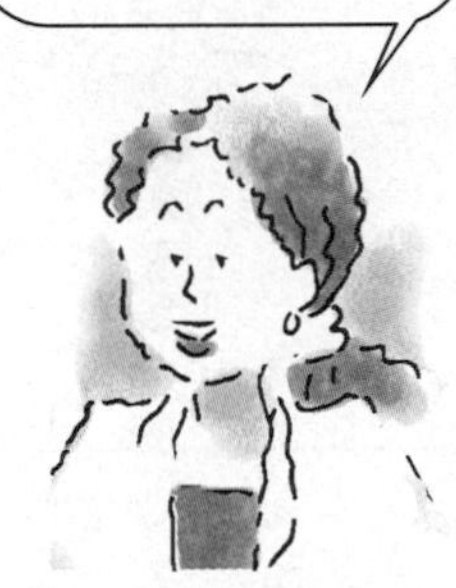

53. 4. Measuring blood pressure in all four extremities is necessary to document hypertension and the blood pressure gradient between the upper and lower extremities. Temperature and heart rate are also important assessments.
NP: Assessment; CN: Physiological integrity; CNS: Physiological adaptation; CL: Application

54. Which of the following interventions is recommended postoperatively for a client with coarctation of the aorta repair?

1. Give a vasoconstrictor.
2. Maintain hypothermia.
3. Maintain a normal to low blood pressure.
4. Give a bolus of I.V. fluids.

54. 3. Blood pressure is tightly managed and kept low so there is no excessive pressure on the fresh suture lines. Normothermia is maintained, and diuretics may be given to decrease fluid volume.
NP: Implementation; CN: Physiological integrity; CNS: Physiological adaptation; CL: Analysis

55. Which of the following assessments is expected when assessing a child with tetralogy of Fallot?

1. Machine-like murmur
2. Eisenmenger's complex
3. Increasing cyanosis with crying or activity
4. Higher pressures in the upper extremities than with the lower extremities

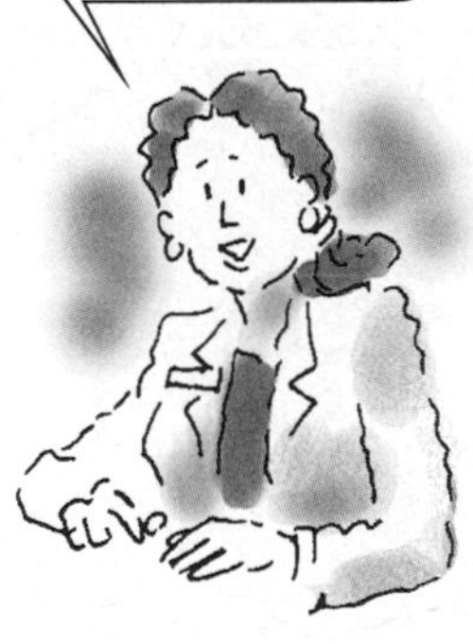

When it comes to assessment, practice makes perfect!

55. 3. A child with tetralogy of Fallot will be mildly cyanotic at rest and have increasing cyanosis with crying, activity, or straining, as with a bowel movement. A machine-like murmur is a characteristic of patent ductus arteriosus. Higher pressures in the upper extremities are characteristic of coarctation of the aorta. Eisenmenger's complex is a complication of ventricular resistance exceeding systemic pressure.
NP: Assessment; CN: Physiological integrity; CNS: Physiological adaptation; CL: Application

56. A child with tetralogy of Fallot has clubbing of the fingers and toes, a finding related to which of the following conditions?

1. Polycythemia
2. Chronic hypoxia
3. Pansystolic murmur
4. Abnormal growth and development

56. 2. Chronic hypoxia longer than 6 months causes clubbing of the fingers and toes when untreated. Hypoxia varies with the degree of pulmonic stenosis. Growth and development may appear normal. Polycythemia is an increased number of red blood cells as a result of the chronic hypoxemia. A pansystolic murmur is heard at the middle to lower left sternal border but has no impact on clubbing.
NP: Assessment; CN: Physiological integrity; CNS: Physiological adaptation; CL: Knowledge

57. A child with tetralogy of Fallot may assume which position of comfort during exercise?

1. Prone
2. Semi-Fowler
3. Side-lying
4. Squat

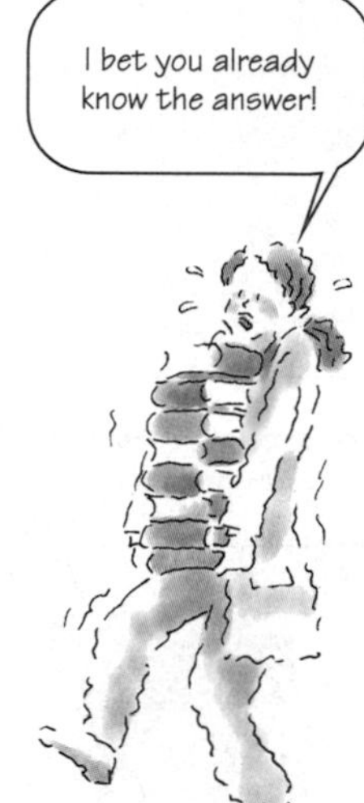

I bet you already know the answer!

57. 4. A child may squat or assume a knee-chest position to reduce venous blood flow from the lower extremities and to increase systemic vascular resistance, which diverts more blood flow into the pulmonary artery. Prone, semi-Fowler, and side-lying positions won't produce this effect.

NP: Evaluation; CN: Physiological integrity; CNS: Physiological adaptation; CL: Analysis

58. Which of the following statements is correct for a child with tetralogy of Fallot?

1. The condition is commonly referred to as "blue tets."
2. They experience hypercyanotic, or "tet," spells.
3. They experience frequent respiratory infections.
4. They experience decreased or absent pulses in the lower extremities.

58. 2. Hypercyanotic, or "tet," spells may occur due to increasing obstruction of right ventricular outflow, resulting in decreased pulmonary blood flow and increased right-to-left shunting. Infants with mild obstruction to blood flow have little or no right-to-left shunting and appear pink, or "pink tets." Frequent respiratory infections are seen in defects with increased pulmonary blood flow such as a patent ductus arteriosus. Decreased or absent pulses in the lower extremities is a sign of coarctation of the aorta.

NP: Assessment; CN: Physiological integrity; CNS: Physiological adaptation; CL: Knowledge

59. Which of the following tests would show the direction and amount of shunting in a child with tetralogy of Fallot?

1. Chest radiography
2. Echocardiography
3. Electrocardiography (ECG)
4. Cardiac catheterization

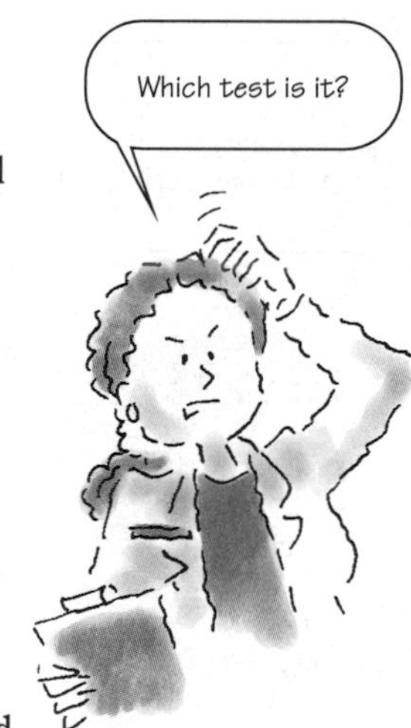

Which test is it?

59. 4. Cardiac catheterization provides specific information about the direction and amount of shunting, coronary anatomy, and each portion of the heart defect. ECG shows right ventricular hypertrophy with tall R waves. Echocardiogram scans define such defects as large ventricular septal defects, pulmonic stenosis, and malposition of the aorta. Chest radiographs will show right ventricular hypertrophy pushing the heart apex upward, resulting in a boot-shaped silhouette.

NP: Analysis; CN: Physiological integrity; CNS: Physiological adaptation; CL: Knowledge

60. A nurse is teaching parents about tricuspid atresia. Which of the following statements indicates the parents understand?

1. "There's a narrowing at the aortic outflow tract."
2. "The pulmonary veins don't return to the left atrium."
3. "There's a narrowing at the entrance of the pulmonary artery."
4. "There's no communication between the right atrium and right ventricle."

60. 4. Tricuspid atresia is failure of the tricuspid valve to develop, leaving no communication between the right atrium and right ventricle. The narrowing at the entrance of the pulmonary artery represents pulmonic stenosis. Narrowing at the aortic outflow tract is aortic stenosis. Total anomalous pulmonary venous return is a defect in which the pulmonary veins don't return to the left atrium but abnormally return to the right side of the heart.

NP: Evaluation; CN: Physiological integrity; CNS: Physiological adaptation; CL: Analysis

61. Which of the following characteristics can be noted during the assessment of a child with tricuspid atresia?

1. Cyanosis
2. Machine-like murmur
3. Decreased respiratory rate
4. Capillary refill more than 2 seconds

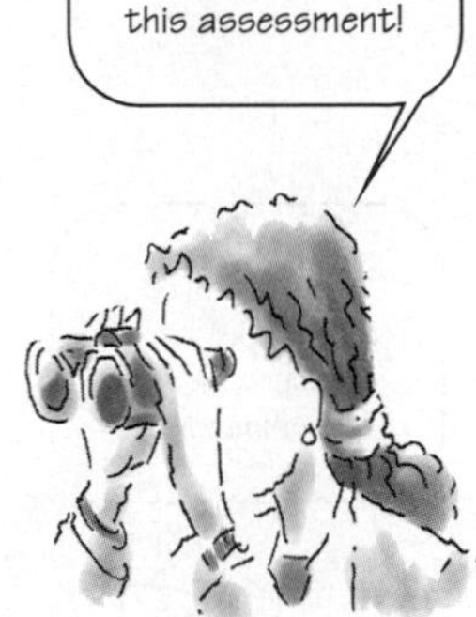

You don't need binoculars for this assessment!

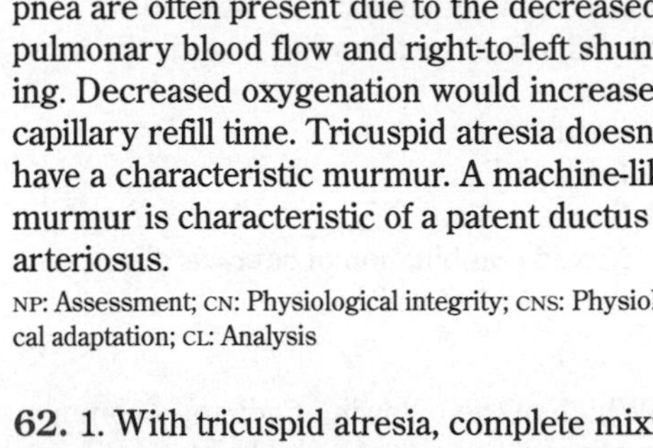

61. 1. Cyanosis is the most consistent clinical sign of tricuspid atresia. Tachypnea and dyspnea are often present due to the decreased pulmonary blood flow and right-to-left shunting. Decreased oxygenation would increase capillary refill time. Tricuspid atresia doesn't have a characteristic murmur. A machine-like murmur is characteristic of a patent ductus arteriosus.

NP: Assessment; CN: Physiological integrity; CNS: Physiological adaptation; CL: Analysis

62. Which of the following laboratory findings is expected in a child with tricuspid atresia?

1. Acidosis
2. Alkalosis
3. Normal red blood cell count
4. Normal arterial oxygen saturation

62. 1. With tricuspid atresia, complete mixing of the oxygenated and deoxygenated blood occurs in the left side of the heart, causing an overall systemic desaturation. The child has chronic hypoxemia due to decreased atrial oxygen saturation. Chronic hypoxemia leads to polycythemia and chronic mild acidosis. Even with repair, the chronic hypoxemia is decreased but continues to exist.

NP: Analysis; CN: Physiological integrity; CNS: Physiological adaptation; CL: Analysis

63. Which of the following operations is recommended to correct tricuspid atresia?

1. Blalock-Taussig operation
2. Fontan procedure
3. Jatene procedure
4. Patch closure

63. 2. The Fontan procedure is used to correct tricuspid atresia. It separates the systemic and pulmonary circulations by closing septal defects and previous shunts and connecting the systemic venous structures with the pulmonary arteries. The Blalock-Taussig operation is used to palliate children with tricuspid atresia. Patch closures are used for defects such as a ventricular or atrial septal defect. The Jatene procedure is used to correct a mixed defect such as transposition of the great arteries.

NP: Planning; CN: Physiological integrity; CNS: Physiological adaptation; CL: Knowledge

64. Which of the following conditions best describes total anomalous pulmonary venous return?

1. Pulmonary veins that don't return to the left atrium
2. Pulmonary veins that are narrowed
3. An acyanotic defect with increased pulmonary blood flow
4. A single large vessel that arises from both ventricles astride a large ventricular septal defect

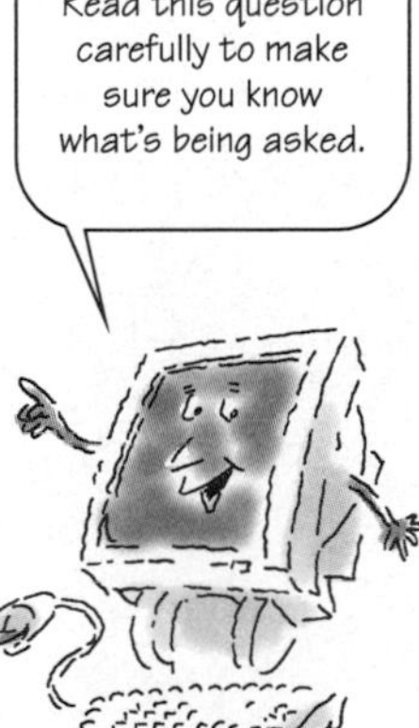

Read this question carefully to make sure you know what's being asked.

64. 1. Total anomalous pulmonary venous return is a condition in which the pulmonary veins don't return to the left atrium; instead, they abnormally return to the right side of the heart. This defect is classified as a cyanotic defect with increased pulmonary blood flow. A single large vessel arising from both ventricles astride a large ventricular septal defect describes truncus arteriosus. Pulmonary veins that are narrowed are referred to as pulmonary vein stenosis.

NP: Assessment; CN: Health promotion and maintenance; CNS: Prevention and early detection of disease; CL: Knowledge

65. There are four different ways the pulmonary veins may be abnormally routed with a total anomalous pulmonary venous return defect. Which of the following types is the most common?

1. Cardiac
2. Infracardiac
3. Supracardiac
4. Mixed combination of supracardiac, cardiac, and infracardiac

65. 3. Supracardiac, the most common type, is characterized by the pulmonary veins draining directly into the superior vena cava. With cardiac, the pulmonary veins drain into the coronary sinuses or directly flow into the right atrium. Infracardiac shows the common pulmonary vein running below the diaphragm into the portals system. The fourth type is a mixed combination.

NP: Analysis; CN: Health promotion and maintenance; CNS: Prevention and early detection of disease; CL: Knowledge

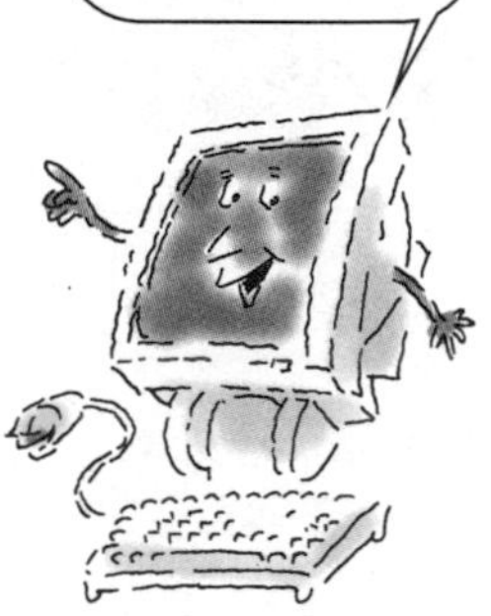

This question asks about what occurs most commonly.

66. Which of the following findings is common during an assessment of a child with a total anomalous pulmonary venous return defect?

1. Hypertension
2. Frequent respiratory infections
3. Normal growth and development
4. Above average weight gain on the growth chart

66. 2. Children with total anomalous pulmonary venous return defects are prone to repeated respiratory infections due to increased pulmonary blood flow. Poor feeding and failure to thrive are also signs. Infants look thin and malnourished. Hypertension usually occurs with coarctation of the aorta, an acyanotic defect with obstructive flow.

NP: Assessment; CN: Physiological integrity; CNS: Physiological adaptation; CL: Application

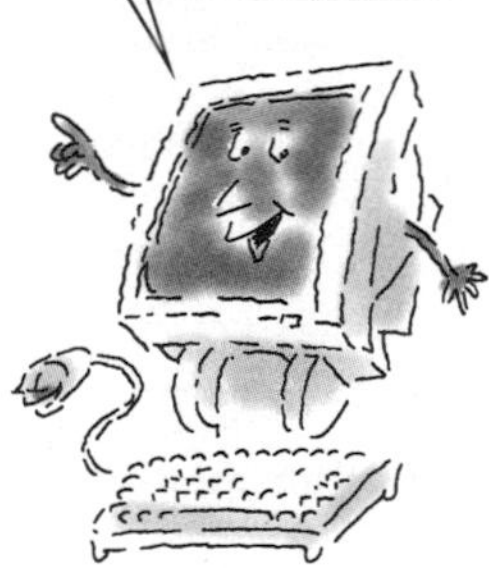

Watch the term *after.* It clues you in to the answer.

67. Which of the following complications may result after the repair of total anomalous pulmonary venous return?

1. Hypotension
2. Pulmonary hypertension
3. Ventricular arrhythmias
4. Pulmonary vein dilatation

67. 2. Pulmonary hypertension, atrial arrhythmias, and pulmonary vein obstruction are complications that may result postoperatively. The left atrium is small and sensitive to fluid volume loading. An increase in the pressure in the right atrium is required to ensure left atrial filling.

NP: Evaluation; CN: Physiological integrity; CNS: Physiological adaptation; CL: Knowledge

68. Which of the following statements about truncus arteriosus is correct?

1. It's classified as an acyanotic defect.
2. Systemic and pulmonary blood mix.
3. It can't be diagnosed until after birth.
4. There are two types of truncus arteriosus.

68. 2. Blood ejects from the left and right ventricles and enters a common trunk, mixing pulmonary and systemic blood. Diagnosis can be made in utero using echocardiography. Truncus arteriosus can be divided into four types or categories. It's classified as a cyanotic defect with increased pulmonary blood flow.

NP: Evaluation; CN: Health promotion and maintenance; CNS: Prevention and early detection of disease; CL: Knowledge

69. Which of the following findings commonly occurs during assessment of a child with truncus arteriosus?

1. Weak, thready pulses
2. Narrowed pulse pressure
3. Pink moist mucous membranes
4. Harsh systolic regurgitant murmur

69. 4. As a result of the ventricular septal defect, a harsh systolic regurgitant murmur is heard along the left sternal border and is usually accompanied by a thrill. Increasing pulmonary blood flow causes bounding pulses and a widened pulse pressure. Systemic and pulmonary blood mixing leads to mild or moderate cyanosis, so mucous membranes may appear dull or gray.

NP: Assessment; CN: Physiological integrity; CNS: Physiological adaptation; CL: Knowledge

NP: Nursing process CN: Client needs category CNS: Client needs subcategory CL: Cognitive level

70. Treatment for truncus arteriosus includes digoxin and diuretics. Which of the following techniques would be best for giving these drugs to an infant?

1. Use a measuring spoon.
2. Use a graduated dropper.
3. Mix the drug with baby food.
4. Mix the drug in a bottle with juice or milk.

70. 2. Using a dropper allows the exact dosage to be given. Mixing drugs with juice, milk, or food may cause a problem if the child doesn't completely finish the meal. Then how much the child received isn't definite. In addition, this may prevent the child from drinking or eating for fear of tasting the drug. A measuring spoon isn't as exact as a dropper.

NP: Evaluation; CN: Physiological integrity; CNS: Pharmacological and parenteral therapies; CL: Application

71. Which of the following statements best describes transposition of the great arteries?

1. The body receives only saturated blood.
2. It's classified as an acyanotic defect with increased pulmonary blood flow.
3. The pulmonary artery leaves the left ventricle, and the aorta exits from the right ventricle.
4. It's a condition in which the right atrium and the left atrium empty into one ventricular chamber.

71. 3. Transposition of the great arteries is a condition in which the pulmonary artery leaves the left ventricle and the aorta exits from the right ventricle. This type of circulation gives the body only desaturated blood. The mixing of blood characterizes this defect as a cyanotic defect with variable pulmonary blood flow or as a mixed defect. A single-ventricle defect is a condition in which the right and left atria empty into one ventricular chamber.

NP: Evaluation; CN: Health promotion and maintenance; CNS: Prevention and early detection of disease; CL: Knowledge

72. Which of the following statements about transposition of the great arteries is correct?

1. Diagnosis is made at birth.
2. Diagnosis can be made in utero.
3. Chest X-ray can show an accurate view of the defect.
4. Heart failure isn't a related complication.

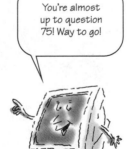

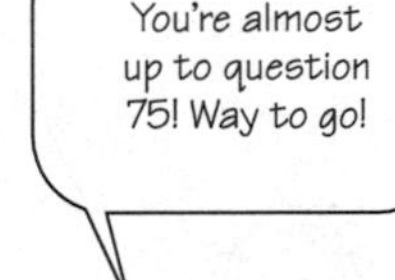

You're almost up to question 75! Way to go!

72. 2. Echocardiography done by a fetal cardiologist can diagnose transposition of the great arteries in utero. The other defects associated with this defect include a patent foramen ovale and a ventricular septal defect that contribute to developing heart failure. Chest X-ray can show cardiomegaly and pulmonary vascular markings only. Echocardiography or cardiac catheterization may be required preoperatively to show the coronary artery anatomy before surgical repair.

NP: Analysis; CN: Physiological integrity; CNS: Physiological adaptation; CL: Analysis

73. Which of the following associated defects is most common with transposition of the great arteries?

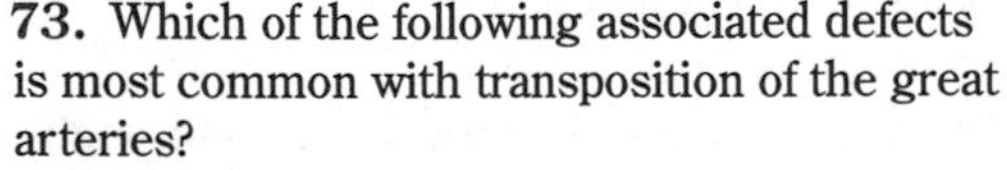

1. Mitral atresia
2. Atrial septal defect
3. Patent foramen ovale
4. Hypoplasia of the left ventricle

73. 3. A patent foramen ovale, patent ductus arteriosus, and ventricular septal defect are associated defects related to transposition of the great arteries. A patent foramen ovale is the most common and is necessary to provide adequate mixing of blood between the two circulations. An atrial septal defect is common in association with total anomalous pulmonary venous return. Hypoplasia of the left ventricle and mitral atresia are two defects associated with hypoplastic left heart syndrome.

NP: Analysis; CN: Physiological integrity; CNS: Physiological adaptation; CL: Knowledge

74. Administration of which of the following drugs would be the most important in treating transposition of the great arteries?

1. Digoxin
2. Diuretics
3. Antibiotics
4. Prostaglandin E_1

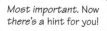

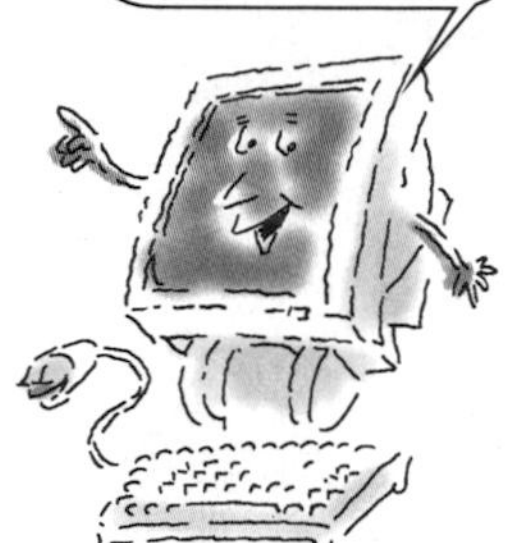

Most important. Now there's a hint for you!

74. 4. Prostaglandin E_1 is necessary to maintain patency of the patent ductus arteriosus and improve systemic arterial flow in children with inadequate intracardiac mixing. Digoxin and diuretics will treat heart failure when present. Antibiotics are given in the immediate preoperative phase.

NP: Planning; CN: Physiological integrity; CNS: Pharmacological and parenteral therapies; CL: Application

75. Which of the following surgical procedures is recommended for repair of transposition of the great arteries?

1. Jatene operation
2. Fontan procedure
3. Balloon atrial septostomy
4. Blalock-Taussig operation

75. 1. The Jatene operation involves transposing the great arteries and mobilizing and reimplanting the coronary arteries. The Fontan procedure is recommended for repair of tricuspid atresia. Balloon atrial septostomy is a palliative procedure used during cardiac catheterization for those children without a coexisting lesion. Blalock-Taussig operation is used to palliate tricuspid atresia and pulmonic atresia.

NP: Planning; CN: Physiological integrity; CNS: Physiological adaptation; CL: Knowledge

76. Which of the following statements best describes a characteristic of valvular pulmonic stenosis?

1. The valve is normal.
2. The right ventricle is hypoplastic.
3. Left ventricular hypertrophy develops.
4. Divisions between the cusps are fused.

76. 4. Blood flow through the valve is restricted by fusion of the divisions between the cusps. The valve may be normal or malformed. Right ventricular hypertrophy develops due to resistance to blood flow.

NP: Assessment; CN: Physiological integrity; CNS: Physiological adaptation; CL: Knowledge

77. During the assessment of a child with pulmonic stenosis, which of the following findings is most common?

1. Hyperactivity
2. Normal respiratory rate
3. Systolic ejection murmur
4. Capillary refill more than 2 seconds

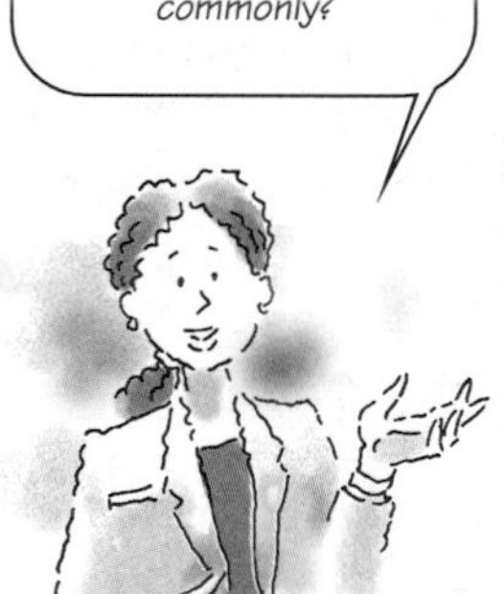

All of these conditions may occur, but which occurs most commonly?

77. 3. A systolic ejection murmur, which may be accompanied by a thrill, can be heard at the upper left sternal border. The decrease in pulmonary blood flow causes fatigue and dyspnea. Systemic cyanosis may result due to right ventricular failure that increases the capillary refill time.

NP: Assessment; CN: Physiological integrity; CNS: Physiological adaptation; CL: Knowledge

78. Which of the following findings is seen during cardiac catheterization of a child with pulmonic stenosis?

1. Right-to-left shunting
2. Left-to-right shunting
3. Decreased pressure in the right side of the heart
4. Increased oxygenation in the left side of the heart

78. 1. Right-to-left shunting develops through a patent foramen ovale due to right ventricular failure and an increase in pressure in the right side of the heart. Decreased oxygenation in the left side of the heart is noted due to the right-to-left shunt and decreased pulmonary blood flow.

NP: Assessment; CN: Physiological integrity; CNS: Physiological adaptation; CL: Analysis

79. Which of the following findings is associated with aortic stenosis?

1. Hypotension
2. Right ventricular failure
3. Increased cardiac output
4. Loud systolic regurgitant murmur with a thrill

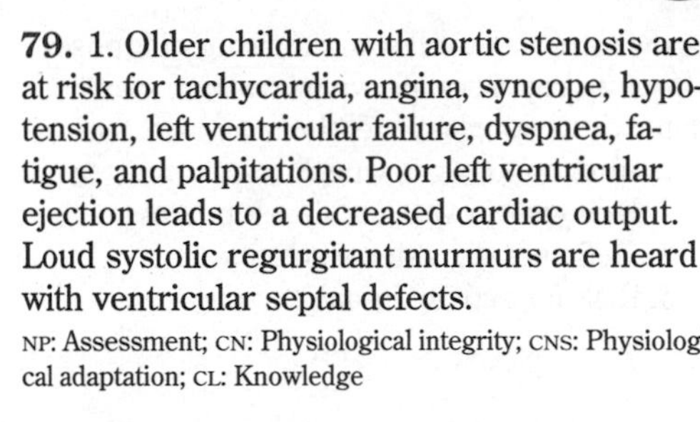

79. 1. Older children with aortic stenosis are at risk for tachycardia, angina, syncope, hypotension, left ventricular failure, dyspnea, fatigue, and palpitations. Poor left ventricular ejection leads to a decreased cardiac output. Loud systolic regurgitant murmurs are heard with ventricular septal defects.

NP: Assessment; CN: Physiological integrity; CNS: Physiological adaptation; CL: Knowledge

80. Which of the following statements about aortic stenosis is correct?

1. It can result from rheumatic fever.
2. It accounts for 25% of all congenital defects.
3. There are two subcategories: valvular and subvalvular.
4. It's classified as an acyanotic defect with increased pulmonary blood flow.

80. 1. Aortic stenosis can result from rheumatic fever, which damages the valve by causing lesions on the leaflets and scar formation to develop over time. It's classified as an acyanotic defect with obstructed flow from the ventricles. It accounts for about 5% of all congenital defects. There are three subcategories; valvular, subvalvular, and supravalvular.

NP: Analysis; CN: Physiological integrity; CNS: Physiological adaptation; CL: Knowledge

81. Which of the following instructions would be most appropriate for a child with aortic stenosis?

1. Restrict exercise.
2. Avoid prostaglandin E_1.
3. Avoid digoxin and diuretics.
4. Allow the child to exercise freely.

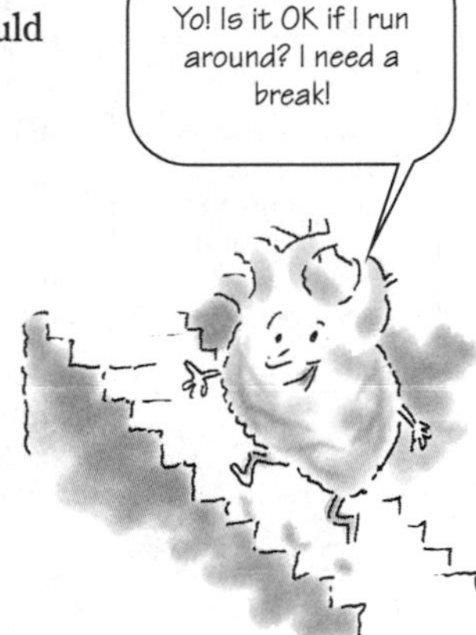

Yo! Is it OK if I run around? I need a break!

81. 1. Exercise should be restricted due to low cardiac output and left ventricular failure. Strenuous activity has been reported to result in sudden death from the development of myocardial ischemia. Digoxin and diuretics may be required for the critically ill infant experiencing heart failure as a result of severe aortic stenosis. Prostaglandin E_1 is recommended to maintain the patency of the ductus arteriosus in the neonate with critical aortic stenosis. This allows for improved systemic blood flow.

NP: Implementation; CN: Physiological integrity; CNS: Physiological adaptation; CL: Application

82. Which of the following statements is correct for hypoplastic left heart syndrome?

1. It can be diagnosed only at birth.
2. It includes a group of related cardiac anomalies.
3. It's classified as 25% of all congenital defects.
4. Surgical intervention is the only option for treatment.

82. 2. Hypoplastic left heart syndrome includes a group of related anomalies, such as hypoplasia of the left ventricle, mitral atresia, aortic atresia, and hypoplasia of the ascending aorta and aortic arch. Treatment options include palliative surgery, cardiac transplantation, or no intervention, in which case death would occur. It can be diagnosed prenatally with a level 2 ultrasound examination. It's classified as about 1% to 2% of all congenital defects.

NP: Evaluation; CN: Health promotion and maintenance; CNS: Prevention and early detection of disease; CL: Knowledge

83. Which of the following nursing diagnoses is the most appropriate when caring for an infant with hypoplastic left heart syndrome?
1. Anticipatory grieving
2. Delayed growth and development
3. Deficient diversional activity
4. Risk for activity intolerance

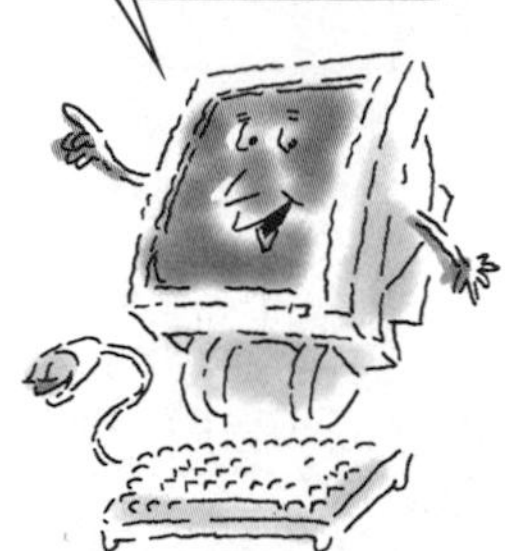

There's that most appropriate phrase again.

83. 1. Without intervention, death usually occurs within the first few days of life due to progressive hypoxia, acidosis, and shock as the ductus closes and systemic perfusion diminishes. If the parents choose cardiac transplantation, the child may die waiting for a donor heart. For those who choose surgery, the child may not survive the three stages of the surgery. The other three choices don't apply to this type of defect due to the low survival rates.
NP: Planning; CN: Physiological integrity; CNS: Physiological adaptation; CL: Analysis

84. Which of the following procedures of heart transplantation leaves the recipient's own heart in place and implants a new heart to act as an additional pump, an arrangement commonly called a "piggyback"?
1. Orthotopic
2. Heterotopic
3. Norwood procedure
4. Modified Fontan procedure

84. 2. This procedure is known as heterotopic. The Norwood procedure and the modified Fontan procedure are stages 1 and 3 of palliative surgery for hypoplastic left heart syndrome. An orthotopic heart transplant refers to the removal of the recipient's own heart and implanting a new heart from a donor.
NP: Planning; CN: Physiological integrity; CNS: Physiological adaptation; CL: Knowledge

85. A child receives prednisone after a heart transplant. Prednisone is in which of the following drug classifications?
1. Antibiotic
2. Cardiac glycoside
3. Corticosteroid
4. Diuretic

85. 3. Prednisone is a corticosteroid used frequently during posttransplantation as part of antirejection therapy. The drug influences the immune system through its strong anti-inflammatory action and immunologic effect. Prednisone isn't an antibiotic, cardiac glycoside, or diuretic.
NP: Evaluation; CN: Physiological integrity; CNS: Pharmacological and parenteral therapies; CL: Knowledge

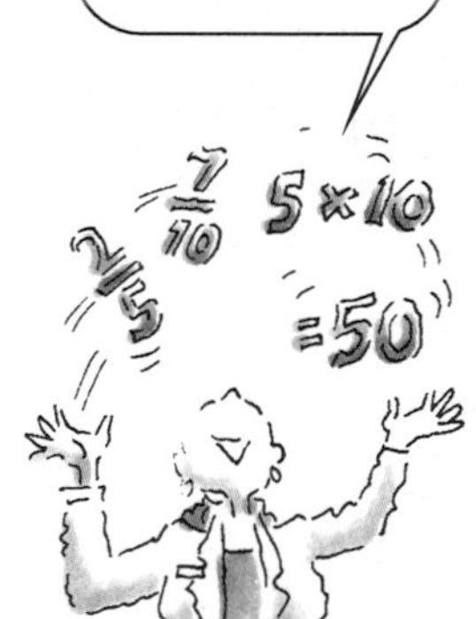

Math problems get you stumped? Just break each problem into manageable pieces, one by one.
5×10
=50

86. A child is given 0.5 mg/kg/day of prednisone divided into two doses. The child weighs 10 kg. How much is given in each dose?
1. 2.5 mg
2. 5 mg
3. 10 mg
4. 1.5 mg

86. 1. $0.5 \text{ mg/kg} \times 10 \text{ kg} = 5 \text{ mg}$
$5 \text{ mg/2 doses} = 2.5 \text{ mg/dose}$
NP: Evaluation; CN: Physiological integrity; CNS: Pharmacological and parenteral therapies; CL: Analysis

87. Which of the following adverse reactions of prednisone is expected in a child after having a heart transplant?
1. Anorexia
2. Hypolipidemia
3. Decreased appetite
4. Poor wound healing

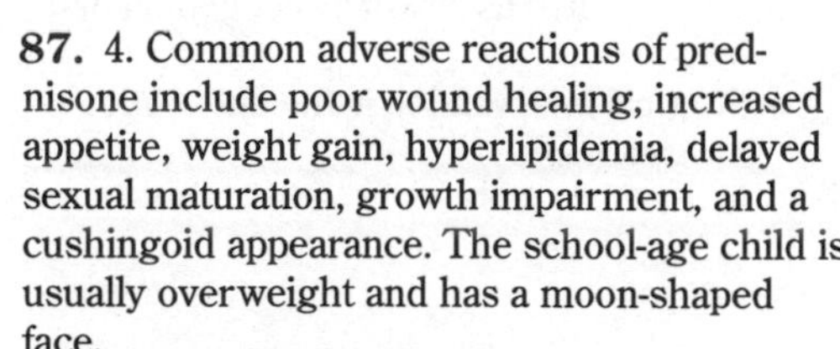

87. 4. Common adverse reactions of prednisone include poor wound healing, increased appetite, weight gain, hyperlipidemia, delayed sexual maturation, growth impairment, and a cushingoid appearance. The school-age child is usually overweight and has a moon-shaped face.
NP: Evaluation; CN: Physiological integrity; CNS: Pharmacological and parenteral therapies; CL: Knowledge

Hey, am *I* to blame for this, or what?

88. Which of the following characteristics best describes bacterial or infective endocarditis?

1. Bacteria invading only tissues of the heart
2. Infection of the valves and inner lining of the heart
3. Inappropriate fusion of the endocardial cushions in fetal life
4. Caused by alterations in cardiac preload, afterload, contractility, or heart rate

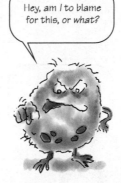

88. 2. Bacterial or infective endocarditis is an infection of the valves and inner lining of the heart. It's usually caused by the bacteria ***Streptococcus viridans*** and frequently affects children with acquired or congenital anomalies of the heart or great vessels. Endocardial cushion defects represent inappropriate fusion of the endocardial cushions in fetal life. Bacteria may grow into adjacent tissues and may break off and embolize elsewhere, such as the spleen, kidney, lung, skin, and central nervous system. Alterations in preload, afterload, contractility, or heart rate refer to heart failure.

NP: Evaluation; CN: Physiological integrity; CNS: Physiological adaptation; CL: Knowledge

89. A child with suspected bacterial endocarditis arrives at the emergency department. Which of the following findings is expected during assessment?

1. Weight gain
2. Bradycardia
3. Low-grade fever
4. Increased hemoglobin level

89. 3. Symptoms may include a low-grade intermittent fever, decrease in hemoglobin level, tachycardia, anorexia, weight loss, and decreased activity level. Bacteremia leads to these signs of an infection.

NP: Assessment; CN: Physiological integrity; CNS: Physiological adaptation; CL: Application

90. Which of the following factors may lead to bacterial endocarditis in a child with underlying heart disease?

1. History of a cold for 3 days
2. Dental work pretreated with antibiotics
3. Peripheral I.V. catheter in place for 1 day
4. Indwelling urinary catheter for 2 days leading to a urinary tract infection

90. 4. Bacterial organisms can enter the bloodstream from any site of infection such as a urinary tract infection. Gram-negative bacilli are common causative agents. A peripheral I.V. catheter is an entry site but only if signs and symptoms of infection are present. Long-term indwelling catheters pose a higher risk for infection. Dental work is a common portal of entry if not pretreated with antibiotics. Colds are usually viral, not bacterial. Heart surgery is also a common cause of endocarditis, especially if synthetic material is used.

NP: Assessment; CN: Physiological integrity; CNS: Physiological adaptation; CL: Analysis

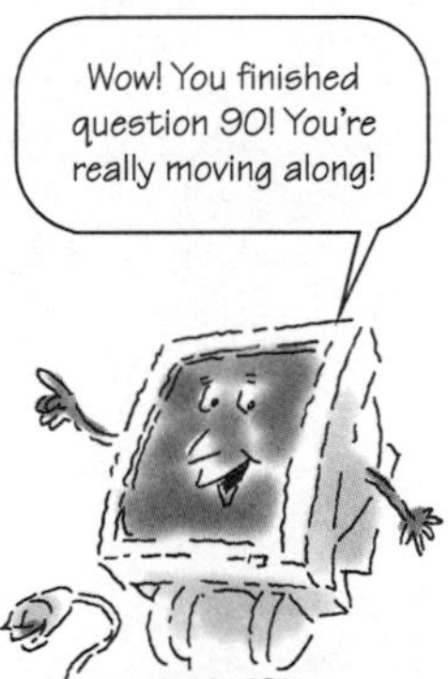

Wow! You finished question 90! You're really moving along!

91. Erythromycin is given to a 6-year-old child before dental work to prevent endocarditis. The child weighs 44 lb. The order is for 20 mg/kg by mouth 2 hours before the procedure. How many milligrams would that be?

1. 200 mg
2. 400 mg
3. 440 mg
4. 880 mg

91. 2. 44 lb/2.2 kg = 20 kg

20 mg/kg $\times$ 20 kg = 400 mg

NP: Evaluation; CN: Physiological integrity; CNS: Pharmacological and parenteral therapies; CL: Analysis

92. Which of the following adverse reactions may occur with the administration of erythromycin?

1. Weight gain
2. Constipation
3. Increased appetite
4. Nausea and vomiting

92. 4. Erythromycin is an antibacterial antibiotic. Common adverse effects include nausea, vomiting, diarrhea, abdominal pain, and anorexia. It should be given with a full glass of water and after meals or with food to lessen GI symptoms.

NP: Evaluation; CN: Physiological integrity; CNS: Pharmacological and parenteral therapies; CL: Knowledge

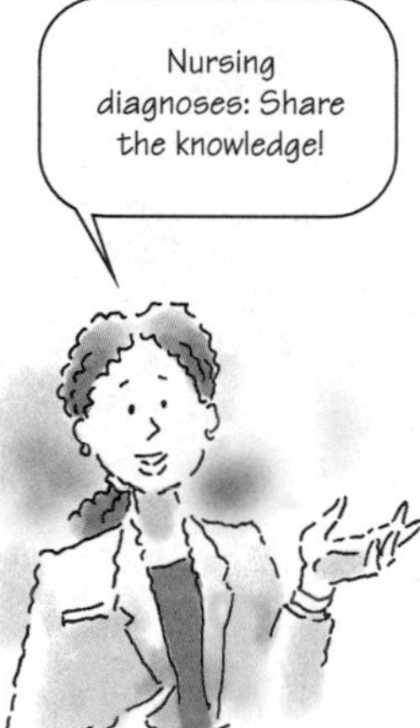
Nursing diagnoses: Share the knowledge!

93. A child is hospitalized with bacterial endocarditis. Which of the following nursing diagnoses is most appropriate?

1. Constipation
2. Excess fluid volume
3. Deficient diversional activity
4. Imbalanced nutrition: More than body requirements

93. 3. Treatment for bacterial endocarditis requires long-term hospitalization or home care for I.V. antibiotics. Children may be bored and depressed, needing age-appropriate activities. Excess fluid volume, diarrhea, and imbalanced nutrition: less than body requirements may be possible nursing diagnoses related to the adverse reactions of antibiotics such as GI upset.

NP: Evaluation; CN: Physiological integrity; CNS: Physiological adaptation; CL: Analysis

94. When assessing a child with suspected Kawasaki disease, which of the following symptoms is common?

1. Low-grade fever
2. "Strawberry" tongue
3. Pink moist mucous membranes
4. Bilateral conjunctival infection with yellow exudate

94. 2. Inflammation of the pharynx and oral mucosa develops, causing red, cracked lips and a "strawberry" tongue in which the normal coating of the tongue sloughs off. A high fever of 5 or more days unresponsive to antibiotics and antipyretics is also part of the diagnostic criteria. The eyes are generally dry without exudation.

NP: Assessment; CN: Physiological integrity; CNS: Physiological adaptation; CL: Knowledge

95. Which of the following statements about Kawasaki disease is the most appropriate?

1. It mostly occurs in the summer and fall.
2. Diagnosis can be made with laboratory testing.
3. It's an acute systemic vasculitis of unknown cause.
4. It manifests in two different stages: acute and subacute.

95. 3. Kawasaki disease can best be described as an acute systemic vasculitis of unknown cause. Diagnosis is based on clinical findings of five of the six diagnostic criteria and associated laboratory results. There's no specific laboratory test for diagnosis. There are three stages: acute, subacute, and convalescent. Most cases are geographic and seasonal, with most occurring in the late winter and early spring.

NP: Evaluation; CN: Physiological integrity; CNS: Physiological adaptation; CL: Knowledge

96. Which of the following characteristics indicates a child with Kawasaki disease has entered the subacute phase?

1. Polymorphous rash
2. Normal blood values
3. Cervical lymphadenopathy
4. Desquamation of the hands and feet

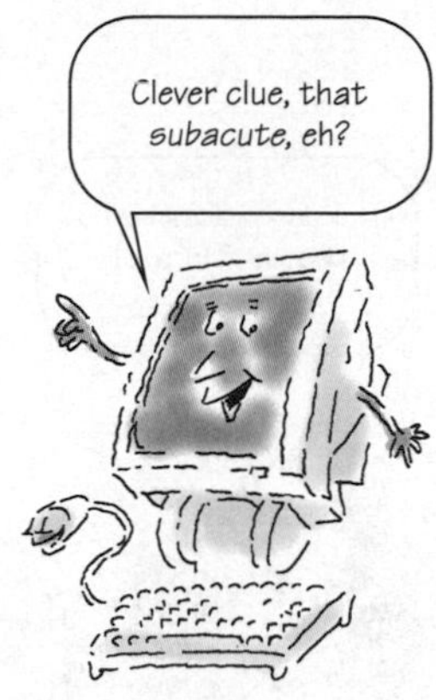

Clever clue, that
subacute, eh?

96. 4. The subacute phase shows characteristic desquamation of the hands and feet. Blood values return to normal at the end of the convalescent phase. Cervical lymphadenopathy and a polymorphous rash can be seen in the acute phase due to the onset of inflammation and fever.

NP: Assessment; CN: Physiological integrity; CNS: Physiological adaptation; CL: Analysis

97. A nurse is caring for a child with Kawasaki disease. Which of the following symptoms concerns the nurse the most?

1. Mild diarrhea
2. Pain in the joints
3. Abdominal pain with vomiting
4. Increased erythrocyte sedimentation rate (ESR)

97. 3. The most serious complication of this disease is cardiac involvement. Abdominal pain, vomiting, and restlessness are the main symptoms of an acute myocardial infarction in children. Pain in the joints is an expected sign of arthritis that usually occurs in the subacute phase. Mild diarrhea can be treated with oral fluids. An increased ESR is a reflection of the inflammatory process and may be seen for 2 to 4 weeks after the onset of symptoms.

NP: Assessment; CN: Physiological integrity; CNS: Physiological adaptation; CL: Analysis

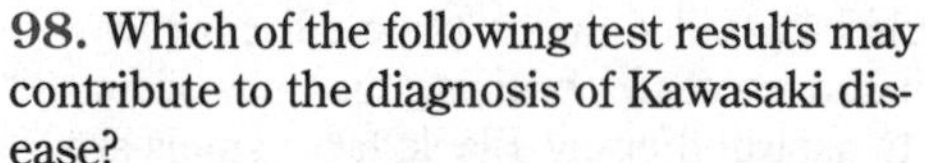

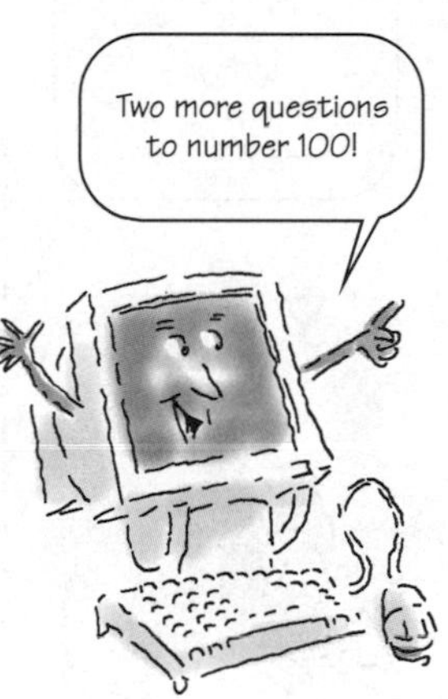

Two more questions
to number 100!

98. Which of the following test results may contribute to the diagnosis of Kawasaki disease?

1. Hematuria
2. Elevated leukocyte count
3. Normal or decreased platelet count
4. Decreased erythrocyte sedimentation rate

98. 2. Inflammation of the small vessels, along with pancarditis, leads to an elevated leukocyte count, increased platelet count, and proteinuria or sterile pyuria. The capillaries, venules, and arterioles are affected first, then the medium-sized muscular arteries. These laboratory results contribute to the clinical presentation and diagnosis of Kawasaki disease.

NP: Assessment; CN: Physiological integrity; CNS: Physiological adaptation; CL: Knowledge

99. Therapy for Kawasaki disease includes I.V. gamma globulin, prescribed at 400 mg/kg/day for 4 days. The child weighs 10 kg. How much is given per dose?

1. 200 mg
2. 400 mg
3. 2,000 mg
4. 4,000 mg

99. 4. 400 mg/kg × 10 kg = 4,000 mg or 4 g

NP: Evaluation; CN: Physiological integrity; CNS: Pharmacological and parenteral therapies; CL: Analysis

100. A child is receiving 8 g of I.V. gamma globulin for treatment of Kawasaki disease. The child weighs 20 kg. The order is for 8 g of gamma globulin over 12 hours. The concentration is 8 g in 300 ml of normal saline. How many milliliters per hour will this child receive?

1. 12 ml/hour
2. 25 ml/hour
3. 50 ml/hour
4. 40 ml/hour

100. 2. 300 ml/12 hours = 25 ml/hour

NP: Evaluation; CN: Physiological integrity; CNS: Pharmacological and parenteral therapies; CL: Analysis

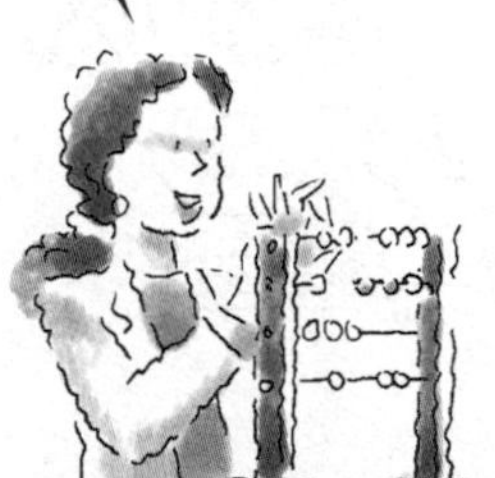

Keep practicing that math! You'll get it!

101. A child is prescribed aspirin as part of the therapy for Kawasaki disease. The order is for 80 mg/kg/day orally in four divided doses until the child is afebrile. The child weighs 15 kg. How much is given in one dose?

1. 60 mg
2. 300 mg
3. 320 mg
4. 1,200 mg

101. 2. 80 mg/kg × 15 kg = 1,200 mg
1,200 mg/4 doses = 300 mg/dose

NP: Evaluation; CN: Physiological integrity; CNS: Pharmacological and parenteral therapies; CL: Analysis

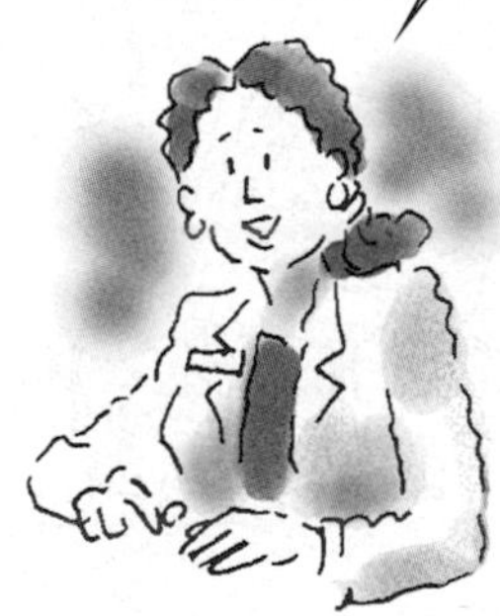

Listen for feedback to find out if your instructions were understood.

102. A nurse is giving discharge instructions to the parents of a child with Kawasaki disease. Which of the following statements shows an understanding of the treatment plan?

1. "A regular diet can be resumed at home."
2. "Black, tarry stools are considered normal."
3. "My child should use a soft-bristled toothbrush."
4. "My child can return to playing football next week."

102. 3. Due to the anticoagulant effects of aspirin therapy, a soft-bristled toothbrush will prevent bleeding of the gums. Contact sports should be avoided due to the cardiac involvement and excessive bruising that may occur due to aspirin therapy. Black, tarry stools are abnormal and are signs of bleeding that should be reported to the physician immediately. A low-cholesterol diet should be followed until coronary artery involvement resolves, usually within 6 to 8 weeks.

NP: Evaluation; CN: Physiological integrity; CNS: Physiological adaptation; CL: Analysis

103. A nurse is preparing the family of a client with Kawasaki disease for discharge. Which of the following instructions is most appropriate?

1. Stop the aspirin when you return home.
2. Immunizations can be given in 2 weeks.
3. The child may return to school in 1 week.
4. Frequent echocardiography will be needed.

103. 4. Due to the risk of coronary artery involvement and possible aneurysm development, repeat echocardiography and electrocardiography will be required the first few weeks and at 6 months. Aspirin therapy may be continued for 2 weeks after the onset of symptoms. If signs of coronary artery involvement are present, aspirin therapy may be continued indefinitely. School should be avoided until cleared by the physician. Live-virus vaccines should be avoided for at least 5 months after gamma globulin therapy due to an increased risk of a cross-sensitivity reaction to the antibodies found in the dose given.

NP: Evaluation; CN: Physiological integrity; CNS: Physiological adaptation; CL: Analysis

122. To which of the following classifications does isoproterenol belong?
1. Adrenergic agonist
2. Anticholinergic
3. Beta-adrenergic blocker
4. Vasopressor

122. 3. Isoproterenol acts as a beta-adrenergic blocker to reduce peripheral resistance and increase the force of cardiac contraction without producing vasoconstriction. It also acts as a bronchodilator, relaxing bronchial smooth muscle and creating peripheral vasodilation.
NP: Evaluation; CN: Physiological integrity; CNS: Pharmacological and parenteral therapies; CL: Analysis

123. Which of the following findings may be seen in a 1-year-old child with supraventricular tachycardia?
1. Heart rate of 100 beats/minute
2. Heart rate of 180 beats/minute
3. Heart rate less than 80 beats/minute
4. Heart rate more than 240 beats/minute

123. 4. Supraventricular tachycardia may be related to increased automaticity of an atrial cell other than the sinoatrial node, or as a reentry mechanism. The rhythm is regular and can occur at rates of 240 beats/minute or more. A heart rate less than 80 beats/minute can be characterized as sinus bradycardia. A heart rate around 180 beats/minute may represent sinus tachycardia. A heart rate of 100 beats/minute is a normal finding for a 1-year-old child.
NP: Analysis; CN: Physiological integrity; CNS: Physiological adaptation; CL: Knowledge

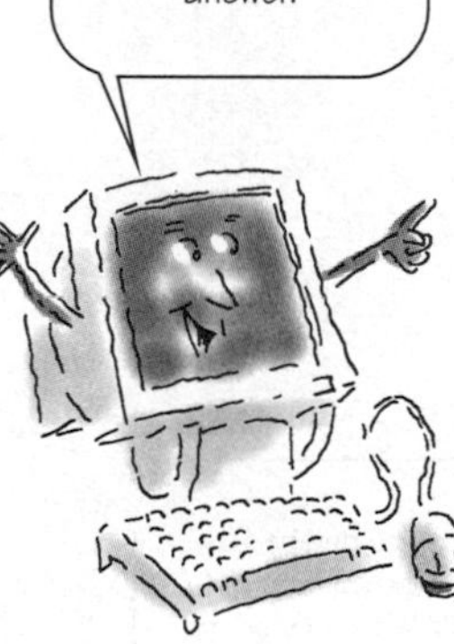

In question 124, the word *first* is your clue to the right answer.

124. A 2-year-old child is experiencing supraventricular tachycardia. Which of the following interventions should be attempted first?
1. Administration of digoxin
2. Administration of verapamil
3. Synchronized cardioversion
4. Immersion of the child's hands in cold water

124. 4. Vagal maneuvers such as immersion of the hands in cold water are often tried first as a mechanism to decrease the heart rate. Other vagal maneuvers include breath-holding, carotid massage, gagging, and placing the head lower than the rest of the body. Synchronized cardioversion may be required if vagal maneuvers and drugs are ineffective. If a child has low cardiac output, cardioversion may be used instead of drugs. Verapamil isn't recommended. Digoxin is one of the most common drugs given to help decrease heart rate by increasing myocardial contractility and automaticity and reducing excitability.
NP: Implementation; CN: Physiological integrity; CNS: Pharmacological and parenteral therapies; CL: Application

125. A 2-month-old infant arrives in the emergency department with a heart rate of 180 beats/minute and a temperature of 103.1° F (39.5° C) rectally. Which of the following interventions is most appropriate?
1. Give acetaminophen (Tylenol).
2. Encourage fluid intake.
3. Apply carotid massage.
4. Place the infant's hands in cold water.

125. 1. Acetaminophen should be given first to decrease the temperature. A heart rate of 180 beats/minute is normal in an infant with a fever. A tepid sponge bath may be given to help decrease the temperature and calm the infant. Carotid massage is an attempt to decrease the heart rate as a vagal maneuver. This won't work in this infant because the source of the increased heart rate is fever. Fluid intake is encouraged after the acetaminophen is given to help replace insensible fluid losses.
NP: Analysis; CN: Physiological integrity; CNS: Physiological adaptation; CL: Application

126. A 1-week-old neonate undergoes cardiovascular surgery for placement of a Blalock-Taussig shunt. During postoperative assessment, which type of murmur should the nurse expect to hear?

1. Diastolic
2. Systolic ejection
3. Continuous
4. Systolic regurgitant

126. 3. A Blalock-Taussig shunt produces a continuous murmur (one that's heard throughout systole and diastole). A diastolic murmur occurs when the aortic or pulmonic valve is incompetent (aortic or pulmonic insufficiency) or when turbulence occurs in the tricuspid or mitral valve. A systolic ejection murmur results from a stenotic or deformed semilunar valve (aortic or pulmonic stenosis) or from increased blood flow through a normal semilunar valve. A systolic regurgitant murmur occurs with ventricular septal defects, tricuspid insufficiency, and mitral insufficiency.

NP: Assessment; CN: Physiological integrity; CNS: Physiological adaptation; CL: Knowledge

127. Which condition is not an innocent heart murmur?

1. Still's murmur
2. Diastolic murmur
3. Pulmonary flow murmur of the neonate
4. Venous hum

127. 2. A diastolic murmur reflects cardiovascular disease and is always pathologic. Still's murmur, pulmonary flow murmur of the neonate, and venous hum are innocent heart murmurs that arise from cardiovascular structures in the absence of anatomic abnormalities.

NP: Assessment; CN: Health promotion and maintenance; CNS: Prevention and early detection of disease; CL: Knowledge

128. Which is the most common cause of heart failure in children?

1. Myocarditis
2. Complete heart block
3. Severe hypoxia
4. Congenital heart disease

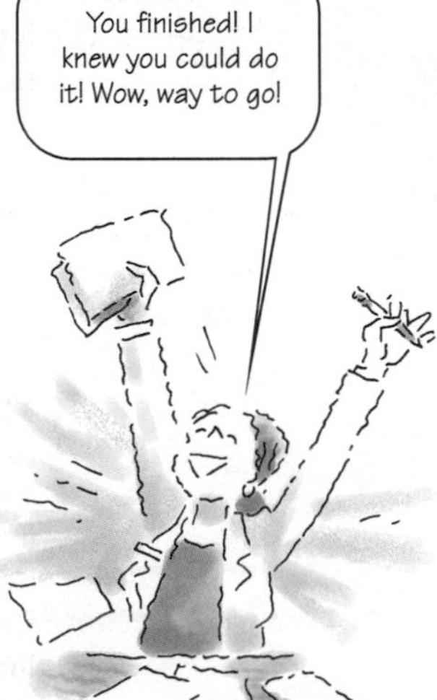
You finished! I knew you could do it! Wow, way to go!

128. 4. Congenital heart disease (especially with volume or pressure overload) is the most common cause of heart failure in children. Cardiovascular disorders, such as moderate to large ventricular septal defects, large patent ductus arteriosus, and endocardial cushion defects, cause heart failure and pulmonary overcirculation as lung pressure falls after birth. Myocarditis, complete heart block, and severe hypoxia are less common causes of heart failure in children.

NP: Evaluation; CN: Physiological integrity; CNS: Physiological adaptation; CL: Analysis

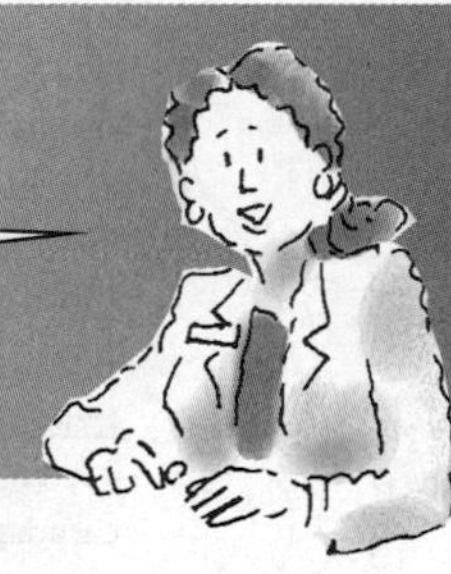

Chapter 28
Hematologic & immune disorders

1. A child comes to the emergency department feeling feverish and lethargic. Which of the following assessment findings suggests Reye's syndrome?

1. Fever, profoundly impaired consciousness, and hepatomegaly
2. Fever, splenogmegaly, and hyperactive reflexes
3. Afebrile, intractable vomiting, and rhinorrhea
4. Malaise, cough, and sore throat

1. 1. Reye's syndrome is defined as toxic encephalopathy, characterized by fever, profoundly impaired consciousness, and disordered hepatic function. Intractable vomiting occurs during the first stage of Reye's syndrome, but rhinorrhea usually precedes the onset of the illness. Reye's syndrome doesn't affect the spleen but causes fatty degeneration of the liver. Hyperactive reflexes occur with central nervous system involvement. Malaise, cough, and sore throat are viral symptoms that often precede the illness.

NP: Assessment; CN: Physiological integrity; CNS: Physiological adaptation; CL: Knowledge

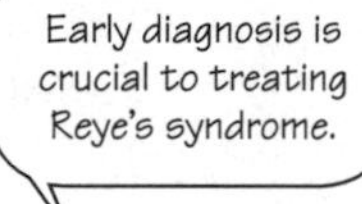

Early diagnosis is crucial to treating Reye's syndrome.

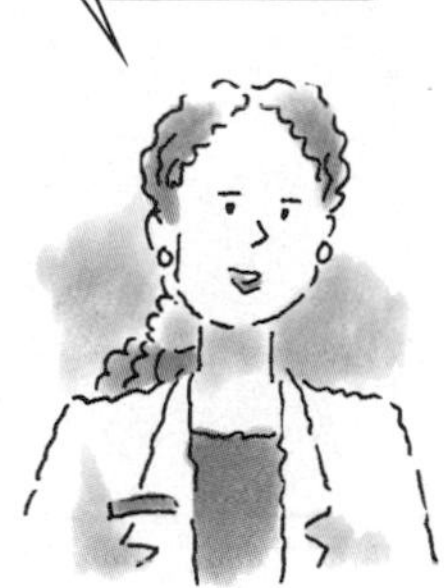

2. Which of the following aspects is most important for successful management of the child with Reye's syndrome?

1. Early diagnosis
2. Initiation of antibiotics
3. Isolation of the child
4. Staging of the illness

2. 1. Early diagnosis and therapy are essential because of the rapid clinical course of the disease and its high mortality. Isolation isn't necessary because the disease isn't communicable. Reye's syndrome is associated with a viral illness and antibiotic therapy isn't crucial to preventing the initial progression of the illness. Staging, although important to therapy, occurs after a differential diagnosis is made.

NP: Assessment; CN: Physiological integrity; CNS: Reduction of risk potential; CL: Knowledge

3. A child with Reye's syndrome is in stage I of the illness. Which of the following measures can be taken to prevent further progression of the illness?

1. Invasive monitoring
2. Endotracheal intubation
3. Hypertonic glucose solution
4. Pancuronium bromide (Pavulon)

3. 3. For children in stage I of Reye's syndrome, treatment is primarily supportive and directed toward restoring blood glucose levels and correcting acid-base imbalances. I.V. administration of dextrose solutions with added insulin helps to replace glycogen stores. Noninvasive monitoring is adequate to assess status at this stage. Endotracheal intubation may be necessary later. Pancuronium bromide is used as an adjunct to endotracheal intubation and wouldn't be used in this stage of Reye's syndrome.

NP: Planning; CN: Physiological integrity; CNS: Reduction of risk potential; CL: Application

NP: Nursing process CN: Client needs category CNS: Client needs subcategory CL: Cognitive level

4. Which of the following group of laboratory results, along with the clinical manifestations, establishes a diagnosis of Reye's syndrome?
1. Elevated liver enzymes and prolonged prothrombin and partial thromboplastin times
2. Increased serum glucose and insulin levels
3. Increased bilirubin and alkaline phosphatase levels
4. Decreased serum glucose and ammonia levels

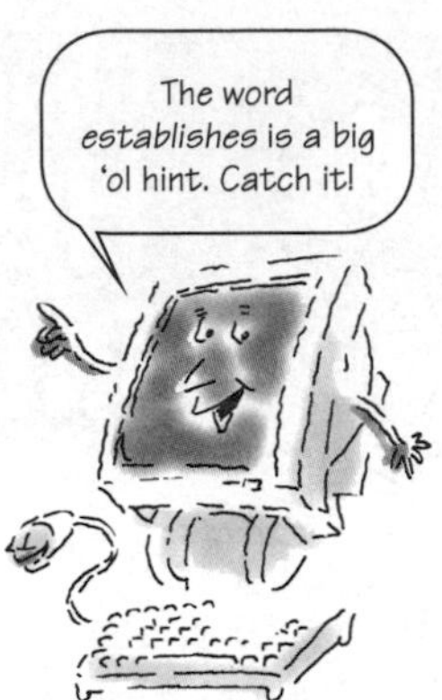

The word *establishes* is a big 'ol hint. Catch it!

4. 1. Reye's syndrome causes fatty degeneration of the liver, altering results of liver function studies. Serum bilirubin and alkaline phosphatase usually aren't affected. Decreased serum glucose levels, with reduced insulin levels, occur secondary to dehydration caused by intractable vomiting.

NP: Assessment; CN: Physiological integrity; CNS: Physiological adaptation; CL: Analysis

5. In the latter stages of Reye's syndrome, which of the following major interventions is directed toward preventing or reducing cerebral edema?
1. Noninvasive pressure monitoring
2. Paralysis and sedation
3. Liberal fluid replacement
4. Nonassisted ventilation

5. 2. Skeletal muscles are paralyzed with the administration of pancuronium (Pavulon). This prevents activity, especially coughing, that might increase intracranial pressure (ICP). Invasive monitoring is essential to detect increased ICP. Liberal fluid replacement may increase cerebral edema and should be strictly monitored. Tracheal intubation is performed as soon as possible to prevent hypoventilation and increased carbon dioxide levels.

NP: Planning; CN: Physiological integrity; CNS: Reduction of risk potential; CL: Analysis

6. Which of the following assessment changes would indicate increased intracranial pressure (ICP) in a child acutely ill with Reye's syndrome?
1. Irritability and quick pupil response
2. Increased blood pressure and decreased heart rate
3. Decreased blood pressure and increased heart rate
4. Sluggish pupil response and decreased blood pressure

6. 2. A marked increase in ICP will trigger the pressure response; increased ICP produces an elevation in blood pressure with a reflex slowing of the heart rate. Irritability is often an early sign but pupillary response becomes more sluggish in response to increased ICP.

NP: Assessment; CN: Physiological integrity; CNS: Physiological adaptation; CL: Application

7. A client with Reye's syndrome is exhibiting signs of increased intracranial pressure (ICP). Which of the following nursing interventions would be contraindicated for this client?
1. Mouth care
2. Scheduled cluster care
3. Suctioning and chest physiotherapy
4. Positioning to avoid neck vein compression

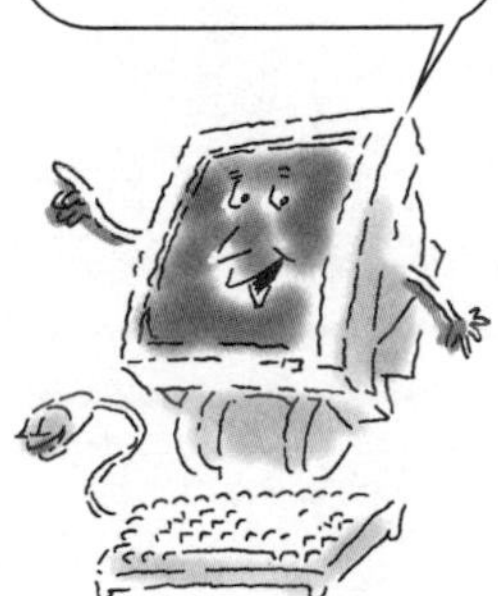

Warning: The word *contraindicated* makes this almost a negative question.

7. 3. Nursing procedures tend to cause reactive pressure waves in many clients. Suctioning and percussion are poorly tolerated; thus, they're contraindicated. Basic mouth care will promote comfort and decrease infection. Care should be provided at an optimal time for the client, clustering care to prevent overstimulation of the client. Neck vein compression may further increase ICP by interfering with venous return.

NP: Implementation; CN: Physiological integrity; CNS: Physiological adaptation; CL: Application

8. The goal of nursing care for a client with Reye's syndrome is to minimize intracranial pressure (ICP). Which of the following nursing interventions help to meet this goal?

1. Keeping the head of bed flat
2. Frequent position changes
3. Positioning to avoid neck flexion
4. Suctioning and chest physiotherapy

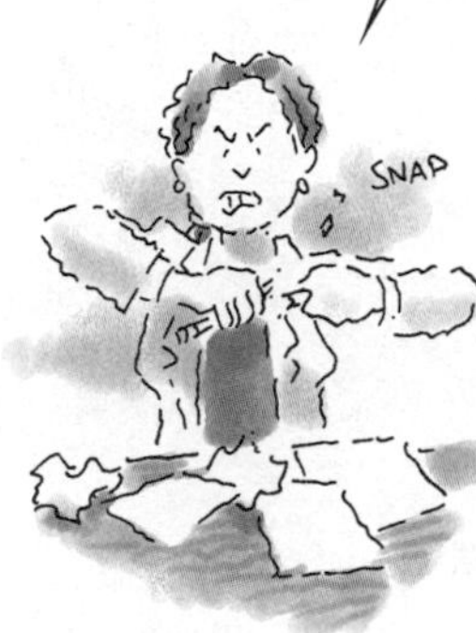

Stay calm when encountering NCLEX questions you're unsure about. That's what I do.
SNAP

8. 3. Neck vein compression can increase ICP by interfering with venous return. The head of the bed should be elevated to help promote venous return. Nursing procedures such as frequent positioning tend to cause overstimulation; therefore, care should be taken to avoid such procedures to prevent increased ICP. Suctioning and percussion are poorly tolerated and are contraindicated, unless concurrent respiratory problems are present.

NP: Implementation; CN: Physiological integrity; CNS: Physiological adaptation; CL: Application

9. Which of the following nursing interventions would be included in the care of an unconscious child with Reye's syndrome?

1. Keep arms and legs flexed
2. Place the child on a sheepskin
3. Avoid using lotions on skin
4. Place the client in a supine position

9. 2. Placing the child on a sheepskin helps to prevent pressure on prominent areas of the body. Rubbing the extremities with lotion stimulates circulation and helps prevent drying of the skin. Keeping extremities in a flexed position can lead to contractures. Placing the child supine would be contraindicated due to the risk of aspiration and increasing intracranial pressure. The supine position puts undue pressure on the sacral and occipital areas.

NP: Implementation; CN: Physiological integrity; CNS: Physiological adaptation; CL: Application

10. Which of the following medications has been connected with the development of Reye's syndrome?

1. Acetaminophen (Tylenol)
2. Aspirin
3. Ibuprofen (Motrin)
4. Guaifenesin (Robitussin)

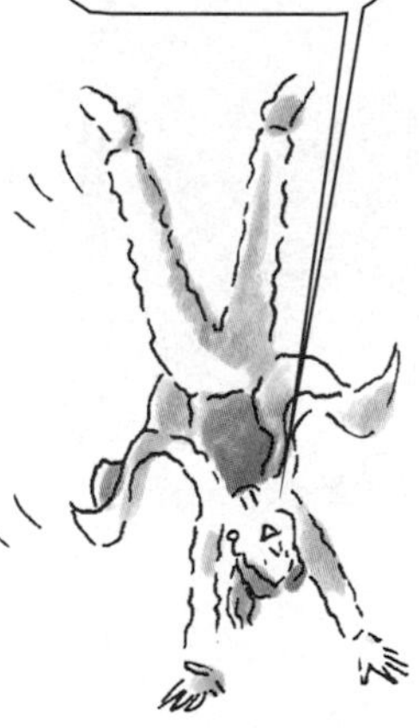

Good job! You've finished 10 questions already! Keep it up!

10. 2. Aspirin administration is associated with the development of Reye's syndrome. Acetaminophen, ibuprofen, and guaifenesin haven't been associated with the development of Reye's syndrome. In fact, there has been a decreased incidence of Reye's syndrome with the increased use of acetaminophen and ibuprofen for management of fevers in children.

NP: Implementation; CN: Physiological integrity; CNS: Pharmacological and parenteral therapies; CL: Knowledge

11. Parents should be told to stop acetylsalicylic acid (aspirin) administration and notify the physician if their child is exposed to which condition?

1. Stress
2. Scabies
3. Influenza
4. Environmental allergies

11. 3. A strong association exists between influenza and aspirin administration and the development of Reye's syndrome. There's no contraindication with the other conditions.

NP: Implementation; CN: Physiological integrity; CNS: Pharmacological and parenteral therapies; CL: Application

12. Which of the following nursing interventions would be included in the care of a client with Reye's syndrome who is receiving pancuronium (Pavulon)?

1. Applying artificial tears as needed
2. Providing regular tactile stimulation
3. Performing active range-of-motion (ROM) exercises
4. Placing the client in a supine position

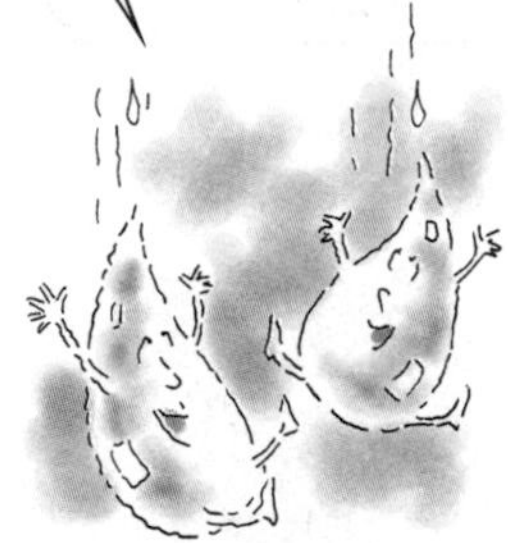

Artificial tears may be necessary when administering paralytic agents.

12. 1. Pancuronium suppresses the corneal reflex, making the eyes prone to irritation. Artificial tears prevent drying. Tactile stimulation isn't appropriate because it may elicit a pressure response. Active ROM exercises may cause an increase in pressure. The head of the bed should be elevated slightly, with the paralyzed client in a side-lying or semi-prone position to prevent aspiration and minimize intracranial pressure.

NP: Implementation; CN: Physiological integrity; CNS: Pharmacological and parenteral therapies; CL: Application

13. Which of the following goals would be achieved by performing a craniotomy on a client with Reye's syndrome?

1. Decrease carbon dioxide levels
2. Determine the extent of brain injury
3. Reduce pressure from an edematous brain
4. Allow continuous monitoring of intracranial pressure (ICP)

13. 3. In severe cases of cerebral edema, creating bilateral bone flaps (craniotomy) is most effective in decreasing ICP. Carbon dioxide levels can be decreased through mechanical ventilation. Most clients with Reye's syndrome recover without any resulting brain injury. Continuous monitoring of ICP is implemented through central venous pressure lines.

NP: Analysis; CN: Physiological integrity; CNS: Reduction of risk potential; CL: Knowledge

14. Parents of a child with Reye's syndrome need a great deal of emotional support. Which of the following nursing interventions should be included to reduce stress and alleviate fears?

1. Not accepting aggressive behavior from parents
2. Encouraging them not to overreact and to hope for the best
3. Letting parents interpret the child's behaviors and responses
4. Explaining therapies and clarifying or reinforcing the information given

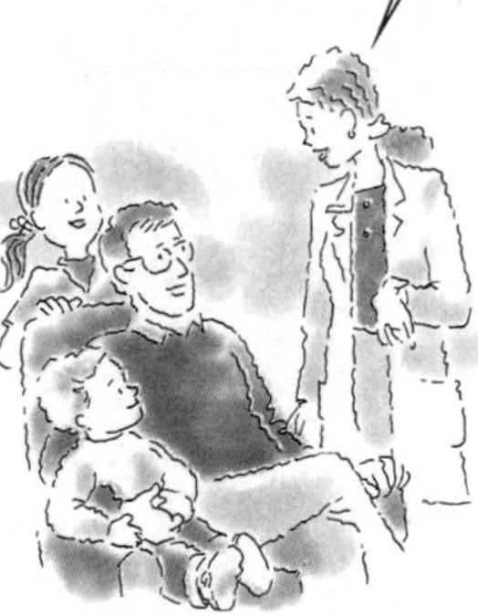

Be sensitive not only to your client's needs but to the family's needs as well.

14. 4. Explaining treatments and therapies will help to alleviate undue stress in the parents. An awareness of the potential for aggressive behaviors provides nurses with the understanding that helps them support the parents in their grief. Being too quick to reassure may block a parent's expression of fears. Parents may need help interpreting their child's behavior to avoid assigning erroneous meanings to the many signs their child exhibits.

NP: Implementation; CN: Psychosocial integrity; CNS: Coping and adaptation; CL: Application

15. Which of the following clinical manifestations would you expect to see in a client in stage V of Reye's syndrome?

1. Vomiting, lethargy, and drowsiness
2. Seizures, flaccidity, and respiratory arrest
3. Hyperventilation and coma
4. Disorientation, aggressiveness, and combativeness

15. 2. Staging criteria were developed to help evaluate the client's progress and to evaluate the efficacy of therapies. The clinical manifestations of stage V include seizures, loss of deep tendon reflexes, flaccidity, and respiratory arrest. Vomiting, lethargy, and drowsiness occur in stage I. Hyperventilation and coma occur in stage III. Disorientation and aggressive behavior occur in stage II.

NP: Assessment; CN: Physiological integrity; CNS: Physiological adaptation; CL: Knowledge

16. Vaccinating a child against preventable diseases represents which of the following types of immunity?
1. Acquired immunity
2. Active immunity
3. Natural immunity
4. Passive immunity

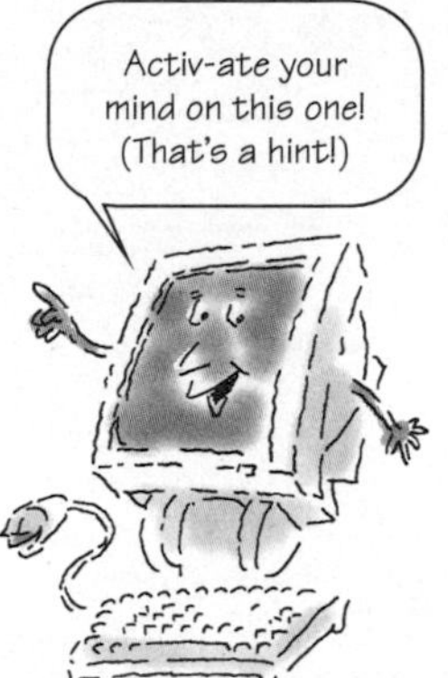
Activ-ate your
mind on this one!
(That's a hint!)

16. 2. Active immunity occurs when the individual forms immune bodies against certain diseases, either by having the disease or by the introduction of a vaccine into the individual. Acquired immunity results from exposure to the bacteria, virus, or toxins. Natural immunity is resistance to infection or toxicity. Passive immunity is a temporary immunity caused by transfusion of immune plasma proteins.

NP: Analysis; CN: Health promotion and maintenance; CNS: Prevention and early detection of disease; CL: Knowledge

17. What is the recommended age for beginning hepatitis B immunization of normal infants?
1. Birth
2. 4 months
3. 6 months
4. 1 year

17. 1. According to the American Academy of Pediatrics, birth to age 2 months is the recommended time for beginning hepatitis B immunizations.

NP: Analysis; CN: Health promotion and maintenance; CNS: Prevention and early detection of disease; CL: Knowledge

18. What is the recommended age to begin receiving the measles vaccine?
1. 6 months
2. 12 months
3. 15 months
4. 18 months

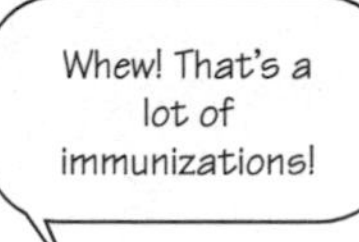

18. 2. According to the American Academy of Pediatrics, the first dose of the measles vaccine should be administered beginning at or after age 12 months.

NP: Analysis; CN: Health promotion and maintenance; CNS: Prevention and early detection of disease; CL: Knowledge

19. Which of the following immunizations should a healthy 2-month-old baby receive?
1. Measles and inactivated polio (IPV)
2. Measles, mumps, and rubella (MMR)
3. Diphtheria, tetanus, and pertussis (DTP)
4. DTP and IPV

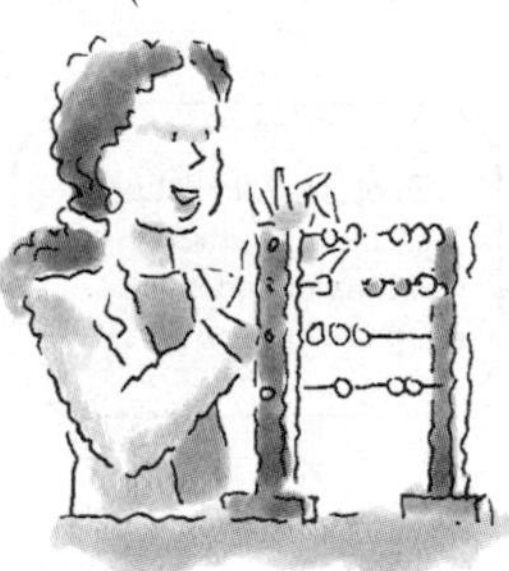

19. 4. At age 2 months, DTP and IPV are the recommended immunizations. DTP and IPV are given again at 4 months and DTP is given again alone at age 6 months. MMR is given at age 12 months.

NP: Analysis; CN: Health promotion and maintenance; CNS: Prevention and early detection of disease; CL: Knowledge

20. The child who is diagnosed with thalassemia major (Cooley's anemia) typically suffers complications from the disease and from the treatment. This child is at risk for which condition?
1. Hypertrophy of the thyroid
2. Hypertrophy of the thymus
3. Polycythemia vera and thrombosis
4. Chronic hypoxia and iron overload

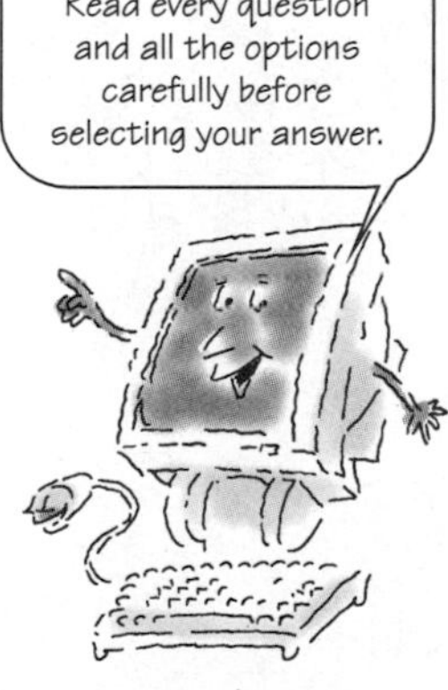
Test-taking tip:
Read every question
and all the options
carefully before
selecting your answer.

20. 4. In thalassemia major, increased destruction of red blood cells (RBCs) causes anemia. RBCs also have a shortened life span. The body responds by increasing the production of RBCs, but it can't adequately produce enough mature cells to meet the body's demands. This process results in chronic hypoxia. Children with the disorder are given multiple transfusions of packed RBCs. The combination of excessive RBC destruction and multiple transfusions causes too much iron to be deposited in organs and tissues and results in damage to the involved organs. The thymus and thyroid aren't involved. Polycythemia vera refers to excessive RBC production, which can result in thrombosis.

NP: Assessment; CN: Physiological integrity; CNS: Reduction of risk potential; CL: Analysis

21. Which is the treatment of choice for severe aplastic anemia?

1. Liver transplantation
2. Exchange transfusion
3. Bone marrow transplantation
4. Administration of intravenous immunoglobulins

21. 3. Aplastic anemia refers to either a congenital or an acquired condition in which severe pancytopenia, or decrease in cellular components of the blood, occurs. Children with the condition have profound anemia, are susceptible to infections, and risk bleeding. When a good match of donor bone marrow is available, transplantation is the treatment of choice. Liver transplantation, exchange transfusion, and the administration of intravenous immunoglobulins aren't treatments for aplastic anemia.

NP: Planning; CN: Safe, effective care environment; CNS: Management of care; CL: Knowledge

22. Which type of transfusion is most likely to be given to a child with sickle cell anemia?

1. Plasma
2. Platelets
3. Whole blood
4. Packed red blood cells (RBCs)

22. 4. Packed RBCs are given to children when their hemoglobin is dangerously low. Severe anemia decreases oxygen perfusion and leads to increased sickling of cells. Packed cells are RBCs with plasma removed. If enough whole blood were given to reach the desired hemoglobin level, fluid overload could occur. Thus, the plasma is removed and packed RBCs are infused. The RBCs are needed to transport oxygen. Platelets are given to children with low platelets, not anemia.

NP: Assessment; CN: Physiological integrity; CNS: Pharmacological and parenteral therapies; CL: Analysis

23. Which of the following directions is most important when administering immunizations?

1. Properly store the vaccine, and follow the recommended procedure for injection.
2. Monitor clients for approximately 1 hour after administration for adverse reactions.
3. Take the vaccine out of refrigeration 1 hour before administration.
4. Inject multiple vaccines at the same injection site.

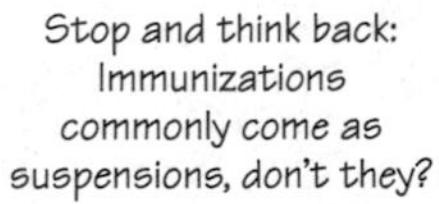

Stop and think back: Immunizations commonly come as suspensions, don't they?

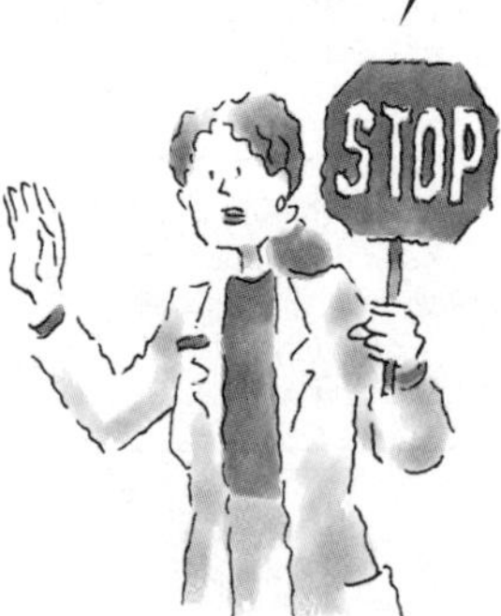

STOP

23. 1. Vaccines must be properly stored to ensure their potency. The nurse must be familiar with the manufacturer's directions for storage and reconstitution of the vaccine. Faulty refrigeration is a major cause of primary vaccine failure. It isn't necessary to monitor the clients but the nurse should teach parents to call the primary care provider and report any adverse effects. Taking the vaccine out of refrigeration too early can affect its potency. If more than one vaccine is to be administered, different injection sites should be used. The nurse should note which vaccine is given and at what site in case of a local reaction.

NP: Implementation; CN: Health promotion and maintenance; CNS: Prevention and early detection of disease; CL: Knowledge

24. Which of the following symptoms is the most common manifestation of severe combined immunodeficiency disease (SCID)?

1. Bruising
2. Failure to thrive
3. Prolonged bleeding
4. Susceptibility to infection

24. 4. SCID is characterized by absence of both humoral and cell-mediated immunity. The most common manifestation is susceptibility to infection early in life, most often by age 3 months. SCID is characterized by chronic infection, failure to completely recover from an infection, and frequent reinfection. The history reveals no logical source for infection. Failure to thrive is a consequence of persistent illnesses. Prolonged bleeding and bruising indicate abnormalities in the clotting system.

NP: Analysis; CN: Physiological integrity; CNS: Physiological adaptation; CL: Knowledge

25. A child is admitted to the hospital for an asthma exacerbation. The nursing history reveals this client was exposed to chickenpox 1 week ago. When would this client require isolation, if he were to remain hospitalized?

1. Isolation isn't required.
2. Immediate isolation is required.
3. Isolation would be required 10 days after exposure.
4. Isolation would be required 12 days after exposure.

25. 2. The incubation period for chickenpox is 2 to 3 weeks, commonly 13 to 17 days. A client is commonly isolated 1 week after exposure to avoid the risk of an earlier breakout. A person is infectious from 1 day before eruption of lesions to 6 days after the vesicles have formed crusts.

NP: Analysis; CN: Safe, effective care environment; CNS: Safety and infection control; CL: Application

26. On assessment of a child's skin, the nurse notes a papular pruritic rash with some vesicles. The rash is profuse on the trunk and sparse on the distal limbs. Based on this assessment, which of the following illnesses does the client have?

1. Measles
2. Mumps
3. Roseola
4. Chickenpox

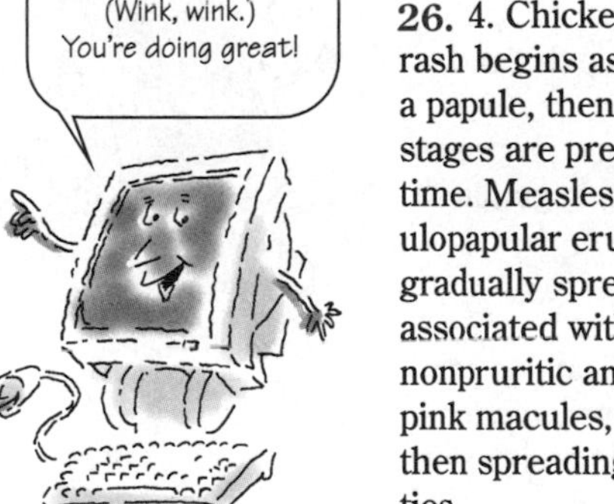
Don't be chicken!
(Wink, wink.)
You're doing great!

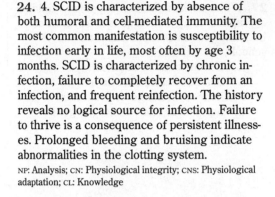

26. 4. Chickenpox rash is highly pruritic. The rash begins as a macule, rapidly progresses to a papule, then becomes a vesicle. All three stages are present in varying degrees at one time. Measles begins as an erythematous maculopapular eruption on the face; the eruption gradually spreads downward. Mumps isn't associated with a skin rash. Roseola rash is nonpruritic and is described as discrete rose-pink macules, appearing first on the trunk and then spreading to the neck, face, and extremities.

NP: Assessment; CN: Health promotion and maintenance; CNS: Prevention and early detection of disease; CL: Knowledge

27. Which of the following responses would be appropriate to a parent inquiring about when her child with chickenpox can return to school?

1. When the child is afebrile
2. When all vesicles have dried
3. When vesicles begin to crust over
4. When lesions and vesicles are gone

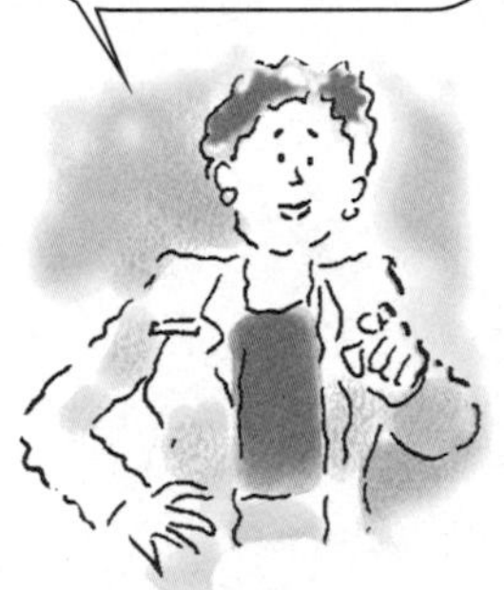

Chickenpox is highly contagious. Teach parents how to assess when it's safe to send kids back to school.

27. 2. Chickenpox is contagious. It's transmitted through direct contact, droplet spread, and contact with contaminated objects. Vesicles break open; therefore, a person is potentially contagious until all vesicles have dried. It isn't necessary to wait until dried lesions have disappeared. Some vesicles may be crusted over, and new ones may have formed. Macules, papules, vesicles, and crusting are present in varying degrees at one time. A child may be free of fever but continue to have vesicles. Isolation is usually necessary only for about 1 week after the onset of the disease.

NP: Implementation; CN: Safe, effective care environment; CNS: Safety and infection control; CL: Knowledge

28. Which of the following symptoms are clinical manifestations associated with roseola?

1. Apparent sickness, fever, and rash
2. Fever for 3 to 4 days, followed by rash
3. Rash, without history of fever or illness
4. Rash for 3 to 4 days, followed by high fevers

28. 2. Roseola is manifested by persistent high fever for 3 to 4 days in a child who appears well. Fever precedes the rash. When the rash appears, a precipitous drop in fever occurs and the temperature returns to normal.

NP: Assessment; CN: Health promotion and maintenance; CNS: Prevention and early detection of disease; CL: Knowledge

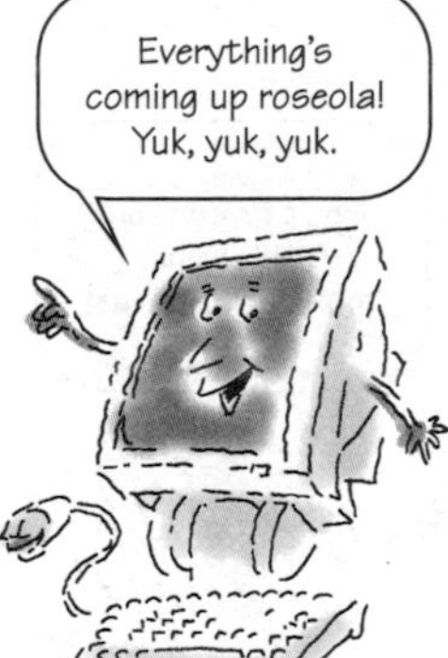

Everything's coming up roseola! Yuk, yuk, yuk.

29. Which of the following assessment findings are consistent with a roseola rash?

1. Maculopapular red spots
2. Macular and pruritic, with papules and vesicles
3. Rose-pink macules that fade on pressure
4. Red maculopapular eruption, beginning on the face

29. 3. Roseola rashes are discrete, rose-pink macules or maculopapules that fade on pressure and usually last 1 to 2 days. Chickenpox rash is macular, with papules and vesicles. Roseola isn't pruritic. Maculopapular red spots may be indicative of fifth disease. Measles begin as a maculopapular eruption on the face.

NP: Assessment; CN: Health promotion and maintenance; CNS: Prevention and early detection of disease; CL: Knowledge

30. Which of the following complications can be caused by a child with chickenpox scratching open and severely irritating the vesicles on his abdomen?

1. Myocarditis
2. Neuritis
3. Obstructive laryngitis
4. Secondary bacterial infection

30. 4. Secondary bacterial infections can occur as a complication of chickenpox. Irritation of skin lesions can lead to cellulitis or even an abscess. Myocarditis isn't considered a complication of chickenpox but has been noted as a complication of mumps. Neuritis has been associated with diphtheria. Obstructive laryngitis occurs as a complication of measles.

NP: Analysis; CN: Physiological integrity; CNS: Reduction of risk potential; CL: Knowledge

31. Which characteristic best describes the cough of an infant who was admitted to the hospital with suspected pertussis?

1. Dry, hacking, more frequent on awakening
2. Loose, nonproductive coughing episodes
3. Occurring more frequently during the day
4. Harsh, associated with a high-pitched crowing sound

31. 4. The cough associated with pertussis is a harsh series of short, rapid coughs, followed by a sudden inspiration and a high-pitched crowing sound. Cheeks become flushed or cyanotic, eyes bulge, and the tongue protrudes. Paroxysm may continue until a thick mucus plug is dislodged. This cough occurs most commonly at night.

NP: Assessment; CN: Physiological integrity; CNS: Physiological adaptation; CL: Knowledge

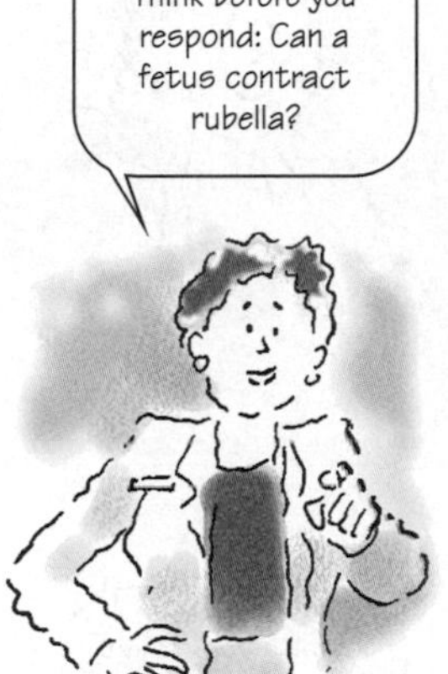

Think before you respond: Can a fetus contract rubella?

32. Which of the following communicable diseases requires isolating an infected child from pregnant women?

1. Pertussis
2. Roseola
3. Rubella
4. Scarlet fever

32. 3. Rubella (German measles) has a teratogenic effect on the fetus. An infected child must be isolated from pregnant women. Pertussis, roseola, and scarlet fever don't have any teratogenic effects on a fetus.

NP: Analysis; CN: Safe, effective care environment; CNS: Safety and infection control; CL: Knowledge

33. Which of the following medications is the treatment of choice for scarlet fever?

1. Acyclovir (Zovirax)
2. Amphotericin B
3. Ibuprofen (Motrin)
4. Penicillin

33. 4. The causative agent of scarlet fever is group A beta-hemolytic streptococci, which is susceptible to penicillin. Erythromycin is used for penicillin-sensitive children. Anti-inflammatory drugs such as ibuprofen aren't indicated for these clients. Acyclovir is used in the treatment of herpes infections. Amphotericin B is used to treat fungal infections.

NP: Implementation; CN: Physiological integrity; CNS: Pharmacological and parenteral therapies; CL: Knowledge

34. Which of the following periods of isolation is indicated for a child with scarlet fever?

1. Until the associated rash disappears
2. Until completion of antibiotic therapy
3. Until the client is fever-free for 24 hours
4. Until 24 hours after initiation of treatment

34. 4. A child requires respiratory isolation until 24 hours after initiation of treatment. Rash may persist for 3 weeks. It isn't necessary to wait until the end of treatment. Fever usually breaks 24 hours after therapy has begun. It isn't necessary to maintain isolation for an additional 24 hours.

NP: Implementation; CN: Safe, effective care environment; CNS: Safety and infection control; CL: Knowledge

35. Which of the following instructions should be included in the teaching about care of a child with chickenpox?

1. Administer penicillin or erythromycin as ordered.
2. Administer local or systemic antipruritics as ordered.
3. Offer periods of interaction with other children to provide distraction.
4. Avoid administering varicella-zoster immune globulin to children receiving long-term salicylate therapy.

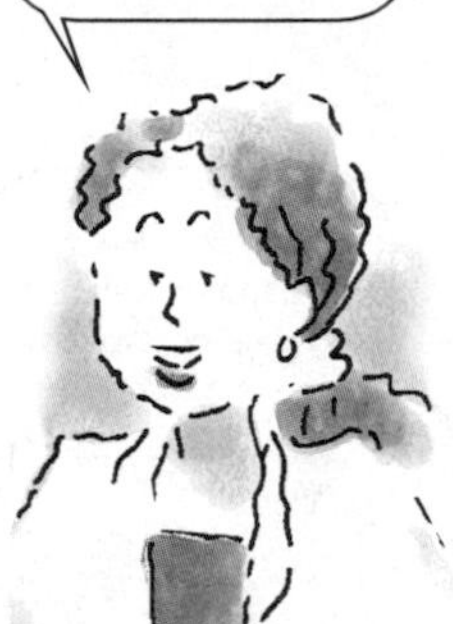

Congratulations! You've finished 35 questions! Keep up the good work!

35. 2. Chickenpox is highly pruritic. Preventing the child from scratching is necessary to prevent scarring and secondary infection caused by irritation of lesions. Penicillin and erythromycin aren't usually used in the treatment of chickenpox. Interaction with other children would be contraindicated due to the risk of communication, unless the other children previously have had chickenpox or been immunized. Varicella-zoster immune globulin *should* be administered to exposed children who are on long-term aspirin therapy because of the possible risk of Reye's syndrome.

NP: Implementation; CN: Physiological integrity; CNS: Pharmacological and parenteral therapies; CL: Knowledge

36. Scarlet fever may result as a complication of which infection?

1. Roseola
2. Staphylococcal parotitis
3. Streptococcal pharyngitis
4. Chickenpox

36. 3. The causative agent of scarlet fever is group A beta-hemolytic streptococci; therefore, scarlet fever may follow a strep throat infection. Roseola, chickenpox, and parotitis aren't strep infections and don't contribute to scarlet fever.

NP: Assessment; CN: Physiological integrity; CNS: Reduction of risk potential; CL: Knowledge

In which body fluids has HIV been isolated?

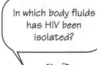

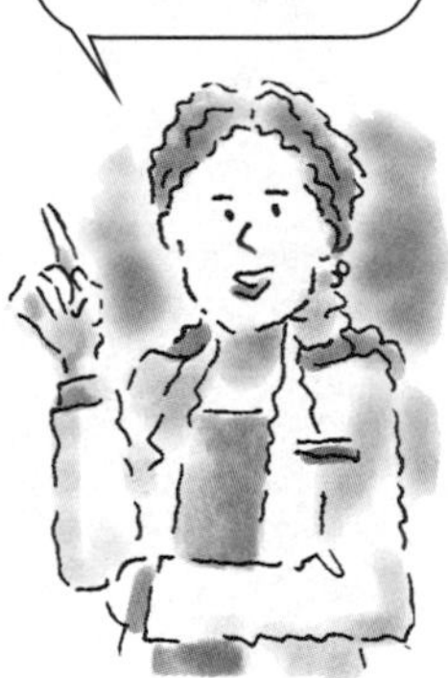

37. A mother infected with human immunodeficiency virus (HIV) inquires about the possibility of breast-feeding her newborn. Which of the following would be a correct response?

1. Breast-feeding isn't an option.
2. Breast-feeding would be best for your baby.
3. Breast-feeding is only an option if the mother is taking zidovudine (Retrovir).
4. Breast-feeding is an option if milk is expressed and fed by a bottle.

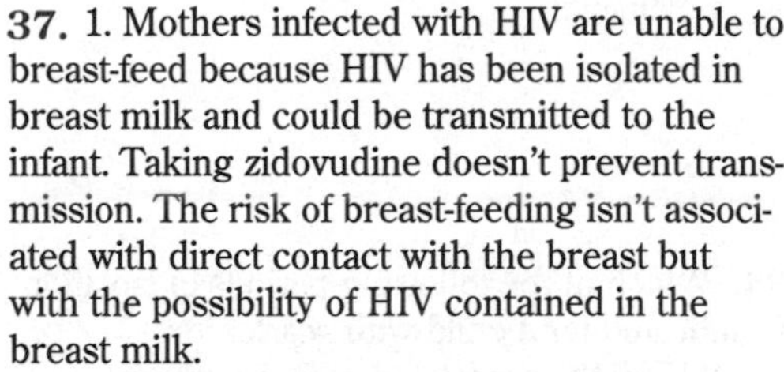

37. 1. Mothers infected with HIV are unable to breast-feed because HIV has been isolated in breast milk and could be transmitted to the infant. Taking zidovudine doesn't prevent transmission. The risk of breast-feeding isn't associated with direct contact with the breast but with the possibility of HIV contained in the breast milk.

NP: Implementation; CN: Health promotion and maintenance; CNS: Prevention and early detection of disease; CL: Application

38. Which of the following subjective assessment findings aids in diagnosing human immunodeficiency virus (HIV) infection in children?

1. Excessive weight gain
2. Arrhythmia
3. Intermittent diarrhea
4. Tolerance of feedings

38. 3. A differential diagnosis may be based on the presence of an underlying cellular immunodeficiency-related disease; symptoms include intermittent episodes of diarrhea, repeated respiratory infections, and the inability to tolerate feedings. Poor weight gain and failure to thrive are objective assessment findings that result from intolerance of feedings and frequent infections. Arrhythmia isn't associated with HIV.

NP: Assessment; CN: Physiological integrity; CNS: Physiological adaptation; CL: Knowledge

39. Which approach should be included in the diagnostic workup for a 12-month-old infant who is suspected of having acquired immunodeficiency syndrome (AIDS)?

1. Sputum culture
2. Esophageal biopsy
3. Parental counseling prior to testing
4. HIV enzyme-linked immunosorbent assay (ELISA)

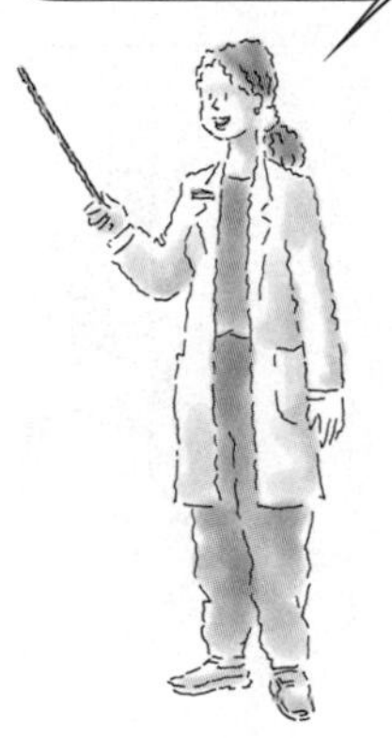

39. 3. AIDS and HIV are devastating diagnoses. Before testing, parents should be counseled regarding the disease, reasons for the tests, confidentiality, and benefits of early treatment. ELISA isn't used diagnostically for children younger than 18 months because of the maternal antibodies in the child's blood. Esophageal biopsy isn't indicated. Sputum culture might help diagnose an upper respiratory infection associated with AIDS but isn't a diagnostic test for AIDS.

NP: Planning; CN: Psychosocial integrity; CNS: Coping and adaptation; CL: Application

40. Parents of a child with Kawasaki disease should be taught the importance of keeping follow-up appointments to monitor and prevent which complication?

1. Encephalitis
2. Glomerulonephritis
3. Myocardial infarction (MI)
4. Idiopathic thrombocytopenia

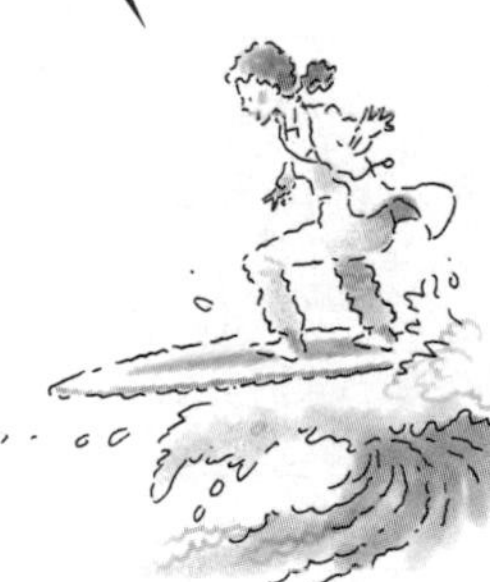

Kowabunga! You're surfing through this test. Keep it up!

40. 3. In Kawasaki disease, inflammation of small and medium blood vessels can result in weakening of the vessels and aneurysm formation, especially in the heart. Blood flow through damaged vessels can cause thrombus formation and MI. Encephalitis, glomerulonephritis, and idiopathic thrombocytopenia aren't associated with Kawasaki disease.

NP: Implementation; CN: Health promotion and maintenance; CNS: Prevention and early detection of disease; CL: Application

41. Sickle cell anemia occurs primarily in which of the following ethnic groups?

1. African-American
2. Asian
3. Hispanic
4. Caucasian

41. 1. Among African-Americans, the incidence is reported to be as high as 45%, and it's estimated that as many as 1 in 12 carries the trait. Sickle cell anemia is rare among Asians and Hispanics; infrequently, it affects Caucasians, especially those of Mediterranean descent.

NP: Assessment; CN: Physiological integrity; CNS: Physiological adaptation; CL: Knowledge

42. A child comes to the emergency department, suspected of being in vaso-occlusive crisis. Which of the following assessment findings would indicate that the client is having a vaso-occlusive crisis?

1. Hypotension, thready pulse
2. Pallor, poor capillary refill
3. Anemia, jaundice, and reticulocytosis
4. Acute leg pain and hand-foot syndrome

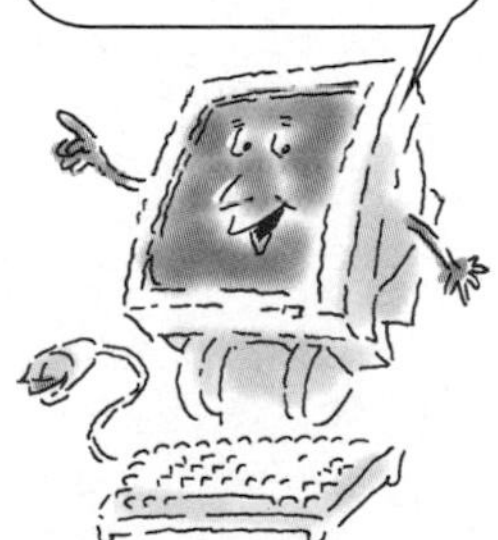

42. 4. There are four types of episodic crises in sickle cell anemia: vaso-occlusive, splenic sequestration, aplastic, and hyperhemolytic. Vaso-occlusive crises are the most common. They're the result of sickled cells obstructing the blood vessels. The major symptoms are fever, acute pain from visceral hypoxia, hand-foot syndrome, and arthralgia. A precipitous drop in blood volume is indicative of a splenic sequestration crisis. Aplastic crisis exhibits diminished red blood cell production and may result in symptoms of shock. Hyperhemolytic crisis is characterized by anemia, jaundice, and reticulocytosis and may also result in symptoms of shock.

NP: Assessment; CN: Physiological integrity; CNS: Physiological adaptation; CL: Knowledge

43. Which of the following responses would be appropriate for the parent inquiring about a child who tests positive for sickle cell trait?

1. Your child has sickle cell anemia.
2. Your child is a carrier of the disorder but doesn't have sickle cell anemia.
3. Your child is a carrier of the disease and will pass the disease to any offspring.
4. Your child doesn't have the disease at present but may show evidence of the disease as he gets older.

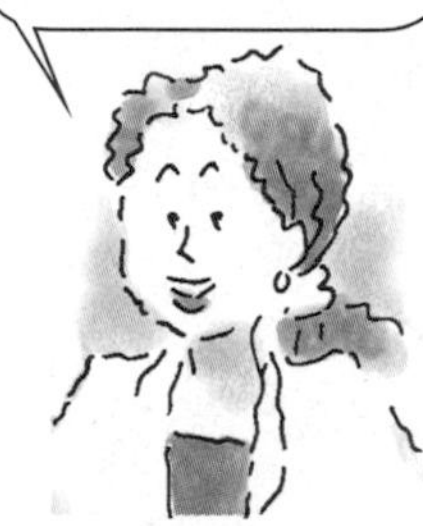

43. 2. A child with sickle cell trait is only a carrier and may never show any symptoms, except under special hypoxic conditions. A child with sickle cell trait doesn't have the disease and will never test positive for sickle cell anemia. Sickle cell anemia would be transmitted to offspring only as the result of a union between two individuals who are positive for the trait.

NP: Implementation; CN: Health promotion and maintenance; CNS: Prevention and early detection of disease; CL: Application

44. What is the primary nursing objective in caring for a child with sickle cell anemia in vaso-occlusive crisis?

1. Managing pain
2. Providing a cool environment
3. Immobilizing the affected part
4. Restricting fluids

44. 1. Pain management is an important aspect in the care of a client with sickle cell anemia in vaso-occlusive crisis. The goal is to prevent sickling. This can be accomplished by promoting tissue oxygenation, hydration, and rest, which minimize energy expenditure and oxygen utilization. A cool environment can cause vasoconstriction and thus more sickling and pain. Immobilization can promote stasis and increase sickling.

NP: Assessment; CN: Physiological integrity; CNS: Basic care and comfort; CL: Analysis

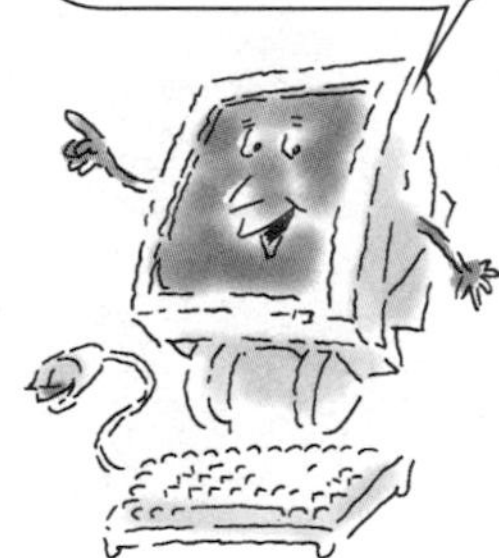

Be careful! The word not is important to the understanding of this question.

45. Which of the following possible complications is the reason for not palpating the abdomen of a child in vaso-occlusive crisis?

1. Risk of splenic rupture
2. Risk of inducing vomiting
3. Presence of abdominal pain
4. Risk of blood cell destruction

45. 1. Palpating a child's abdomen in vaso-occlusive crisis should be avoided because sequestered red blood cells may precipitate splenic rupture. Abdominal pain alone wouldn't be a reason to avoid palpation. Vomiting or blood cell destruction wouldn't occur from palpation of the abdomen.

NP: Implementation; CN: Physiological integrity; CNS: Reduction of risk potential; CL: Knowledge

46. Which of the following nursing measures would be included in the care of a child in vaso-occlusive crisis to maximize tissue perfusion?

1. Administering analgesics
2. Monitoring fluid restrictions
3. Limiting foods containing folic acid
4. Administering oxygen as prescribed

46. 4. Administering oxygen on a short-term basis helps to prevent hypoxia, which leads to metabolic acidosis, causing sickling. Long-term oxygen therapy will depress erythropoiesis. Analgesics are used to control pain. Hydration is essential to promote hemodilution and maintain electrolyte balance. Folic acid is needed to support red blood cell production.

NP: Implementation; CN: Physiological integrity; CNS: Reduction of risk potential; CL: Application

47. Which of the following nursing measures is most important to decrease the postoperative complications of a client with sickle cell anemia?

1. Increasing fluids
2. Preparing the child psychologically
3. Discouraging coughing
4. Limiting the use of analgesics

47. 1. The main surgical risk from anesthesia is hypoxia; however, emotional stress, demands of wound healing, and the potential for infection can each increase the sickling phenomenon. Increased fluids are encouraged because keeping the child well-hydrated is important for hemodilution to prevent sickling. Preparing the child psychologically to decrease fear will minimize undue emotional stress. Deep coughing is encouraged to promote pulmonary hygiene and prevent respiratory tract infection. Analgesics are used to control wound pain and to prevent abdominal splinting and decreased ventilation.

NP: Implementation; CN: Health promotion and maintenance; CNS: Prevention and early detection of disease; CL: Application

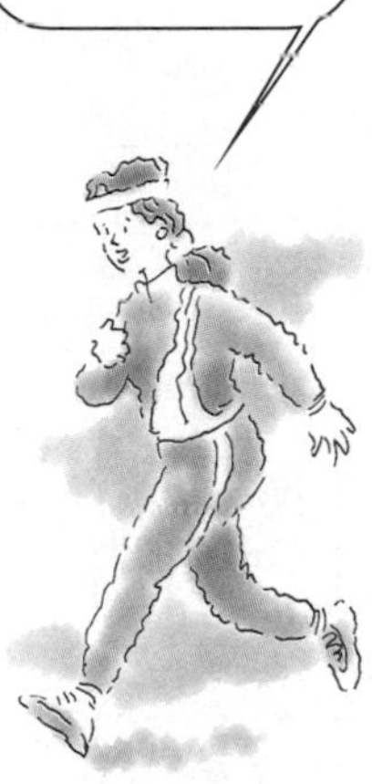

Don't let question 48 trip you up! It's asking you to prioritize.

48. Which of the following factors should be included as a priority in teaching parents about prevention of infection in children with sickle cell anemia?

1. Providing adequate nutrition
2. Avoiding emotional stress
3. Visiting the physician when sick
4. Avoiding strenuous physical exertion

48. 1. The nurse must stress adequate nutrition. Frequent medical supervision is imperative to prevention because infection is often a predisposing factor toward development of a crisis. Avoiding strenuous physical exertion and emotional stress are important aspects to prevent sickling but adequate nutrition remains a priority.

NP: Implementation; CN: Health promotion and maintenance; CNS: Prevention and early detection of disease; CL: Application

49. Thalassemia is seen predominantly in which of the following ethnic groups?

1. African-Americans
2. Asians
3. Greeks
4. Hispanics

49. 3. The disease is highly prevalent in people living near the Mediterranean Sea, namely Greeks, Italians, and Syrians. Evidence suggests that the high prevalence among these groups is a result of selective damage of the trait as a result of malaria.

NP: Assessment; CN: Health promotion and maintenance; CNS: Prevention and early detection of disease; CL: Knowledge

50. Which assessment findings would indicate vaso-occlusive crisis in a child with sickle cell anemia?

1. Painful urination
2. Pain with ambulation
3. Complaints of throat pain
4. Fever with associated rash

50. 2. Bone pain is one of the major symptoms of vaso-occlusive crisis in clients with sickle cell anemia. Hand-foot syndrome, characterized by edematous painful extremities, is usually exhibited in the refusal of the child to bear weight and ambulate. Painful urination doesn't occur but sickle cell anemia can cause kidney abnormalities. Throat pain isn't a symptom of vaso-occlusive crisis. Fever commonly accompanies vaso-occlusive crisis but isn't associated with rash.

NP: Assessment; CN: Physiological integrity; CNS: Physiological adaptation; CL: Knowledge

51. Which of the following bone-related complications can occur in sickle cell anemia?
1. Arthritis
2. Osteoporosis
3. Osteogenic sarcoma
4. Spontaneous fractures

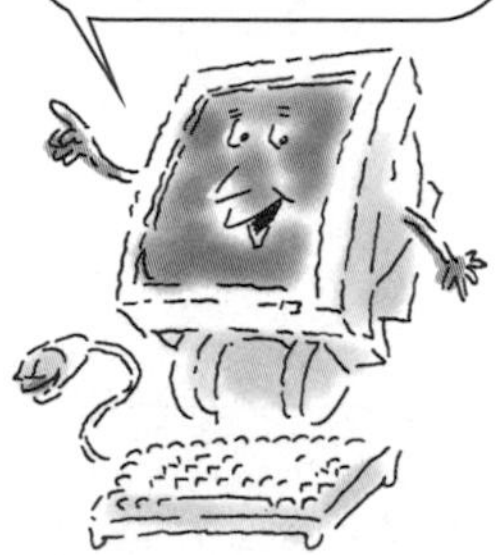

Would I be giving away the answer if I suddenly blurted out, "Poor ol' Oh, Sis, eh?"

51. 2. Sickle cell anemia causes hyperplasia and congestion of the bone marrow, resulting in osteoporosis. Arthritis doesn't occur secondary to sickle cell anemia; however, a crisis can cause localized swelling over joints, resulting in arthralgia. Osteogenic sarcoma is bone cancer; sickle cell anemia isn't a contributing factor to bone cancer. Bones do become weakened but spontaneous fractures don't occur as a result.

NP: Analysis; CN: Physiological integrity; CNS: Physiological adaptation; CL: Knowledge

52. What is the nurse's role with the parents of a child who has been diagnosed with sickle cell anemia?
1. Encouraging selective birth methods or abortion
2. Referring only sickle cell positive parents for counseling
3. Rendering support to parents of newly diagnosed children
4. Reinforcing that transmission is unlikely in subsequent pregnancies

52. 3. The nurse can be instrumental in providing genetic counseling. She can give parents correct information about the disease and render support to parents of newly diagnosed children. Alternative birth methods are discussed but parents make their own decisions. All heterozygous, or trait-positive, parents should be referred for genetic counseling. The risk of transmission in subsequent pregnancies remains the same.

NP: Implementation; CN: Health promotion and maintenance; CNS: Prevention and early detection of disease; CL: Application

53. A child with sickle cell anemia is admitted to the emergency department; her symptoms include a distended, boardlike, painful abdomen and symptoms of hypovolemic shock. These symptoms are indicative of which type of sickle cell crisis?
1. Aplastic
2. Hyperhemolytic
3. Vaso-occlusive
4. Splenic sequestration

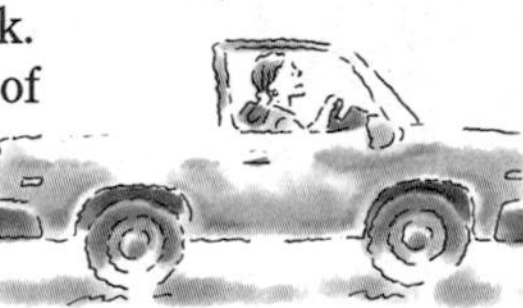

Excellent! You're covering the terrain well! Keep on truckin'!

53. 3. The primary symptom — severe pain — of a vaso-occlusive crisis is caused by the obstruction and ischemia of cells. Symptoms of splenic sequestration are caused by sudden massive pooling of blood in the spleen and other major organs. Aplastic and hyperhemolytic crises are from a lack of red blood cell (RBC) production or increased destruction of RBCs, either of which can lead to symptoms of shock, but not to the abdominal symptoms.

NP: Assessment; CN: Physiological integrity; CNS: Reduction of risk potential; CL: Analysis

54. The nurse is administering a blood transfusion to a client with sickle cell anemia. Which of the following assessment findings would indicate that the client is having a transfusion reaction?
1. Diaphoresis and hot flashes
2. Urticaria, flushing, and wheezing
3. Fever, urticaria, and red raised rash
4. Fever, disorientation, and abdominal pain

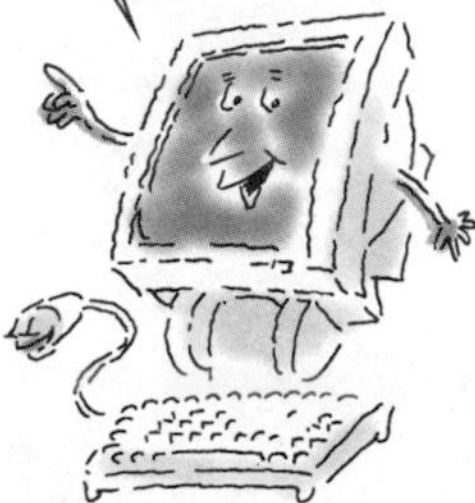

One wrong part of an option makes the entire option wrong.

54. 2. Allergic reactions may occur when the recipient reacts to allergens in the donor's blood; this reaction causes urticaria, flushing, and wheezing. A febrile reaction can occur, causing fever and urticaria, but it isn't accompanied by rash. Diaphoresis, hot flashes, disorientation, and abdominal pain aren't symptoms of a transfusion reaction.

NP: Assessment; CN: Physiological integrity; CNS: Reduction of risk potential; CL: Knowledge

55. How often should a child receive the influenza virus vaccine?

1. Annually
2. Twice a year
3. Contraindicated in children
4. Only with the outbreak of illness

55. 1. The influenza virus vaccine is usually administered annually. The vaccine isn't contraindicated in children but is targeted at clients with chronic cardiac, pulmonary, hematologic, and neurologic problems. The vaccine is given to prevent the onset of illness before an outbreak occurs.

NP: Analysis; CN: Health promotion and maintenance; CNS: Prevention and early detection of disease; CL: Knowledge

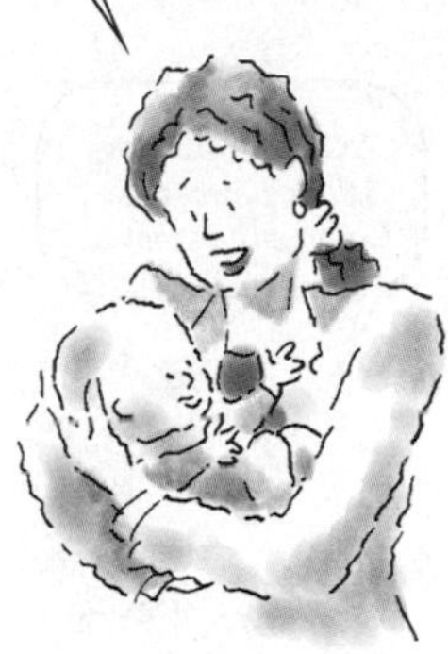

Prevention is often the best medicine!

56. A 3-year-old sister of a newborn baby is diagnosed with pertussis. The mother has a history of having been immunized as a child. Which of the following information should be included in teaching the mother about possible infection of her neonate?

1. The baby will inevitably contract pertussis.
2. Immune globulin is effective in protecting the infant.
3. The risk to the infant depends on the mother's immune status.
4. Erythromycin should be administered prophylactically to the infant.

56. 4. In exposed, high-risk persons such as neonates, erythromycin may be effective in preventing or lessening severity of the disease if administered during the preparoxysmal stage. Immune globulin isn't indicated as it's used as an immunization against hepatitis A. Neonates exposed to pertussis are at considerable risk for infections, regardless of the mother's immune status; however, infection isn't inevitable.

NP: Implementation; CN: Health promotion and maintenance; CNS: Prevention and early detection of disease; CL: Application

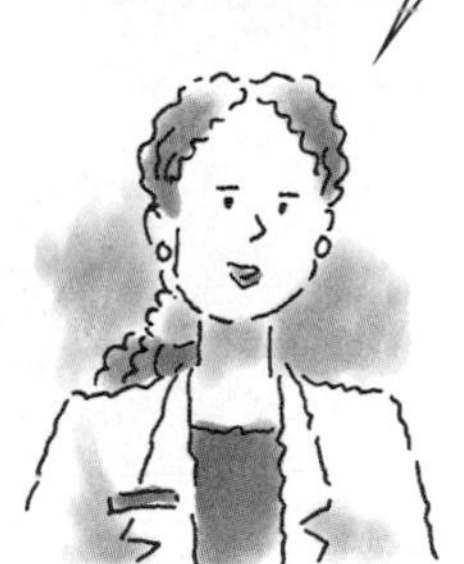

You beta get this one right!

57. An imbalance in one of the four chains of amino acids that make up hemoglobin is found in children with which of the following disorders?

1. Beta-thalassemia trait
2. Iron deficiency anemia
3. Lead poisoning
4. Sickle cell anemia

57. 1. Beta-thalassemia is caused by an imbalance in the beta chain of the amino acids that produce hemoglobin. Iron deficiency anemia, lead poisoning, and sickle cell anemia aren't related to the imbalance.

NP: Analysis; CN: Physiological integrity; CNS: Physiological adaptation; CL: Knowledge

58. A 4-year-old child has a petechial rash but is otherwise well. The platelet count is 20,000/μl and the hemoglobin level and white blood cell (WBC) count are normal. Which of the following diagnoses is most likely?

1. Acute lymphoblastic leukemia (ALL)
2. Disseminated intravascular coagulation (DIC)
3. Idiopathic thrombocytopenic purpura (ITP)
4. Systemic lupus erythematosus (SLE)

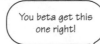

58. 3. The onset of ITP typically occurs between ages 1 and 6. Clients look well, except for a petechial rash. ALL is associated with a low platelet count but an *abnormal* hemoglobin level and WBC count. DIC is secondary to a severe underlying disease. SLE is rare in a 4-year-old child.

NP: Analysis; CN: Physiological integrity; CNS: Physiological adaptation; CL: Knowledge

59. Which of the following instructions would be included in the nurse's discharge teaching for the parents of a newborn diagnosed with sickle cell anemia?

1. Stressing the importance of iron supplementation
2. Stressing the importance of monthly vitamin B_{12} injections
3. Reviewing signs of abdominal pain in infants and demonstrating how to take a temperature
4. Explaining that immunizations are contraindicated

59. 3. Acute splenic sequestration is a serious complication of sickle cell anemia. Early detection of splenomegaly by parents is an important aspect of client management. Parents should be able to take the temperature and identify abdominal pain. A temperature of 101.3° F to 102.2° F (38.5° C to 39° C) calls for emergency evaluation, even if the child appears well. Folic acid requirement is increased; therefore, supplementation may be indicated. Vitamin B_{12} supplementation and iron supplementation aren't necessary. Parents should be encouraged to keep immunizations up to date.

NP: Implementation; CN: Health promotion and maintenance; CNS: Reduction of risk potential; CL: Knowledge

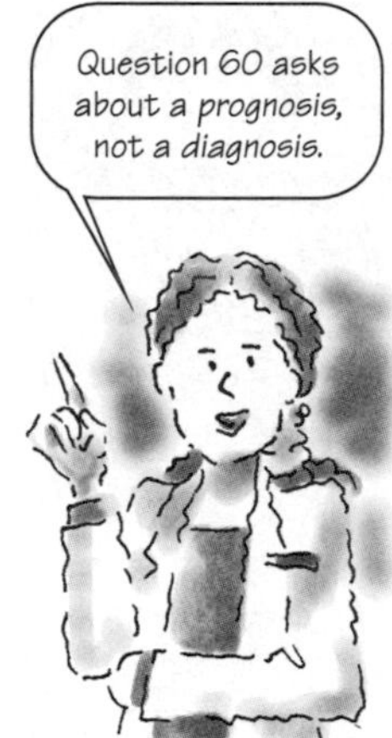
Question 60 asks about a *prognosis*, not a *diagnosis*.

60. Which of the following findings yields a poor prognosis for a child with leukemia?

1. Presence of a mediastinal mass
2. Late central nervous system (CNS) leukemia
3. Normal white blood cell (WBC) count at diagnosis
4. Disease presents between ages 2 and 10

60. 1. The presence of a mediastinal mass indicates a poor prognosis for children with leukemia. The prognosis is poorer if age at onset is less than 2 years or greater than 10 years. A WBC count of 100,000/µl or higher and early CNS leukemia also indicate a poor prognosis for a child with leukemia.

NP: Assessment; CN: Physiological integrity; CNS: Physiological adaptation; CL: Knowledge

61. A 1-year-old boy in the pediatrician's office for an examination is noted to be pale. He's in the 75th percentile for weight and the 25th percentile for length. His physical examination is normal but his hematocrit is 24%. Which question would be most helpful in establishing a diagnosis of anemia?

1. Is the child on any medications?
2. What's the child's usual daily diet?
3. Did the child receive phototherapy for jaundice?
4. What's the pattern and appearance of bowel movements?

61. 2. Iron deficiency anemia is the most common nutritional deficiency in children between ages 9 months and 15 months. Anemia in a 1-year-old child is mostly nutritional in origin, and its cause will be suggested by a detailed nutritional history. None of the other selections would be helpful in diagnosing anemia.

NP: Assessment; CN: Health promotion and maintenance; CNS: Prevention and early detection of disease; CL: Knowledge

62. Which of the following statements regarding Hodgkin's disease is true?

1. Staging laparotomy is mandatory for every client.
2. Edema and chills can be symptoms.
3. Hodgkin's disease is rare before age 5.
4. Incidence of Hodgkin's disease peaks between ages 11 and 15.

62. 3. Hodgkin's disease is rare before age 5. Systemic symptoms of Hodgkin's disease include fever, night sweats, malaise, weight loss, and pruritus. The peak incidence of Hodgkin's disease occurs in late adolescence and young adulthood (ages 15 to 34). Staging laparotomy is *not* recommended for clients who have obvious intra-abdominal disease by noninvasive studies.

NP: Analysis; CN: Physiological integrity; CNS: Physiological adaptation; CL: Knowledge

63. Children with perinatally acquired human immunodeficiency virus (HIV) usually demonstrate symptoms of acquired immunodeficiency syndrome (AIDS) at what age?

1. Within the first month of life
2. At 1 to 3 months of age
3. At 18 to 24 months of age
4. At 3 to 5 years of age

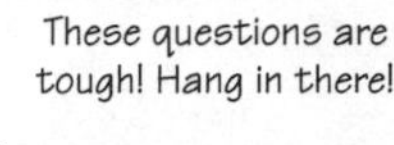

These questions are tough! Hang in there!

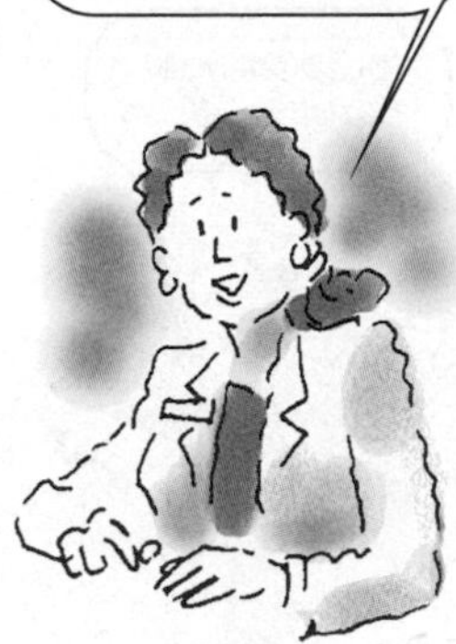

63. 3. The majority of children with perinatally transmitted AIDS appear normal in early infancy. Symptoms usually develop at 18 to 24 months of age.

NP: Assessment; CN: Physiological integrity; CNS: Physiological adaptation; CL: Knowledge

64. Which factors may make adolescent girls at risk for iron deficiency anemia?

1. Menses
2. Vegetarian diet
3. Weight loss diets
4. All of the above

64. 4. All the options make adolescent girls, who are still growing, at risk for iron deficiency anemia. That's because these girls lose blood monthly with menstrual periods, and they often consume inadequate amounts of nutrients because of their eating patterns, which include hurried meals, vegetarian diets, and weight-loss diets.

NP: Assessment; CN: Health promotion and maintenance; CNS: Prevention and early detection of disease; CL: Analysis

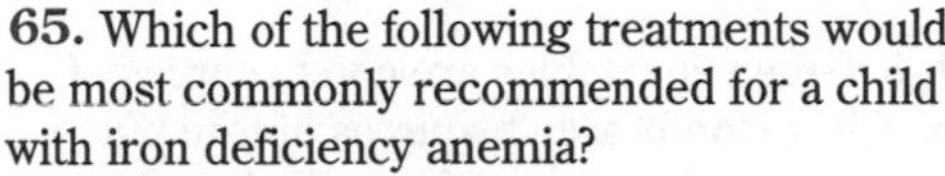

65. Which of the following treatments would be most commonly recommended for a child with iron deficiency anemia?

1. Blood transfusion
2. Oral ferrous sulfate
3. An iron-fortified cereal
4. Intramuscular iron dextran

65. 2. A prompt rise in hemoglobin level and hematocrit follow the administration of oral ferrous sulfate. Blood transfusion is rarely indicated unless a child becomes symptomatic or is further compromised by a superimposed infection. Dietary modifications are appropriate long-term measures but they won't make enough iron available to replenish iron stores. Intramuscular dextran is reserved for situations in which compliance can't be achieved because it's expensive, painful, and no more effective than oral iron.

NP: Analysis; CN: Physiological integrity; CNS: Pharmacological and parenteral therapies; CL: Knowledge

66. Which of the following infections is not associated with human parvovirus B-19 infection?

1. Roseola
2. Fifth disease
3. Transient aplastic anemia
4. Persistent infection in immunodeficient clients

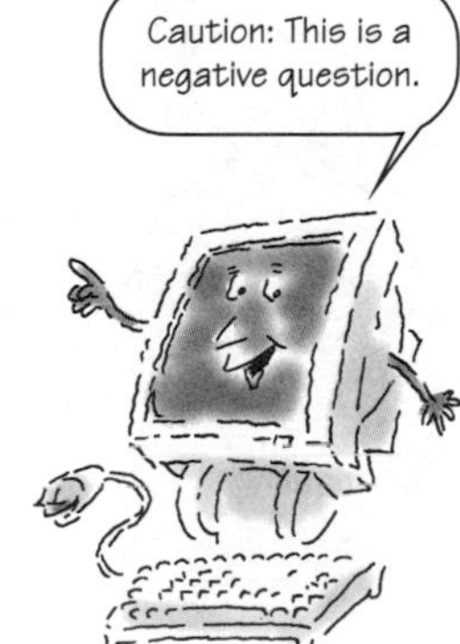

Caution: This is a negative question.

66. 1. Roseola is thought to be caused by the human herpes virus 6. Fifth disease is known to be caused by human parvovirus B-19. In clients with immunodeficiency, parvovirus infection may be persistent and lead to chronic anemia. In a compromised client, parvovirus can cause serious anemia (for example, a sickle cell client may develop transient aplastic anemia).

NP: Analysis; CN: Physiological integrity; CNS: Physiological adaptation; CL: Knowledge

67. A 6-year-old child has been diagnosed with Rocky Mountain spotted fever. In teaching the parents about the cause of the illness, the nurse would be correct in telling them that a bite by which of the following animals or insects caused the illness?

1. Cat
2. Mosquito
3. Spider
4. Tick

67. 4. Rocky Mountain spotted fever is caused by *Rickettsia rickettsii,* which is transmitted by the bite of a tick. Spider, mosquito, and cat bites haven't been known to transmit *R. rickettsii.*

NP: Implementation; CN: Safe, effective care environment; CNS: Management of care; CL: Knowledge

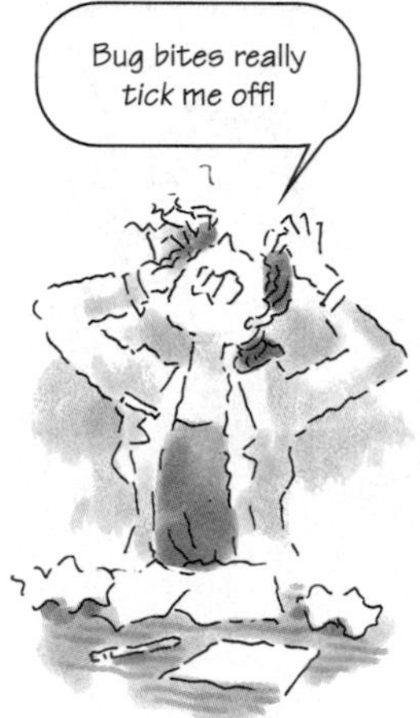

Bug bites really
tick me off!

68. An iron dextran (Imferon) injection has been ordered for an 8-month-old child with iron-deficiency anemia whose parents haven't been compliant with oral supplements. What is the correct method of injection for Imferon?

1. Intradermally
2. Subcutaneously
3. Intramuscularly
4. Intramuscularly, using the Z-track method

68. 4. If iron dextran is ordered, it must be injected deeply into a large muscle mass, using the Z-track method to minimize skin staining and irritation. Neither a subcutaneous nor an intradermal injection would inject the dextran into the muscle. The Z-track method is preferred over a normal intramuscular injection.

NP: Implementation; CN: Physiological integrity; CNS: Pharmacological and parenteral therapies; CL: Application

69. Which of the following foods are appropriate sources of dietary iron for the prevention of nutritional anemia?

1. Citrus fruits
2. Fish
3. Green vegetables
4. Milk products

69. 3. Green vegetables are good sources of iron. Citrus foods aren't sources of iron but help with the absorption of iron. Fish isn't a good source of dietary iron. Milk is deficient in iron and should be limited in cases of nutritional anemia.

NP: Implementation; CN: Health promotion and maintenance; CNS: Prevention and early detection of disease; CL: Knowledge

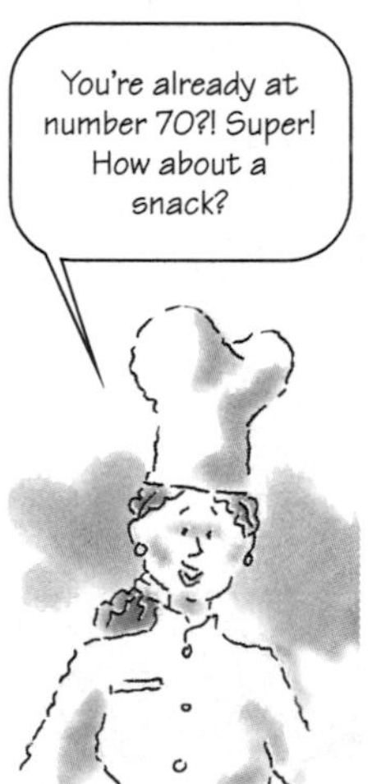

You're already at
number 70?! Super!
How about a
snack?

70. Which of the following instructions should the nurse provide when teaching parents the proper administration of liquid oral iron supplements?

1. Give the supplements with food.
2. Stop medication if vomiting occurs.
3. Decrease dose if constipation occurs.
4. Give the medicine via a dropper or through a straw.

70. 4. Liquid iron preparations may temporarily stain the teeth; therefore, the drug should be given by dropper or through a straw. Supplements should be given between meals, when the presence of free hydrochloric acid is greatest. Constipation can be decreased by increasing intake of fruits and vegetables. If vomiting occurs, supplementation shouldn't be stopped; instead, it should be administered with food.

NP: Implementation; CN: Physiological integrity; CNS: Pharmacological and parenteral therapies; CL: Knowledge

71. Which of the following symptoms is the primary clinical manifestation of hemophilia?

1. Petechiae
2. Prolonged bleeding
3. Decreased clotting time
4. Decreased white blood cell count

71. 2. The effect of hemophilia is prolonged bleeding, anywhere from or within the body. With severe deficiencies, hemorrhage can occur as a result of minor trauma. Petechiae are uncommon in persons with hemophilia because repair of small hemorrhages depends on platelet function, not on blood clotting mechanisms. Clotting time is increased in a client with hemophilia. A decrease in white blood cells is *not* indicative of hemophilia.

NP: Analysis; CN: Physiological integrity; CNS: Physiological adaptation; CL: Knowledge

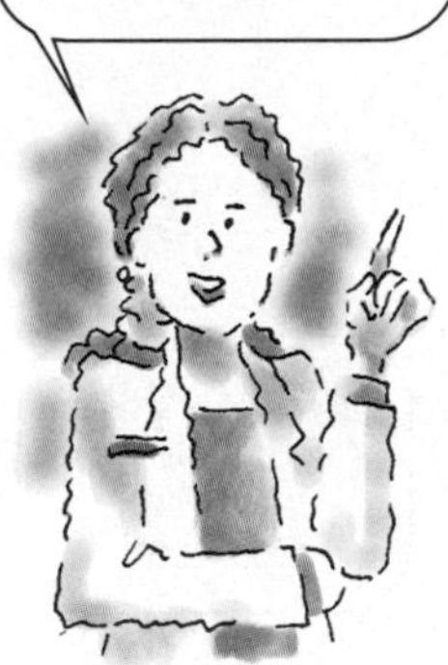
Careful! All of these answers may be accurate, but this question is asking for the most frequent site.

72. Which of the following areas is the most frequent site of internal bleeding associated with hemophilia?

1. Brain tissue
2. GI tract
3. Joint cavities
4. Spinal cord

72. 3. The joint cavities, especially the knees, ankles, and elbows, are the most frequent site of internal bleeding. This bleeding often results in bone changes and crippling, disabling deformities. Intracranial hemorrhage occurs less frequently than expected because the brain tissue has a high concentration of thromboplastin. Hemorrhage along the GI tract and spinal cord can occur but are less common.

NP: Analysis; CN: Physiological integrity; CNS: Physiological adaptation; CL: Knowledge

73. Which of the following measures should parents of a hemophilic child be taught to prepare them to initiate immediate treatment before blood loss is excessive?

1. Apply heat to the area.
2. Withhold factor replacement.
3. Apply pressure for at least 5 minutes.
4. Immobilize and elevate the affected area.

73. 4. Elevating the area above the level of the heart will decrease blood flow. Pressure should be applied to the area for at least 10 to 15 minutes to allow clot formation. Cold, not heat, should be applied to promote vasoconstriction. Factor replacement should *not* be delayed.

NP: Implementation; CN: Physiological integrity; CNS: Physiological adaptation; CL: Application

74. A 2-year-old child with hemophilia who sustains a joint injury is best treated promptly in which location?

1. Home
2. Clinic
3. Hospital unit
4. Emergency department

74. 1. Prompt treatment to prevent joint injury and other complications is best delivered in the home. After the child reaches age 2 or 3 years, parents can learn venipuncture techniques so treatment can be done at home and further injury avoided. The life of the child and family is also less disrupted. The child may be transfused on a regular basis to prevent bleeding and will be given additional doses of the missing factor when an injury occurs. By mid- to late-school age, children can learn to administer their own treatment.

NP: Planning; CN: Physiological integrity; CNS: Reduction of risk potential; CL: Knowledge

75. Which of the following nursing measures is an important aid in prevention of the crippling effects of joint degeneration caused by hemophilia?

1. Avoiding the use of analgesics
2. Using aspirin for pain relief
3. Administering replacement factor
4. Using active range-of-motion (ROM) exercises

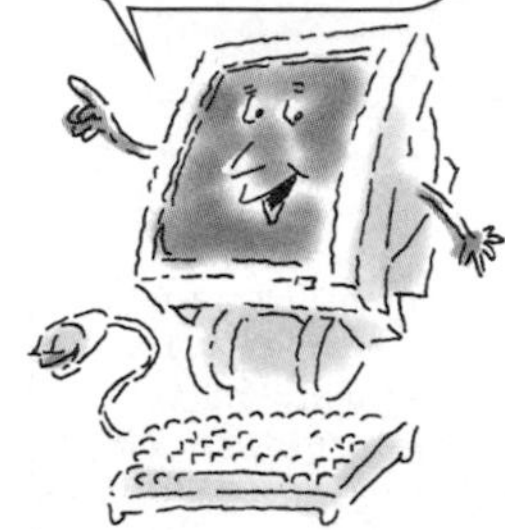

Read carefully. This question is looking for a preventive measure.

75. 3. Prevention of bleeding is the goal and is achieved by factor replacement therapy. Passive ROM exercises are contraindicated after a bleeding episode because the joint capsule can be stretched, causing bleeding. Acetaminophen should be used for pain relief because aspirin has anticoagulant effects. Analgesics should be administered before physical therapy to control pain and provide the maximum benefit.

NP: Implementation; CN: Physiological integrity; CNS: Physiological adaptation; CL: Application

76. Increased tendency to bleed in which of the following areas differentiates von Willebrand's disease from hemophilia?

1. Brain tissue
2. GI tract
3. Mucous membranes
4. Spinal cord

76. 3. The most characteristic clinical feature of von Willebrand's disease is an increased tendency to bleed from mucous membranes, which may be seen as frequent nosebleeds or menorrhagia. In hemophilia, the joint cavities are the most common site of internal bleeding. Bleeding into the GI tract, spinal cord, and brain tissue can occur but these are *not* the most common sites for bleeding.

NP: Analysis; CN: Physiological integrity; CNS: Physiological adaptation; CL: Knowledge

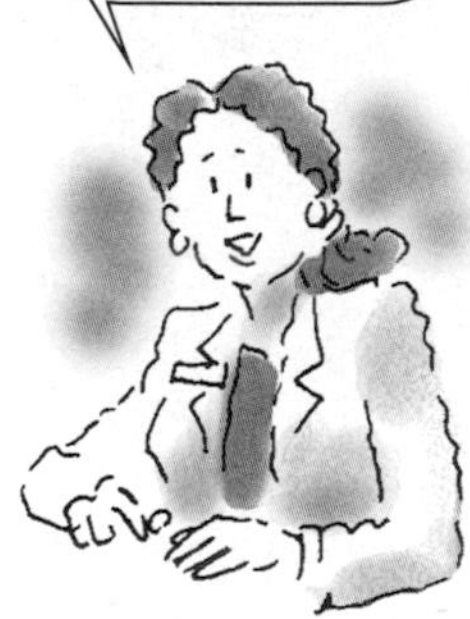

Epistaxis is a term from early in your schooling. Remember?

77. Which of the following nursing measures should be implemented for a client with von Willebrand's disease who is having epistaxis?

1. Lying the child supine
2. Avoiding packing of nostrils
3. Avoiding pressure to the nose
4. Applying pressure to the nose

77. 4. Applying pressure to the nose may stop bleeding because most bleeds occur in the anterior part of the nasal septum. Encourage mouth breathing at this time. The child should be instructed to sit up and lean forward to avoid aspiration of blood. Pressure should be maintained for at least 10 minutes to allow clotting to occur. Packing with tissue or cotton may be used to help stop bleeding, although care must be taken in removing packing to avoid dislodging the clot.

NP: Implementation; CN: Physiological integrity; CNS: Physiological adaptation; CL: Application

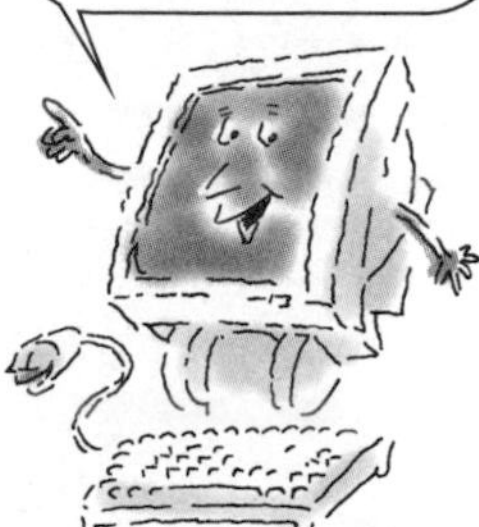

Some of the same factors appear in more than one answer. Select your final answer carefully.

78. What are the three most important prognostic factors in determining long-term survival for children with acute leukemia?

1. Histologic type of disease, initial platelet count, and type of treatment
2. Type of treatment and client's sex
3. Histologic type of disease, initial white blood cell (WBC) count, and client's age at diagnosis
4. Progression of illness, WBC at time of diagnosis, and client's age at time of diagnosis

78. 3. The factor whose prognostic value is considered to be of greatest significance in determining long-range outcome is the histologic type of leukemia. Children with a normal or low WBC count appear to have a much better prognosis than those with a high WBC count. Children diagnosed between ages 2 and 10 have consistently demonstrated a better prognosis than those diagnosed before age 2 or after age 10.

NP: Analysis; CN: Physiological integrity; CNS: Physiological adaptation; CL: Knowledge

79. Which of the following complications are three main consequences of leukemia?

1. Bone deformities, spherocytosis, and infection
2. Anemia, infection, and bleeding tendencies
3. Lymphocytopoesis, growth delays, and hirsutism
4. Polycythemia, decreased clotting time, and infection

79. 2. The three main consequences of leukemia are anemia, caused by decreased erythrocyte production; infection secondary to neutropenia; and bleeding tendencies, from decreased platelet production. Bone deformities don't occur with leukemia although bones may become painful because of the proliferation of cells in the bone marrow. Spherocytosis refers to erythrocytes taking on a spheroid shape and isn't a feature in leukemia. Lymphocytopoesis is production of lymphocytes with leukemia. Mature cells aren't produced in adequate numbers. Hirsutism and growth delay can be a result of large doses of steroids but isn't common in leukemia. Anemia, not polycythemia, occurs. Clotting times would be prolonged.

NP: Analysis; CN: Physiological integrity; CNS: Physiological adaptation; CL: Knowledge

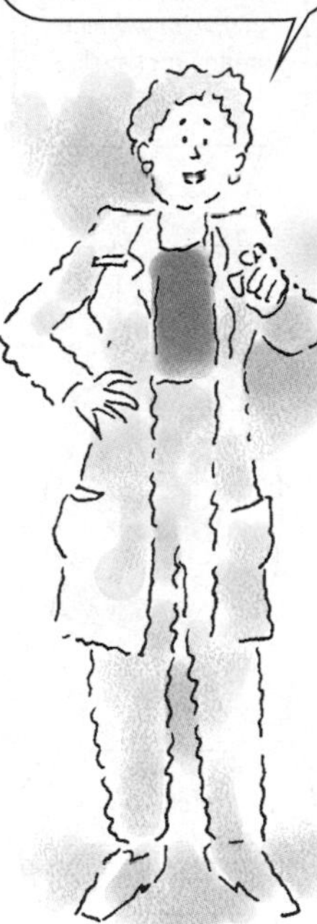

You, my friend, are doing extraordinarily well. Keep up the good work!

80. A child is seen in the pediatrician's office for complaints of bone and joint pain. Which of the following other assessment findings may suggest leukemia?

1. Abdominal pain
2. Increased activity level
3. Increased appetite
4. Petechiae

80. 4. The most frequent signs and symptoms of leukemia are a result of infiltration of the bone marrow. These include fever, pallor, fatigue, anorexia, and petechiae, along with bone and joint pain. Increased appetite can occur but it usually isn't a presenting symptom. Abdominal pain may be caused by areas of inflammation from normal flora within the GI tract or any number of other causes.

NP: Analysis; CN: Physiological integrity; CNS: Physiological adaptation; CL: Knowledge

81. Which of the following assessment findings in a client with leukemia would indicate that the cancer has invaded the brain?

1. Headache and vomiting
2. Restlessness and tachycardia
3. Hypervigilant and anxious behavior
4. Increased heart rate and decreased blood pressure

81. 1. The usual effect of leukemic infiltration of the brain is increased intracranial pressure. The proliferation of cells interferes with the flow of cerebrospinal fluid in the subarachnoid space and at the base of the brain. The increased fluid pressure causes dilation of the ventricles, which creates symptoms of severe headache, vomiting, irritability, lethargy, increased blood pressure, decreased heart rate, and, eventually, coma. Often children with a variety of illnesses are hypervigilant and anxious when hospitalized.

NP: Analysis; CN: Physiological integrity; CNS: Physiological adaptation; CL: Knowledge

82. Which of the following types of leukemia carries the best prognosis?

1. Acute lymphoblastic leukemia
2. Acute myelogenous leukemia
3. Basophilic leukemia
4. Eosinophilic leukemia

82. 1. Acute lymphoblastic leukemia, which accounts for more than 80% of all childhood cases, carries the best prognosis. Acute myelogenous leukemia, with several subtypes, accounts for most of the other leukemias affecting children. Basophilic and eosinophilic leukemia are named for the specific cells involved. These are much rarer and carry a poorer prognosis.

NP: Analysis; CN: Physiological integrity; CNS: Physiological adaptation; CL: Knowledge

83. Which of the following is the reason to perform a spinal tap on a client newly diagnosed with leukemia?

1. To rule out meningitis
2. To decrease intracranial pressure
3. To aid in classification of the leukemia
4. To assess for central nervous system infiltration

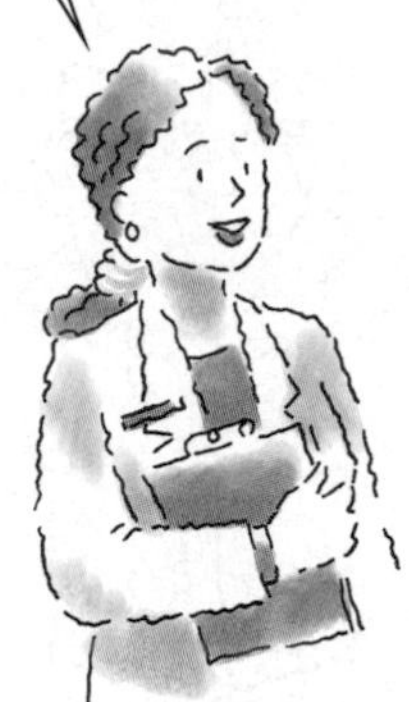

Think back to basic physiology. Which organs metabolize drugs?

83. 4. A spinal tap is performed to assess for central nervous system infiltration. It wouldn't be done to decrease intracranial pressure nor does it aid in the classification of the leukemia. Spinal taps can result in brain stem herniation in cases of increased intracranial pressure. A spinal tap can be done to rule out meningitis but this isn't the indication for the test on a leukemic client.

NP: Analysis; CN: Physiological integrity; CNS: Physiological adaptation; CL: Knowledge

84. Which of the following tests is performed on a client with leukemia before initiation of therapy to evaluate the child's ability to metabolize chemotherapeutic agents?

1. Lumbar puncture
2. Liver function studies
3. Complete blood count (CBC)
4. Peripheral blood smear

84. 2. Liver and kidney function studies are done before initiation of chemotherapy to evaluate the child's ability to metabolize the chemotherapeutic agents. A CBC is performed to assess for anemia and white blood cell count. A peripheral blood smear is done to assess the maturity and morphology of red blood cells. A lumbar puncture is performed to assess for central nervous system infiltration.

NP: Analysis; CN: Physiological integrity; CNS: Pharmacological and parenteral therapies; CL: Knowledge

85. Which of the following immunizations should not be given to a 4-month-old sibling of a client with leukemia?

1. Diphtheria and tetanus and pertussis (DTP) vaccine
2. Hepatitis B vaccine
3. *Haemophilus influenzae* type b vaccines (Hib)
4. Oral poliovirus vaccine (OPV)

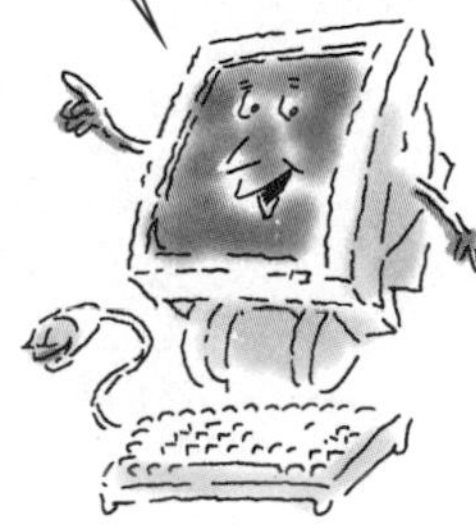

Careful. This is another negative question.

85. 4. OPV is a live attenuated virus excreted in the stool. The excreted virus can be communicated to the immunosuppressed child, resulting in an overwhelming infection. Inactivated polio vaccine would be indicated because it isn't a live virus and wouldn't pose the threat of infection. DTP, Hib, and hepatitis B vaccines can be given according to the recommended schedule.

NP: Analysis; CN: Health promotion and maintenance; CNS: Prevention and early detection of disease; CL: Application

86. Which of the following medications usually is given to a client with leukemia as prophylaxis against *Pneumocystic carinii* pneumonia?

1. Co-trimoxazole (Bactrim)
2. Oral nystatin suspension
3. Prednisone (Deltasone)
4. Vincristine (Oncovin)

86. 1. The most frequent cause of death from leukemia is overwhelming infection. *P. carinii* infection is lethal to a child with leukemia. As prophylaxis against *P. carinii* pneumonia, continuous low dosages of co-trimoxazole are frequently prescribed. Oral nystatin suspension would be indicated for the treatment of thrush. Prednisone isn't an antibiotic and increases susceptibility to infection. Vincristine is an antineoplastic agent.

NP: Analysis; CN: Physiological integrity; CNS: Pharmacological and parenteral therapies; CL: Knowledge

87. In which of the following diseases would bone marrow transplantation not be indicated in a newly diagnosed client?

1. Acute lymphocytic leukemia
2. Chronic myeloid leukemia
3. Severe aplastic anemia
4. Severe combined immunodeficiency

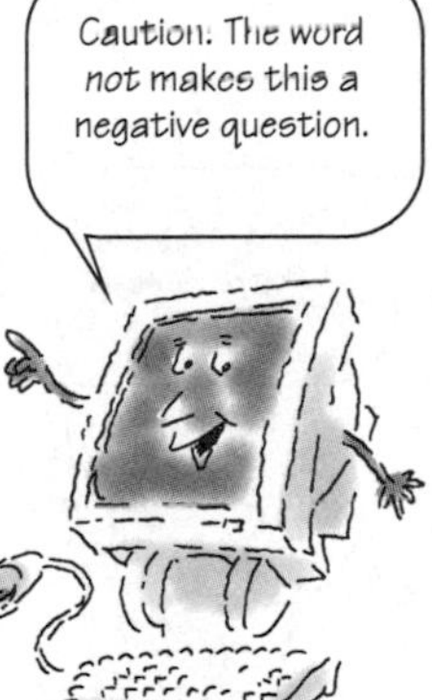

Caution: The word not makes this a negative question.

87. 1. For the first episode of acute lymphocytic leukemia, conventional therapy is superior to bone marrow transplantation. In severe combined immunodeficiency and in severe aplastic anemia, bone marrow transplantation has been employed to replace abnormal stem cells with healthy cells from the donor's marrow. In myeloid leukemia, bone marrow transplantation is done after chemotherapy to infuse healthy marrow and to replace marrow stem cells ablated during chemotherapy.

NP: Analysis; CN: Physiological integrity; CNS: Pharmacological and parenteral therapies; CL: Knowledge

88. Which of the following treatment measures should be implemented for a child with leukemia who has been exposed to chickenpox?

1. No treatment is indicated.
2. Acyclovir (Zovirax) should be started on exposure.
3. Varicella-zoster immune globulin (VZIG) should be given with evidence of the disease.
4. VZIG should be given within 72 hours of exposure.

88. 4. Varicella is a lethal organism to a child with leukemia. VZIG, given within 72 hours, may favorably alter the course of the disease. Giving the vaccine at the onset of symptoms wouldn't likely decrease the severity of the illness. Acyclovir may be given if the child develops the disease but not if the child has just been exposed.

NP: Analysis; CN: Health promotion and maintenance; CNS: Prevention and early detection of disease; CL: Knowledge

89. Nausea and vomiting are common adverse effects of radiation and chemotherapy. When should a nurse administer antiemetics?

1. 30 minutes before initiation of therapy
2. With the administration of therapy
3. Immediately after nausea begins
4. When therapy is completed

89. 1. Antiemetics are most beneficial if given before the onset of nausea and vomiting. To calculate the optimum time for administration, the first dose is given 30 minutes to 1 hour before nausea is expected, and then every 2, 4, or 6 hours for approximately 24 hours after chemotherapy. If the antiemetic was given with the medication or after the medication, it could lose its maximum effectiveness when needed.

NP: Implementation; CN: Physiological integrity; CNS: Pharmacological and parenteral therapies; CL: Application

90. Which route of medication administration is contraindicated in children receiving chemotherapy?

1. Oral
2. Rectal
3. Intravenous
4. Intrathecal

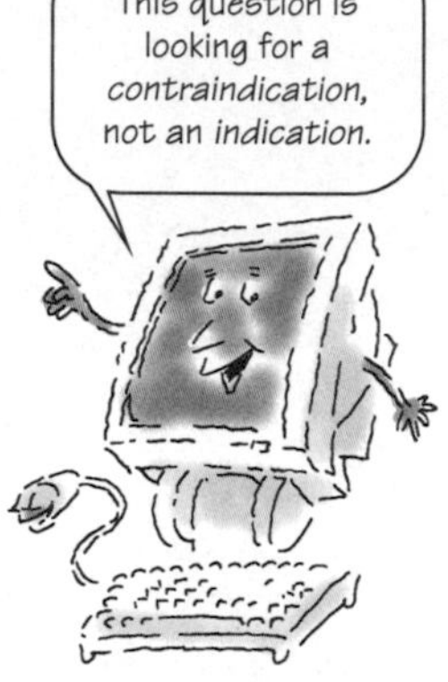

This question is looking for a contraindication, not an indication.

90. 2. Rectal medications and rectal thermometers are contraindicated in children receiving chemotherapy because of the risk of developing rectal ulcers with cytotoxic drug administration. Medications given intravenously enter the bloodstream directly, often into a central line so that the medication can mix with a large volume of blood. The intrathecal route is used to deliver specific medication directly into the spinal fluid to treat or prevent central nervous system leukemia.

NP: Analysis; CN: Physiological integrity; CNS: Pharmacological and parenteral therapies; CL: Application

91. Which of the following nursing measures are helpful when mouth ulcers develop as an adverse effect of chemotherapy?

1. Using lemon glycerin swabs
2. Administering milk of magnesia
3. Providing a bland, moist, soft diet
4. Frequently washing the mouth with full-strength hydrogen peroxide

91. 3. Oral ulcers are red, eroded, and painful. Providing a bland, moist, soft diet will make chewing and swallowing less painful. The use of lemon glycerin swabs and milk of magnesia should be avoided. Glycerin, a trihydric alcohol, absorbs water and dries the membranes. Milk of magnesia also has a drying effect because unabsorbed magnesium salts exert an osmotic pressure on tissue fluids. Many children also find the taste unpleasant. Frequent mouthwashes without alcohol are indicated. Peroxide shouldn't be used because it's irritating to tissues.

NP: Implementation; CN: Physiological integrity; CNS: Basic care and comfort; CL: Application

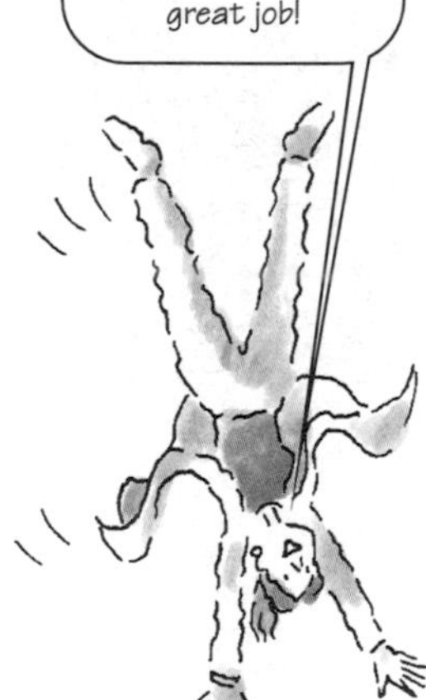

Don't stop now! You're doing a great job!

92. Parents of pediatric clients who undergo irradiation involving the central nervous system (CNS) should be warned about postirradiation somnolence. When does this neurologic syndrome usually occur?

1. Immediately
2. Within 1 to 2 weeks
3. Within 5 to 8 weeks
4. Within 3 to 6 months

92. 3. Postirradiation somnolence may develop 5 to 8 weeks after CNS irradiation and may last 3 to 15 days. It's characterized by somnolence with or without fever, anorexia, nausea, and vomiting. Although the syndrome isn't thought to be clinically significant, parents should be prepared to expect such symptoms and encouraged to allow the child needed rest.

NP: Analysis; CN: Physiological integrity; CNS: Physiological adaptation; CL: Knowledge

93. Which of the following interventions can prevent hemorrhagic cystitis caused by bladder irritation from chemotherapeutic medications?

1. Giving antacids
2. Giving antibiotics
3. Restricting fluid intake
4. Increasing fluid intake

93. 4. Sterile hemorrhagic cystitis is an adverse effect of chemical irritation of the bladder from cyclophosphamide. It can be prevented by liberal fluid intake (at least 1½ times the recommended daily fluid requirement). Antibiotics don't aid in the prevention of sterile hemorrhagic cystitis. Restricting fluids would only increase the risk of developing cystitis. Antacids wouldn't be indicated for treatment.

NP: Implementation; CN: Physiological integrity; CNS: Reduction of risk potential; CL: Application

94. Which of the following characteristics explains why aspirin is contraindicated for pain relief for a child with leukemia?
1. Decreases platelet production
2. Promotes bleeding tendencies
3. Not a strong enough analgesic
4. Decreases the effects of methotrexate

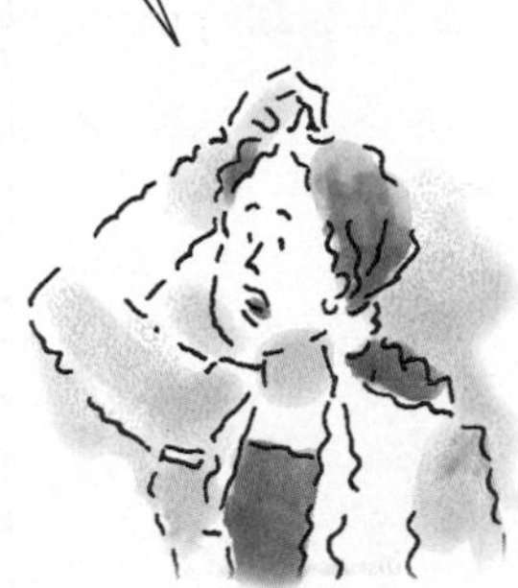
What other conditions is aspirin used for?

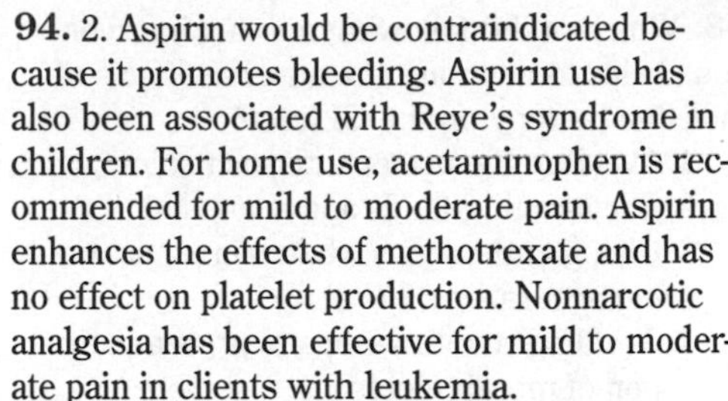

94. 2. Aspirin would be contraindicated because it promotes bleeding. Aspirin use has also been associated with Reye's syndrome in children. For home use, acetaminophen is recommended for mild to moderate pain. Aspirin enhances the effects of methotrexate and has no effect on platelet production. Nonnarcotic analgesia has been effective for mild to moderate pain in clients with leukemia.
NP: Analysis; CN: Physiological integrity; CNS: Pharmacological and parenteral therapies; CL: Application

95. Which of the following nursing measures helps prepare the parent and child for alopecia, a common adverse effect of several chemotherapeutic agents?
1. Introducing the idea of a wig after hair loss occurs
2. Explaining that hair typically begins to regrow in 6 to 9 months
3. Stressing that hair loss during a second treatment with the same medication will be more severe
4. Explaining that, as hair thins, keeping it clean, short, and fluffy may camouflage partial baldness

95. 4. The nurse must prepare parents and children for possible hair loss. Cutting the hair short lessens the impact of seeing large quantities of hair on bed linens and clothing. Sometimes, keeping the hair short and fuller can make a wig unnecessary. Hair usually regrows in 6 months, depending upon the treatment protocol. A child should be encouraged to pick out a wig similar to his own hair style and color before the hair falls out to foster adjustment to hair loss. Hair loss during a second treatment with the same medication is usually less severe.
NP: Implementation; CN: Psychosocial integrity; CNS: Coping and adaptation; CL: Application

96. Which of the following areas is the most common site of cancer in children?
1. Lungs
2. Genitalia
3. Bone marrow
4. GI tract

96. 3. Childhood cancers occur most commonly in rapidly growing tissue, especially in the bone marrow. Tumors of the lungs, genitalia, and GI tract are rarely seen in children.
NP: Analysis; CN: Physiological integrity; CNS: Physiological adaptation; CL: Knowledge

97. Which of the following symptoms are early warning signs of childhood cancer?
1. Difficulty in swallowing
2. Frequent upper respiratory infections or hoarseness
3. Slight change in bowel and bladder habits
4. Swellings, lumps, or masses anywhere on the body

You're doing swell! Keep going!
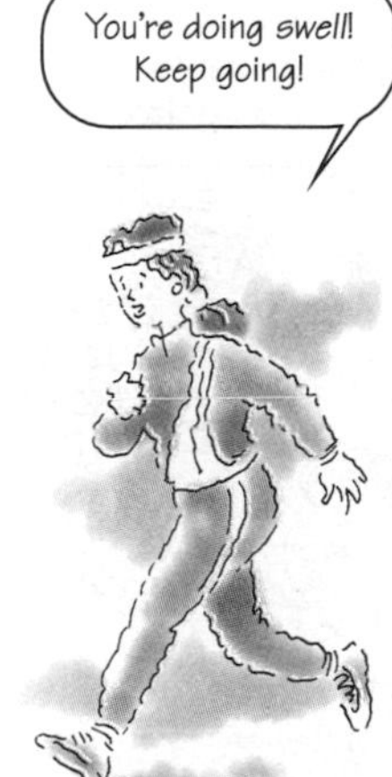

97. 4. By being aware of early signs of childhood cancer, nurses can refer children for further evaluation. Swellings, lumps, or masses anywhere on the body are early warning signals of childhood cancer. Difficulty swallowing, cough, and hoarseness are early signs of cancer in adults. Frequent upper respiratory infections are common in carly childhood. Usually there's also a marked change in bowel or bladder habits, not associated with dietary intake.
NP: Analysis; CN: Health promotion and maintenance; CNS: Prevention and early detection of disease; CL: Knowledge

98. Which of the following nursing interventions helps to decrease the adverse effects of radiation therapy on the GI tract?

1. Avoiding the use of antispasmodics
2. Encouraging fluids and a soft diet
3. Giving antiemetics when nausea or vomiting occurs
4. Avoiding mouthwashes to prevent irritation of mouth ulcers

98. 2. Radiation therapy can cause adverse effects such as nausea and vomiting, anorexia, mucosal ulceration, and diarrhea. Encouraging fluids and a soft diet will help with anorexia. Antiemetics should be given before the onset of nausea. Antispasmodics are used to help reduce diarrhea. Frequent mouthwashes are indicated to prevent mycosis.

NP: Implementation; CN: Physiological integrity; CNS: Pharmacological and parenteral therapies; CL: Application

99. Which of the following types of cancer is most common in children?

1. Hodgkin's disease
2. Leukemia
3. Osteogenic sarcoma
4. Wilms' tumor

99. 2. Leukemia, cancer of the blood-forming tissues, is the most common form of childhood cancer. The annual incidence in children under age 15 is approximately 4 in every 100,000. Hodgkin's disease occurs almost as frequently as leukemia. Osteogenic sarcoma is the most frequently encountered malignant bone cancer in children but the incidence isn't as high as leukemia. Wilms' tumor is the most frequent intra-abdominal tumor of childhood but leukemia is most prevalent when comparing all types of childhood cancers.

NP: Analysis; CN: Health promotion and maintenance; CNS: Prevention and early detection of disease; CL: Knowledge

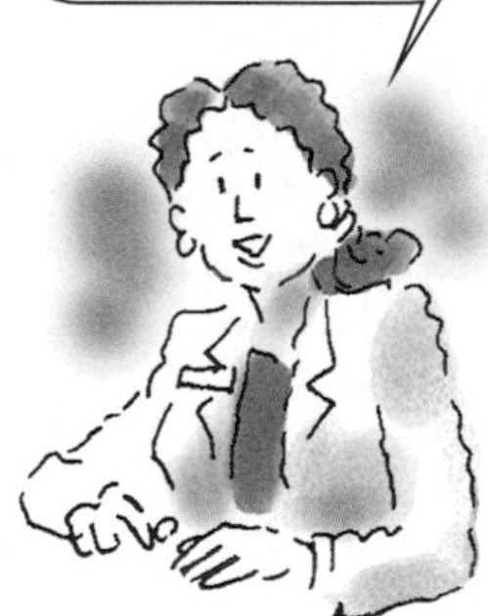
One hundred questions! You must be proud!

100. Teaching children with leukemia and their families should include potential side effects of treatments. Which is not an adverse effect of prednisone?

1. Increased appetite
2. Decreased blood glucose
3. Increased risk for infection
4. Peptic and esophageal irritation and ulceration

100. 2. Prednisone may cause an increase in blood glucose requiring doses of insulin, especially when other factors are involved. Increased appetite, increased risk for infection, and peptic and esophageal irritation and ulceration are all adverse effects of prednisone.

NP: Implementation; CN: Physiological integrity; CNS: Pharmacological and parenteral therapies; CL: Application

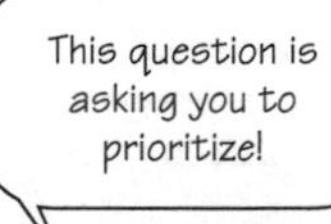
This question is asking you to prioritize!

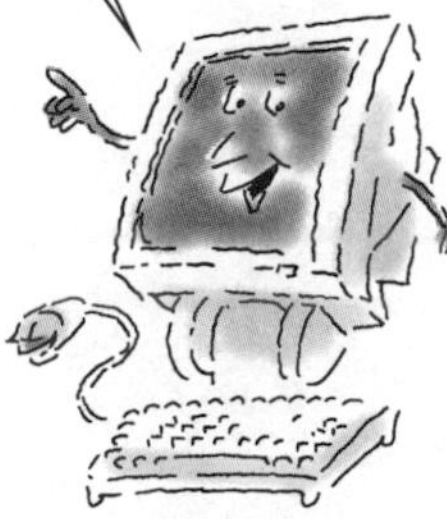

101. Which of the following interventions is a priority for a hemophiliac child who has fallen and badly bruised his leg?

1. Appropriate dose of aspirin and rest
2. Immobilization of the leg and a dose of ibuprofen
3. Heating pad and administration of factor VIII concentrate
4. Pressure on the site and administration of required clotting factor

101. 4. With any bleeding injury in a client with hemophilia, the first line of treatment is always to replace the clotting factor. Pressure is applied along with cool compresses and the extremity is immobilized. Heat isn't used because it increases bleeding. Aspirin isn't used because of its anticoagulant properties and the risk of Reye's syndrome in children. Immobilizing the leg and giving ibuprofen would be done after applying pressure and administering the necessary clotting factor.

NP: Planning; CN: Physiological integrity; CNS: Physiological adaptation; CL: Application

102. When teaching an adolescent with iron deficiency anemia about diet choices, which of the following menu selections would indicate that more instruction is necessary?

1. Caesar salad and pretzels
2. Cheeseburger with milkshake
3. Red beans and rice with sausage
4. Egg sandwich and snack peanuts

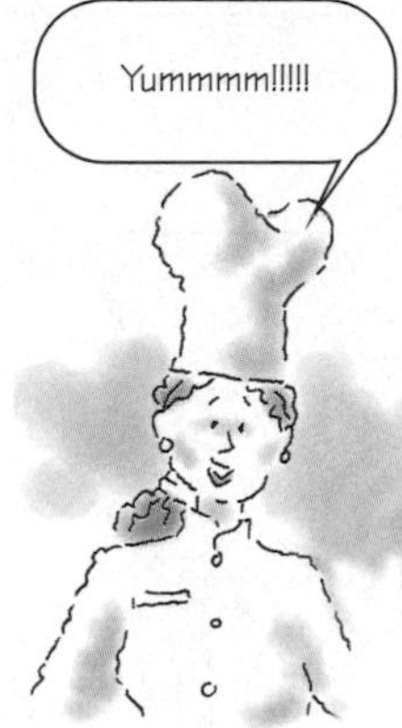
Yummmm!!!!!

102. 1. Caesar salad and pretzels aren't foods high in iron and protein. Meats (especially organ meats), eggs, and nuts have high protein and iron.

NP: Evaluation; CN: Health promotion and maintenance; CNS: Prevention and early detection of disease; CL: Analysis

103. The nurse is speaking to the mother of a child with leukemia who wants to know why her child is so susceptible to infection if he has too many white blood cells (WBCs). Which of the following responses would be most accurate?

1. This is an adverse effect of the medication he has to take.
2. He hasn't been able to eat a proper diet since he's been sick.
3. Leukemia is a problem of tumors in the internal organs that prevent his ability to fight infection.
4. Leukemia causes production of too many immature WBCs, which can't fight infection very well.

103. 4. Leukemia is an unrestricted proliferation of immature WBCs that don't function properly and are a poor defense against infection. Diet contributes to overall health but doesn't cause the overproduction of WBCs. There are no solid tumors in the internal organs in leukemia. Medications such as chemotherapy can diminish the immune system's effectiveness; however, they don't cause the overproduction of immature WBCs and the poor resistance to infection that the mother asked about.

NP: Implementation; CN: Physiological integrity; CNS: Physiological adaptation; CL: Application

104. The nurse is developing a teaching plan for parents of a toddler who was just diagnosed with sickle cell anemia. Which of the following statements is important to emphasize in the teaching plan?

1. If they have any more children, those children will also have sickle cell anemia.
2. Knowing how to prevent vaso-occlusive crisis is an important part of the parent's role.
3. The child will have a greater tendency to bleed and should avoid contact sports.
4. Vaso-occlusive crisis will occur eventually, requiring medical care.

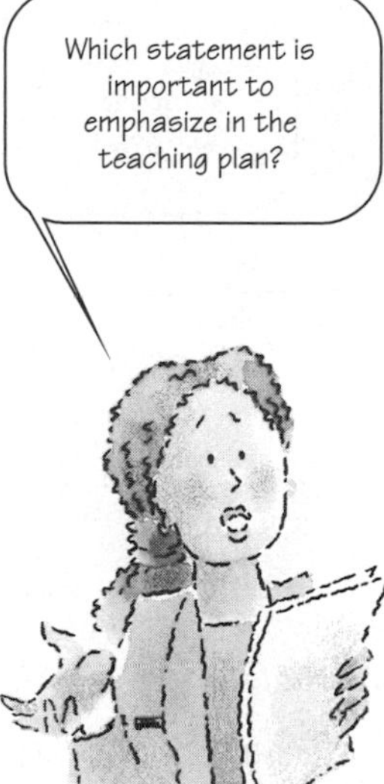
Which statement is important to emphasize in the teaching plan?

104. 2. Prevention is the key to teaching a family of a child with sickle cell anemia. The nurse should emphasize the daily use of prescribed oral antibiotics and avoidance of dehydration, high altitudes, and cold. These interventions can dramatically reduce the incidence of crisis. The disease is autosomal recessive, so each pregnancy has a 1 in 4 chance of the child having the disease, a 1 in 4 chance of not having the disease, and a 2 in 4 chance of carrying the trait. Abnormal bleeding and the need to avoid contact sports is associated with hemophilia.

NP: Planning; CN: Health promotion and maintenance; CNS: Prevention and early detection of disease; CL: Application

105. A grandmother calls the pediatric children's clinic to find out if her 3-year-old grandson can get shingles from her. Which of the following responses would be appropriate?

1. No, shingles don't occur in small children.
2. Yes, the grandson can get shingles from her. Shingles are caused by the herpes zoster virus.
3. The grandson could develop shingles if the lesions are on exposed skin areas and are weeping.
4. No, but the grandson would be exposed to the varicella-zoster virus, which could lead to the development of chickenpox.

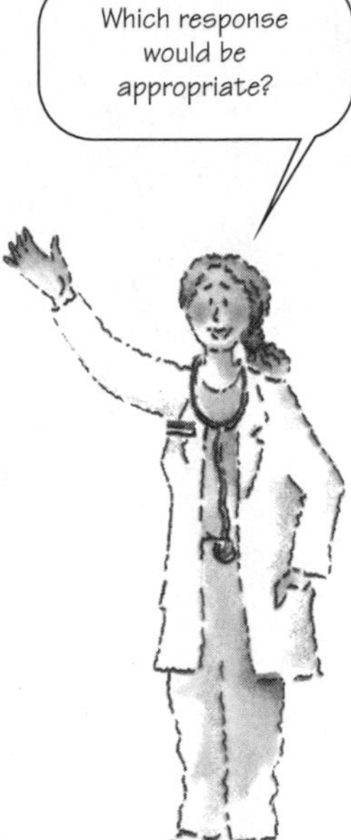

Which response would be appropriate?

105. 4. Shingles occur when a dormant varicella-zoster virus in a nerve becomes inflamed. The vesicles of shingles contain the virus and would expose others to it. The grandson couldn't develop shingles from such exposure. Shingles can occur in children, but only if they previously had chickenpox. The impetus for the inflammation is internal, not external. A herpes virus doesn't cause shingles.

NP: Implementation; CN: Safe, effective care environment; CNS: Safety and infection control; CL: Analysis

106. A child with idiopathic thrombocytopenic purpura (ITP) is admitted to the hospital with a platelet count of 20,000/mm^3. She should be closely monitored for which condition?

1. Hyperactivity
2. Proteinuria
3. Hand-foot syndrome
4. Change in level of consciousness (LOC)

106. 4. When the platelet count drops to 20,000/mm^3, the child is at risk for spontaneous bleeding, including intracranially. A change in LOC is an important sign of increased intracranial pressure. This child is likely to become somnolent and difficult to arouse—not hyperactive. Proteinuria is more common in glomerulonephritis. With blood in the urine, protein also increases—but this isn't the primary concern. Hand-foot syndrome occurs in a child with sickle cell disease.

NP: Analysis; CN: Physiological integrity; CNS: Reduction of risk potential; CL: Application

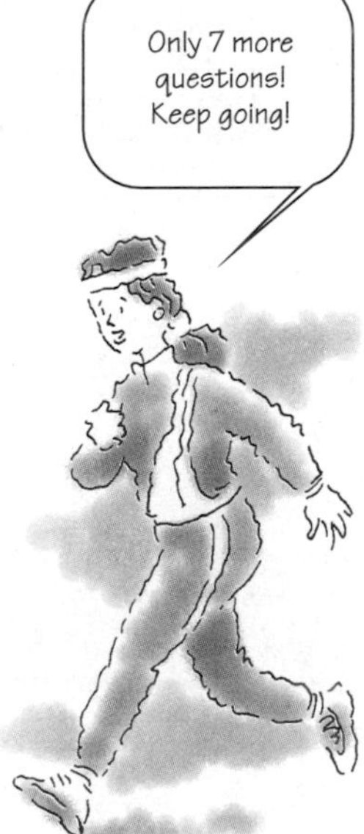

Only 7 more questions! Keep going!

107. Infants must be monitored closely because they can't report changes in their condition. In a 1-month-old infant, which are the signs of increased intracranial pressure (ICP)?

1. Bulging fontanels, a high-pitched cry, vomiting
2. Frequent crying, sunken fontanel, pulse rate above 120 beats/minute
3. Blood-tinged vomitus, legs flexed to the abdomen, frequent crying
4. Falling asleep during feeding, pulse rate above 120 beats/minute when fussing, irregular arm and leg movements

107. 1. Because fontanels haven't closed by the age of 1 month, they bulge with increasing ICP. A high-pitched cry and vomiting also signal increased ICP. Quality of the cry is an important sign in an infant. Vomiting should be distinguished from a small amount of formula regurgitation, which is normal. A pulse rate of 120 beats/minute is normal for a 1-month infant at rest; in fact, the pulse may increase to 200 beats/minute during stress. Frequent crying may result from various stressors, and quality of the cry should be assessed. Blood-tinged vomitus, flexed legs, and crying indicate an abdominal disorder and pain. Infants normally have irregular arm and leg movements.

NP: Assessment; CN: Physiological integrity; CNS: Reduction of risk potential; CL: Analysis

108. Discharge teaching for the family of a school-age child with idiopathic thrombocytopenia should include restriction of which activity?

1. Swimming
2. Bicycle riding
3. Computer games
4. Exposure to large crowds

108. 2. When routine blood counts reveal the platelet level is 100,000/mm^3 or less, the child shouldn't engage in contact sports, bicycle or scooter riding, climbing, or other activities that could lead to injury (especially to the head). Swimming releases energy, builds muscle, and allows the child to compete without risking injury, as long as she follows normal safety precautions. Computer games don't cause physical injury. This child need not avoid large crowds because idiopathic thrombocytopenia doesn't suppress the immune system.

NP: Planning; CN: Safe, effective care environment; CNS: Safety and infection control; CL: Application

109. A 17-year-old boy with classic hemophilia (hemophilia A) is admitted to the hospital for surgery. His preoperative preparation should include which treatment?

1. Bed rest
2. Transfusion of clotting factor 8
3. I.V. analgesics given around the clock
4. Hydration at 50% above the normal fluid requirement

109. 2. In classic hemophilia or hemophilia A, clotting factor 8 is deficient. This factor must be transfused before surgery and at intervals afterward to prevent bleeding during and after surgery. Analgesics would be indicated if the child experienced bleeding, especially into the joints. Hydration above the normal requirement isn't needed. Because the child wasn't admitted for bleeding, bed rest isn't necessary.

NP: Planning; CN: Physiological integrity; CNS: Pharmacological and parenteral therapies; CL: Application

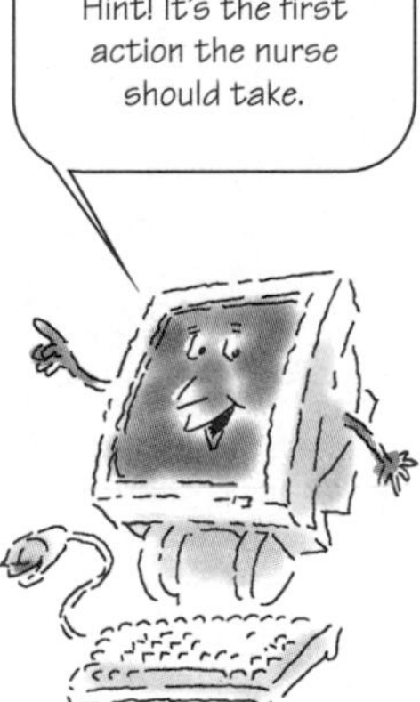

Hint! It's the first action the nurse should take.

110. A child with hemophilia is hospitalized with bleeding into the knee. Which action should the nurse take *first*?

1. Prepare to administer a whole blood transfusion.
2. Prepare to administer a plasma transfusion.
3. Perform active range-of-motion (ROM) exercise on the affected part.
4. Elevate the affected part.

110. 4. Bleeding into the joints is the most common type of bleeding episode in the more severe hemophilia forms. Elevating the affected part and applying pressure and cold are indicated. The nurse should anticipate transfusing the missing clotting factor—not whole blood or plasma, which won't stop the bleeding promptly and may pose a risk of fluid overload. Active ROM exercises are contraindicated because they may cause more bleeding, injury, and pain.

NP: Implementation; CN: Physiological integrity; CNS: Reduction of risk potential; CL: Application

111. Which of the following measures is indicated for a child in sickle cell vaso-occlusive crisis?

1. Immobilizing the affected part
2. Applying warm packs to the affected part
3. Applying cool packs to the affected part
4. Performing active range-of-motion (ROM) exercises to the affected part

111. 2. Applying warm packs promotes vasodilation and perfusion and provides pain relief and comfort. Cool packs are contraindicated because they cause vasoconstriction and may precipitate red blood cell sickling. Immobilization leads to stasis, which promotes sickling. A child in vaso-occlusive crisis experiences acute pain and limits movement of the affected part. Once the acute crisis passes, the child should be encouraged to ambulate. Active ROM exercises increase pain in the affected part.

NP: Analysis; CN: Physiological integrity; CNS: Basic care and comfort; CL: Application

112. A child with sickle cell disease is admitted to the hospital for a splenectomy. Which of the following assessment data is most important to collect preoperatively?

1. Dietary intake
2. Grade level in school
3. Previous admissions
4. Immunization history

112. 4. Spleen removal places the child at higher risk for infection—which is already high in clients with sickle cell disease. Because infection may trigger a crisis, all immunizations must be up to date. Although the other assessment data are important, they're less critical than the client's immunization history.

NP: Assessment; CN: Physiological integrity; CNS: Reduction of risk potential; CL: Application

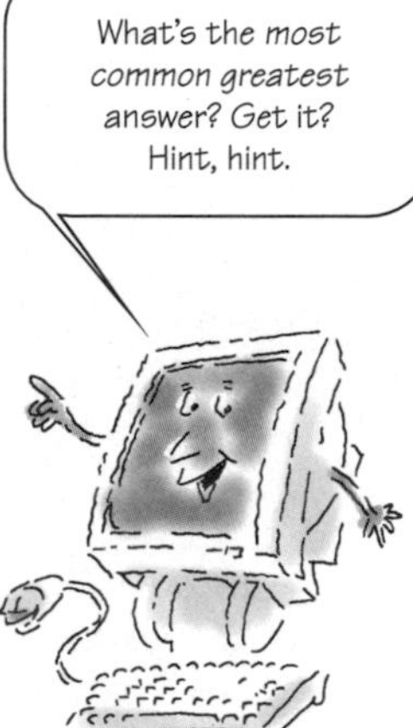

What's the most common greatest answer? Get it? Hint, hint.

113. Which of the following signs is a common early sign of acquired immunodeficiency syndrome (AIDS) in a toddler?

1. Enuresis
2. Poor appetite
3. Short attention span
4. Loss of previously acquired developmental milestones

113. 4. Loss of previously acquired developmental milestones (which reflects viral invasion of the central nervous system) is commonly the first indication that a child has AIDS. Enuresis, poor appetite, and short attention span occur during normal toddler development (although anorexia and malnutrition may become major problems as AIDS progresses).

NP: Analysis; CN: Health promotion and maintenance; CNS: Growth and development through the life span; CL: Knowledge

114. In a child receiving treatment for leukemia, which of the following conditions poses the greatest risk of death?

1. Bleeding
2. Infection
3. Electrolyte imbalance
4. Chronic anemia with heart failure

114. 2. Infection is the main cause of death in children treated for leukemia. The treatment destroys both abnormal and normal bone marrow cells, and immunity declines. Also, these children are commonly hospitalized, meaning they're exposed to multiple caregivers, breaks in skin integrity, and separation from a familiar routine, family, and friends. Poor appetite, nausea and vomiting, pain or discomfort, fatigue, and malaise compound the risk of infection. Bleeding, electrolyte imbalance, and chronic anemia with heart failure can be managed through blood and platelet transfusions and fluid and electrolyte administration.

NP: Planning; CN: Physiological integrity; CNS: Reduction of risk potential; CL: Analysis

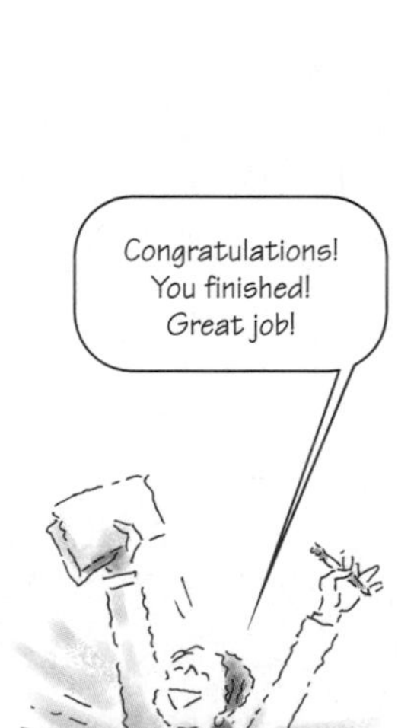

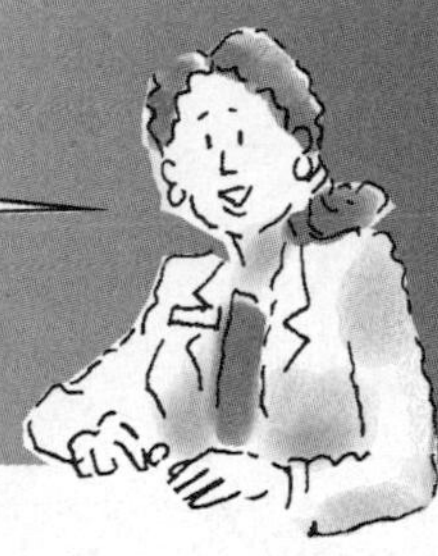

Chapter 29 Respiratory disorders

1. Which of the following definitions best describes the etiology of sudden infant death syndrome (SIDS)?

1. Cardiac arrhythmias
2. Apnea of prematurity
3. Unexplained death of an infant
4. Apparent life-threatening event

1. 3. SIDS can best be defined as the sudden death of an infant under age 1 that remains unexplained after autopsy. Apnea of prematurity occurs in infants less than 32 weeks' gestation who have periodic breathing lapses for 20 seconds or more. Apparent life-threatening events usually have some combination of apnea, color change, marked change in muscle tone, choking, or gagging.

NP: Assessment; CN: Physiological integrity; CNS: Physiological adaptation; CL: Knowledge

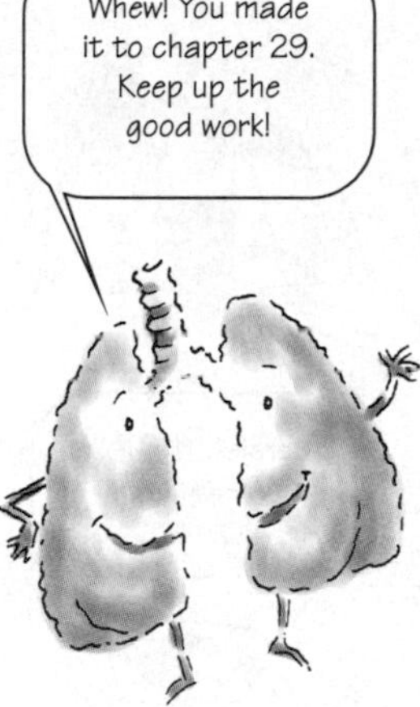

Whew! You made it to chapter 29. Keep up the good work!

2. Which of the following children has an increased risk of sudden infant death syndrome (SIDS)?

1. Premature infant with low birth weight
2. A healthy 2-year-old
3. Infant hospitalized for fever
4. Firstborn child

2. 1. Premature infants, especially those with low birth weight, have an increased risk for SIDS. Hospitalization for fever is insignificant. Infants with apnea, central nervous system disorders, or respiratory disorders have a higher risk of SIDS. Peak age for SIDS is 2 to 4 months. There's an increased risk of SIDS in subsequent siblings of two or more SIDS victims.

NP: Assessment; CN: Physiological integrity; CNS: Reduction of risk potential; CL: Knowledge

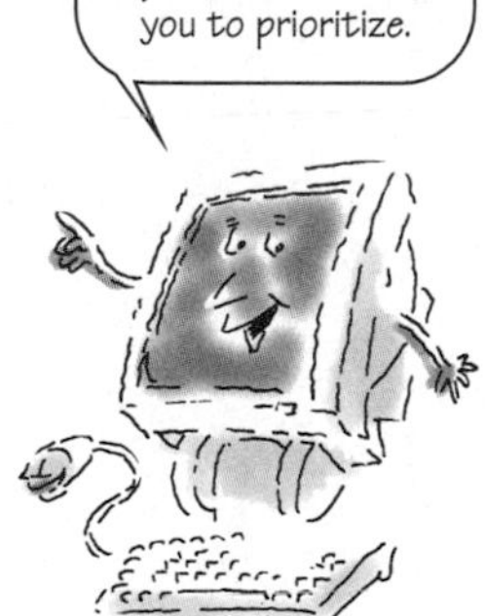

3. A 6-week-old infant is brought to the emergency department not breathing; a preliminary finding of sudden infant death syndrome (SIDS) is made to the parents. Which of the following interventions should the nurse take initially?

1. Call their spiritual advisor.
2. Explain the etiology of SIDS.
3. Allow them to see their infant.
4. Collect the infant's belongings and give them to the parents.

3. 3. The parents need time with their infant to assist with the grieving process. Calling their pastor and collecting the infant's belongings are also important steps in the plan of care but aren't priorities. The parents will be too upset to understand an explanation of SIDS at this time.

NP: Implementation; CN: Psychosocial integrity; CNS: Coping and adaptation; CL: Application

4. Which of the following risk factors is related to sudden infant death syndrome (SIDS)?
1. Feeding habits
2. Gestational age of 42 weeks
3. Immunizations
4. Low birth weight

4. 4. Prematurity, low birth weight, and multiple births are important risk factors associated with SIDS. Immunizations have been disproved to be associated with the disorder. Feeding habits and a gestational age of 42 weeks aren't significant.
NP: Assessment; CN: Physiological integrity; CNS: Reduction of risk potential; CL: Knowledge

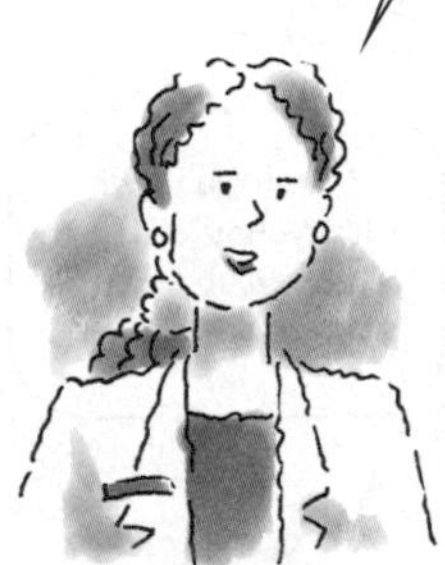

It's important to be sensitive to a family's feelings when they've lost a child to SIDS.

5. An infant is brought to the emergency department and pronounced dead with the preliminary finding of sudden infant death syndrome (SIDS). Which of the following questions to the parents is appropriate?
1. Did you hear the infant cry out?
2. Was the infant's head buried in a blanket?
3. Were any of the siblings jealous of the new baby?
4. How did the infant look when you found him?

5. 4. Only factual questions should be asked during the initial history in the emergency department. The other questions imply blame, guilt, or neglect.
NP: Implementation; CN: Physiological integrity; CNS: Physiological adaptation; CL: Application

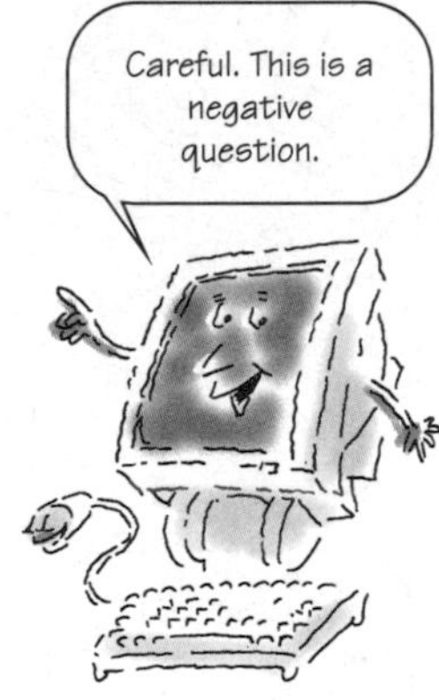

6. Which of the following interventions is not recommended for children with an increased risk of sudden infant death syndrome (SIDS)?
1. Pneumogram
2. Home apnea monitor
3. Respiratory stimulant drugs
4. Chest X-ray at 1 month of age

6. 4. No diagnostic test such as a chest X-ray can predict which infants will survive or die from SIDS. A home apnea monitor or the use of respiratory stimulant drugs is recommended. A pneumogram may be ordered to check for periods of apnea or reflux during sleep.
NP: Assessment; CN: Physiological integrity; CNS: Reduction of risk potential; CL: Knowledge

7. Which of the following reactions are usually exhibited by the family of an infant who has died from sudden infant death syndrome (SIDS)?
1. Feelings of blame or guilt
2. Acceptance of the diagnosis
3. Requests for the infant's belongings
4. Questions regarding the etiology of the diagnosis

7. 1. During the first few moments, the parents often are in shock and have overwhelming feelings of blame or guilt. Acceptance of the diagnosis and questions regarding the etiology may not occur until the parents have had time to see the child. The infant's belongings are usually packaged for the family to take home but some parents may see this as a painful reminder.
NP: Assessment; CN: Psychosocial integrity; CNS: Coping and adaptation; CL: Application

8. Sudden infant death syndrome (SIDS) is confirmed by which of the following procedures?
1. Autopsy
2. Chest X-ray
3. Skeletal survey
4. Laboratory analysis

8. 1. Autopsies reveal consistent pathological findings, such as pulmonary edema and intrathoracic hemorrhages, that confirm the diagnosis of SIDS. Chest X-rays are used to diagnose respiratory complications. Skeletal surveys are used with cases of suspected child abuse. Laboratory analysis will show no characteristics to confirm the diagnosis of SIDS.
NP: Evaluation; CN: Physiological integrity; CNS: Physiological adaptation; CL: Knowledge

9. Which of the following plans is most appropriate for a nurse scheduling a home visit to parents who lost an infant to sudden infant death syndrome (SIDS)?

1. One visit in 2 weeks
2. No visit is necessary
3. As soon after death as possible
4. One visit with parents only, no siblings

9. 3. When parents return home, a visit is necessary as soon after the death as possible. The nurse should assess what the parents have been told, what they think happened, and how they've explained this to the other siblings. Not all of these issues will be resolved in one visit. The number of visits and plan for intervention must be flexible. The needs of the siblings must always be considered.

NP: Planning; CN: Psychosocial integrity; CNS: Coping and adaptation; CL: Analysis

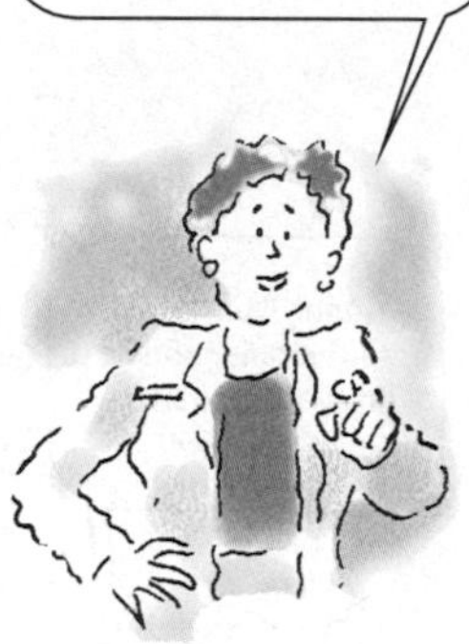

Make sure you understand the grieving process necessary for SIDS parents.

10. About 1 week after the death of an infant from sudden infant death syndrome (SIDS), which of the following behaviors would the nurse expect to observe in a parent?

1. Disorganized thinking
2. Feelings of guilt
3. Repressed thoughts
4. Structured thinking

10. 4. One week after the death, the parent of the infant would most likely be in the turmoil phase. In the turmoil phase, structured thinking is common. Almost immediately, at the time of death, parents may have repressed thoughts and feelings of guilt or blame. Within a day or two, the parents enter the impact phase of crisis. This consists of disorganized thoughts in which they can't deal with the crisis in concrete terms.

NP: Analysis; CN: Psychosocial integrity; CNS: Coping and adaptation; CL: Comprehension

11. Which of the following positions is recommended for placing an infant to sleep?

1. Prone position
2. Supine position
3. Side-lying position
4. With head of bed elevated 30 degrees

11. 2. The American Academy of Pediatrics endorses placing infants face-up in their cribs as a way to reduce sudden infant death syndrome (SIDS). Raising the head of the bed 30 degrees is recommended for infants with gastroesophageal reflux. The side-lying position promotes gastric emptying. Placing infants on their stomach is thought to make an attack of apnea harder to fight off but how exactly the sleeping position predisposes a child to SIDS is still unclear.

NP: Implementation; CN: Health promotion and maintenance; CNS: Growth and development through the life span; CL: Application

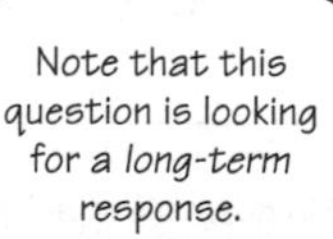

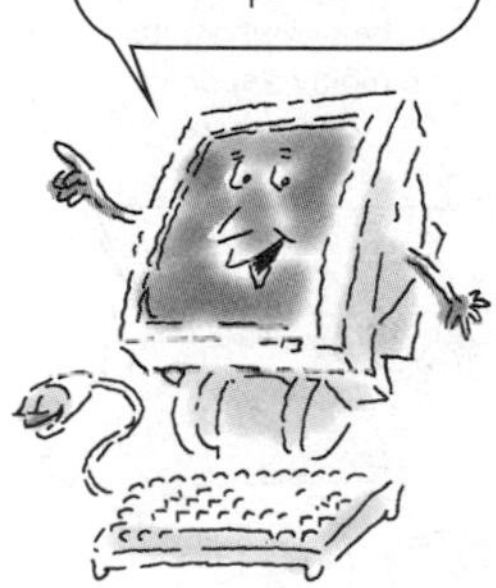

12. Which of the following activities should be recommended for long-term support of parents with an infant who has died of sudden infant death syndrome (SIDS)?

1. Attending support groups
2. Attending church regularly
3. Attending counseling sessions
4. Discussing feelings with family and friends

12. 1. The best support will come from parents who have had the same experience. Attending church and discussing feelings with family and friends can offer support but they may not understand the experience. Counseling sessions are usually a short-term support.

NP: Evaluation; CN: Psychosocial integrity; CNS: Coping and adaptation; CL: Application

13. Which of the following interventions is best to help a 2-year-old child adapt to hospitalization?

1. Allow the child to have favorite toys.
2. Allow the child to play with equipment used on him.
3. Explain procedures in simple terms.
4. Ask one or both parents to stay with the child.

13. 4. The most important factor in helping a child cope with new and strange surroundings is to have the security of the parents being present. This is the hallmark of family-centered care. Placing the child's favorite toys in the room provides distraction and allows the child to have something of his own with him but may *not* alleviate fears. Allowing the child to play with the equipment may pose a safety hazard and isn't appropriate. Explaining procedures in simple terms is important but a 2-year-old has limited understanding.

NP: Implementation; CN: Psychosocial integrity; CNS: Coping and adaptation; CL: Application

14. A 2-year-old child comes to the emergency department with inspiratory stridor and a barking cough. A preliminary diagnosis of croup has been made. Which of the following actions should be an initial intervention?

1. Administer I.V. antibiotics.
2. Provide oxygen by facemask.
3. Establish and maintain the airway.
4. Ask the mother to go to the waiting room.

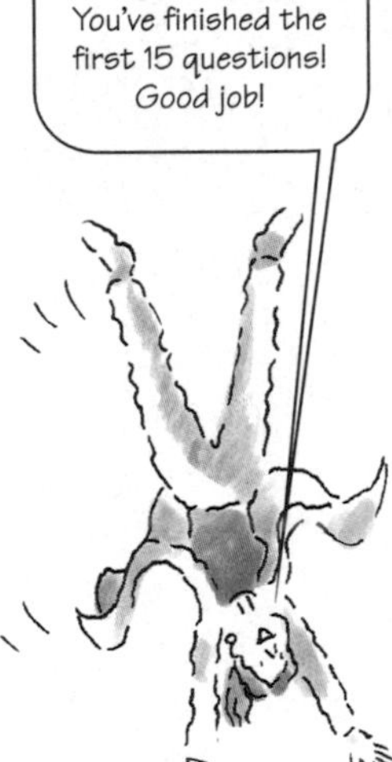

Congratulations! You've finished the first 15 questions! Good job!

14. 3. The initial priority is to establish and maintain the airway. Edema and accumulation of secretions may contribute to airway obstruction. Oxygen should be administered by tent as soon as possible to decrease the child's distress. Allowing the child to stay with the mother reduces anxiety and distress. Antibiotics aren't indicated for viral illnesses.

NP: Assessment; CN: Physiological integrity; CNS: Physiological adaptation; CL: Application

15. Which of the following is the best intervention for parents to take if their child is experiencing an episode of "midnight croup," or acute spasmodic laryngitis?

1. Give warm liquids.
2. Raise the heat on the thermostat.
3. Provide humidified air with cool mist.
4. Take the child into the bathroom with a warm running shower.

15. 3. High humidity with cool mist provides the most relief. A warm, running shower provides a mist that may be helpful to moisten and decrease the viscosity of airway secretions and may also decrease laryngeal spasm, but cool liquids would be best for the child. If unable to take liquid, the child needs to be in the emergency unit. Raising the heat on the thermostat will result in dry, warm air, which may cause secretions to adhere to the airway wall.

NP: Evaluation; CN: Physiological integrity; CNS: Physiological adaptation; CL: Application

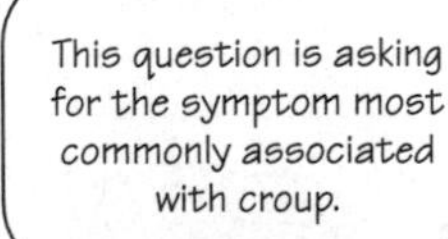

This question is asking for the symptom most commonly associated with croup.

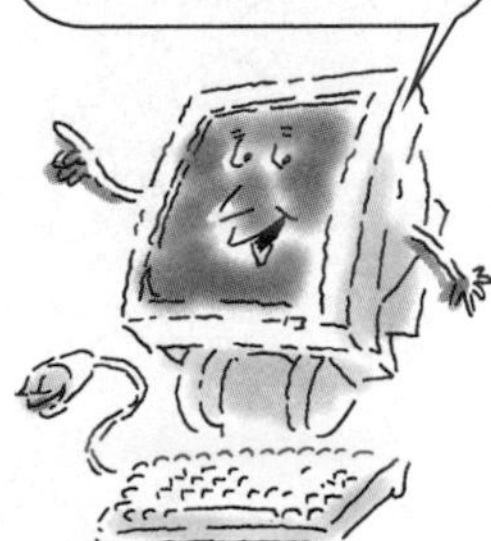

16. Which of the following signs is most characteristic of a child with croup?

1. "Barking" cough
2. Fever
3. Low heart rate
4. Respiratory distress

16. 1. A resonant cough described as "barking" is the most characteristic sign of croup. The child may have varying degrees of respiratory distress related to swelling or obstruction. The child may present with a low-grade or high fever depending on whether the etiologic agent is viral or bacterial. Usually the heart rate is rapid.

NP: Assessment; CN: Physiological integrity; CNS: Physiological adaptation; CL: Knowledge

17. Which of the following characteristics best describes croup?

1. Inflammation of the palatine tonsils
2. Acute, highly contagious respiratory infection
3. Infection of supraglottic area with involvement of the epiglottis
4. Clinical syndrome of laryngitis and laryngotracheobronchitis

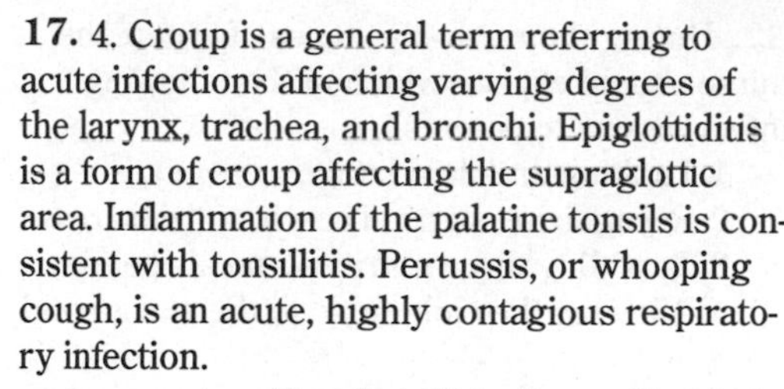

17. 4. Croup is a general term referring to acute infections affecting varying degrees of the larynx, trachea, and bronchi. Epiglottiditis is a form of croup affecting the supraglottic area. Inflammation of the palatine tonsils is consistent with tonsillitis. Pertussis, or whooping cough, is an acute, highly contagious respiratory infection.

NP: Assessment; CN: Physiological integrity; CNS: Physiological adaptation; CL: Knowledge

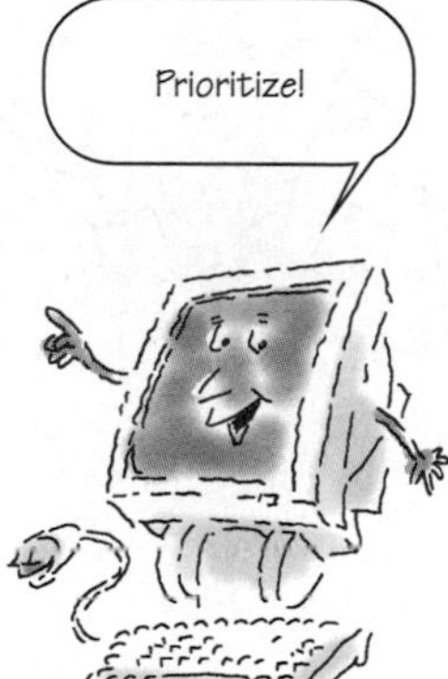

18. Which of the following interventions is the most important goal for a child with ineffective airway clearance?

1. Reducing the child's anxiety
2. Maintaining a patent airway
3. Providing adequate oral fluids
4. Administering medications as ordered

18. 2. The most important goal is to maintain a patent airway. Reducing anxiety and administering medications will follow after the airway is secure. The child shouldn't be allowed to eat or drink anything to prevent the risk of aspiration.

NP: Assessment; CN: Physiological integrity; CNS: Physiological adaptation; CL: Application

19. A 2-year-old child with croup suffering respiratory distress may show which of the following signs on initial assessment?

1. Capillary refill time less than 3 seconds
2. Elevated temperature
3. Grunting or nasal flaring
4. Respiratory rate of 28 breaths/minute

19. 3. Grunting or nasal flaring is seen in a child in respiratory distress. A respiratory rate of 28 breaths/minute and capillary refill time less than 3 seconds are normal findings. The child's temperature may be elevated if infection is present.

NP: Assessment; CN: Physiological integrity; CNS: Physiological adaptation; CL: Knowledge

20. Which of the following precautions is recommended when caring for children with respiratory infections such as croup?

1. Enforce hand washing.
2. Place the child in isolation.
3. Teach children to use tissues.
4. Keep siblings in the same room.

20. 1. Hand washing helps prevent the spread of infections. Ill children should be placed in separate bedrooms if possible but don't need to be isolated. Teaching children to use tissues properly is important, but the key is disposal and hand washing after use.

NP: Implementation; CN: Health promotion and maintenance; CNS: Prevention and early detection of disease; CL: Application

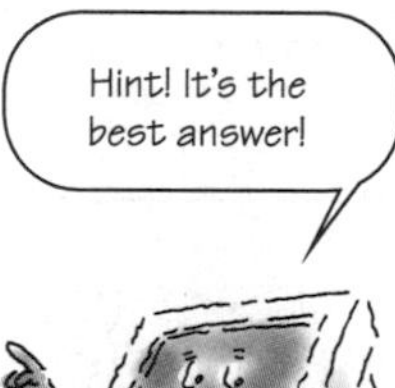

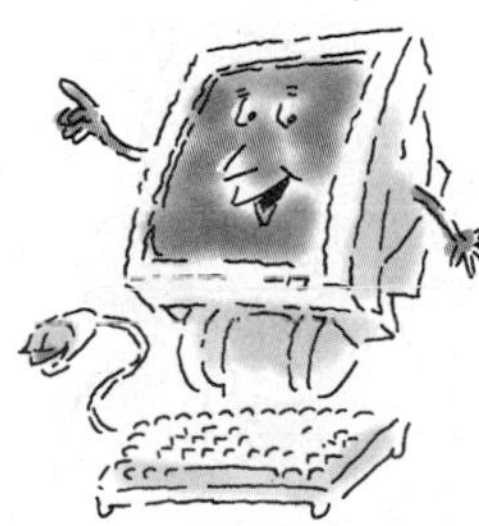

21. What is the best time to administer a nebulizer treatment to a child with croup?

1. During naptime
2. During playtime
3. After the child eats
4. After the parents leave

21. 1. The nurse should administer nebulizer treatments at prescribed intervals. During naptime allows for as little disruption as possible. A child should be given a treatment before eating so the airway will be open and the work of eating will be decreased. Administering treatment during playtime will disrupt the child's daily pattern. Parents are usually helpful when administering treatments. The child can sit on the parents' lap to help decrease anxiety or fear.

NP: Planning; CN: Physiological integrity; CNS: Pharmacological and parenteral therapies; CL: Application

22. During the recovery stages of croup, the nurse should explain which of the following interventions to parents?

1. Limiting oral fluid intake
2. Recognizing signs of respiratory distress
3. Providing three nutritious meals per day
4. Allowing the child to go to the playground

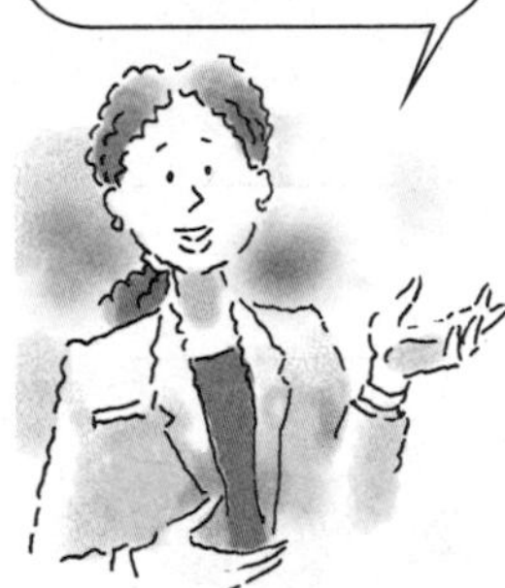

Adequate parent teaching is essential for managing a child with croup.

22. 2. Although most children recover without complications, the parents should be able to recognize signs and symptoms of respiratory distress and know how to access emergency services. Oral fluids should be encouraged because fluids help to thin secretions. Although nutrition is important, frequent small nutritious snacks are usually more appealing than an entire meal. Children should have optimal rest and engage in quiet play. A comfortable environment free of noxious stimuli lessens respiratory distress.
NP: Evaluation; CN: Physiological integrity; CNS: Physiological adaptation; CL: Application

23. Which of the following agents is related to acute epiglottiditis?

1. Allergen
2. Bacteria
3. Virus
4. Yeast

23. 2. ***Haemophilus influenzae*** type B is usually the bacterial agent responsible for acute epiglottiditis. Viral and allergen agents can be seen with acute laryngotracheobronchitis and acute spasmodic croup. Yeast infections in the oral cavity cause thrush.
NP: Assessment; CN: Physiological integrity; CNS: Physiological adaptation; CL: Knowledge

24. Which of the following clinical observations is predictive of epiglottiditis?

1. Decreased secretions
2. Drooling
3. Low-grade fever
4. Spontaneous cough

24. 2. Drooling of saliva is common due to the pain of swallowing, excessive secretions, and sore throat. The child usually has a high fever and the absence of a spontaneous cough. The classic picture is the child in a tripod position with mouth open and tongue protruding.
NP: Assessment; CN: Physiological integrity; CNS: Physiological adaptation; CL: Knowledge

25. Which of the following strategies is the best plan of care for a child with acute epiglottiditis?

1. Encourage oral fluids for hydration.
2. Maintain the client in semi-Fowler's position.
3. Administer I.V. antibiotic therapy.
4. Maintain respiratory isolation for 48 hours.

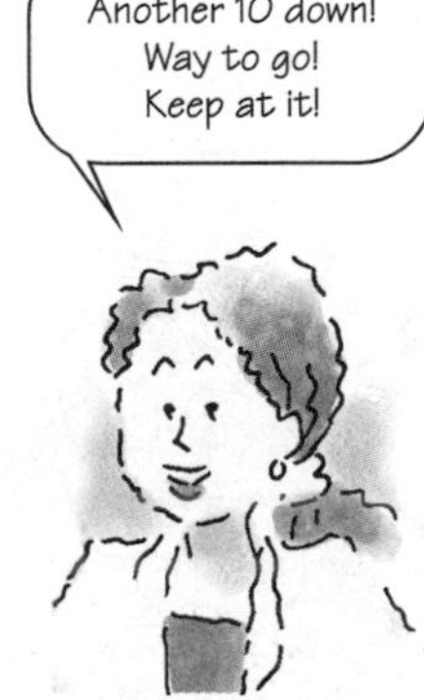

Another 10 down! Way to go! Keep at it!

25. 3. The etiologic agent for epiglottiditis is usually bacterial; therefore, the treatment consists of I.V. antibiotic therapy. The client shouldn't be allowed anything by mouth during the initial phases of the infection to prevent aspiration. The client should be placed in Fowler's position or any position that provides the most comfort and security. Respiratory isolation isn't required.
NP: Planning; CN: Physiological integrity; CNS: Physiological adaptation; CL: Application

26. A 2-year-old child is found on the floor next to his toy chest. After first determining unresponsiveness and calling for help, which of the following steps should be taken next?

1. Start mouth-to-mouth resuscitation.
2. Begin chest compressions.
3. Check for a pulse.
4. Open the airway.

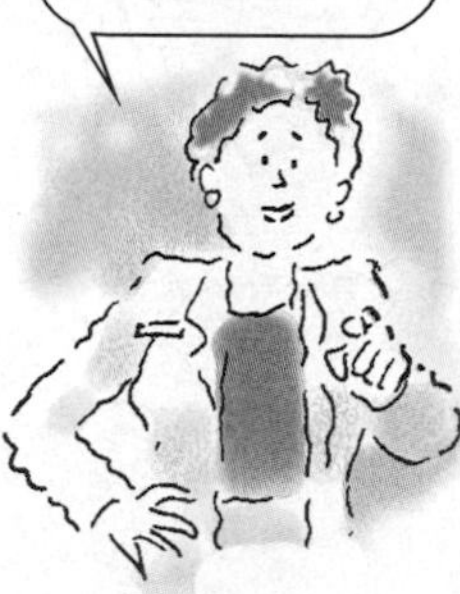

It's important to prioritize in an emergency situation.

26. 4. The airway should be opened by using the chin thrust and breathlessness should be determined at the start of cardiopulmonary resuscitation. The sequence of airway, breathing, and circulation needs to be followed.

NP: Implementation; CN: Physiological integrity; CNS: Physiological adaptation; CL: Application

27. A 10-month-old infant is found in respiratory arrest and cardiopulmonary resuscitation is started. Which of the following sites is best to check for a pulse?

1. Brachial
2. Carotid
3. Femoral
4. Radial

27. 1. Palpation of the brachial artery is recommended. The short, chubby neck of infants makes rapid location of the carotid artery difficult. After age 1, the carotid would be used. The femoral pulse, often palpated in a hospital setting, may be difficult to assess because of the infant's position, fat folds, and clothing. The radial pulse isn't a good indicator of central artery perfusion.

NP: Implementation; CN: Physiological integrity; CNS: Physiological adaptation; CL: Application

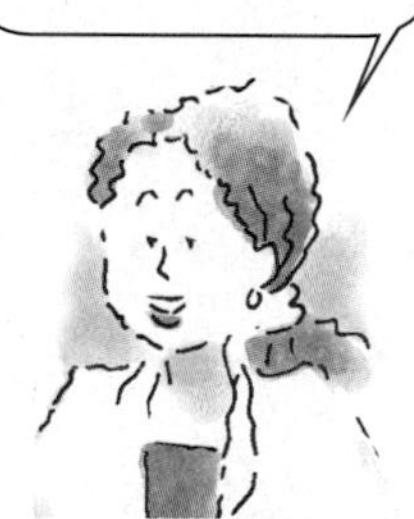

The procedure for rescue breathing for infants is different from that for adults.

28. When giving rescue breathing to an infant under age 1, what is the ratio of breaths per second?

1. 1 breath every 2 seconds
2. 1 breath every 3 seconds
3. 1 breath every 4 seconds
4. 1 breath every 5 seconds

28. 2. Rescue breathing should be performed once every 3 seconds until spontaneous breathing resumes. This provides 20 breaths/minute. One breath every 5 seconds is recommended for adults. One breath every 2 seconds may cause gastric distention.

NP: Implementation; CN: Physiological integrity; CNS: Physiological adaptation; CL: Application

29. When performing chest compressions on a 2-year-old child, which of the following depths is correct?

1. ½″ to 1″ (1 to 2.5 cm)
2. 1″ to 1½″ (2.5 to 3.5 cm)
3. 1½″ to 2″ (3.5 to 5 cm)
4. 2″ to 2½″ (5 to 6.5 cm)

29. 2. The chest compressions should equal approximately one-third to one-half the total depth of the chest. This corresponds to about 1 to 1½″ in a child age 1 to 8, ½″ to 1″ for an infant younger than age 1, and 1½″ to 2″ for an adult.

NP: Implementation; CN: Physiological integrity; CNS: Physiological adaptation; CL: Application

30. Chest compressions must be coordinated with ventilations. Which of the following ratios is accurate for a 3-year-old child?

1. 5 compressions to 1 ventilation
2. 5 compressions to 2 ventilations
3. 15 compressions to 1 ventilation
4. 15 compressions to 2 ventilations

30. 1. A ratio of 5:1 is recommended for children under age 8. A ratio of 15:2 is recommended for adults. Ratios of 5:2 and 15:1 won't provide optimal compression and ventilation.

NP: Implementation; CN: Physiological integrity; CNS: Physiological adaptation; CL: Application

31. A 10-month-old child is found choking and soon becomes unconscious. Which of the following interventions should the nurse attempt first after opening the airway?

1. Look inside the child's mouth for a foreign object.
2. Give five back blows and five chest thrusts.
3. Attempt a blind finger sweep.
4. Attempt rescue breathing.

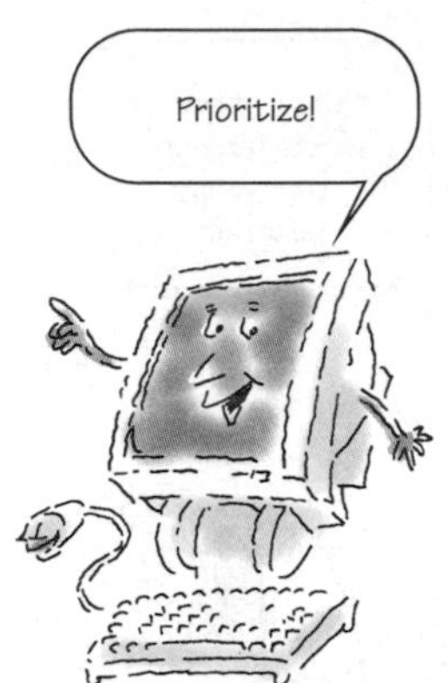
Prioritize!

31. 1. After the airway is open, the nurse should check for the foreign object and remove it with a finger sweep if it can be seen. After this step, rescue breathing should be attempted. If ventilation is unsuccessful, the nurse should then give five back blows and five chest thrusts in an attempt to dislodge the object. Blind finger sweeps should never be performed because this may push the object further back into the airway.

NP: Implementation; CN: Physiological integrity; CNS: Physiological adaptation; CL: Application

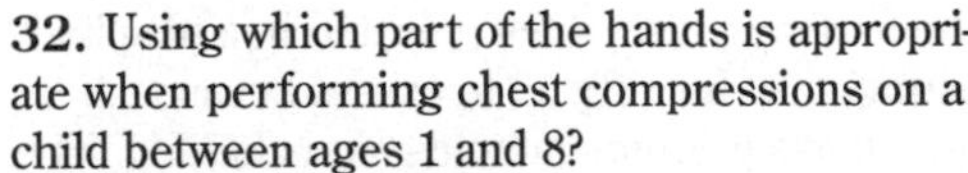

32. Using which part of the hands is appropriate when performing chest compressions on a child between ages 1 and 8?

1. Heels of both hands
2. Heel of one hand
3. Index and middle fingers
4. Thumbs of both hands

32. 2. The heel of one hand is recommended for performing chest compressions on children between ages 1 and 8. Two hands are used for adult cardiopulmonary resuscitation. Chest thrusts administered with the middle and third fingers, and in some cases the thumbs of each hand, are used on infants under age 1.

NP: Implementation; CN: Physiological integrity; CNS: Physiological adaptation; CL: Application

33. A 3-year-old child is brought to the emergency department not breathing, cyanotic, and lethargic. The mother states that she thinks he swallowed a penny. Which of the following interventions is the first the nurse should take?

1. Give 100% oxygen.
2. Administer five back blows.
3. Attempt a blind finger sweep.
4. Administer abdominal thrusts.

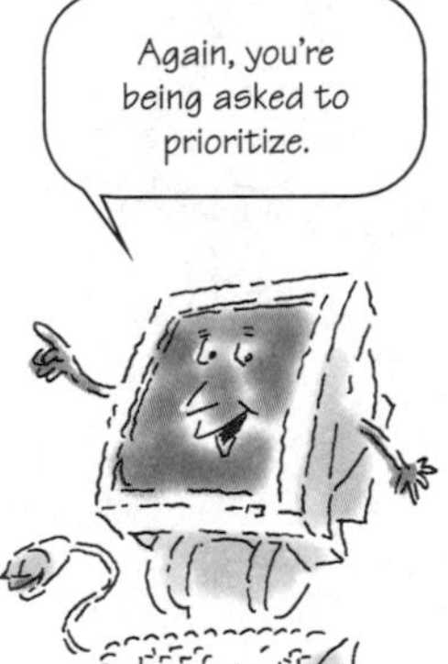
Again, you're
being asked to
prioritize.

33. 4. A child between ages 1 and 8 should receive abdominal thrusts to help dislodge the object. Blind finger sweeps should never be performed because this could push the object further back into the airway. Administering 100% oxygen won't help if the airway is occluded. Infants younger than age 1 should receive back blows before chest thrusts.

NP: Implementation; CN: Physiological integrity; CNS: Physiological adaptation; CL: Application

34. A 1-year-old child is brought to the emergency department with a mild respiratory infection and a temperature of 101.3° F (38.5° C). Otitis media is diagnosed. Which of the following signs is characteristic of otitis media?

1. Excessive drooling
2. Tugging on the ears
3. High-pitched, barking cough
4. Pearl-gray tympanic membrane

34. 2. Tugging on the ears is a common sign for a child with ear pain. Pearl-gray tympanic membranes are a normal finding. A child with otitis media usually exhibits a discolored membrane (bright red, yellow, or dull gray). A high-pitched, barking cough and excessive drooling indicate croup.

NP: Assessment; CN: Physiological integrity; CNS: Physiological adaptation; CL: Knowledge

35. A 7-month-old child is diagnosed with otitis media; the physician orders amoxicillin 40 mg/kg/day to be administered three times per day. The child weighs 9 kg. How much amoxicillin should the child receive per dose?

1. 120 mg
2. 180 mg
3. 200 mg
4. 360 mg

35. 1. The child should receive 120 mg per dose. Here are the calculations: 40 mg × 9 kg = 360 mg/day; 360 mg/3 doses = 120 mg/dose.

NP: Implementation; CN: Physiological integrity; CNS: Pharmacological and parenteral therapies; CL: Knowledge

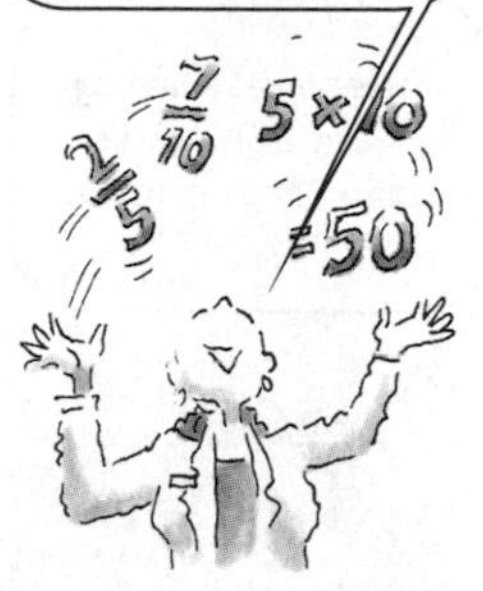

Make sure you understand this formula. You'll use it again later in this chapter.
5×10
=50

36. Children with chronic otitis media often require surgery for a myringotomy and ear tube placement. Which of the following management strategies explains the purpose of the ear tubes?

1. To administer antibiotics
2. To flush the middle ear
3. To increase pressure
4. To drain fluid

36. 4. Ear tubes allow normal fluid to drain (not flush) from the middle ear. They also allow ventilation. The purpose isn't to administer medication. The tubes also allow pressure to equalize in the middle ear.

NP: Implementation; CN: Physiological integrity; CNS: Physiological adaptation; CL: Application

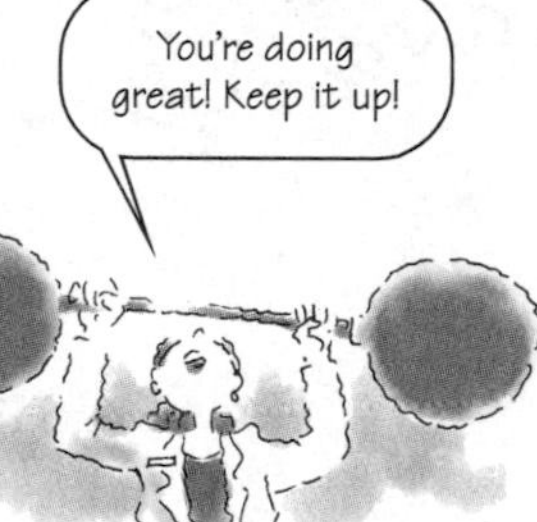

37. The nurse is discharging a 10-month-old client with eardrops. Which of the following information should she give the parent about how to administer the drops?

1. Pull the earlobe upward.
2. Pull the earlobe up and back.
3. Pull the earlobe down and back.
4. Pull the earlobe down and forward.

37. 3. For infants, the parent should be told to gently pull the earlobe down and back to visualize the external auditory canal. For children over age 3 and for adults, the earlobe is gently pulled slightly up and back.

NP: Evaluation; CN: Physiological integrity; CNS: Pharmacological and parenteral therapies; CL: Knowledge

38. A child is diagnosed as having right chronic otitis media. After the child returns from surgery for myringotomy and placement of ear tubes, which of the following interventions is appropriate?

1. Apply gauze dressings.
2. Position the child on the left side.
3. Position the child on the right side.
4. Apply warm compresses to both ears.

38. 3. The child should be positioned on the right side to facilitate drainage. The left side isn't an area of concern for drainage. Warm compresses may help to facilitate drainage only when used on the affected ear. Gauze dressings aren't necessary after surgery. Some physicians may prefer a loose cotton wick.

NP: Implementation; CN: Physiological integrity; CNS: Physiological adaptation; CL: Application

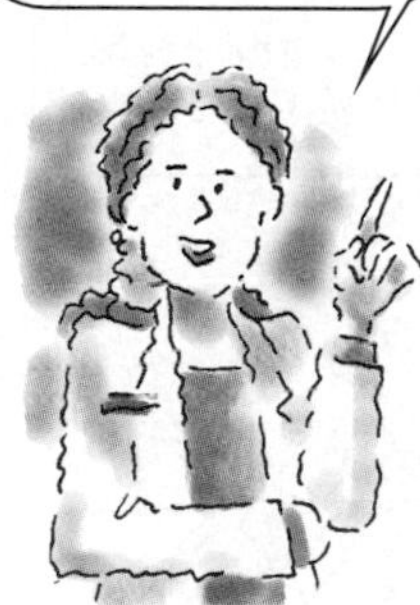

Question 39 is testing your knowledge of the different types of otitis media.

39. Which of the following durations would cause otitis media to be classified as chronic?

1. Approximately 2 weeks
2. Approximately 3 weeks
3. 3 weeks to 3 months
4. Longer than 3 months

39. 4. Otitis media is considered chronic when it lasts longer than 3 months. Subacute otitis media lasts 3 weeks to 3 months. Acute otitis media has a rapid onset and lasts approximately 2 to 3 weeks.

NP: Evaluation; CN: Physiological integrity; CNS: Physiological adaptation; CL: Knowledge

40. Which of the following descriptions best matches the findings of otoscopy in acute otitis media?

1. Pearl-gray tympanic membrane
2. Bright red, bulging tympanic membrane
3. Dull gray membrane with fluid behind the eardrum
4. Bright red or yellow bulging or retracted tympanic membrane

40. 4. With acute otitis media, the tympanic membrane may present as bright red or yellow, bulging or retracted. Dull gray membrane fluid is consistent with subacute or chronic otitis media. A pearl-gray tympanic membrane is a normal finding.

NP: Assessment; CN: Physiological integrity; CNS: Physiological adaptation; CL: Knowledge

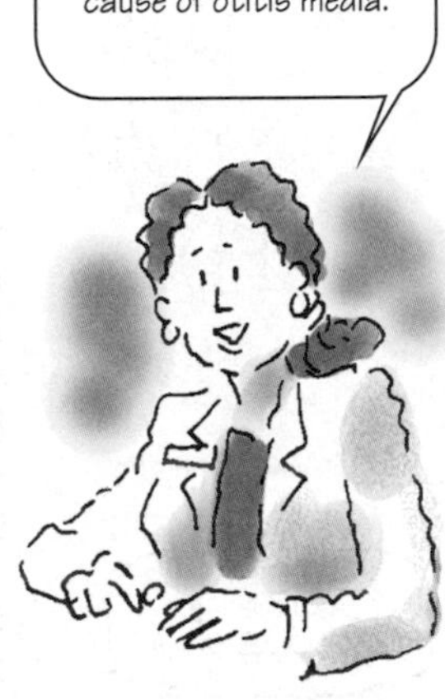

Question 41 is asking about a proximate cause of otitis media.

41. Which of the following conditions is a predisposing factor for development of otitis media in children?

1. The cartilage lining is overdeveloped.
2. When infants sit up, it favors the pooling of fluid.
3. Humoral defense mechanisms decrease the risk of infection.
4. Eustachian tubes are short, wide, and straight and lie in a horizontal plane.

41. 4. In an infant or child, the eustachian tubes are short, wide, and straight and lie in a horizontal plane. Cartilage lining is underdeveloped, making the tubes more distensible and more likely to open inappropriately. Immature humoral defense mechanisms increase the risk of infection. The usual lying-down position of infants favors the pooling of fluid such as formula in the pharyngeal cavity.

NP: Assessment; CN: Physiological integrity; CNS: Physiological adaptation; CL: Knowledge

42. Which of the following complications is most commonly related to acute otitis media?

1. Eardrum perforation
2. Hearing loss
3. Meningitis
4. Tympanosclerosis

42. 1. Eardrum perforation is the most common complication as the exudate accumulates and pressure increases. Hearing loss in most cases is conductive in nature and mild in severity but is less common than eardrum perforation. Hearing tests aren't usually performed during episodes of otitis media. Tympanosclerosis and meningitis are possible but uncommon when adequate antibiotic therapy is implemented.

NP: Assessment; CN: Physiological integrity; CNS: Physiological adaptation; CL: Application

43. Which of the following interventions is recommended for children with chronic otitis media with effusion?

1. Antihistamines
2. Corticosteroids
3. Decongestants
4. Surgical intervention

43. 4. The most common treatment for chronic otitis media is the surgical placement of tympanostomy tubes. They allow drainage of fluid and ventilation of the middle ear. Decongestants and antihistamines are used to shrink mucous membranes but are of unproven benefit. Corticosteroids have also proved to be of limited value.

NP: Implementation; CN: Physiological integrity; CNS: Reduction of risk potential; CL: Knowledge

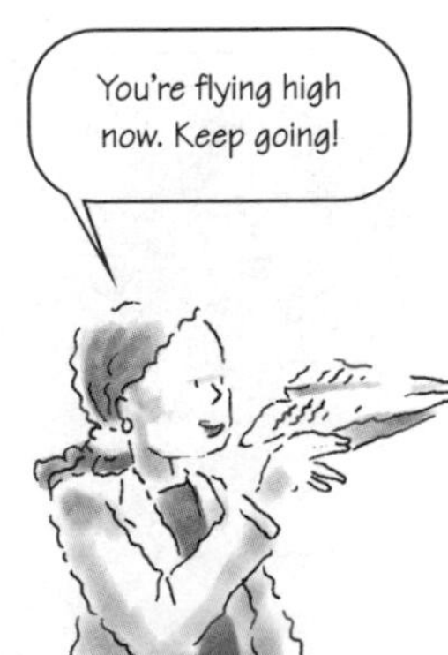

You're flying high now. Keep going!

61. Which of the following outcomes should be anticipated of parental care of a child with bronchopulmonary dysplasia?

1. Reports increased levels of stress
2. Makes safe decisions with professional assistance only
3. Participates in routine, but not complex, caretaking activities
4. Verbalizes the causes, risks, therapy options, and nursing care

61. 4. The parents should understand the causes, risks, and care of their infant by the time of discharge. Having the parents verbalize this information is the only way to assess their understanding. The parents should report decreased levels of stress, be capable of making decisions independently, and participate in routine and complex care.

NP: Evaluation; CN: Physiological integrity; CNS: Basic care and comfort; CL: Analysis

62. Bronchopulmonary dysplasia can be classified into four categories. Which of the following characteristics is noted during the early or first stage of the disease?

1. Interstitial fibrosis
2. Signs of emphysema
3. Hyperexpansion on chest X-ray
4. Resemblance to respiratory distress syndrome

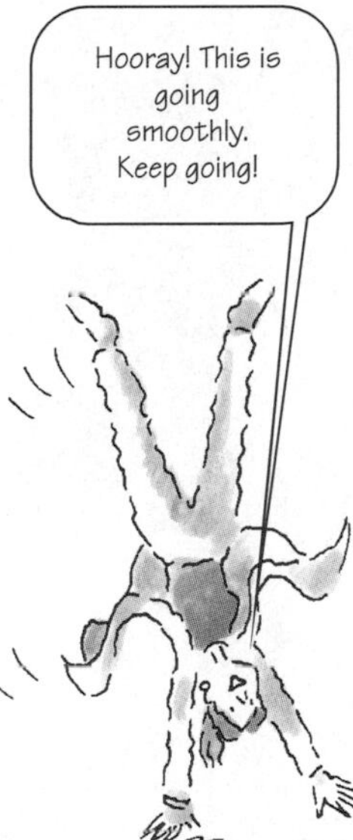

Hooray! This is going smoothly. Keep going!

62. 4. Stage I can be characterized by early interstitial changes and resembles respiratory distress syndrome. Stage III shows signs of the beginning of chronic disease with interstitial edema, signs of emphysema, and pulmonary hypertension. Stage IV shows interstitial fibrosis and hyperexpansion on chest X-ray.

NP: Assessment; CN: Physiological integrity; CNS: Physiological adaptation; CL: Knowledge

63. Bronchopulmonary dysplasia can cause increased fluid in the lungs due to disruption of the alveolar-capillary membrane, and the client may begin receiving furosemide (Lasix). Which of the following adverse effects is possible?

1. Hypercalcemia
2. Hyperkalemia
3. Hypernatremia
4. Irregular heart rhythm

63. 4. An irregular heart rhythm and muscle cramps are adverse effects related to hypokalemia and hypocalcemia. Diuretics cause volume depletion by inhibiting reabsorption of sodium and chloride. Hypokalemia can occur with excessive fluid loss or as part of contraction alkalosis. Hypocalcemia is related to the urinary excretion of calcium.

NP: Evaluation; CN: Physiological integrity; CNS: Pharmacological and parenteral therapies; CL: Knowledge

64. A pediatric client is to receive furosemide (Lasix) 4 mg/kg/day in one daily dose. The client weighs 20 kg. How many milligrams should be administered in each dose?

1. 20 mg
2. 40 mg
3. 80 mg
4. 160 mg

64. 3. The child should receive 80 mg per dose. Here are the calculations: 4 mg/kg × 20 kg = 80 mg.

NP: Evaluation; CN: Physiological integrity; CNS: Pharmacological and parenteral therapies; CL: Application

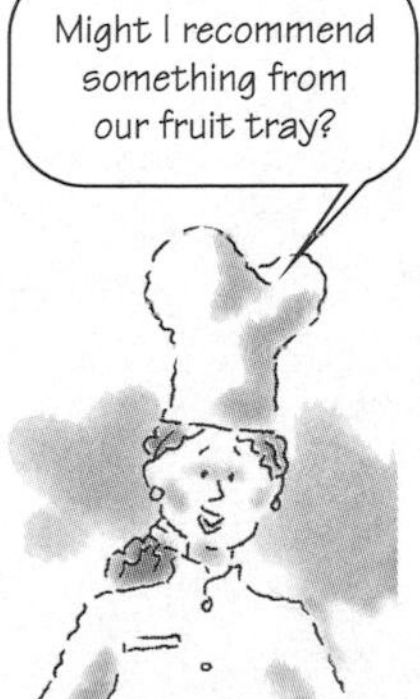

Might I recommend something from our fruit tray?

65. A 2-year-old child with bronchopulmonary dysplasia is placed on furosemide (Lasix) once per day. The parents are being educated on foods that are rich in potassium. Which of the following foods should the nurse recommend?

1. Apples
2. Oranges
3. Peaches
4. Raisins

65. 4. Raisins, dates, figs, and prunes are among the highest potassium-rich foods. They average 17 to 20 mEq of potassium. Apples, oranges, and peaches have very low amounts of potassium. They average 3 to 4 mEq.

NP: Evaluation; CN: Physiological integrity; CNS: Pharmacological and parenteral therapies; CL: Knowledge

66. Which of the following reasons necessitates tracheostomy tube placement in long-term care of infants with bronchopulmonary dysplasia?

1. Increased risk of tracheomalacia
2. Inability to wean from the ventilator
3. Need to allow for gastrostomy tube feedings
4. Increased signs of respiratory distress

66. 2. Tracheostomy may be required after a child has been ventilator dependent for 6 to 8 weeks and is unable to wean from the ventilator. This will allow for oral feedings and reduce the risks of tracheomalacia and bronchomalacia.

NP: Planning; CN: Physiological integrity; CNS: Physiological adaptation; CL: Analysis

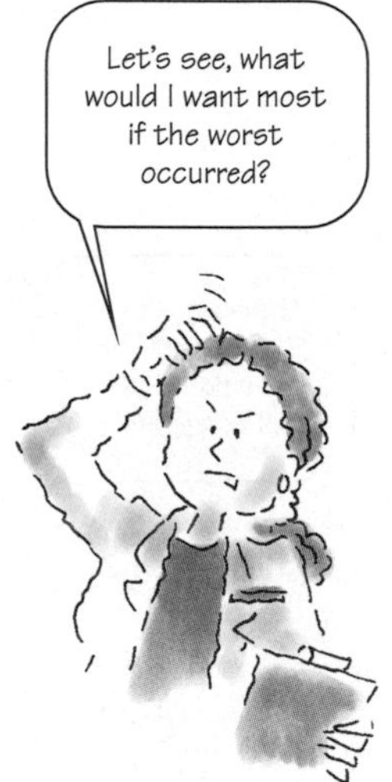

Let's see, what would I want most if the worst occurred?

67. A 1-year-old infant with bronchopulmonary dysplasia has just received a tracheostomy. Which of the following interventions is appropriate?

1. Keep extra tracheostomy tubes at the bedside.
2. Secure ties at the side of the neck for easy access.
3. Change the tracheostomy tube 2 weeks after surgery.
4. Secure the tracheostomy ties tightly to prevent dislodgment of the tube.

67. 1. Extra tracheostomy tubes should be kept at the bedside in case of an emergency, including one size smaller in case the appropriate size doesn't fit due to edema or lack of a tract formation. The ties should be placed securely but allow the width of a little finger for room to prevent excessive pressure or skin breakdown. The first tracheostomy tube change is usually performed by the physician after 7 days. Ties are usually placed at the back of the neck.

NP: Implementation; CN: Physiological integrity; CNS: Physiological adaptation; CL: Application

68. An 11-month-old infant with bronchopulmonary dysplasia and a tracheostomy experiences a decline in oxygen saturation from 97% to 88%. He appears anxious and his heart rate is 180 beats/minute. Which of the following interventions is most appropriate?

1. Change the tracheostomy tube.
2. Suction the tracheostomy tube.
3. Obtain an arterial blood gas (ABG) level.
4. Increase the oxygen flow rate.

68. 2. Tracheostomy tubes, particularly in small children, require frequent suctioning to remove mucus plugs and excessive secretions. The tracheostomy tube can be changed if suctioning is unsuccessful. Obtaining an ABG level may be beneficial if oxygen saturation remains low and the child appears to be in respiratory distress. Increasing the oxygen flow rate will only help if the airway is patent.

NP: Implementation; CN: Physiological integrity; CNS: Physiological adaptation; CL: Analysis

69. Which of the following interventions is most appropriate when suctioning a tracheostomy tube?

1. Hypoventilate the child before suctioning.
2. Repeat the suctioning process for two intervals.
3. Insert the catheter 1 to 2 cm below the tracheostomy tube.
4. Inject a small amount of normal saline solution into the tube before suctioning.

69. 4. Injecting a small amount of normal saline solution helps to loosen secretions for easier aspiration. Preservative-free normal saline solution should be used. If the catheter is inserted too far, it will irritate the carina and may cause blood-tinged secretions. The suctioning process should be repeated until the trachea is clear. The child should be hyperventilated before and after suctioning to prevent hypoxia. The catheter should be inserted *0.5 cm beyond* the tracheostomy tube.

NP: Analysis; CN: Physiological integrity; CNS: Physiological adaptation; CL: Application

78. A 10-year-old client with asthma has recently started receiving I.V. aminophylline. He begins to vomit and complains of his stomach hurting. Which of the following nursing interventions is appropriate?

1. Check the theophylline level.
2. Increase the infusion rate of the aminophylline.
3. Take no action; aminophylline can cause nausea.
4. Stop the aminophylline infusion and call the physician.

78. 1. Although nausea and GI upset are adverse effects of aminophylline, they can also represent signs of toxicity. The theophylline level should be checked to make sure the blood level is in the therapeutic range of 10 to 20 μg/ml. The aminophylline drip may need to be decreased based on the blood level. The infusion shouldn't be stopped until a theophylline level is obtained.

NP: Evaluation; CN: Physiological integrity; CNS: Pharmacological and parenteral therapies; CL: Analysis

79. Which of the following findings would you expect on a typical X-ray of a child with asthma?

1. Atelectasis
2. Hemothorax
3. Infiltrates
4. Pneumothoraces

79. 1. Hyperexpansion, atelectasis, and a flattened diaphragm are typical X-ray findings for a child with asthma. Air becomes trapped behind the narrowed airways and the residual capacity rises, leading to hyperinflation. Hypoxemia results from areas of the lung not being well perfused. Infiltrates and pneumothoraces are uncommon. A hemothorax isn't a finding related to asthma.

NP: Assessment; CN: Physiological integrity; CNS: Physiological adaptation; CL: Analysis

80. Which of the following interventions is most appropriate for a client with atelectasis?

1. Perform chest physiotherapy.
2. Give increased I.V. fluids.
3. Administer oxygen.
4. Obtain arterial blood gas (ABG) levels.

80. 1. Chest physiotherapy and incentive spirometry help to enhance the clearance of mucus and open the alveoli. Administration of oxygen will *not* give enough pressure to open the alveoli. I.V. and oral fluids are recommended to help liquefy and thin secretions. Obtaining ABG levels isn't necessary.

NP: Implementation; CN: Physiological integrity; CNS: Physiological adaptation; CL: Application

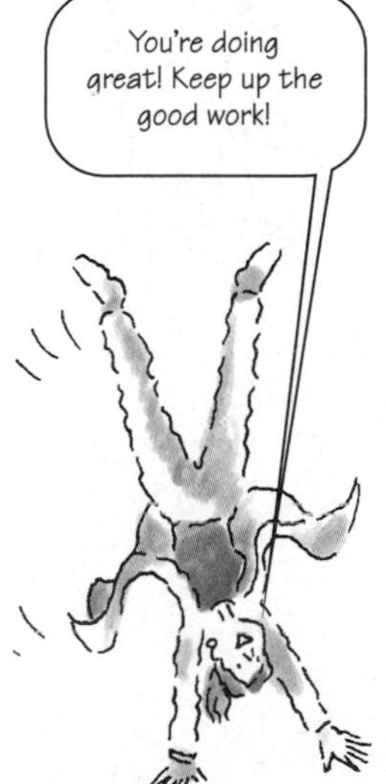
You're doing great! Keep up the good work!

81. The parents of a 10-year-old child recently diagnosed with asthma ask if the child can continue to play sports. Which of the following responses is most appropriate?

1. Sports can cause asthma attacks.
2. You should limit activities to quiet play.
3. It's okay to play some sports but swimming isn't recommended.
4. Physical activity and sports are encouraged provided the asthma is under control.

81. 4. Participation in sports is encouraged but should be evaluated on an individual basis provided the asthma is under control. Exercise-induced asthma is an example of the airway hyperactivity common to asthmatics. Swimming is well-tolerated related to the type of breathing and the moisture in the air. Exclusion from sports or activities may hamper peer interaction.

NP: Evaluation; CN: Physiological integrity; CNS: Physiological adaptation; CL: Analysis

82. What is the normal therapeutic range of aminophylline?

1. 2 to 4 μg/ml
2. 5 to 15 μg/ml
3. 10 to 20 μg/ml
4. 20 to 30 μg/ml

82. 3. The normal therapeutic range of aminophylline is considered to be 10 to 20 μg/ml. Levels below 10 μg/ml are considered to be less than therapeutic. Symptoms of toxicity such as nausea, tachycardia, and irritability can appear when levels exceed 20 μg/ml. Levels greater than 30 μg/ml can cause seizures and arrhythmias.

NP: Evaluation; CN: Physiological integrity; CNS: Pharmacological and parenteral therapies; CL: Knowledge

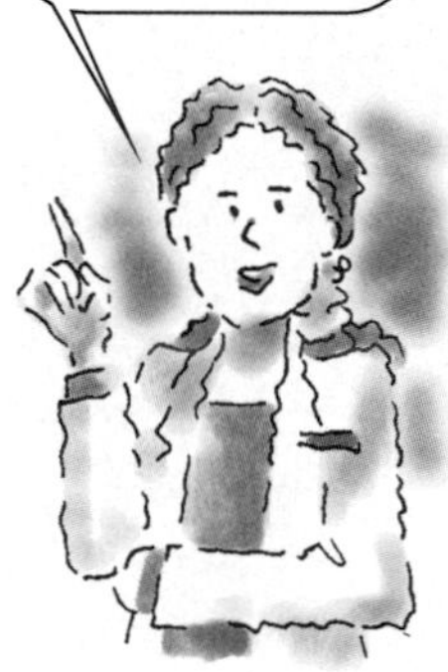

Keep this client's age in mind when answering question 83.

83. Which of the following nursing interventions is appropriate to correct dehydration for a 2-year-old client with asthma?

1. Give warm liquids.
2. Give cold juice or ice pops.
3. Provide three meals and three snacks.
4. Give I.V. fluid boluses.

83. 1. Liquids are best tolerated if they're warm. Cold liquids may cause bronchospasm and should be avoided. Dehydration should be corrected slowly. Overhydration may increase interstitial pulmonary fluid and exacerbate small airway obstruction. Small, frequent meals should be provided to avoid abdominal distention that may interfere with diaphragm excursion.

NP: Implementation; CN: Physiological integrity; CNS: Physiological adaptation; CL: Application

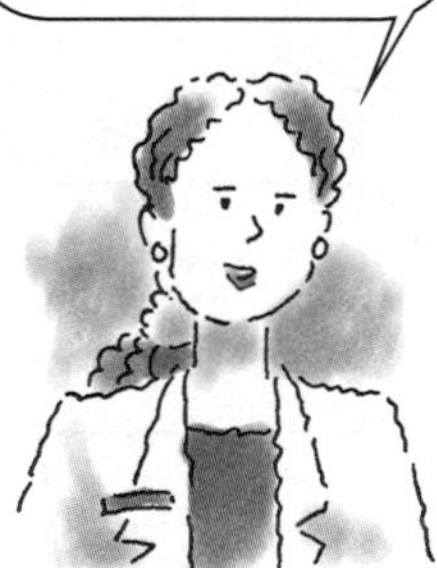

"Allergy proofing" a home can be just as important as "kid proofing" it.

84. Which of the following interventions by the parents is appropriate to "allergy proof" the home?

1. Cover floors with carpeting.
2. Designate the basement as the play area.
3. Dust and clean the house thoroughly twice a month.
4. Use foam rubber pillows and synthetic blankets.

84. 4. Bedding should be free of allergens with nonallergenic covers. Unnecessary rugs should be removed and floors should be bare and mopped a few times a week to reduce dust. Dusting and cleaning should occur daily or at least weekly. Basements or cellars should be avoided to lessen the child's exposure to molds and mildew.

NP: Planning; CN: Physiological integrity; CNS: Physiological adaptation; CL: Knowledge

85. Which of the following nursing diagnoses is appropriate for a client with acute asthma?

1. Imbalanced nutrition: More than body requirements
2. Excess fluid volume
3. Activity intolerance
4. Constipation

85. 3. Ineffective oxygen supply and demand may lead to activity intolerance. The nurse should promote rest and encourage developmentally appropriate activities. Nutrition may be decreased due to respiratory distress and GI upset. Dehydration is common due to diaphoresis, insensible water loss, and hyperventilation. Medications given to treat asthma may cause nausea, vomiting, and diarrhea, *not* constipation.

NP: Analysis; CN: Physiological integrity; CNS: Physiological adaptation; CL: Analysis

86. Which of the following definitions best describes bronchiolitis?

1. Acute inflammation and obstruction of the bronchioles
2. Airway obstruction from aspiration of a solid object
3. Inflammation of the pulmonary parenchyma
4. Acute highly contagious croup-like syndrome

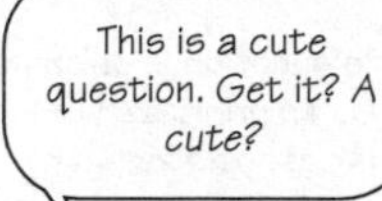

This is a cute question. Get it? A cute?

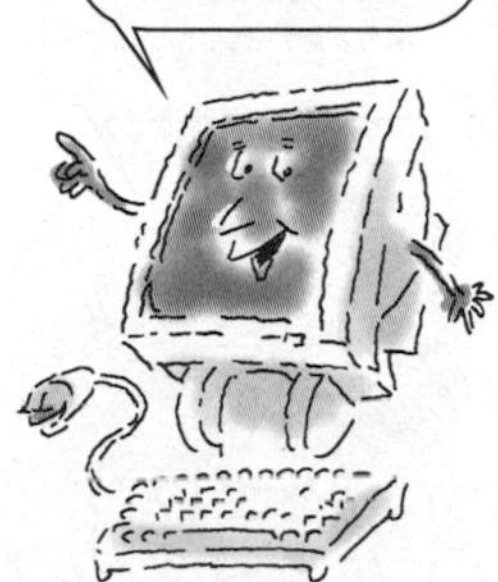

86. 1. Bronchiolitis is an infection of the bronchioles, causing the mucosa to become edematous, inflamed, and full of mucus. Pneumonia is characterized by inflammation of the pulmonary parenchyma. Lower airway obstruction from a solid object is a form of a foreign body aspiration. Croup syndromes are generally upper airway infections or obstructions.

NP: Assessment; CN: Physiological integrity; CNS: Physiological adaptation; CL: Knowledge

87. A 2-month-old infant is brought to the emergency department and a preliminary diagnosis of bronchiolitis is given. Which of the following symptoms would the nurse expect to find on assessment?

1. Bradycardia
2. Increased appetite
3. Wheezing on auscultation
4. No signs of an upper respiratory infection

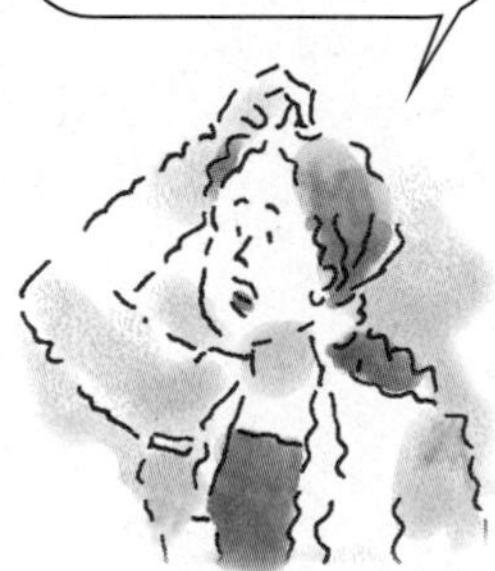

Consider the pathology of bronchiolitis when answering question 87.

87. 3. In bronchiolitis, the bronchioles become narrowed and edematous. This can cause wheezing. These infants typically have a 2- to 3-day history of an upper respiratory infection and feeding difficulties with loss of appetite due to nasal congestion and increased work of breathing. This combination leads to respiratory distress with tachypnea and tachycardia.

NP: Assessment; CN: Physiological integrity; CNS: Physiological adaptation; CL: Application

88. In most cases, bronchiolitis is caused by a viral agent, most commonly respiratory syncytial virus (RSV). Which of the following characteristics is associated with RSV?

1. Prevalence in the summer and fall months
2. High affinity for respiratory tract mucosa
3. Most common in children over age 5
4. Infected children aren't contagious

88. 2. RSV attacks the respiratory tract mucosa. The virus is most prevalent in the winter and early spring months. Most children develop the infection between ages 2 and 6 months, and RSV generally occurs during the first 3 years of life. RSV is a highly contagious respiratory virus.

NP: Assessment; CN: Physiological integrity; CNS: Physiological adaptation; CL: Knowledge

89. Which of the following precautions should a nurse caring for a 2-month-old infant with respiratory syncytial virus (RSV) take to prevent the spread of infection?

1. Gloves only
2. Gown, gloves, and mask
3. No precautions are required; the virus isn't contagious
4. Proper hand washing between clients

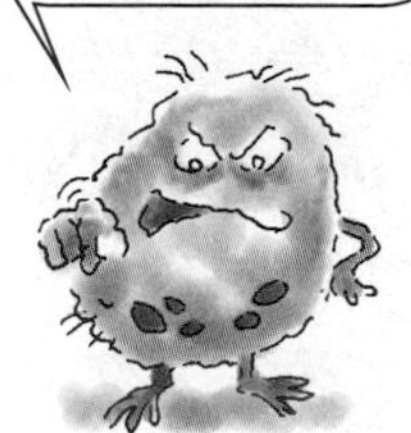

What precautions should you take when treating a highly contagious agent such as my none-too-lovable self?

89. 2. RSV is highly contagious and is spread through direct contact with infectious secretions via hands, droplets, and fomites. Gowns, gloves, and masks should be worn for client care to prevent the spread of infection.

NP: Implementation; CN: Safe, effective care environment; CNS: Safety and infection control; CL: Application

90. Which of the following tests gives a positive diagnosis of respiratory syncytial virus (RSV)?

1. Blood test
2. Nasopharyngeal washings
3. Sputum culture
4. Throat culture

90. 2. RSV can only be diagnosed with direct aspiration of nasal secretions or nasopharyngeal washings. Positive identification is accomplished using the enzyme-linked immunosorbent assay. Blood, throat, and sputum cultures can't definitively diagnose RSV.

NP: Analysis; CN: Physiological integrity; CNS: Physiological adaptation; CL: Knowledge

91. Which of the following children would be at increased risk for a respiratory syncytial virus (RSV) infection?

1. A 2-month-old child managed at home
2. A 2-month-old child with bronchopulmonary dysplasia
3. A 3-month-old child requiring low-flow oxygen
4. A 2-year-old child

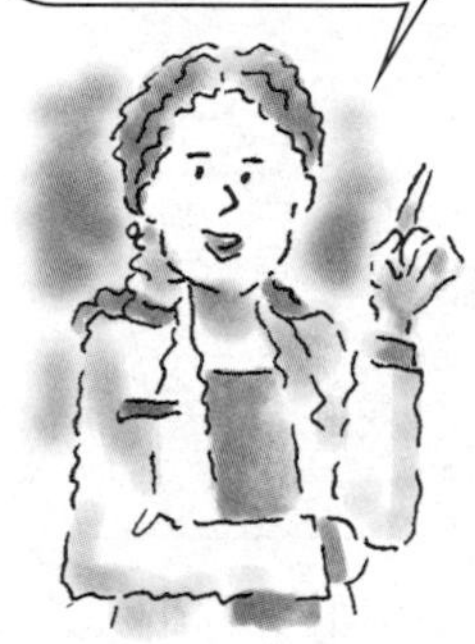

This question is asking you to prioritize the risk associated with RSV infection.

91. 2. Infants with cardiac or pulmonary conditions are at highest risk for RSV. Because of their underlying conditions, they more commonly require mechanical ventilation. Many infants can be managed at home; few require hospitalization. A 2-year-old child has built up the immune system and can tolerate the infection without major problems. A 3-month-old on low-flow oxygen has some risks of progression but is *not* at a high risk.

NP: Assessment; CN: Physiological integrity; CNS: Reduction of risk potential; CL: Analysis

92. Which of the following medications can help to prevent respiratory syncytial virus (RSV)?

1. Aminophylline
2. Bronchodilators
3. Corticosteroids
4. Respigam

92. 4. Respigam is I.V. RSV immune globulin. It can help to prevent serious lower respiratory tract infections caused by RSV. The first dose is given before RSV season, with monthly doses given throughout the season for protection. This agent is indicated for children younger than age 24 months with bronchopulmonary dysplasia or a history of prematurity. Bronchodilators, aminophylline, and corticosteroids are sometimes used for treatment.

NP: Planning; CN: Health promotion and maintenance; CNS: Prevention and early detection of disease; CL: Analysis

93. Which of the following medications is an antiviral agent used to treat bronchiolitis caused by respiratory syncytial virus (RSV)?

1. Albuterol
2. Aminophylline
3. Cromolyn sodium
4. Ribavirin (Virazole)

93. 4. Ribavirin is an antiviral agent sometimes used to reduce the severity of bronchiolitis caused by RSV. Aminophylline and albuterol are bronchodilators and haven't been proven effective in viral bronchiolitis. Cromolyn sodium is an inhaled anti-inflammatory agent.

NP: Evaluation; CN: Physiological integrity; CNS: Pharmacological and parenteral therapies; CL: Analysis

94. Which of the following interventions is most important when monitoring dehydration in an infant with bronchiolitis?

1. Measurement of intake and output
2. Blood levels every 4 hours
3. Urinalysis every 8 hours
4. Weighing each diaper

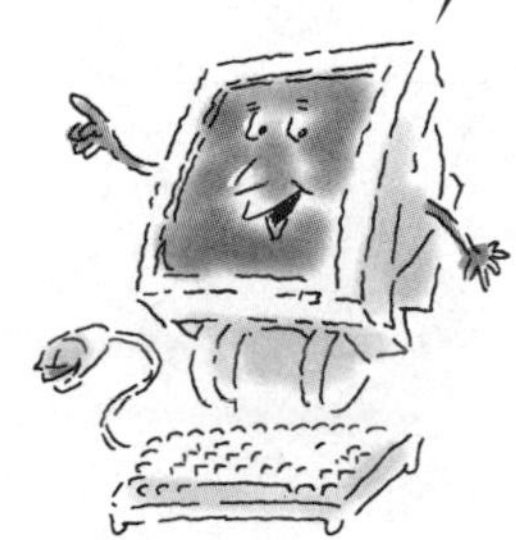

This one is tricky. Pay attention to the frequency of the measurements.

94. 1. Accurate measurement of intake and output is essential to assess for dehydration. Blood levels may be obtained daily or every other day. A urinalysis every 8 hours isn't necessary. Urine specific gravities are recommended but can be obtained with diaper changes. Weighing diapers is a way of measuring output only.

NP: Analysis; CN: Physiological integrity; CNS: Physiological adaptation; CL: Application

95. Which of the following nursing diagnoses is appropriate for an infant with bronchiolitis?

1. Imbalanced nutrition: More than body requirements
2. Deficient diversional activity
3. Impaired gas exchange
4. Social isolation

95. 3. Infants with bronchiolitis will have impaired gas exchange related to bronchiolar obstruction, atelectasis, and hyperinflation. Deficient diversional activity and social isolation usually aren't priorities. These infants are too uncomfortable to respond to social stimuli and need quiet, soothing activities that minimize energy. Nutrition may be seen as less than body requirements. If respiratory distress is present, these infants should have nothing by mouth and fluids given I.V. only.

NP: Planning; CN: Physiological integrity; CNS: Physiological adaptation; CL: Analysis

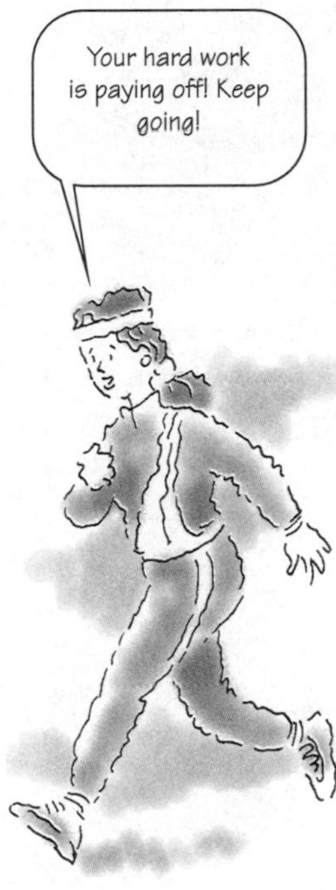

Your hard work is paying off! Keep going!

96. Which of the following teaching points is essential for parents caring for a child with bronchiolitis at home?

1. Place the child in a prone position for comfort.
2. Use warm mist to replace insensible fluid loss.
3. Recognize signs of increasing respiratory distress.
4. Engage the child in many activities to prevent developmental delay.

96. 3. It's essential for parents to be able to recognize signs of increasing respiratory distress and know how to count the respiratory rate. Use of cool mist may help to replace insensible fluid loss. The child should be positioned with the head of the bed elevated for comfort and to facilitate removal of secretions. Quiet play activities are required only as the child's energy level permits. These infants show clinical improvement in 3 to 4 days; therefore, developmental delay isn't an issue.

NP: Planning; CN: Physiological integrity; CNS: Physiological adaptation; CL: Analysis

97. Which of the following definitions best describes pneumonia?

1. Inflammation of the large airways
2. Severe infection of the bronchioles
3. Inflammation of the pulmonary parenchyma
4. Acute viral infection with maximum effect at the bronchiolar level

97. 3. Pneumonia is an inflammation of the pulmonary parenchyma. Bronchiolitis is a severe infection of the bronchioles. Bronchitis is inflammation of the large airways. Bronchiolitis and respiratory syncytial virus are terms for an acute viral infection with maximum effect at the bronchiolar level.

NP: Assessment; CN: Physiological integrity; CNS: Physiological adaptation; CL: Knowledge

98. Pneumonias can be classified by four etiologic processes. Which of the following causative agents is responsible for bacterial pneumonia?

1. Mycoplasma
2. Parainfluenza virus
3. Pneumococci
4. Respiratory syncytial virus (RSV)

98. 3. Pneumococcal pneumonia is the most common causative agent accounting for about 90% of bacterial pneumonia. Parainfluenza virus and RSV account for viral pneumonia. Mycoplasma is a causative agent for primary atypical pneumonia.

NP: Assessment; CN: Physiological integrity; CNS: Physiological adaptation; CL: Knowledge

99. Which of the following types of pneumonias is most common in children ages 5 to 12?

1. Enteric bacilli
2. Mycoplasma pneumonia
3. Staphylococcal pneumonia
4. Streptococcal pneumonia

99. 2. Mycoplasma pneumonia is a primary atypical pneumonia seen in children between ages 5 and 12. Streptococcal pneumonia, enteric bacilli, and staphylococcal pneumonia are mostly seen in children in the 3 month to 5 year age-group.

NP: Assessment; CN: Physiological integrity; CNS: Physiological adaptation; CL: Knowledge

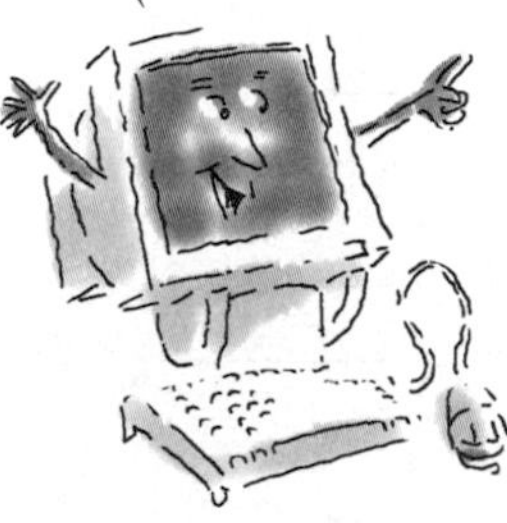

Whoopee! You reached 100! Can you believe it?

100. Which of the following characteristics is commonly seen in a child with pertussis?

1. Barking cough
2. Whooping cough
3. Abrupt high fever
4. Inspiratory stridor

100. 2. Pertussis is characterized by consistent short, rapid coughs followed by a sudden inspiration with a high-pitched whooping sound. A barking cough and inspiratory stridor are noted with croup. Pertussis is usually accompanied by a low-grade fever.

NP: Assessment; CN: Physiological integrity; CNS: Physiological adaptation; CL: Knowledge

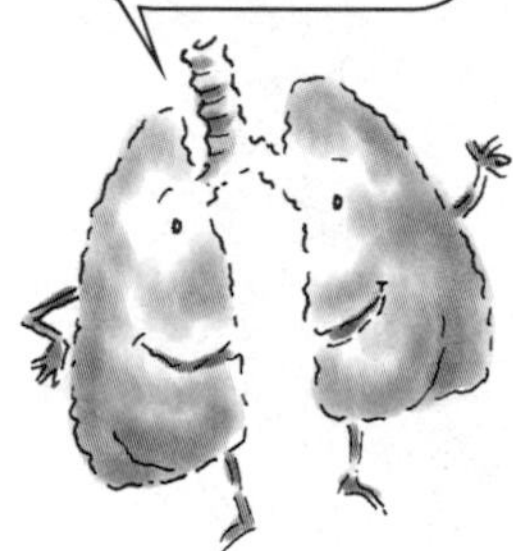

Psssst! The name of the disorder is your hint on this one!

101. Which of the following tests is the definitive means of diagnosing tuberculosis (TB)?

1. Chest X-ray
2. Sputum sample
3. Tuberculin test
4. Urine culture

101. 2. A sputum culture is the definitive test. The tuberculin test is the most accurate but not necessarily the most reliable test for TB in children. X-rays usually appear normal in children with TB. Stool cultures and gastric washings will show positive results on acid-fast smears but aren't specific for *Mycobacterium tuberculosis*. Sputum samples are difficult to obtain from children, so gastric washings commonly replace them.

NP: Assessment; CN: Physiological integrity; CNS: Physiological adaptation; CL: Analysis

102. Which of the following symptoms is a characteristic sign of tuberculosis?

1. Chills
2. Hyperactivity
3. Lymphadenitis
4. Weight gain

102. 3. Children are usually asymptomatic and often don't manifest the usual pulmonary symptoms, but lymphadenitis is more likely in infants and children than in adults. Weight loss, anorexia, night sweats, fatigue, and malaise are general responses to the disease.

NP: Assessment; CN: Physiological integrity; CNS: Physiological adaptation; CL: Knowledge

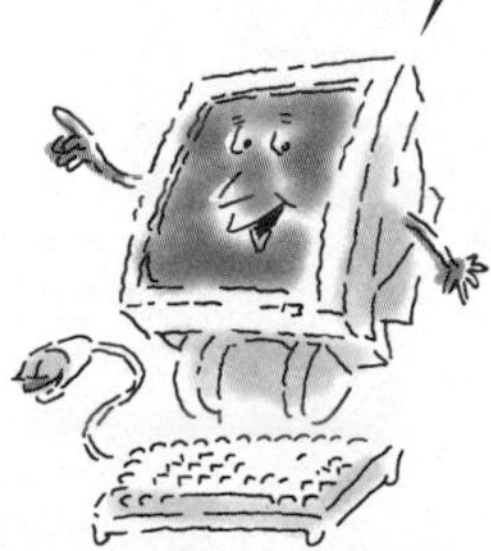

Orange you glad you're almost finished! (Hahahahaha! I slay myself.)

103. Which of the following adverse effects can be expected by the parents of a 2-year-old child who has been started on rifampin (Rifadin) after testing positive for tuberculosis?

1. Hyperactivity
2. Orange body secretions
3. Decreased bilirubin levels
4. Decreased levels of liver enzymes

103. 2. Rifampin and its metabolites will turn urine, feces, sputum, tears, and sweat an orange color. This isn't a serious adverse effect. Rifampin may also cause GI upset, headache, drowsiness, dizziness, visual disturbances, and fever. Liver enzyme and bilirubin levels increase because of hepatic metabolism of the drug. Parents should be taught the signs and symptoms of hepatitis and hyperbilirubinemia such as jaundice of the sclera or skin.

NP: Evaluation; CN: Physiological integrity; CNS: Pharmacological and parenteral therapies; CL: Application

104. Children under age 3 are prone to aspirating foreign bodies. Which of the following actions is recommended to prevent aspiration?

1. Cut hot dogs in half.
2. Limit popcorn and peanuts.
3. Cut grapes into small pieces.
4. Limit hard candy to special occasions.

104. 3. Grapes, hotdogs, and sausage should be cut into many small pieces. Hard candy, raisins, popcorn, and peanuts should be avoided for children age 4 and younger.

NP: Evaluation; CN: Physiological integrity; CNS: Reduction of risk potential; CL: Application

105. Which of the following groups of clinical findings suggests a foreign body located in the trachea?

1. Cough, dyspnea, and drooling
2. Cough, stridor, and changes in phonation
3. Expiratory wheeze and inspiratory stridor
4. Cough, asymmetric breath sounds, and wheeze

105. 3. Expiratory and inspiratory noise indicates that the foreign body is in the trachea. Cough, dyspnea, drooling, and gagging indicate supraglottic obstruction. A cough with stridor and changes in phonation would occur if the foreign body were in the larynx. Asymmetric breath sounds indicate that the object may be located in the bronchi.

NP: Assessment; CN: Physiological integrity; CNS: Physiological adaptation; CL: Knowledge

106. Which of the following activities is recommended to prevent foreign body aspiration during meals?

1. Insist that children are seated.
2. Give children toys to play with.
3. Allow children to watch television.
4. Allow children to eat in a separate room.

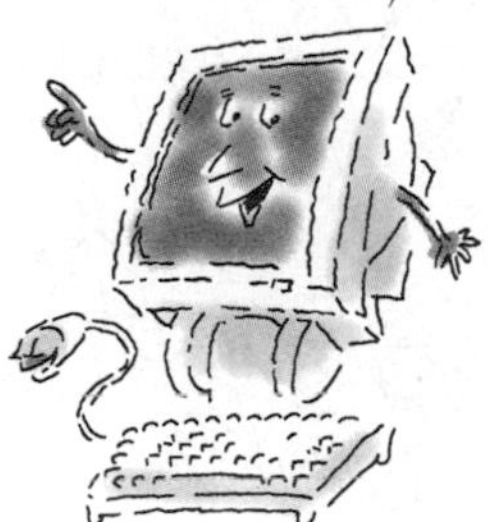

Here are two more questions that address foreign body aspiration.

106. 1. Children should remain seated while eating. The risk of aspiration increases if the child is running, jumping, or talking with food in their mouth. Television and toys are a dangerous distraction to toddlers and young children and should be avoided. Children need constant supervision and should be monitored while eating snacks and meals.

NP: Planning; CN: Safe, effective care environment; CNS: Safety and infection control; CL: Application

107. Which of the following diagnostic tools is best for general diagnosis of foreign body aspiration?

1. Bronchoscopy
2. Chest X-ray
3. Fluoroscopy
4. Lateral neck X-ray

107. 1. Bronchoscopy can give a definitive diagnosis of the presence of foreign bodies and is also the best choice for removal of the object with direct visualization. Chest X-ray and lateral neck X-ray may also be used but findings vary. Some films may appear normal or show changes such as inflammation related to the presence of the foreign body. Fluoroscopy is valuable in detecting and localizing foreign bodies in the bronchi.

NP: Assessment; CN: Physiological integrity; CNS: Physiological adaptation; CL: Knowledge

108. Which of the following definitions best describes cystic fibrosis?

1. An inflammation of the pulmonary parenchyma
2. A chromosomal abnormality inherited as an autosomal-dominant trait
3. A multisymptom disorder affecting the exocrine or mucus-producing glands
4. A chronic lung disease related to high concentrations of oxygen and ventilation

109. Which of the following clinical features would be found in a child with cystic fibrosis?

1. Increase of pancreatic secretions of bicarbonate and chloride
2. Decrease in sodium and chloride in both saliva and sweat
3. Increased viscosity of mucous gland secretions
4. Decreased mucous gland secretions

110. Which of the following signs would the nurse most likely see on assessment of an infant with cystic fibrosis?

1. Constipation
2. Decreased appetite
3. Hyperalbuminemia
4. Meconium ileus

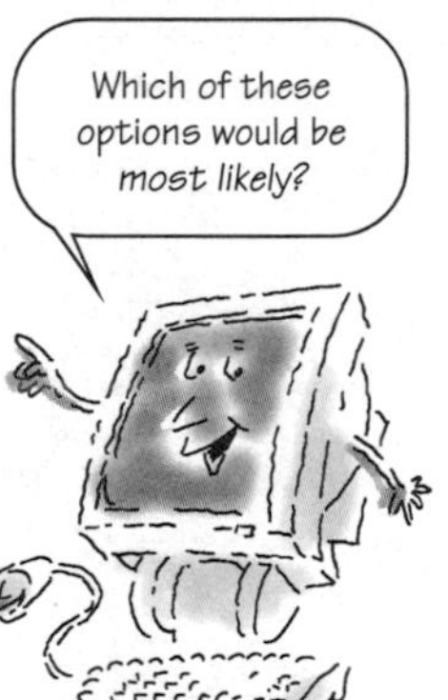

Which of these options would be most likely?

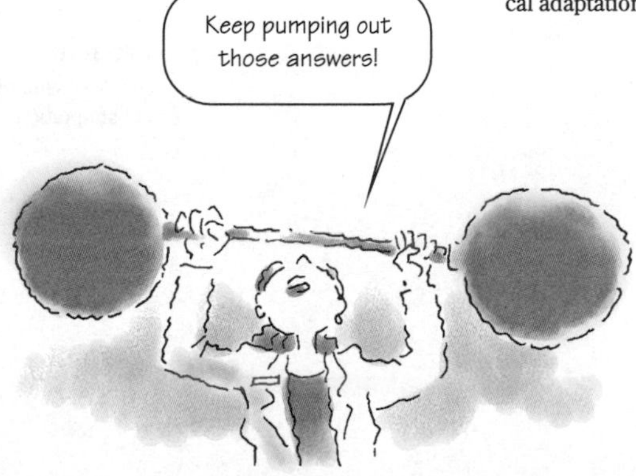

Keep pumping out those answers!

108. 3. Cystic fibrosis affects many organs as well as the exocrine or mucus-producing glands. In cystic fibrosis, an autosomal-recessive chromosomal abnormality, the child inherits its defective genes from both parents. Inflammation of the pulmonary parenchyma describes pneumonia. Bronchopulmonary dysplasia is related to high concentrations of oxygen and ventilation.

NP: Assessment; CN: Physiological integrity; CNS: Physiological adaptation; CL: Knowledge

109. 3. A primary feature of children with cystic fibrosis includes the increased viscosity of mucous gland secretions. Instead of thin, free-flowing secretions, the mucous glands produce a thick mucoprotein that accumulates and dilates them. The electrolytes sodium and chloride are increased in sweat; this forms the basis of the diagnosis of the disorder. Pancreatic enzymes are decreased because mucus secretions block the pancreatic ducts.

NP: Assessment; CN: Physiological integrity; CNS: Physiological adaptation; CL: Knowledge

110. 4. Meconium ileus is commonly a presenting sign of cystic fibrosis. Thick, mucilaginous meconium blocks the lumen of the small intestine, causing intestinal obstruction, abdominal distention, and vomiting. These infants may have an increased appetite related to poor absorption from the intestine. Large-volume, loose, frequent, foul-smelling stools are common. The undigested food is excreted, increasing the bulk of feces. Hypoalbuminemia is a common result from the decreased absorption of protein.

NP: Assessment; CN: Physiological integrity; CNS: Physiological adaptation; CL: Knowledge

111. Which of the following tools are most frequently used to diagnose cystic fibrosis?

1. Chest X-ray
2. Pulmonary function test
3. Stool culture
4. Sweat test

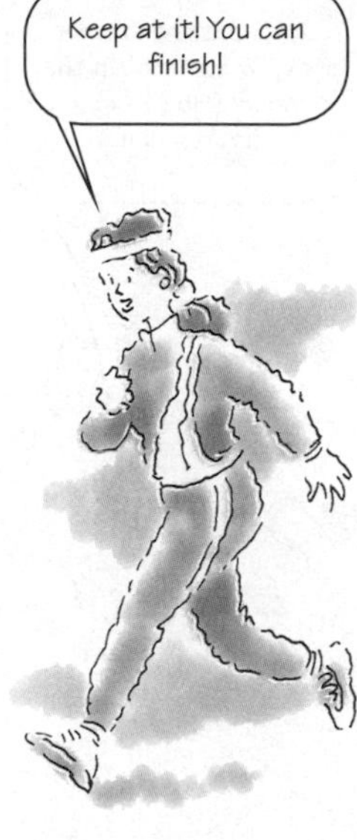

Keep at it! You can finish!

111. 4. A sweat test is the most reliable diagnostic procedure for cystic fibrosis. It involves stimulating the production of sweat, collecting the sweat, and measuring electrolytes in the sweat. Two separate samples are collected to assure reliability of the test. Chest X-rays can show characteristic atelectasis and obstructive emphysema. Pulmonary function tests can show lung function and abnormal small airway function in cystic fibrosis. Stool analysis requires a 72-hour sample with an accurate food intake record.

NP: Analysis; CN: Physiological integrity; CNS: Physiological adaptation; CL: Knowledge

112. Which of the following chloride levels is a diagnostic criteria for cystic fibrosis?

1. Below 20 mEq/L
2. Below 40 mEq/L
3. 40 to 60 mEq/L
4. Above 60 mEq/L

112. 4. A chloride concentration greater than 60 mEq/L is diagnostic of cystic fibrosis. Normal sweat chloride content is less than 40 mEq/L, with the average being 18 mEq/L. Levels between 40 and 60 mEq/L are highly suggestive of cystic fibrosis.

NP: Analysis; CN: Physiological integrity; CNS: Physiological adaptation; CL: Knowledge

113. Which of the following diets is recommended for a child with cystic fibrosis?

1. Fat-restricted diet
2. High-calorie diet
3. Low-protein diet
4. Sodium-restricted diet

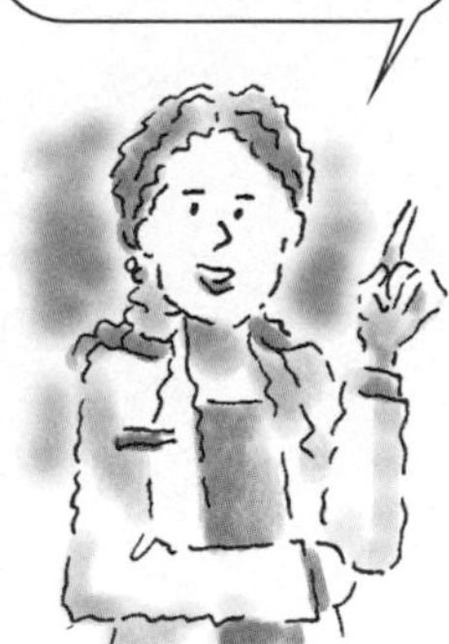

In light of the pathology of cystic fibrosis, which is the only diet that makes sense?

113. 2. A well-balanced high-calorie, high-protein diet is recommended for a child with cystic fibrosis due to the impaired intestinal absorption. Fat restriction isn't required because digestion and absorption of fat in the intestine are impaired. The child usually increases enzyme intake when high-fat foods are eaten. Low-sodium foods can lead to hyponatremia; therefore, high-salt foods are recommended, especially during hot weather or when the child has a fever.

NP: Planning; CN: Safe, effective care environment; CNS: Management of care; CL: Application

114. Which of the following statements concerning pancreatic enzymes for a cystic fibrosis client is correct?

1. Capsules may not be opened.
2. Microcapsules can be crushed.
3. Encourage eating throughout the day.
4. Administer enzymes at each meal and with snacks.

114. 4. Enzymes are administered with each feeding, meal, and snack to optimize absorption of the nutrients consumed. Microcapsules can't be crushed due to the enteric coating. Regular capsules may be opened and the contents mixed with a small amount of applesauce or other nonalkaline food. Eating throughout the day should be discouraged. Three meals and two or three snacks per day are recommended.

NP: Planning; CN: Physiological integrity; CNS: Physiological adaptation; CL: Application

115. Ranitidine (Zantac) is ordered for a 2-year-old child with cystic fibrosis. Which of the following classifications accurately describes this drug?

1. Aluminum salt
2. Antacid
3. Anticholinergic
4. Histamine-2 (H_2) receptor antagonist

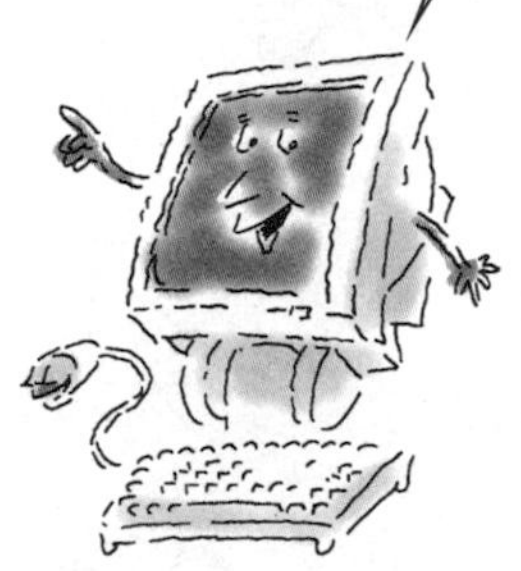

Don't antagonize me, now, I'm just not in the mood! (Hey, Bubba, that's a hint!)

115. 4. Ranitidine acts as an H_2-receptor antagonist. It helps to decrease duodenal acidity and enhance pancreatic enzyme activity. Antacids are used to neutralize gastric acid. Anticholinergics may be used to decrease gastric emptying and to decrease gastric acid secretions. Aluminum salts are used as antacids.

NP: Evaluation; CN: Physiological integrity; CNS: Pharmacological and parenteral therapies; CL: Knowledge

116. The nurse is caring for a client with cystic fibrosis. Ranitidine (Zantac) 4 mg/kg/day every 12 hours is ordered. The child weighs 20 kg. How many milligrams are given per dose?

1. 16 mg
2. 20 mg
3. 40 mg
4. 80 mg

116. 3. The child should receive 40 mg per dose. Here are the calculations: 20 kg × 4 mg/kg = 80 mg; 24 hr/12 hr = 2 doses; 80 mg/2 doses = 40 mg.

NP: Evaluation; CN: Physiological integrity; CNS: Pharmacological and parenteral therapies; CL: Application

117. Which of the following interventions is appropriate for care of the child with cystic fibrosis?

1. Decrease exercise and limit physical activity.
2. Administer cough suppressants and antihistamines.
3. Administer chest physiotherapy two to four times per day.
4. Administer bronchodilator or nebulizer treatments after chest physiotherapy.

117. 3. Chest physiotherapy is recommended two to four times per day to help loosen and move secretions to facilitate expectoration. Exercise and physical activity is recommended to stimulate mucus secretion and to establish a good habitual breathing pattern. Cough suppressants and antihistamines are contraindicated. The goal is for the child to be able to cough and expectorate mucus secretions. Bronchodilator or nebulizer treatments are given before chest physiotherapy to help open the bronchi for easier expectoration.

NP: Implementation; CN: Safe, effective care environment; CNS: Management of care; CL: Application

118. Which of the following statements is appropriate for the nurse to address to the parents of a child with cystic fibrosis who are planning to have a second child?

1. Genetic counseling is recommended.
2. There's a 50% chance the child will be normal.
3. There's a 50% chance of the child being affected.
4. There's a 25% chance the child will only be a carrier.

118. 1. Genetic counseling should be recommended. Cystic fibrosis is an autosomal-recessive disease. Therefore, there's a 25% chance of the child having the disease, a 25% chance of the child being normal, and a 50% chance of the child being a carrier.

NP: Planning; CN: Health promotion and maintenance; CNS: Prevention and early detection of disease; CL: Application

119. Which of the following statements best describes an autosomal-recessive disorder such as cystic fibrosis?
1. The genetic disorder is carried on the X chromosome.
2. Both parents must pass the defective gene or set of genes.
3. Only one defective gene or set of genes is passed by one parent.
4. The child has an extra chromosome, resulting in an XXY karyotype.

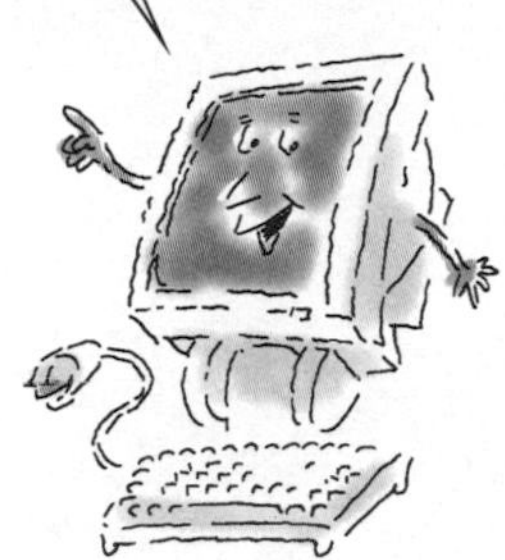

Here's a hint: X doesn't mark the spot on this one!

119. 2. In recessive disorders such as cystic fibrosis, both parents must pass the defective gene or set of genes to the child. Dominant disorders are characterized by only one defective gene or set of genes passed by one parent. Sex-linked genetic disorders are carried on the X chromosome. A child with an XXY karyotype would have Klinefelter's syndrome.

NP: Assessment; CN: Health promotion and maintenance; CNS: Prevention and early detection of disease; CL: Knowledge

120. A 2-year-old client with cystic fibrosis has been diagnosed as having a respiratory infection caused by *Pseudomonas* and ceftazidime (Fortaz) has been ordered. Which of the following classifications is accurate for this drug?
1. Aminoglycoside
2. Cephalosporin
3. Penicillin
4. Sulfonamide

120. 2. Ceftazidime is a third-generation cephalosporin, a class of drugs with extended activity against gram-negative bacteria such as *Pseudomonas.* Aminoglycosides such as gentamicin are also useful in treating gram-negative bacteria. Penicillin can be used to treat gram-positive and gram-negative infections, including pneumonia. Sulfonamides are commonly used to treat urinary tract infections.

NP: Analysis; CN: Physiological integrity; CNS: Pharmacological and parenteral therapies; CL: Knowledge

121. Ceftazidime (Fortaz) has been ordered for a client with cystic fibrosis. The order states to give 40 mg/kg every 8 hours. The child is 2 years old and weighs 38.5 lb. How many milligrams of the ceftazidime is given in one dose?
1. 116 mg
2. 233 mg
3. 260 mg
4. 466 mg

121. 2. The child should receive 233 mg per dose. Here are the calculations: 38.5 lb/2.2 kg = 17.5 kg (1 lb equals 2.2 kg); 40 mg/kg × 17.5 kg = 700 mg; 24 hours/8 hours = 3 doses; 700 mg/3 doses = 233 mg.

NP: Evaluation; CN: Physiological integrity; CNS: Pharmacological and parenteral therapies; CL: Application

122. A child with cystic fibrosis is placed on an oral antibiotic to be given in four equally divided doses per day for 14 days. Which of the following time schedules is most appropriate?
1. 8 a.m., 12 p.m., 4 p.m., 8 p.m.
2. 8 a.m., 2 p.m., 8 p.m., 2 a.m.
3. 9 a.m., 1 p.m., 5 p.m., 9 p.m.
4. 10 a.m., 2 p.m., 6 p.m., 10 p.m.

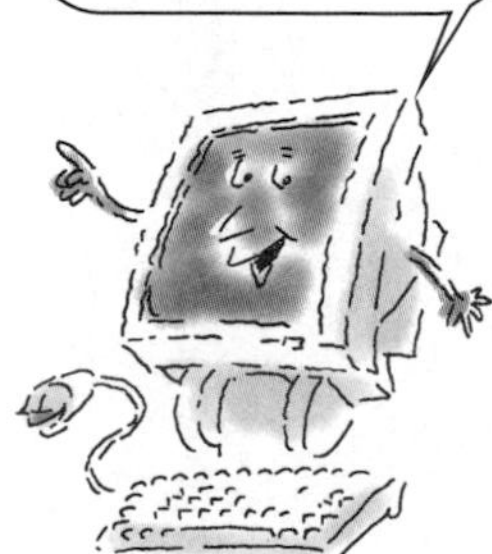

Pay attention to the intervals between doses when answering this one!

122. 2. The doses should be given routinely every 6 hours. This helps to maintain a therapeutic blood level of the antibiotic. The other answers have doses only every 4 hours during the day and then no doses for 12 hours at night.

NP: Planning; CN: Physiological integrity; CNS: Pharmacological and parenteral therapies; CL: Analysis

123. Which of the following complications of cystic fibrosis may eventually lead to death?

1. Rectal prolapse
2. Pulmonary obstruction
3. Gastroesophageal reflux
4. Reproductive system obstruction

123. 2. Pulmonary obstruction related to thickened mucus secretions can lead to a progressive pulmonary disturbance and secondary infections that can lead to death. Obstruction of the reproductive system can lead to infertility due to increased mucus blocking sperm entry in the female or blockage of the vas deferens in the male. Rectal prolapse is managed with enzyme replacement therapy and manipulation of the rectum back into place. Gastroesophageal reflux can be managed with medications and proper reflux precautions.

NP: Evaluation; CN: Physiological integrity; CNS: Physiological adaptation; CL: Analysis

124. Which of the following methods is best for evaluation of a 6-year-old child with cystic fibrosis who has been placed on an aerosol inhaler?

1. Ask if the parents have any questions.
2. Ask if the child can explain the procedure.
3. Ask the parents if they understand the usage.
4. Ask the client to perform a return demonstration.

124. 4. A return demonstration is the best evaluation. It will show if the client can repeat the steps shown and appropriately use the inhaler. The child may have difficulty explaining the procedure at age 6. The parents should understand how the inhaler should be used and ask questions, but the child must be able to correctly demonstrate usage first.

NP: Evaluation; CN: Physiological integrity; CNS: Pharmacological and parenteral therapies; CL: Application

125. Which of the following interventions is appropriate for a 2-year-old client with chest trauma who has a left lower chest tube in place?

1. Stripping or milking the tubing
2. Requiring routine dressing changes
3. Clamping the chest tube during transport
4. Inspecting tubing for kinks or obstructions

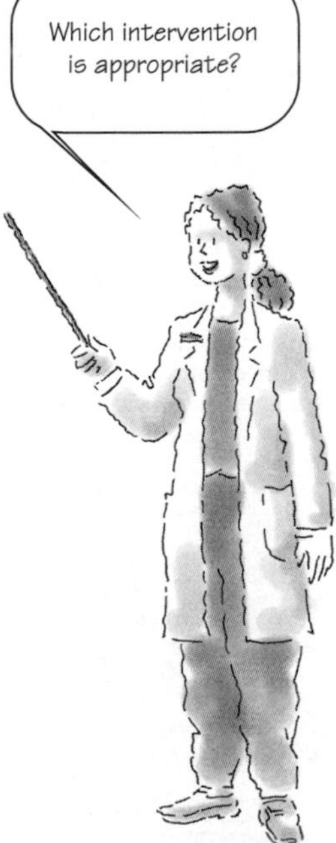
Which intervention is appropriate?

125. 4. Tubing should be inspected for kinks or obstructions so that drainage can flow freely. Manipulation of the tubing should be avoided. The pressure created from stripping can damage the pleural space or mediastinum. There's no need for routine dressing changes if the dressing isn't soiled and there's no evidence of infection. Inspect and palpate around the dressing routinely. The chest tube should never be clamped because it may lead to a tension pneumothorax. Waterseal will protect the client during transit.

NP: Implementation; CN: Physiological integrity; CNS: Physiological adaptation; CL: Application

126. A toddler in respiratory distress is admitted to the pediatric intensive care unit. When he refuses to keep his oxygen face mask on, his mother tries to help. Which action by the nurse is most appropriate?

1. Giving the child his favorite toy to play with
2. Having the mother read the child's favorite book to him
3. Administering a strong sedative so the child will sleep
4. Telling the child that the face mask will help him breathe better

126. 2. Having the mother read the child's favorite book will ease his anxiety and provide comfort to the child. Although giving the child a favorite toy is also appropriate, the child needs his mother's comfort because the face mask is frightening. Sedation is contraindicated because it can hide signs of respiratory distress. A toddler is too young to understand that something will make him feel better.

NP: Implementation; CN: Safe, effective environment; CNS: Management of care; CL: Application

Which is *not* a symptom? Remember the word *not*.

127. A 12-year-old girl is discharged from the hospital after an acute asthma attack. She has received a prescription for theophylline (Theo-Dur). Which is not a symptom of theophylline toxicity?

1. Vomiting
2. Increased wheezing
3. Diarrhea
4. Headache

127. 2. Increased wheezing and respiratory distress aren't signs and symptoms of theophylline toxicity but rather herald subtherapeutic levels. Vomiting, diarrhea, and headache are signs of theophylline toxicity.

NP: Evaluation; CN: Physiological integrity; CNS: Pharmacological and parenteral therapies; CL: Analysis

128. A 6-year-old with a history of asthma is being evaluated by an allergist, who orders skin testing to be done at the next visit. Which action by the nurse will help ensure accurate skin testing results?

1. Making sure the child doesn't have a runny nose
2. Making sure the child hasn't received antihistamines in the past 7 days
3. Using the child's posterior legs for testing
4. Limiting testing to environmental allergens

128. 2. Antihistamines may alter results of skin testing and should be withheld at least 1 week before testing. A runny nose won't alter test results. The forearm and upper back are the best sites for allergy testing. Testing only for environmental allergens precludes diagnosis of allergies to other substances.

NP: Assessment; CN: Physiological integrity; CNS: Pharmacological and parenteral therapies; CL: Application

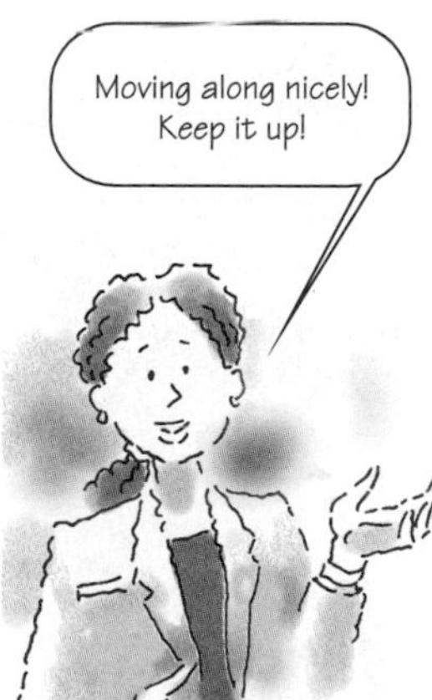
Moving along nicely! Keep it up!

129. For 30 minutes after receiving an allergy shot, a child must be observed for signs and symptoms of anaphylaxis. Which condition may result from anaphylactic shock?

1. Anuria
2. Bradycardia
3. Hypotension
4. Rash

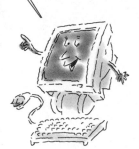

129. 3. Anaphylaxis can cause hypotension and tachycardia (not bradycardia). Urinary urgency and incontinence, not anuria, may also be reported. A rash may signal an allergic reaction, but not a severe one such as anaphylaxis.

NP: Assessment; CN: Physiological integrity; CNS: Physiological adaptation; CL: Knowledge

130. A child is diagnosed with an allergy to dust mites. To limit her exposure to dust mites, which measure should the nurse recommend to the family?

1. Removing all stuffed animals from the child's room
2. Getting rid of the family dog or keeping it away from the child
3. Forbidding smoking in the home
4. Using the air conditioner instead of opening windows

130. 1. Stuffed animals are notorious dust collectors and should be removed from the child's room. Getting rid of the family dog would eliminate animal dander but not dust mites. Smoking is an irritant, not an allergen. Using the air conditioner decreases exposure to pollen, not dust mites.

NP: Implementation; CN: Health promotion and maintenance; CNS: Prevention and early detection of disease; CL: Application

131. A 6-year-old child is admitted after falling from a jungle gym. He has bruising over the left rib cage and is in respiratory distress. Which assessment finding supports the nurse's suspicion that he has pneumothorax from blunt chest trauma?

1. Productive cough
2. Wheezing
3. Diminished breath sounds on the affected side
4. Clubbing of the fingers and toes

131. 3. In pneumothorax, breath sounds are diminished on the affected side as air collects between the pleural layers, causing the lung to collapse. A productive cough accompanies a respiratory infection such as pneumonia. Wheezing signals airway obstruction such as in asthma. Clubbing of the fingers and toes is a long-term effect of chronic hypoxia.

NP: Assessment; CN: Physiological integrity; CNS: Physiological adaptation; CL: Knowledge

132. A 6-year-old child undergoes thoracostomy and insertion of a chest tube attached to a closed-chest drainage system. For which purpose is water in the closed-chest drainage system?

1. It decreases the risk of a sudden pressure change in the tube.
2. It prevents air from entering the pleural cavity.
3. It allows faster removal of chest secretions from the pleural cavity.
4 It promotes emptying of bloody drainage from the pleural space.

132. 2. The water prevents entrance of air into the pleural cavity. Checking and taping connections prevents sudden pressure changes. Suction promotes faster removal of chest secretions, including blood.

NP: Planning; CN: Physiological integrity; CNS: Reduction of risk potential; CL: Analysis

133. A 2-year-old toddler is admitted to a pediatric unit for a lower respiratory tract infection. Because this is the third infection he has had within the last year, the physician orders a tuberculin skin test. Which site is best for this intradermal test?

1. Upper thigh
2. Scapular area
3. Back
4. Ventral forearm

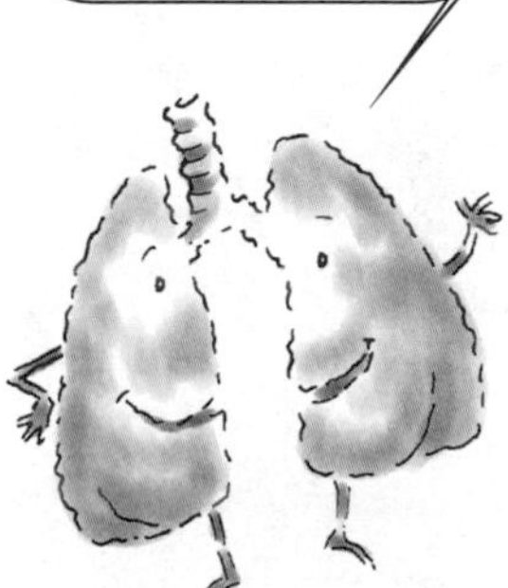

You finished chapter 29! Now you can breathe easier.

133. 4. The ventral forearm is the preferred site for the tuberculin skin test. The upper thigh is used for subcutaneous and I.M. injections. The scapular area and back are used for allergy skin testing.

NP: Implementation; CN: Physiological integrity; CNS: Pharmacological and parenteral therapies; CL: Application

Here are three Internet sites you can check for more information about neurosensory disorders in children: **www.add.org** (Attention Deficit Disorder Association), **www.ndss.org** (National Down Syndrome Society), and **www.sbaa.org** (Spina Bifida Association of America).

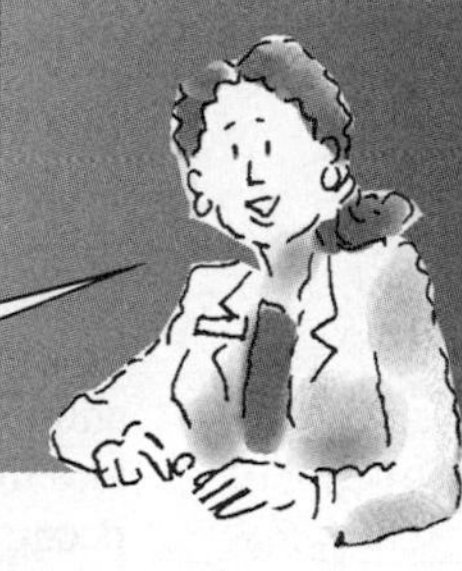

Chapter 30 Neurosensory disorders

1. The mother of a 3-year-old with a myelomeningocele is thinking about having another baby. The nurse should inform the woman that she should increase her intake of which of the following acids?

1. Folic acid to 0.4 mg/day
2. Folic acid to 4.0 mg/day
3. Ascorbic acid to 0.4 mg/day
4. Ascorbic acid to 4.0 mg/day

1. 2. The American Academy of Pediatrics recommends that a woman who has had a child with a neural tube defect increase her intake of folic acid to 4.0 mg per day one month before becoming pregnant and continue this regimen through the first trimester. A woman who has no family history of neural tube defects should take 0.4 mg. All women of childbearing age should be encouraged to take a folic acid supplement because the majority of pregnancies in the United States are unplanned. Ascorbic acid hasn't been shown to have any effect on preventing neural tube defects.

NP: Implementation; CN: Health promotion and maintenance; CNS: Prevention and early detection of disease; CL: Application

Most relevant — that's the key phrase for question 2.

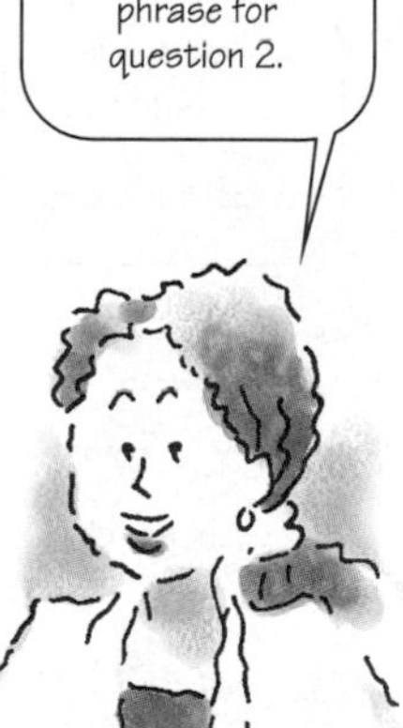

2. Which of the following nursing diagnoses is most relevant in the first 12 hours of life for a neonate born with a myelomeningocele?

1. Risk for infection
2. Colonic constipation
3. Impaired physical mobility
4. Delayed growth and development

2. 1. All of these diagnoses are important for a child with a myelomeningocele. However, during the first 12 hours of life, the most life-threatening event would be an infection. The other diagnoses will be addressed as the child develops.

NP: Planning; CN: Physiological integrity; CNS: Reduction of risk potential; CL: Application

3. Which of the following conditions would the nurse expect when assessing a neonate for hydrocephalus?

1. Bulging fontanel, low-pitched cry
2. Depressed fontanel, low-pitched cry
3. Bulging fontanel, eyes rotated downward
4. Depressed fontanel, eyes rotated downward

3. 3. Hydrocephalus is caused from the alteration in circulation of the cerebrospinal fluid (CSF). The amount of CSF increases, causing the fontanel to bulge. This also causes an increase in intracranial pressure. This increase in pressure causes the neonate's eyes to deviate downward (the "setting sun sign"), and the neonate's cry becomes high-pitched.

NP: Assessment; CN: Health promotion and maintenance; CNS: Prevention and early detection of disease; CL: Knowledge

4. A 2-year-old child is admitted to the hospital for revision of a ventriculoperitoneal shunt. Which of the following complications is the most common reason for a revision?

1. Shunt infection
2. A broken shunt
3. Growth of the child
4. Heart failure

4. 3. This type of shunt has to be replaced periodically as the child grows and the tubing becomes too short. Shunt infection usually occurs within 2 to 3 months of insertion, not at 2 years. The shunts rarely break, unless there's head trauma. The fluid from a ventriculoperitoneal shunt goes into the peritoneal cavity and not into the heart; therefore, heart failure shouldn't occur.

NP: Analysis; CN: Health promotion and maintenance; CNS: Growth and development through the life span; CL: Knowledge

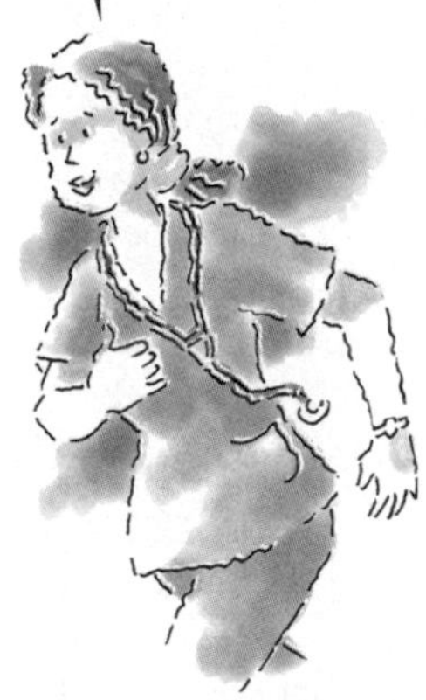

Remember, in emergency situations, your first priority is to ensure the client's safety.

5. Which of the following nursing actions is appropriate when a child has a seizure?

1. Inserting a nasogastric tube to prevent emesis
2. Restraining the extremities with a pillow or blanket
3. Inserting a tongue blade to prevent injury to the tongue
4. Padding the side rails of the bed to protect the child from injury

5. 4. A child having a seizure could fall out of bed or injure himself on anything, including the side rails of the bed. Attempts to insert anything into the child's mouth may injure the child. Attempting to restrain the child can't stop seizures. In fact, tactile stimulation may increase the seizure activity; therefore, it must be limited as much as possible.

NP: Implementation; CN: Safe, effective care environment; CNS: Safety and infection control; CL: Application

6. A mother brings her infant to the emergency department and says he had a seizure. While the nurse is obtaining a history, the mother says she was running out of formula so she stretched the formula by adding three times the normal amount of water. Electrolytes and blood glucose levels are drawn on the infant. The nurse would expect which of the following laboratory values?

1. Blood glucose: 120 mg/dl
2. Chloride: 104 mmol/L
3. Potassium: 4.0 mmol/L
4. Sodium: 125 mmol/L

6. 4. Diluting formula in a different manner than is recommended alters the infant's electrolyte levels. Normal serum sodium for an infant is 135 to 145 mmol/L. When formula is diluted, the infant's sodium is also diluted and will decrease. Hyponatremia is one of the causes of seizures in infants. The other values are all within normal limits.

NP: Evaluation; CN: Physiological integrity; CNS: Physiological adaptation; CL: Analysis

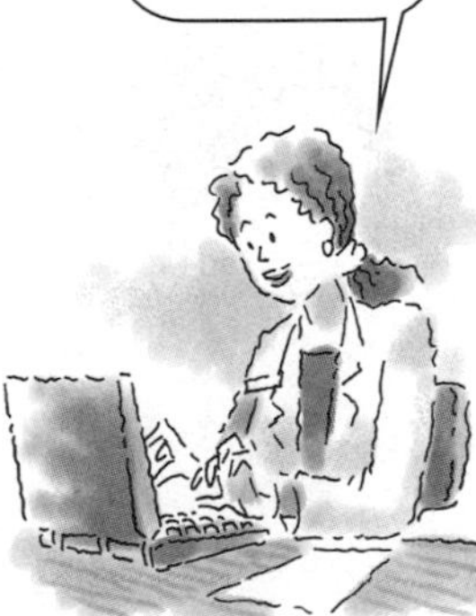

For the NCLEX, you need to be familiar with normal lab values.

7. For which of the following symptoms will the nurse assess a neonate diagnosed with bacterial meningitis?

1. Temperature instability, irritability, and poor feeding
2. Positive Babinski's reflex, mottling, and pallor
3. Headache, nuchal rigidity, and developmental delays
4. Positive Moro's embrace reflex, hyperthermia, and sunken fontanel

7. 1. The clinical appearance of a neonate with meningitis is different from that of a child or an adult. Neonates may be either hypothermic or hyperthermic. The irritation to the meninges causes the neonates to be irritable and to have a decreased appetite. They may be pale and mottled with a bulging, full fontanel. Older children and adults with meningitis have headaches, nuchal rigidity, and hyperthermia as clinical manifestations. Normal neonates have positive Moro's embrace and Babinski's reflexes.

NP: Assessment; CN: Physiological integrity; CNS: Physiological adaptation; CL: Comprehension

16. A preschool-age child has just been admitted to the pediatric unit with a diagnosis of bacterial meningitis. The nurse would include which of the following recommendations in the nursing plan?

1. Take vital signs every 4 hours.
2. Monitor temperature every 4 hours.
3. Decrease environmental stimulation.
4. Encourage the parents to hold the child.

16. 3. A child with the diagnosis of meningitis is much more comfortable with decreased environmental stimuli. Noise and bright lights stimulate the child and can be irritating, causing the child to cry, in turn increasing intracranial pressure. Vital signs would be taken initially every hour and temperature monitored every two hours. Children are usually much more comfortable if allowed to lie flat because this position doesn't cause increased meningeal irritation.

NP: Planning; CN: Physiological integrity; CNS: Physiological adaptation; CL: Application

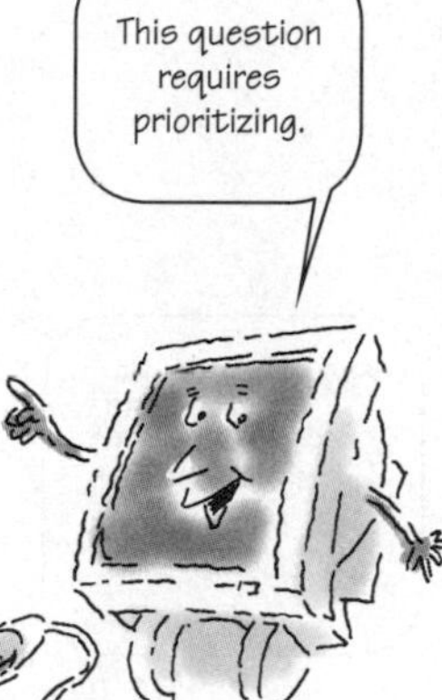
This question requires prioritizing.

17. A child has just returned to the pediatric unit following ventriculoperitoneal shunt placement for hydrocephalus. Which of the following interventions would the nurse perform first?

1. Assess intake and output.
2. Place the child on the side opposite the shunt.
3. Offer fluids because the child has a dry mouth.
4. Administer pain medication by mouth as ordered.

17. 2. Following shunt placement surgery, the child should be placed on the side opposite of the surgical site to prevent pressure on the shunt valve. Intake and output will be assessed, but that isn't the priority nursing intervention. Many children are nauseated after a general anesthetic, and ice chips or clear liquids would be introduced after the nurse had determined if the child was nauseated. Pain medication should be administered by an I.V. route initially postoperatively.

NP: Implementation; CN: Physiological integrity; CNS: Basic care and comfort; CL: Application

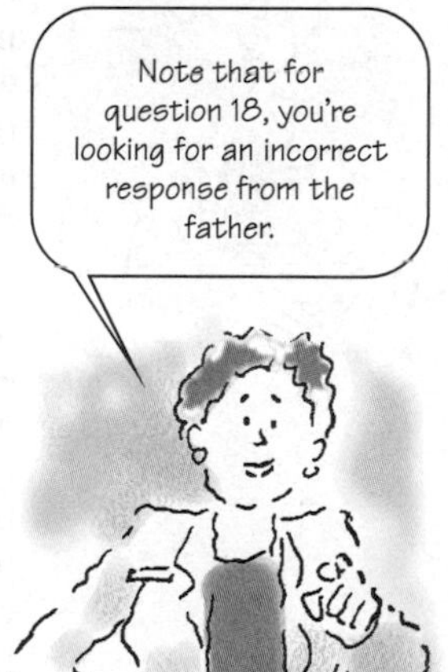
Note that for question 18, you're looking for an incorrect response from the father.

18. An otherwise healthy 18-month-old child has a history of febrile seizures and is in the well-child clinic today. Which of the following statements by the father would indicate to the nurse that additional teaching needs to be done?

1. "I have ibuprofen available in case it's needed."
2. "My child will outgrow these seizures by age 5."
3. "I always keep phenobarbital with me in case of a fever."
4. "The most likely time for a seizure is when the fever is rising."

18. 3. Anticonvulsant drugs, such as phenobarbital, are administered to children with prolonged seizures or neurologic abnormalities. Ibuprofen, not phenobarbital, is given for fever. Febrile seizures usually occur after 6 months of age and are unusual after 5 years of age. Treatment is to decrease the temperature because seizures occur as the temperature rises.

NP: Evaluation; CN: Health promotion and maintenance; CNS: Prevention and early detection of disease; CL: Application

19. When assessing a 5-month-old infant, which of the following symptoms would alert the nurse that the infant needs further follow-up?

1. Absent grasp reflex
2. Rolls from back to side
3. Balances head when sitting
4. Moro's embrace reflex present

19. 4. Moro's embrace reflex should be absent at 4 months. Grasp reflex begins to fade at 2 months and should be absent at 3 months. A 4-month-old infant should be able to roll from back to side and balance his head when sitting.

NP: Assessment; CN: Health promotion and maintenance; CNS: Prevention and early detection of disease; CL: Application

20. An adolescent is started on valproic acid to treat seizures. Which of the following statements should be included when educating the adolescent?

1. This medication has no adverse effects.
2. A common adverse effect is weight gain.
3. Drowsiness and irritability occur frequently.
4. Early morning dosing is recommended to decrease insomnia.

20. 2. Weight gain is a common adverse effect of valproic acid. Drowsiness and irritability are adverse effects more commonly associated with phenobarbital. Felbamate (Felbatol) more commonly causes insomnia.

NP: Application; CN: Physiological integrity; CNS: Pharmacological and parenteral therapies; CL: Application

21. Which of the following statements about cerebral palsy would be accurate?

1. Cerebral palsy is a condition that runs in families.
2. Cerebral palsy means there will be many disabilities.
3. Cerebral palsy is a condition that doesn't get worse.
4. Cerebral palsy occurs because of too much oxygen to the brain.

21. 3. By definition, cerebral palsy is a nonprogressive neuromuscular disorder. It can be mild or quite severe and is believed to be the result of a hypoxia event during the pregnancy or the birth process.

NP: Evaluation; CN: Physiological integrity; CNS: Physiological adaptation; CL: Application

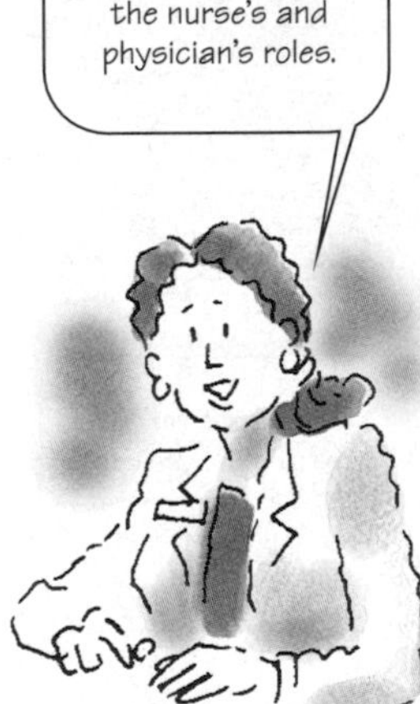

For question 22, keep in mind the difference between the nurse's and physician's roles.

22. An older child has a craniotomy for removal of a brain tumor. Which of the following statements would be appropriate for the nurse to say to the parents?

1. "Your child really had a close call."
2. "I'm sure your child will be back to normal soon."
3. "I'm so glad to hear your child doesn't have cancer."
4. "It may take some time for your child to return to normal."

22. 4. When comforting parents, it's best to first ascertain what the primary health care provider has told them about the tumor. Final pathology results won't be available for several days, so refrain from making premature statements about whether the tumor is malignant or not. Usually after a craniotomy, it takes several weeks or longer before the child is back to normal.

NP: Implementation; CN: Psychosocial integrity; CNS: Coping and adaptation; CL: Application

23. A 6-month-old infant is being admitted with a diagnosis of bacterial meningitis. The nurse would place the infant in which of the following rooms?

1. A room with a 12-month-old infant with urinary tract infection
2. A room with an 8-month-old infant with failure to thrive
3. An isolation room near the nurses' station
4. A two-bed room in the middle of the hall

23. 3. A child who has the diagnosis of bacterial meningitis will need to be placed in isolation near the nurses' station until that child has received I.V. antibiotics for 24 hours. The child is considered contagious. Additionally, bacterial meningitis can be quite serious; therefore, the child should be placed near the nurse's station for close monitoring and easier access in case of a crisis.

NP: Implementation; CN: Safe, effective care environment; CNS: Management of care; CL: Application

40. Diagnosis of meningitis can be established based on which of the following findings of cerebrospinal fluid (CSF) analysis and blood cultures?

1. Increased glucose content in spinal fluid
2. Decreased protein content in spinal fluid
3. Consistently elevated spinal fluid pressure
4. Positive blood culture in greater than 90% of the cases

40. 3. Spinal fluid pressure is consistently increased in bacterial meningitis. Depending on the age of the client and the type of organism involved, blood cultures are positive in 40% to 60% of the cases. The CSF sample typically reveals an increase in protein levels and a decrease in the glucose levels.

NP: Assessment; CN: Physiological integrity; CNS: Physiological adaptation; CL: Knowledge

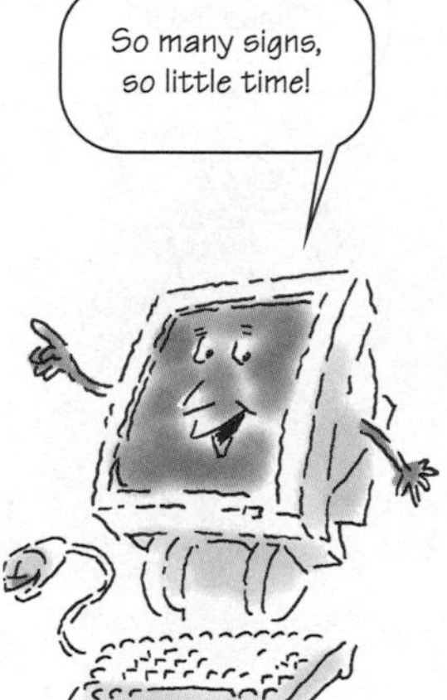
So many signs,
so little time!

41. Which of the following assessment data indicates nuchal rigidity?

1. Positive Kernig's sign
2. Negative Brudzinski's sign
3. Positive Homans' sign
4. Negative Kernig's sign

41. 1. A positive Kernig's sign indicates nuchal rigidity, caused by an irritative lesion of the subarachnoid space. Brudzinski's sign is also indicative of the condition. Homans' sign indicates venous inflammation of the lower leg, not nuchal rigidity.

NP: Analysis; CN: Physiological integrity; CNS: Physiological adaptation; CL: Knowledge

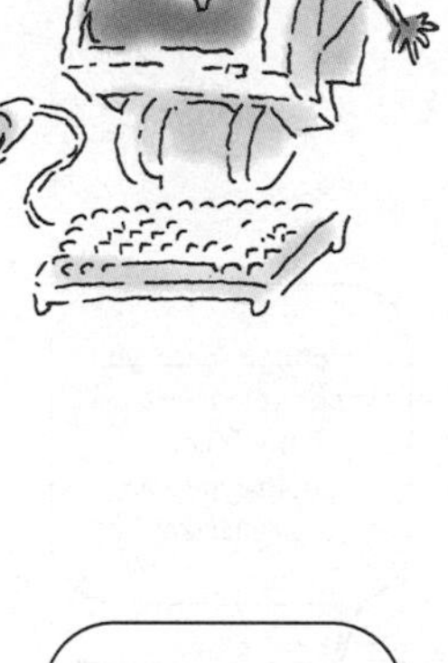

42. Meningitis occurs as an extension of a variety of bacterial infections due to which of the following conditions?

1. Congenital anatomic abnormality of the meninges
2. Lack of acquired resistance to the various etiologic organisms
3. Occlusion or narrowing of the cerebrospinal fluid pathway
4. Natural affinity of the central nervous system (CNS) to certain pathogens

42. 2. Extension of a variety of bacterial infections is a major causative factor of meningitis and occurs as a result of a lack of acquired resistance to the etiologic organisms. Preexisting CNS anomalies are factors that contribute to susceptibility. Certain specific organisms have been identified as causative, such as *H. influenzae, S. pneumoniae, N. meningitidis, S. aureus, E. coli,* and *L. monocytogenes.*

NP: Analysis; CN: Physiological integrity; CNS: Physiological adaptation; CL: Comprehension

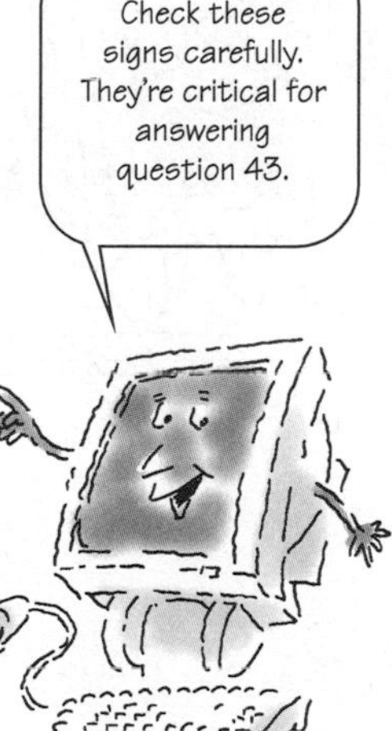
Check these
signs carefully.
They're critical for
answering
question 43.

43. A child with a diagnosis of meningococcal meningitis develops signs of sepsis and a purpuric rash over both lower extremities. The primary health care provider should be notified immediately because these signs could be indicative of which of the following complications?

1. A severe allergic reaction to the antibiotic regimen with impending anaphylaxis
2. Onset of the syndrome of inappropriate antidiuretic hormone (SIADH)
3. Meningococcemia
4. Adhesive arachnoiditis

43. 3. Meningococcemia is a serious complication usually associated with meningococcal infection. Anaphylactic shock would need to be differentiated from septic shock. SIADH can be an acute complication, but it wouldn't be accompanied by the purpuric rash. Adhesive arachnoiditis occurs in the chronic phase of the disease and leads to obstruction of the flow of cerebrospinal fluid.

NP: Implementation; CN: Physiological integrity; CNS: Reduction of risk potential; CL: Application

44. Which of the following pathologic processes is often associated with aseptic meningitis?
1. Ischemic infarction of cerebral tissue
2. Childhood diseases of viral causation such as mumps
3. Brain abscess caused by a variety of pyogenic organisms
4. Cerebral ventricular irritation from a traumatic brain injury

44. 2. Aseptic meningitis is caused principally by viruses and is often associated with other diseases such as measles, mumps, herpes, and leukemia. Incidence of brain abscess is high in bacterial meningitis, and ischemic infarction of cerebral tissue can occur with tubercular meningitis. Traumatic brain injury could lead to bacterial (not viral) meningitis.

NP: Assessment; CN: Physiological integrity; CNS: Physiological adaptation; CL: Knowledge

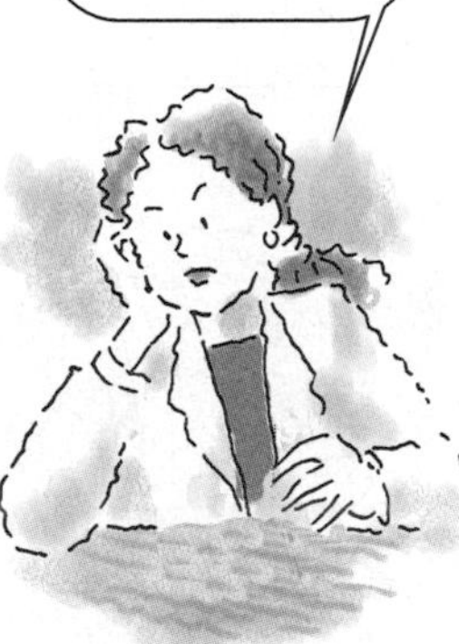

I see you've finished 44 questions. Super! Are we having fun yet? I know I am. (Chaaa, as if.)

45. To alleviate the child's pain and fear of lumbar puncture, which of the following interventions should the nurse perform?
1. Sedate the child with fentanyl citrate (Sublimaze).
2. Apply a topical anesthetic to the skin 5-10 minutes prepuncture.
3. Have a parent hold the child in their lap during the tap procedure.
4. Have the child inhale small amounts of nitrous oxide gas prepuncture.

45. 1. Sedation with fentanyl citrate or other drugs can alleviate the pain and fear associated with a lumbar puncture. A topical anesthetic can be applied, but it should be done 1 hour before the procedure to be fully effective. Parents holding a child in their lap increases the risk of neurologic injury due to the inability to assume and maintain the proper anatomic position required for a safe lumbar puncture. Use of nitrous oxide gas isn't recommended.

NP: Implementation; CN: Physiological integrity; CNS: Basic care and comfort; CL: Application

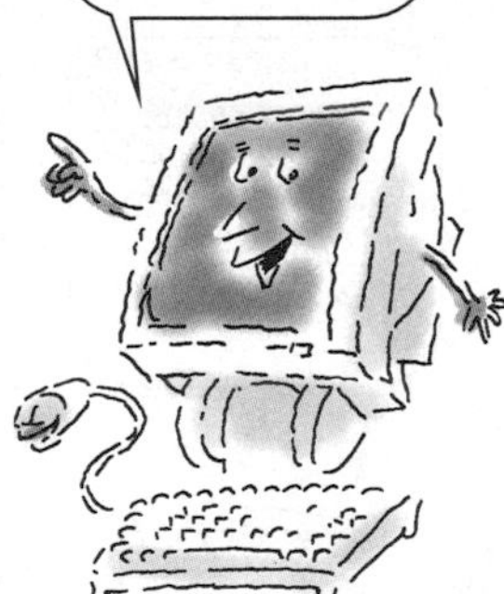

Hear ye, hear ye, hear ye! Prioritize, my fellow countrypeople, prioritize!

46. Antimicrobial therapy to treat meningitis should be instituted immediately after which of the following events?
1. Admission to the nursing unit
2. Initiation of I.V. therapy
3. Identification of the causative organism
4. Collection of cerebrospinal fluid (CSF) and blood for culture

46. 4. Antibiotics are always begun immediately after the collection of CSF and blood cultures. After the specific organism is identified, bacteria-specific antibiotics can be administered if the organism isn't covered by the initial choice of antibiotic therapy. Admission and initiation of I.V. therapy aren't, by themselves, appropriate times to begin antimicrobial therapy.

NP: Planning; CN: Physiological integrity; CNS: Pharmacological and parenteral therapies; CL: Analysis

47. Steroid therapy (dexamethasone) is commonly used in conjunction with antimicrobial therapy in treating a child with meningitis for which of the following reasons?
1. Treatment of choice in aseptic meningitis
2. Prevention of GI hemorrhage
3. Management of problems related to blood pressure
4. Prevention of deafness with *Haemophilus influenzae* meningitis

47. 4. Dexamethasone may play a role in the prevention of bilateral deafness in children with *H. influenzae* type b meningitis, and its use is recommended by the American Academy of Pediatrics. Use of dexamethasone could complicate rather than prevent GI bleeding and problems related to blood pressure. Treatment of aseptic meningitis is primarily symptomatic with acetaminophen for headache and muscle pain and positioning for comfort.

NP: Implementation; CN: Physiological integrity; CNS: Pharmacological and parenteral therapies; CL: Knowledge

48. Which of the following descriptions is accurate about the incidence of sequelae in a client with bacterial meningitis?
1. Occur during the first 2 months of life
2. Occur in children with meningococcal meningitis
3. Primarily involve the fourth ventricle of the brain
4. Tend to affect the ocular nerves, leading to retinal damage

48. 1. In infants under age 2 months with bacterial meningitis, communicating hydrocephalus and the effects of cerebritis on the immature brain leads to the frequent occurrence of sequelae. Sequelae are least often seen in children experiencing meningococcal meningitis. Meningitis primarily affects the nerves for hearing rather than vision.

NP: Planning; CN: Physiological integrity; CNS: Physiological adaptation; CL: Application

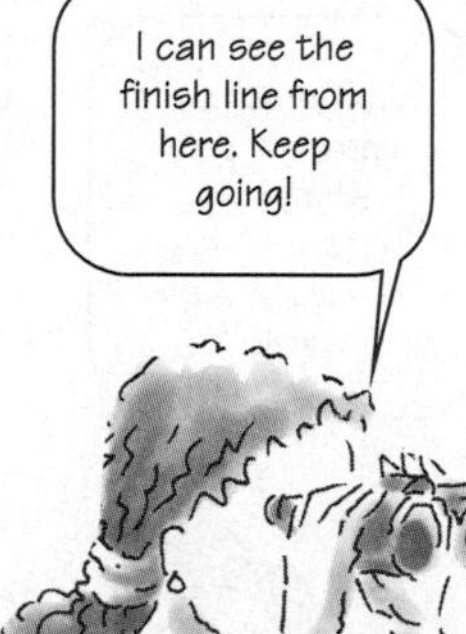

49. Which of the following goals of nursing care is the most difficult to accomplish in caring for a child with meningitis?
1. Protecting self and others from possible infection
2. Avoiding actions that increase discomfort such as lifting the head
3. Keeping environmental stimuli to a minimum such as reduced light and noise
4. Maintaining I.V. infusion to administer adequate antimicrobial therapy

49. 4. One of the most difficult problems in the nursing care of children with meningitis is maintaining the I.V. infusion for the length of time needed to provide adequate therapy. All of the other options are important aspects in the provision of care to the child with meningitis, but they're secondary to antimicrobial therapy.

NP: Implementation; CN: Physiological integrity; CNS: Basic care and comfort; CL: Application

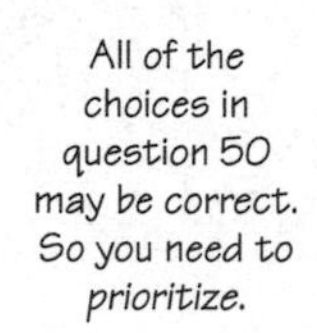

All of the choices in question 50 may be correct. So you need to prioritize.

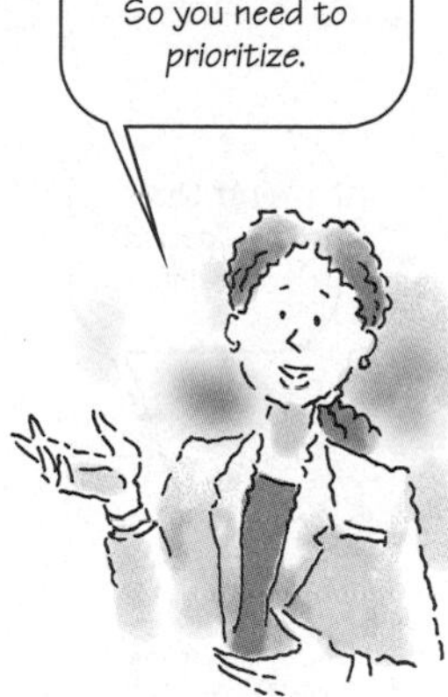

50. Which of the following nursing assessment data should be given the highest priority for a child with clinical findings related to tubercular meningitis?
1. Onset and character of fever
2. Degree and extent of nuchal rigidity
3. Signs of increased intracranial pressure (ICP)
4. Occurrence of urine and fecal contamination

50. 3. Assessment of fever and evaluation of nuchal rigidity are important aspects of care, but assessment for signs of increasing ICP should be the highest priority due to the life-threatening implications. Urinary and fecal incontinence can occur in a child who's ill from nearly any cause but don't pose a great danger to life.

NP: Implementation; CN: Physiological integrity; CNS: Reduction of risk potential; CL: Analysis

51. The clinical manifestations of acute bacterial meningitis are dependent on which of the following factors?
1. Age of the child
2. Length of the prodromal period
3. Time span from bacterial invasion to onset of symptoms
4. Degree of elevation of cerebrospinal fluid (CSF) glucose compared to serum glucose level

51. 1. Clinical manifestations of acute bacterial meningitis depend largely on the age of the child. Clinical manifestations aren't dependent on the prodromal or initial period of the disease nor the time from invasion of the host to the onset of the symptoms. The glucose level of the CSF is reduced, not elevated. A serum glucose level is drawn one-half hour before lumbar puncture so that the relationship between the CSF glucose and the serum glucose levels can be determined.

NP: Assessment; CN: Physiological integrity; CNS: Physiological adaptation; CL: Application

52. Which of the following responses is most appropriate for a mother who asks why her son would begin having seizures without warning and in the absence of injury?

1. Clonic seizure activity is usually interpreted as falling.
2. A delay between head injury and the development of seizures isn't unusual.
3. Focal discharge in the brain may lead to absence seizures that go unnoticed.
4. The epileptogenic focus in the brain needs multiple stimuli before it will discharge to cause a seizure.

52. 2. Stimuli from an earlier injury may eventually elicit seizure activity, a process known as kindling. Atonic seizures, not clonic, are frequently accompanied by falling. Focal seizures are partial seizures; absence seizures are generalized seizures. Focal seizures don't lead to absence seizures. The epileptogenic focus consists of a group of hyperexcitable neurons responsible for initiating synchronous, high-frequency discharges leading to a seizure rather than needing multiple stimuli.

NP: Analysis; CN: Physiological integrity; CNS: Physiological adaptation; CL: Comprehension

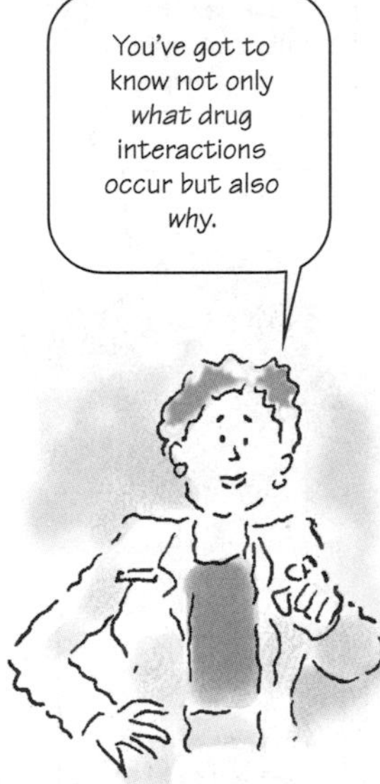

You've got to know not only what drug interactions occur but also why.

53. Which of the following actions describe how anticonvulsant drugs work?

1. Suppression of sodium influx through the gated pores in the cell membrane
2. Enhancement of calcium influx through the gated pores in the cell membrane
3. Potentiation of dopamine, facilitating passage across the neuronal cell membrane
4. Suppression of potassium removal from the neuronal intracellular compartment

53. 1. Anticonvulsant drugs, such as phenytoin (Dilantin), suppress the influx of sodium, thereby decreasing the ability of the neurons to fire. Some anticonvulsant drugs, such as valproate sodium (Depakene) used for absence seizures, suppress the influx of calcium. The role of potassium and dopamine in the generation of seizure activity hasn't been identified.

NP: Analysis; CN: Physiological integrity; CNS: Pharmacological and parenteral therapies; CL: Knowledge

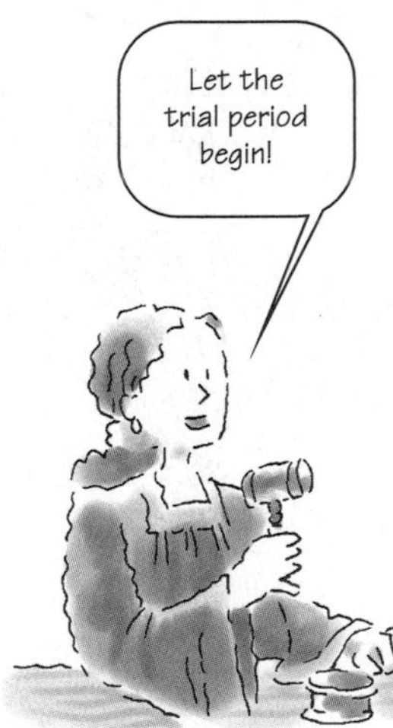

Let the trial period begin!

54. During the trial period to determine the efficacy of an anticonvulsant drug, which of the following cautions should be explained to the parents?

1. Plasma levels of the drug will be monitored on a daily basis.
2. Drug dosage will be adjusted depending on the frequency of seizure activity.
3. Drug must be discontinued immediately if even the slightest problem occurs.
4. Child shouldn't participate in activities that could be hazardous if a seizure occurs.

54. 4. Until seizure control is certain, clients shouldn't participate in activities (such as riding a bicycle) that could be hazardous if a seizure were to occur. Anticonvulsant drugs should be withdrawn over a period of 6 weeks to several months, never immediately, as this could precipitate status epilepticus. Plasma levels need to be monitored periodically over the course of drug therapy; daily monitoring isn't necessary. Dosage changes are usually based on plasma drug levels as well as seizure control.

NP: Implementation; CN: Physiological integrity; CNS: Pharmacological and parenteral therapies; CL: Analysis

55. Phenytoin (Dilantin) is a commonly used anticonvulsant drug that interacts with warfarin sodium (Coumadin) and the glucocorticoids. This drug interaction is the result of which of the following mechanisms of action?

1. Increased blood level of phenytoin
2. Decreased blood level of phenytoin
3. An interference with the metabolism of vitamin D
4. An increase in synthesis of hepatic drug-metabolizing enzymes

55. 4. By increasing drug metabolism, phenytoin decreases the effects of other drugs, such as warfarin and the glucocorticoids, and the dosages of these drugs may need to be increased to be effective. The blood level of phenytoin isn't altered by interactions with these drugs and has no known effect on the metabolism of vitamin D.

NP: Planning; CN: Physiological integrity; CNS: Pharmacological and parenteral therapies; CL: Knowledge

56. Maintaining plasma phenytoin levels within the therapeutic range is difficult for which of the following reasons?

1. A drop in the plasma drug level will lead to a toxic state.
2. The capacity to metabolize the drug becomes overwhelmed over time.
3. Small increments in dosage lead to sharp increases in plasma drug levels.
4. Large increments in dosage lead to a more rapid stabilizing therapeutic effect.

56. 3. Within the therapeutic range for phenytoin, small increments in dosage produce sharp increases in plasma drug levels. The capacity of the liver to metabolize phenytoin is affected by slight changes in the dosage of the drug, not necessarily the length of time the client has been taking the drug. Large increments in dosage will greatly increase plasma levels leading to drug toxicity.

NP: Implementation; CN: Physiological integrity; CNS: Pharmacological and parenteral therapies; CL: Comprehension

57. Client teaching should stress which of the following rules in relation to the differences in bioavailability of different forms of phenytoin?

1. Use the cheapest formulation the pharmacy has on hand at the time of refill.
2. Shop around to get the least expensive formulation.
3. There's no difference in one formulation from another, regardless of price.
4. Avoid switching formulations without the primary health care provider's approval.

57. 4. Differences in bioavailability exist among different formulations (tablets and capsules) and among the same formulations produced by different manufacturers. Clients shouldn't switch from one formulation to another or from one brand to another without primary health care provider approval and supervision.

NP: Implementation; CN: Physiological integrity; CNS: Pharmacological and parenteral therapies; CL: Application

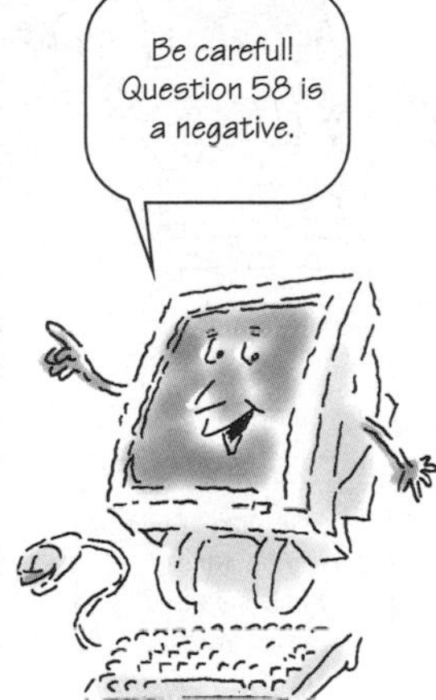
Be careful! Question 58 is a negative.

58. In contrast to other barbiturates, the anticonvulsant barbiturate phenobarbital ultimately has the action of seizure suppression without which of the following adverse effects?

1. Causing sedation
2. Development of ataxia and nystagmus
3. Development of significant dependence
4. Risk of developing acute intermittent porphyria

58. 1. Phenobarbital is able to suppress seizure activity at doses that produce minimal disruption to central nervous system function. During the initial phase, some drowsiness may occur, but with continued use, tolerance to sedation occurs. Exacerbation of intermittent porphyria is an adverse effect. Ataxia and nystagmus can be signs of overdose or toxicity and, like all other barbiturates, physical dependence can develop but is dosage-related.

NP: Planning; CN: Physiological integrity; CNS: Pharmacological and parenteral therapies; CL: Comprehension

59. Which of the following instructions should be included in client teaching specifically related to anticonvulsant drug efficacy?

1. Wear a medical identification bracelet
2. Maintain a seizure frequency chart
3. Avoid potentially hazardous activities
4. Discontinue the drug immediately if adverse effects are suspected

59. 2. Ongoing evaluation of the therapeutic effects can be accomplished by maintaining a frequency chart that indicates the date, time, and nature of all seizure activity. These data may be helpful in making dosage alterations and specific drug selection. Avoidance of hazardous activities and wearing a medical identification bracelet are ways to minimize danger related to seizure activity, but these factors don't affect drug efficacy. Anticonvulsant drugs should never be discontinued abruptly due to the potential for the development of status epilepticus.

NP: Planning; CN: Physiological integrity; CNS: Pharmacological and parenteral therapies; CL: Comprehension

60. I.V. administration of phenytoin would be contraindicated if which of the following conditions was identified in the preadmission assessment?

1. Episodic nose bleeds
2. History of Stokes-Adams syndrome
3. History of bone marrow depression
4. Attention deficit disorder

60. 2. I.V. administration of phenytoin can lead to arrhythmia and hypotension and is contraindicated in a history of sinus bradycardia, sinoatrial block, second- or third-degree heart block, or Stokes-Adams syndrome. Phenytoin would be administered cautiously in clients with episodic nosebleeds or bone marrow depression due to its adverse effects of leukopenia, anemia, and thrombocytopenia. Phenytoin has no known effect on attention deficit disorder but can interfere with cognitive function in excessive doses.

NP: Implementation; CN: Physiological integrity; CNS: Pharmacological and parenteral therapies; CL: Analysis

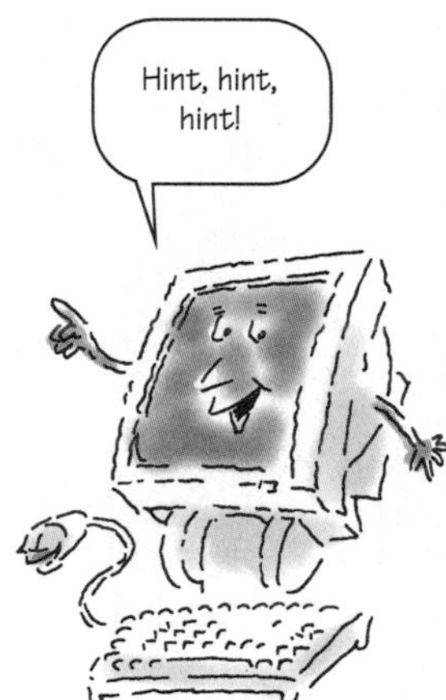

61. At which of the following times is seizure activity most likely to occur?

1. During the rapid eye movement (REM) stage of sleep
2. During long periods of excitement
3. While falling asleep and on awakening
4. While eating, particularly if the client is hurried

61. 3. Falling asleep or awakening from sleep are periods of functional instability of the brain; seizure activity is more likely to occur during these times. Eating quickly, excitement without undo fatigue, and REM sleep haven't been identified as contributing factors.

NP: Planning; CN: Physiological integrity; CNS: Physiological adaptation; CL: Knowledge

62. Emergency medical services should be called for a child experiencing a seizure only if which of the following complications occurs?

1. Continuous vomiting for 30 minutes following the seizure
2. Stereotypic or automatous body movements during the onset
3. Lack of expression, pallor, or flushing of the face during the seizure
4. Unilateral or bilateral posturing of one or more extremities during the onset

62. 1. Continuous vomiting after a seizure has ended can be a sign of an acute problem and indicates that the child requires an immediate medical evaluation. All of the other manifestations are normally present in various types of seizure activity and don't indicate a need for immediate medical evaluation.

NP: Assessment; CN: Physiological integrity; CNS: Reduction of risk potential; CL: Analysis

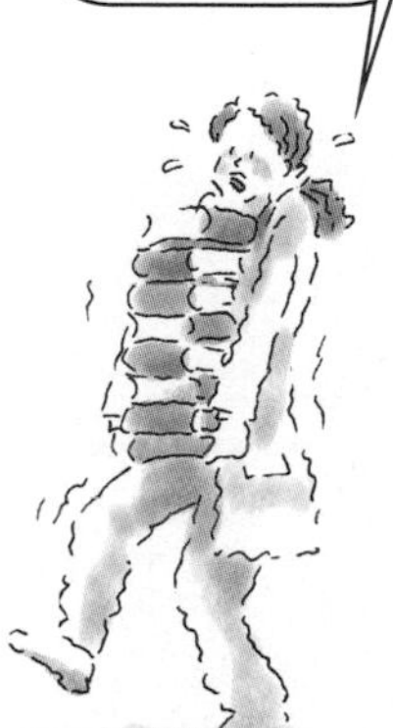

It's important to know which activities and environmental factors can trigger seizures.

63. Identifying factors that trigger seizure activity could lead to which of the following alterations in the child's environment or activities of daily living?

1. Avoiding striped wallpaper and ceiling fans
2. Having the child sleep alone to prevent sleep interruption
3. Including extended periods of intense physical activity daily
4. Allowing the child to drink soda only between noon and 5 p.m.

63. 1. Striped wallpaper, ceiling fans, and blinking lights on a Christmas tree can all be triggers to seizure activity if the child is photosensitive. Sleep interruption hasn't been identified as a triggering factor. Avoidance of fatigue can reduce seizure activity; therefore, intense physical activity for extended periods of time should be avoided. Restricting caffeine intake by using caffeine-free soda is a dietary modification that may prevent seizures.

NP: Implementation; CN: Physiological integrity; CNS: Physiological adaptation; CL: Application

64. Which of the following nursing interventions would be included to support the goal of avoiding injury, respiratory distress, or aspiration during a seizure?

1. Positioning the child with the head hyperextended
2. Placing a hand under the child's head for support
3. Using pillows to prop the child into the sitting position
4. Working a padded tongue blade or small plastic airway between the teeth

64. 2. Placing a hand or a small cushion or blanket under the child's head will help prevent injury. Position the child with the head in midline, not hyperextended, to promote a good airway and adequate ventilation. Don't attempt to prop the child up into a sitting position, but ease him to the floor to prevent falling and unnecessary injury. Don't put *anything* in the child's mouth because it could cause infection or obstruct the airway.

NP: Planning; CN: Physiological integrity; CNS: Reduction of risk potential; CL: Application

65. Which of the following factors can aid in neural tube defect detection?

1. Flat plate of the lower abdomen after the 23rd week of gestation
2. Significant level of alpha-fetoprotein present in the amniotic fluid
3. Amniocentesis for lecithin-sphingomyelin (L/S) ratio
4. Presence of high maternal levels of albumin after 12th week of gestation

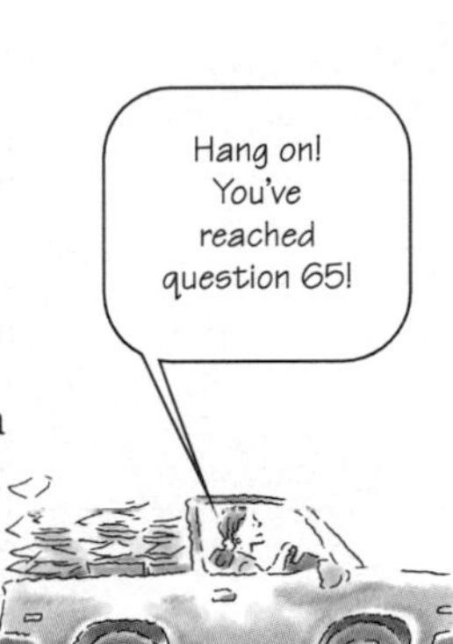
Hang on! You've reached question 65!

65. 2. Significant levels of alpha-fetoprotein have been effective in detecting neural tube defects. Prenatal screening includes a combination of maternal serum and amniotic fluid levels, amniocentesis, amniography, and ultrasonography and has been relatively successful in diagnosing the defect. Flat plate X-rays of the abdomen, L/S ratio, and maternal serum albumin levels aren't diagnostic for the defect.

NP: Assessment; CN: Health promotion and maintenance; CNS: Prevention and early detection of disease; CL: Knowledge

66. Spina bifida, a congenital spinal cord injury, may be characterized by which of the following descriptions?

1. It has little influence on the intellectual and perceptual abilities of the child.
2. It's a simple neurologic defect that is completely corrected surgically within 1 to 2 days after birth.
3. Its presence predisposes that many areas of the central nervous system (CNS) may not develop or function adequately.
4. It's a complex neurologic disability that involves a collaborative health team effort for the entire first year of life.

66. 3. When a spinal cord lesion exists at birth, it often leads to altered development or function of other areas of the CNS. Spina bifida is a complex neurologic defect that heavily impacts the physical, cognitive, and psychosocial development of the child and involves a collaborative, life-long management due to the chronicity and multiplicity of the problems involved.

NP: Assessment; CN: Physiological integrity; CNS: Physiological adaptation; CL: Knowledge

67. Common deformities occurring in the child with spina bifida are related to the muscles of the lower extremities that are active or inactive. These may include which of the following complications?

1. Club feet
2. Hip extension
3. Ankylosis of the knee
4. Abduction and external rotation of the hip

67. 1. The type and extent of deformity in the lower extremities depends on the muscles that are active or inactive. Passive positioning *in utero* may result in deformities of the feet such as equinovarus (club foot), knee flexion and extension contractures, hip flexion with adduction and internal rotation leading to subluxation or dislocation of the hip.

NP: Assessment; CN: Physiological integrity; CNS: Physiological adaptation; CL: Analysis

68. A mother asks the nurse what role she had in causing her child's spina bifida. Which of the following explanations is most appropriate?

1. Exact causative factors of this defect remain in question.
2. This defect is a hereditary problem transmitted through the autosomal recessive process.
3. Incidence of spina bifida is associated with a consistently high intake of alcohol during pregnancy.
4. Development of this defect is related to some type of maternal traumatic injury during the pregnancy.

68. 1. The exact cause of spina bifida remains unknown although environmental factors such as hyperthermia in the first weeks of pregnancy or dietary factors, such as canned meats, potatoes, and peas, have been implicated but not substantiated. Nutritional deficiencies, such as folic acid and vitamin A, have also been implicated. A genetic predisposition, along with certain environmental factors, may trigger the development; currently, there's no definitive evidence to support this theory. There's no evidence to support a connection with intake of alcohol or maternal trauma.

NP: Implementation; CN: Health promotion and maintenance; CNS: Prevention and early detection of disease; CL: Application

69. Infants with myelomeningocele must be closely observed for manifestations of Chiari II malformation, including which of the following symptoms?

1. Rapidly progressing scoliosis
2. Changes in urologic functioning
3. Back pain below the site of the sac closure
4. Respiratory stridor, apneic periods, and difficulty swallowing

69. 4. Children with a myelomeningocele have a 90% chance of having a Chiari II malformation. This may lead to a possibility of respiratory function problems, such as respiratory stridor associated with paralysis of the vocal cords, apneic episodes of unknown cause, difficulty swallowing, and an abnormal gag reflex. Lower back pain doesn't occur due to the loss of sensory function related to the cord defect. Urologic function changes and scoliosis occur with myelomeningocele, but these complications aren't specifically related to Chiari II malformation.

NP: Assessment; CN: Physiological integrity; CNS: Reduction of risk potential; CL: Knowledge

70. A child with myelomeningocele and hydrocephalus may demonstrate problems related to damage of the white matter caused by ventricular enlargement. This damage may manifest itself in which of the following conditions?

1. Inability to speak
2. Early hand dominance
3. Impaired intellectual functions
4. Flaccid paralysis of the lower extremities

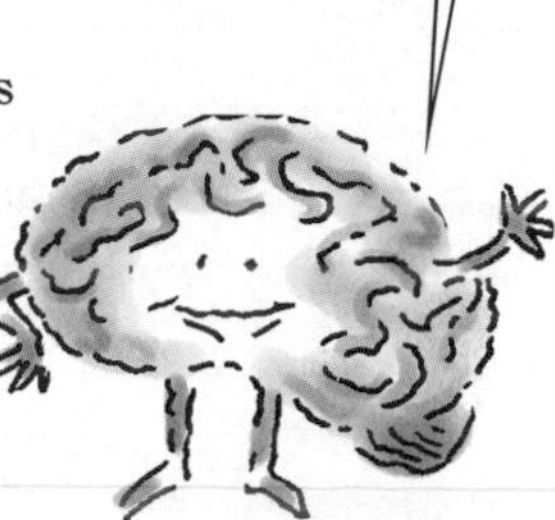
For question 70, it helps to know that my white matter is also known as the "association area."

70. 3. Damage to the white matter (association area) caused by ventricular enlargement has been linked to impairment of intellectual and perceptual abilities often seen in children with spina bifida. It hasn't been related to hand dominance development, flaccid paralysis of the lower extremities, or the ability to speak, though it may affect the semantics of speech dependent upon the association areas.

NP: Assessment; CN: Physiological integrity; CNS: Physiological adaptation; CL: Analysis

71. Myelomeningocele requires nearly immediate surgical repair for which of the following purposes?

1. Rapid restoration of the neural pathways to the legs
2. Decreased possibility of infection and further cord damage
3. Exposure of the spinal cord defect to individualize the therapeutic strategy
4. Removal of excess nerve tissue from the vertebral canal to decrease pressure on the cord

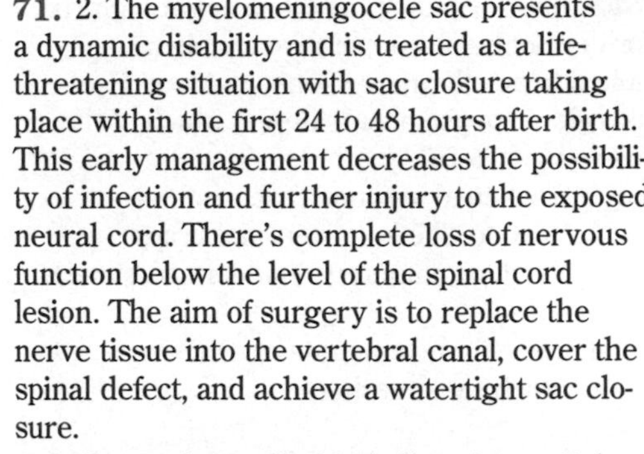

71. 2. The myelomeningocele sac presents a dynamic disability and is treated as a life-threatening situation with sac closure taking place within the first 24 to 48 hours after birth. This early management decreases the possibility of infection and further injury to the exposed neural cord. There's complete loss of nervous function below the level of the spinal cord lesion. The aim of surgery is to replace the nerve tissue into the vertebral canal, cover the spinal defect, and achieve a watertight sac closure.

NP: Implementation; CN: Physiological integrity; CNS: Reduction of risk potential; CL: Comprehension

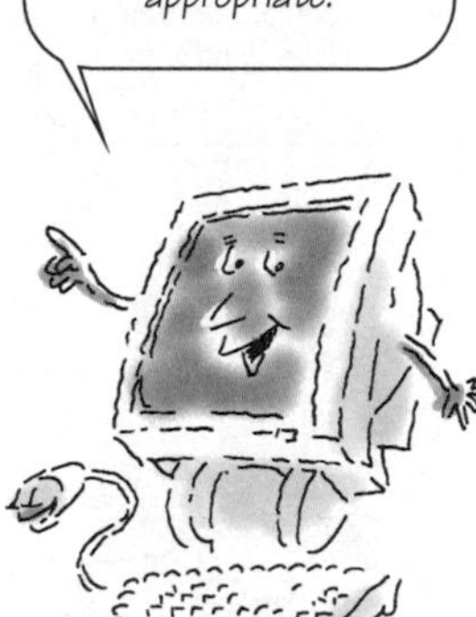

72. One of the most important aspects of preoperative care with myelomeningocele is the positioning of the infant. Which of the following positions is the most appropriate?

1. Prone position with head turned to the side for feeding
2. Side-lying position with the head at a 30-degree angle to the feet
3. Prone position with a nasogastric (NG) tube inserted for feedings
4. Supported by diaper rolls, both anterior and posterior, in the side-lying position

72. 1. Prone position is used preoperatively because it minimizes tension on the sac and the risk of trauma. The head is turned to one side for feeding. There's no advantage to positioning the body with a 30-degree head elevation. Side-lying or partial side-lying positions are better used *after* the repair has been accomplished unless it permits undesirable hip flexion. Although feeding can be a problem in the prone position, it can be accomplished without the need for an NG tube.

NP: Implementation; CN: Physiological integrity; CNS: Basic care and comfort; CL: Application

73. Large body areas of sensory and motor impairment associated with myelomeningocele necessitate which of the following nursing interventions?

1. Gentle stretching of contractures
2. Vigorous active range-of-motion exercises
3. Frequent turning side-to-side and prone-to-supine
4. Keeping skin dry and avoiding the use of emollients and lubricants

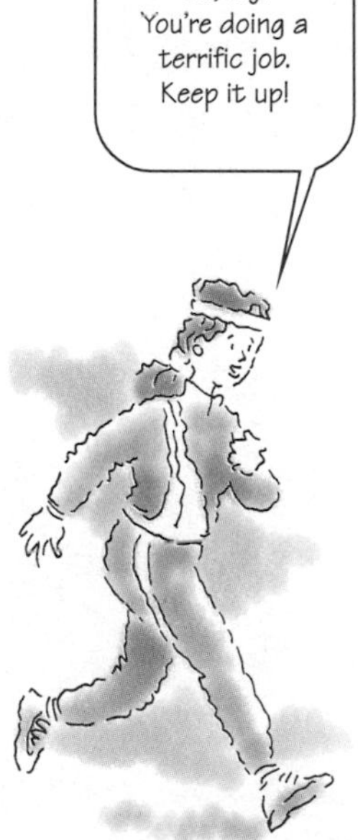

Oh, my.
You're doing a terrific job.
Keep it up!

73. 1. Areas of sensory and motor impairment require meticulous care, including range-of-motion exercises to prevent contractures as well as stretching of contractures when indicated. Vigorous exercise is avoided in contrast to the gentle range of motion that is recommended. Frequent turning is indicated in order to maintain skin integrity, but the supine position shouldn't be used to avoid pressure on the surgical site. Skin should be kept clean and dry, but lubrication can be used to facilitate massage, which increases circulation to the areas involved.

NP: Planning; CN: Physiological integrity; CNS: Basic care and comfort; CL: Application

74. Children with spina bifida are at high risk for developing intraoperative anaphylaxis linked to an allergic response to latex. This allergic response occurs due to which of the following factors?

1. Weakened immune response
2. Need for life-long steroid therapy
3. Need for numerous bladder catheterizations
4. Use of large amounts of adhesive tape to attach sac dressings

74. 3. Children with spina bifida are at high risk for developing a latex allergy because of repeated exposure to latex products during multiple surgeries and from numerous bladder catheterizations related to lack of bladder function. A weakened immune response wouldn't elicit an anaphylactic reaction due to the reduced functioning of the immune response. Steroid therapy isn't indicated in the management of spina bifida and also wouldn't support an anaphylactic reaction. Sac removal is accomplished as quickly as possible after birth, and the sac usually isn't covered with any type of dressing because it may contribute to trauma to the sac.

NP: Analysis; CN: Physiological integrity; CNS: Reduction of risk potential; CL: Comprehension

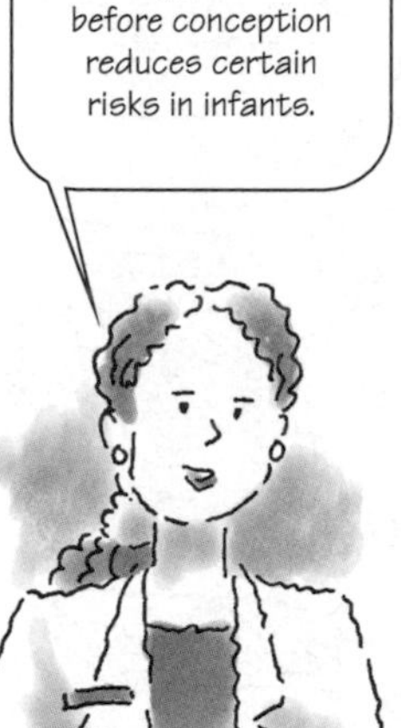
Taking folic acid before conception reduces certain risks in infants.

75. Which of the following explanations of how to avoid the incidence of a second child with spina bifida is most accurate?

1. There's no known way to avoid it; adoption is recommended.
2. A previous pregnancy affected by a neural tube defect isn't a factor.
3. Prepregnancy intake of 4 mg of folic acid daily reduces the recurrence rate.
4. Aerobic exercise in the first trimester to decrease the chances of a positive alpha-fetoprotein (AFP).

75. 3. Studies have shown that women at high risk for having an infant with a neural tube defect, demonstrated by a previously delivered infant or fetus with spina bifida, significantly reduced the recurrence rate by taking supplements of folic acid before conception. The chances of having a second affected child are low (between 1% and 2%), but still greater than the chances of the general population. Aerobic exercise won't decrease the chances of a positive AFP.

NP: Implementation; CN: Health promotion and maintenance; CNS: Prevention and early detection of disease; CL: Analysis

76. A school-age child with a diagnosis of epilepsy is admitted to the pediatric unit of a local hospital for evaluation of his anticonvulsant medications. As the nurse enters the child's room, the child begins to have a seizure. Which nursing action should the nurse do first?

1. Push the call bell and ask for help.
2. Hold the child down so he doesn't injure himself.
3. Loosen any restrictive clothing.
4. Force the jaw open to maintain an open airway.

76. 3. The primary nursing goal during a seizure is to protect the client from physical injury and maintain a patent airway. Loosening clothing will allow free movement and aid in keeping the airway open. After making sure the client is safe from injury, the nurse should push the call bell only if further assistance is needed. The nurse should never forcibly hold a client down and shouldn't force the jaw open; the jaw could be injured or break.

NP: Implementation; CN: Physiological integrity; CNS: Reduction of risk potential; CL: Application

77. The nurse is evaluating a 10-month-old infant for possible developmental delay and cerebral palsy. A 10-month-old infant should have mastered which of the following tasks?

1. Holding a spoon and cup
2. Speaking 10 to 20 words
3. Throwing a ball
4. Sitting without support

77. 4. By age 10 months an infant should be able to sit without support. Holding a spoon and cup, speaking 10 to 20 words, and throwing a ball are developmental milestones for a 12- to 18-month-old.

NP: Assessment; CN: Health promotion and maintenance; CNS: Growth and development through the life span; CL: Comprehension

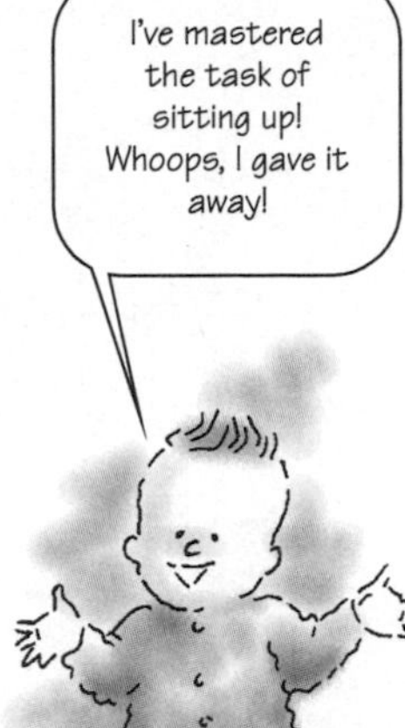

I've mastered the task of sitting up! Whoops, I gave it away!

78. A nurse is caring for a child with a brain tumor who's scheduled for a craniotomy. Which preoperative nursing task is important for this client?

1. Giving a complete bath
2. Shampooing the hair
3. Familiarizing the child and family with the recovery room, intensive care unit, and hospital personnel.
4. Administering an enema

78. 3. Preoperative emphasis should be on explaining procedures and alleviating fears for the child and family. Although a complete bath is usually given and the hair shampooed, these tasks aren't the highest priority. An enema shouldn't be given because it may increase intracranial pressure.

NP: Implementation; CN: Physiological integrity; CNS: Reduction of risk potential; CL: Analysis

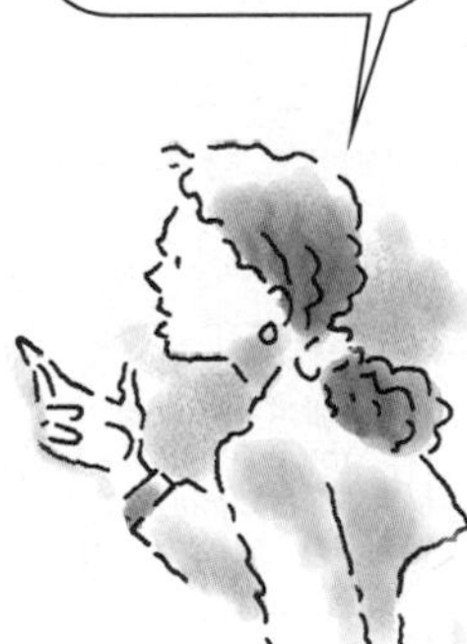

79. A child has just undergone a craniotomy. Which postoperative nursing care procedure is included?

1. Placing the child in Trendelenburg's position
2. Administering morphine for pain
3. Placing the child in a vest restraint and soft wrist restraints
4. Recording rectal temperatures frequently

79. 4. Hyperthermia is a complication of brain surgery, so the client's temperature needs to be monitored frequently. Rectal temperatures are the safest and most accurate because the child isn't fully awake and oriented. Trendelenburg's position is contraindicated postcraniotomy because of the risk of increasing intracranial pressure. Morphine may depress respirations and impede accurate neurologic assessments. Restraints aren't usually necessary.

NP: Implementation; CN: Physiological integrity; CNS: Physiological adaptation; CL: Analysis

80. A 6-year-old child is unconscious with a head injury from a bicycle accident. The nurse is assessing him for increased intracranial pressure (ICP). His baseline vital signs are respirations 20 breaths/minute; blood pressure 100/56 mm Hg; pulse 100 beats/minute. Which set of vital signs would indicate increased ICP?

1. Respirations 12 breaths/minute; blood pressure 90/45 mm Hg; pulse 80 beats/minute
2. Respirations 14 breaths/minute; blood pressure 130/40 mm Hg; pulse 70 beats/minute
3. Respirations 30 breaths/minute; blood pressure 80/45 mm Hg; pulse 130 beats/minute
4. Respirations 14 breaths/minute; blood pressure 70/58 mm Hg; pulse 102 beats/minute

80. 2. Classic signs of increased ICP are a decrease in respirations, an increase in blood pressure, and a decrease in pulse rate. Option 1 may indicate normal vital signs. Options 3 and 4 may indicate shock.

NP: Assessment; CN: Physiological integrity; CNS: Physiological adaptation; CL: Analysis

81. An 8-year-old child has been admitted to the emergency department. The physician suspects a head injury and skull fracture in which cerebrospinal fluid (CSF) leakage may occur. Which condition should the nurse assess?

1. Tearing of the eyes and drainage of mucus from the nose
2. Draining of clear fluid from the nose or ears
3. Draining of purulent, thick yellow mucus from the nose or ears
4. Bleeding from the nose or ears

81. 2. CSF is clear fluid and may drain from the nose or ears of a client with a head injury. To positively identify the drainage as CSF, the nurse should test the fluid for glucose. Tearing and mucus from the nose can be caused by allergies or an upper respiratory infection. Purulent, thick mucus is indicative of an infection. Bleeding may indicate an intracranial bleed or skull fracture.

NP: Assessment; CN: Physiological integrity; CNS: Physiological adaptation; CL: Application

82. A 9-year-old child with a possible skull fracture was admitted to the hospital. During the admission assessment, the nurse noted the child's religious affiliation as Jehovah's Witness. Which beliefs about health and medicine are common in this religion?

1. Members may not have blood transfusions.
2. Diseases are treated either with cold or hot food.
3. Members should avoid tea, coffee, chocolate, and other products containing caffeine.
4. Diseases are treated based on the ying and yang theory

82. 1. A Jehovah's Witness doesn't believe in receiving blood or blood products. Hispanics treat disease with hot or cold foods. Members of the Mormon faith avoid products containing caffeine. The Asian populations practice ying and yang.

NP: Assessment; CN: Health promotion and maintenance; CNS: Prevention and early detection of disease; CL: Knowledge

83. The father of a Hispanic child with meningitis places a necklace made of herbs around the child's neck. What should the nurse do?

1. Prohibit the father from being alone with his child.
2. Ask the father to remove the necklace immediately, and dispose of it.
3. Forbid this practice while the child is in the hospital.
4. Recognize that this is a traditional healing method among Hispanics.

83. 4. The use of herb necklaces is a common practice among Hispanics. The father isn't hurting the child, so there's no reason for him to leave. The father can leave the necklace on; it isn't interfering with other therapies.

NP: Planning; CN: Psychosocial integrity; CNS: Coping and adaptation; CL: Analysis

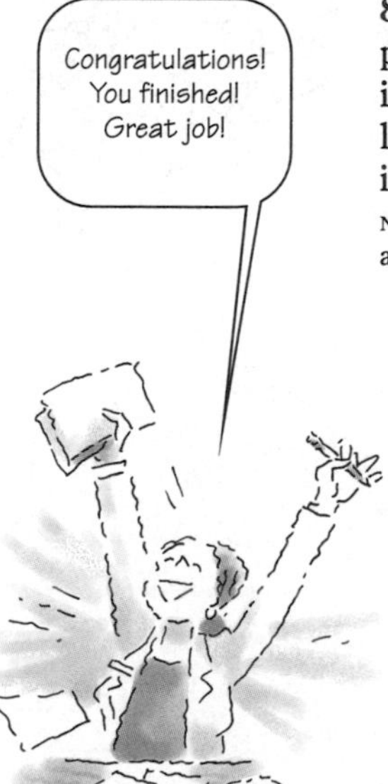
Congratulations!
You finished!
Great job!

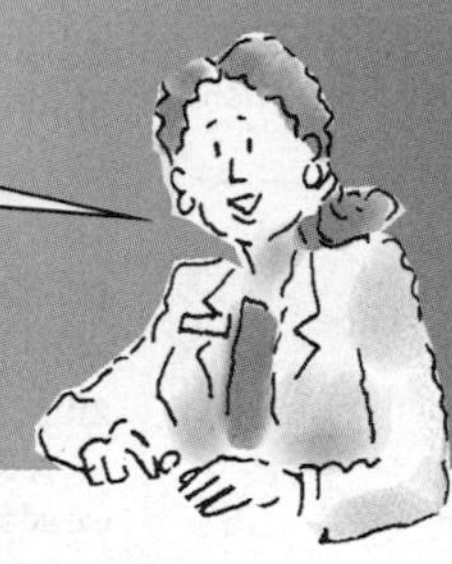

Chapter 31 Musculoskeletal disorders

1. Which of the following definitions best describes the form of clubfoot called talipes varus?
1. Inversion of the foot
2. Eversion of the foot
3. Plantar flexion
4. Dorsiflexion

1. 1. Talipes varus is an inversion of the foot. Talipes valgus is an eversion of the foot. Talipes equinus is plantar flexion of the foot, and talipes calcaneus is dorsiflexion of the foot.
NP: Assessment; CN: Physiological integrity; CNS: Physiological adaptation; CL: Knowledge

2. Which of the following types of clubfoot is the one most commonly treated by primary health care providers?
1. Talipes calcaneus
2. Talipes equinovarus
3. Talipes valgus
4. Talipes varus

2. 2. Ninety-five percent of treated clubfoot cases are for feet that point downward and inward (talipes equinovarus) in varying degrees. Talipes valgus, talipes calcaneus, and talipes varus aren't as common.
NP: Assessment; CN: Physiological integrity; CNS: Physiological adaptation; CL: Knowledge

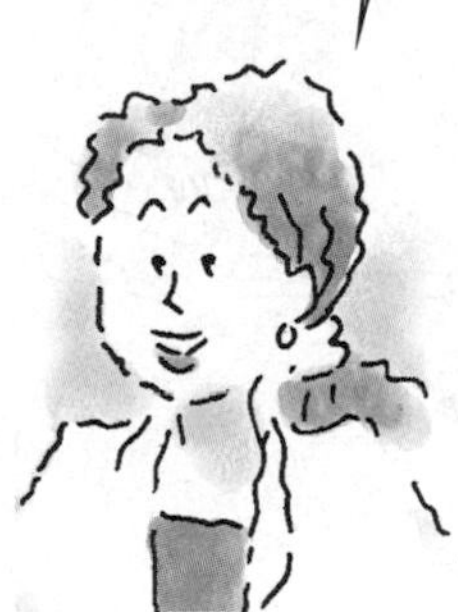

Knowing how to treat a disorder is only part of the NCLEX. Question 3 asks you for the cause of the disorder as well.

3. The mother of a neonate with clubfoot feels guilty because she believes she did something to cause the condition. The nurse should explain that the cause of clubfoot in neonates is due to which of the following factors?
1. Unknown
2. Hereditary
3. Restricted movement in utero
4. Anomalous embryonic development

3. 1. The definitive cause of clubfoot is unknown. In some families, there's an increased incidence. Some postulate that anomalous embryonic development or restricted fetal movement are the reasons. Currently, there's no way to predict the occurrence of clubfoot.
NP: Assessment; CN: Psychosocial integrity; CNS: Coping and adaptation; CL: Knowledge

4. Which of the following statements about clubfoot is true?
1. It's hereditary.
2. More girls are affected.
3. More boys are affected.
4. It occurs once in every 500 births.

4. 3. Boys are affected twice as often as girls. Clubfoot occurs once in every 700 to 1,000 births. It isn't known if the condition is hereditary.
NP: Assessment; CN: Physiological integrity; CNS: Physiological adaptation; CL: Knowledge

5. Congenital torticollis usually involves which of the following muscles?

1. Platysma
2. Lower trapezius
3. Middle trapezius
4. Sternocleidomastoid

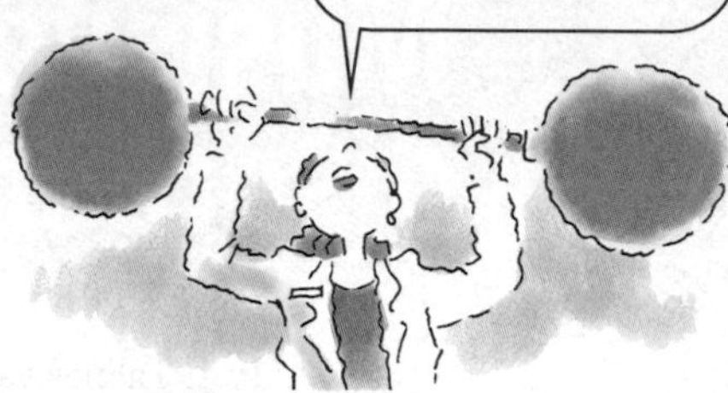
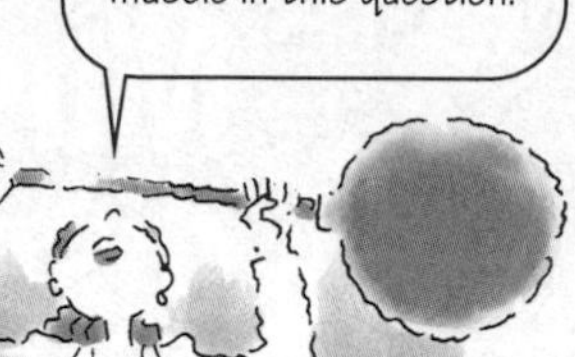

There sure is a lot of muscle in this question!

5. 4. Congenital torticollis usually involves a shortening of the sternocleidomastoid muscle. Rotation is *away* from the side of shortening, and side bending is *toward* the side of the contraction. The platysma is shortened if the head is held in flexion. The middle and lower trapezius aren't associated with torticollis.

NP: Assessment; CN: Physiological integrity; CNS: Physiological adaptation; CL: Knowledge

6. A 3-month-old infant who has severe torticollis presents with the head rotated to the left and the side bent to the right. Which of the following muscles is shortened?

1. Left upper trapezius
2. Right middle trapezius
3. Left sternocleidomastoid
4. Right sternocleidomastoid

6. 4. The right sternocleidomastoid is shortened with the head in this position. The left upper trapezius isn't shortened; the right one is. The middle trapezius isn't affected, and the left sternocleidomastoid is in a lengthened position.

NP: Assessment; CN: Physiological integrity; CNS: Physiological adaptation; CL: Knowledge

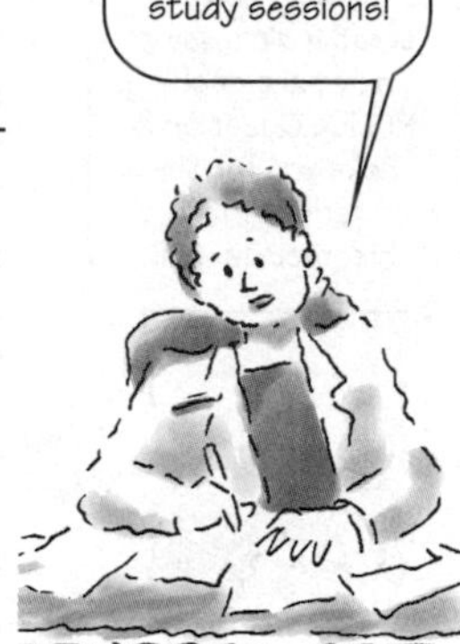

Muscle lengthening? Maybe I'd better lengthen my study sessions!

7. A 9-month-old infant has torticollis with rotation of the head to the left and side bending to the right. Placing the infant in which of the following positions would be most effective for developing muscle lengthening?

1. Prone
2. Supine
3. Left side-lying
4. Right side-lying

7. 3. The left side-lying position will help assist with lengthening of the muscles because this position will make it easier to stretch the sternocleidomastoid and upper trapezius. No other positions will assist in increasing muscle length.

NP: Implementation; CN: Physiological integrity; CNS: Reduction of risk potential; CL: Application

8. Scoliosis can be described by which of the following definitions?

1. An increase in the lumbar lordosis
2. A decrease in the thoracic kyphosis
3. Lateral curves in the spinal column described as right or left concavities
4. Lateral curves in the spinal column described as right or left convexities

8. 4. Scoliosis is described along the longitudinal axis of the body and curves are described according to the convexity, *not* the concavity. Lordosis and kyphosis describe the back in the frontal plane.

NP: Assessment; CN: Physiological integrity; CNS: Physiological adaptation; CL: Knowledge

9. Which of the following surgical interventions could be used in the treatment of scoliosis?

1. Segmental diskectomy
2. Austin Moore procedure
3. Segmented spine instrumentation
4. Thoracic and lumbar laminectomy

9. 3. In segmented spine instrumentation, flexible rods are placed on the transverse processes of the spine, and wires are threaded through the laminae so the spinal column is stabilized. Segmental diskectomy won't cure or help scoliosis. Austin Moore procedure is used in fractured hips. Thoracic and lumbar laminectomies are performed for herniated disks.

NP: Implementation; CN: Physiological integrity; CNS: Basic care and comfort; CL: Knowledge

10. Upon physical examination, which of the following conditions may be a warning sign of scoliosis?
1. Scapula winging
2. Forward head posture
3. Raised right iliac crest
4. Forward flexion of the cervical spine

10. 3. A raised iliac crest may be a warning sign of some curvature secondary to the attachment of the pelvis to the spine. Scapula winging could be caused by muscle paralysis. Forward head posture isn't a result of scoliosis. Forward flexion doesn't describe lateral curves in the spine.

NP: Assessment; CN: Physiological integrity; CNS: Physiological adaptation; CL: Knowledge

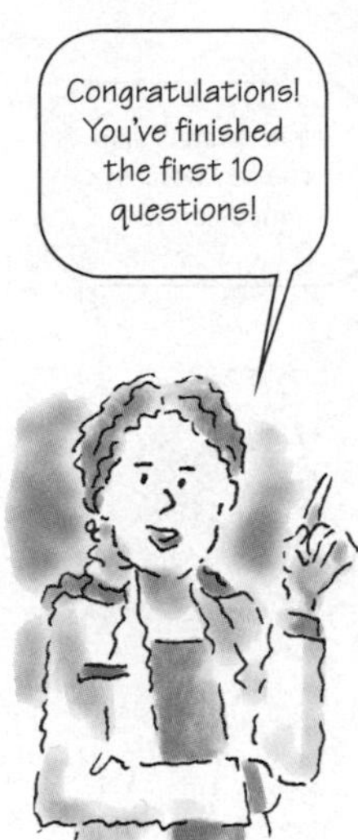
Congratulations!
You've finished
the first 10
questions!

11. Which of the following braces is used in the treatment of scoliosis?
1. Don Joy braces
2. Long leg braces
3. Milwaukee brace
4. Knee-ankle-foot orthosis

11. 3. The Milwaukee brace is used to place lateral pressure on the back in hopes of halting or slowing the progression of the curves in the back. It isn't curative. Don Joy braces are used following knee reconstruction. Long leg braces are used for lower extremity weakness or partial paralysis. Knee-ankle-foot orthosis is used for lower extremity and foot weakness.

NP: Assessment; CN: Physiological integrity; CNS: Reduction of risk potential; CL: Knowledge

12. The Milwaukee brace is used often in the treatment of scoliosis. Which of the following positions best describes the placement of the pressure rods?
1. Laterally on the convex portion of the curve
2. Laterally on the concave portion of the curve
3. Posteriorly on the convex portion of the curve
4. Posteriorly along the spinal column at the exact level of the curve

12. 1. Lateral pressure applied to the convex portion of the curve will help best in reducing the curvature. Pressure pads applied posteriorly will help maintain erect posture. Pressure applied to the concave portion of the curve will increase the lordosis.

NP: Assessment; CN: Physiological integrity; CNS: Reduction of risk potential; CL: Application

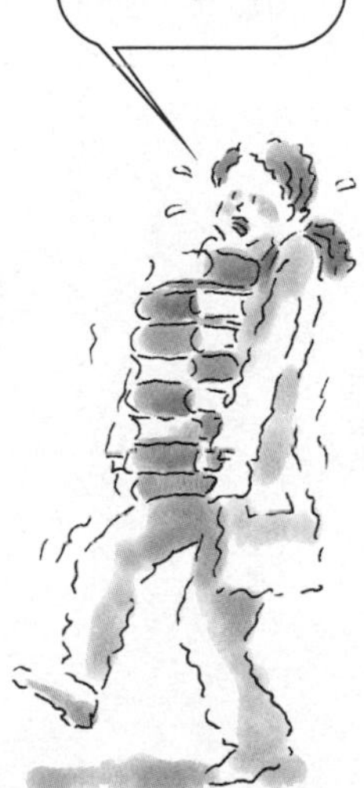
All this studying
is strengthening
my muscle
groups.
Oh, goody.

13. Strengthening of which of the following muscle groups is important in a client diagnosed with talipes equinovarus?
1. Evertors
2. Invertors
3. Plantar flexors
4. Plantar fascia musculature

13. 1. Because the foot is held in inversion, it's important to strengthen the evertors to counter the inversion present in the foot. Inversion is incorrect because the foot is already held in this position. Plantar musculature and plantar flexors aren't important because the foot is already in a plantar flexed position.

NP: Assessment; CN: Physiological integrity; CNS: Reduction of risk potential; CL: Analysis

14. Torticollis describes scoliosis in which of the following areas of the spine?
1. Cervical
2. Lumbar
3. Sacral
4. Thoracic

14. 1. Torticollis describes only the cervical spine. No other areas apply.

NP: Assessment; CN: Physiological integrity; CNS: Physiological adaptation; CL: Knowledge

15. Which of the following conditions describes a structural scoliosis?

1. Muscular dystrophy with muscle weakness
2. Cerebral palsy with muscle weakness
3. Leg length discrepancy
4. Spina bifida

16. Nonstructural scoliosis can be caused by which of the following complications?

1. Wedge vertebrae
2. Hemivertebrae
3. Poor posture
4. Tumor

17. Idiopathic scoliosis accounts for which of the following percentages of cases of scoliosis?

1. 50% to 60%
2. 65% to 75%
3. 75% to 85%
4. 85% to 95%

18. Which of the following techniques may assist a 3-month-old client diagnosed with torticollis?

1. Lying supine
2. Gentle massage
3. Range-of-motion (ROM) exercises
4. Lying on the side

19. A physical therapist has instructed the nursing staff in range-of-motion exercises for an infant with torticollis. Which of the following interventions should the nurse perform if she feels uncomfortable performing the stretches that result in crying and grimacing of the client?

1. Check the primary health care provider's orders.
2. Call the primary health care provider.
3. Call the physical therapist.
4. Discontinue the exercises.

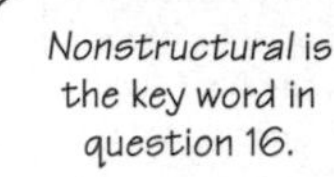

Nonstructural is the key word in question 16.

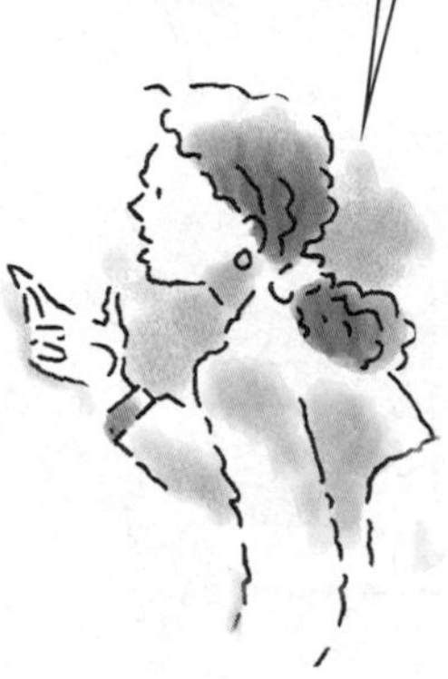

15. 3. Leg length discrepancy is a structural deformity that can be associated with scoliosis. Cerebral palsy, muscular dystrophy, and spina bifida are disease processes that may cause scoliosis.

NP: Assessment; CN: Physiological integrity; CNS: Physiological adaptation; CL: Knowledge

16. 3. Poor posture is a nonstructural problem that may be a cause of scoliosis. Hemivertebrae, wedge vertebrae, and tumor are all structural causes of scoliosis.

NP: Assessment; CN: Physiological integrity; CNS: Physiological adaptation; CL: Knowledge

17. 3. Studies have shown that idiopathic scoliosis accounts for 75% to 85% of all cases.

NP: Assessment; CN: Physiological integrity; CNS: Physiological adaptation; CL: Knowledge

18. 4. Side-lying opposite the affected side may help elongate shortened muscles. Lying supine won't assist with elongation of muscles. Gentle massage won't assist with elongation of muscles. ROM exercises won't assist with shortened muscles unless in specific patterns and with stretching.

NP: Implementation; CN: Health promotion and maintenance; CNS: Growth and development through the life span; CL: Application

19. 3. The only cure for the torticollis is exercise or surgery. The therapist is the expert in exercise and should be called for assistance in this situation. The primary health care provider would be called only if there was concern over the orders written or an abnormal development in the child.

NP: Implementation; CN: Physiological integrity; CNS: Physiological adaptation; CL: Analysis

20. A client has developed a right torticollis with side-bending to the right and rotation to the left. Which of the following exercises may assist in reduction of the torticollis?

1. Rotation exercises to the right
2. Rotation exercises to the left
3. Cervical extension exercises
4. Cervical flexion exercises

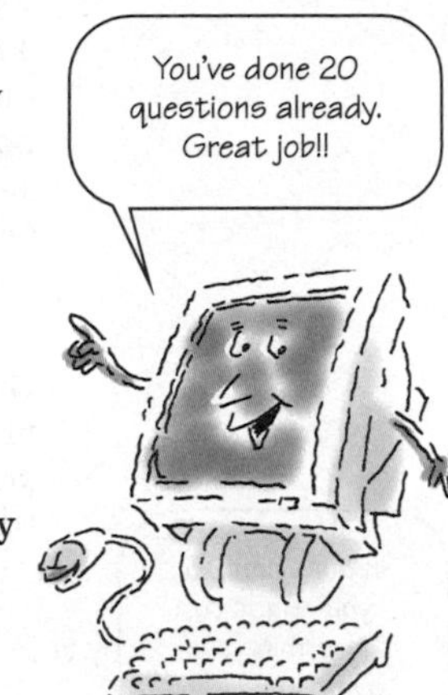

You've done 20 questions already. Great job!!

20. 1. Performing rotation exercises to the right will help increase the length of the shortened right sternocleidomastoid. Rotation to the left will just add to the torticollis as the head is already rotated in that direction. Cervical extension exercises won't lengthen tightened muscles. Cervical flexion will add to shortening of the muscles.

NP: Implementation; CN: Physiological integrity; CNS: Reduction of risk potential; CL: Application

21. Which of the following complications may occur due to severe scoliosis?

1. Increased vital capacity
2. Increased oxygen uptake
3. Diminished vital capacity
4. Decreased residual volume

21. 3. Scoliosis of greater than 60 degrees can cause shifting of organs and decreased ability for the ribs to expand, thus decreasing vital capacity. An increase in oxygen uptake won't occur secondary to a decrease in chest expansion. An increase in vital capacity also won't occur secondary to a decrease in chest expansion. Residual volume will increase secondary to decreased ability of the lungs to expel air.

NP: Assessment; CN: Physiological integrity; CNS: Physiological adaptation; CL: Knowledge

22. A 4-year-old child is diagnosed with cerebral palsy and resultant thoracic scoliosis. Which of the following conditions may be the cause of the scoliosis?

1. Hypotonia
2. Mental retardation
3. Autonomic dysreflexia
4. Increased thoracic kyphosis

22. 1. Cerebral palsy is usually associated with some degree of hypotonia or hypertonia. Poor muscle tone may result in scoliosis. Mental retardation isn't a cause of scoliosis. Autonomic dysreflexia is described in spinal cord injury and involves abnormal muscle spasms secondary to abnormal inhibitory neurons present during stretch reflexes. Increased thoracic kyphosis won't result in scoliosis.

NP: Assessment; CN: Physiological integrity; CNS: Physiological adaptation; CL: Knowledge

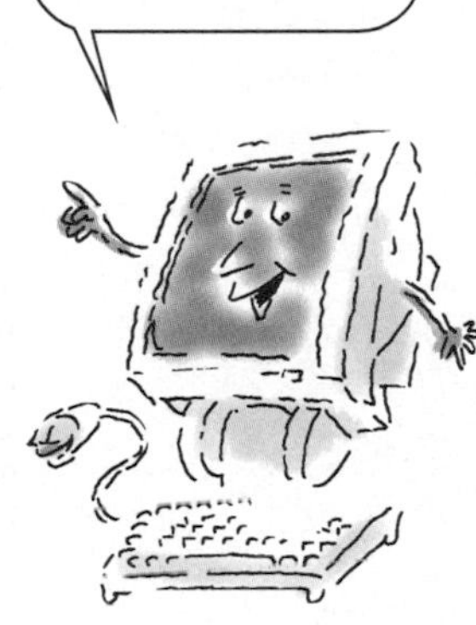

Do you know what myopathic means? I knew you would!

23. Which of the following disease processes is myopathic in nature?

1. Cerebral palsy
2. Marfan syndrome
3. Muscular dystrophy
4. Spinal muscular atrophy

23. 3. Muscular dystrophy is myopathic in nature. Cerebral palsy occurs from prenatal, perinatal, or postnatal central nervous system damage. An upper motor neuron lesion may be the cause. Marfan syndrome is mesenchymal in nature. Spinal muscular atrophy is related to lower motor neurons.

NP: Assessment; CN: Physiological integrity; CNS: Physiological adaptation; CL: Knowledge

24. During a scoliosis screening, the school nurse notices a raised iliac crest height, indicating which of the following conditions?

1. Forward head posture
2. Leg length discrepancy
3. Increased lumbar lordosis
4. Increased thoracic kyphosis

24. 2. A raised iliac crest may be indicative of a leg length discrepancy or a curvature in the lumbar spine. It isn't indicative of forward head posture, lumbar lordosis, or thoracic kyphosis.

NP: Assessment; CN: Physiological integrity; CNS: Physiological adaptation; CL: Knowledge

25. Scoliosis is most common in which of the following groups?

1. Preteenage girls
2. Preteenage boys
3. Adolescent girls
4. Adolescent boys

25. 3. Scoliosis is eight times more prominent in adolescent girls than boys.

NP: Assessment; CN: Physiological integrity; CNS: Physiological adaptation; CL: Knowledge

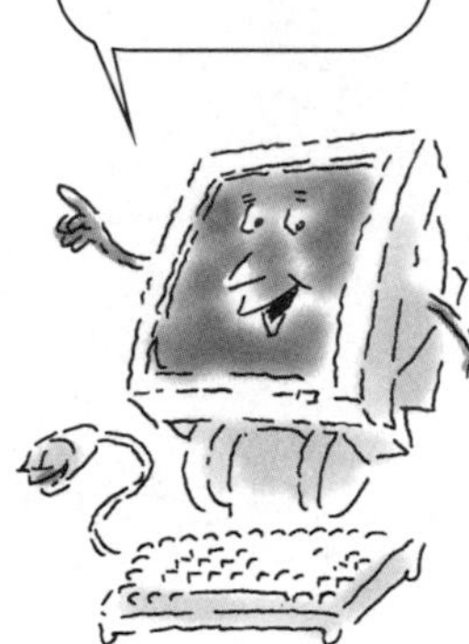

In question 26, you've got to determine the symptom that causes the most concern.

26. In caring for a child with a Harrington instrumentation rod placement, which of the following symptoms would be of greatest concern two days postoperatively?

1. Fever of 99.5° F (37.5° C)
2. Pain along the incision
3. Decreased urinary output
4. Hypoactive bowel sounds

26. 3. Because of extensive blood loss during surgery and possible renal hypoperfusion, decreased urinary output could indicate decreased renal function. A fever of 99.5° F is of concern, but it may be due to decreased chest expansion secondary to anesthesia, surgery, and pain. A paralytic ileus is common after this surgery, and the client may have a nasogastric tube for the first 48 hours.

NP: Assessment; CN: Physiological integrity; CNS: Reduction of risk potential; CL: Analysis

27. Observing which of the following structures will serve the nurse best when screening a child for scoliosis?

1. Iliac crests
2. Spinous processes
3. Acromion processes
4. Posterior superior iliac spines

27. 2. Spinous processes are the best bony landmark to identify when attempting to screen for scoliosis because this will show lateral deviation of the column. Abnormalities in the acromion process, iliac crests, and posterior superior iliac spines may not be indicative of scoliosis.

NP: Assessment; CN: Physiological integrity; CNS: Physiological adaptation; CL: Knowledge

28. Which of the following interventions may be a possible treatment choice for talipes equinovarus?

1. Traction
2. Serial casting
3. Short leg braces
4. Inversion range-of-motion exercises

28. 2. Serial casting is a treatment choice in attempts to change the length of soft tissue. Traction isn't an option. Corrective shoes are used instead of short leg braces. Inversion exercises won't help; eversion exercise will.

NP: Assessment; CN: Physiological integrity; CNS: Reduction of risk potential; CL: Knowledge

29. When performing stretches with a child who has scoliosis, which of the following techniques should be used?

1. Slow and sustained
2. Until a change in muscle length is seen
3. Quick movements to the end range of pain
4. Slow movements for brief, 3- to 4-second periods

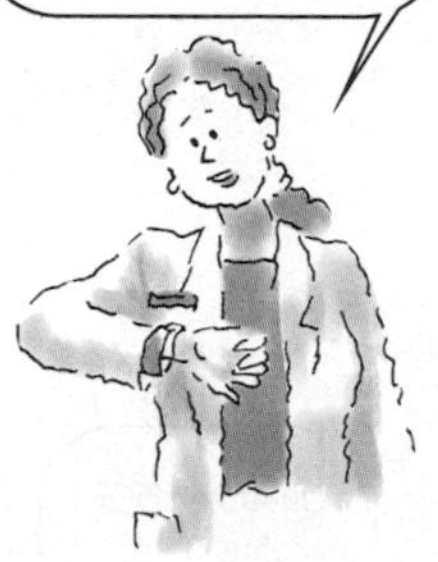

You might need a stretch right now. Why not take a brief one and then get right back to work?

29. 1. Stretches should be slow and sustained. It's difficult to see changes in muscle length. Stretches should be performed for longer than a few seconds. Stretches shouldn't be performed with quick movements.
NP: Implementation; CN: Safe, effective care environment; CNS: Management of care; CL: Application

30. Congenital hip dislocation is most commonly found in which of the following groups?

1. Males
2. Females
3. First-born males
4. First-born females

30. 4. Studies have shown that first-born females are six times more likely to have a congenital hip dislocation than males.
NP: Assessment; CN: Physiological integrity; CNS: Physiological adaptation; CL: Knowledge

31. Diagnosis of congenital hip dislocation can best be confirmed by which of the following diagnostic techniques?

1. X-ray
2. Positive Ortolani's sign
3. Positive Trendelenburg gait
4. Audible clicking with adduction

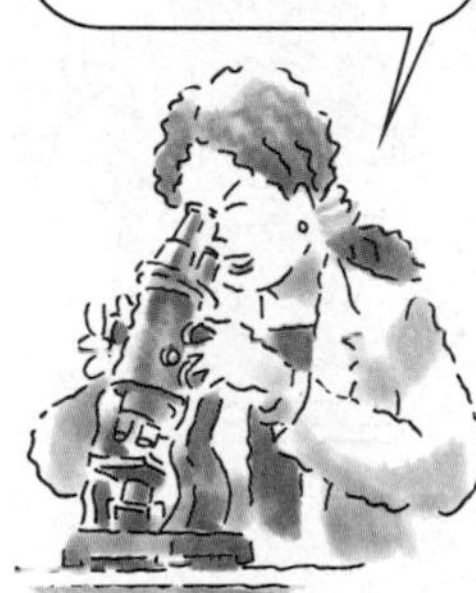

31. 1. X-ray will confirm the diagnosis of congenital hip dislocation. All of the options are positive signs of dislocation, but only the X-ray will confirm the diagnosis.
NP: Assessment; CN: Physiological integrity; CNS: Physiological adaptation; CL: Knowledge

32. Which of the following hip positions should be avoided in an 8-month-old infant who has been diagnosed with congenital hip dysplasia?

1. Extension
2. Abduction
3. Internal rotation
4. External rotation

32. 3. Internal rotation of the hip is an unstable position and should be avoided in infants with hip instability. Hip extension is a relatively stable position. Often the child is placed in slight abduction while in a hip spica cast. External rotation isn't necessarily an unstable position, as long as it isn't externally rotated too far.
NP: Implementation; CN: Physiological integrity; CNS: Reduction of risk potential; CL: Knowledge

33. Based on knowledge of the progression of muscular dystrophy, which of the following activities would a nurse anticipate the client having difficulty with first?

1. Breathing
2. Sitting
3. Standing
4. Swallowing

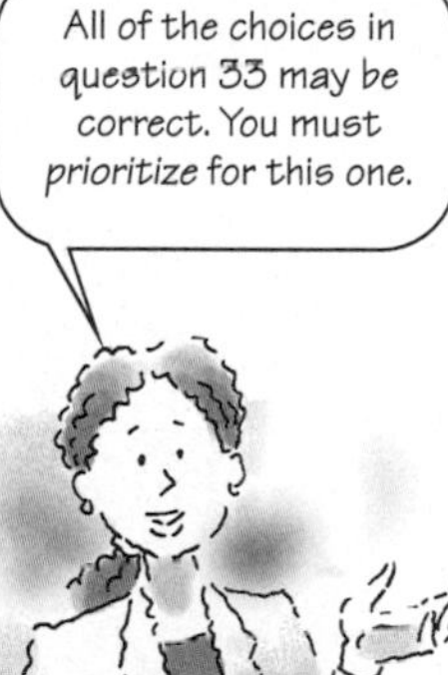
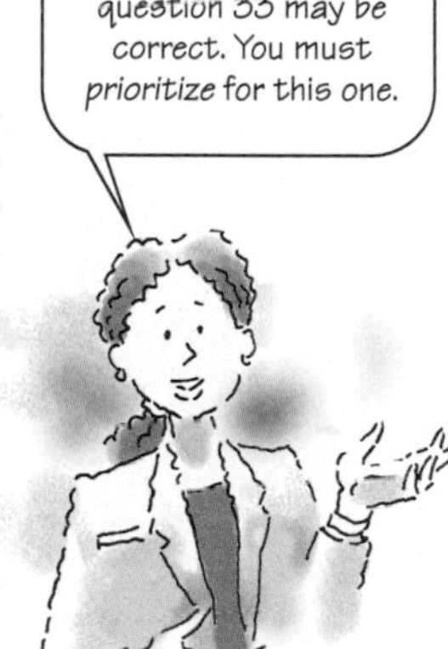

All of the choices in question 33 may be correct. You must *prioritize* for this one.

33. 3. Muscular dystrophy usually affects postural muscles of the hip and shoulder first. Swallowing and breathing are usually affected last. Sitting may be affected, but a client would have difficulty standing before having difficulty sitting.
NP: Assessment; CN: Physiological integrity; CNS: Physiological adaptation; CL: Knowledge

34. Ortolani-Barlow test is used to diagnose hip dislocation in which of the following age groups?
1. 0 to 3 months
2. 3 to 18 months
3. 18 to 36 months
4. 0 to 4 years

34. 1. Ortolani-Barlow test is most effective up to age 3 months. After age 3 months, development of adduction contractures causes the hip "click" to disappear.
NP: Assessment; CN: Physiological integrity; CNS: Physiological adaptation; CL: Knowledge

35. Galeazzi sign is used to assist in the diagnosis of hip dislocation. Which of the following definitions best describes the sign?
1. Raised iliac crest
2. Pelvic downward tilt on weight bearing
3. Knees are flexed to 90 degrees, one knee higher
4. Involved leg flexed to 90 degrees, audible click with external rotation

35. 3. Positive Galeazzi sign is exhibited as one knee being higher than the other. Raised iliac crest isn't indicative of specific hip pathology. A downward pelvic tilt with weight bearing is Trendelenburg gait. External rotation of the hip with audible click is Ortolani-Barlow test.
NP: Assessment; CN: Health promotion and maintenance; CNS: Prevention and early detection of disease; CL: Knowledge

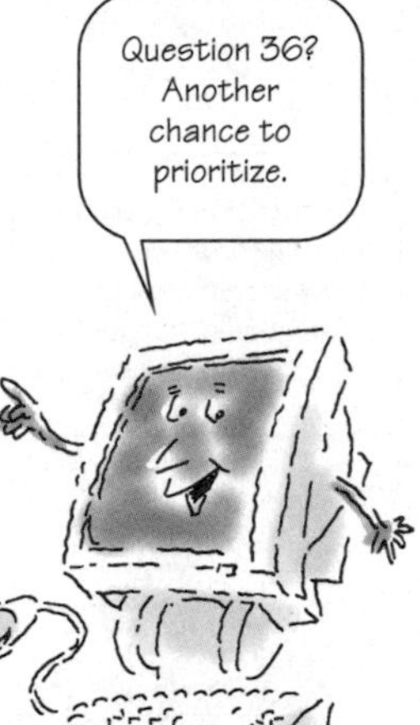
Question 36? Another chance to prioritize.

36. A young child sustains a dislocated hip as well as a subcapital fracture. Which of the following complications is of greatest concern?
1. Avascular necrosis
2. Postsurgical infection
3. Hemorrhage during surgery
4. Poor postsurgical ambulation

36. 1. Avascular necrosis is common with fractures to the subcapital region secondary to possible compromise of blood supply to the femoral head. Postsurgical infection is always a concern but not a priority at first. Hemorrhage shouldn't occur. Poor postsurgical ambulation is of concern but not as much as the possibility of avascular necrosis.
NP: Assessment; CN: Physiological integrity; CNS: Reduction of risk potential; CL: Knowledge

37. Which of the following positions of the femur is accurate in relation to the acetabulum in a child with congenital hip dislocation?
1. Anterior
2. Inferior
3. Posterior
4. Superior

37. 1. The head of the femur is anterior to the acetabulum in a congenital hip dislocation. All other positions are inaccurate.
NP: Assessment; CN: Physiological integrity; CNS: Physiological adaptation; CL: Knowledge

38. Which of the following definitions best describes muscular dystrophy?
1. A demyelinating disease
2. Lesions of the brain cortex
3. Upper motor neuron lesions
4. Degeneration of muscle fibers

38. 4. Degeneration of muscle fibers with progressive weakness and wasting best describes muscular dystrophy. Demyelination of myelin sheaths is a description of multiple sclerosis. Lesions within the cortex and in upper motor neurons suggest a neurologic, not a muscular, disease.
NP: Assessment; CN: Physiological integrity; CNS: Physiological adaptation; CL: Knowledge

39. Which of the following muscles are affected first with muscular dystrophy?
1. Muscles of the hip
2. Muscles of the foot
3. Muscles of the hand
4. Muscles of respiration

39. 1. Positional muscles of the hip and shoulder are affected first. Progression later advances to muscles of the foot and hand. Involuntary muscles, such as the muscles of respiration, are affected last.

NP: Assessment; CN: Physiological integrity; CNS: Physiological adaptation; CL: Knowledge

40. Which of the following tests is most frequently used in assisting with the diagnosis of muscular dystrophy?
1. X-ray
2. Muscle biopsy
3. Electroencephalogram
4. Assessment of ambulation

40. 2. A muscle biopsy shows the degeneration of muscle fibers and infiltration of fatty tissue. It is used for diagnostic confirmation. X-ray is best for osseous deformity. Electroencephalogram wouldn't be appropriate in this case. Ambulation assessment alone wouldn't confirm the diagnosis.

NP: Assessment; CN: Health promotion and maintenance; CNS: Prevention and early detection of disease; CL: Knowledge

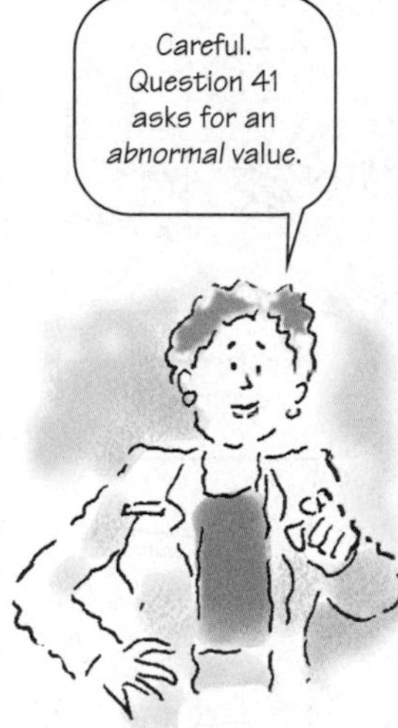

Careful. Question 41 asks for an *abnormal* value.

41. Which of the following laboratory values would be most abnormal in a client diagnosed with muscular dystrophy?
1. Bilirubin
2. Creatinine
3. Serum potassium
4. Sodium

41. 2. Creatinine is a by-product of muscle metabolism as it hypertrophies. Bilirubin is a by-product of liver function. Potassium and sodium levels can change due to a variety of factors and aren't indicators of muscular dystrophy.

NP: Assessment; CN: Health promotion and maintenance; CNS: Prevention and early detection of disease; CL: Knowledge

42. Which of the following forms of muscular dystrophy is the most common?
1. Duchenne's
2. Becker's
3. Limb girdle
4. Myotonic

42. 1. Duchenne's accounts for 50% of all cases of muscular dystrophy.

NP: Assessment; CN: Physiological integrity; CNS: Physiological adaptation; CL: Knowledge

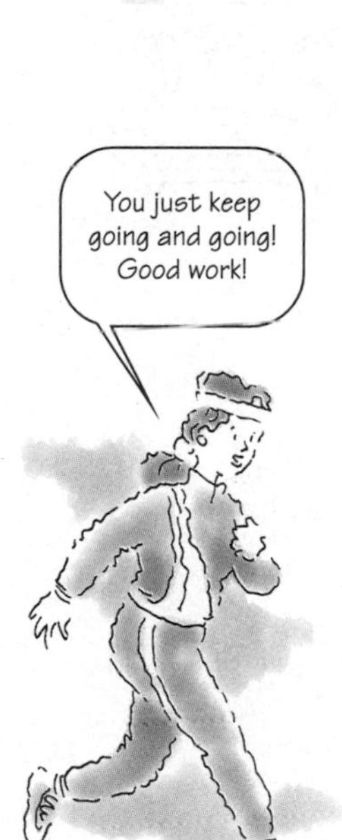

You just keep going and going! Good work!

43. Which of the following conditions may be indicative of a child suffering from muscular dystrophy?
1. Hypertonia of extremities
2. Increased lumbar lordosis
3. Upper extremity spasticity
4. Hyperactive lower extremity reflexes

43. 2. An increased lumbar lordosis occurs secondarily to paralysis of lower lumbar postural muscles; it also occurs to increase lower extremity support. Upper extremity spasticity isn't seen because this disease isn't due to upper motor neuron lesions. Hyperactive reflexes aren't indications of muscular dystrophy. Hypertonia isn't seen in this disease.

NP: Assessment; CN: Physiological integrity; CNS: Physiological adaptation; CL: Knowledge

44. Through which of the following mechanisms is Duchenne's muscular dystrophy acquired?
1. Virus
2. Hereditary
3. Autoimmune factors
4. Environmental toxins

44. 2. Muscular dystrophy is hereditary and acquired through a recessive sex-linked trait. Therefore, it isn't viral, autoimmune, or caused by toxins.

NP: Assessment; CN: Physiological integrity; CNS: Physiological adaptation; CL: Knowledge

45. A client with muscular dystrophy has lost complete control of his lower extremities. He has some strength bilaterally in the upper extremities, but poor trunk control. Which of the following mechanisms would be the most important to have on the wheelchair?

1. Antitip device
2. Extended breaks
3. Headrest support
4. Wheelchair belt

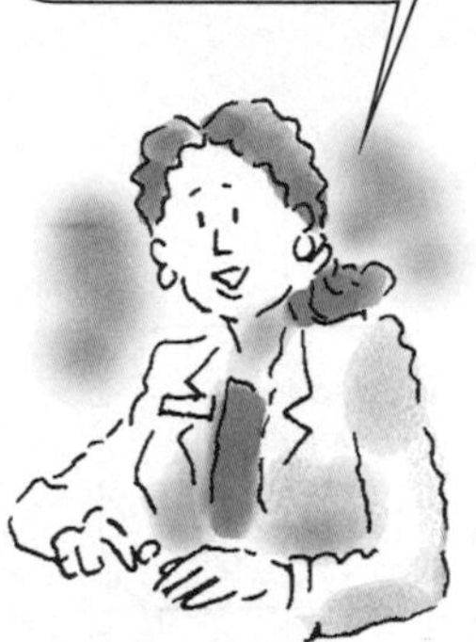

Question 45 tests your ability to ensure the client's safety.

45. 4. This client has poor trunk control; a belt will prevent him from falling out of the wheelchair. Antitip devices, head rest supports, and extended breaks are all important options but aren't the best choice in this situation.
NP: Planning; CN: Safe, effective care environment; CNS: Safety and infection control; CL: Application

46. A 2-year-old infant has muscular dystrophy. His legs are held together with the knees touching. Which of the following muscles are contracted?

1. Hip abductors
2. Hip adductors
3. Hip extensors
4. Hip flexors

46. 2. The hip adductors are in a shortened position. The abductors are in a lengthened position. This position isn't indicative of hip flexor or hip extensor shortening.
NP: Assessment; CN: Health promotion and maintenance; CNS: Prevention and early detection of disease; CL: Knowledge

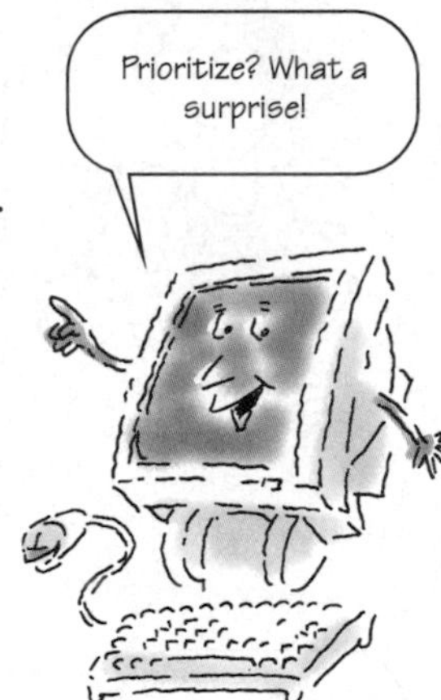

Prioritize? What a surprise!

47. A 12-year-old child diagnosed with muscular dystrophy is hospitalized secondary to a fall. Surgery is necessary as well as skeletal traction. Which of the following complications would be of greatest concern to the nursing staff?

1. Skin integrity
2. Infection of pin sites
3. Respiratory infection
4. Nonunion healing of the fracture

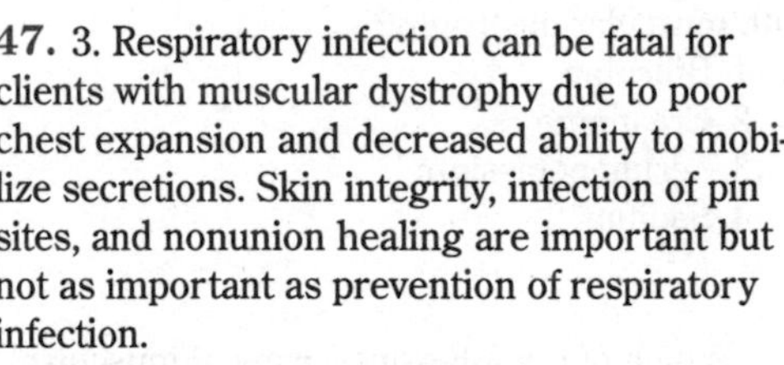

47. 3. Respiratory infection can be fatal for clients with muscular dystrophy due to poor chest expansion and decreased ability to mobilize secretions. Skin integrity, infection of pin sites, and nonunion healing are important but not as important as prevention of respiratory infection.
NP: Assessment; CN: Physiological integrity; CNS: Reduction of risk potential; CL: Application

48. Which of the following components replaces necrotic muscle tissue in clients diagnosed with muscular dystrophy?

1. Fat
2. Bone
3. New muscle fibers
4. Calcified soft tissue

48. 1. Fat and connective tissue replace muscle fibers. New muscle fibers don't develop, calcification of soft tissue doesn't occur, and bone doesn't replace the tissue.
NP: Assessment; CN: Physiological integrity; CNS: Physiological adaptation; CL: Knowledge

49. Which of the following portions of a shoe is raised to attempt a correction of the deformity of clubfoot?

1. Forefoot
2. Lateral
3. Medial
4. Rearfoot

49. 2. Raising the lateral portion of the foot will help pull the foot into eversion. Raising the medial portion will pull the foot into increased inversion. Raising the forefoot or rearfoot won't help in correction of the problem.
NP: Assessment; CN: Physiological integrity; CNS: Reduction of risk potential; CL: Application

50. A child has developed difficulty ambulating and tends to walk on his toes. Which of the following surgical techniques may benefit the client?
1. Adductor release
2. Hamstring release
3. Plantar fascia release
4. Achilles tendon release

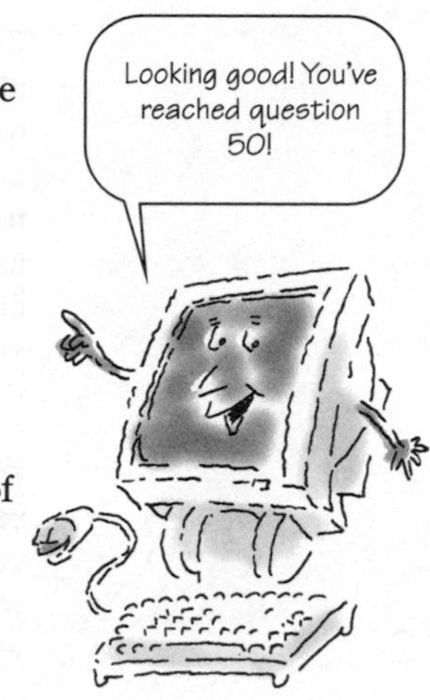

Looking good! You've reached question 50!

50. 4. A shortened Achilles tendon may cause a child to walk on his toes. A release of the tendon may assist the child in walking. An adductor release is often performed if the legs are held together. A plantar fascia release won't help, and a hamstring release is done only when there's a knee flexion contracture.
NP: Evaluation; CN: Physiological integrity; CNS: Reduction of risk potential; CL: Application

51. Muscular dystrophy is a result of which of the following causes?
1. Gene mutation
2. Chromosomal aberration
3. Unknown nongenetic origin
4. Genetic and environmental factors

51. 1. Muscular dystrophy is a result of a gene mutation. It isn't from a chromosome aberration or environmental factors. It's genetic, and there's a known origin of the disease.
NP: Assessment; CN: Physiological integrity; CNS: Physiological adaptation; CL: Knowledge

52. Evidence of muscle weakness associated with muscular dystrophy usually appears at which of the following ages?
1. Age 1
2. Age 2
3. Age 3
4. Age 4

52. 3. Studies have shown that children diagnosed with muscular dystrophy usually show some form of weakness around age 3.
NP: Assessment; CN: Health promotion and maintenance; CNS: Prevention and early detection of disease; CL: Knowledge

53. Which of the following muscle groups is most important in maintaining maximum function in regards to lower extremity strength in a client diagnosed with muscular dystrophy?
1. Gastrocnemius
2. Gluteus maximus
3. Hamstrings
4. Quadriceps

53. 2. Gluteus maximus is the strongest muscle in the body and is important for standing as well as for transfers. All of the named muscles are important, but the maintenance of the gluteus maximus will enable maximum function.
NP: Assessment; CN: Health promotion and maintenance; CNS: Growth and development through the life span; CL: Knowledge

54. Which of the following strategies would be the last choice in attempting to maximize function in a child with muscular dystrophy?
1. Long leg braces
2. Straight cane
3. Wheelchair
4. Walker

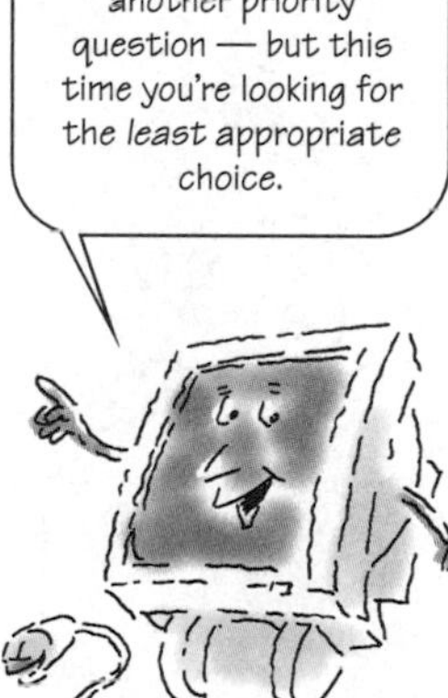

Question 54 is another priority question — but this time you're looking for the least appropriate choice.

54. 3. A wheelchair provides decreased independence and decreased use of upper extremity and lower extremity function. It should be used only when absolutely necessary. A straight cane, long leg braces, and a walker are functional assistive devices, much more so than a wheelchair.
NP: Evaluation; CN: Physiological integrity; CNS: Basic care and comfort; CL: Application

55. A child is having increased difficulty getting out of his chair at school. Which of the following recommendations may the nurse make to assist the child?

1. A seat cushion
2. Long leg braces
3. Powered wheelchair
4. Removable arm rests on wheelchair

55. 1. A seat cushion will put the hip extensors at an advantage and make it somewhat easier to get up. Long leg braces wouldn't be the first choice. A powered wheelchair wouldn't be important in assisting with the transfer. Removable armrests have no bearing on assisting the client.

NP: Implementation; CN: Physiological integrity; CNS: Basic care and comfort; CL: Application

56. Muscles in a child with muscular dystrophy will have which of the following characteristics?

1. Soft on palpation
2. Firm or woody on palpation
3. Extremely hard on palpation
4. No muscle consistency on palpation

56. 2. Muscles will often be firm on palpation secondary to the infiltration of fatty tissue and connective tissue into the muscle. The muscles won't be soft secondary to the infiltration and won't be hard upon palpation. There's some consistency to the muscle although, in advanced stages, atrophy is present.

NP: Assessment; CN: Physiological integrity; CNS: Physiological adaptation; CL: Knowledge

57. Nurses should instruct wheelchair-bound clients with muscular dystrophy in which of the following exercises to best prevent skin breakdown?

1. Wheelchair push-ups
2. Leaning side-to-side
3. Leaning forward
4. Gluteal sets

57. 1. A wheelchair push-up will alleviate the most pressure off the buttocks. Leaning side-to-side will help but not as much as wheelchair push-ups. Gluteal sets won't help with pressure relief.

NP: Planning; CN: Health promotion and maintenance; CNS: Prevention and early detection of disease; CL: Application

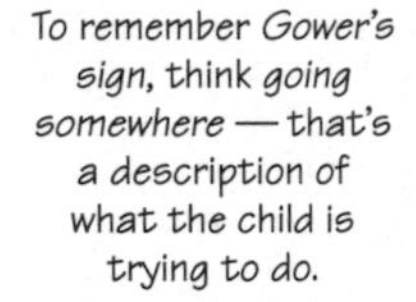

To remember Gower's sign, think going somewhere — that's a description of what the child is trying to do.

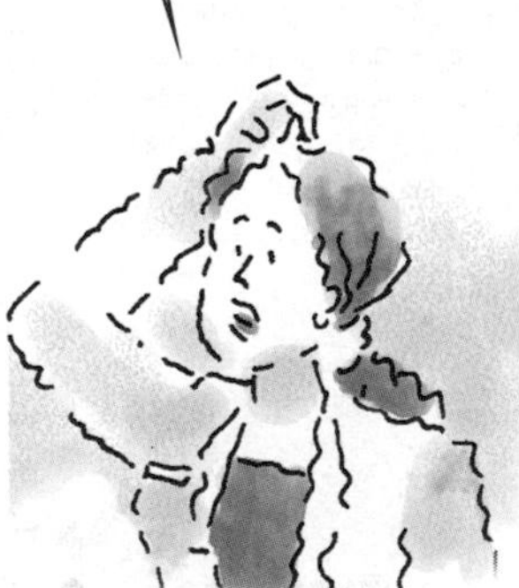

58. Which of the following definitions best describes Gower's sign?

1. A transfer technique
2. A waddling-type gait
3. The pelvis position during gait
4. Muscle twitching present during a quick stretch

58. 1. Gower's sign is a description of a transfer technique present during some phases of muscular dystrophy. The child turns on the side or abdomen, extends the knees, and pushes on the torso to an upright position by walking his hands up the legs. Waddling-type gait doesn't describe Gower's sign. The position of the pelvis during gait isn't described by Gower's sign. Muscle twitching present after a quick stretch is described as *clonus*.

NP: Assessment; CN: Physiological integrity; CNS: Physiological adaptation; CL: Knowledge

59. Which of the following definitions best describes pseudohypertrophy?

1. Increased muscle hypertrophy secondary to increased muscle mass
2. Increased muscle hypertrophy secondary to fat infiltration
3. Decreased muscle secondary to muscle degeneration
4. Decreased muscle mass secondary to disease

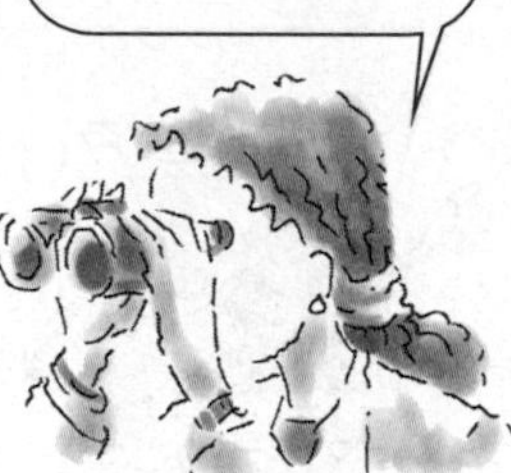

Focus in on the right definition — and on the prefix *pseudo*.

59. 2. Pseudohypertrophy is present secondary to fat infiltration. Increased muscle mass is called hypertrophy. Pseudohypertrophy isn't due to degeneration or decreased muscle mass.

NP: Assessment; CN: Physiological integrity; CNS: Physiological adaptation; CL: Knowledge

60. Which of the following characteristics best describes the rate of onset of facioscapulohumeral muscular dystrophy?

1. Fast
2. Slow
3. Present at birth
4. Present in late adolescence

60. 2. The progression of this disease is slow, not fast. It's difficult to detect at birth and is present in early adolescence.

NP: Assessment; CN: Physiological integrity; CNS: Physiological adaptation; CL: Knowledge

61. Facioscapulohumeral muscular dystrophy is characterized initially by which of the following conditions?

1. Complete upper extremity and lower extremity paralysis
2. Difficulty raising the arms overhead
3. Poor ambulation
4. Blindness

61. 2. This form of muscular dystrophy is characterized by difficulty raising the arms overhead and lack of facial muscles. Complete paralysis isn't usually present with this deformity. Poor ambulation and blindness aren't initial characteristics of the disease.

NP: Assessment; CN: Physiological integrity; CNS: Physiological adaptation; CL: Knowledge

62. Which of the following forms of muscular dystrophy is the most severe?

1. Duchenne's
2. Facioscapulohumeral
3. Limb girdle
4. Myotonia

62. 1. Studies have shown that Duchenne's is the most severe form of muscular dystrophy. Myotonia isn't a form of the disease; it's a symptom.

NP: Assessment; CN: Physiological integrity; CNS: Physiological adaptation; CL: Knowledge

63. Which of the following definitions best describes acetabular dysplasia?

1. Partial dislocation of the head of the femur
2. Delay in acetabular development
3. Ligamentous laxity of the joint
4. Audible clicking of the femur

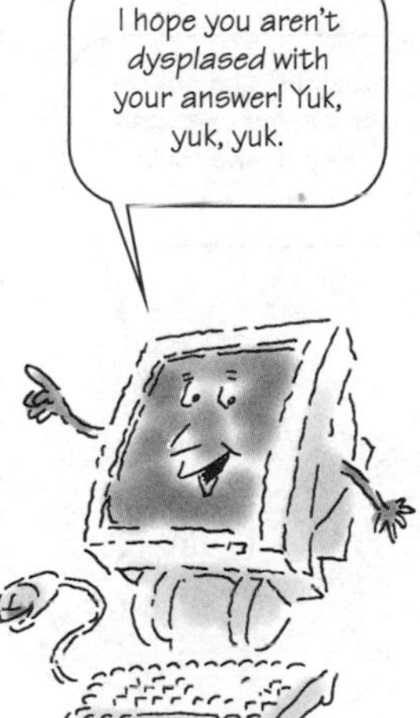

I hope you aren't *dysplased* with your answer! Yuk, yuk, yuk.

63. 2. Acetabular dysplasia is characterized by an underdevelopment of the acetabular ridge. Partial dislocation is described as a subluxation. Ligamentous laxity can be described in a number of ways, but isn't appropriate here. Audible clicking is indicative of some degree of subluxation or dislocation.

NP: Assessment; CN: Physiological integrity; CNS: Physiological adaptation; CL: Knowledge

64. Which of the following complications accounts for the greatest number of cases of congenital hip dysplasia?

1. Dislocation
2. Subluxation
3. Acetabular dysplasia
4. Dislocation with fracture

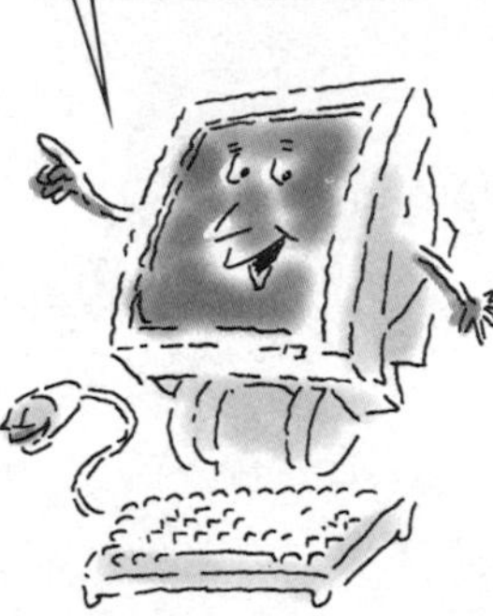

Key here: *greatest number*. Use it, or lose it.

64. 2. Studies show that subluxation accounts for the greatest number of cases of congenital hip dysplasia.

NP: Assessment; CN: Physiological integrity; CNS: Physiological adaptation; CL: Knowledge

65. Which of the following positions of the hip best describes the condition of a client diagnosed with congenital hip dysplasia?

1. Ligamentum teres is shortened.
2. Femoral head loses contact with acetabulum and is displaced inferiorly.
3. Femoral head loses contact with the acetabulum and is displaced posteriorly.
4. Femoral head maintains contact with acetabulum, but there's noted capsular rupture.

65. 3. The femoral head loses contact with the acetabulum and is displaced posteriorly, not inferiorly. Ligamentum teres is lengthened.

NP: Assessment; CN: Physiological integrity; CNS: Physiological adaptation; CL: Knowledge

66. Which of the following percentages represents cases of congenital hip dysplasia involving both hips?

1. 10%
2. 25%
3. 50%
4. 75%

66. 2. Studies show that 25% of all cases of congenital hip dysplasia involve both hips.

NP: Assessment; CN: Physiological integrity; CNS: Physiological adaptation; CL: Knowledge

67. Which of the following choices is best for handling a client's hip-spica cast that has been soiled?

1. Clean with damp cloth and dry cleanser.
2. Clean with soap and water.
3. Don't do anything.
4. Change the cast.

67. 1. A damp cloth is best to use rather than water. Water will break the cast down. Changing the cast isn't an option. If nothing is done, the cast will give off an odor.

NP: Assessment; CN: Physiological integrity; CNS: Basic care and comfort; CL: Application

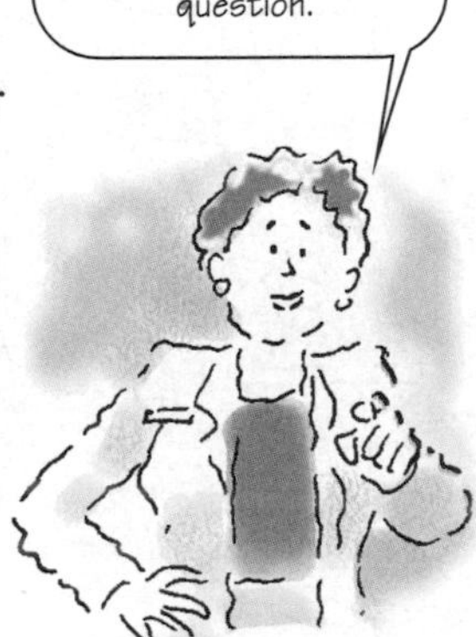

Knowing the shape of a spica cast can help answer this question.

68. Which of the following positions is best for a child in a hip-spica cast who needs to be toileted?

1. Supine
2. Sitting in a toilet chair
3. Shoulder lower than buttocks
4. Buttocks lower than shoulder

68. 4. The buttocks need to be lowered to toilet the child. This will keep the cast from being soiled. Supine will cause soiling of the cast. The child isn't able to use a toilet chair.

NP: Planning; CN: Physiological integrity; CNS: Basic care and comfort; CL: Knowledge

69. Congenital hip dysplasia is most common in which of the following ethnic groups?

1. Blacks
2. Whites
3. Native Americans
4. Chinese

70. Which of the following characteristics indicates a positive Trendelenburg gait?

1. Pelvis tilts downward upon weight bearing
2. Pelvis tilts upward upon weight bearing
3. Abnormal height of the iliac crests
4. Leg length discrepancy

71. Which of the following complications involving leg length is seen with a congenital hip dislocation?

1. Increased hip abduction
2. Increased leg length on the affected side
3. Decreased leg length on the affected side
4. No change in muscle length or leg length

72. Which of the following positions should be avoided in a child suspected of congenital hip dysplasia?

1. Hip abduction
2. Knee extension
3. External rotation
4. Tightly wrapped blankets

73. Immediately after a spinal fusion, which of the following restrictions is usually put on the child's activity?

1. Bed rest
2. Non-weight bearing
3. No restriction
4. Limited weight bearing

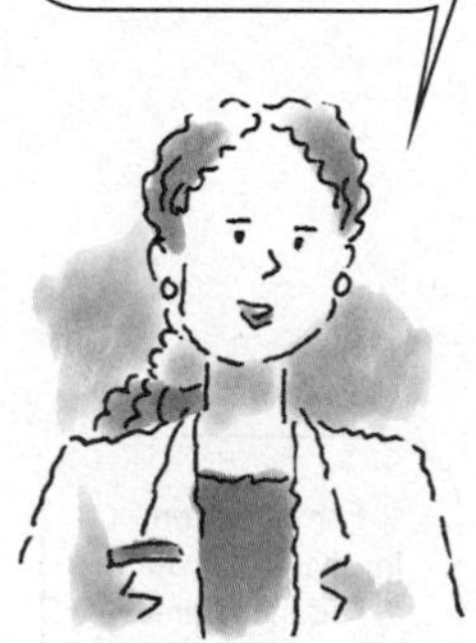

You've completed 70 questions. You're awesome!

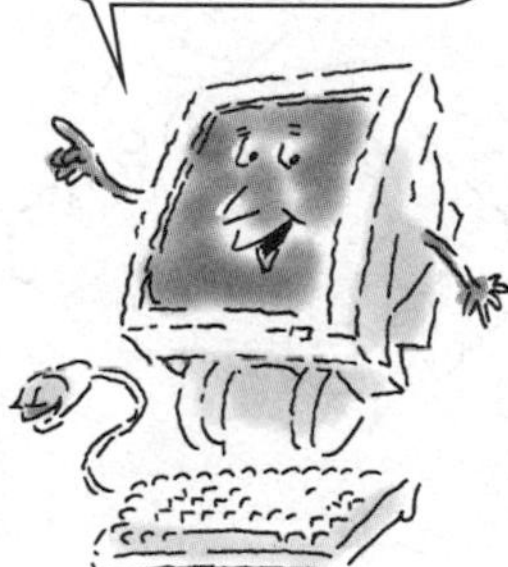

The word avoided makes this a negative question.

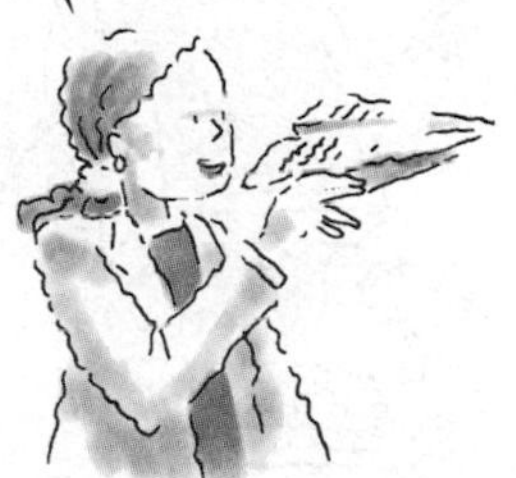

At the rate you're going, the sky's the limit!

69. 3. Native Americans traditionally wrap their neonates in tight blankets that increase internal rotation in the hip. This condition isn't as common in other ethnic groups.

NP: Assessment; CN: Physiological integrity; CNS: Physiological adaptation; CL: Knowledge

70. 1. The pelvis will tilt downward upon weight bearing secondary to a weakness of the abductors on the affected side. The pelvis doesn't tilt upward. Leg length and iliac crest height aren't indicative of Trendelenburg gait.

NP: Assessment; CN: Physiological integrity; CNS: Physiological adaptation; CL: Knowledge

71. 3. The internal rotation with subsequent dislocation will cause the leg to be shorter, not longer. There's usually *decreased* abduction as well as muscle and leg length changes.

NP: Assessment; CN: Physiological integrity; CNS: Physiological adaptation; CL: Knowledge

72. 4. Tightly wrapped blankets force the hip into internal rotation. Abduction, external rotation, and knee extension won't increase the risk of dislocation.

NP: Implementation; CN: Health promotion and maintenance; CNS: Prevention and early detection of disease; CL: Application

73. 1. After a spinal fusion, the child is usually placed on bed rest and ordered to lie flat. In 2 to 4 days, the child is allowed to sit up in and get out of bed. Other activities are gradually reintroduced.

NP: Implementation; CN: Physiological integrity; CNS: Basic care and comfort; CL: Knowledge

74. Which of the following interventions would a nurse expect to use to prevent venous stasis after skeletal traction application?

1. Bed rest only
2. Eggcrate mattress
3. Vigorous pulmonary care
4. Antiembolism stockings or an intermittent compression device

74. 4. To prevent venous stasis after skeletal traction application, antiembolism stockings or an intermittent compression device is used on the unaffected leg. Eggcrate mattresses and pulmonary care don't prevent venous stasis. Bed rest can *cause* venous stasis.

NP: Implementation; CN: Health promotion and maintenance; CNS: Prevention and early detection of disease; CL: Application

75. A 13-year-old girl is suspected of having structural scoliosis by her school nurse. What should the nurse ask the girl to do to help confirm her suspicion?

1. Bend over and touch her toes while the nurse observes from the back.
2. Stand sideways while the nurse observes her profile.
3. Assume a knee-chest position on the examination table.
4. Arch her back while the nurse observes her from the back.

75. 1. As the child bends over, the curvature of the spine is more apparent. The scapula on one side becomes more prominent, and the opposite side hollows. Scoliosis can't be properly assessed from the side or the front. The knee-chest position is used for lumbar pucture.

NP: Assessment; CN: Health promotion and maintenance; CNS: Prevention and early detection of disease; CL: Comprehension

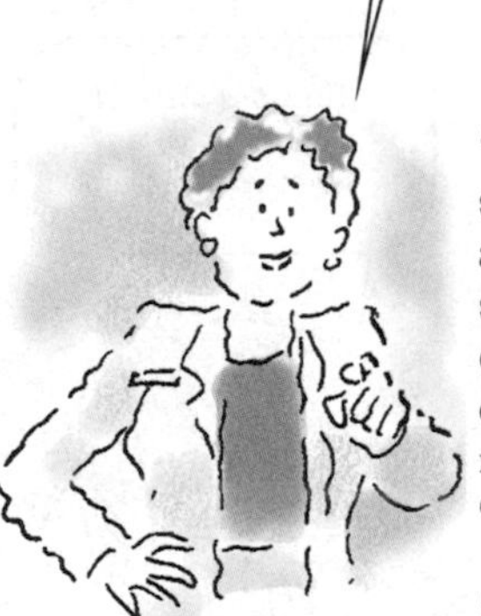

For questions involving a trauma scene, think safety first!

76. At the scene of a trauma, which of the following nursing interventions is appropriate for a child with a suspected fracture?

1. Never move the child.
2. Sit the child up to facilitate breathing.
3. Move the child to a safe place immediately.
4. Immobilize the extremity and then move child to a safe place.

76. 4. At the scene of a trauma, the nurse should immobilize the extremity of a child with a suspected fracture and then move him to a safe place. If the child is already in a safe place, don't attempt to move him. Never try to sit the child up; this could make the fracture worse.

NP: Implementation; CN: Safe, effective care environment; CNS: Safety and infection control; CL: Application

77. Which of the following statements is true about fracture reduction?

1. All fractures can be reduced
2. Fracture reduction restores alignment
3. Undisplaced fractures may be reduced
4. Fracture reduction is usually performed with minimal discomfort

77. 2. Fracture reduction restores alignment. All fractures can't be reduced. Undisplaced fractures can't be reduced. Fracture reduction is usually very painful.

NP: Implementation; CN: Physiological integrity; CNS: Reduction of risk potential; CL: Knowledge

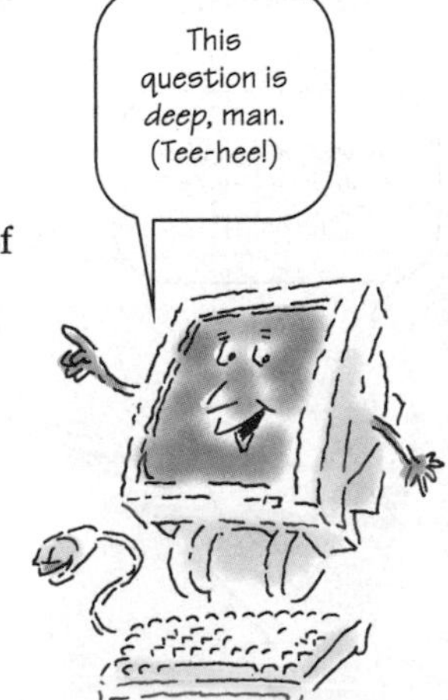

This question is deep, man. (Tee-hee!)

78. A child in skeletal traction for a fracture of the right femur exhibits a positive Homans' sign, complains of left-sided leg pain, and has edema in the left leg. Which condition should be expected?

1. A fat emboli
2. An infection
3. A pulmonary embolism
4. Deep vein thrombosis (DVT)

78. 4. Unilateral leg pain and edema with a positive Homans' sign (not always present) should lead you to suspect DVT. Symptoms of fat emboli include restlessness, tachypnea, and tachycardia and are more common in long bone injuries. It's unlikely that an infection would occur on the opposite side of the fracture without cause. Tachycardia, chest pain, and shortness of breath may be symptoms of a pulmonary embolism.

NP: Implementation; CN: Physiological integrity; CNS: Reduction of risk potential; CL: Knowledge

NP: Nursing process CN: Client needs category CNS: Client needs subcategory CL: Cognitive level

79. Nursing care for a client in traction may include which of the following interventions?

1. Assessing pin sites every shift and as needed
2. Ensuring that the rope knots catch on the pulley
3. Adding and removing weights per client's request
4. Placing all joints through range of motion every shift

79. 1. Nursing care for a client in traction may include assessing pin sites every shift and as needed and ensuring that the knots in the rope don't catch on the pulley. Weights should be added and removed per the primary health care provider's order, and all joints, except those immediately proximal and distal to the fracture, should be placed through range of motion every shift.

NP: Implementation; CN: Physiological integrity; CNS: Basic care and comfort; CL: Application

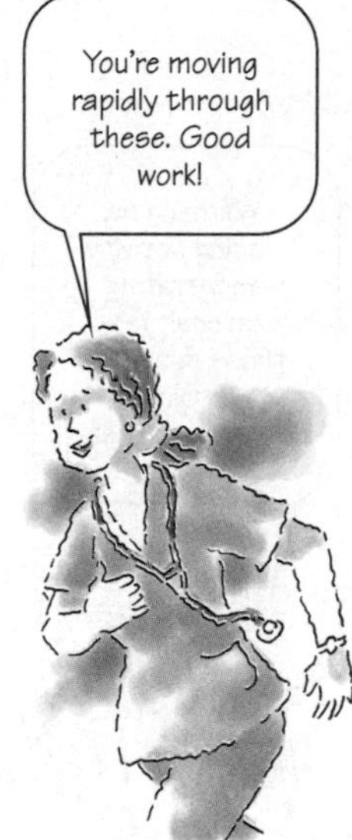

You're moving rapidly through these. Good work!

80. After assisting the primary health care provider in applying a cast, the nurse should include which of the following interventions in the immediate cast care?

1. Rest the cast on the bedside table
2. Dispose of the plaster water in the sink
3. Support the cast with the palms of her hands
4. Wait until the cast dries before cleansing surrounding skin

80. 3. After a cast has been applied, it should be immediately supported with the palms of the nurse's hands. Later, the nurse should dispose of the plaster water in a sink with a plaster trap or in a garbage bag, cleanse the surrounding skin before the cast dries, and make sure that the cast isn't resting on a hard or sharp surface.

NP: Implementation; CN: Safe, effective care environment; CNS: Management of care; CL: Comprehension

81. Which of the following time periods best represents approximately how long it takes a synthetic cast to set?

1. Immediately
2. 20 minutes
3. 45 minutes
4. 2 hours

81. 2. Synthetic casts take about 20 minutes to set.

NP: Implementation; CN: Safe, effective care environment; CNS: Management of care; CL: Knowledge

82. Which of the following nursing interventions should be taken if, as a cast is drying, the client complains of heat from the cast?

1. Remove the cast immediately.
2. Notify the primary health care provider.
3. Assess the client for other signs of infection.
4. Explain to the client that this is a normal sensation.

82. 4. Normally, as the cast is drying, the client may complain of heat from the cast. The nurse should offer reassurance but doesn't need to notify the primary health care provider or remove the cast. Heat from the cast isn't a sign of infection.

NP: Implementation; CN: Safe, effective care environment; CNS: Management of care; CL: Comprehension

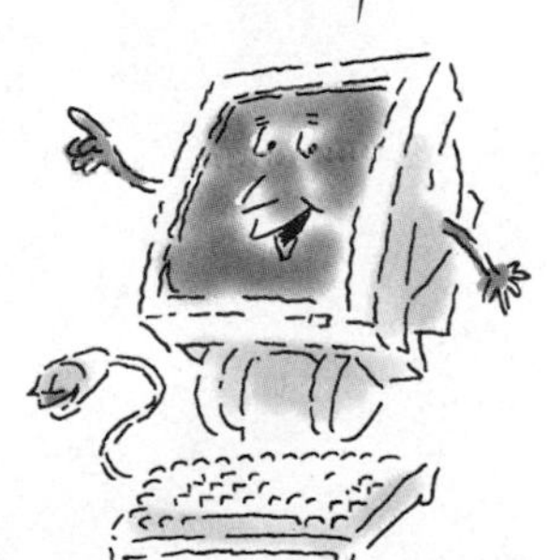

In question 83, you're trying to prevent a problem, not react to it.

83. Which of the following nursing interventions can be implemented to prevent foot drop in a casted leg?

1. Encourage bed rest.
2. Support the foot with 45 degrees of flexion.
3. Support the foot with 90 degrees of flexion.
4. Place a stocking on the foot to provide warmth.

83. 3. To prevent foot drop in a casted leg, the foot should be supported with 90 degrees of flexion. Bed rest can cause foot drop. Keeping the extremity warm won't prevent foot drop.

NP: Implementation; CN: Health promotion and maintenance; CNS: Prevention and early detection of disease; CL: Comprehension

84. A client with a hip-spica cast should avoid gas-forming foods for which of the following reasons?

1. To prevent flatus
2. To prevent diarrhea
3. To prevent constipation
4. To prevent abdominal distention

84. 4. A client with a hip-spica cast should avoid gas-forming foods. The rationale for this is to prevent abdominal distention. Gas-forming foods may cause flatus, but that isn't a reason to avoid them. Gas-forming foods don't generally cause diarrhea or constipation.

NP: Implementation; CN: Physiological integrity; CNS: Reduction of risk potential; CL: Comprehension

85. Which of the following actions does touch-down weight bearing allow the client to perform?

1. Allows full weight bearing on the affected extremity
2. Allows 30% to 50% weight bearing on the affected extremity
3. Allows no weight on the extremity, which must be kept elevated at all times
4. Allows no weight on the extremity, but the client may touch the floor with the affected extremity

85. 4. Touch-down weight bearing allows the client to put no weight on the extremity, but the client may touch the floor with the affected extremity. Full weight bearing allows for full weight bearing on the affected extremity. Partial weight bearing allows for only 30% to 50% weight bearing on the affected extremity. Non-weight bearing is no weight on the extremity, and the extremity must remain elevated.

NP: Implementation; CN: Safe, effective care environment; CNS: Management of care; CL: Knowledge

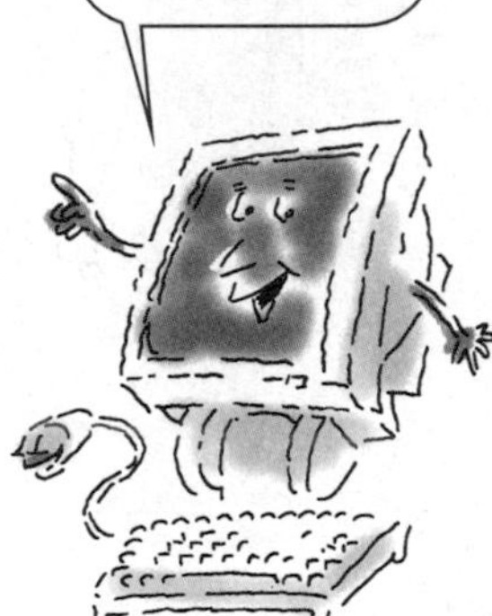
Warming up, pacing activity, moderating intensity — those sound like study instructions!

86. Which of the following strategies is best for preventing sports-related injuries?

1. Warming up
2. Pacing activity
3. Building strength
4. Moderating intensity

86. 1. To prevent sports-related injuries, instruct your client that the best prevention is warming up. Pacing activity, building strength, and using moderate intensity are also prevention measures.

NP: Planning; CN: Safe, effective care environment; CNS: Management of care; CL: Knowledge

87. Which of the following activities may be most helpful for a child who's allowed full activity after repair of a clubfoot?

1. Playing catch
2. Standing
3. Swimming
4. Walking

87. 4. Walking will stimulate all of the involved muscles and help with strengthening. All of the options are good exercises, but walking is the best choice.

NP: Planning; CN: Physiological integrity; CNS: Physiological adaptation; CL: Application

88. Which of the following joints is involved most with clubfoot?

1. Midtarsal
2. Subtalar
3. Talocrural
4. Transmetatarsal

88. 2. The subtalar joint is involved most with clubfoot. It's primarily responsible for adduction and inversion of the foot, the greatest defect. The midtarsal and transmetatarsal joints aren't affected.

NP: Assessment; CN: Physiological integrity; CNS: Physiological adaptation; CL: Knowledge

89. Which of the following complications may occur secondary to a mild talipes equinovarus deformity?

1. Medial ankle sprain
2. Irritation of the fifth metatarsal
3. Lengthening of the Achilles tendon
4. Lengthening of medial joint structures

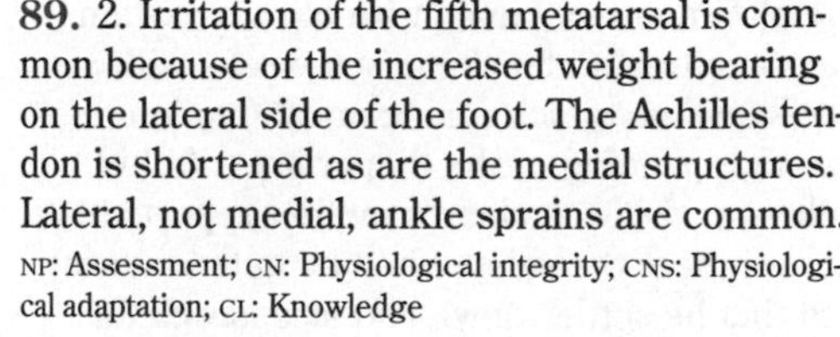

89. 2. Irritation of the fifth metatarsal is common because of the increased weight bearing on the lateral side of the foot. The Achilles tendon is shortened as are the medial structures. Lateral, not medial, ankle sprains are common.

NP: Assessment; CN: Physiological integrity; CNS: Physiological adaptation; CL: Knowledge

90. Which of the following diseases may be associated with a congenital clubfoot?

1. Spina bifida
2. Muscular dystrophy
3. Osteogenesis imperfecta
4. Juvenile rheumatoid arthritis

90. 1. Studies have shown that there's an increased incidence of clubfoot with spina bifida. This doesn't occur at an increased rate with the other conditions.

NP: Assessment; CN: Physiological integrity; CNS: Physiological adaptation; CL: Knowledge

91. Which of the following findings in a history related to congenital hip dislocation is most significant?

1. Mother's activity during the third trimester
2. Breech presentation at birth
3. Infant's serum calcium level at birth
4. Apgar score of 4 at 1 minute and 6 at 5 minutes

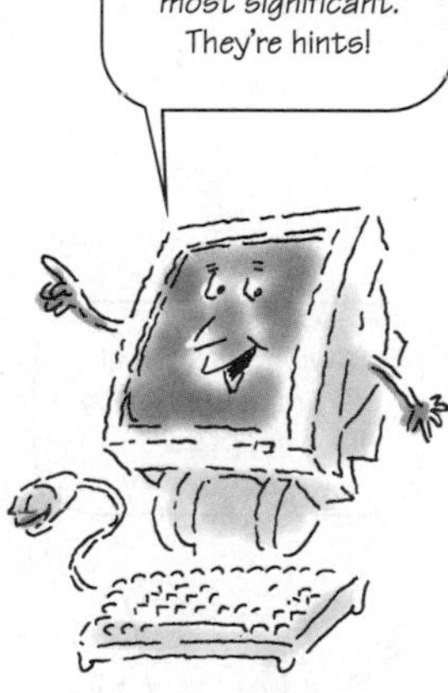

Watch the words most significant. They're hints!

91. 2. Breech presentation is a factor frequently associated with congenital hip dislocation. The mother's activity during the third trimester, the infant's serum calcium level at birth, and Apgar scores have no bearing on hip dislocation.

NP: Assessment; CN: Health promotion and maintenance; CNS: Growth and development through the life span; CL: Application

92. A 13-year-old with structural scoliosis has Harrington rods inserted. Which of the following positions would be best during the postoperative period?

1. Supine in bed
2. Side-lying
3. Semi-Fowler
4. High Fowler

92. 1. After placement of Harrington rods, the client must remain flat in bed. The gatch on a manual bed should be taped, and electric beds should be unplugged to prevent the client from raising the head or foot of the bed. Other positions, such as side-lying, semi-Fowler, or high Fowler, could prove damaging because the rods may not be able to maintain the spine in a straight position.

NP: Implementation; CN: Physiological integrity; CNS: Reduction of risk potential; CL: Application

93. A client with structural scoliosis has been fitted for a Milwaukee brace. How many hours a day should the nurse tell the client that the brace must be worn?

1. 8 hours
2. 12 hours
3. 23 hours
4. 24 hours

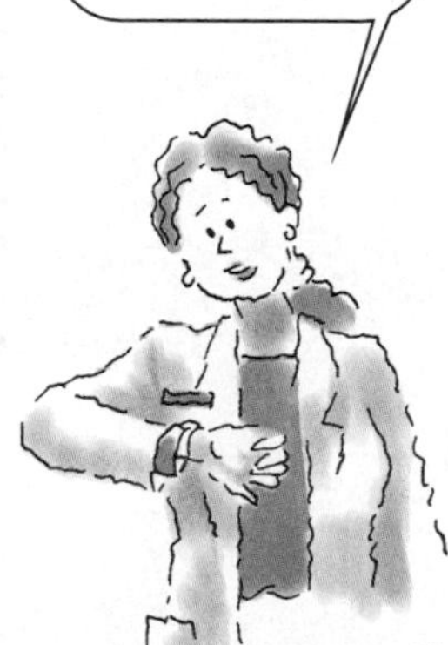

Let's see, if it's 10 o'clock in Milwaukee, how long does the child need to wear the brace?

93. 3. The brace can be removed only 1 hour per day for bathing and hygiene; otherwise, it must remain in place. Wearing the brace for 8 or 12 hours per day isn't enough time to provide the necessary correction. Wearing the brace 24 hours per day doesn't allow for bathing or skin integrity checks.

NP: Implementation; CN: Physiological integrity; CNS: Reduction of risk potential; CL: Knowledge

94. A 6-month-old male with hip dislocation has been treated for the past 6 weeks with a Frejka splint, which maintains abduction through padding of the diaper area. At his follow-up visit, the client's mother reports that she removes the splint when he gets too fussy and that he settles down and sleeps well for several hours after the padding is removed. Which of the following responses by the nurse would be most appropriate?

1. "I can tell you're concerned about his comfort, but he must wear the padded splint except during the three times a day when you perform range-of-motion exercises on his legs."
2. "I'm pleased that you recognize that the padding is too thick and have adjusted it so he can sleep comfortably."
3. "I realize that seeing him uncomfortable is difficult for you, but he needs to keep his splint on except when you bathe him or change his diaper."
4. "If he seems uncomfortable while wearing the splint, it's important that you call us immediately."

94. 3. Soft abduction devices, such as the Frejka splint, must be worn continually except for diaper changes and skin care. The abduction position must be maintained to establish a deep hip socket. Discomfort is anticipated; appropriate responses including changing position, holding, cuddling, and providing diversion.

NP: Evaluation; CN: Physiological integrity; CNS: Physiological adaptation; CL: Application

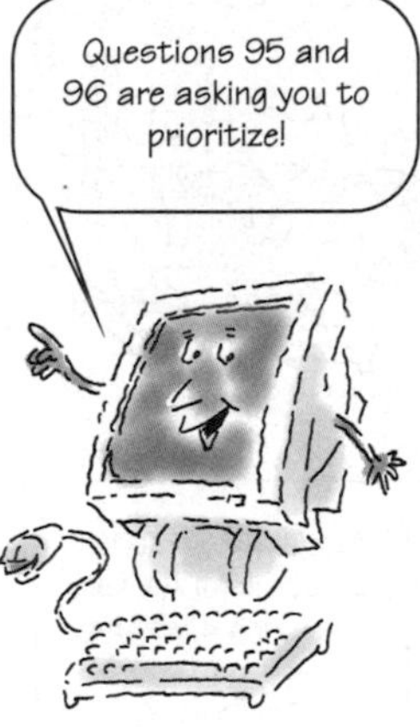
Questions 95 and
96 are asking you to
prioritize!

95. The nurse is caring for a 2-year-old child who weighs 25 lb (11.3 kg) and has a simple fracture of his femur. For this client, which initial treatment is most likely?

1. Setting the fracture with a pin during surgery
2. Placing the child in skeletal traction
3. Immediately setting and casting the fractured leg
4. Putting the child in Bryant's traction

95. 4. Bryant's traction is the usual method for treating a child younger than age 3 and weighing less than 35 lb (15.9 kg). Surgery and pin placement is an invasive treatment that isn't usually needed. Skeletal traction is used for older children. For a femur fracture to heal properly, it usually requires traction before casting.

NP: Implementation; CN: Physiological integrity; CNS: Reduction of risk potential; CL: Application

96. A female client, age 15 months, has just had a hip-spica cast applied. Which nursing intervention is a priority for this client?

1. Limit fluids so she won't urinate often and won't risk getting the cast wet.
2. Instruct the parents on how to get their child home in the car.
3. Assess sensation, circulation, and motion of her feet and toes.
4. Avoid giving her pain medication so she won't become constipated.

96. 3. Assessing sensation, circulation, and motion is necessary in all children with a cast. Fluids should be encouraged; careful diapering and padding will keep the cast dry. Instructions about discharge can be shared with the parents at a later date. Children experiencing pain should receive medication as needed.

NP: Implementation; CN: Physiological integrity; CNS: Reduction of risk potential; CL: Application

97. A male client, age 16, was injured in a motorcycle accident and fractured his left tibia and fibula. He's in a long leg cast and complains of deep pain unrelieved by analgesics. The physician must be notified immediately because the client may be exhibiting the signs and symptoms of which condition?

1. Volkmann's contracture
2. Dupuytren's contracture
3. Compartment syndrome
4. Peroneal nerve compression

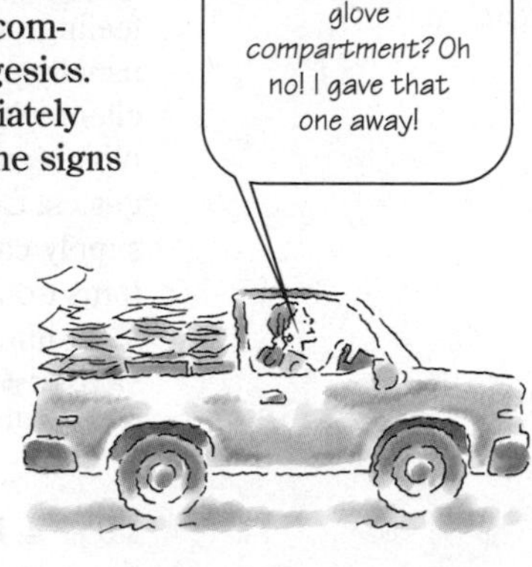

What's in the glove compartment? Oh no! I gave that one away!

97. 3. Deep pain unrelieved by analgesics is an important sign of compartment syndrome, which may occur with a crush injury or when a fracture is reduced. Compartment syndrome occurs when swelling associated with inflammation reduces blood flow to the affected areas; casting causes additional constriction of blood flow. Volkmann's contracture is a contraction of the fingers and sometimes the wrist that occurs after severe injury or improper use of a tourniquet or cast. Dupuytren's contracture is a flexion deformity of the fingers or toes caused by shortening, thickening, and fibrosis of the palmar or plantar fascia. Peroneal nerve compression is compression of the nerve that innervates the calf and foot.

NP: Assessment; CN: Physiological integrity; CNS: Physiological adaptation; CL: Analysis

98. A 6-year-old boy is admitted to a pediatric unit for treatment of osteomyelitis. The nurse knows that the peak incidence in children is between ages 1 and 12 and that boys are affected two to three times more commonly than girls. Which organism most commonly causes osteomyelitis?

1. *Staphylococcus epidermidis*
2. *Escherichia coli* 157
3. *Pneumocystis carinii*
4. *S. aureus*

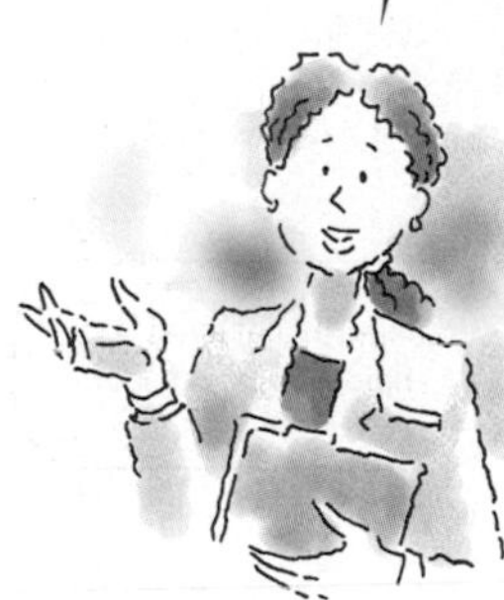

Question 98 gives you the hint, now you need to find the most common cause.

98. 4. ***S. aureus*** is the most common causative pathogen of osteomyelitis; the usual source of the infection is an upper respiratory infection. *S. epidermidis* is a microorganism found on the skin of healthy individuals. *E. coli* 157, which is in uncooked meat, can cause a severe case of diarrhea. *P. carinii* causes pneumonia in clients with human immunodeficiency virus or acquired immunodeficiency syndrome but doesn't normally cause healthy individuals to become ill.

NP: Planning; CN: Physiological integrity; CNS: Physiological adaptation; CL: Application

99. A 14-year-old girl was recently fitted with a full back brace for scoliosis. Which response by the girl indicates the need for further teaching?

1. "I can leave the brace off for school parties."
2. "I have to wear the brace all the time, even when bathing."
3. "I can take the brace off for a couple of hours if my back starts to hurt."
4. "I only have to wear the brace for a couple of weeks."

99. 2. A brace must be worn at all times except for bathing. It can't be removed for other reasons including parties and discomfort. Most braces must be worn for several months to 1 year.

NP: Evaluation; CN: Physiological integrity; CNS: Reduction of risk potential; CL: Analysis

100. A 16 year-old-client had a full body cast applied 3 days ago. She's diaphoretic, tachycardic, and tachypneic. Which condition is the client **most likely** experiencing?

1. Pneumonia
2. Compartment syndrome
3. Anxiety
4. Decreased intestinal motility

100. 3. The client is exhibiting signs and symptoms of anxiety most likely caused by the feeling of being claustrophobic. Pneumonia usually presents with fever and coughing. A client with compartment syndrome would exhibit signs of intense pain unrelieved by analgesics. Compression of the mesenteric blood supply can cause constipation, but the symptoms don't indicate that constipation is the most likely condition.

NP: Assessment; CN: Psychological integrity; CNS: Psychological adaptation; CL: Analysis

101. A 15-year-old boy broke his right forearm during a skateboard accident 6 weeks ago. He has had the arm in a cast since then but has returned to the physician complaining of continued discomfort in the arm. The physician orders an X-ray because he suspects which condition?

1. Compartment syndrome
2. Thrombophlebitis
3. New fracture
4. Delayed union

101. 4. Delayed union may cause pain beyond the expected healing time. Symptoms of compartment syndrome usually occur within 48 hours after the cast is applied. Thrombophlebitis in an extremity in a cast is rare. A new fracture could occur if there was trauma to the arm while in the cast.

NP: Assessment; CN: Physiological integrity; CNS: Reduction of risk potential; CL: Application

102. A 10-year-old girl fell off her bicycle and fractured her right radius. The physician applied a short-arm cast. Which instruction concerning cast care should the nurse include when teaching the parents?

1. Elevate the hand above the level of the heart.
2. Keep the cast clean by wrapping it in a plastic bag.
3. If itching occurs, insert a flat object, such as knitting needle, to scratch the area.
4. After the cast hardens, she can shower.

102. 1. Elevating the arm above the heart can prevent swelling. If the cast is made of plaster, enclosing it may cause burns because the plaster generates heat when drying. Nothing should be inserted into a cast because of the risk of breaking skin integrity. Water will cause the cotton lining to crumble and cause irritation; the client should take baths rather than showers and should keep the cast dry.

NP: Planning; CNS: Physiological integrity; CNS: Reduction of risk potential; CL: Application

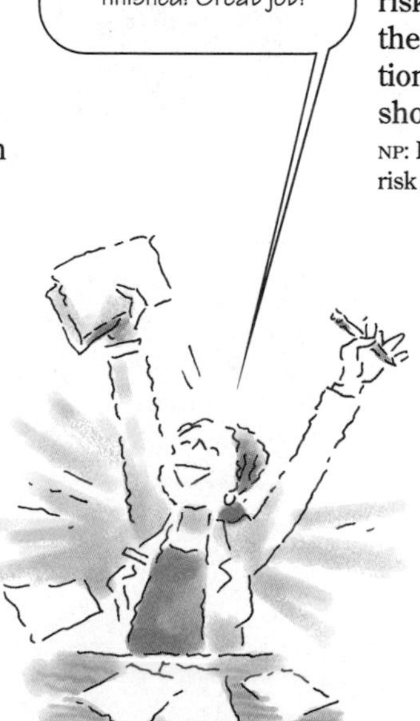
Congratulations! You finished! Great job!

I'll bet that when you started nursing school, you had no idea kids could be subject to so many GI disorders. I know I didn't. This chapter tests you on the most common ones. Good luck!

Chapter 32 Gastrointestinal disorders

1. Which substance in the following list is the part of the protein gluten that children with celiac disease are unable to digest?
1. Gliadin
2. Glucagon
3. Glycogen
4. Thyroxine

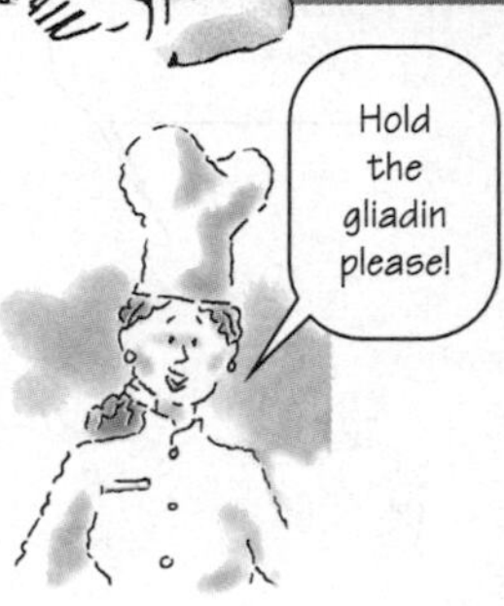

Hold the gliadin please!

1. 1. When broken down, gliadin is toxic to epithelial cells, eventually causing villi to atrophy and reducing the absorption of the small intestine. Thyroxine is a hormone, not a protein. Glucagon increases blood sugar levels. Glycogen is a storage form of glucose.
NP: Analysis; CN: Physiological integrity; CNS: Physiological adaptation; CL: Knowledge

2. Which of the following goals is most important when teaching the parents of a child diagnosed with celiac disease?
1. Promote a normal life for the child.
2. Stress the importance of good health in preventing infection.
3. Introduce the parents and child to another peer with celiac disease.
4. Help the parents and child follow the prescribed dietary restrictions.

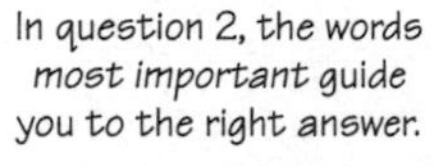

In question 2, the words *most important* guide you to the right answer.

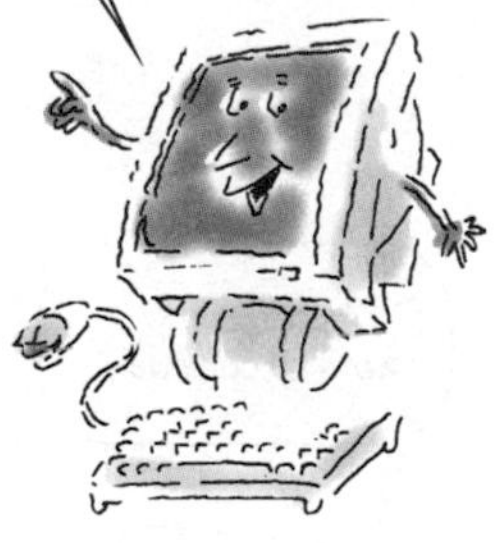

2. 4. It takes a long time to describe the disease process, the specific role of gluten, and the foods that must be restricted. Gluten is added to many foods but is obscurely listed on labels. To avoid hidden sources of gluten, parents need to read labels carefully. Promoting a normal life for the child, stressing good health in preventing infection, and meeting a peer with celiac disease are also important nursing considerations, but they would come after the dietary means of dealing with this chronic disease.
NP: Planning; CN: Psychosocial integrity; CNS: Coping and adaptation; CL: Knowledge

3. Which of the following characteristics or conditions would the nurse expect to find in a child diagnosed with celiac disease?
1. Constipation
2. Pleasant disposition
3. Proper weight gain
4. Steatorrhea

3. 4. Steatorrhea (fatty, foul-smelling, frothy, bulky stools) is common due to the inability to absorb fat. Profuse watery diarrhea, not constipation, is usually a sign of celiac crisis. Behavior changes, such as irritability, uncooperativeness, and apathy, are common, and they usually aren't pleasant. Poor weight gain would be a symptom of celiac disease because impaired absorption leads to malnutrition.
NP: Assessment; CN: Physiological integrity; CNS: Physiological adaptation; CL: Knowledge

4. A client with celiac disease is being discharged from the hospital. Which of the following food items would be included in his diet?
1. Cereal
2. Luncheon meat
3. Pizza
4. Rice

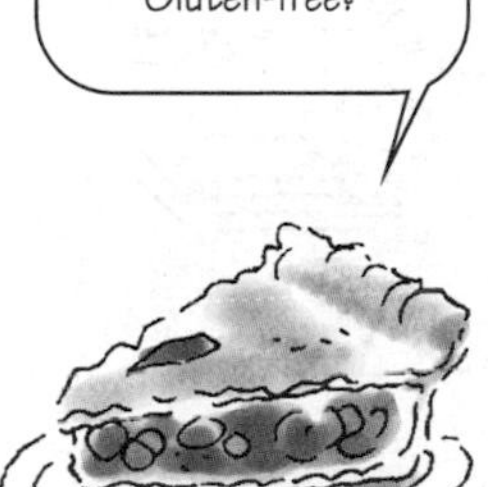

Gluten-free?

4. 4. Sources of gluten found in wheat, rye, barley, and oats should be avoided. Rice and corn are suitable substitutes because they don't contain gluten. Pizza, luncheon meat, and cereal contain gluten and, when broken down, can't be digested by people with celiac disease.
NP: Planning; CN: Psychosocial integrity; CNS: Coping and adaptation; CL: Knowledge

NP: Nursing process CN: Client needs category CNS: Client needs subcategory CL: Cognitive level

5. To help promote a normal life for children with celiac disease, which of the following interventions should the parents use?

1. Treat the child differently than other siblings.
2. Focus on restrictions that make him feel different.
3. Introduce the child to another peer with celiac disease.
4. Don't allow the child to express doubt in keeping with dietary restrictions.

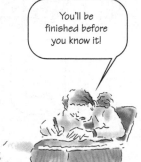

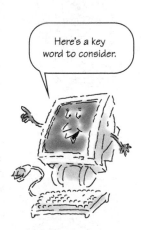

5. 3. Introducing the child to another child with celiac disease will let him know he isn't alone. It will show him how other people live a normal life with similar restrictions. Instead of focusing on restrictions that make him feel different, the nurse should encourage the parents to focus on ways he can be normal. Treat the child no differently than other siblings, but stress appropriate limit setting. Allow the child with celiac disease to express his feelings about dietary restrictions.

NP: Implementation; CN: Psychosocial integrity; CNS: Coping and adaptation; CL: Application

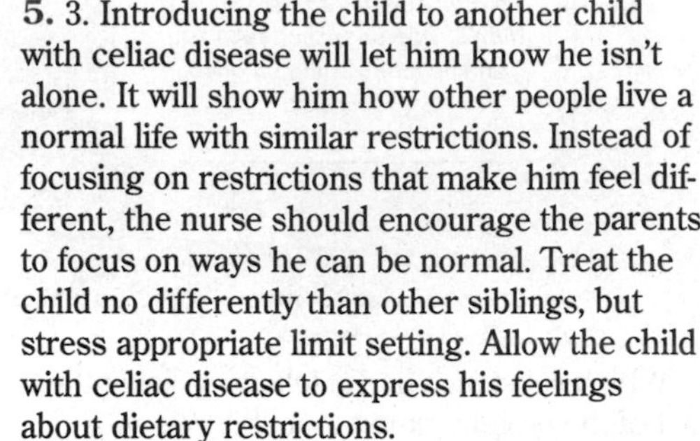

6. Which of the following conditions would be considered a malabsorption disease of the GI system?

1. Addison's disease
2. Celiac disease
3. Crohn's disease
4. Hirschsprung's disease

6. 2. In celiac disease, the absorptive surface of the small intestine is impaired. Addison's disease involves dysfunction of the adrenal cortex. Crohn's disease is an inflammatory disease of the bowel. Hirschsprung's disease is an obstructive defect in part of the intestine.

NP: Analysis; CN: Physiological integrity; CNS: Physiological adaptation; CL: Knowledge

7. Within a day or two after starting their prescribed diet, most children with celiac disease show which of the following characteristics?

1. Diarrhea
2. Foul-smelling stools
3. Improved appetite
4. Weight loss

7. 3. Within a day or two of starting their diet, most children show improved appetite, weight gain, and disappearance of diarrhea. Steatorrhea (fatty, oily, foul-smelling stools) usually doesn't occur for several days or weeks.

NP: Evaluation; CN: Physiological integrity; CNS: Physiological adaptation; CL: Application

8. In caring for a neonate with cleft lip and palate, which of the following issues is first encountered by the nurse?

1. Feeding difficulties
2. Operative care
3. Pain management
4. Parental reaction

8. 4. Parents typically show strong negative responses to this deformity. They may mourn the loss of the perfect child. Helping the parents cope with their child's condition is the first step. Feeding issues are important, but parents must first cope with the reality of their neonate's condition. Surgical repair is usually delayed until 6 to 12 weeks of age. This deformity isn't painful.

NP: Assessment; CN: Psychosocial integrity; CNS: Coping and adaptation; CL: Analysis

9. To prevent trauma to the suture line of an infant who underwent cleft lip repair, the nurse would perform which of the following interventions?

1. Place mittens on the infant's hands.
2. Maintain arm restraints.
3. Not allow the parents to touch the infant.
4. Remove the lip device from the infant after surgery.

9. 2. Arm restraints are used to prevent the infant from rubbing the sutures. Placing mittens alone won't prevent the infant from rubbing the suture line. Parental contact will increase the infant's comfort. The lip device shouldn't be removed.

NP: Implementation; CN: Physiological integrity; CNS: Reduction of risk potential; CL: Analysis

10. To prevent tissue infection and breakdown after cleft palate or lip repair, the nurse would use which of the following interventions?

1. Keep the suture line moist at all times.
2. Allow the infant to suck on his pacifier.
3. Rinse the infant's mouth with water after each feeding.
4. Follow orders from the physician to not feed the infant by mouth.

10. 3. To prevent formula buildup around the suture line, the mouth is usually rinsed. The sutures should be kept dry at all times. Objects placed in the mouth are generally avoided after surgery. Infants are fed by mouth using the Asepto-syringe technique.

NP: Implementation; CN: Physiological integrity; CNS: Physiological adaptation; CL: Analysis

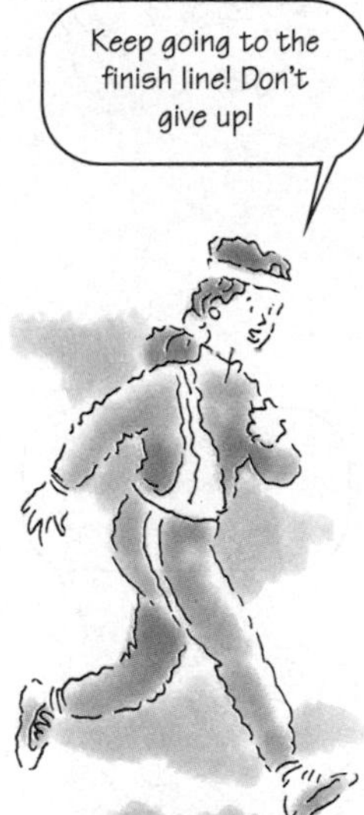

Keep going to the finish line! Don't give up!

11. Which of the following structural defects involves the use of the Logan bow postoperatively?

1. Cleft lip or palate
2. Esophageal atresia
3. Hiatal hernia
4. Tracheoesophageal fistula

11. 1. Immediately after surgery for cleft lip or palate, the Logan bow, a thin arched metal device, is used to protect the suture line from tension. Esophageal atresia, hiatal hernia, or tracheoesophageal fistula repairs don't need a device to protect sutures after surgery.

NP: Implementation; CN: Physiological integrity; CNS: Reduction of risk potential; CL: Knowledge

12. When feeding an infant with a cleft palate or lip, gentle steady pressure should be applied to the base of the bottle for which of the following reasons?

1. Reduce the risk for choking or coughing.
2. Prevent further damage to the affected area.
3. Decrease the amount of formula lost while eating.
4. Decrease the amount of noise the infant makes when eating.

12. 1. Children with cleft palate or lip have a greater risk for choking while eating, so all measures are used to reduce this risk. Steady pressure creates a seal when the nipple is against the cleft palate or lip, reducing the risk of aspiration. The nurse can't cause more damage to an infant's cleft lip or palate unless proper precautions aren't followed postoperatively. If the nipple is cut correctly and proper procedures are followed, the infant won't lose a lot of formula during a feeding. Infants with cleft palate or lip usually make more noise while eating.

NP: Implementation; CN: Physiological integrity; CNS: Reduction of risk potential; CL: Knowledge

13. Which of the following nursing interventions should be used when feeding an infant with cleft lip and palate?

1. Burp the infant often.
2. Limit the amount the infant eats.
3. Feed the infant at scheduled times.
4. Remove the nipple if the infant is making loud noises.

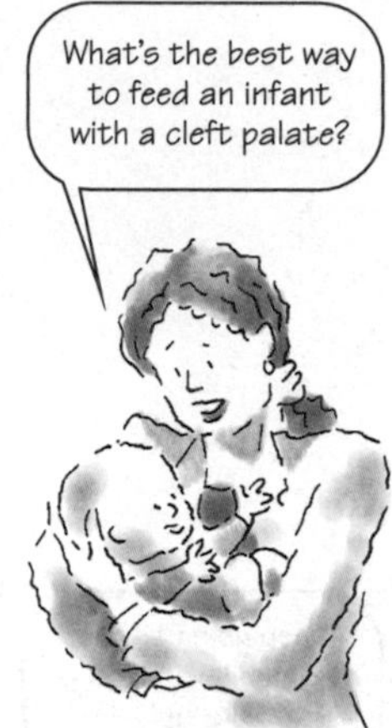
What's the best way to feed an infant with a cleft palate?

13. 1. Infants with cleft lip and palate have a tendency to swallow an excessive amount of air. The amount of formula they eat at each feeding is the same as an infant without cleft lip or palate. Loud noises are common when these infants eat, and scheduled feedings aren't necessary.

NP: Implementation; CN: Physiological integrity; CNS: Physiological adaptation; CL: Knowledge

14. Nursing care for an infant with cleft lip or palate would include which of the following interventions?

1. Discourage breast-feeding.
2. Hold the infant flat while feeding.
3. Involve the parents as soon as possible.
4. Use a normal nursery nipple for feedings.

14. 3. The sooner the parents become involved, the quicker they're able to determine the method of feeding best suited for them and the infant. There are a variety of special nipples devised for infants with cleft lip or palate; a normal nursery nipple isn't effective. Feedings are usually given in the upright position to prevent formula from coming through the nose. Breastfeeding, like bottle-feeding, may be difficult but can be facilitated if the mother intends to breast-feed. Sometimes, especially if the cleft isn't severe, breast-feeding may be easier because the human nipple conforms to the shape of the infant's mouth.

NP: Implementation; CN: Physiological integrity; CNS: Physiological adaptation; CL: Knowledge

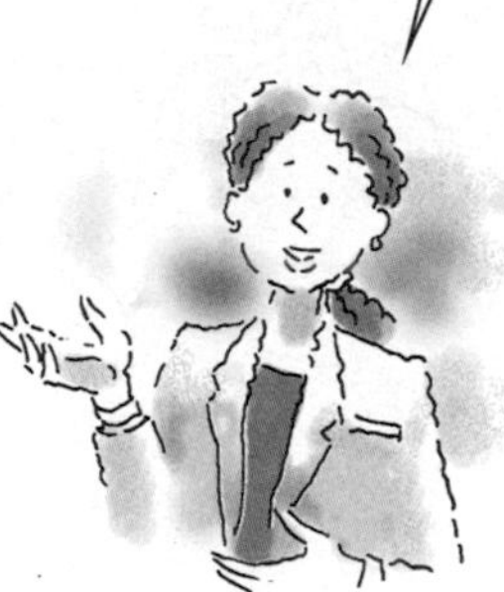
Here's where to show your compassion.

15. The parents of an infant born with cleft lip and palate are seeing the infant for the first time. The nurse caring for the infant should focus on which of the following areas?

1. The infant's positive features
2. Irritation with how the infant eats
3. Ambivalence in caring for an infant with this defect
4. Dissatisfaction with the infant's physical appearance

15. 1. To relieve the parents' anxiety, positive aspects of the infant's physical appearance need to be emphasized. Showing optimism toward surgical correction and showing a photograph of possible cosmetic improvements may be helpful.

NP: Implementation; CN: Psychosocial integrity; CNS: Coping and adaptation; CL: Application

16. Which of the following long-term physical problems might occur after cleft palate surgery?

1. Deviated septum
2. Recurring tonsillitis
3. Tooth decay
4. Varying degrees of hearing loss

16. 4. Improper draining of the middle ear causes recurrent otitis media and scarring of the tympanic membrane, which lead to varying degrees of hearing loss. Cleft palate doesn't cause problems with the tonsils. Improper tooth alignment is common, not tooth decay. The septum remains intact with cleft palate repair.

NP: Evaluation; CN: Physiological integrity; CNS: Reduction of risk potential; CL: Knowledge

17. The mother of a neonate born with a cleft lip and palate is preparing to feed her neonate for the first time. When giving her instructions, which of the following interventions should be taught first?

1. Burp the neonate.
2. Clean the mouth.
3. Hold the neonate in an upright position.
4. Prepare the bottle using a normal nursery nipple.

17. 3. When neonates are held in the upright position, the formula is less likely to leak out the nose or mouth. Neonates need to be burped frequently but not before a feeding. There's no need to clean the mouth before eating. After surgical repair, the mouth is cleaned at the suture site to prevent infection. The bottle should be prepared using a special nipple or feeding device.

NP: Planning; CN: Physiological integrity; CNS: Physiological adaptation; CL: Comprehension

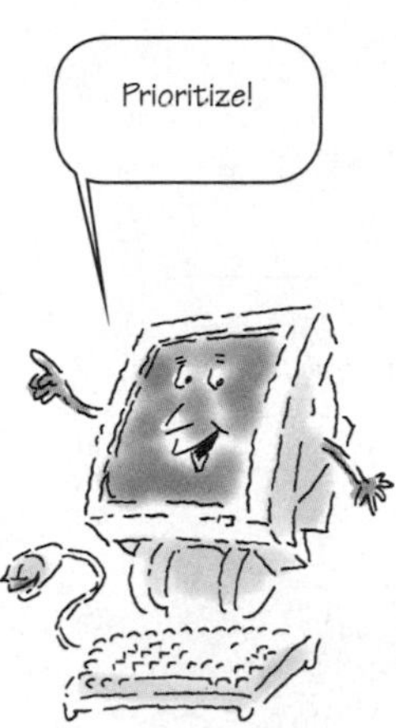

18. An infant returns from surgery after repair of a cleft palate. Which of the following nursing interventions should be done first?

1. Offer a pacifier for comfort.
2. Position the infant on his side.
3. Suction the mouth and nose of all secretions.
4. Remove the arm restraints placed on infant after surgery.

18. 2. The infant should be positioned on his side to allow oral secretions to drain from the mouth so suctioning is avoided. Arm restraints should be kept on to protect the suture line. The restraints should be removed periodically to allow for full range of motion during this time. Only one restraint should be removed at a time, and the infant should be closely supervised. Pacifiers shouldn't be used because they can damage the suture line.

NP: Implementation; CN: Physiological integrity; CNS: Reduction of risk potential; CL: Analysis

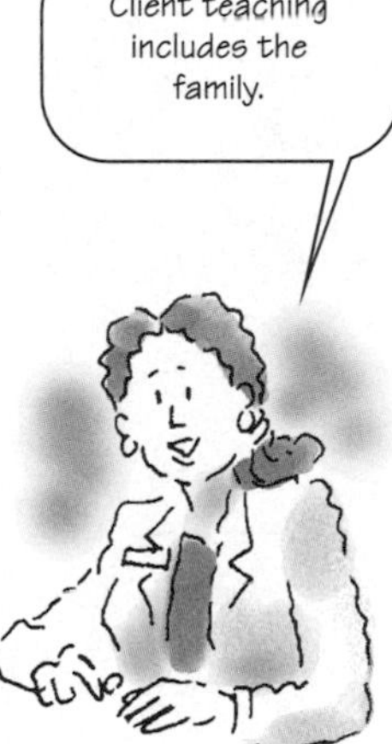

19. A small child has just had surgical repair of a cleft palate. Which of the following instructions should be included in the discharge teaching to the parents?

1. Continue a normal diet.
2. Continue using arm restraints at home.
3. Don't allow the child to drink from a cup.
4. Establish good mouth care and proper brushing.

19. 2. Arm restraints are also used at home to keep the child's hands away from the mouth until the palate is healed. A soft diet is recommended. No food harder than mashed potatoes can be eaten. Proper mouth care is encouraged after the palate is healed. Fluids are best taken from a cup.

NP: Planning; CN: Physiological integrity; CNS: Physiological adaptation; CL: Application

20. Most cleft palates are repaired at what age?

1. Immediately after birth
2. 1 to 2 months
3. 3 to 4 months
4. 1 to 2 years

20. 4. Most surgeons will correct the cleft at age 1 to 2 years, before faulty speech patterns develop. To take advantage of palatal changes, surgical repair is usually postponed until this time.

NP: Assessment; CN: Physiological integrity; CNS: Physiological adaptation; CL: Knowledge

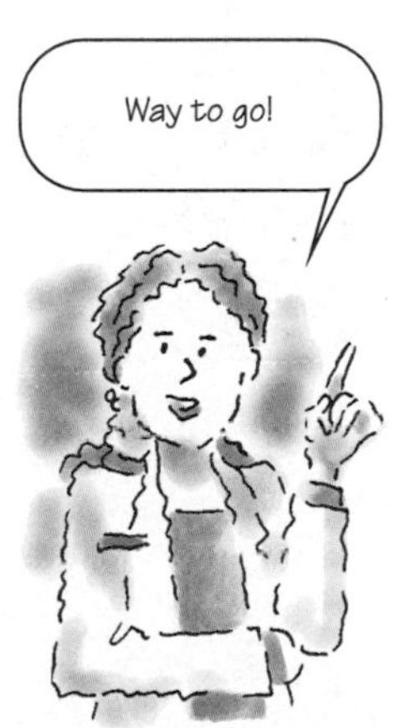

21. After an infant with a cleft lip has surgical repair and heals, the parents can expect to see which of the following results?

1. A large scar
2. An abnormally large upper lip
3. Distorted jaw
4. Some scarring

21. 4. If there's no trauma or infection to the site, healing occurs with little scar formation. There may be some inflammation right after surgery, but after healing, the lip is a normal size. No jaw malformation occurs with cleft lip repair.

NP: Evaluation; CN: Psychosocial integrity; CNS: Coping and adaptation; CL: Comprehension

22. Which of the following specialists are involved in the management of a neonate born with cleft lip or palate?

1. Cardiologist
2. Neurologist
3. Nutritionist
4. Otolaryngologist

23. Which of the following conditions or factors is the major cause of esophageal atresia and tracheoesophageal fistula?

1. Genetic
2. Prematurity
3. Poor nutrition during pregnancy
4. Unknown

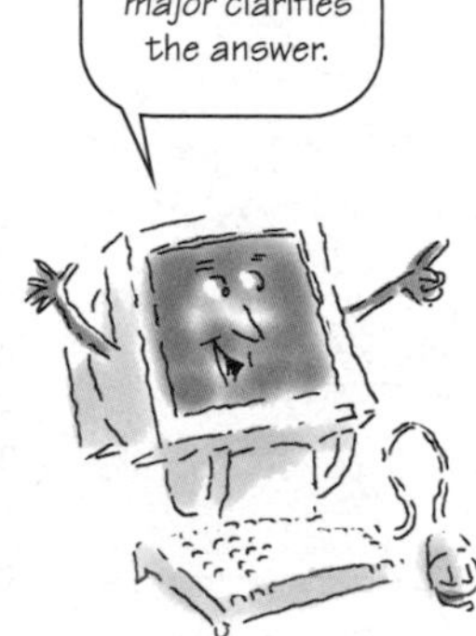
The word major clarifies the answer.

24. Which of the following types of tracheoesophageal fistula and esophageal atresia is the most commonly encountered?

1. A cleft from the trachea to the upper esophagus
2. A normal trachea and esophagus connected by a common fistula
3. A blind pouch at each end, widely separated, with no involvement of the trachea
4. Proximal esophageal segment terminated in a blind pouch, distal segment connected to the trachea

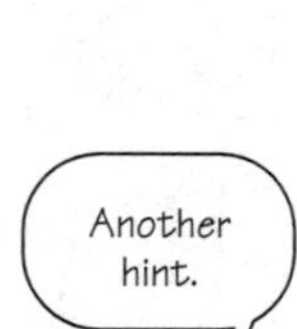
Another hint.

25. Which of the following findings is common in neonates born with esophageal atresia?

1. Cyanosis
2. Decreased production of saliva
3. Inability to cough
4. Inadequate swallow

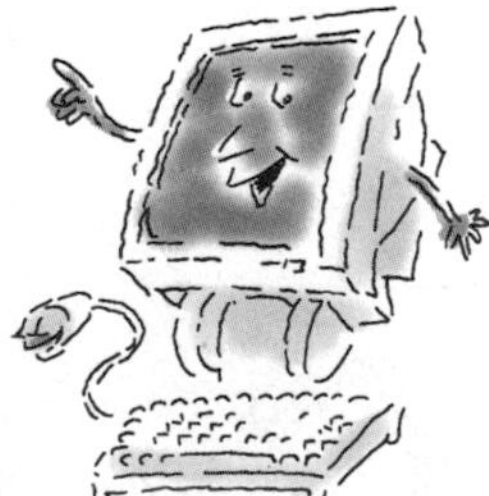

26. For a neonate suspected of having esophageal atresia, a definitive diagnostic evaluation would include which of the following factors?

1. Decreased breath sounds
2. Absence of bowel sounds
3. How a neonate tolerates eating
4. Ability to pass a catheter down the esophagus

22. 4. An otolaryngologist is used because ear infections are common, along with hearing loss. Brain and cardiac function are usually normal. A nutritionist isn't needed unless the neonate becomes malnourished.

NP: Implementation; CN: Safe, effective care environment; CNS: Management of care; CL: Knowledge

23. 4. The cause of these malformations is unknown. Genetics isn't an issue with these structural defects. A premature neonate isn't necessarily born with either malformation. These defects occur much earlier in the process of development than viability (23 to 24 weeks' gestation). Poor nutrition could contribute to other factors in a neonate, such as iron deficiency anemia.

NP: Assessment; CN: Physiological integrity; CNS: Physiological adaptation; CL: Knowledge

24. 4. In 80% to 90% of all cases, these malformations have the proximal esophageal segment terminated in a blind pouch and the distal segment connected to the trachea. A normal trachea and esophagus connected by a common fistula represents the rarest form. A blind pouch at each end, widely separated, with no involvement of the trachea is the second most common type of tracheoesophageal fistula, making up 5% to 8% of all cases. A cleft doesn't occur in the trachea.

NP: Assessment; CN: Physiological integrity; CNS: Physiological adaptation; CL: Knowledge

25. 1. Cyanosis occurs when fluid from the blind pouch is aspirated into the trachea. Increased drooling is common, along with choking, coughing, and sneezing. The ability to swallow isn't affected by this disorder.

NP: Assessment; CN: Physiological integrity; CNS: Physiological adaptation; CL: Knowledge

26. 4. A moderately stiff catheter will meet resistance if the esophagus is blocked and will pass unobstructed if the esophagus is patent. If a neonate doesn't tolerate eating, it doesn't mean he has an esophageal atresia. The intestinal tract isn't affected with this anomaly, so bowel sounds are present. Breath sounds are normal unless aspiration occurs.

NP: Assessment; CN: Physiological integrity; CNS: Physiological adaptation; CL: Knowledge

27. For a neonate diagnosed with a tracheoesophageal fistula, which of the following interventions would be needed?

1. Start antibiotic therapy.
2. Keep the neonate lying flat.
3. Continue feedings.
4. Remove the diagnostic catheter from the esophagus.

27. 1. Antibiotic therapy is started because aspiration pneumonia is inevitable and appears early. The neonate's head is usually kept in an upright position to prevent aspiration. I.V. fluids are started, and the neonate isn't allowed oral intake. The catheter is left in the upper esophageal pouch to easily remove fluid that collects there.

NP: Implementation; CN: Physiological integrity; CNS: Pharmacological and parenteral therapies; CL: Analysis

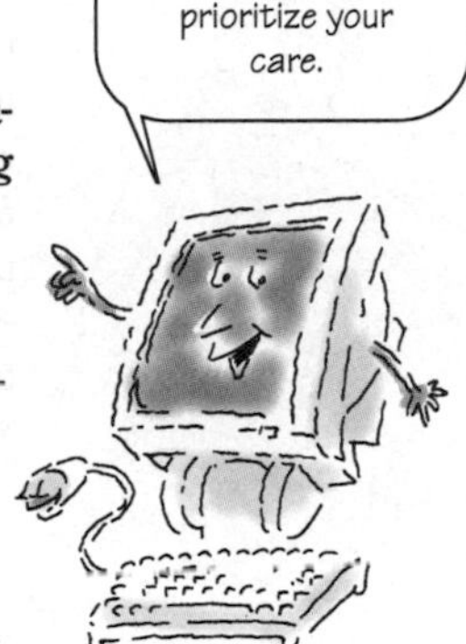

Question 28 asks you to prioritize your care.

28. When tracheoesophageal fistula or esophageal atresia is suspected, which of the following nursing interventions would be done first?

1. Give oxygen.
2. Tell the parents.
3. Put the neonate in an isolette or on a radiant warmer.
4. Report the suspicion to the physician.

28. 4. The physician needs to be told so immediate diagnostic tests can be done for a definitive diagnosis and surgical correction. Oxygen should be given only after notifying the physician except in the case of an emergency. It isn't the nurse's responsibility to inform the parents of the suspected finding. By the time tracheoesophageal fistula or esophageal atresia is suspected, the neonate would have already been placed in an isolette or a radiant warmer.

NP: Implementation; CN: Physiological integrity; CNS: Physiological adaptation; CL: Analysis

29. Which of the following complications may follow the surgical repair of a tracheoesophageal fistula?

1. Atelectasis
2. Choking during feeding attempts
3. Damaged vocal cords
4. Infection

29. 1. Respiratory complications (atelectasis) are a threat to the neonate's life preoperatively and postoperatively due to the continual risk for aspiration. Vocal cord damage isn't common after this repair. The neonate is generally given antibiotics preoperatively to prevent infection. Choking is more likely to occur preoperatively, although careful attention is paid postoperatively when neonates begin to eat to make sure they can swallow without choking.

NP: Assessment; CN: Physiological integrity; CNS: Physiological adaptation; CL: Analysis

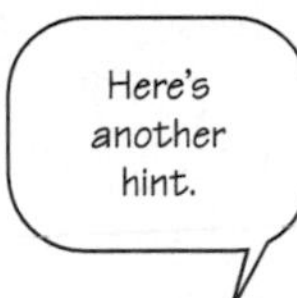

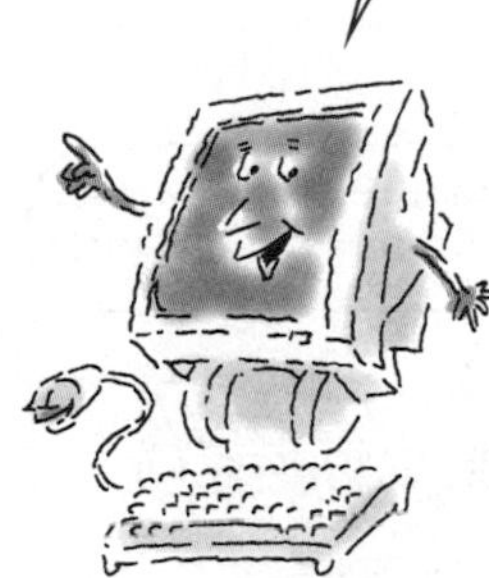

30. Which of the following signs of esophageal atresia with distal tracheoesophageal fistula would appear the earliest?

1. Abdominal distention
2. Decreased oral secretions
3. Normal respiratory effort
4. Scaphoid abdomen

30. 1. Crying may force air into the stomach, causing distention. Secretions in a client with this condition may be more visible, though normal in quantity, due to the client's inability to swallow effectively. Respiratory effort is usually more difficult. When no distal fistula is present, the abdomen will appear scaphoid.

NP: Assessment; CN: Physiological integrity; CNS: Physiological adaptation; CL: Knowledge

31. Dietary management in a child diagnosed with ulcerative colitis would include which of the following diets?

1. High-calorie diet
2. High-residue diet
3. Low-protein diet
4. Low-salt diet

31. 1. A high-calorie diet is given to combat weight loss and restore nitrogen balance. A low-residue or residue-free diet is encouraged to decrease bowel irritation. A high-protein diet is also encouraged. Salt reduction isn't a factor in this disease.

NP: Implementation; CN: Physiological integrity; CNS: Physiological adaptation; CL: Analysis

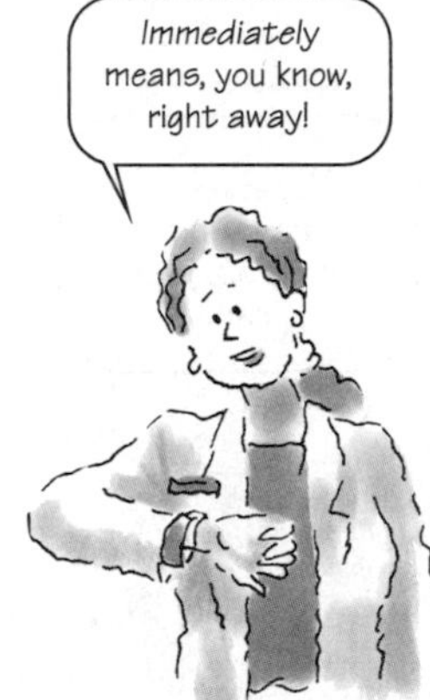

Immediately means, you know, right away!

32. A neonate comes back from the operating room after surgical repair of a tracheoesophageal fistula and esophageal atresia. Which of the following interventions is done immediately?

1. Maintain a patent airway.
2. Start feedings right away.
3. Let the parents hold the neonate right away.
4. Suction the endotracheal tube, stopping when resistance is met.

32. 1. Maintaining a patent airway is essential until sedation from surgery wears off. Feedings usually aren't started for at least 48 hours after surgery. The catheter should be measured before suctioning so the tube doesn't meet resistance, which could cause damage. Parents are encouraged to participate in the neonate's care, but not immediately after surgery.

NP: Implementation; CN: Physiological integrity; CNS: Physiological adaptation; CL: Knowledge

33. Before discharging a neonate with a repaired tracheoesophageal fistula and esophageal atresia, the nurse would give the parents or caregivers instructions in which of the following areas?

1. Giving antibiotics
2. Preventing infection
3. Positioning techniques
4. Giving solid food as soon as possible

33. 3. Positioning instructions should be given during hospitalization and before the neonate returns home. For optimum effective respiration and because gastroesophageal reflux is a common complication, solid food usually isn't started until liquid feedings are tolerated. Preventing infection, especially at the operative sites, is a responsibility of the nurse postoperatively. Antibiotics are usually discontinued before discharge.

NP: Planning; CN: Psychosocial integrity; CNS: Coping and adaptation; CL: Comprehension

34. Which of the following nursing interventions would be done postoperatively for a neonate after repair of tracheoesophageal fistula and esophageal atresia?

1. Withhold mouth care.
2. Offer a pacifier frequently.
3. Decrease tactile stimulation.
4. Use restraints to prevent injury to the repair.

34. 2. Meeting the neonate's oral needs is important because he can't drink from a bottle. The nurse should provide tactile stimulation. Restraints should be avoided if possible. The nurse should give mouth care to these neonates.

NP: Implementation; CN: Physiological integrity; CNS: Physiological adaptation; CL: Application

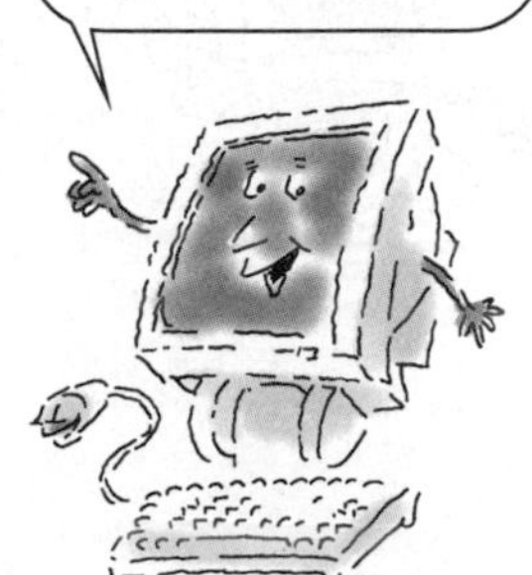

Yet another classic clue. Don'tcha just love 'em?

35. Which of the following conditions would be a long-term postoperative complication of a tracheoesophageal fistula and esophageal atresia repair?

1. Oral aversion
2. Gastroesophageal reflux
3. Inability to tolerate feedings
4. Strictures

35. 4. Strictures of the anastomosis occur in 40% to 50% of the cases. Oral aversion can be a problem, but it occurs quickly after surgery. Reflux is a common complication but appears when feedings are started. If the neonate is having problems tolerating feedings, it's quickly noted.

NP: Assessment; CN: Physiological integrity; CNS: Physiological adaptation; CL: Knowledge

36. Which of the following structural defects is suspected when a neonate has excessive salivation and drooling, accompanied by coughing, choking, and sneezing?

1. Cleft lip
2. Cleft palate
3. Gastroschisis
4. Tracheoesophageal fistula and esophageal atresia

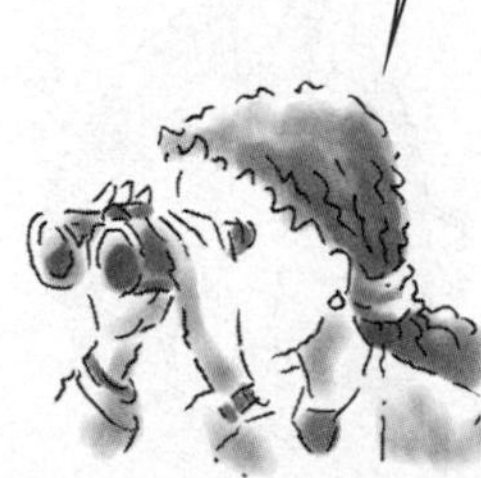

Looking for the end of these questions? Hang in there!

36. 4. Because of an ineffective swallow, saliva and secretions appear in the mouth and around the lips. Coughing, choking, and sneezing occur for the same reason and usually after an attempt at eating. Cleft lip and palate don't produce excessive salivation. None of these symptoms occur with gastroschisis.

NP: Assessment; CN: Physiological integrity; CNS: Physiological adaptation; CL: Knowledge

37. Esophageal atresia and tracheoesophageal fistula are usually associated with which of the following factors?

1. Female sex
2. Higher then average birth weight
3. Male sex
4. Prematurity

37. 4. The cause of these defects is unknown, but an unusually high percentage of cases occurs in premature infants. The birth weight is significantly less than average. There are no sex differences noted.

NP: Assessment; CN: Physiological integrity; CNS: Physiological adaptation; CL: Knowledge

38. Which of the following structural defects involves a portion of an organ protruding through an abnormal opening?

1. Cleft lip
2. Cleft palate
3. Gastroschisis
4. Tracheoesophageal fistula

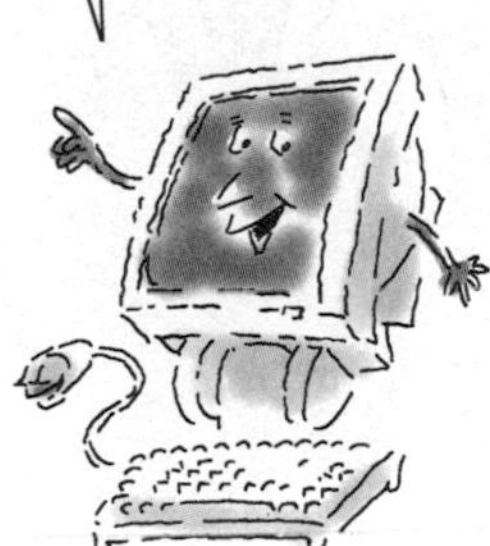

There's nothing tricky about this hint.

38. 3. Gastroschisis is a herniation of the bowel through an abnormal opening in the abdominal wall. Tracheoesophageal fistula is a malformation of the trachea and esophagus. Cleft lip and palate are facial malformations, not hernias.

NP: Assessment; CN: Physiological integrity; CNS: Physiological adaptation; CL: Knowledge

39. When an infant is diagnosed with a diaphragmatic hernia on the left side, which of the following abdominal organs may be found in the thorax?

1. Appendix
2. Descending colon
3. Right kidney
4. Spleen

39. 4. The spleen has often been seen in the thorax of infants with this defect. The right kidney wouldn't be seen with a left-sided defect. The appendix and descending colon usually don't protrude into the thorax due to limited space from the other organs present.

NP: Assessment; CN: Physiological integrity; CNS: Physiological adaptation; CL: Knowledge

40. In which direction does the mediastinum shift in an infant diagnosed with a diaphragmatic hernia?

1. No shift
2. Shifts to the affected side
3. Shifts to the unaffected side
4. Partial shifts to the affected or unaffected sides

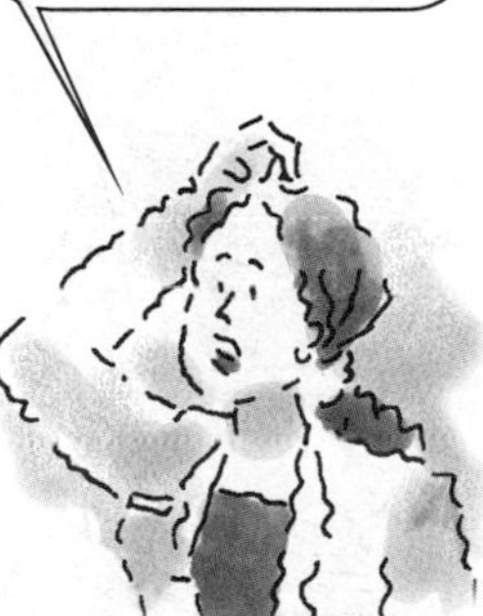

40. 3. The increased volume in the chest cavity from the abdominal organs causes the mediastinum to shift to the unaffected side, which causes a partial collapse of that lung. Due to the increased volume on the affected side, the mediastinum can't shift that way.

NP: Assessment; CN: Physiological integrity; CNS: Physiological adaptation; CL: Analysis

41. Which of the following ways is best to position an infant with a diaphragmatic hernia before surgery?

1. On the affected side
2. On the unaffected side
3. Supine
4. Trendelenburg's position

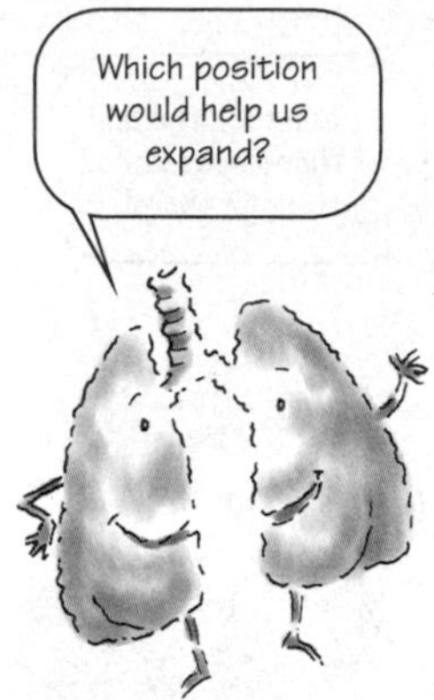

Which position would help us expand?

41. 1. Positioning the infant on the affected side lets the lung on the unaffected side expand, making breathing easier. Positioning the infant on the unaffected side or in Trendelenburg's position will further diminish respiration and would increase pressure in the chest cavity, compromising respirations. Supine position doesn't facilitate lung expansion.

NP: Implementation; CN: Physiological integrity; CNS: Physiological adaptation; CL: Analysis

42. Before surgery, which of the following interventions would be used for an infant with a diaphragmatic hernia?

1. Feed the infant.
2. Provide tactile stimulation.
3. Prevent the infant from crying.
4. Place the infant on the unaffected side.

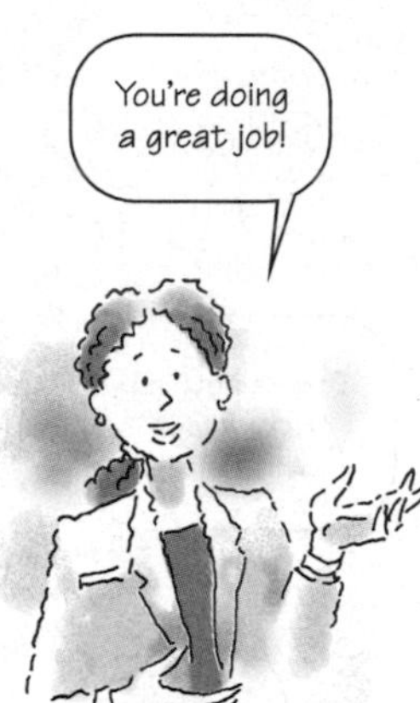

42. 3. The stomach and intestine in the chest cavity become distended with swallowed air from crying. Negative pressure from crying pulls the intestines into the chest cavity, increasing the amount of distension. The infant usually isn't fed until after surgery. Tactile stimulation is limited because it may disturb the infant's fragile condition. The infant is always placed on the affected side.

NP: Assessment; CN: Physiological integrity; CNS: Physiological adaptation; CL: Knowledge

43. The nursing care of a neonate born with an omphalocele would include which of the following interventions?

1. Keep the malformation dry.
2. Don't let the parents see it.
3. Carefully position and handle it.
4. Touch it often to assess any changes.

43. 3. Careful positioning and handling prevent infection and rupture of the sac. The omphalocele is kept moist until the neonate is taken to the operating room. The parents can see the defect if they so choose. Touching it often increases the risk of infection.

NP: Analysis; CN: Physiological integrity; CNS: Physiological adaptation; CL: Knowledge

44. What is the treatment for a diagnosed omphalocele?

1. Immediate surgical repair
2. Surgical repair after the sac ruptures
3. Use sterile technique and manual manipulation
4. No treatment is necessary; it goes away by itself

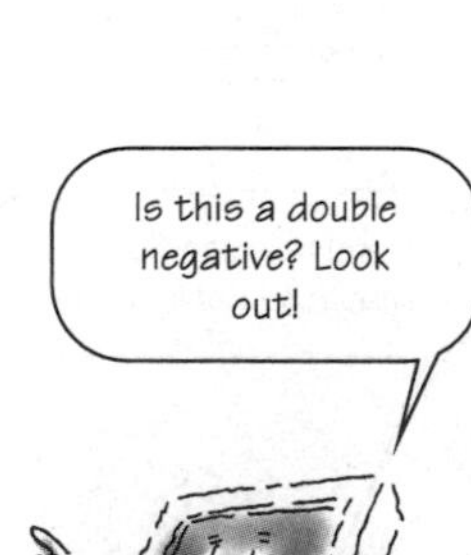

Is this a double negative? Look out!

44. 1. Surgical repair is done immediately to prevent infection and possible tissue damage. The omphalocele is covered and kept moist until the infant goes to the operating room. Careful positioning and handling techniques are used to prevent rupture of the sac and damage to the abdominal contents.

NP: Assessment; CN: Physiological integrity; CNS: Physiological adaptation; CL: Knowledge

45. Which of the following abdominal defects isn't covered by a protective sac and doesn't cause damage to the umbilical cord?

1. Diaphragmatic hernia
2. Gastroschisis
3. Omphalocele
4. Umbilical hernia

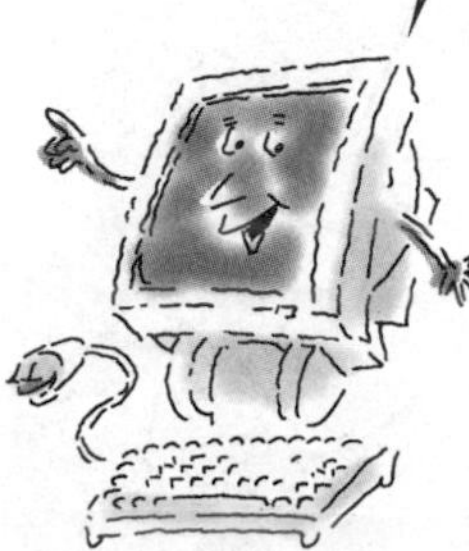

45. 2. Gastroschisis is always located to the right of an intact umbilical cord and isn't enclosed in a protective sac. Diaphragmatic hernia is a protrusion of abdominal organs into the thoracic cavity. The omphalocele is covered by only a translucent sac of amnion. Umbilical hernia is a protrusion of the intestine into the umbilicus, which is covered by skin.

NP: Assessment; CN: Physiological integrity; CNS: Physiological adaptation; CL: Knowledge

46. Which of the following statements is true about pyloric stenosis?
1. It's more common in girls.
2. It's diagnosed by severe diarrhea.
3. It's more frequent in Blacks and Asians.
4. It's more common in full-term than preterm neonates.

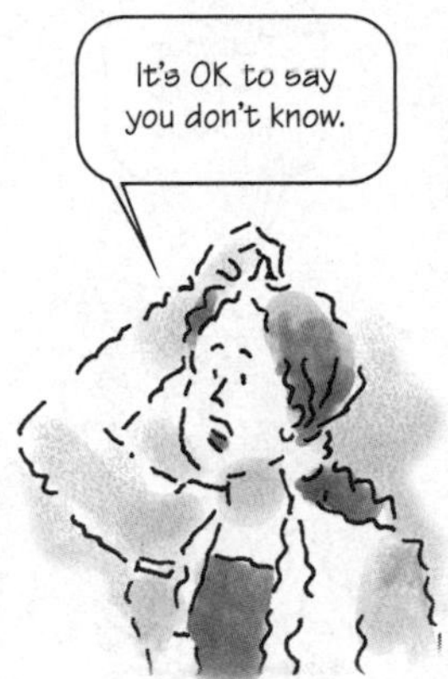

It's OK to say
you don't know.

46. 4. Pyloric stenosis is more likely to affect a full-term than a preterm neonate. It's more common in boys and is usually diagnosed by vomiting. It occurs more commonly in white neonates.

NP: Assessment; CN: Physiological integrity; CNS: Physiological adaptation; CL: Knowledge

47. Which of the following factors is the cause of pyloric stenosis?
1. Unknown
2. Hereditary
3. Poor nutrition in pregnancy
4. Usually directly related to poor muscle development in the stomach

47. 1. The cause of the narrowing of the pyloric musculature is unknown. A hereditary factor hasn't been established. Poor nutrition in pregnancy and poor muscle development in the stomach may relate to this defect, but at present, they haven't been established as definitive causes.

NP: Assessment; CN: Physiological integrity; CNS: Physiological adaptation; CL: Knowledge

48. In which of the following areas does the pyloric canal narrow in clients with pyloric stenosis?
1. Stomach and esophagus
2. Stomach and duodenum
3. Both the stomach and esophagus and the stomach and duodenum
4. Neither the stomach and esophagus nor the stomach and duodenum

48. 2. The narrowing of the pyloric canal occurs between the stomach and duodenum, where the pyloric sphincter is located. Hyperplasia and hypertrophy cause narrowing and possibly obstruction of the circular muscle of the pylorus.

NP: Analysis; CN: Physiological integrity; CNS: Physiological adaptation; CL: Knowledge

49. Which of the following signs and symptoms is classic for an infant with pyloric stenosis?
1. Loss of appetite
2. Chronic diarrhea
3. Projectile vomiting
4. Occasional nonprojectile vomiting

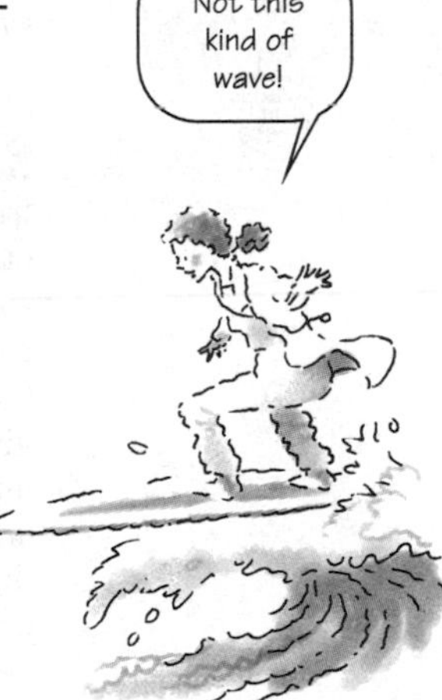

49. 3. The obstruction doesn't allow food to pass through to the duodenum. Once the stomach becomes full, the infant vomits for relief. Chronic hunger is often seen. There's no diarrhea because food doesn't pass the stomach. Occasional nonprojectile vomiting may occur initially if the obstruction is only partial.

NP: Assessment; CN: Physiological integrity; CNS: Physiological adaptation; CL: Knowledge

50. When assessing a neonate, the nurse notes visible peristaltic waves across the epigastrium. This characteristic is indicative of which of the following disorders?
1. Hypertrophic pyloric stenosis
2. Imperforate anus
3. Intussusception
4. Short-gut syndrome

50. 1. The diagnosis of pyloric stenosis can be established from a finding of hypertrophic pyloric stenosis. Intussusception, imperforate anus, and short-gut syndromes are diagnosed by other characteristics.

NP: Assessment; CN: Physiological integrity; CNS: Physiological adaptation; CL: Knowledge

51. After surgical repair of pyloric stenosis, at which of the following times will the infant return to a normal feeding regimen?

1. 4 to 6 hours after surgery
2. 24 hours after surgery
3. 48 hours after surgery
4. 1 week after surgery

51. 3. Small frequent feedings of clear fluids are usually started 4 to 6 hours after surgery. If clear fluids are tolerated, formula feedings are started 24 hours after surgery, in gradually increasing amounts. It usually takes 48 hours to reach a normal full feeding regimen in this manner. The infant usually goes home on the fourth postoperative day.

NP: Assessment; CN: Physiological integrity; CNS: Physiological adaptation; CL: Knowledge

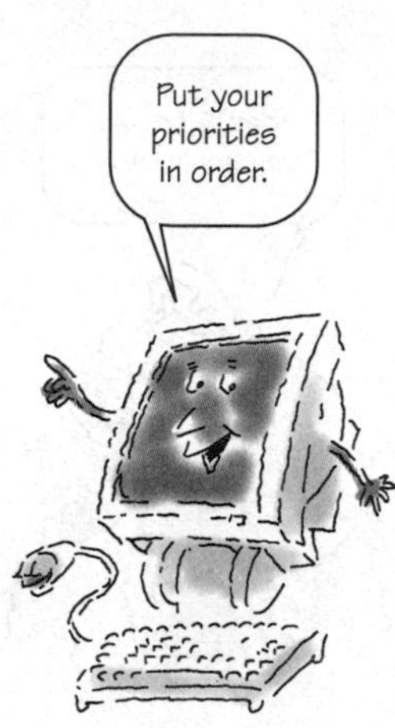

Put your priorities in order.

52. A nurse admits an infant diagnosed with pyloric stenosis. Which of the following nursing interventions would most likely be done first?

1. Weigh the infant.
2. Check urine specific gravity.
3. Place an I.V. catheter.
4. Change the infant and weigh the diaper.

52. 1. Weighing the infant would be done first so a baseline weight can be established and weight changes can be assessed. After a baseline weight is obtained, an I.V. catheter can be placed because oral feedings generally aren't given. These infants are usually dehydrated, so while checking the diaper and specific gravity are important tools to help assess their status, they aren't the first priority.

NP: Implementation; CN: Physiological integrity; CNS: Physiological adaptation; CL: Analysis

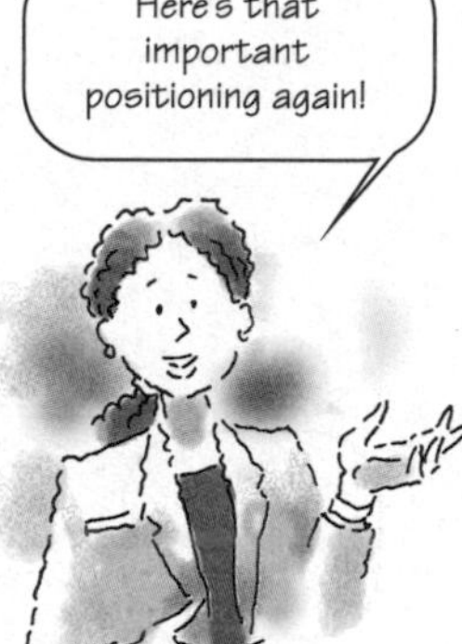

Here's that important positioning again!

53. A nurse is caring for an infant with pyloric stenosis. After feeding the infant, he should be placed in which of the following positions?

1. Prone in Fowler's position
2. On his back without elevation
3. On the left side in Fowler's position
4. Slightly on the right side in high semi-Fowler's position

53. 4. Positioning the infant slightly on the right side in high semi-Fowler's position will help facilitate gastric emptying. The other positions won't facilitate gastric emptying and may cause the infant to vomit.

NP: Implementation; CN: Physiological integrity; CNS: Physiological adaptation; CL: Knowledge

54. When preparing to feed an infant with pyloric stenosis before surgical repair, which of the following interventions is important?

1. Give feedings quickly.
2. Burp the infant frequently.
3. Discourage parental participation.
4. Don't give more feedings if the infant vomits.

54. 2. These infants usually swallow a lot of air from sucking on their hands and fingers because of their intensive hunger (feedings aren't easily tolerated). Burping frequently will lessen gastric distention and increase the likelihood the infant will retain the feeding. Feedings are given slowly with the infant lying in a semi-upright position. Record the type, amount, and character of the vomit as well as its relation to the feeding. The amount of feeding volume lost is usually refed. Parental participation should be encouraged and allowed to the extent possible.

NP: Analysis; CN: Physiological adaptation; CNS: Physiological adaptation; CL: Application

55. Which of the following symptoms is common up to 48 hours after the surgical repair of pyloric stenosis?
1. Dysuria
2. Oral aversion
3. Scaphoid abdomen
4. Vomiting

55. 4. Even with successful surgery, most infants have some vomiting during the first 24 to 48 hours. Dysuria isn't a complication with this surgical procedure. Oral aversion doesn't occur because these infants may be fed up until surgery. Scaphoid abdomen isn't characteristic of this condition. The abdomen may appear distended, not scaphoid.

NP: Assessment; CN: Physiological integrity; CNS: Physiological adaptation; CL: Knowledge

56. Which of the following interventions will help prevent vomiting in an infant diagnosed with pyloric stenosis?
1. Hold the infant for 1 hour after feeding.
2. Handle the infant minimally after feedings.
3. Space the feedings out, and give them in large amounts.
4. Lay the infant prone with the head of the bed elevated.

56. 2. Minimal handling, especially after a feeding, will help prevent vomiting. Feedings are given frequently and slowly in small amounts. Holding the infant would provide too much stimulation, which might increase the risk of vomiting. An infant should be positioned in a semi-Fowler's position and slightly on the right side after a feeding.

NP: Implementation; CN: Physiological integrity; CNS: Physiological adaptation; CL: Knowledge

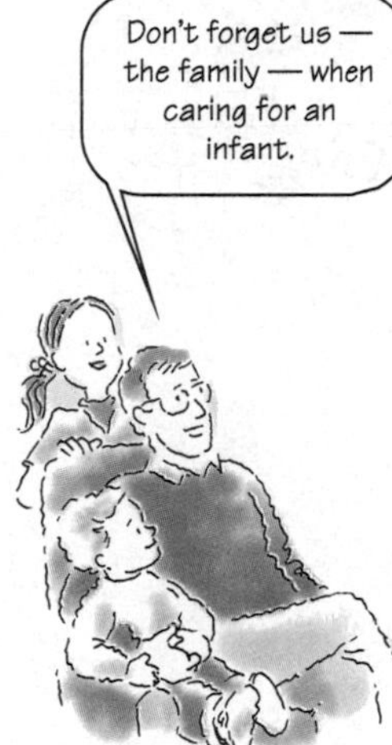

57. It's an important nursing function to give support to the parents of an infant diagnosed with pyloric stenosis. Which of the following nursing interventions best serves that purpose?
1. Keep the parents informed of the infant's progress.
2. Provide all care for the infant, even when the parents visit.
3. Tell the parents to minimize handling of the infant at all times.
4. Tell the physicians to keep the parents informed of the infant's progress.

57. 1. Keeping the parents informed will decrease their anxiety. The nurse should encourage the parents to be involved with the infant's care. Telling the parents to minimize handling of the infant isn't appropriate because parent-child contact is important. The physician is responsible for updating the parents on the infant's medical condition, and the nurse is responsible for updating the parents on the day-to-day activities of the infant and his improvement with the day's activities.

NP: Assessment; CN: Psychosocial integrity; CNS: Coping and adaptation; CL: Analysis

58. Which of the following symptoms would be likely in an infant diagnosed with pyloric stenosis?
1. Apathy
2. Arrhythmia
3. Dry lips and skin
4. Hypothermia

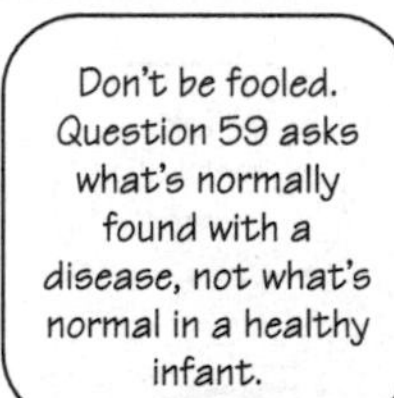

Don't be fooled. Question 59 asks what's normally found with a disease, not what's normal in a healthy infant.

58. 3. Dry lips and skin are signs of dehydration, which is common in infants with pyloric stenosis. These infants are constantly hungry due to their inability to retain feedings. Apathy, arrhythmias, and hypothermia aren't clinical findings with pyloric stenosis.

NP: Assessment; CN: Physiological integrity; CNS: Physiological adaptation; CL: Application

59. When assessing an infant diagnosed with pyloric stenosis, which of the following findings would be considered normal?
1. Decreased or diminished bowel sounds
2. Heart murmur
3. Normal respiratory effort
4. Positive bowel sounds

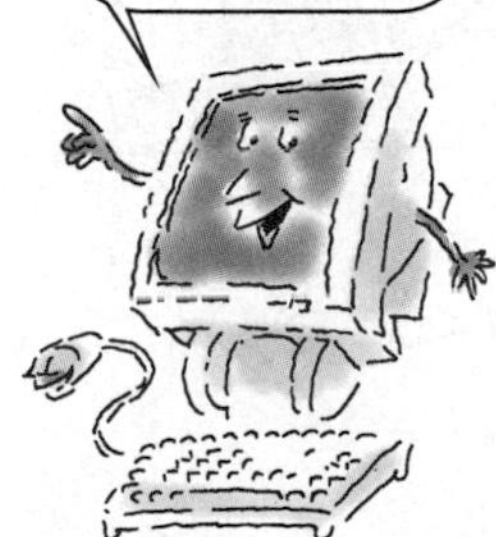

59. 1. Bowel sounds decrease because food can't pass into the intestines. Normal respiratory effort is affected due to the abdominal distension that pushes the diaphragm up into the pleural cavity. Heart murmurs may be present but aren't directly associated with pyloric stenosis.

NP: Assessment; CN: Physiological integrity; CNS: Physiological adaptation; CL: Knowledge

60. Which of the following abdominal organs is directly affected when pyloric stenosis is diagnosed?

1. Colon and rectum
2. Stomach and duodenum
3. Stomach and esophagus
4. Liver and bile ducts

60. 2. This defect occurs at the pyloric sphincter, which is located between the stomach and duodenum. The stomach and esophagus, liver and bile ducts, and colon and rectum aren't affected by this obstructive disorder.
NP: Assessment; CN: Physiological integrity; CNS: Physiological adaptation; CL: Knowledge

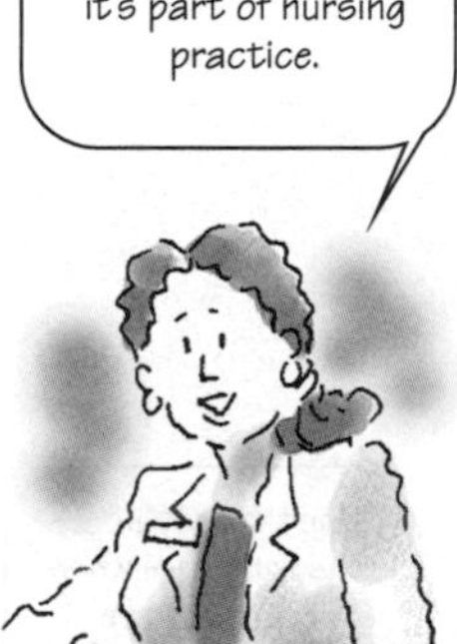

Practice setting priorities because it's part of nursing practice.

61. Which of the following nursing interventions is the most important in dealing with a child who has been poisoned?

1. Stabilize the child.
2. Notify the parents.
3. Identify the poison.
4. Determine when the poisoning took place.

61. 1. Stabilization and the initial emergency treatment of the child (such as respiratory assistance, circulatory support, or control of seizures) will prevent further damage to the body from the poison. Identification of the poison is crucial and should begin at the same time as the stabilization of the child, although the initial ABCs should be assessed first. If the parents didn't bring the child in, they can be notified as soon as the child is stabilized or treated. Determining when the poisoning took place is an important consideration, but emergency stabilization and treatment are priorities.
NP: Assessment; CN: Physiological integrity; CNS: Physiological adaptation; CL: Analysis

62. For a child who has ingested a poisonous substance, the initial step in emergency treatment is to stop the exposure to the substance. Which of the following methods would best achieve this?

1. Make the child vomit.
2. Call 911 as soon as possible.
3. Give large amounts of water to flush the system.
4. Empty the mouth of pills, plant parts, or other material.

62. 4. Emptying the mouth of pills, plant parts, or other material will stop exposure to the poison. Calling 911 is important, but removing any further sources of the poison would come first. Only small amounts of water are recommended so the poison is confined to the smallest volume. Large amounts of water will let the poison pass the pylorus. The small intestines absorb fluid rapidly, increasing the potential toxicity. Making the child vomit is important, but won't remove exposure to the substance; it's also contraindicated with some poisons.
NP: Implementation; CN: Physiological integrity; CNS: Physiological adaptation; CL: Analysis

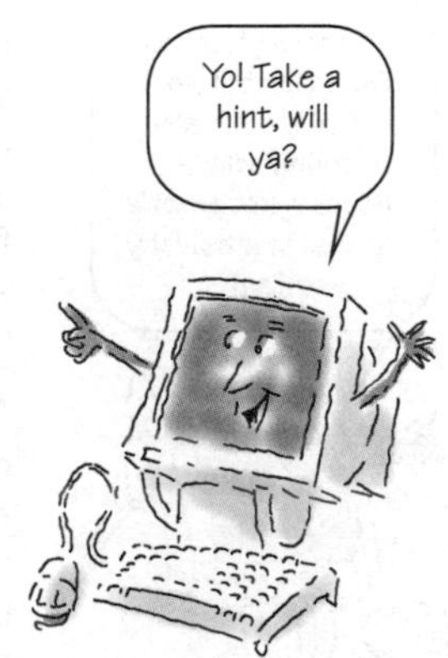

Yo! Take a hint, will ya?

63. An ingested poison can be removed by inducing vomiting. Which of the following methods is preferred?

1. Give syrup of ipecac.
2. Have the child smell something offensive to cause vomiting.
3. Put a finger down the throat of the child who ingested the poison.
4. Do nothing because ingesting the poison may cause vomiting in some children.

63. 1. If vomiting is indicated, syrup of ipecac should be given instead of waiting for the child to vomit by himself. This syrup causes stimulation of the vomiting center and an irritant effect on gastric mucosa. Vomiting should occur within 20 minutes. Smelling something offensive may not work because it's difficult to get the child to comply. Putting a finger down his throat could cause damage to the oropharynx. Waiting for the child to vomit may allow the poison to enter systemic circulation.
NP: Implementation; CN: Physiological integrity; CNS: Pharmacological and parenteral therapies; CL: Analysis

64. Under which of the following circumstances is emetic treatment indicated for a child who ingested a poison?
1. The child refuses to take the emetic.
2. The child is in severe shock.
3. The child is experiencing seizures.
4. The poison is a low-viscosity hydrocarbon.

64. 1. The child shouldn't be given a choice; the emetic must be given if indicated. Severe shock increases the risk for aspiration, so emetic treatment is contraindicated when a child is in severe shock. An emetic shouldn't be administered to a child experiencing seizures. If the poison is a low-viscosity hydrocarbon, it can cause severe chemical pneumonitis if aspirated.
NP: Assessment; CN: Physiological integrity; CNS: Physiological adaptation; CL: Knowledge

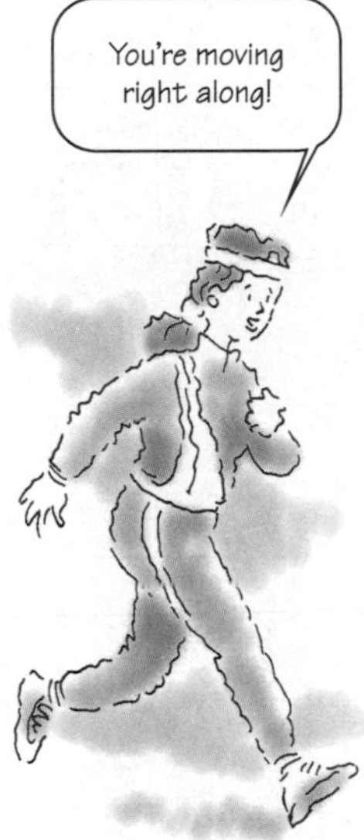

65. Which of the following inflammatory diseases most commonly affects the terminal ileum?
1. Acute appendicitis
2. Crohn's disease
3. Meckel's diverticulum
4. Ulcerative colitis

65. 2. Crohn's disease affects the terminal ileum. Ulcerative colitis affects the entire bowel. Acute appendicitis affects the blind sac at the end of the cecum. Meckel's diverticulum is a sac that becomes inflamed.
NP: Assessment; CN: Physiological integrity; CNS: Physiological adaptation; CL: Knowledge

66. If a child ingests poisonous hydrocarbons, an important nursing intervention would include which of the following actions?
1. Induce vomiting.
2. Keep the child calm and relaxed.
3. Scold the child for the wrongdoing.
4. Keep the parents away from the child.

66. 2. Keeping the child calm and relaxed will help prevent vomiting. If vomiting occurs, there's a great chance the esophagus will be damaged from regurgitation of the gastric poison. Additionally, the risk for chemical pneumonitis exists if vomiting occurs. The parents should remain with the child to help keep him calm. Scolding the child may upset him.
NP: Implementation; CN: Physiological integrity; CNS: Physiological adaptation; CL: Analysis

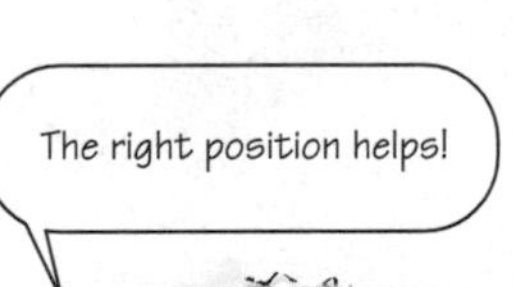

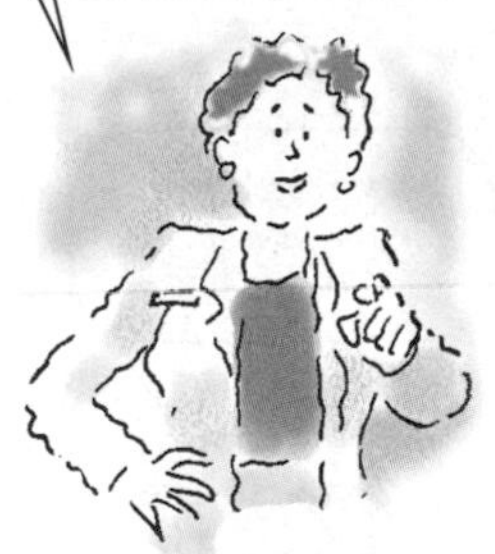

67. Shock is a complication of several types of poisoning. Which of the following measures would help reduce the risk of shock?
1. Keep the child on his right side.
2. Let the child maintain normal activity as possible.
3. Elevate the head and legs to the level of the heart.
4. Keep the head flat, and raise the legs to the level of the heart.

67. 3. Elevating the head and legs to the level of the heart will promote venous drainage and decrease the chance of the child going into shock. The child should be encouraged to get plenty of rest. The child may safely lie on the side he prefers.
NP: Assessment; CN: Physiological integrity; CNS: Physiological adaptation; CL: Knowledge

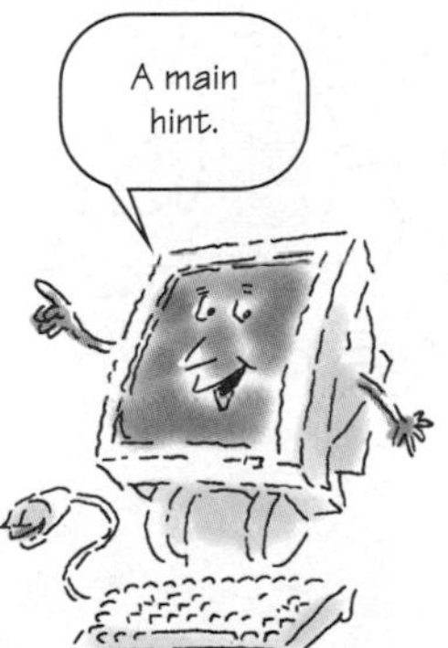

68. A 7-year-old child ingested several leaves of a poinsettia plant. After arrival in the emergency department, which of the following interventions would be the main nursing function for this client?
1. Begin teaching accident prevention.
2. Provide emotional support to the child.
3. Be prepared for immediate intervention.
4. Provide emotional support to the parents.

68. 3. Time and speed are critical factors in recovery from poisonings. The remaining three answers are important nursing functions but don't require the immediate attention that first stabilizing the child does.
NP: Assessment; CN: Health promotion and maintenance; CNS: Prevention and early detection of disease; CL: Analysis

69. Which of the following drugs is most commonly ingested by children?

1. Acetaminophen (Tylenol)
2. Aspirin
3. Ibuprofen (Motrin)
4. Acetaminophen and oxycodone hydrochloride (Percocet)

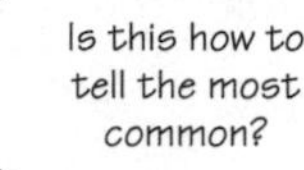

Is this how to tell the most common?

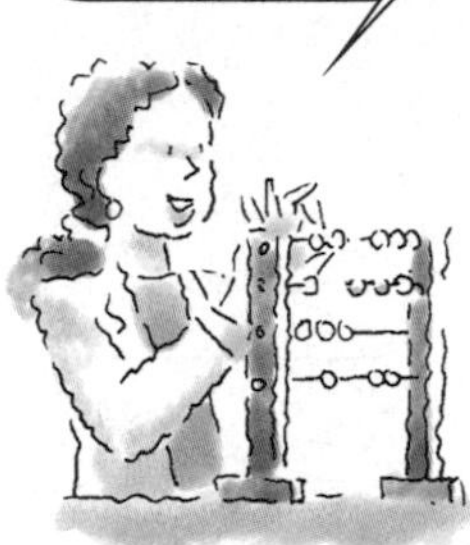

69. 2. Aspirin is the most readily available drug in many homes, thus increasing the likelihood of poisoning by this drug. Acetaminophen would be the second most readily available drug. Motrin may or may not be used in the home. Percocet isn't a common household drug.

NP: Analysis; CN: Physiological integrity; CNS: Physiological adaptation; CL: Knowledge

70. Which of the following symptoms helps in the initial diagnosis of ulcerative colitis?

1. Constipation
2. Diarrhea
3. Vomiting
4. Weight loss

70. 2. Recurrent or persistent diarrhea is a common feature of ulcerative colitis. Constipation doesn't occur because the bowel becomes smooth and inflexible. Vomiting isn't common in this disease. Weight loss will occur after or during the episode, but not initially.

NP: Assessment; CN: Physiological integrity; CNS: Physiological adaptation; CL: Knowledge

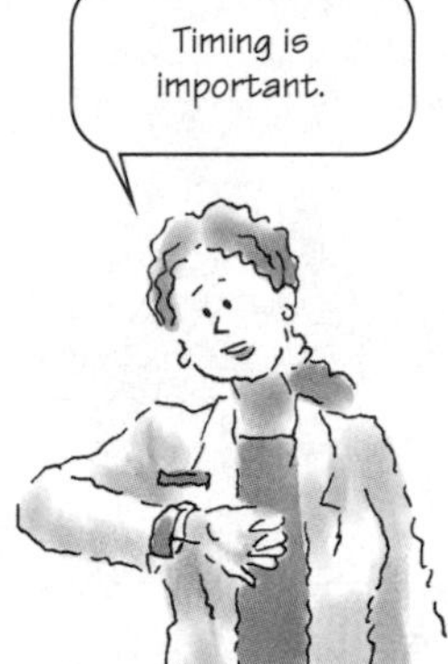

71. If a child ingests poisonous amounts of salicylates, how soon after ingestion would signs of toxicity become obvious?

1. Immediately
2. 2 to 4 hours after ingestion
3. 6 hours after ingestion
4. 18 hours after ingestion

71. 3. There's usually a delay of 6 hours before evidence of toxicity is noted. Aspirin will exert its peak effect in 2 to 4 hours. The effect of aspirin may last as long as 18 hours. Toxic evidence is rarely immediate.

NP: Assessment; CN: Health promotion and maintenance; CNS: Prevention and early detection of disease; CL: Knowledge

72. In extreme cases of salicylate poisoning, which of the following treatments is used?

1. Forced emesis
2. Hypothermia blankets
3. Peritoneal dialysis
4. Vitamin K injection

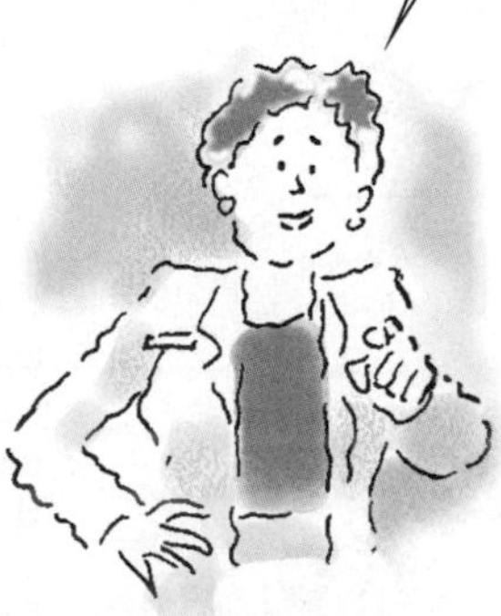

72. 3. Peritoneal dialysis is usually reserved for cases of life-threatening salicylism. Forced emesis is the immediate treatment for salicylate poisoning because the stomach contents and salicylates will move from the stomach to the remainder of the GI tract, where vomiting will no longer result in the removal of the poison. Vitamin K may be used to decrease bleeding tendencies but only if evidence of this exists. Hypothermia blankets may be used to reduce the possibility of seizures.

NP: Analysis; CN: Health promotion and maintenance; CNS: Prevention and early detection of disease; CL: Knowledge

73. When a child has been poisoned, identifying the ingested poison is an important treatment goal. Which of the following actions would help determine which poison was ingested?

1. Call the local poison control center.
2. Ask the child.
3. Ask the parents.
4. Save all evidence of poison.

73. 4. Saving all evidence of poison (container, vomitus, urine) will help determine which drug was ingested and how much. The parent may be helpful in some instances, although the parent may not have been home or with the child when the ingestion occurred. Asking the child may help, but the child may fear punishment and may not be honest about the incident. Calling the local poison control center may help get information on specific poisons or if a certain household placed a call, although rarely can they help determine which poison has been ingested.

NP: Assessment; CN: Health promotion and maintenance; CNS: Prevention and early detection of disease; CL: Analysis

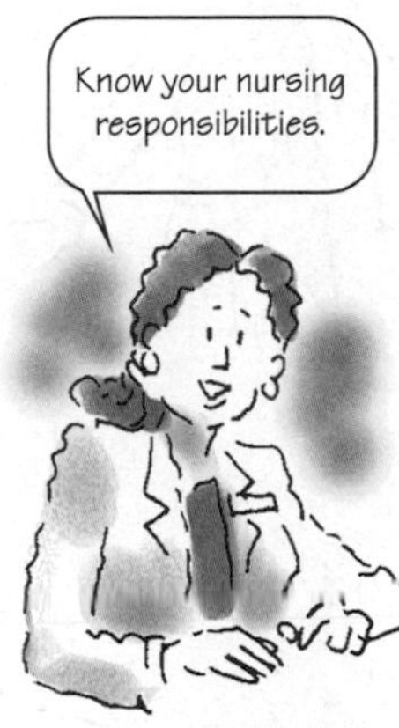

Know your nursing responsibilities.

74. One of the most important nursing responsibilities to help prevent salicylate poisoning would include which of the following actions?

1. Identify salicylate overdose.
2. Teach children the hazards of ingesting nonfood items.
3. Decrease curiosity; teach parents to keep aspirin and drugs in clear view.
4. Teach parents to keep large amounts of drugs on hand but out of reach of children.

74. 2. Teaching children the hazards of ingesting nonfood items will help prevent ingestion of poisonous substances. Identifying the overdose won't prevent it from occurring. Aspirin and drugs should be kept out of the sight of children. Parents should be warned about keeping large amounts of drugs on hand.

NP: Implementation; CN: Health promotion and maintenance; CNS: Prevention and early detection of disease; CL: Comprehension

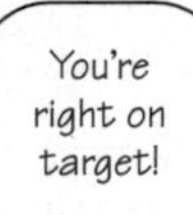

You're right on target!

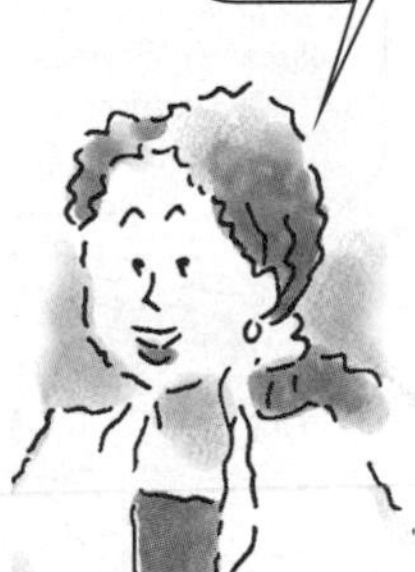

75. Which of the following conditions can result from an acute overdose of acetaminophen?

1. Brain damage
2. Heart failure
3. Hepatic damage
4. Kidney damage

75. 3. The damage to the hepatic system isn't from the drug, but from one of its metabolites. This metabolite binds to liver cells in large quantities. Brain damage, heart failure, and kidney damage may develop but not initially.

NP: Assessment; CN: Physiological integrity; CNS: Physiological adaptation; CL: Knowledge

76. Which of the following symptoms is a sign of acetaminophen poisoning?

1. Hyperthermia
2. Increased urine output
3. Profuse sweating
4. Rapid pulse

76. 3. During the first 12 to 24 hours, profuse sweating is a significant sign of acetaminophen poisoning. Weak pulse, hypothermia, and decreased urine output are also common findings.

NP: Assessment; CN: Physiological integrity; CNS: Physiological adaptation; CL: Knowledge

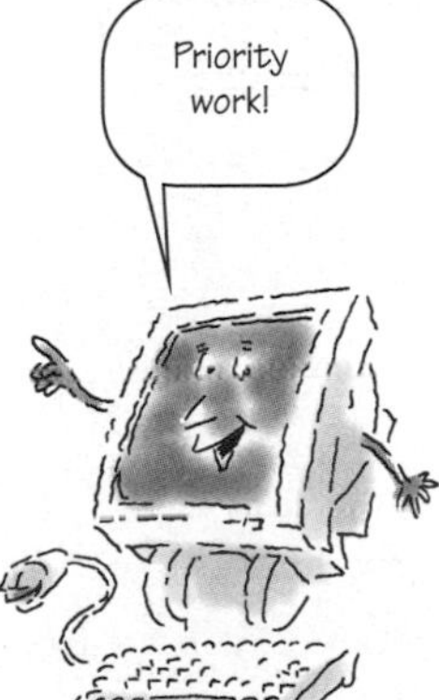

Priority work!

77. In a client diagnosed with acetaminophen poisoning, the initial therapeutic management would include which of the following actions?

1. Induce vomiting.
2. Obtain blood work.
3. Give I.V. fluid.
4. Use activated charcoal.

77. 1. Inducing vomiting using syrup of ipecac would be the initial treatment after acetaminophen poisoning has been confirmed. Blood work would be obtained but wouldn't be the first priority. Caution is taken when fluids are administered. Activated charcoal isn't used because it interferes with the antidote *N*-acetylcysteine, which helps protect the liver.

NP: Assessment; CN: Physiological integrity; CNS: Physiological adaptation; CL: Knowledge

78. Which of the following ethnic groups has the highest prevalence of lead poisoning in children?
1. Black
2. Hispanic
3. Asian
4. White

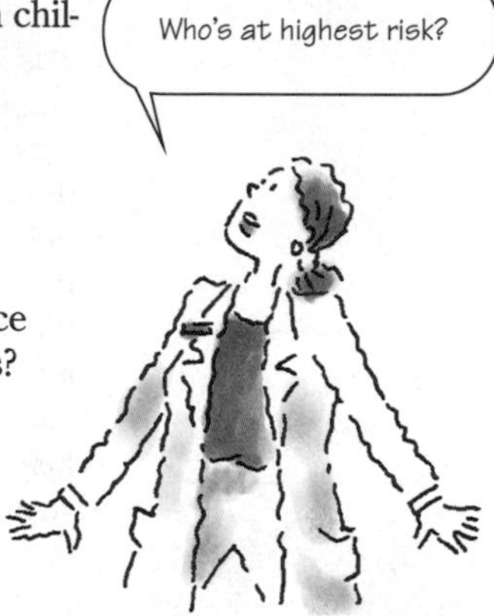

Who's at highest risk?

78. 1. Black children have a six times greater risk for lead poisoning compared with white children. Lead poisoning isn't common in Asian or Hispanic populations.
NP: Assessment; CN: Health promotion and maintenance; CNS: Prevention and early detection of disease; CL: Knowledge

79. Which of the following factors influence the ingestion of lead-containing substances?
1. Child's age
2. Child's sex
3. Child's nationality
4. A parent with the same habit

79. 1. The highest risk for lead poisoning occurs in young children who have a tendency to put things in their mouth. In older homes that contain lead-based paint, paint chips may be eaten directly by the child or they may cling to toys or hands that are then put into the child's mouth. Poisoning isn't sex-related. Blacks have a higher incidence of lead poisoning, but it can happen in any race. Children of low socioeconomic status are more likely to eat lead-based paint chips. Most parents don't eat lead-based paint on purpose.
NP: Assessment; CN: Health promotion and maintenance; CNS: Prevention and early detection of disease; CL: Knowledge

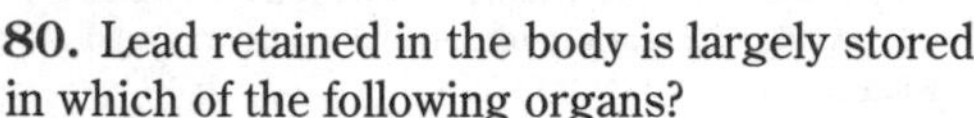

80. Lead retained in the body is largely stored in which of the following organs?
1. Bone
2. Brain
3. Kidney
4. Liver

80. 1. Ingested lead is initially absorbed by bone. If chronic ingestion occurs, then the hematologic, renal, and central nervous systems are affected.
NP: Assessment; CN: Physiological integrity; CNS: Physiological adaptation; CL: Knowledge

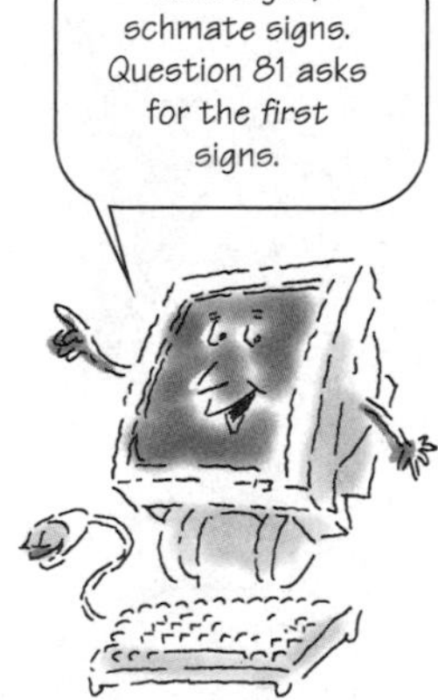

Late signs, schmate signs. Question 81 asks for the first signs.

81. Which of the following conditions is one of the initial signs of lead poisoning?
1. Anemia
2. Diarrhea
3. Overeating
4. Paralysis

81. 1. Lead is dangerously toxic to the biosynthesis of heme. The reduced heme molecule in red blood cells causes anemia. Constipation and anorexia are vague, nonspecific symptoms. Paralysis may occur as toxic damage to the brain progresses.
NP: Assessment; CN: Physiological integrity; CNS: Physiological adaptation; CL: Knowledge

82. The most serious and irreversible adverse effects of lead intoxication affect which of the following systems?
1. Central nervous system
2. Hematologic system
3. Renal system
4. Respiratory system

82. 1. Damage that occurs to the central nervous system is difficult to repair. Damage to the renal and hematologic systems can be reversed if treated early. The respiratory system isn't affected until coma and death occur.
NP: Assessment; CN: Physiological integrity; CNS: Physiological adaptation; CL: Analysis

83. Black lines along the gums indicate which of the following types of poisoning?
1. Acetaminophen
2. Lead
3. Plants
4. Salicylates

84. Which of the following procedures is the main treatment for lead poisoning?
1. Blood transfusion
2. Bone marrow transplant
3. Chelation therapy
4. Dialysis

85. Which of the following nursing objectives would be the most important for a child with lead poisoning who must undergo chelation therapy?
1. Prepare the child for complete bedrest.
2. Prepare the child for I.V. fluid therapy.
3. Prepare the child for an extended hospital stay.
4. Prepare the child for a large number of injections.

86. Which of the following conditions may occur during chelation therapy in a child with lead-poisoning?
1. Hypercalcemia
2. Hypocalcemia
3. Hyperglycemia
4. Hypoglycemia

87. Which of the following interventions is the best way to prevent lead poisoning in children?
1. Educate the child.
2. Educate the public.
3. Identify high-risk groups.
4. Provide home chelation kits.

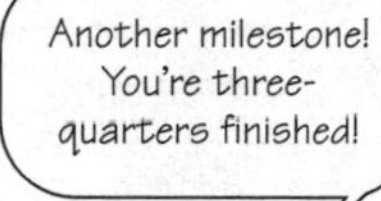

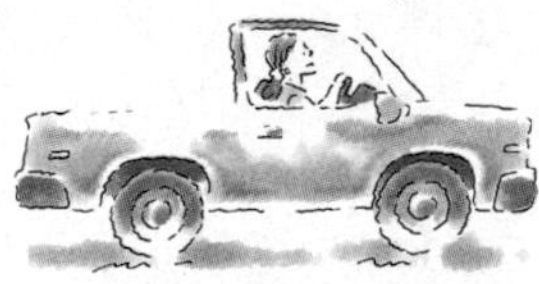

Another milestone! You're three-quarters finished!

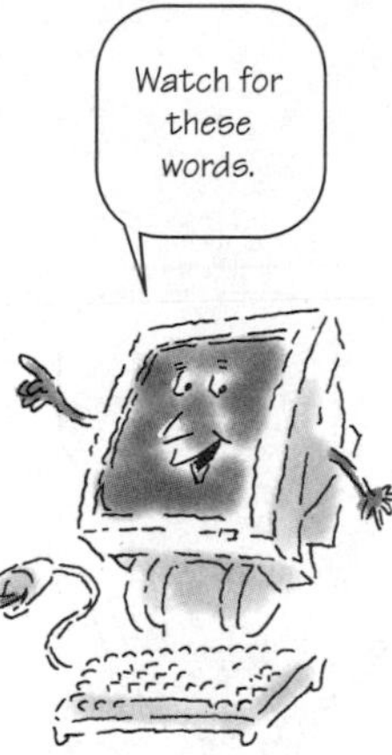
Watch for these words.

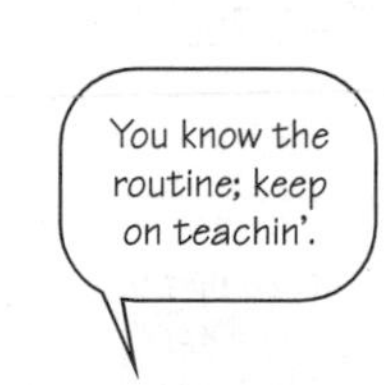
You know the routine; keep on teachin'.

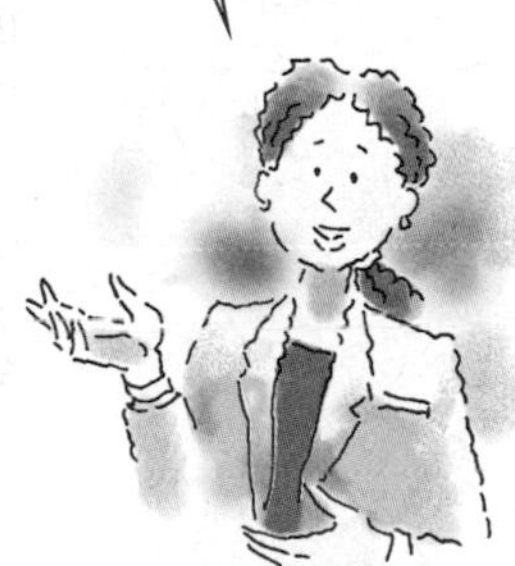

83. 2. One diagnostic characteristic of lead poisoning is black lines along the gums. Black lines don't occur along the gums with acetaminophen, plant, or salicylate poisoning.
NP: Assessment; CN: Physiological integrity; CNS: Physiological adaptation; CL: Knowledge

84. 3. Chelation therapy involves the removal of metal by combining it with another substance. Sometimes exchange transfusions are used to rid the blood of lead quickly. Bone marrow transplants usually aren't needed. Dialysis usually isn't part of the treatment.
NP: Implementation; CN: Physiological integrity; CNS: Physiological adaptation; CL: Knowledge

85. 4. Chelation therapy involves getting a large number of injections in a relatively short period of time. It's traumatic to the majority of children, and they need some preparation for the treatment. The other components of the treatment plan are important, but not as likely to cause the same anxiety as multiple injections. Receiving I.V. fluid isn't as traumatizing as 60 injections. Physical activity is usually limited. Allowing adequate rest to not aggravate the painful injection sites is important.
NP: Implementation; CN: Physiological integrity; CNS: Physiological adaptation; CL: Analysis

86. 2. A calcium chelating agent is used for the treatment of lead-poisoning, so calcium is removed from the body with the lead. Hypocalcemia, not hypercalcemia, occurs. Hyperglycemia and hypoglycemia don't occur as a result of this therapy.
NP: Assessment; CN: Physiological integrity; CNS: Physiological adaptation; CL: Analysis

87. 2. By educating others about lead poisoning, including the danger signs, symptoms, and treatment, identification can be determined quickly. Very young children may not understand the dangers of lead poisoning. Home chelation kits currently aren't available. Identifying high-risk groups will help, but won't prevent the poisoning.
NP: Implementation; CN: Health promotion and maintenance; CNS: Prevention and early detection of disease; CL: Analysis

88. Which of the following terms describes a purposeful ingestion of a nonfood substance?

1. Patent ductus arteriosus (PDA)
2. RDSI
3. Pica
4. Plumbism

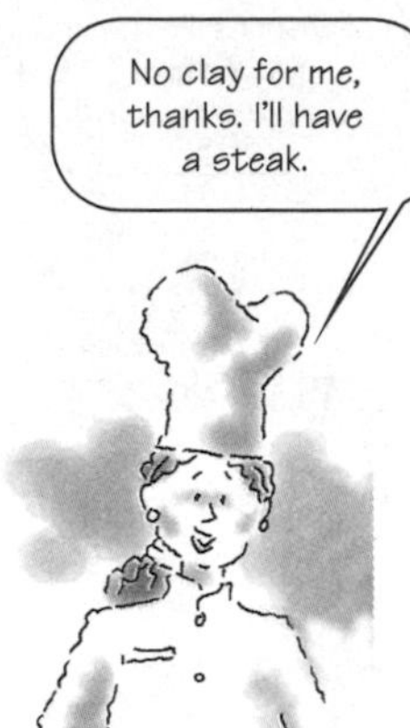

No clay for me, thanks. I'll have a steak.

88. 3. Pica is a Latin word for magpie, a bird with a voracious appetite. Today, pica refers to the purposeful ingestion of a nonfood substance. PDA is a term for a heart murmur. RDSI stands for revised developmental screening inventory, a developmental screening test. Plumbism is another term for lead poisoning.

NP: Analysis; CN: Health promotion and maintenance; CNS: Prevention and early detection of disease; CL: Knowledge

89. Certain forms of pica are caused by a deficiency of which of the following nutrients?

1. Minerals
2. Vitamin B complex
3. Vitamin C
4. Vitamin D

89. 1. Eating clay is related to zinc deficiency, and eating chalk to calcium deficiency. Vitamin deficiencies aren't related to pica.

NP: Analysis; CN: Health promotion and maintenance; CNS: Prevention and early detection of disease; CL: Knowledge

90. Which of the following helminthic infections caused by nematodes is the most common?

1. Flukes
2. Hookworms
3. Roundworms
4. Tapeworms

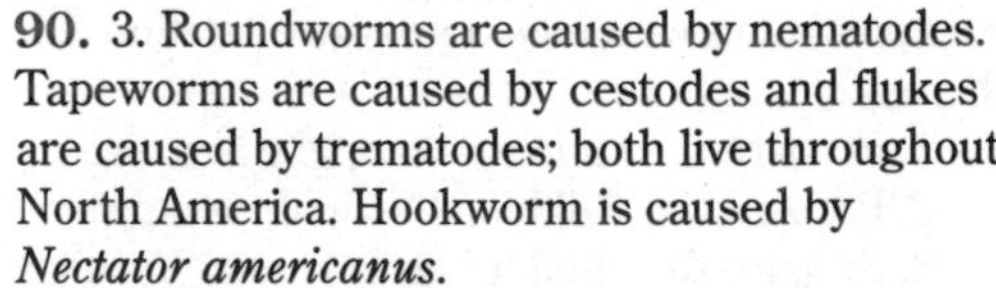

90. 3. Roundworms are caused by nematodes. Tapeworms are caused by cestodes and flukes are caused by trematodes; both live throughout North America. Hookworm is caused by *Nectator americanus.*

NP: Assessment; CN: Health promotion and maintenance; CNS: Prevention and early detection of disease; CL: Knowledge

91. Which of the following inflammatory conditions requiring surgery during childhood would be the most common?

1. Acute appendicitis
2. Necrotizing enterocolitis
3. Tonsillitis
4. Ulcerative colitis

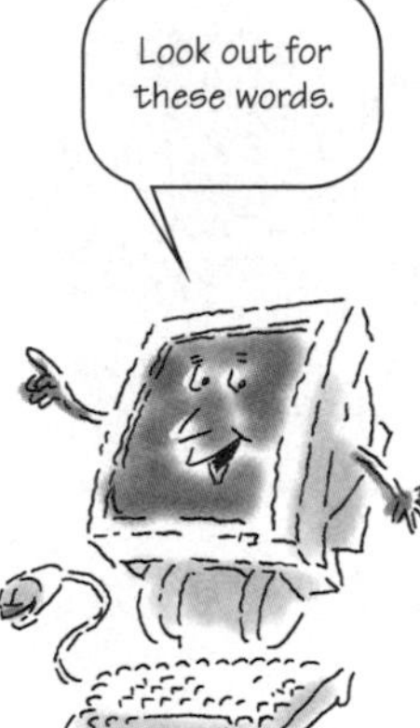

91. 1. Acute appendicitis is the most common inflammatory condition requiring surgery in childhood. Ulcerative colitis occurs in prepubescent and adolescent children and generally doesn't require surgery. Necrotizing enterocolitis is seen in ill neonates. Tonsillitis can occur at any age but doesn't always require surgery.

NP: Analysis; CN: Physiological integrity; CNS: Physiological adaptation; CL: Knowledge

92. Which of the following symptoms is the most common for acute appendicitis?

1. Bradycardia
2. Fever
3. Pain descending to the lower left quadrant
4. Pain radiating down the legs

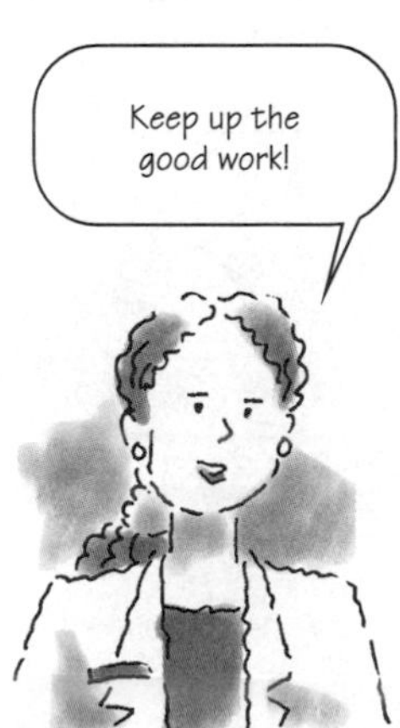

92. 2. Fever, abdominal pain, and tenderness are the first signs of appendicitis. Tachycardia, not bradycardia, is seen. Pain can be generalized or periumbilical. It usually descends to the lower right quadrant, not the left.

NP: Assessment; CN: Physiological integrity; CNS: Physiological adaptation; CL: Analysis

93. Which of the following nursing interventions would be important to do preoperatively in a child with appendicitis?

1. Give clear fluids.
2. Apply heat to the abdomen.
3. Maintain complete bed rest.
4. Administer an enema if ordered.

93. 3. Bed rest will prevent aggravating the condition. Clients with appendicitis aren't allowed anything by mouth. Cold applications are placed on the abdomen as heat would increase blood flow to the area and possibly spread any infectious disease. Enemas may aggravate the condition.

NP: Implementation; CN: Physiological integrity; CNS: Physiological adaptation; CL: Analysis

94. Postoperative care of a child with a ruptured appendix would include which of the following treatments or interventions?
1. Liquid diet
2. Oral antibiotics for 7 to 10 days
3. Position the child on the left side
4. Parenteral antibiotics for 7 to 10 days

94. 4. Parenteral antibiotics are used for 7 to 10 days postoperatively to help prevent the spread of infection. The child is kept on I.V. fluids and isn't allowed anything by mouth. Oral antibiotics may continue after the parenteral antibiotics are discontinued. The child is positioned on the right side after surgery.
NP: Implementation; CN: Physiological integrity; CNS: Physiological adaptation; CL: Analysis

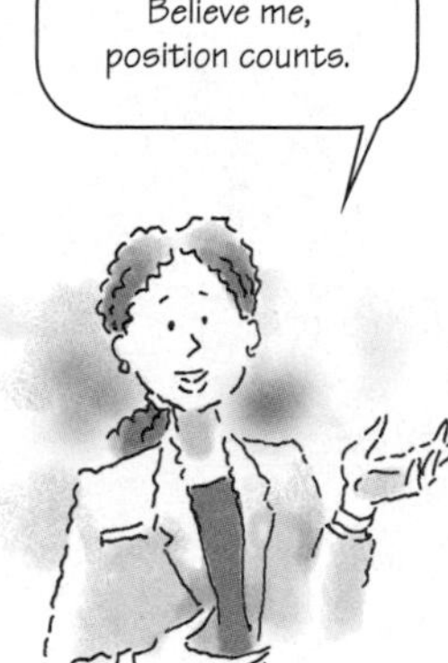

Believe me, position counts.

95. After surgical repair of a ruptured appendix, which of the following positions would be the most appropriate?
1. High Fowler's position
2. Left side
3. Semi-Fowler's position
4. Supine

95. 3. Using the semi-Fowler's or right side-lying positions will facilitate drainage from the peritoneal cavity and prevent the formation of a subdiaphragmatic abscess. High Fowler's, left side, and prone positions won't facilitate drainage from the peritoneal cavity.
NP: Implementation; CN: Physiological integrity; CNS: Physiological adaptation; CL: Analysis

96. In which of the following inflammatory diseases do the majority of children show signs of painless bright or dark red rectal bleeding?
1. Crohn's disease
2. Meckel's diverticulum
3. Ruptured appendix
4. Ulcerative colitis

96. 2. Acute and sometimes massive hemorrhage may occur in Meckel's diverticulum. Children with ulcerative colitis present with recurring diarrhea. There's no rectal bleeding with a ruptured appendix or Crohn's disease.
NP: Assessment; CN: Physiological integrity; CNS: Physiological adaptation; CL: Knowledge

97. Ulcerative colitis is a disease that affects which of the following groups?
1. Both sexes
2. Boys
3. Girls
4. Neonates

97. 1. Ulcerative colitis occurs in both sexes and all ages. The peak onset of this disease is between ages 10 and 19.
NP: Assessment; CN: Physiological integrity; CNS: Physiological adaptation; CL: Knowledge

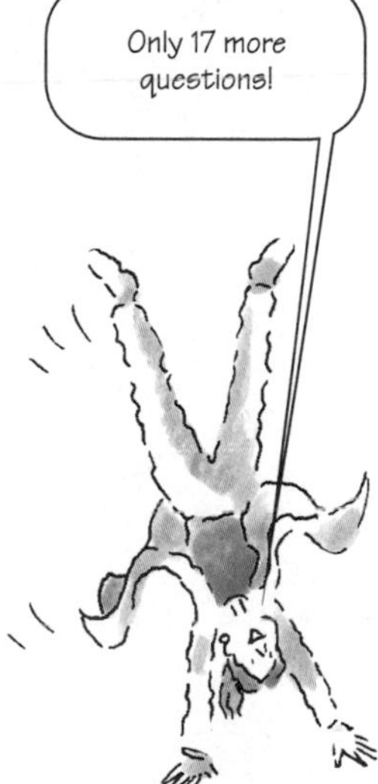

Only 17 more questions!

98. A neonate has been diagnosed with a unilateral complete cleft lip and cleft palate. The nurse formulating the care plan for this neonate will have which of the following nursing diagnoses as a priority?
1. Risk for infection
2. Impaired skin integrity
3. Risk for aspiration
4. Delayed growth and development

98. 3. Although all these diagnoses are important for the neonate with a cleft lip and cleft palate, the most important diagnosis relates to airway. Neonates with a cleft lip and a cleft palate may have an excessive amount of saliva and usually have a difficult time with feedings. Special feeding techniques, such as using a flanged nipple, may be necessary to prevent aspiration.
NP: Planning; CN: Physiological integrity; CNS: Reduction of risk potential; CL: Analysis

99. A neonate is suspected of having a tracheoesophageal fistula (type III/C). Which of the following symptoms would be seen on the initial assessment?

1. Excessive drooling
2. Excessive vomiting
3. Mottling
4. Polyhydramnios

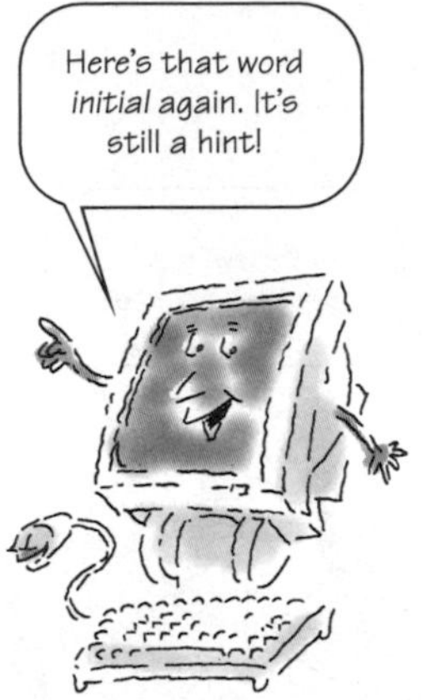

initial again. It's
still a hint!

99. 1. In type III/C tracheoesophageal fistula, the proximal end of the esophagus ends in a blind pouch and a fistula connects the distal end of the esophagus to the trachea. Saliva will pool in this pouch and cause the child to drool. Mottling is a netlike reddish blue discoloration of the skin usually due to vascular contraction in a response to hypothermia. The mother of a neonate with tracheoesophageal fistula may have had polyhydramnios. Because the distal end of the esophagus is connected to the trachea, the neonate can't vomit, but he can aspirate, and stomach acid may go into the lungs through this fistula, causing pneumonitis.

NP: Assessment; CN: Physiological integrity; CNS: Reduction of risk potential; CL: Analysis

100. When assessing a client suspected of having pyloric stenosis, which of the following findings would be seen?

1. An "olive" mass in the right upper quadrant
2. An "olive" mass in the left upper quadrant
3. A "sausage" mass in the right upper quadrant
4. A "sausage" mass in the left upper quadrant

100. 1. Pyloric stenosis involves hypertrophy of the circular muscle fibers of the pylorus. This hypertrophy is palpable in the right upper quadrant of the abdomen. A "sausage" mass is palpable in the right upper quadrant in children with intussusception. A "sausage" mass in the left upper quadrant wouldn't indicate pyloric stenosis.

NP: Assessment; CN: Physiological integrity; CNS: Physiological adaptation; CL: Comprehension

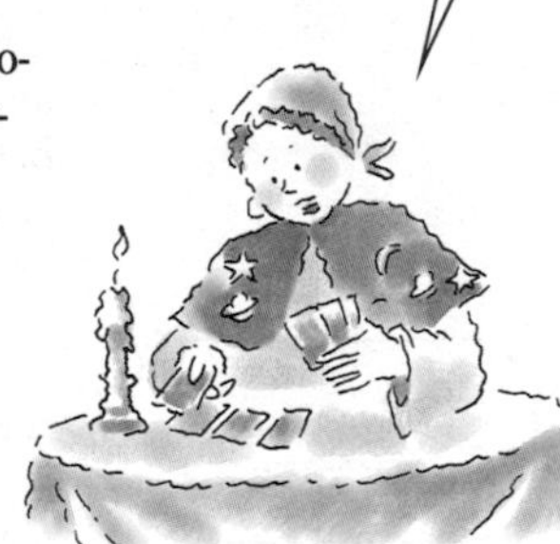

Lab results will tell
you waaaay more
than these cards.

101. The nurse caring for an infant with pyloric stenosis would expect which of the following laboratory values?

1. pH, 7.30; chloride, 120 mEq/L
2. pH, 7.38; chloride, 110 mEq/L
3. pH, 7.43; chloride, 100 mEq/L
4. pH, 7.49; chloride, 90 mEq/L

101. 4. Infants with pyloric stenosis vomit hydrochloric acid. This causes them to become alkalotic and hypochloremic. Normal serum pH is 7.35 to 7.45; levels above 7.45 represent alkalosis. The normal serum chloride level is 99 to 111 mEq/L; levels below 99 mEq/L represent hypochloremia.

NP: Assessment; CN: Physiological integrity; CNS: Physiological adaptation; CL: Analysis

102. A 1-day-old neonate hasn't passed meconium. The nurse would assess this neonate for which of the following conditions?

1. Biliary atresia
2. Gastroesophageal reflux
3. Gastroschisis
4. Hirschsprung's disease

102. 4. Hirschsprung's disease is an absence of the autonomic parasympathetic ganglion cells of a section of colon. The lack of neural intervention prevents peristalsis, so the neonate can't pass meconium. Biliary atresia is a malformation of the biliary drainage system, causing the baby to eventually develop liver failure; the neonate appears normal at birth. Gastroesophageal reflux is caused by stomach contents entering the esophagus secondary to a weak lower esophageal sphincter. Gastroschisis is an abdominal wall defect through which the intestines herniate. This defect is obvious at birth.

NP: Assessment; CN: Physiological integrity; CNS: Physiological adaptation; CL: Comprehension

103. A nurse assessing a client with necrotizing enterocolitis would expect which of the following findings?

1. Abdominal distention and gastric retention
2. Gastric retention and guaiac-negative stools
3. Metabolic alkalosis and abdominal distention
4. Guaiac-negative stools and metabolic alkalosis

103. 1. Necrotizing enterocolitis is an ischemic disorder of the gut. The cause is unknown, but it's more common in premature neonates who had a hypoxic episode. The neonate's intestines become dilated and necrotic, and the abdomen becomes very distended. Paralytic ileus develops, causing the neonate to have gastric retention. These retained gastric contents, along with any passed stool, will be guaiac-positive. The neonate also develops metabolic acidosis.

NP: Assessment; CN: Physiological integrity; CNS: Physiological adaptation; CL: Comprehension

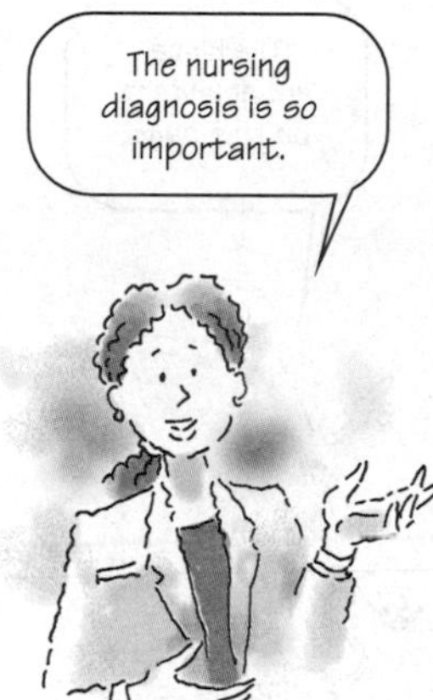
The nursing
diagnosis is so
important.

104. An infant has been admitted to the hospital with gastroenteritis. The nursing care plan for this infant will consider which of the following nursing diagnoses first?

1. Acute pain
2. Diarrhea
3. Deficient fluid volume
4. Imbalanced nutrition: Less than body requirements

104. 3. Young children with gastroenteritis are at high risk for developing a fluid volume deficit. Their intestinal mucosa allows for more fluid and electrolytes to be lost when they have gastroenteritis. The main goal of the health care team should be to rehydrate the infant. The other nursing diagnoses are important, but deficient fluid volume is more life-threatening.

NP: Planning; CN: Physiological integrity; CNS: Physiological adaptation; CL: Application

105. Which of the following symptoms are consistent with the diagnosis of pyloric stenosis?

1. Projectile vomiting, metabolic alkalosis, hunger
2. Projectile vomiting, metabolic acidosis, dehydration, hunger
3. Frequent vomiting of formula, respiratory alkalosis, weight gain
4. Frequent vomiting of bilious emesis, metabolic acidosis, poor appetite

105. 1. Classic signs of pyloric stenosis include projectile vomiting of nonbilious emesis, metabolic alkalosis (because acid is lost in vomit), hunger, dehydration, and failure to thrive. The problem is a too-tight pylorus, which causes projectile nonbilious vomiting. The infants are hungry because they continue to lose their feedings; it isn't an absorption or digestion problem. The problem results in metabolic imbalances, not problems with the respiratory system, and weight loss instead of weight gain.

NP: Analysis; CN: Physiological integrity; CNS: Physiological adaptation; CL: Comprehension

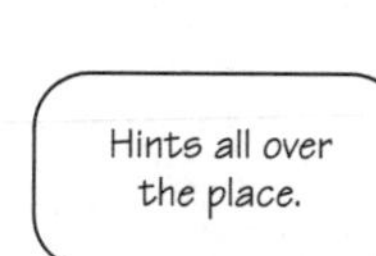
Hints all over
the place.

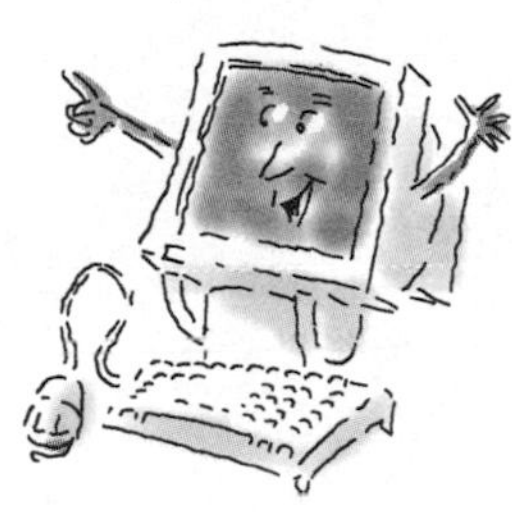

106. A mother calls the children's clinic, says she found her toddler with an open and empty bottle of acetaminophen (Tylenol), and wants to know what to do. What's the priority intervention for this situation?

1. Ask the mother if she has any syrup of ipecac.
2. Ask the mother to give the child a large glass of milk.
3. Ask the mother to rush the child to the emergency department.
4. Ask the mother if she knows cardiopulmonary resuscitation (CPR).

106. 1. The emergency treatment for acute acetaminophen poisoning is syrup of ipecac. The mother doesn't need to delay treatment that may be available in the home such as syrup of ipecac. Asking about CPR isn't appropriate as the priority intervention; it would distract from the immediate interventions needed. Milk isn't an antidote for acetaminophen toxicity.

NP: Implementation; CN: Safe, effective care environment; CNS: Safety and infection control; CL: Analysis

107. Which of the following facts should be emphasized in the teaching plan for the parents of a child with celiac disease?

1. The gluten-free diet alterations must be continued for a lifetime.
2. The diet needs to be free of lactose because the child is intolerant.
3. Diet alterations are necessary when the child reports cramping and bloating.
4. The diet needs to be low in fats because of the malabsorption problem in the intestines.

107. 1. Celiac disease is the inability to digest gluten. The treatment is a gluten-free diet for life. It's important the diet is continued to avoid symptoms and the associated risk colon cancer. The disease isn't caused by lactose intolerance or a problem digesting fats.

NP: Planning; CN: Health promotion and maintenance; CNS: Prevention and early detection of disease; CL: Knowledge

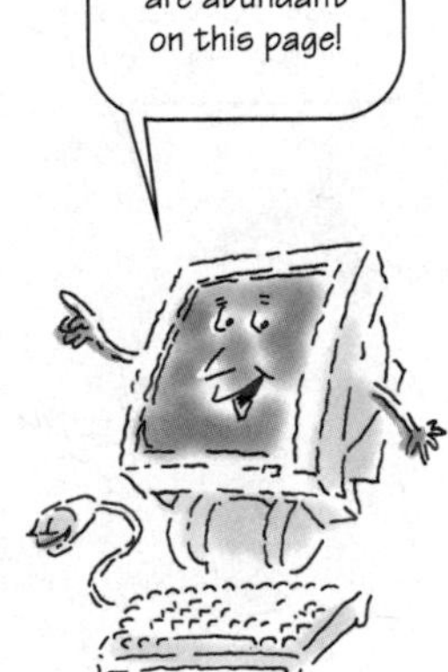
The hints
are abundant
on this page!

108. A pediatrician suspects that a child has pinworms and instructs the nurse to assess the child for their presence. Which is the most reliable method of assessing for pinworms?

1. A history of itching at the anal area and of restlessness at night
2. A blood culture
3. Eggs retrieved from the anal edge on a piece of cellophane tape
4. A stool culture

108. 3. Cellophane tape placed near the anal edge will capture the eggs. A history of itching and of restlessness aren't enough to definitely diagnosis pinworms. Neither a blood culture nor a stool culture would be helpful.

NP: Assessment; CN: Physiological integrity; CNS: Reduction of risk potential; CL: Application

109. A male infant, age 1 month, is brought to the pediatrician's office. His mother states that he's fussy and cries as if in pain. He's tolerating normal amounts of formula, gaining weight, and having episodes of paroxysmal abdominal cramping after feedings. These signs and symptoms indicate that the infant most likely has which condition?

1. Intussusception
2. Meconium ileus
3. Colic
4. Pyloric stenosis

109. 3. An infant with colic exhibits symptoms of abdominal cramping after feedings, cries as if in pain, and is fussy. An intussusception begins suddenly and leads to bloody stools and vomiting. A meconium ileus is nonpassage of meconium by 24 hours of age. Signs of pyloric stenosis include projectile vomiting and weight loss.

NP: Assessment; CN: Physiological integrity; CNS: Physiological adaptation; CL: Analysis

110. A 16-year-old black student visits the school nurse with complaints of nausea and fatigue. The nurse determines a need to check for jaundice. Which area of the body should the nurse examine?

1. Sclera of the eye
2. Overall skin color
3. The outer ears and back of the neck
4. The tongue and inside the cheek area

110. 1. The sclera is the best place to check for jaundice, especially in a person of darker color. The outer ears and back of the neck and the tongue and inside of the cheek aren't appropriate places to check for jaundice.

NP: Assessment; CN: Physiological integrity; CNS: Physiological adaptation; CL: Application

111. A mother brings her 4-week-old son to the clinic. She states that he hasn't been eating well and is lethargic when she holds and cuddles him. He has lost 7 oz since birth. He's otherwise healthy and has no congenital defects. Which condition is the pediatrician most likely to diagnose?

1. Celiac disease
2. Failure to thrive
3. Hirschsprung's disease
4. Imperforate anus

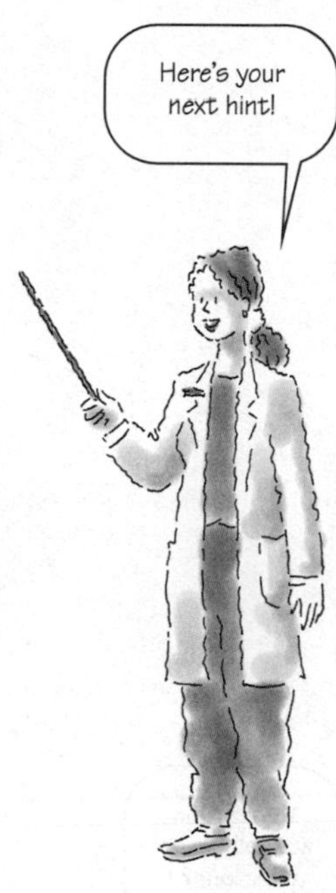
Here's your next hint!

111. 2. These signs and symptoms are classic of the condition failure to thrive. Celiac disease presents with steatorrhea, weight loss, and inability to digest gluten foods. Hirschsprung's disease and imperforate anus present with abdominal distention and absence of stool; no anal opening is present in imperforate anus.

NP: Implementation; CN: Physiological integrity; CNS: Physiological adaptation; CL: Application

112. A 15-year-old client needs a nasogastric tube inserted because of peritonitis caused by a ruptured appendix. The client is afraid that the procedure will hurt. Which statement would most help decrease the client's anxiety?

1. "Breathe deeply through your mouth and relax. It will be over soon."
2. "This is a simple procedure, and it won't hurt."
3. "You'll feel pressure and be uncomfortable for a few minutes, but it shouldn't be painful."
4. "You're a man now and need to be able to handle pain."

112. 3. Discussing the procedure will help the client understand the extent of discomfort. Breathing deeply will help relieve discomfort, but the statement may also imply that the procedure will be painful and will, thus, increase the client's anxiety. By saying the procedure is simple, the nurse isn't acknowledging the client's concerns. Calling the client a man and telling him that he should be able to handle pain is condescending, No matter what the client's age, he has a right to express his fears and to have those fears acknowledged.

NP: Implementation; CN: Psychosocial integrity; CNS: Coping and adaptation; CL: Analysis

113. A mother brings her 18-month-old daughter to the emergency department and tells the nurse that her daughter has been ill for the past 2 days. The daughter has a fever of 104° F (40° C), is irritable, has had diarrhea, and hasn't been wetting her diaper much in the past 24 hours. The child is admitted to the pediatric unit for treatment of moderate dehydration and gastroenteritis. I.V. therapy and strict intake and output are ordered. As rehydration occurs, the child is started on oral feedings of a rehydration fluid. When caring for this child during the later stage of rehydration, the nurse should take which action?

1. Force fluids.
2. Allow the client to drink as much as she wants.
3. Monitor the client's intake and output.
4. Monitor the client's ability to retain fluids.

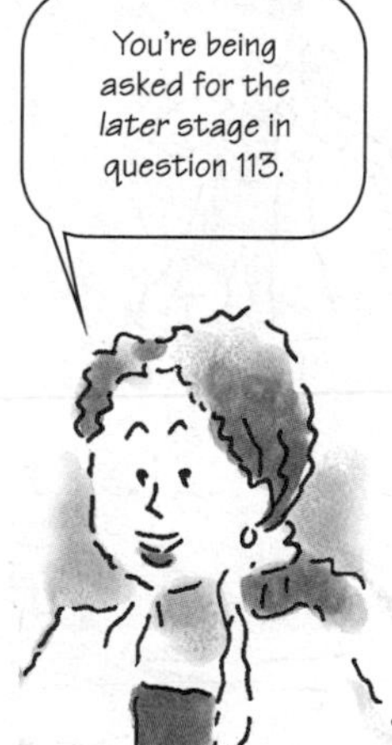
You're being asked for the later stage in question 113.

113. 4. The GI tract may tolerate a full liquid diet immediately. Allowing only clear liquids gives the intestine time to heal, but the fluids should be reintroduced slowly to determine the child's ability to tolerate and retain them. The GI tract won't tolerate forcing fluids. Don't allow the client to drink as much as she wants; instead, offer small amounts of fluid every couple of hours. Monitoring intake and output is important and was *initially* ordered; it will continue until discharge.

NP: Planning; CN: Physiological integrity; CNS: Basic care and comfort; CL: Analysis

114. The nurse is developing a teaching plan for a parent of a 2-week-old infant with gastroesophageal reflux disease (GERD). Which intervention would alleviate some of the infant's discomfort and be included in the nurse's plan?

1. Apply warmth to the abdominal area.
2. Schedule feedings every 4 hours.
3. Elevate the head of the bed after meals.
4. Feed rice cereal by spoon before each feeding.

114. 3. Infants with GERD should be held upright for at least 30 minutes after each feeding. An infant placed in a crib should be laid with his head toward the head of the crib, which has been elevated. Applying warmth to the abdomen will help ease abdominal spasms, but GERD doesn't produce spasms. Small, frequent feedings—more often than every 4 hours—will help decrease reflux. Rice cereal is sometimes added to formula to help reduce refluxing; however, a 2-week-old infant should never be fed with a spoon because his suck and swallow reflex isn't developed and he could aspirate the food.

NP: Planning; CN: Physiological integrity; CNS: Basic care and comfort; CL: Analysis

115. A 6-year-old client is seen in the clinic. Her mother states that the child hasn't had a bowel movement in 3 days. The nurse should instruct the mother to encourage the child to eat which foods?

1. Scrambled eggs with cheese and toast
2. Fruit juice and bran cereal
3. An apple and carrot sticks
4. Chicken and mashed potatoes

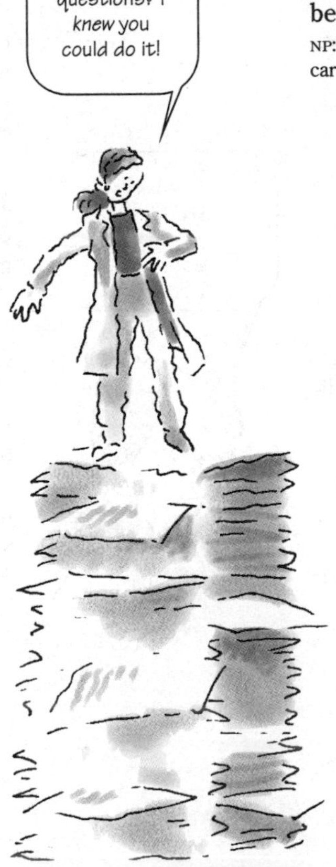

You're done with all those questions? I knew you could do it!

115. 2. Increasing fluids and fiber in the diet will aid in softening stool and will facilitate bowel movement. The other options don't include enough fluid or fiber, so they wouldn't be the best choices.

NP: Implementation; CN: Physiological integrity; CNS: Basic care and comfort; CL: Application

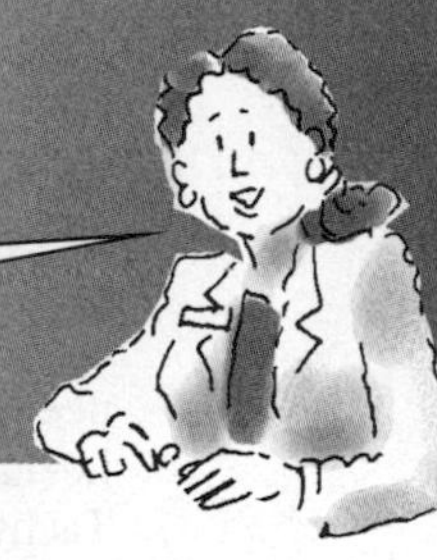

Caring for a child with an endocrine system disorder can be overwhelming. To get started on the right track, check out the Internet site of the Juvenile Diabetes Research Foundation International at **www.jdrf.org/**. Go for it!

Chapter 33 Endocrine disorders

1. When explaining the causes of hypothyroidism to the parents of a newly diagnosed infant, the nurse should recognize that further education is needed when the parents ask which of the following questions?

1. "So, hypothyroidism can be only temporary, right?"
2. "Are you saying that hypothyroidism is caused by a problem in the way the thyroid gland develops?"
3. "Do you mean that hypothyroidism may be caused by a problem in the way the body makes thyroxine?"
4. "So, hypothyroidism can be treated by exposing our baby to a special light, right?"

1. 4. Congenital hypothyroidism can be permanent or transient and may result from a defective thyroid gland or an enzymatic defect in thyroxine synthesis. Only the last question, which refers to phototherapy for physiologic jaundice, indicates that the parents need more information.

NP: Implementation; CN: Psychosocial integrity; CNS: Coping and adaptation; CL: Knowledge

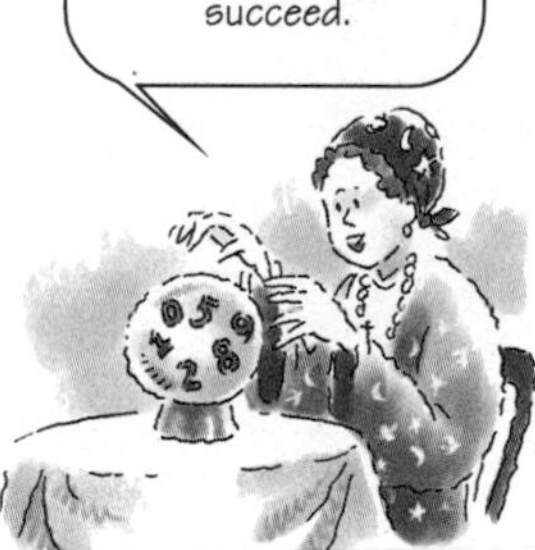

Don't let your studying be transient. Concentrate and know you can succeed.

2. The nurse understands that transient hypothyroidism can result from which of the following factors?

1. Intrauterine transfer of insulin
2. Placental transfer of antibodies
3. Placental transfer of teratogens
4. Intrauterine transfer of expectorants

2. 4. Intrauterine transfer of antithyroid drugs and expectorants given for asthma are factors associated with transient hypothyroidism. The other choices don't affect hypothyroidism.

NP: Assessment; CN: Health promotion and maintenance; CNS: Prevention and early detection of disease; CL: Knowledge

3. When a nurse is teaching parents of a neonate newly diagnosed with hypothyroidism, which of the following statements should be included?

1. A large goiter in a neonate doesn't present a problem.
2. Preterm neonates usually aren't affected by hypothyroidism.
3. Usually the neonate exhibits obvious signs of hypothyroidism.
4. The severity of the disorder depends on the amount of thyroid tissue present.

3. 4. The severity of the disorder depends on the amount of thyroid tissue present. The more thyroid tissue present, the less severe the disorder. A large goiter in a neonate could possibly occlude the airway and lead to obstruction. Preterm neonates are usually affected by hypothyroidism due to hypothalamic and pituitary immaturity. Usually the neonate doesn't exhibit obvious signs of the disorder due to maternal circulation.

NP: Implementation; CN: Health promotion and maintenance; CNS: Prevention and early detection of disease; CL: Application

4. Which of the following conditions is a subtle sign of hypothyroidism?
1. Diarrhea
2. Lethargy
3. Severe jaundice
4. Tachycardia

4. 2. Subtle signs of this disorder that may be seen shortly after birth include lethargy, poor feeding, prolonged jaundice, respiratory difficulty, cyanosis, constipation, and bradycardia. Diarrhea in the neonate isn't normal and isn't associated with this disorder. Severe jaundice needs immediate attention by the primary health care provider and isn't a subtle sign. Tachycardia typically occurs in hyperthyroidism, not hypothyroidism.
NP: Implementation; CN: Health promotion and maintenance; CNS: Prevention and early detection of disease; CL: Application

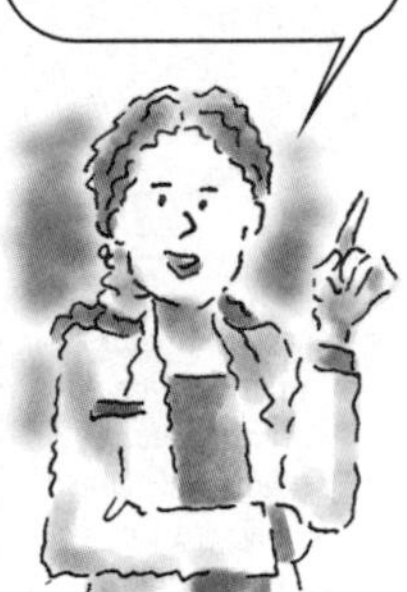

In question 5, the phrase most serious means you must prioritize.

5. In an assessment of a neonate with congenital hypothyroidism, the nurse understands that which of the following complications is the most serious consequence of this condition?
1. Anemia
2. Cyanosis
3. Retarded bone age
4. Delayed central nervous system (CNS) development

5. 4. The most serious consequence of congenital hypothyroidism is delayed development of the CNS, which leads to severe mental retardation. The other choices occur but aren't the most serious consequences.
NP: Assessment; CN: Safe, effective care environment; CNS: Management of care; CL: Knowledge

6. When counseling parents of a neonate with congenital hypothyroidism, the nurse understands that the severity of the intellectual deficit is related to which of the following parameters?
1. Duration of condition before treatment
2. Degree of hypothermia
3. Cranial malformations
4. T_4 level at diagnosis

6. 1. The severity of the intellectual deficit is related to the degree of hypothyroidism and the duration of the condition before treatment. Cranial malformations don't affect the severity of the intellectual deficit nor does the degree of hypothermia as it relates to hypothyroidism. It isn't the specific T_4 level at diagnosis that affects the intellect but how long the client has been hospitalized that will affect the intellect.
NP: Implementation; CN: Health promotion and maintenance; CNS: Prevention and early detection of disease; CL: Application

7. Which of the following statements should be included in an explanation of the diagnostic evaluation of neonates for congenital hypothyroidism?
1. Tests are mandatory in all states.
2. An arterial blood test is preferred.
3. Tests shouldn't be performed until after discharge.
4. Blood tests should be done after the first month of life.

7. 1. Heel stick blood tests are mandatory in all states and are usually taken on neonates between 2 and 6 days of age. Typically, specimens are taken before the neonate is discharged from the hospital; the test is included with other tests that screen the neonate for errors of metabolism.
NP: Implementation; CN: Health promotion and maintenance; CNS: Prevention and early detection of disease; CL: Application

8. Which of the following results would indicate to the nurse the possibility that a neonate has congenital hypothyroidism?

1. High level T_4 and low level TSH
2. Low level T_4 and high level TSH
3. Normal TSH and high level T_4
4. Normal T_4 and low level TSH

8. 2. Screening results that show a low level of T_4 and a high level of TSH indicate congenital hypothyroidism and the need for further tests to determine the cause of the disease.

NP: Implementation; CN: Physiological integrity; CNS: Reduction of risk potential; CL: Application

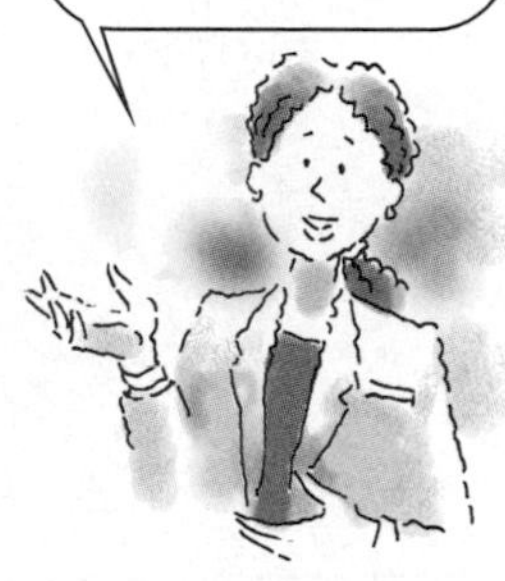

In question 9, the phrase *further teaching* indicates that you're looking for an *incorrect* statement.

9. The nurse is teaching parents about therapeutic management of their neonate diagnosed with congenital hypothyroidism. Which of the following responses by a parent would indicate the need for further teaching?

1. "My baby will need regular measurements of his thyroxine levels."
2. "Treatment involves lifelong thyroid hormone replacement therapy."
3. "Treatment should begin as soon as possible after diagnosis is made."
4. "As my baby grows, his thyroid gland will mature, and he won't need medications."

9. 4. Treatment involves lifelong thyroid hormone replacement therapy that begins as soon as possible after diagnosis to abolish all signs of hypothyroidism and to reestablish normal physical and mental development. The drug of choice is synthetic levothyroxine (Synthroid or Levothroid). Regular measurements of thyroxine levels are important in ensuring optimum treatment.

NP: Evaluation; CN: Health promotion and maintenance; CNS: Prevention and early detection of disease; CL: Application

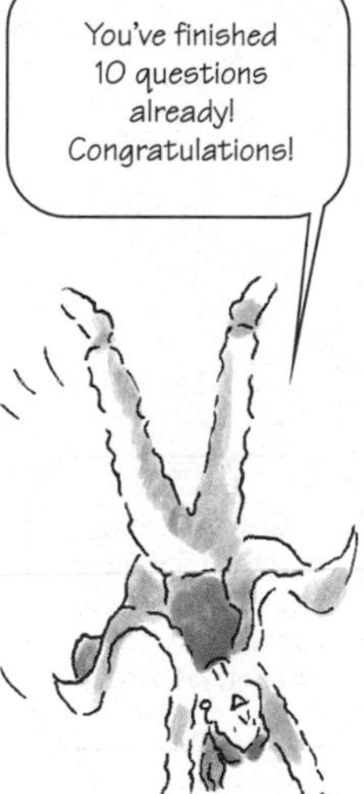

You've finished 10 questions already! Congratulations!

10. Which of the following comments made by the mother of a neonate at her 2-week office visit should alert the nurse to suspect congenital hypothyroidism?

1. "My baby is unusually quiet and good."
2. "My baby seems to be a yellowish color."
3. "After feedings, my baby pulls her legs up and cries."
4. "My baby seems to really look at my face during feeding time."

10. 1. Parental remarks about an unusually "quiet and good" neonate together with any of the early physical manifestations should lead to a suspicion of hypothyroidism, which requires a referral for specific tests. The neonate likes looking at the human face and should show interest in this at two weeks of age. If the neonate is pulling her legs up and crying after feedings, she might be showing signs of colic. If a neonate begins to look yellow in color, hyperbilirubinemia may be the cause.

NP: Assessment; CN: Health promotion and maintenance; CNS: Prevention and early detection of disease; CL: Application

11. Which of the following statements should be included when educating a mother about giving levothyroxine (Synthroid) to her neonate after a diagnosis of hypothyroidism is made?

1. The drug has a bitter taste.
2. The pill shouldn't be crushed.
3. Never put the medication in formula or juice.
4. If a dose is missed, double the dose the next day.

11. 4. If a dose is missed, twice the dose should be given the next day. The importance of compliance with the drug regimen for the neonate to achieve normal growth and development must be stressed. Because the drug is tasteless, it can be crushed and added to formula, water, or food.

NP: Implementation; CN: Physiological integrity; CNS: Pharmacological and parenteral therapies; CL: Application

12. When teaching the parents about signs that indicate levothyroxine (Synthroid) overdose, which of the following comments by a parent indicates the need for further teaching?

1. "Irritability is a sign of overdose."
2. "If my baby's heart beat is fast, I should count it."
3. "If my baby loses weight, I should be concerned."
4. "I shouldn't worry if my baby doesn't sleep very much."

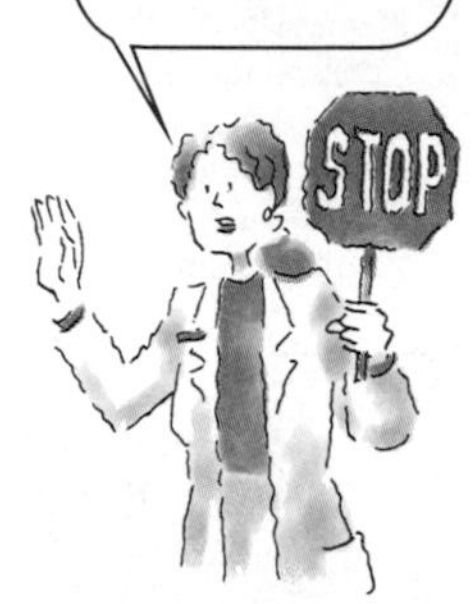

Watch out! Question 12 is another further teaching question.
STOP

12. 4. Parents need to be aware of signs indicating overdose, such as rapid pulse, dyspnea, irritability, insomnia, fever, sweating, and weight loss. The parents would be given acceptable parameters for the heart rate and weight loss or gain. If the baby is experiencing a heart rate or weight loss outside of the acceptable parameters, the primary health care provider should be called.

NP: Evaluation; CN: Physiological integrity; CNS: Pharmacological and parenteral therapies; CL: Analysis

13. A nurse should recognize that exophthalmos (protruding eyeballs) may occur in children with which of the following conditions?

1. Hypothyroidism
2. Hyperthyroidism
3. Hypoparathyroidism
4. Hyperparathyroidism

13. 2. Exophthalmos occurs when there's an overproduction of thyroid hormone. This sign should alert the primary health care provider to follow up with further testing.

NP: Assessment; CN: Health promotion and maintenance; CNS: Prevention and early detection of disease; CL: Application

14. A nurse should understand that which of the following symptoms is a common clinical manifestation of juvenile hypothyroidism?

1. Accelerated growth
2. Diarrhea
3. Dry skin
4. Insomnia

14. 3. Children with hypothyroidism will have dry skin. The other choices aren't evident in children with juvenile hypothyroidism.

NP: Assessment; CN: Health promotion and maintenance; CNS: Prevention and early detection of disease; CL: Knowledge

15. A nurse should understand that manifestations of thyroid hormone deficiency in infancy include which of the following symptoms?

1. Tachycardia, profuse perspiration, and diarrhea
2. Lethargy, feeding difficulties, and constipation
3. Hypertonia, small fontanels, and moist skin
4. Dermatitis, dry skin, and round face

15. 2. Hypothyroidism results from inadequate thyroid production to meet an infant's needs. Clinical signs include feeding difficulties, prolonged physiologic jaundice, lethargy, and constipation.

NP: Assessment; CN: Health promotion and maintenance; CNS: Prevention and early detection of disease; CL: Comprehension

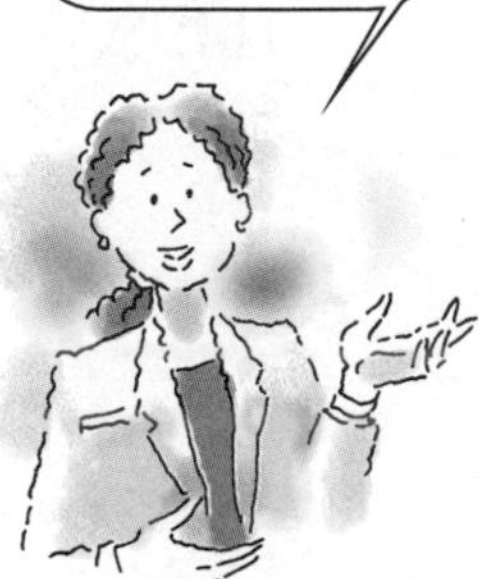

Question 16 is asking for the most appropriate behavior. In other words, prioritize!

16. When counseling parents of a neonate with congenital hypothyroidism, the nurse should encourage which of the following behaviors?

1. Seeking professional genetic counseling
2. Retracing the family tree for others born with this condition
3. Talking to relatives who have gone through a similar experience
4. Waiting until the neonate is 1 year old before obtaining counseling

16. 1. Seeking professional genetic counseling is the best option for parents who have a neonate with a genetic disorder. Retracing the family tree and talking to relatives won't help the parents to become better educated about the disorder. Education about the disorder should occur as soon as the parents are ready so they will understand the genetic implications for future children.

NP: Implementation; CN: Safe, effective care environment; CNS: Management of care; CL: Application

NP: Nursing process CN: Client needs category CNS: Client needs subcategory CL: Cognitive level

17. While teaching an adolescent about giving insulin injections, the adolescent questions the nurse about the reuse of disposable needles and syringes. Which of the following responses from the nurse is most appropriate?

1. This is an unsafe practice.
2. This is acceptable for up to 7 days.
3. This is acceptable for only 48 hours.
4. This is acceptable only if the family has very limited resources.

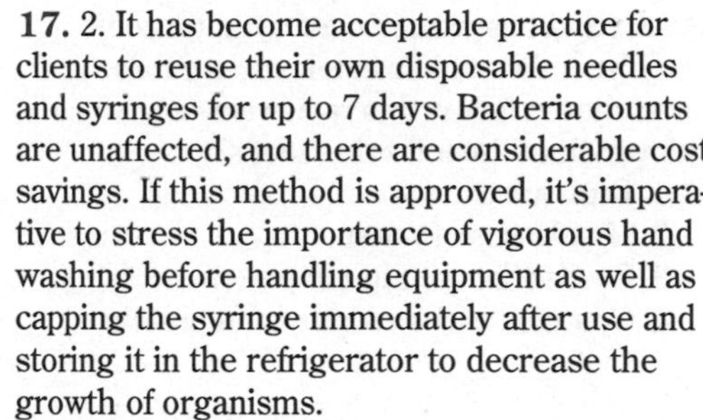

17. 2. It has become acceptable practice for clients to reuse their own disposable needles and syringes for up to 7 days. Bacteria counts are unaffected, and there are considerable cost savings. If this method is approved, it's imperative to stress the importance of vigorous hand washing before handling equipment as well as capping the syringe immediately after use and storing it in the refrigerator to decrease the growth of organisms.

NP: Implementation; CN: Safe, effective care environment; CNS: Safety and infection control; CL: Application

18. When children are more physically active, which of the following changes in the management of the child with diabetes should the nurse expect?

1. Increased food intake
2. Decreased food intake
3. Decreased risk of insulin shock
4. Increased risk of hyperglycemia

18. 1. If a child is more active at one time of the day than another, food or insulin can be altered to meet the activity pattern of the individual. Food should be increased when children are more physically active.

NP: Planning; CN: Safe, effective care environment; CNS: Management of care; CL: Knowledge

19. When the nurse is helping the adolescent deal with diabetes, which of the following characteristics of adolescence should be considered?

1. Wanting to be an individual
2. Needing to be like their peers
3. Being preoccupied with future plans
4. Teaching peers that this is a serious disease

19. 2. Adolescents appear to have the most difficulty in adjusting to diabetes. Adolescence is a time when there's much stress on being "perfect" and being like one's peers and, to adolescents, having diabetes is being different.

NP: Implementation; CN: Health promotion and maintenance; CNS: Growth and development through the life span; CL: Knowledge

20. An adolescent with diabetes tells the community nurse that he has recently started drinking alcohol on the weekends. Which of the following actions would be most appropriate for the nurse to take?

1. Recommend referral to counseling.
2. Make the adolescent promise to stop drinking.
3. Discuss with the adolescent why he has started drinking.
4. Teach the adolescent about the effects of alcohol on diabetes.

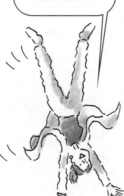

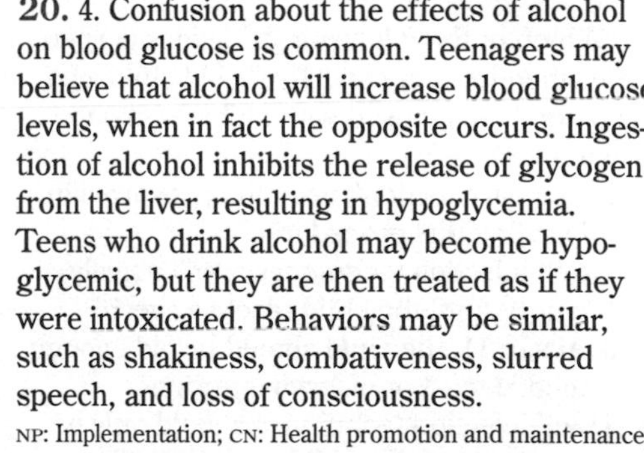
20 questions completed? That's cause for celebration!

20. 4. Confusion about the effects of alcohol on blood glucose is common. Teenagers may believe that alcohol will increase blood glucose levels, when in fact the opposite occurs. Ingestion of alcohol inhibits the release of glycogen from the liver, resulting in hypoglycemia. Teens who drink alcohol may become hypoglycemic, but they are then treated as if they were intoxicated. Behaviors may be similar, such as shakiness, combativeness, slurred speech, and loss of consciousness.

NP: Implementation; CN: Health promotion and maintenance; CNS: Growth and development through the life span; CL: Application

21. A child has experienced symptoms of hypoglycemia and has eaten sugar cubes. The nurse should follow this rapid-releasing sugar with which of the following foods?

1. Fruit juices
2. Six glasses of water
3. Foods that are high in protein
4. Complex carbohydrates and protein

21. 4. When a child exhibits signs of hypoglycemia, the majority of cases can be treated with a simple concentrated sugar, such as honey, that can be held in the mouth for a short time. This will elevate the blood glucose level and alleviate the symptoms. The simpler the carbohydrate, the more rapidly it will be absorbed. A complex carbohydrate and protein, such as a slice of bread or a cracker spread with peanut butter, should follow the rapid-releasing sugar or the client may become hypoglycemic again.

NP: Evaluation; CN: Health promotion and maintenance; CNS: Prevention and early detection of disease; CL: Application

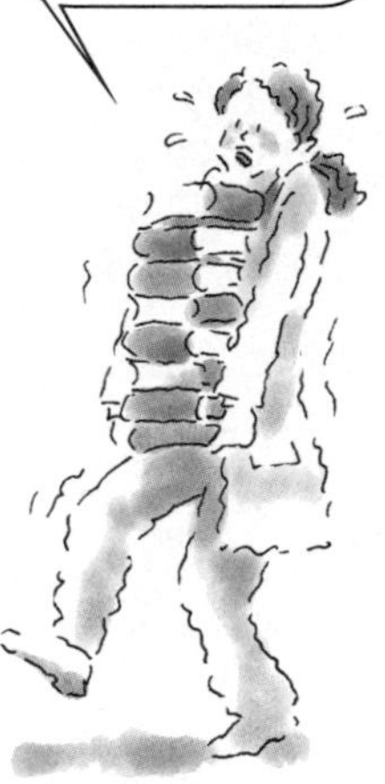

If you know the definitions of hypo and hyper, it can help you with a bunch of questions.

22. Which of the following symptoms is indicative of hypoglycemia?

1. Irritability
2. Drowsiness
3. Abdominal pain
4. Nausea and vomiting

22. 1. Signs of hypoglycemia include irritability, shaky feeling, hunger, headache, and dizziness. Drowsiness, abdominal pain, nausea, and vomiting are signs of *hyper*glycemia.

NP: Assessment; CN: Physiological integrity; CNS: Physiological adaptation; CL: Knowledge

23. Which of the following assessments is accurate for a child with diabetes who develops ketoacidosis?

1. Normal outcome
2. Life-threatening situation
3. Situation that can easily be treated at home
4. Situation best treated in the pediatrician's office

23. 2. Diabetic ketoacidosis, the most complete state of insulin deficiency, is a life-threatening situation. The child should be admitted to an intensive care facility for management, which consists of rapid assessment, adequate insulin to reduce the elevated blood glucose level, fluids to overcome dehydration, and electrolyte replacement (especially potassium).

NP: Evaluation; CN: Safe, effective care environment; CNS: Management of care; CL: Knowledge

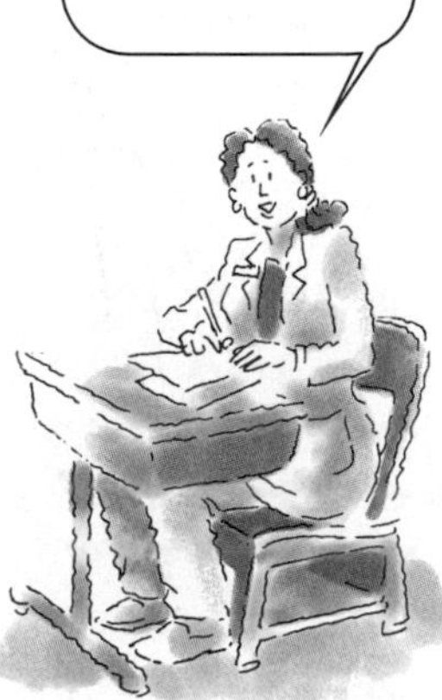

Knowing blood glucose values is a must for sitting for the NCLEX.

24. Which of the following guidelines is appropriate when teaching an 11-year-old child who was recently diagnosed with diabetes about insulin injections?

1. The parents don't need to be involved in learning this procedure.
2. Self-injection techniques aren't usually taught until the child reaches age 16.
3. At age 11, the child should be old enough to give most of his own injections.
4. Self-injection techniques should only be taught when the child can reach all injection sites.

24. 3. The parents must supervise and manage the child's therapeutic program, but the child should assume responsibility for self-management as soon as he is capable. Children can learn to collect their own blood for glucose testing at a relatively young age (4 to 5 years), and most are able to check their blood glucose level and administer insulin at about age 9. Some children may be able to do it earlier.

NP: Implementation; CN: Health promotion and maintenance; CNS: Growth and development through the life span; CL: Application

NP: Nursing process CN: Client needs category CNS: Client needs subcategory CL: Cognitive level

25. A nurse should understand that hyperglycemia associated with diabetic ketoacidosis is defined as a blood glucose measurement equal to or greater than which of the following values?

1. 150 mg/dl
2. 300 mg/dl
3. 450 mg/dl
4. 600 mg/dl

25. 2. Diabetic ketoacidosis is determined by the presence of hyperglycemia (blood glucose measurement of 300 mg/dl or higher), accompanied by acetone breath, dehydration, weak and rapid pulse, and decreased level of consciousness.

NP: Assessment; CN: Physiological integrity; CNS: Physiological adaptation; CL: Knowledge

26. A nurse should recognize which of the following symptoms as a cardinal sign of diabetes mellitus?

1. Nausea
2. Seizure
3. Hyperactivity
4. Frequent urination

26. 4. Polyphagia, polyuria, polydipsia, and weight loss are cardinal signs of diabetes mellitus. Other signs include irritability, shortened attention span, lowered frustration tolerance, fatigue, dry skin, blurred vision, sores that are slow to heal, and flushed skin.

NP: Assessment; CN: Health promotion and maintenance; CNS: Prevention and early detection of disease; CL: Knowledge

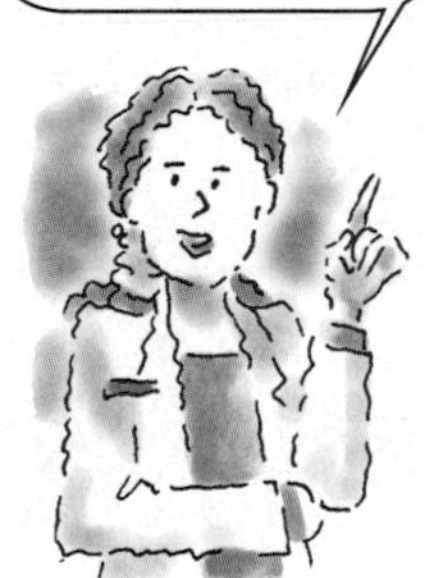

Teaching clients how to help manage their own conditions is a common subject on the NCLEX.

27. The parent of a child with diabetes asks a nurse why blood glucose monitoring is needed. The nurse should base her reply on which of the following premises?

1. This is an easier method of testing.
2. This is a less expensive method of testing.
3. This allows children the ability to better manage their diabetes.
4. This gives children a greater sense of control over their diabetes.

27. 3. Blood glucose monitoring improves diabetes management and is used successfully by children from the onset of their diabetes. By testing their own blood, children are able to change their insulin regimen to maintain their glucose level in the normoglycemic range of 80 to 120 mg/dl. This allows them better management of their diabetes.

NP: Implementation; CN: Health promotion and maintenance; CNS: Prevention and early detection of disease; CL: Application

28. To increase the adolescent's compliance with treatment for diabetes mellitus, the nurse should attempt which of the following strategies?

1. Provide for a special diet in the high school cafeteria.
2. Clarify the adolescent's values to promote involvement in care.
3. Identify energy requirements for participation in sports activities.
4. Educate the adolescent about long-term consequences of poor metabolic control.

28. 2. Adolescent compliance with diabetes management may be hampered by dependence versus independence conflicts and ego development. Attempts to have the adolescent clarify personal values fosters compliance.

NP: Planning; CN: Health promotion and maintenance; CNS: Growth and development through the life span; CL: Application

29. A child with diabetes type 1 tells the nurse she feels shaky. The nurse assesses the child's skin color to be pale and sweaty. Which of the following actions should the nurse initiate immediately?

1. Give supplemental insulin.
2. Have the child eat a glucose tablet.
3. Administer glucagon S.C.
4. Offer the child a complex carbohydrate snack.

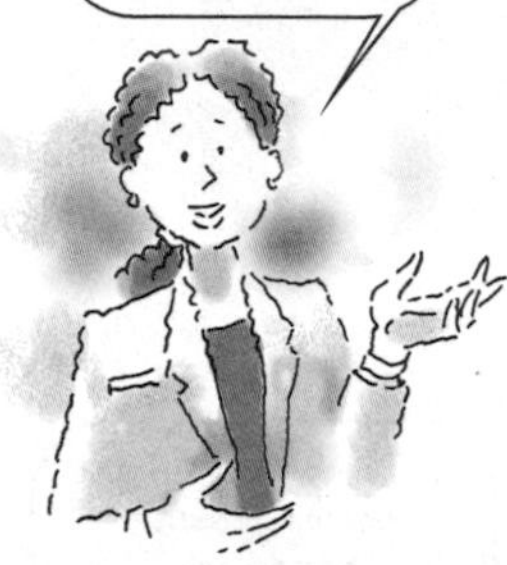

The word immediately signals a need for you to prioritize.

29. 2. These are symptoms of hypoglycemia. Rapid treatment involves giving the alert child a glucose tablet (4 mg of dextrose) or, if unavailable, a glass of glucose-containing liquid. It would be followed by a complex carbohydrate snack and protein. Giving supplemental insulin would be contraindicated because that would lower the blood glucose even more. Glucagon would be given only if there was a risk of aspiration with oral glucose, such as if the child was semiconscious.

NP: Implementation; CN: Safe, effective care environment; CNS: Management of care; CL: Application

30. The parents of a child diagnosed with diabetes ask the nurse about maintaining metabolic control during a minor illness with loss of appetite. Which of the following nursing responses is appropriate?

1. Decrease the child's insulin by half the usual dose during the course of the illness.
2. Call your primary health care provider to arrange hospitalization.
3. Give increased amounts of clear liquids to prevent dehydration.
4. Substitute calorie-containing liquids for uneaten solid food.

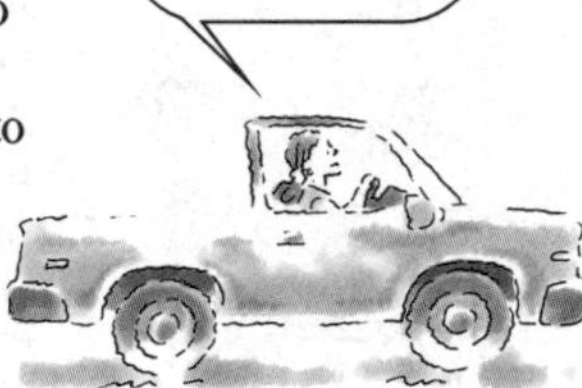

Another 10 down! You're cruisin' now!

30. 4. Calorie-containing liquids can help to maintain more normal blood sugar levels as well as decrease the danger of dehydration. The child with diabetes should always take *at least* the usual dose of insulin during an illness based on more frequent blood sugar checks. During an illness where there's vomiting or loss of appetite, NPH insulin is cut in half or stopped altogether, and regular insulin is given according to home glucose monitoring results.

NP: Implementation; CN: Safe, effective care environment; CNS: Management of care; CL: Application

31. Which of the following criteria would the nurse use to measure good metabolic control in a child with diabetes mellitus?

1. Fewer than eight episodes of severe hyperglycemia in a month
2. Infrequent occurrences of mild hypoglycemia reactions
3. Hemoglobin A values less than 12%
4. Growth below the 15th percentile

31. 2. Criteria for good metabolic control generally includes few episodes of hypoglycemia or hyperglycemia, hemoglobin A values less than 8%, and normal growth and development.

NP: Assessment; CN: Health promotion and maintenance; CNS: Prevention and early detection of disease; CL: Application

32. Which of the following congenital anomalies is most commonly associated with poorly controlled maternal diabetes?

1. Cataracts
2. Low-set ears
3. Cardiac malformations
4. Cleft lip and palate deformities

32. 3. Cardiac and central nervous system anomalies, along with neural tube defects, skeletal, and GI anomalies, are most likely to occur in uncontrolled maternal diabetes.

NP: Assessment; CN: Health promotion and maintenance; CNS: Prevention and early detection of disease; CL: Knowledge

33. Which of the following conditions could possibly cause hypoglycemia?

1. Too little insulin
2. Mild illness with fever
3. Excessive exercise without a carbohydrate snack
4. Eating ice cream and cake to celebrate a birthday

34. A nurse should recognize which of the following assessment factors as one of the best indicators of a client's control of his diabetes during the preceding 2 to 3 months?

1. A fasting glucose level
2. Oral glucose tolerance test
3. A glycosylated hemoglobin level
4. The client's verbal report of his symptoms

35. A client has received diet instruction as part of his treatment plan for diabetes type 1. Which of the following statements by the client indicates to the nurse that he needs additional instructions?

1. "I will need a bedtime snack because I take an evening dose of NPH insulin."
2. "I can eat whatever I want as long as I cover the calories with sufficient insulin."
3. "I can have an occasional low-calorie drink as long as I include it in my meal plan."
4. "I should eat meals as scheduled, even if I'm not hungry, to prevent hypoglycemia."

36. Which of the following symptoms are signs of hyperglycemia?

1. Rapid heart rate
2. Headache
3. Hunger
4. Thirst

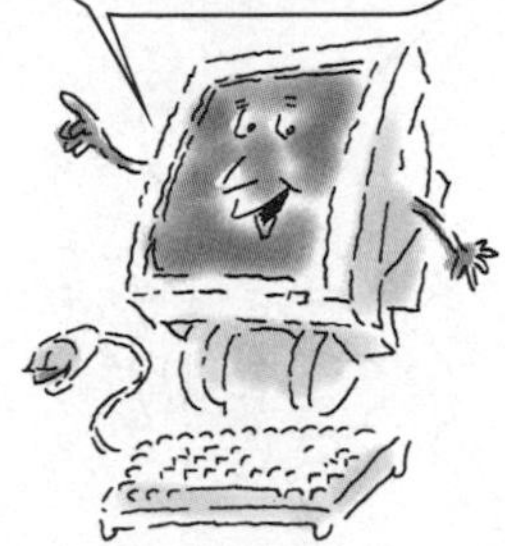

Comparing signs of hypoglycemia and hyperglycemia is a common NCLEX subject.

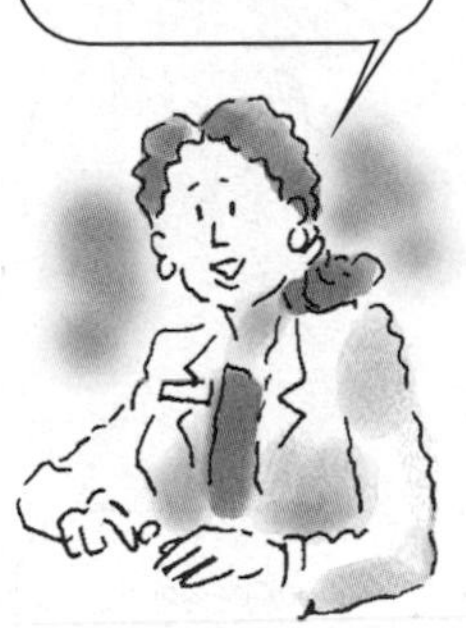

Additional instructions is another way of saying further teaching. Both types of questions ask you to find an incorrect statement.

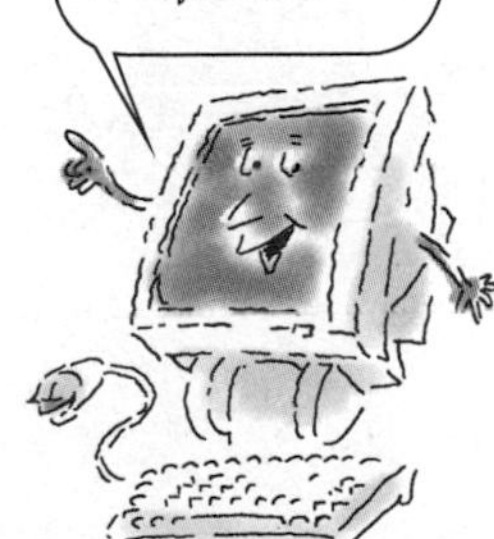

What did I tell you? Another hyperglycemia versus hypoglycemia question.

33. 3. Excessive exercise without a carbohydrate snack could cause hypoglycemia. The other options describe situations that cause *hyper*glycemia.

NP: Evaluation; CN: Health promotion and maintenance; CNS: Prevention and early detection of disease; CL: Application

34. 3. A glycosylated hemoglobin level provides an overview of a person's blood glucose level over the previous 2 to 3 months. Glycosylated hemoglobin values are reported as a percentage of the total hemoglobin within an erythrocyte. The time frame is based on the fact that the usual life span of an erythrocyte is 2 to 3 months; a random blood sample, therefore, will theoretically give samples of erythrocytes for this same period. The other options won't indicate a true picture of the person's blood glucose level over the previous 2 to 3 months.

NP: Evaluation; CN: Health promotion and maintenance; CNS: Prevention and early detection of disease; CL: Knowledge

35. 2. The goal of diet therapy in diabetes mellitus is to attain and maintain ideal body weight. Each client will be prescribed a specific caloric intake and insulin regimen to help accomplish this goal.

NP: Evaluation; CN: Physiological integrity; CNS: Basic care and comfort; CL: Analysis

36. 4. Thirst (polydipsia) is one of the symptoms of hyperglycemia. Rapid heart rate, headache, and hunger are signs and symptoms of *hypo*glycemia.

NP: Evaluation; CN: Physiological integrity; CNS: Physiological adaptation; CL: Knowledge

37. A client is learning to mix regular insulin and NPH insulin in the same syringe. Which of the following actions, if performed by the client, would indicate the need for further teaching?

1. Withdraws the NPH insulin first
2. Injects air into NPH insulin bottle first
3. After drawing up first insulin, removes air bubbles
4. Injects an amount of air equal to the desired dose of insulin

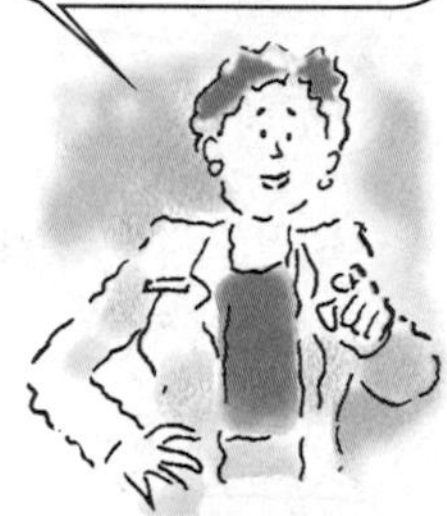

In question 37, you're looking for an incorrect action, rather than an incorrect statement.

37. 1. Regular insulin is *always* withdrawn first so it won't become contaminated with NPH insulin. The client is instructed to inject air into the NPH insulin bottle equal to the amount of insulin to be withdrawn because there will be regular insulin in the syringe and he won't be able to inject air when he needs to withdraw the NPH. It's necessary to remove the air bubbles to be assured of a correct dosage before drawing up the second insulin.

NP: Assessment; CN: Physiological integrity; CNS: Pharmacological and parenteral therapies; CL: Application

38. A client is diagnosed with diabetes type 1. The primary health care provider prescribes an insulin regimen of regular insulin and NPH insulin administered S.C. each morning. How soon after administration will the onset of regular insulin begin?

1. Within 5 minutes
2. ½ to 1 hour
3. 1 to 1½ hours
4. 4 to 8 hours

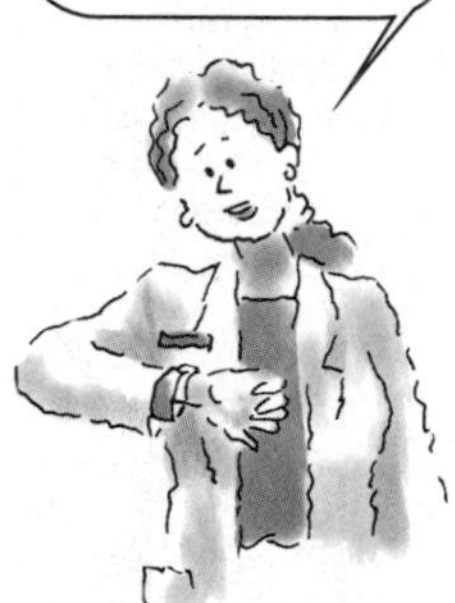

It's important to know how and when different types of insulin react.

38. 2. Regular insulin's onset is ½ to 1 hour, peak is 2 to 4 hours, and duration is 8 to 12 hours. Lispro insulin has an onset within 5 minutes. NPH insulin has an onset within 1 to 1½ hours, and ultralente insulin is the longest acting with an onset of 4 to 8 hours.

NP: Evaluation; CN: Physiological integrity; CNS: Pharmacological and parenteral therapies; CL: Application

39. When assessing a neonate for signs of diabetes insipidus, a nurse should recognize which of the following symptoms as signs of this disorder?

1. Hypocalcemia
2. Hyperaldosteronism
3. Polyuria and polydipsia
4. Diminished or absent skin pigmentation

39. 3. The cardinal signs of diabetes insipidus are polyuria and polydipsia. All of the other options are signs and symptoms for other disorders.

NP: Assessment; CN: Physiological integrity; CNS: Physiological adaptation; CL: Application

40. Which of the following complications is an initial symptom of diabetes insipidus in the neonate?

1. Dehydration
2. Inability to arouse the neonate
3. Extreme hunger relieved by frequent feedings of milk
4. Irritability relieved with feedings of water but not milk

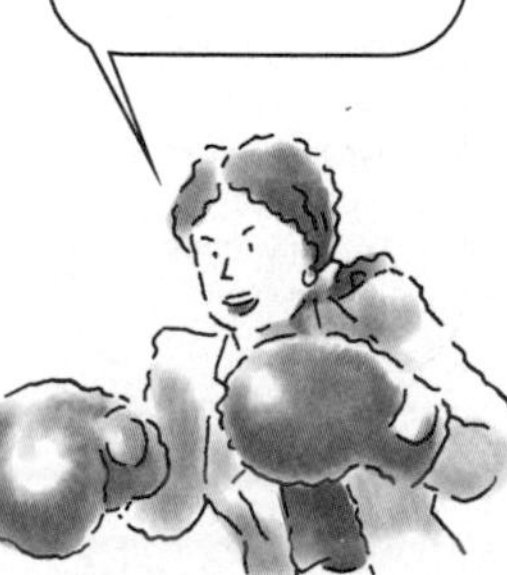

Looking good, champ! Hang in there!

40. 4. One of the initial symptoms of diabetes insipidus in the neonate is irritability relieved with feedings of water but not milk.

NP: Assessment; CN: Health promotion and maintenance; CNS: Prevention and early detection of disease; CL: Knowledge

41. A nurse is helping parents understand when treatments of growth hormone replacement will end. Which of the following statements should be included?

1. The dosage of growth hormone will decrease as the child's age increases.
2. The dosage of growth hormone will increase as time of epiphyseal closure nears.
3. After giving growth hormone replacement for one year, the dose will be tapered down.
4. Growth hormone replacement can't be abruptly stopped; it must be spread out over several months.

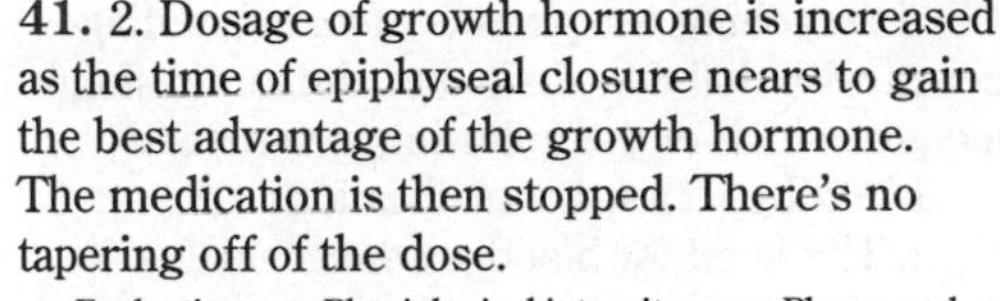

41. 2. Dosage of growth hormone is increased as the time of epiphyseal closure nears to gain the best advantage of the growth hormone. The medication is then stopped. There's no tapering off of the dose.

NP: Evaluation; CN: Physiological integrity; CNS: Pharmacological and parenteral therapies; CL: Application

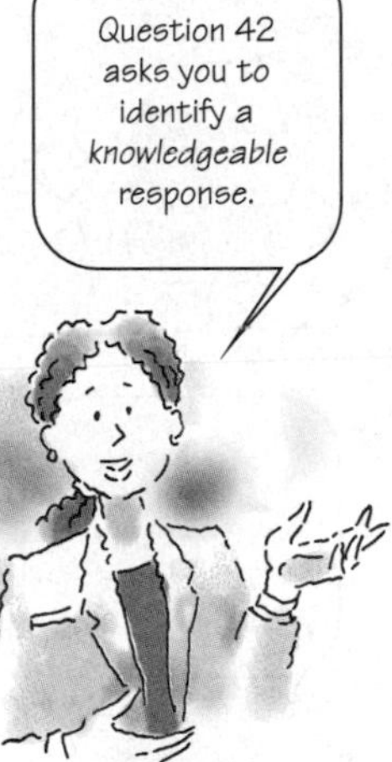

Question 42 asks you to identify a knowledgeable response.

42. The nurse is explaining diabetes insipidus to parents of an infant. When explaining the diagnostic test that is used, which of the following comments by the parents would indicate an understanding of the diagnostic test?

1. "Fluids will be offered every 2 hours."
2. "My infant's fluid intake will be restricted."
3. "I won't change anything about my infant's intake."
4. "Formula will be restricted, but glucose water is okay."

42. 2. The simplest test used to diagnose diabetes insipidus is restriction of oral fluids and observation of consequent changes in urine volume and concentration. A weight loss of 3% to 5% indicates severe dehydration, and the test should be terminated at this point. This is done in the hospital, and the infant is watched closely.

NP: Implementation; CN: Health promotion and maintenance; CNS: Prevention and early detection of disease; CL: Application

43. A nurse should anticipate which of the following physiologic responses in an infant being tested for diabetes insipidus?

1. Increase in urine output
2. Decrease in urine output
3. No effect on urine output
4. Increase in urine specific gravity

43. 3. In diabetes insipidus, fluid restriction for diagnostic testing has little or no effect on urine formation but causes weight loss from dehydration.

NP: Assessment; CN: Physiological integrity; CNS: Physiological adaptation; CL: Application

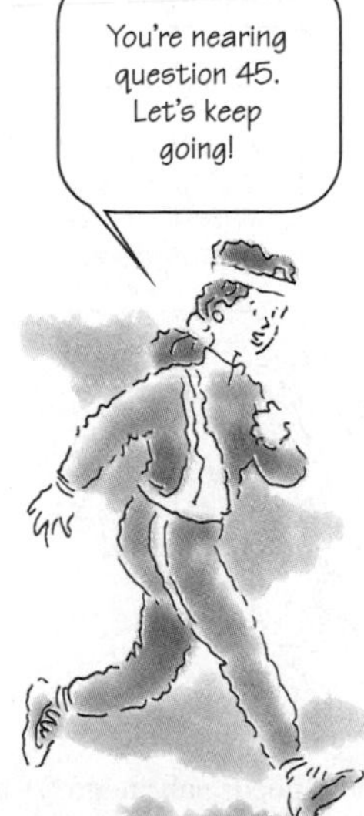

You're nearing question 45. Let's keep going!

44. If an infant has a positive test result for diabetes insipidus, the nurse should anticipate the primary health care provider ordering a test dose of which of the following medications?

1. Antidiuretic hormone
2. Biosynthetic growth hormone
3. Adrenocorticotropic hormone
4. Aqueous vasopressin (Pitressin Synthetic)

44. 4. If the fluid restriction test is positive, the child should be given a test dose of injected aqueous vasopressin (Pitressin), which should alleviate the polyuria and polydipsia. Unresponsiveness to exogenous vasopressin usually indicates nephrogenic diabetes insipidus. The other choices are used to determine other types of endocrine disorders.

NP: Evaluation; CN: Physiological integrity; CNS: Pharmacological and parenteral therapies; CL: Knowledge

45. In teaching the parents of an infant diagnosed with diabetes insipidus, the nurse should include which of the following treatments?

1. Antihypertensive medications
2. The need for blood products
3. Hormone replacement
4. Fluid restrictions

45. 3. The usual treatment for diabetes insipidus is hormone replacement with vasopressin or desmopressin acetate (DDAVP). Blood products shouldn't be needed. No problem with hypertension is associated with this condition, and fluids shouldn't be restricted.

NP: Implementation; CN: Health promotion and maintenance; CNS: Prevention and early detection of disease; CL: Knowledge

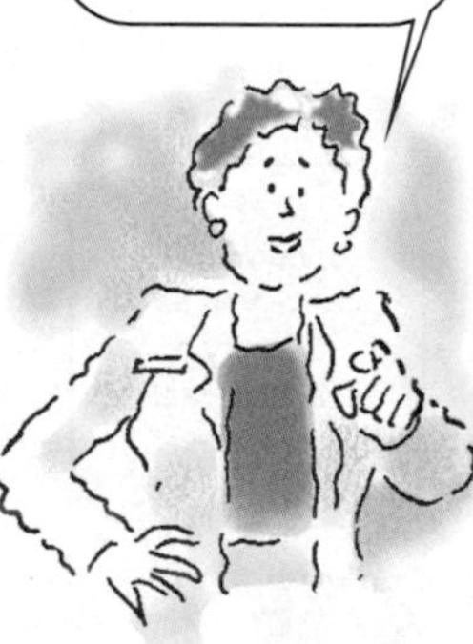

Although the word deter sounds like a negative, question 46 actually asks you to identify a true characteristic of nasal sprays.

46. When providing information about treatments for diabetes insipidus to parents, a nurse explains the use of nasal spray and injections. Which of the following indications might deter a parent from choosing nasal spray treatment?

1. Applications must be repeated every 8 to 12 hours.
2. Applications must be repeated every 2 to 4 hours.
3. Nasal sprays can't be used in infants.
4. Measurements are too difficult.

46. 1. Applications of nasal spray used to treat diabetes insipidus must be repeated every 8 to 12 hours; injections last for 48 to 72 hours. The nasal spray must be timed for adequate night sleep. However, the injections are oil-based and quite painful. Nasal sprays have been used in infants with diabetes insipidus and are dispensed in premeasured intranasal inhalers, eliminating the need for measuring doses.

NP: Implementation; CN: Physiological integrity; CNS: Pharmacological and parenteral therapies CL: Analysis

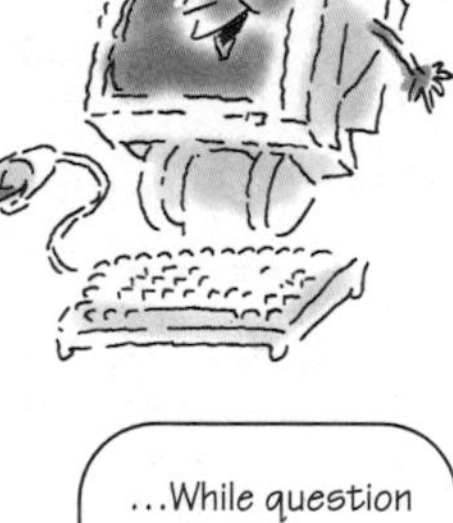

Caution! Question 47 is looking for an inaccurate statement...

47. A nurse is teaching the parents of an infant with diabetes insipidus about an injectable drug used to treat the disorder. Which of the following statements made by a parent would indicate the need for further teaching?

1. "I must hold the medication under warm running water for 10 to 15 minutes before administering it."
2. "The medication must be shaken vigorously before being drawn up into the syringe."
3. "Small brown particles must be seen in the suspension."
4. "I will store this medication in the refrigerator."

47. 4. The medication should be stored at room temperature. When giving injectable vasopressin, it must be thoroughly resuspended in the oil by being held under warm running water for 10 to 15 minutes and shaken vigorously before being drawn into the syringe. If this isn't done, the oil may be injected minus the drug. Small brown particles, which indicate drug dispersion, must be seen in the suspension.

NP: Implementation; CN: Physiological integrity; CNS: Pharmacological and parenteral therapies; CL: Application

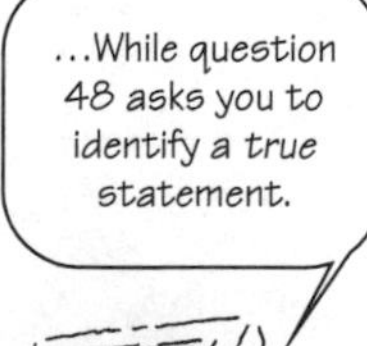

...While question 48 asks you to identify a true statement.

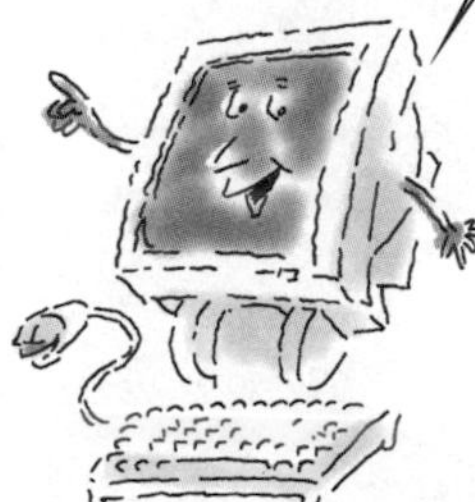

48. When teaching parents of an infant newly diagnosed with diabetes insipidus, which of the following statements by a parent indicates a good understanding of this condition?

1. "When my infant stabilizes, I won't have to worry about giving hormone medication."
2. "I don't have to measure the amount of fluid intake that I give my infant."
3. "I realize that treatment for diabetes insipidus is lifelong."
4. "My infant will outgrow this condition."

48. 3. Diabetes insipidus is a condition that will need lifelong treatment. The amount of fluid intake is very important and must be measured with the infant's output to monitor the medication regime. The infant won't outgrow this condition.

NP: Implementation; CN: Safe, effective care environment; CNS: Management of care; CL: Application

49. The nurse understands that diabetes insipidus is the principal disorder of which of the following glands?

1. Thyroid hyperfunction
2. Pituitary hypofunction
3. Pituitary hyperfunction
4. Parathyroid hypofunction

49. 2. The principle disorder of posterior pituitary hypofunction is diabetes insipidus. The disorder results from hyposecretion of antidiuretic hormone, producing a state of uncontrolled diuresis.

NP: Assessment; CN: Health promotion and maintenance; CNS: Prevention and early detection of disease; CL: Knowledge

50. After the nurse has explained the causes of diabetes insipidus to the parents, which of the following statements made by a parent indicates the need for further teaching?

1. "This condition could be familial or congenital."
2. "Drinking alcohol during my pregnancy caused this condition."
3. "My child might have a tumor that's causing these symptoms."
4. "An infection such as meningitis may be the reason my child has diabetes insipidus."

50. 2. Drinking alcohol during pregnancy can lead to a neonate born with fetal alcohol syndrome, but has no known affect with diabetes insipidus. The other options are possible causes of diabetes insipidus.

NP: Implementation; CN: Health promotion and maintenance; CNS: Prevention and early detection of disease; CL: Application

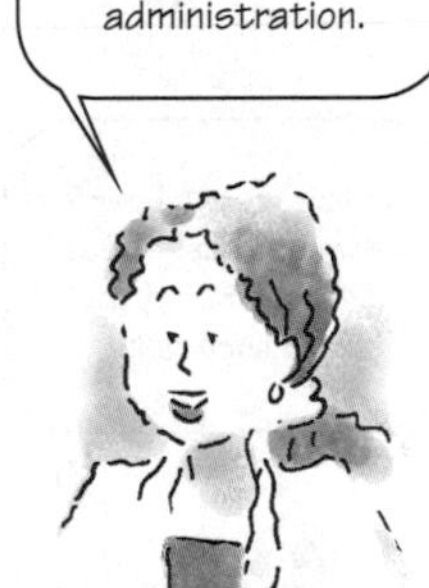

Question 51 asks for a common adverse effect of vasopressin administration.

51. Which of the following assessment findings would alert the nurse to change the intranasal route for vasopressin administration?

1. Mucous membrane irritation
2. Severe coughing
3. Nosebleeds
4. Pneumonia

51. 1. Mucous membrane irritation caused by a cold or allergy renders the intranasal route unreliable. Severe coughing, pneumonia, or nosebleeds shouldn't interfere with the intranasal route.

NP: Assessment; CN: Physiological integrity; CNS: Pharmacological and parenteral therapies; CL: Application

52. The nurse should include which of the following in-home management instructions for a child who's receiving desmopressin acetate (DDAVP) for symptomatic control of diabetes insipidus?

1. Give DDAVP only when urine output begins to decrease.
2. Cleanse skin with alcohol before application of the DDAVP dermal patch.
3. Increase the DDAVP dose if polyuria occurs just before the next scheduled dose.
4. Call the primary health care provider for an alternate route of DDAVP when the child has an upper respiratory infection (URI) or allergic rhinitis.

52. 4. Excessive nasal mucus associated with URI or allergic rhinitis may interfere with DDAVP absorption because it's given intranasally. Parents should be instructed to contact the primary health care provider for advice in altering the hormone dose during times when nasal mucus may be increased. The DDAVP dose should remain unchanged, even if there's polyuria just before the next dose. This is to avoid overmedicating the child.

NP: Implementation; CN: Safe, effective care environment; CNS: Management of care; CL: Application

53. The nurse is assessing a client with suspected hypopituitarism. Which of the following conditions is the chief complaint associated with this condition?

1. Insomnia
2. Polyuria
3. Polydipsia
4. Short stature

53. 4. The chief complaint in most instances of hypopituitarism is short stature. All other choices are complaints of other metabolic disorders.

NP: Assessment; CN: Health promotion and maintenance; CNS: Prevention and early detection of disease; CL: Knowledge

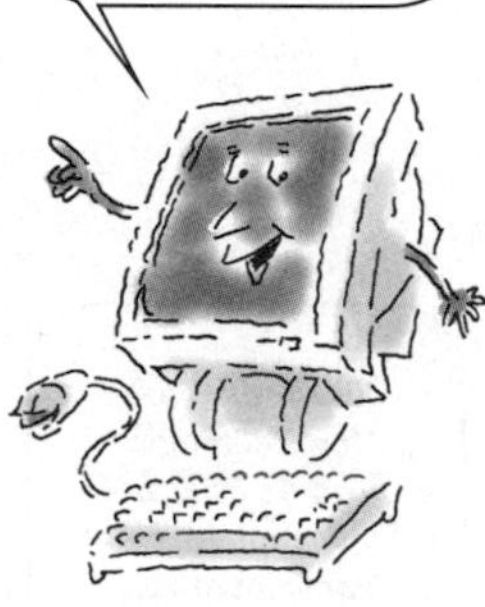

54. Which of the following statements made to the nurse by the parents of a child with idiopathic growth hormone deficiency would indicate the need for further teaching?

1. "This disorder may be familial."
2. "There's no genetic basis for this disorder."
3. "This disorder might be secondary to hypothalamic deficiency."
4. "There may be other disorders related to pituitary hormone deficiencies."

54. 2. The cause of idiopathic growth hormone deficiency is unknown. The condition is commonly associated with other pituitary hormone deficiencies, such as deficiencies of thyroid-stimulating hormone and corticotropin, and may be secondary to hypothalamic deficiency. There's also a higher-than-average occurrence of the disorder in some families, which indicates a possible genetic cause.

NP: Implementation; CN: Psychosocial integrity; CNS: Coping and adaptation; CL: Application

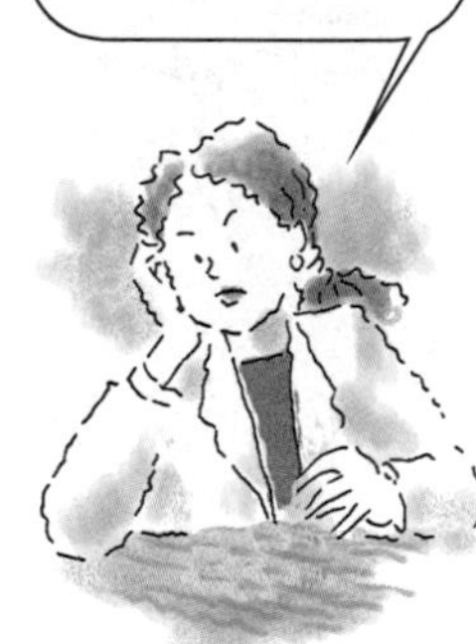

I'm tired, but I can't stop at 55 — and neither should you! Let's keep going!

55. A nurse is teaching health to a class of fifth graders. Which of the following statements related to growth should be included?

1. "There's nothing that you can do to influence your growth."
2. "Intensive physical activity that begins before puberty might stunt growth."
3. "All children who are short in stature also have parents who are short in stature."
4. "Because this is a time of tremendous growth, being concerned about calorie intake isn't important."

55. 2. Intensive physical activity (greater than 18 hours per week) that begins before puberty may stunt growth so that the child doesn't reach full adult height. During the school-age years, growth slows and doesn't accelerate again until adolescence. Nutrition and environment influence a child's growth. All children who are short in stature don't necessarily have parents who are short in stature.

NP: Implementation; CN: Health promotion and maintenance; CNS: Growth and development through the life span; CL: Application

56. A nurse should understand that familial short stature refers to which of the following children?

1. Children who are members of a very large family with limited resources
2. Children who have no siblings and who moved a great deal during their early childhood
3. Children with delayed linear growth and skeletal and sexual maturation that is behind that of age mates
4. Children who have ancestors with adult height in the lower percentiles and whose height during childhood is appropriate

56. 4. Familial short stature refers to otherwise healthy children who have ancestors with adult height in the lower percentiles and whose height during childhood is appropriate for genetic background. Children with delayed linear growth and skeletal and sexual maturation that's behind that of age mates is considered constitutional growth delay. Children who are members of very large families with limited resources or who are only children don't fit the description of familial short stature.

NP: Assessment; CN: Health promotion and maintenance; CNS: Prevention and early detection of disease; CL: Knowledge

57. When assessing a 2-year-old, which of the following findings would indicate to the nurse the possibility of growth hormone deficiency?

1. The child had normal growth during the first year of life but showed a slowed growth curve below the 3rd percentile for the second year of life.
2. The child fell below the 5th percentile for growth during the first year of life but, at this check-up, only falls below the 50th percentile.
3. There has been a steady decline in growth over the 2 years of this toddler's life that has accelerated during the past 6 months.
4. There was delayed growth below the 5th percentile for the first and second years of life.

57. 1. Children generally grow normally during the first year and then follow a slowed growth curve that's below the 3rd percentile. If growth is consistently below the 5th percentile; it may be an indication of failure to thrive.

NP: Assessment; CN: Health promotion and maintenance; CNS: Prevention and early detection of disease; CL: Application

58. When assessing a child with growth hormone deficiency, the nurse would expect to observe which of the following characteristics?

1. Decreased weight with no change in height
2. Decreased weight with increased height
3. Increased weight with decreased height
4. Increased weight with increased height

58. 3. Height may be retarded more than weight because, with good nutrition, children with growth hormone deficiency can become overweight or even obese. Their well-nourished appearance is an important diagnostic clue to differentiation from other disorders such as failure to thrive.

NP: Assessment; CN: Health promotion and maintenance; CNS: Prevention and early detection of disease; CL: Knowledge

59. The nurse should find which of the following characteristics in her assessment of a child with growth hormone deficiency?

1. Normal skeletal proportions
2. Abnormal skeletal proportions
3. Child's appearing older than his age
4. Longer than normal upper extremities

59. 1. Skeletal proportions are normal for the age, but these children appear younger than their chronological age. However, later in life, premature aging is evident.

NP: Assessment; CN: Physiological integrity; CNS: Physiological adaptation; CL: Application

60. When counseling the parents of a child with growth hormone deficiency, the nurse should encourage which of the following sports?

1. Basketball
2. Field hockey
3. Football
4. Gymnastics

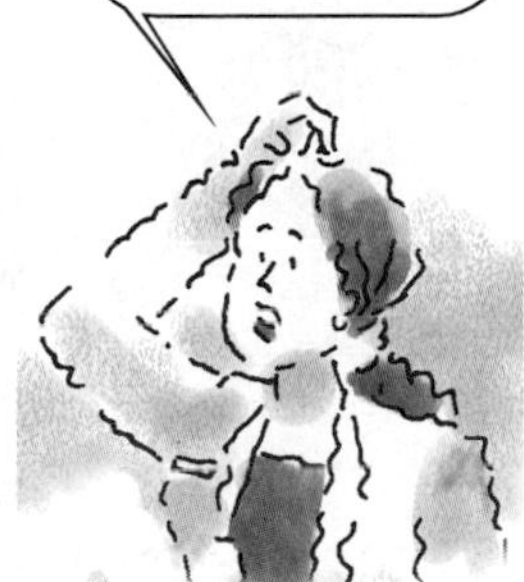
Which of these sports would be best for a child with growth hormone deficiency?

60. 4. Children with growth hormone deficiency can be no less active than other children if directed to size-appropriate sports, such as gymnastics, swimming, wrestling, or soccer.

NP: Planning; CN: Psychosocial integrity; CNS: Coping and adaptation; CL: Application

61. In explaining the social behavior of children with hypopituitarism to parents, a nurse should recognize which of the following statements as a need for further teaching?

1. "I realize that my child might have school anxiety and a low self-esteem."
2. "Because my child is short in stature, people expect less of him than his peers."
3. "Because of my child's short stature, he may not be pushed to perform at his chronological age by others."
4. "My child's vocabulary is very well developed, so even though he's short in stature, no one will treat him differently."

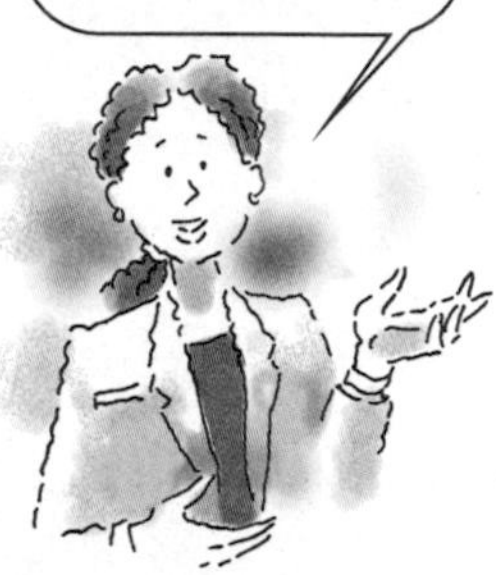

It's important that parents have realistic expectations about their child's disorder.

61. 4. Height discrepancy has been significantly correlated with emotional adjustment problems and may be a valuable predictor of the extent to which growth hormone-delayed children will have trouble with anxiety, social skills, and positive self-esteem. Also, academic problems aren't uncommon. These children aren't usually pushed to perform at their chronological age, but are often subjected to juvenilization (related to in an infantile or childish manner).

NP: Evaluation; CN: Psychosocial integrity; CNS: Psychosocial adaptation; CL: Application

62. The mother of a child diagnosed with hypopituitarism states to the nurse that she feels guilty because she feels that she should have recognized this disorder. Which of the following statements by the nurse about children with hypopituitarism would be the most helpful?"

1. "They're usually large for gestational age at birth."
2. "They're usually small for gestational age at birth."
3. "They usually exhibit signs of this disorder soon after birth."
4. "They're usually of normal size for gestational age at birth."

62. 4. Children with hypopituitarism are usually of normal size for gestational age at birth. Clinical features develop slowly and vary with the severity of the disorder and the number of deficient hormones.

NP: Implementation; CN: Psychosocial integrity; CNS: Coping and adaptation; CL: Knowledge

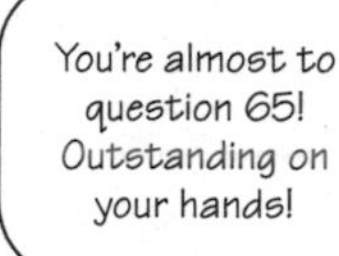

You're almost to question 65! Outstanding on your hands!

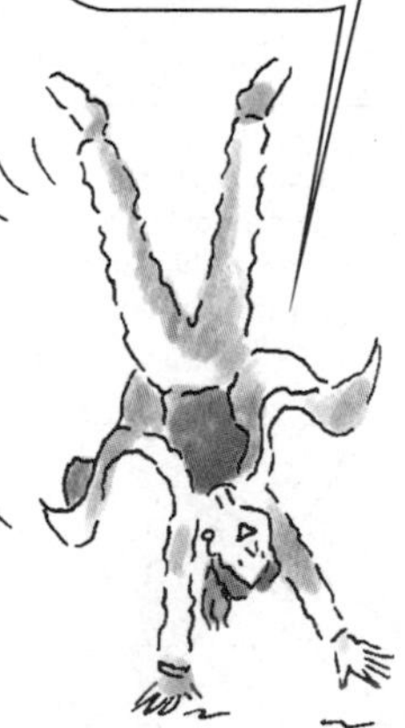

63. Which of the following observations when plotting height and weight on a growth chart would indicate that a child who's 4 years old has a growth hormone deficiency?

1. Upward shift of 1 percentile or more
2. Upward shift of 5 percentiles or more
3. Downward shift of 2 percentiles or more
4. Downward shift of 5 percentiles or more

63. 3. When the primary health care provider evaluates the results of plotting height and weight, upward or downward shifts of 2 percentiles or more in children older than 3 years may indicate a growth abnormality.

NP: Assessment; CN: Health promotion and maintenance; CNS: Prevention and early detection of disease; CL: Analysis

64. When reviewing the results of radiographic examinations of a child with hypopituitarism, which of the following characteristics should the nurse expect to observe?

1. Bone age near normal
2. Epiphyseal maturation normal
3. Epiphyseal maturation retarded
4. Bone maturation greatly retarded

64. 3. Epiphyseal maturation is retarded in hypopituitarism consistent with retardation in height. This is in contrast to hypothyroidism, in which bone maturation is greatly retarded, or Turner syndrome, in which bone age is near normal.

NP: Assessment; CN: Health promotion and maintenance; CNS: Prevention and early detection of disease; CL: Knowledge

65. Which of the following tests is used for a definitive diagnosis of hypopituitarism?

1. Hypersecretion of thyroid hormone
2. Increased reserves of growth hormone
3. Hyposecretion of antidiuretic hormone
4. Decreased reserves of growth hormone

65. 4. Definitive diagnosis is based on absent or subnormal levels of pituitary growth hormone. Antidiuretic hormone and thyroid hormone levels aren't affected.

NP: Assessment; CN: Health promotion and maintenance; CNS: Prevention and early detection of disease; CL: Knowledge

66. The parents of a child who's going through testing for hypopituitarism ask the nurse what test results they should expect. The nurse's response should be based on which of the following factors?

1. Measurement of growth hormone will occur only one time.
2. Growth hormone levels are decreased after strenuous exercise.
3. There will be increased overnight urine growth hormone concentration.
4. Growth hormone levels are elevated 45 to 90 minutes following the onset of sleep.

66. 4. Growth hormone levels are elevated 45 to 90 minutes following the onset of sleep. Low growth hormone levels following the onset of sleep would indicate the need for further evaluation. Exercise is a natural and benign stimulus for growth hormone release, and elevated levels can be detected after 20 minutes of strenuous exercise in normal children. Also, growth hormone levels will need to be checked frequently related to the type of therapy instituted.

NP: Evaluation; CN: Physiological integrity; CNS: Physiological adaptation; CL: Application

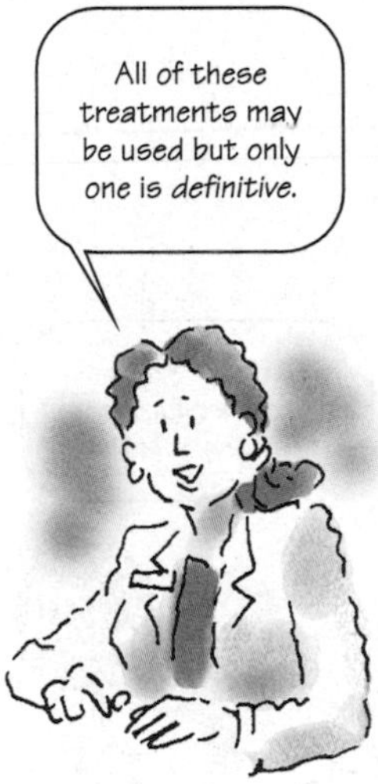

67. Which of the following methods is considered the definitive treatment for hypopituitarism due to growth hormone deficiency?

1. Treatment with desmopressin acetate (DDAVP)
2. Replacement of antidiuretic hormone
3. Treatment with testosterone or estrogen
4. Replacement with biosynthetic growth hormone

67. 4. The definitive treatment of growth hormone deficiency is replacement of growth hormone and is successful in 80% of affected children. DDAVP is used to treat diabetes insipidus. Antidiuretic hormone deficiency causes diabetes insipidus and isn't related to hypopituitarism. Testosterone or estrogen may be given during adolescence for normal sexual maturation but aren't the definitive treatment for hypopituitarism.

NP: Evaluation; CN: Physiological integrity; CNS: Pharmacological and parenteral therapies; CL: Application

68. When obtaining information about a child, which of the following comments made by a parent to the nurse would indicate the possibility of hypopituitarism in a child?

1. "I can pass down my child's clothes to his younger brother."
2. "Usually my child wears out his clothes before his size changes."
3. "I have to buy bigger size clothes for my child about every 2 months."
4. "I have to buy larger shirts more frequently than larger pants for my child."

68. 2. Parents of children with hypopituitarism frequently comment that the child wears out clothes before growing out of them or that, if the clothing fits the body, it's often too long in the sleeves or legs.

NP: Assessment; CN: Health promotion and maintenance; CNS: Growth and development through the life span; CL: Application

69. In helping parents who are planning to give growth hormone at home, the nurse should explain that optimum dosing is achieved when growth hormone is administered at which of the following times?

1. At bedtime
2. After dinner
3. In the middle of the day
4. First thing in the morning

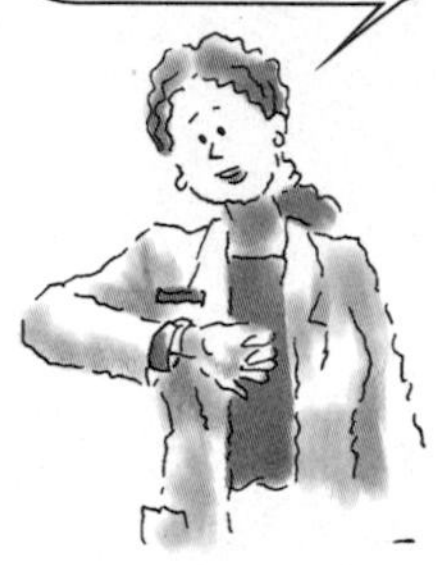

The point at which a drug is most effective is information to know for the NCLEX.

69. 1. Optimum dosing is often achieved when growth hormone is administered at bedtime. Pituitary release of growth hormone occurs during the first 45 to 90 minutes after the onset of sleep so normal physiological release is mimicked with bedtime dosing.

NP: Implementation; CN: Physiological integrity; CNS: Pharmacological and parenteral therapies; CL: Knowledge

70. In educating parents of a child with hypopituitarism about realistic expectations of height for their child who's successfully responding to growth hormone replacement, a nurse should include which of the following statements?

1. "Your child will never reach a normal adult height."
2. "Your child will attain his eventual adult height at a faster rate."
3. "Your child will attain his eventual adult height at a slower rate."
4. "The rate of your child's growth will be the same as children without this disorder."

70. 3. Even when hormone replacement is successful, these children attain their eventual adult height at a slower rate than their peers do; therefore, they need assistance in setting realistic expectations regarding improvement.

NP: Implementation; CN: Psychosocial integrity; CNS: Coping and adaptation; CL: Application

71. Which of the following statements made by a parent of a child with short stature would indicate to the nurse the need for further teaching?

1. "Obtaining blood studies won't aid in proper diagnosis."
2. "A history of my child's growth patterns should be discussed."
3. "X-rays should be included in my child's diagnostic procedures."
4. "A family history is important information for me to share with my primary health care provider."

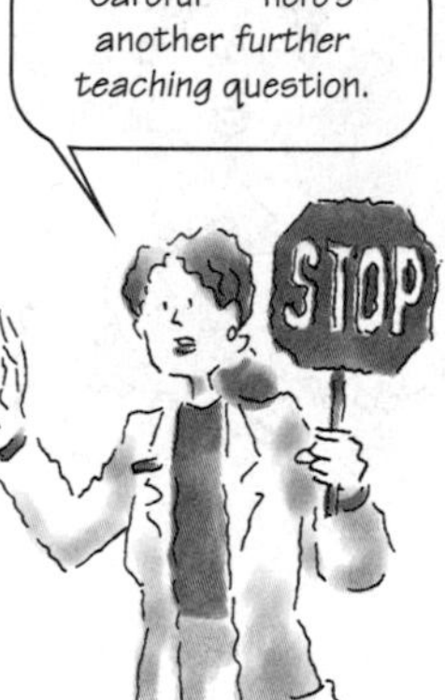

71. 1. A complete diagnostic evaluation should include a family history, a history of the child's growth patterns and previous health status, physical examination, physical evaluation, radiographic survey, and endocrine studies that may involve blood samples.

NP: Evaluation; CN: Health promotion and maintenance; CNS: Prevention and early detection of disease; CL: Application

72. If hypersecretion of growth hormone occurs after epiphyseal closure, which of the following conditions might be observed by the nurse?

1. Acromegaly
2. Cretinism
3. Dwarfism
4. Gigantism

72. 1. If excessive growth hormone is evident after epiphyseal closure, growth is in the transverse direction, producing a condition known as acromegaly. The other options aren't seen as a result of excess growth hormone after epiphyseal closure.

NP: Assessment; CN: Physiological integrity; CNS: Physiological adaptation; CL: Knowledge

73. Which of the following metabolic alteration characteristics might be associated with growth hormone deficiency?

1. Galactosemia
2. Homocystinuria
3. Hyperglycemia
4. Hypoglycemia

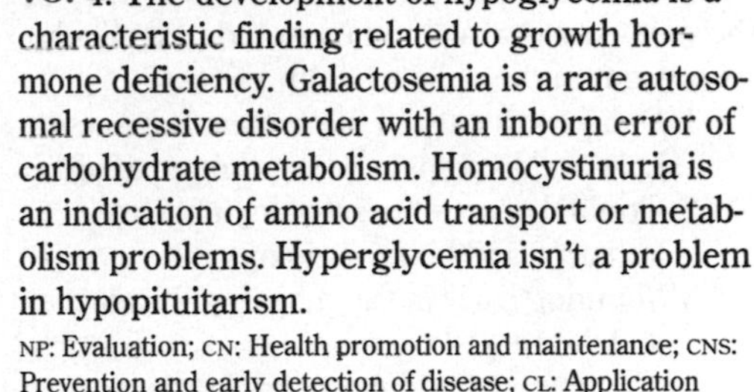

73. 4. The development of hypoglycemia is a characteristic finding related to growth hormone deficiency. Galactosemia is a rare autosomal recessive disorder with an inborn error of carbohydrate metabolism. Homocystinuria is an indication of amino acid transport or metabolism problems. Hyperglycemia isn't a problem in hypopituitarism.

NP: Evaluation; CN: Health promotion and maintenance; CNS: Prevention and early detection of disease; CL: Application

74. When providing information to support home management of a child receiving growth hormone replacement therapy for hypopituitarism, the nurse should include which of the following interventions?

1. Explaining that growth in height and weight won't begin until puberty
2. Teaching how to perform venipuncture for administration of the growth hormone
3. Helping parents recognize the importance of interacting with the child according to age rather than size
4. Advising parents to hold the child back in school until linear growth begins to approximate the normal patterns

74. 3. Recognizing potential threats to self-esteem and healthy development are important aspects of nursing care for the child with growth hormone deficiency. Growth hormone administration is S.C., and a child shouldn't be held back in school because of his size. Growth in height and weight will begin soon after treatment with growth hormone begins.

NP: Implementation; CN: Psychosocial integrity; CNS: Coping and adaptation; CL: Application

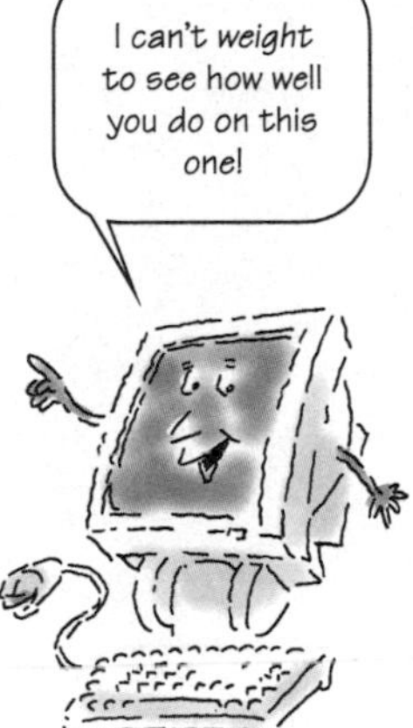

I can't weight to see how well you do on this one!

75. When assessing a neonate diagnosed with diabetes insipidus, which of the following findings would indicate the need for intervention?

1. Edema
2. Increased head circumference
3. Weight gain
4. Weight loss

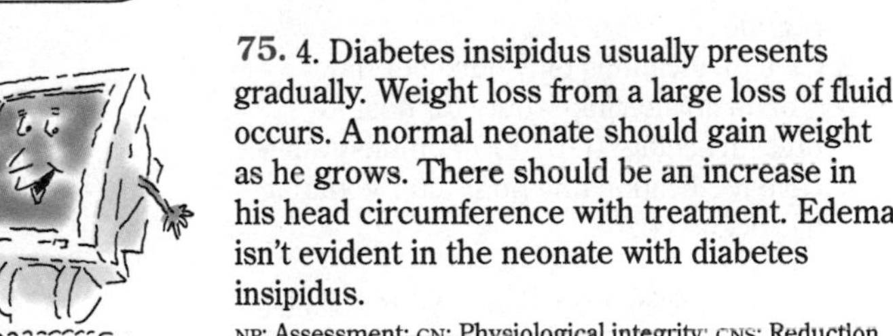

75. 4. Diabetes insipidus usually presents gradually. Weight loss from a large loss of fluid occurs. A normal neonate should gain weight as he grows. There should be an increase in his head circumference with treatment. Edema isn't evident in the neonate with diabetes insipidus.

NP: Assessment; CN: Physiological integrity; CNS: Reduction of risk potential; CL: Application

76. In a client with diabetes insipidus, a nurse could expect which of the following characteristics of the urine?

1. Pale in color; specific gravity less than 1.006
2. Concentrated; specific gravity less than 1.006
3. Concentrated; specific gravity less than 1.030
4. Pale in color; specific gravity more than 1.030

76. 1. With diabetes insipidus, the client has difficulty with excessive urine output; therefore, the urine will be pale in color and the specific gravity will fall below the low normal of 1.010.

NP: Assessment; CN: Physiological integrity; CNS: Physiological adaptation; CL: Analysis

77. In a child with diabetes insipidus, which of the following characteristics would most likely be present in the child's health history?

1. Delayed closure of the fontanels, coarse hair, and hypoglycemia in the morning
2. Gradual onset of personality changes, lethargy, and blurred vision
3. Vomiting early in the morning, headache, and decreased thirst
4. Abrupt onset of polyuria, nocturia, and polydipsia

77. 4. Diabetes insipidus is characterized by deficient secretion of antidiuretic hormone leading to diuresis. Most children with this disorder experience an abrupt onset of symptoms, including polyuria, nocturia, and polydipsia. The other choices reflect symptoms of pituitary hyperfunction.

NP: Evaluation; CN: Health promotion and maintenance; CNS: Prevention and early detection of disease; CL: Application

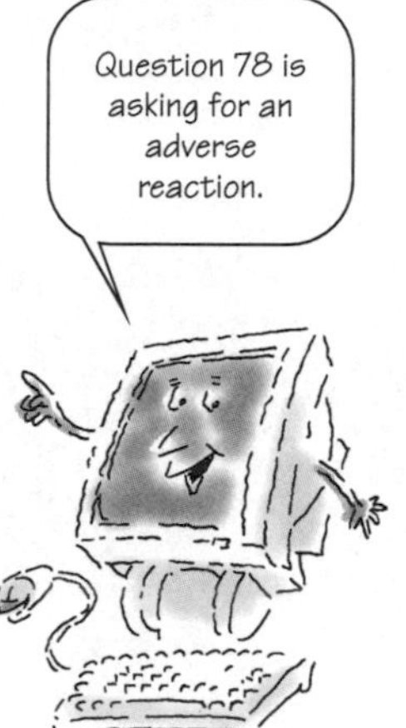

Question 78 is asking for an adverse reaction.

78. Which of the following conditions in a client on fluid restriction for diabetes insipidus diagnostic testing would indicate a need for the nurse to discontinue fluid restriction?

1. Weight gain of 3% to 5%
2. Weight loss of 3% to 5%
3. Increase in urine output
4. Generalized edema

78. 2. A weight loss between 3% to 5% indicates significant dehydration and requires termination of the fluid restriction. Weight gain would be a good sign. Generalized edema wouldn't occur with fluid restriction, nor would increased urine output.

NP: Assessment; CN: Physiological integrity; CNS: Physiological adaptation; CL: Analysis

79. When a child with diabetes insipidus has a viral illness that includes congestion, nausea, and vomiting, the nurse should instruct the parents to take which of the following actions?

1. Make no changes in the medication regime.
2. Give medications only once per day.
3. Obtain an alternate route for desmopressin acetate (DDAVP) administration.
4. Give medication one hour after vomiting has occurred.

79. 3. An alternate route for administration of DDAVP would be needed for absorption due to nasal congestion. The other options reflect actions that need to be covered by a medical order.

NP: Implementation; CN: Health promotion and maintenance; CNS: Prevention and early detection of disease; CL: Application

80. A nurse is preparing a child with diabetes insipidus who will be taking injectable vasopressin for hospital discharge. Which of the following actions is best for the nurse to take in regards to teaching injection techniques?

1. Teach injection techniques to the primary caregiver.
2. Teach injection techniques to anyone who will provide care for the child.
3. Teach injection techniques to anyone who will provide care for the child as well as to the child if he's old enough to understand.
4. Provide information about the nearest home health agency so the parents can arrange for the home health nurse to come and give the injection.

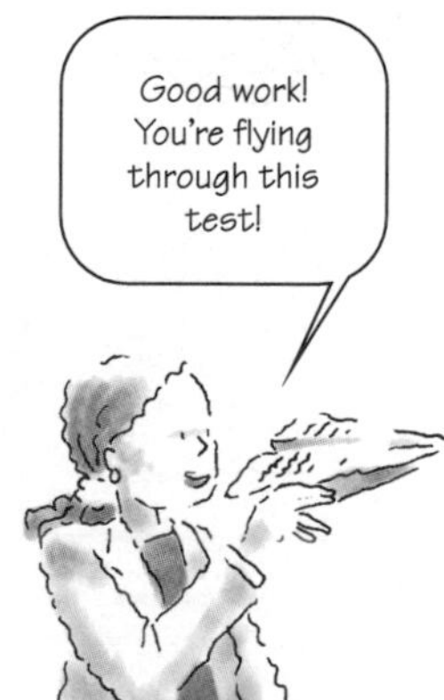

Good work! You're flying through this test!

80. 3. The best response is to teach all those who will provide care for the child. The child should be included if age-appropriate. It's unrealistic to arrange home health nurses to give injections that are required throughout the life span.

NP: Implementation; CN: Health promotion and maintenance; CNS: Prevention and early detection of disease; CL: Application

81. When providing care for a school-age client with diabetes insipidus, the nurse understands that which of the following behaviors might be difficult related to this child's growth and development?

1. Taking desmopressin acetate (DDAVP) at school
2. Taking DDAVP before bedtime
3. Letting his mother administer the vasopressin injection
4. Giving himself a vasopressin injection before school starts

81. 1. Anything that singles a child out and makes him feel different from his peers will result in possible noncompliance with the medical regimen. It's important for the nurse to help the client schedule the need for medications around the times he will be in school.
NP: Implementation; CN: Health promotion and maintenance; CNS: Growth and development through the life span; CL: Application

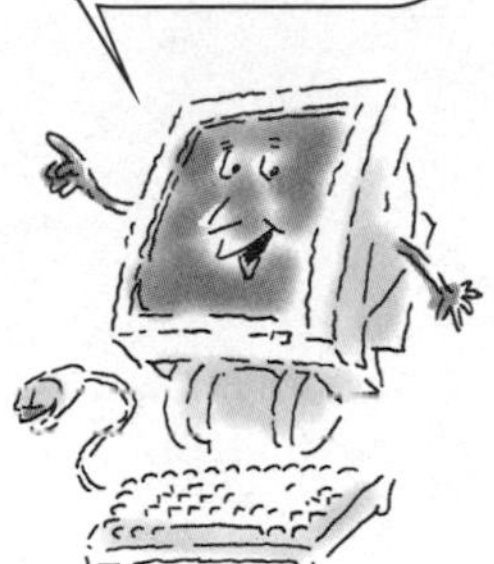

Question 82 asks you to rank monitoring methods for appropriateness. Can you do it? I knew you could!

82. Which of the following monitoring methods would be best for a client newly diagnosed with diabetes insipidus?

1. Measuring abdominal girths every day
2. Measuring intake, output, and urine specific gravity
3. Checking daily weights, measuring intake
4. Checking for pitting edema in the lower extremities

82. 2. Measuring intake and output with related specific gravity results will enable the nurse to closely monitor the client's condition along with daily weights. All other options aren't as accurate for a child with diabetes insipidus.
NP: Assessment; CN: Health promotion and maintenance; CNS: Prevention and early detection of disease; CL: Application

83. When assessing a neonate for signs of congenital hypothyroidism, which of the following characteristics would the nurse observe?

1. Hyperreflexia
2. Long forehead
3. Puffy eyelids
4. Small tongue

83. 3. Assessment findings would include depressed nasal bridge, short forehead, puffy eyelids, and large tongue; thick, dry, mottled skin that feels cold to the touch; coarse, dry, lusterless hair; abdominal distention; umbilical hernia; hyporeflexia; bradycardia; hypothermia; hypotension; anemia; and wide cranial sutures.
NP: Assessment; CN: Health promotion and maintenance; CNS: Prevention and early detection of disease; CL: Knowledge

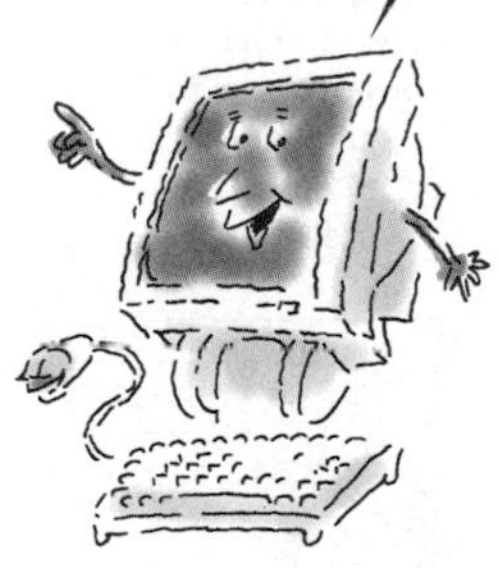

Question 84 is almost a negative question. It asks about adverse effects.

84. Which of the following factors is most significant in adversely affecting eventual intelligence of a neonate with hypothyroidism?

1. Overtreatment
2. Inadequate treatment
3. Educational level of the parents
4. Socioeconomic level of the family

84. 2. The most significant factor adversely affecting eventual intelligence appears to be inadequate treatment, which may be related to noncompliance. Parental factors such as educational and socioeconomic level will affect only the environmental stimulation, not the child's basic intellect. Overtreatment could cause physical problems and possibly death. It would be treated before the intellect was affected.
NP: Implementation; CN: Health promotion and maintenance; CNS: Prevention and early detection of disease; CL: Application

85. Which of the following nursing objectives is most important when working with neonates who are suspected of having congenital hypothyroidism?
1. Early identification
2. Promoting bonding
3. Allowing rooming in
4. Encouraging fluid intake

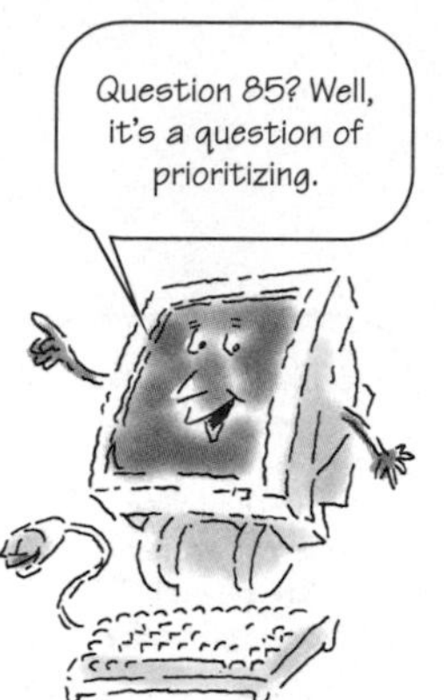

Question 85? Well, it's a question of prioritizing.

85. 1. The most important nursing objective is early identification of the disorder. Nurses caring for neonates must be certain that screening is performed, especially in neonates who are preterm, discharged early, or born at home. Promoting bonding, allowing rooming in, and encouraging fluid intake are all important but are less important than early identification.
NP: Assessment; CN: Physiological integrity; CNS: Basic care and comfort; CL: Knowledge

86. When the parents of an infant diagnosed with hypothyroidism have been taught to count the pulse, which of the following interventions should the nurse teach them in case they obtain a high pulse rate?
1. Allow the infant to take a nap, and then give the medication.
2. Withhold the medication, and give a double dose the next day.
3. Hold the medication, and call the primary health care provider.
4. Give the medication, and then consult the primary health care provider.

86. 3. If parents have been taught to count the infant's pulse, they should be instructed to withhold the dose and consult their primary health care provider if the pulse rate is above a certain value.
NP: Evaluation; CN: Health promotion and maintenance; CNS: Prevention and early detection of disease; CL: Application

87. In an infant receiving inadequate treatment for congenital hypothyroidism, the nurse would expect to observe which of the following symptoms?
1. Irritability and jitteriness
2. Fatigue and sleepiness
3. Increased appetite
4. Diarrhea

87. 2. Signs of inadequate treatment are fatigue, sleepiness, decreased appetite, and constipation.
NP: Assessment; CN: Health promotion and maintenance; CNS: Prevention and early detection of disease; CL: Application

88. Which of the following characteristics best describes congenital hypothyroidism?
1. It's sex-linked.
2. It has no genetic basis.
3. It's an autosomal dominant gene.
4. It's caused by an inborn error of metabolism.

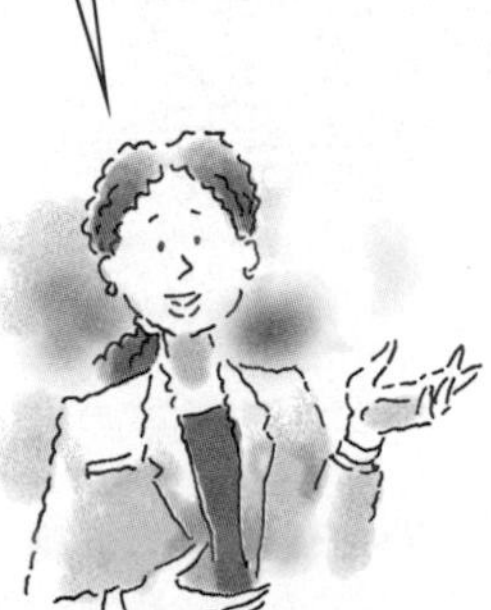

Question 90 is just around the corner. Have I told you lately how proud of you I am? Well, I am!

88. 4. The disorder is caused by an inborn error of thyroid hormone synthesis, which is autosomal recessive. Therefore, genetic counseling is important. There's no evidence that this disorder is sex-linked.
NP: Assessment; CN: Health promotion and maintenance; CNS: Prevention and early detection of disease; CL: Knowledge

89. Which of the following recommendations for preventing hypoglycemia in an adolescent with diabetes type 1 should the nurse make?

1. Limit participation in planned exercise activities that involve competition.
2. Carry crackers or fruit to eat before or during periods of increased activity.
3. Increase the insulin dosage before planned or unplanned strenuous exercise.
4. Check blood sugar before exercising, and eat a protein snack if the level is elevated.

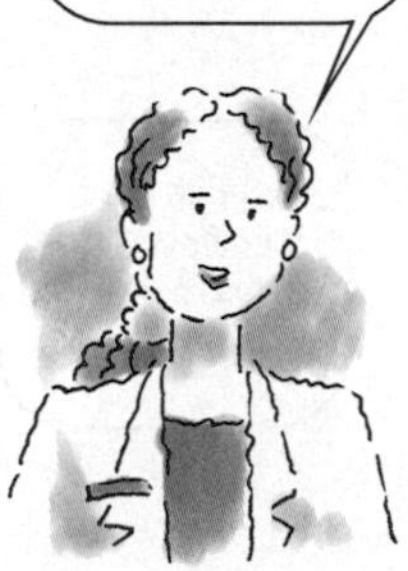
Let's discuss some steps for preventing hypoglycemia.

89. 2. Hypoglycemia can usually be prevented if a child with diabetes eats more food before or during exercise. Because exercise with adolescents isn't commonly planned, carrying additional carbohydrate foods is a good preventative measure.

NP: Implementation; CN: Health promotion and maintenance; CNS: Prevention and early detection of disease; CL: Application

90. Which of the following statements accurately describes the incidence of type 1 diabetes mellitus?

1. It's the most common endocrine disease of childhood.
2. Diabetes mellitus is an inherited disease caused by a recessive gene.
3. Diabetes mellitus is more commonly seen in children who are obese.
4. The prevalence of diabetes mellitus is decreasing due to early detection.

90. 1. Diabetes mellitus is the most common endocrine disease in childhood. There's a higher incidence of type 2 diabetes when there's a strong family history of diabetes, but the genetic predisposition for type 1 diabetes isn't known. Obesity is also a predisposing factor for type 2 diabetes; there's no link to obesity in type 1 diabetes. Early detection of a disease doesn't affect its prevalence.

NP: Assessment; CN: Health promotion and maintenance; CNS: Prevention and early detection of disease; CL: Knowledge

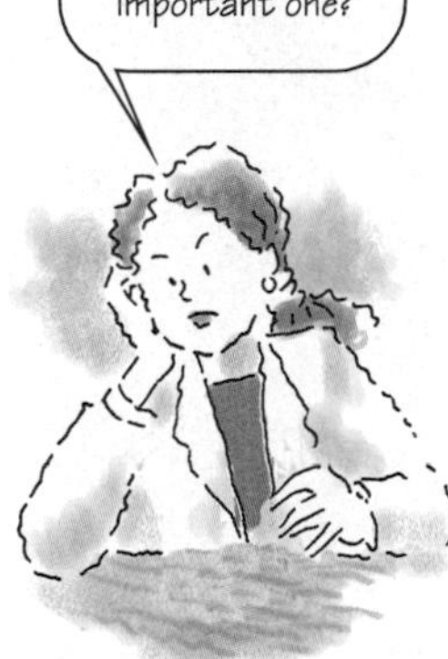
Hmmm, which of these questions is the most important one?

91. An adolescent girl is admitted to the hospital with type 1 diabetes and unstable blood glucose levels. Which of the following questions is most important to include in the history?

1. Does she play any team sports?
2. Does she refrigerate her insulin?
3. Is she satisfied with her weight?
4. Does she use recreational drugs?

91. 3. It's important to ascertain the adolescent's feelings about her body, in particular, her weight. Some adolescents skip their insulin because they know it will result in weight loss. The other issues of sports, drug use, and technique of administering her insulin are all relevant but not as important as knowing what she's thinking about her own body.

NP: Implementation; CN: Psychosocial integrity; CNS: Coping and adaptation; CL: Application

92. A 14-year-old boy with type 1 diabetes mellitus plans to join the basketball team at his school. The practices are twice a week with games on Saturdays. He calls the nurse at his clinic for advice. The nurse should respond with which of the following statements?

1. "Delay eating a meal until after practice or a game."
2. "Time your insulin to peak at the time of practice and games."
3. "Monitor your blood sugar before, during, and after exercise."
4. "Increase your daily calorie intake by 10% and up your insulin dose by 10%."

92. 3. For increases in activity, a client with type 1 diabetes would require a snack before the activity and increased insulin. The amount of insulin is the most difficult determination. Monitoring is required for accurate regulation before, during, and after the activity. The client shouldn't delay eating until afterwards because the body needs the calories to provide energy to the muscles and tissues. Extreme hypoglycemia may occur if the insulin peaks without extra calories. There's no standard of 10% increase in calories and insulin. Every person would require individualization of the insulin and calories needed.

NP: Planning; CN: Health promotion and maintenance; CNS: Prevention and early detection of disease; CL: Application

93. A nurse is collecting a history from the parents of a 12-month-old infant being evaluated for possible hypopituitarism. Which of the following components of the history is important to establish the diagnosis?

1. Did the mother drink alcohol while pregnant?
2. Does the infant receive multivitamins?
3. What's the infant's growth pattern?
4. Was the infant premature?

93. 3. Hypopituitarism presents with a retarded growth pattern, appearance younger than chronological age, and normal skeletal proportions and intelligence. It's related to tumors, irradiation, infection, and head trauma. Therefore, serial growth patterns will be crucial to the diagnosis process. It isn't related to fetal alcoholism, use of multivitamins, or prematurity.
NP: Assessment; CN: Physiological integrity; CNS: Physiological adaptation; CL: Application

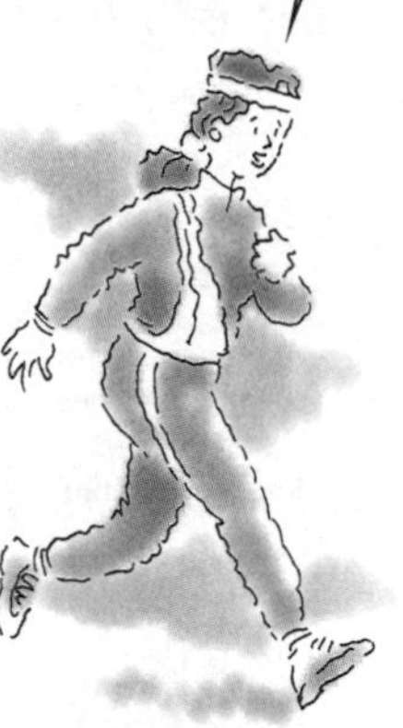
I can see the finish line! You're doing great!

94. The nurse has just completed teaching a family about hypothyroidism. Which actions would indicate the parents understand their child's diagnosis?

1. Providing a diet including whole grains, produce, and water
2. Anticipating their child outgrowing hypothyroidism
3. Providing a white diet for their child
4. Providing a diet high in fat for their child to encourage growth

94. 1. A diet including fruits, vegetables, whole grains and water will help counteract the trend toward obstinate constipation, the result of a slowed metabolism and hypotonic bowel. Congenital hypothyroidism isn't outgrown, and thyroid replacement is necessary throughout the life span. A white diet involves foods low in fiber, which leads to constipation. Hypothyroid individuals tend to have elevated cholesterol and triglyceride levels; therefore, a diet high in fat is contraindicated.
NP: Assessment; CN: Health promotion and maintenance; CNS: Prevention and early detection of disease; CL: Application

95. A client asks the nurse about her chances of developing diabetes. Which statement is true of diabetes mellitus?

1. Development of type 1 diabetes is gradual.
2. If both parents have type 1 diabetes, all of their children will too.
3. Management of type 2 diabetes may include oral medication, controlled diet, and exercise.
4. Type 2 diabetes isn't seen in people under age 40.

95. 3. Balancing medication, caloric intake, and activity level is essential for the long-term survival of clients with diabetes. Type 1 diabetes develops suddenly, and no genetic predisposition has been identified at this time. In recent years as diets contain increased amounts of fat and people are more sedentary, type 2 diabetes has become a problem of people of all ages, including children.
NP: Analysis; CN: Physiological integrity; CNS: Physiological adaptation; CL: Knowledge

96. The nurse is caring for a client with hyperfunctioning of the adrenal gland. Which nursing intervention is appropriate for this client with pheochromocytoma?

1. Promoting an environment free from emotional distress
2. Avoiding analgesia administration
3. Advising a low-calorie, high-nutrient diet
4. Avoiding parents rooming in because they make the client less dependent on staff

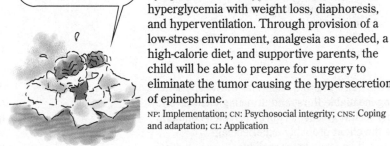

Promote a stress-free environment for your clients with pheochromocytoma.

96. 1. The child experiencing hyperfunctioning of the adrenal gland, or pheochromocytoma, is in a chronic state of "fight or flight" related to excessive exogenous epinephrine. Therefore, the child has an accelerated metabolism. Symptoms include hypertension, headaches, hyperglycemia with weight loss, diaphoresis, and hyperventilation. Through provision of a low-stress environment, analgesia as needed, a high-calorie diet, and supportive parents, the child will be able to prepare for surgery to eliminate the tumor causing the hypersecretion of epinephrine.

NP: Implementation; CN: Psychosocial integrity; CNS: Coping and adaptation; CL: Application

97. The nurse is instructing a family about promoting the health of their child with diabetes. Which teaching point should be included?

1. Avoid daily bathing so skin doesn't become too dry.
2. Cuts and scratches on the playground are of little concern.
3. Children with diabetes need few immunizations.
4. Regular dental care and annual ophthalmologic appointments should be kept.

97. 4. Regular dental care will preserve oral health, and ophthalmologic examinations will ensure visual acuity for reading. Because of their impaired immune system, children with diabetes need to maintain a high level of health to avoid infection. Daily bathing and application of lotion, cleaning minor playground scrapes and applying antibiotic ointments, and keeping immunizations up-to-date are all important.

NP: Implementation; CN: Health promotion and maintenance; CNS: Prevention and early detection of disease; CL: Application

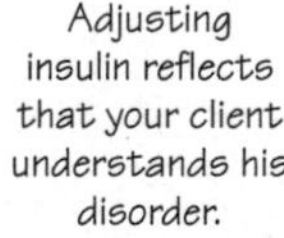

Adjusting insulin reflects that your client understands his disorder.

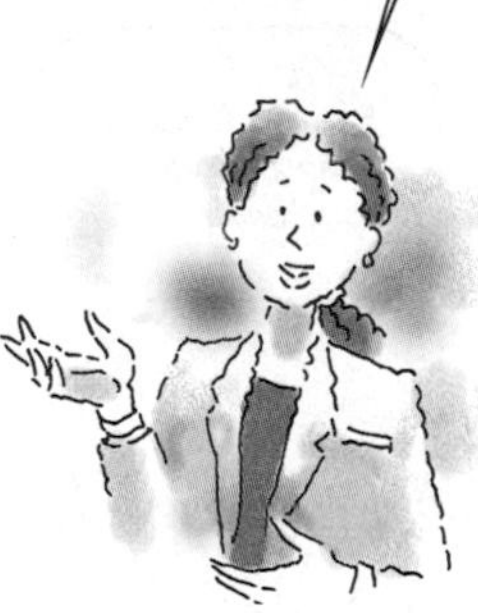

98. A 10-year-old child monitors and adjusts his own insulin. Which response reflects an understanding of appropriate adjustment of insulin dosage when the child has the flu?

1. "I withhold all insulin because I'm not eating."
2. "I'll take my usual dose of regular and NPH insulin."
3. "I'll perform fingerstick blood sugar testing and adjust my insulin according to results."
4. "I'll perform fingerstick blood sugar testing and record the results."

98. 3. Because of the stress of illness, serum glucose will likely be elevated during an episode of the flu. Appropriate adjustment of insulin dosage will help prevent the child from becoming hypoglycemic or ketoacidotic.

NP: Implementation; CN: Physiological integrity; CNS: Physiological adaptation; CL: Analysis

99. The parents of a child with hypopituitary dwarfism have many questions about their son's diagnosis. Which statement is true about children with hypopituitary dwarfism?

1. They're usually low birth weight babies.
2. Symptoms aren't apparent until puberty.
3. Symptoms include early primary dentition.
4. They grow normally the first 2 years then fall below the 3rd percentile.

99. 4. Generally, hypopituitary children are of average birth weight and grow at a normal pace the first 2 or 3 years then fall behind their peers in height, usually below the 3rd percentile. Dentition of primary teeth is normal; permanent teeth are delayed.

NP: Assessment; CN: Health promotion and maintenance; CNS: Growth and development through the life span; CL: Knowledge

100. A 10-year-old client has been experiencing insatiable thirst and urinating excessively; his serum glucose is normal. Which condition is the client probably experiencing?

1. Type 2 diabetes mellitus
2. Type 1 diabetes mellitus
3. Hyperthyroidism
4. Diabetes insipidus

100. 4. Polydipsia and polyuria with normal serum glucose may be indicative of diabetes insipidus. Interview and laboratory results can determine whether the origin is neurogenic or nephrogenic. Type 1 or 2 diabetes mellitus requires an elevated serum glucose. A child with hyperthyroidism may present as dehydrated from the excessive sweating and rapid respirations that accompany this hypermetabolic state.

NP: Assessment; CN: Physiological integrity; CNS: Physiological adaptation; CL: Analysis

101. Last evening at swim practice, the lifeguard had to help a 12-year-old client with diabetes out of the pool when she felt she was too weak to move. Her fingerstick glucose was low. Which action will help prevent weakness in the future?

1. Consuming a balanced meal prior to swim practice
2. Eating two string cheeses part way through practice
3. Eating an apple and a peanut butter sandwich before swimming
4. Eating a good lunch

101. 3. The apple contains simple sugars, which are available for a fast release of energy, and the peanut butter sandwich provides complex carbohydrates, fats, and protein for a stable, long-term release of glucose. Eating an entire meal so close to exercise may be too filling and might cause abdominal upset. The cheese, which contains mostly fat and protein, won't give the immediate glucose boost needed during exercise. Practices are usually in the evening, too long after lunch for simple sugars to be available.

NP: Implementation; CN: Physiological integrity; CNS: Reduction of risk potential; CL: Application

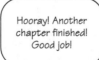

Hooray! Another chapter finished! Good job!

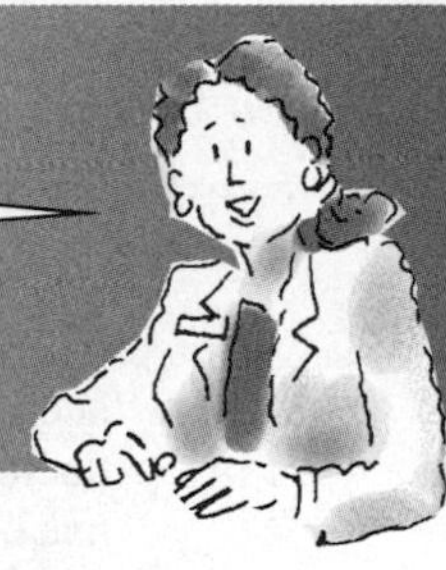

This chapter covers altered
patterns of urinary elimination
in children and includes
glomerulonephritis, hypospadias,
and — oh, a whole lot of other
conditions. Ready? Let's go!

Chapter 34
Genitourinary disorders

1. A child with acute glomerulonephritis has a nursing diagnosis of ***Impaired urinary elimination*** related to fluid retention and impaired glomerular filtration. The child should have which of the following expected outcomes?

1. Exhibits no evidence of infection
2. Engages in activities appropriate to capabilities
3. Demonstrates no periorbital, facial, or body edema
4. Maintains a fluid intake of more than 2,000 ml in 24 hours

1. 3. The goal of this diagnosis involves interventions, such as decreased fluid and salt intake, designed to minimize or prevent fluid retention and edema. These interventions may be evaluated through observations for edema. The other options are appropriate outcomes for other nursing diagnoses, not the diagnosis in question.

NP: Evaluation; CN: Health promotion and maintenance; CNS: Prevention and early detection of disease; CL: Analysis

2. An important nursing intervention to support the therapeutic management of the child with acute glomerulonephritis would include which of the following?

1. Measuring daily weight
2. Increasing oral fluid intake
3. Providing sodium supplements
4. Monitoring client for signs of hypokalemia

2. 1. The child with acute glomerulonephritis should be monitored for fluid imbalance, which is done through daily weights. Increasing oral intake, monitoring for hypokalemia, and providing sodium supplements aren't part of the therapeutic management of acute glomerulonephritis.

NP: Implementation; CN: Physiological integrity; CNS: Basic care and comfort; CL: Application

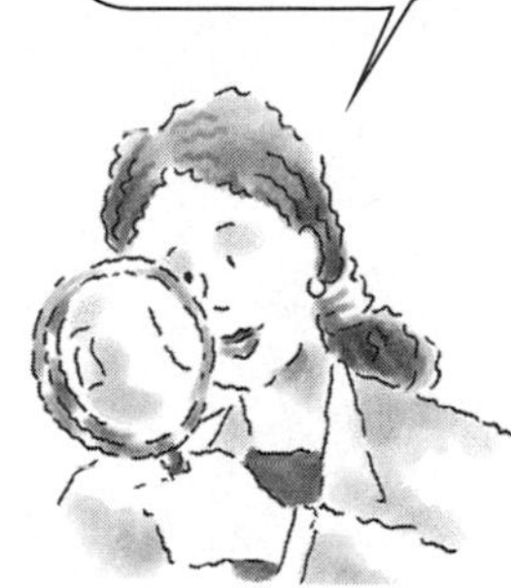

trouble deciding
on an answer,

ones you know

3. A child has been diagnosed with acute glomerulonephritis. Which of the following components should the nurse expect the child's urine to contain?

1. Blood
2. Calcium casts
3. Cystine crystals
4. Glucose

3. 1. Urinalysis findings consistent with glomerulonephritis should include specific gravity less than 1.030, positive blood and protein casts, and white and red blood cell casts. Calcium casts and glucose aren't usually found in the urine of a client with acute glomerulonephritis. The presence of cystine crystals typically indicate a congenital metabolic problem.

NP: Assessment; CN: Physiological integrity; CNS: Physiological adaptation; CL: Knowledge

4. The nurse is taking frequent blood pressure readings on a child diagnosed with acute glomerulonephritis. The parents ask the nurse why this is necessary. The nurse's reply should be based on which of the following factors?

1. Blood pressure fluctuations are a sign that the condition has become chronic.
2. Blood pressure fluctuations are a common adverse effect of antibiotic therapy.
3. Hypotension leading to sudden shock can develop at any time.
4. Acute hypertension must be anticipated and identified.

4. 4. Regular measurement of vital signs, body weight, and intake and output is essential to monitor the progress of the disease and to detect complications that may appear at any time during the course of the disease. Hypertension is more likely than hypotension to occur with glomerulonephritis. Blood pressure fluctuations don't indicate that the condition has become chronic and aren't common adverse reactions to antibiotic therapy.

NP: Assessment; CN: Safe, effective care environment; CNS: Management of care; CL: Comprehension

5. When evaluating the urinalysis report of a child with acute glomerulonephritis, the nurse would expect which of the following results?

1. Proteinuria and decreased specific gravity
2. Bacteriuria and increased specific gravity
3. Hematuria and proteinuria
4. Bacteriuria and hematuria

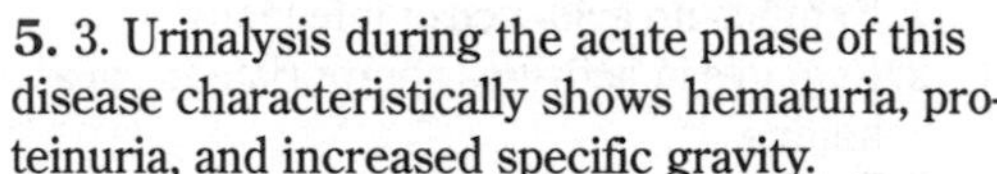

5. 3. Urinalysis during the acute phase of this disease characteristically shows hematuria, proteinuria, and increased specific gravity.

NP: Evaluation; CN: Physiological integrity; CNS: Physiological adaptation; CL: Analysis

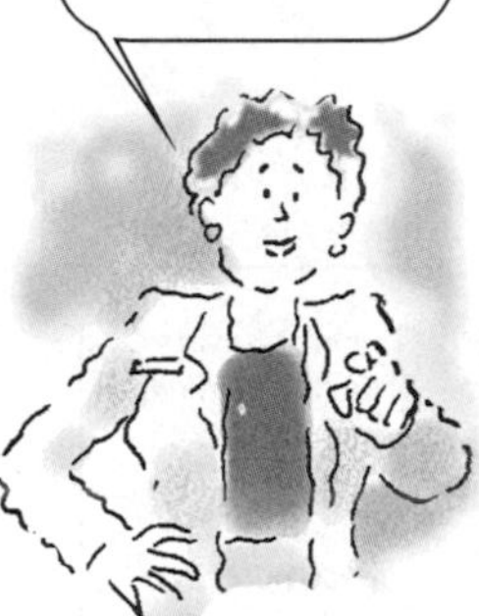

More than one answer may seem correct. It's your job to choose the best answer.

6. Which of the following statements by the nurse would be the best response to a mother who wants to know the first indication that acute glomerulonephritis is improving?

1. Urine output will increase.
2. Urine will be free of protein.
3. Blood pressure will stabilize.
4. The child will have more energy.

6. 1. One of the first signs of improvement during the acute phase of glomerulonephritis is an increase in urine output. It will take time for the urine to be free of protein. Antihypertensive drugs may be needed to stabilize the blood pressure. Children generally don't have much energy during the acute phase of this disease.

NP: Assessment; CN: Health promotion and maintenance; CNS: Prevention and early detection of disease; CL: Analysis

7. Which of the following statements best describes acute glomerulonephritis?

1. This disease occurs after a urinary tract infection.
2. This disease is associated with renal vascular disorders.
3. This disease occurs after an antecedent streptococcal infection.
4. This disease is associated with structural anomalies of the genitourinary tract.

7. 3. Acute glomerulonephritis is an immune-complex disease that occurs as a by-product of an antecedent streptococcal infection. Certain strains of the infection are usually a beta-hemolytic streptococcus.

NP: Assessment; CN: Health promotion and maintenance; CNS: Prevention and early detection of disease; CL: Knowledge

8. When obtaining daily weights on a client, the nurse notes that a child has lost 6 lb (2.7 kg) after 3 days of hospitalization for acute glomerulonephritis. This is most likely the result of which of the following factors?

1. Poor appetite
2. Reduction of edema
3. Decreased salt intake
4. Restriction to bed rest

8. 2. When there is reduction of edema, the client will lose weight. This should normally occur after treatment for acute glomerulonephritis has been followed for several days. It will take longer for the child's appetite to improve, but this shouldn't lead to such a dramatic weight loss in a child this age.

NP: Evaluation; CN: Physiological integrity; CNS: Basic care and comfort; CL: Application

9. A nurse should make which of the following dietary recommendations to a client who has been newly diagnosed with acute glomerulonephritis?

1. Decrease calories
2. Increase potassium
3. Severely restrict sodium
4. Moderately restrict sodium

9. 4. Moderate sodium restriction with a diet that has no added salt after cooking is usually effective. Calorie consumption doesn't need to decrease and potassium consumption shouldn't increase due to the decrease in urinary output. *Severe* sodium restriction isn't needed and will make it more difficult to ensure adequate nutrition.

NP: Implementation; CN: Physiological integrity; CNS: Basic care and comfort; CL: Application

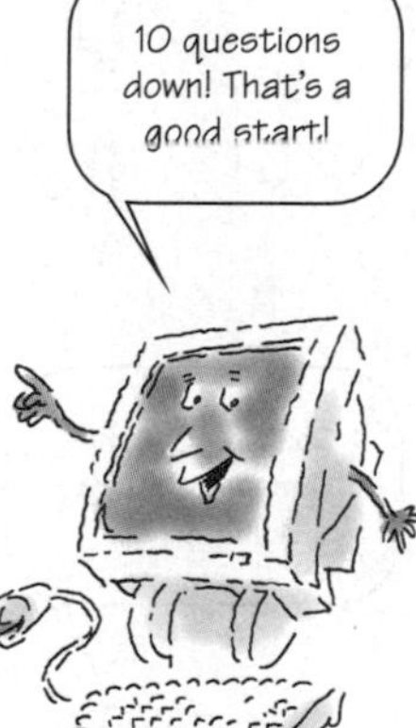
10 questions down! That's a good start!

10. The nurse is evaluating a group of children for acute glomerulonephritis. Which of the following clients would be most likely to develop the disease?

1. A client who had pneumonia a month ago
2. A client who was bitten by a brown spider
3. A client who shows no signs of periorbital edema
4. A client who had a streptococcal infection 2 weeks ago

10. 4. A latent period of 10 to 14 days occurs between the streptococcal infection of the throat or skin and the onset of clinical manifestations. The peak incidence of disease corresponds to the incidence of streptococcal infections. Pneumonia isn't a precursor to glomerulonephritis, nor is a bite from a brown spider. A sign of periorbital edema would lead the nurse to investigate the possibility of glomerulonephritis, especially if reported to be worse in the morning.

NP: Evaluation; CN: Safe, effective care environment; CNS: Management of care; CL: Analysis

11. At which of the following ages would the nurse observe a higher incidence of acute glomerulonephritis?

1. 1 to 2 years
2. 6 to 7 years
3. 12 to 13 years
4. 18 to 20 years

11. 2. Acute glomerulonephritis can occur at any age, but it primarily affects early school-age children with a peak age of onset of 6 to 7 years. It is uncommon in children younger than 2 years old.

NP: Assessment; CN: Health promotion and maintenance; CNS: Growth and development through the life span; CL: Knowledge

12. In understanding the recurrence of glomerulonephritis, the nurse should know which of the following characteristics to be true?

1. Second attacks are quite common.
2. A recessive gene transfers this disease.
3. Multiple cases tend to occur in families.
4. Overcrowding in the schoolroom leads to higher incidence.

12. 3. Multiple cases tend to occur in families. Second attacks are rare. Acute glomerulonephritis isn't transmitted through a recessive gene and overcrowding in the schoolroom should have no influence on this disease.

NP: Assessment; CN: Health promotion and maintenance; CNS: Prevention and early detection of disease; CL: Application

13. Which of the following tests is the most familiar and most readily available test for streptococcal antibodies?

1. Antistreptolysin-O test (ASOT)
2. Blood culture
3. Blood urea nitrogen (BUN)
4. Mono spot

13. 1. The ASOT is the most familiar and most readily available test for streptococcal antibodies. ASO appears in the serum approximately 10 days after the initial infection; however, there is no correlation between the degree of elevation and the severity or prognosis of the glomerulonephritis. The mono spot test is done to detect mononucleosis. Blood cultures are drawn to determine sepsis and a BUN will indicate renal function.

NP: Planning; CN: Physiological integrity; CNS: Physiological adaptation; CL: Comprehension

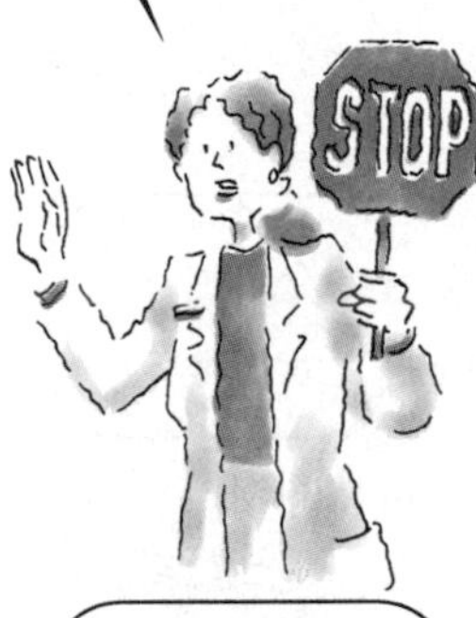

The phrase *further education* indicates that question 14 is looking for an *inaccurate* statement.
STOP

14. When teaching families of children with acute glomerulonephritis about complications, which of the following comments made by a parent would indicate to the nurse the need for further education?

1. "Dizziness is expected and I should have my child lie down."
2. "I should let the nurse know every time my child urinates."
3. "I need to ask my child if he has a headache."
4. "I shouldn't force my child to eat."

14. 1. Dizziness is a sign of encephalopathy and must be reported to the nurse. Hypertensive encephalopathy, acute cardiac decompensation, and acute renal failure are the major complications that tend to develop during the acute phase of glomerulonephritis.

NP: Implementation; CN: Physiological integrity; CNS: Reduction of risk potential; CL: Application

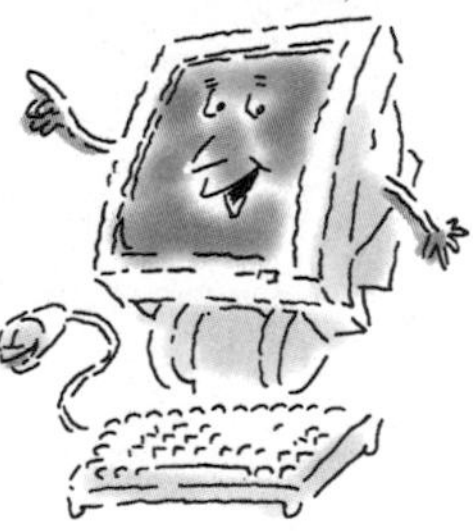

Don't a-*void* this question. You're doing great!

15. When teaching an 8-year-old child to obtain a clean-catch urine specimen, which of the following techniques should be included by the nurse?

1. Collect the specimen right after a nap.
2. Never use the first voided specimen of the day.
3. Collect the specimen at the beginning of urination.
4. You don't need to wash your perineal area before collecting the specimen.

15. 2. When collecting a clean-catch urine specimen, the first voided specimen of the day should never be used due to urinary stasis; this also applies after a nap. Washing the perineal area before collecting a specimen is very important to make sure there are no contaminants from the skin in the specimen.

NP: Implementation; CN: Health promotion and maintenance; CNS: Growth and development through the life span; CL: Application

16. Which of the following therapies should the nurse expect to incorporate into the care of the child with acute glomerulonephritis?

1. Antibiotic therapy
2. Dialysis therapy
3. Diuretic therapy
4. Play therapy

16. 4. Play therapy is an important aspect of care to help the child understand what is happening to him. Unless the child has the ability to express concerns and fears, he may have night terrors and regress in his stage of growth and development.

NP: Implementation; CN: Health promotion and maintenance; CNS: Prevention and early detection of disease; CL: Application

17. In explaining treatment for glomerulonephritis, the nurse should include which of the following statements?
1. All children who have signs of glomerulonephritis are hospitalized for approximately 1 week.
2. Parents should expect children to have a normal energy level during the acute phase.
3. Children who have normal blood pressure and a satisfactory urinary output can generally be treated at home.
4. Children with gross hematuria and significant oliguria should be brought to the primary health care provider's office about every 2 days for monitoring.

17. 3. Children who have normal blood pressure and a satisfactory urinary output can generally be treated at home. Those with gross hematuria and significant oliguria will probably be hospitalized for monitoring. Parents should expect children to have a decrease in energy levels during the acute phase of the disease.
NP: Implementation; CN: Health promotion and maintenance; CNS: Prevention and early detection of disease; CL: Comprehension

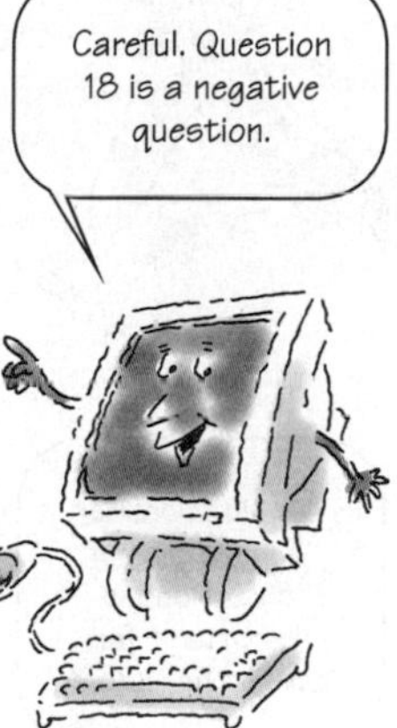

Careful. Question 18 is a negative question.

18. Which of the following reasons accounts for why bed rest isn't recommended during the acute phase of glomerulonephritis?
1. It's too difficult to keep a child on bed rest.
2. Children on bed rest lose too much muscle tone due to lack of movement.
3. Parents find enforcing bed rest causes them to feel guilty about the disease.
4. Ambulation doesn't seem to have an adverse effect on the course of the disease.

18. 4. Ambulation doesn't seem to have an adverse effect on the course of the disease once the gross hematuria, edema, hypertension, and azotemia have abated. Because they're generally listless and experience fatigue and malaise, most children voluntarily restrict their activities during the most active phase of the disease. Children on short-term bed rest don't lose muscle tone because they usually move around in the bed. Parents don't feel guilty enforcing bed rest; but they may find it challenging.
NP: Assessment; CN: Physiological integrity; CNS: Reduction of risk potential; CL: Application

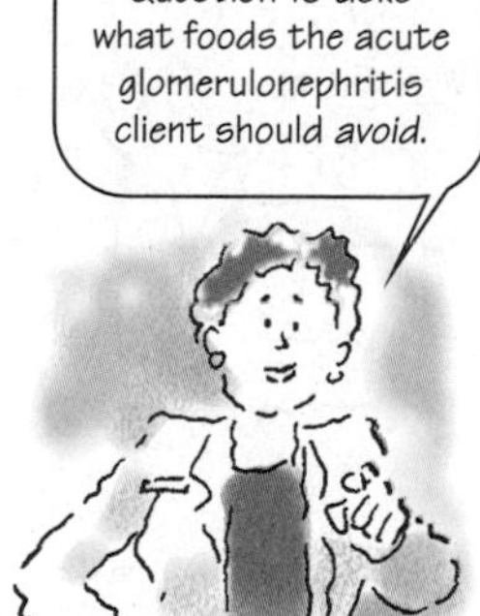

Question 19 asks what foods the acute glomerulonephritis client should avoid.

19. Which of the following foods should the nurse eliminate from the child's diet who is diagnosed with acute glomerulonephritis?
1. Turkey sandwich with mayonnaise
2. Hot dog with ketchup and mustard
3. Chocolate cake with white icing
4. Apple with peanut butter

19. 2. Foods that are high in sodium content should be eliminated from the child's diet. Snacks such as pretzels and potato chips should be discouraged. Any other foods that the child likes should be encouraged. Because hot dogs contain a great deal of sodium, they should be eliminated from the child's diet.
NP: Evaluation; CN: Physiological integrity; CNS: Basic care and comfort; CL: Application

20. The nurse understands that hypospadias refers to which of the following conditions?
1. Absence of a urethral opening
2. Penis shorter than usual for age
3. Urethral opening along dorsal surface of penis
4. Urethral opening along ventral surface of penis

20. 4. Hypospadias refers to a condition in which the urethral opening is located below the glans penis or anywhere along the ventral surface of the penile shaft.
NP: Assessment; CN: Health promotion and maintenance; CNS: Prevention and early detection of disease; CL: Knowledge

21. After the acute phase of glomerulonephritis is over, which of the following discharge instructions should the nurse include?

1. Every 6 months, a cystogram will be needed for evaluation of progress.
2. Weekly visits to the primary health care provider may be needed for evaluation.
3. It will be acceptable to keep the regular yearly check-up appointment for the next evaluation.
4. There is no need to worry about further evaluations by the primary health care provider related to this disease.

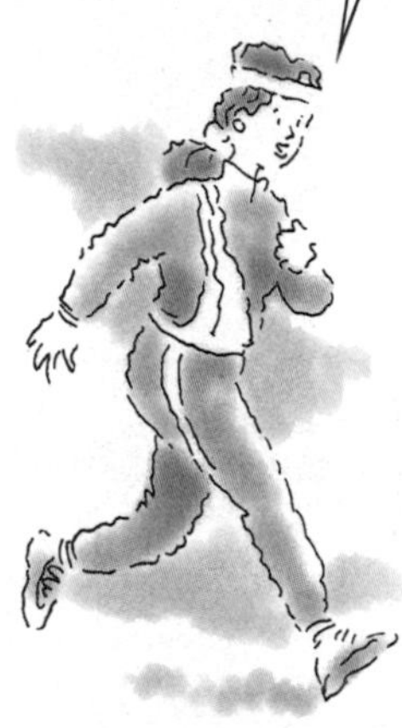
Twenty-one
questions done!
Keep plugging along!

21. 2. Weekly or monthly visits to the primary health care provider will be needed for evaluation of improvement and will usually involve the collection of a urine specimen for urinalysis. A cystogram isn't helpful in determining the progression of this disease; it's used to review the anatomic structures of the urinary tract.

NP: Implementation; CN: Physiological integrity; CNS: Reduction of risk potential; CL: Application

22. The nurse understands that chordee refers to which of the following conditions?

1. Ventral curvature of the penis
2. Dorsal curvature of the penis
3. No curvature of the penis
4. Misshapen penis

22. 1. Chordee, or ventral curvature of the penis, results from the replacement of normal skin with a fibrous band of tissue and usually accompanies more severe forms of hypospadias.

NP: Assessment; CN: Health promotion and maintenance; CNS: Prevention and early detection of disease; CL: Knowledge

23. Which of the following anomalies commonly accompanies hypospadias?

1. Undescended testicles
2. Ambiguous genitalia
3. Umbilical hernias
4. Inguinal hernias

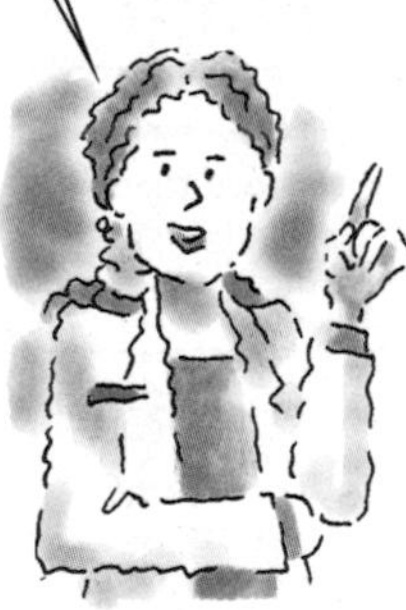
Knowing common
accompanying
conditions is
important for
taking the NCLEX.

23. 1. Because undescended testes may also be present, the small penis may appear to be an enlarged clitoris. This shouldn't be mistaken for ambiguous genitalia. If there is any doubt, more tests should be performed. Hernias don't generally accompany hypospadias.

NP: Assessment; CN: Health promotion and maintenance; CNS: Prevention and early detection of disease; CL: Knowledge

24. Which of the following reasons explains why surgical repair of a hypospadias is done as early as possible?

1. Prevent separation anxiety.
2. Prevent urinary complications.
3. Promote acceptance of hospitalization.
4. Promote development of normal body image.

24. 4. Whenever there are defects of the genitourinary tact, surgery should be performed early to promote development of a normal body image. Hypospadias doesn't put the child at a greater risk for urinary complications. A child with normal emotional development shows separation anxiety at 7 to 9 months. Within a few months, he understands the mother's permanence, and separation anxiety diminishes.

NP: Implementation; CN: Health promotion and maintenance; CNS: Prevention and early detection of disease; CL: Application

25. The nurse should counsel parents to postpone which of the following actions until after their son's hypospadias has been repaired?

1. Circumcision
2. Infant baptism
3. Getting hepatitis B vaccine
4. Checking blood for inborn errors of metabolism

25. 1. Circumcision shouldn't be performed until after the hypospadias has been repaired. The foreskin might be needed to help in the repair of the hypospadias. None of the other choices have any bearing on the repair of the hypospadias.

NP: Evaluation; CN: Health promotion and maintenance; CNS: Prevention and early detection of disease; CL: Application

NP: Nursing process CN: Client needs category CNS: Client needs subcategory CL: Cognitive level

26. Which of the following statements made about the principal objective of surgical correction by the parents of a child undergoing hypospadias repair implies a need for further teaching?
1. "The purpose is to improve the physical appearance of the genitalia for psychological reasons."
2. "The purpose is to enhance the child's ability to void in the standing position."
3. "The purpose is to decrease the chances of urinary tract infections."
4. "The purpose is to preserve a sexually adequate organ."

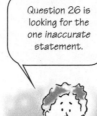

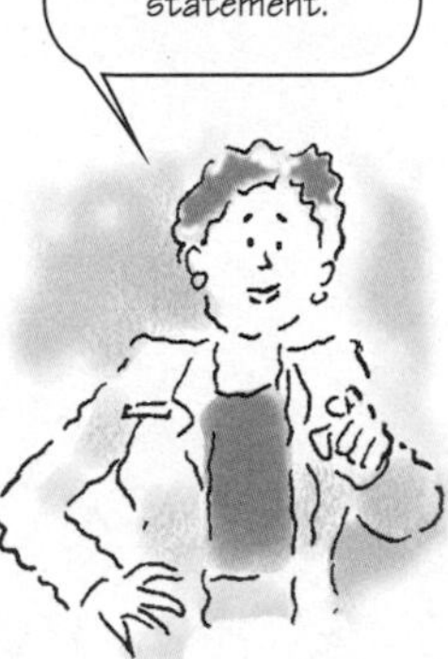

Question 26 is looking for the one inaccurate statement.

26. 3. A child with hypospadias isn't at greater risk for urinary tract infections. The principal objectives of surgical corrections are to enhance the child's ability to void in the standing position with a straight stream, to improve the physical appearance of the genitalia for psychological reasons, and to preserve a sexually adequate organ.

NP: Implementation; CN: Health promotion and maintenance; CNS: Prevention and early detection of disease; CL: Application

27. Which of the following nursing interventions should be included in the plan of care for a male infant following surgical repair of hypospadias?
1. Sterile dressing changes every 4 hours
2. Frequent inspection of the tip of the penis
3. Removal of the suprapubic catheter on the second postoperative day
4. Urethral catheterization if voiding doesn't occur over an 8-hour period

27. 2. Following hypospadias repair, a pressure dressing is applied to the penis to reduce bleeding and tissue swelling. The penile tip should then be assessed frequently for signs of circulatory impairment. The dressing around the penis shouldn't be changed as frequently as every 4 hours. The primary health care provider will determine when the suprapubic catheter will be removed. Urethral catheterization should be avoided after repair of hypospadias to prevent injury to the urethra.

NP: Assessment; CN: Physiological integrity; CNS: Basic care and comfort; CL: Application

28. When explaining to the parents the optimum time for repair of hypospadias, the nurse should indicate which of the following as the age of choice?
1. 1 week
2. 6 to 18 months
3. 2 years
4. 4 years

28. 2. The preferred time for surgical repair is 6 to 18 months of age, before the child has developed body image and castration anxiety. Surgical repair of hypospadias as early as 3 months old has been successful but with a high incidence of complications.

NP: Implementation; CN: Health promotion and maintenance; CNS: Prevention and early detection of disease; CL: Comprehension

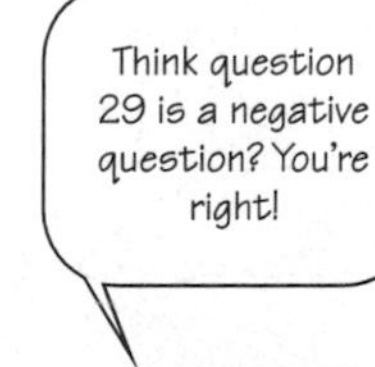

Think question 29 is a negative question? You're right!

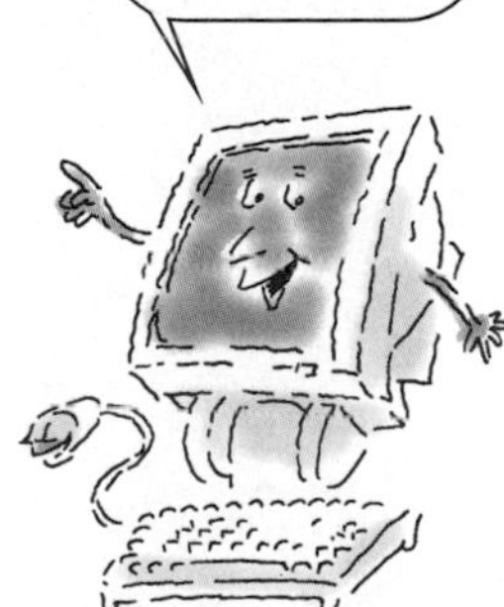

29. When providing discharge information to parents of a child with a hypospadias repair, which of the following instructions would be inappropriate?
1. Irrigation techniques, if indicated
2. Techniques for providing tub baths
3. Care for the indwelling catheter or stent
4. Techniques for avoiding kinking, twisting, or blockage of the catheter or stent

29. 2. A tub bath should be avoided to prevent infection until the stent has been removed. Parents are taught to care for the indwelling catheter or stent and irrigation techniques if indicated. They need to know how to empty the urine bag and how to avoid kinking, twisting, or blockage of the catheter or stent.

NP: Evaluation; CN: Safe, effective care environment; CNS: Management of care; CL: Analysis

30. When providing discharge instructions to parents of an older child who has had hypospadias repair, which of the following activities shouldn't be avoided?
1. Finger painting
2. Playing in sandboxes
3. Increased fluid intake
4. Playing with the family pet

30. 3. The family is advised to encourage the child to increase fluid intake. Sandboxes, straddle toys, swimming, and rough activities are avoided until allowed by the surgeon.
NP: Implementation; CN: Physiological integrity; CNS: Physiological adaptation; CL: Application

31. The mother of a neonate born with hypospadias is sharing her feelings of guilt about this anomaly with a nurse. The nurse should explain which of the following facts about the defect?
1. It occurs around the third month of fetal development.
2. It occurs around the sixth month of fetal development.
3. It's carried by an autosomal recessive gene.
4. It's hereditary.

31. 1. The defect of hypospadias occurs around the end of the third month of fetal development. Many women don't even know that they're pregnant at this time. This defect isn't hereditary, nor is it carried by an autosomal recessive gene.
NP: Implementation; CN: Health promotion and maintenance; CNS: Prevention and early detection of disease; CL: Application

32. The discovery of hypospadias is usually made by which of the following people?
1. By the primary health care provider when doing a neonatal assessment
2. By the primary health care provider, just before circumcision
3. By the mother when she sees her neonate for the first time
4. By the nurse doing the neonatal assessment

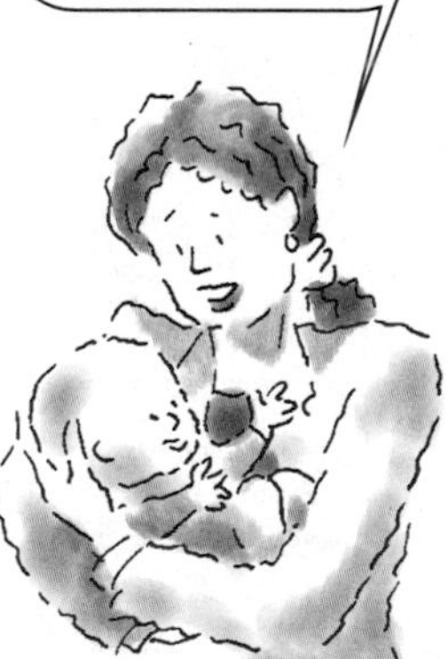

Question 32 asks you to think about the *typical* sequence of events for a neonate.

32. 4. After delivery, neonates bond with their mothers for a period of time and then are taken to the neonate nursery. The nurse who admits the neonate does a thorough assessment and should recognize hypospadias and alert the primary health care provider. The pediatrician who examines the neonate may not come to the nursery for hours after the delivery.
NP: Assessment; CN: Health promotion and maintenance; CNS: Prevention and early detection of disease; CL: Knowledge

33. A 3-year-old had a hypospadias repair yesterday; he has a suprapubic catheter in place and an I.V. Which of the following rationales is appropriate for administering propantheline bromide (Pro-Banthine) on an as-needed basis?
1. To decrease the chance of infection at the suture line
2. To decrease the number of organisms in the urine
3. To prevent bladder spasms while the catheter is present
4. To increase urine flow from the kidney to the ureters

33. 3. Propantheline bromide is an antispasmodic that works effectively on children. It isn't an antibiotic and therefore won't decrease the chance of infection or the number of organisms in the urine. The drug has no diuretic effect and won't increase urine flow.
NP: Planning; CN: Physiological integrity; CNS: Pharmacological and parenteral therapies; CL: Application

34. Which of the following interventions by the nurse would be most helpful when discussing hypospadias with the parents of an infant with this defect?

1. Refer the parents to a counselor.
2. Be there to listen to the parents' concerns.
3. Notify the primary health care provider, and have him talk to the parents.
4. Suggest a support group of other parents who have gone through this experience.

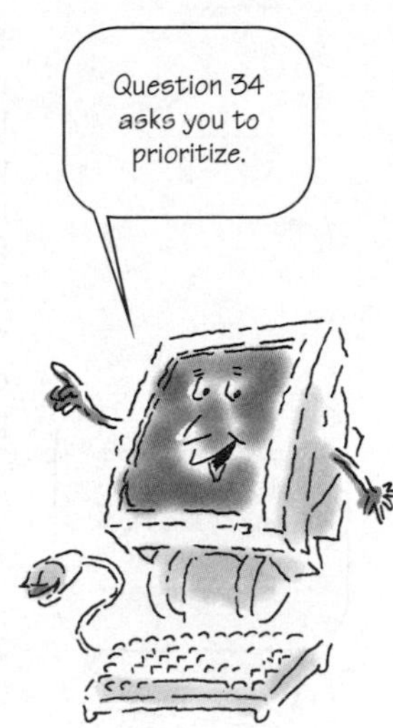

Question 34 asks you to prioritize.

34. 2. The nurse must recognize that parents are going to grieve the loss of the normal child when they have a neonate born with a birth defect. Initially, the parents need to have a nurse who will listen to their concerns for their neonate's health. Suggesting a support group or referring the parents to a counselor might be good actions, but not initially. The primary health care provider will need to spend time with the parents but, again, the nurse is in the best position to allow the parents to vent their grief and anger.

NP: Evaluation; CN: Psychosocial integrity; CNS: Coping and adaptation; CL: Application

35. The nurse should understand that hypospadias defects take the greatest emotional toll on which of the following persons?

1. The father
2. The mother
3. The grandfather
4. The grandmother

35. 1. Because the penis is involved, studies have shown that fathers have a great deal of difficulty dealing with a birth defect like hypospadias.

NP: Assessment; CN: Psychosocial integrity; CNS: Coping and adaptation; CL: Knowledge

36. The difference between hypospadias and epispadias is defined by which of the following characteristics?

1. Epispadias defects can only occur in males.
2. The difference between the defects is the length of the urethra.
3. Hypospadias is an abnormal opening on the ventral side of the penis; epispadias is an abnormal opening on the dorsal side.
4. Hypospadias is an abnormal opening on the dorsal side of the penis; epispadias is an abnormal opening on the ventral side.

36. 3. Hypospadias results from the incomplete closure of the urethral folds along the ventral surface of the developing penis. Epispadias results when the urinary meatus is on the dorsal surface of the penis. Epispadias defects can occur in males and females. The difference is where the opening of the urinary meatus is located, not the length of the urethra.

NP: Assessment; CN: Health promotion and maintenance; CNS: Prevention and early detection of disease; CL: Comprehension

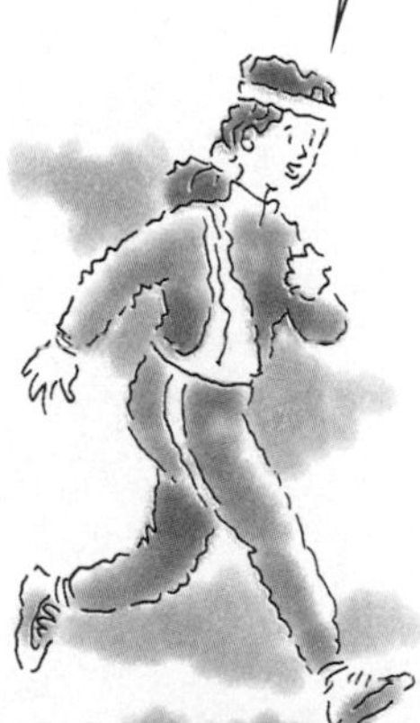

Don't *alter* your course. You're on the road to success!

37. Which of the following nursing diagnoses would be most appropriate for a client with hypospadias?

1. Deficient fluid volume
2. Impaired urinary elimination
3. Delayed growth and development
4. Risk for infection

37. 2. The most appropriate diagnosis for a client with hypospadias is *Impaired urinary elimination.* A client with hypospadias should have no problems with the ingestion of fluids. The child's growth and development isn't affected with this defect, and he doesn't have any problem with infection until possibly after a repair of the hypospadias is performed.

NP: Planning; CN: Health promotion and maintenance; CNS: Prevention and early detection of disease CL: Analysis

38. When a nurse is teaching the parent how to care for the penis after a hypospadias repair with a skin graft, which of the following statements made by the parent would indicate the need for further teaching?

1. "My infant won't be able to take baths until healing has occurred."
2. "I will change the dressing around the penis daily."
3. "I will make sure I change my infant's diaper often."
4. "If there is a color change in the penis, I will notify my primary care provider."

38. 2. Dressing changes after a hypospadias repair with a skin graft are generally performed by the primary health care provider and aren't performed every day because the skin graft needs time to heal and adhere to the penis. Changing the infant's diapers often helps keep the penis dry. Baths aren't given until postoperative healing has taken place. If the penis color changes, it might be evidence of circulation problems and should be reported.

NP: Evaluation; CN: Psychosocial integrity; CNS: Psychosocial adaptation; CL: Analysis

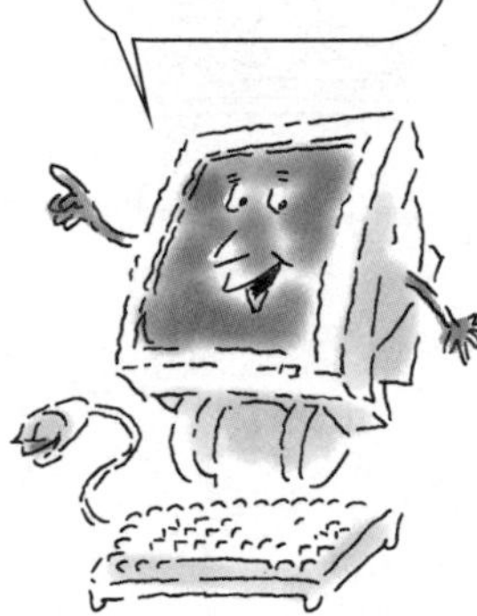

Lots of negative questions here. Remember to look for *incorrect* statements.

39. The nurse is preparing the parents of an infant with hypospadias for surgery. Which of the following statements made by the parents would indicate the need for further teaching?

1. "Skin grafting might be involved in my infant's repair."
2. "After surgery, my infant's penis will look perfectly normal."
3. "Surgical repair may need to be performed in several stages."
4. "My infant will probably be in some pain after the surgery and might need to take some medication for relief."

39. 2. It's important to stress to the parents that, even after a repair of hypospadias, the outcome isn't a completely "normal-looking" penis. The goals of surgery are to allow the child to void from the tip of his penis, void with a straight stream, and stand up while voiding.

NP: Evaluation; CN: Psychosocial integrity; CNS: Coping and adaptation; CL: Application

40. Which of the following assessment data collected by the nurse would indicate to the primary care provider the need for a staged repair of a hypospadias rather than a single repair?

1. There is chordee present with the hypospadias.
2. The urinary meatus opens between the scrotum.
3. The urinary meatus is just below the tip of the penis.
4. The infant has been circumcised before the defect was discovered.

40. 2. Increased surgical experience and improvements in technique have reduced the number of staged procedures applied to hypospadias defects; however, a staged procedure is indicated in particularly severe defects with marked deficits of available skin for mobilization of flaps. If an infant has been circumcised but has a relatively minor hypospadias, the repair can still occur in one stage. Having a chordee present doesn't require a staged hypospadias repair.

NP: Assessment; CN: Physiological integrity; CNS: Physiological adaptation; CL: Analysis

41. A nurse should understand that prevention of pelvic inflammatory disease (PID) in adolescents is important due to which of the following reasons?
1. PID is easily prevented by proper personal hygiene.
2. PID is easily prevented by compliance with any form of contraception.
3. PID can have devastating effects on the reproductive tract of affected adolescents.
4. PID can cause life-threatening defects in infants born to affected adolescents.

41. 3. Long-term complications of PID include abscess formation in the fallopian tubes and adhesion formation leading to increased risk for ectopic pregnancy or infertility. It isn't prevented by proper personal hygiene or any form of contraception; some forms of contraception such as the male or female condom do help to decrease the incidence of it.
NP: Evaluation; CN: Health promotion and maintenance; CNS: Prevention and early detection of disease; CL: Comprehension

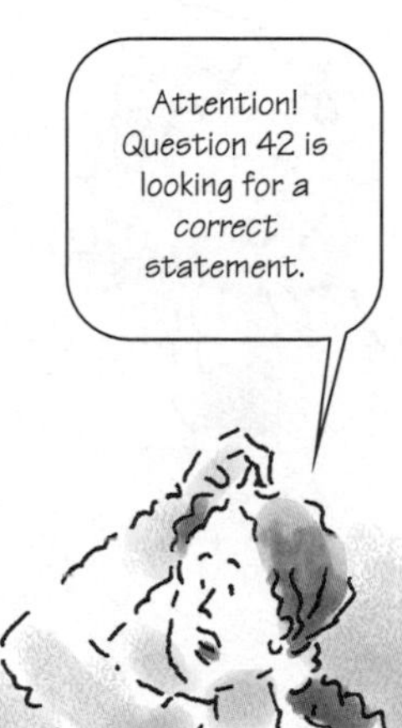

Attention! Question 42 is looking for a correct statement.

42. After the nurse has completed discharge teaching, which of the following statements made by the client treated for a sexually transmitted disease would indicate that discharge instructions were understood?
1. "I don't need those condoms because I'm not allergic to penicillin and I'll come for a shot at the first sign of infection."
2. "I will notify my sex partners and not have unprotected sex from now on."
3. "I will be careful not to have intercourse with someone who isn't clean."
4. "If you're going to get it, you're going to get it."

42. 2. Goal achievement is indicated by the client's ability to describe preventive behaviors and health practices. The other options indicate that the client doesn't understand the need to take preventive measures.
NP: Evaluation; CN: Health promotion and maintenance; CNS: Prevention and early detection of disease; CL: Analysis

43. Which of the following statements regarding chlamydial infections is correct?
1. The treatment of choice is oral penicillin.
2. The treatment of choice is nystatin or miconazole.
3. Clinical manifestations include dysuria and urethral itching in males.
4. Clinical manifestations include small, painful vesicles on genital areas.

43. 3. Clinical manifestations of chlamydia include meatal erythema, tenderness, itching, dysuria, and urethral discharge in the male and mucopurulent cervical exudate with erythema, edema, and congestion in the female. The treatment of choice is doxycycline or azithromycin.
NP: Implementation; CN: Health promotion and maintenance; CNS: Prevention and early detection of disease; CL: Application

44. Before a client with syphilis can be treated, the nurse must determine which of the following factors?
1. Portal of entry
2. Size of the chancre
3. Names of sexual contacts
4. Existence of medication allergies

44. 4. The treatment of choice for syphilis is penicillin; clients allergic to penicillin must be given another antibiotic. The other choices aren't necessary before treatment can begin.
NP: Assessment; CN: Health promotion and maintenance; CNS: Prevention and early detection of disease; CL: Comprehension

45. Which of the following techniques should the nurse consider when she is discussing sex and sexual activities with adolescents?

1. Break down all the information into scientific terminology.
2. Refer the adolescent to their parents for sexual information.
3. Only answer questions that are asked; don't present any other content.
4. Present sexual information using the proper terminology and in a straightforward manner.

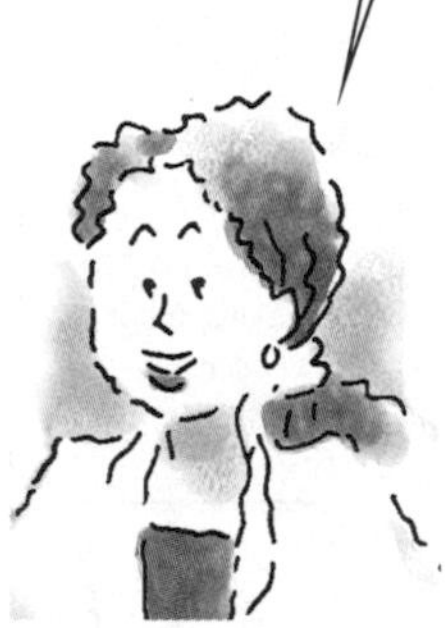

The NCLEX tests your ability to teach clients at different life-stages.

45. 4. Although many adolescents have received sex education from parents and school throughout childhood, they aren't always adequately prepared for the impact of puberty. A large portion of their knowledge is acquired from peers, television, movies, and magazines. Consequently, much of the sex information they have is incomplete, inaccurate, riddled with cultural and moral values, and not very helpful. The public perceives nurses as having authoritative information and being willing to take time with parents. To be effective teachers, nurses need to be honest and open with sexual information.
NP: Implementation; CN: Health promotion and maintenance; CNS: Growth and development through the life span; CL: Application

46. Without proper treatment, anogenital warts caused by the human papillomavirus (HPV) increases the risk of which of the following illnesses in adolescent females?

1. Gonorrhea
2. Cervical cancer
3. Chlamydial infections
4. Urinary tract infections

46. 2. All external lesions are treated because of concern regarding the relationship of HPV to cancer. HPV doesn't increase the risk for gonorrhea, chlamydia, or urinary tract infections.
NP: Implementation; CN: Health promotion and maintenance; CNS: Prevention and early detection of disease; CL: Application

47. Which of the following statements should the nurse include when teaching an adolescent about gonorrhea?

1. It's caused by *Treponema pallidum.*
2. Treatment of sexual partners is an essential part of treatment.
3. It's most often treated by multidose administration of penicillin.
4. It may be contracted through contact with a contaminated toilet bowl.

47. 2. Adolescents should be taught that treatment is needed for all sexual partners. The medication of choice is a single dose of I.M. ceftriaxone sodium (Rocephin) in males and a single oral dose of cefixime (Suprax) in females. Gonorrhea can't be contracted from a contaminated toilet bowl.
NP: Implementation; CN: Health promotion and maintenance; CNS: Prevention and early detection of disease; CL: Application

48. When planning sex education and contraceptive teaching for adolescents, which of the following factors should the nurse consider?

1. Neither sexual activity nor contraception requires planning.
2. Most teenagers today are knowledgeable about reproduction.
3. Most teenagers use pregnancy as a way to rebel against their parents.
4. Most teenagers are open about contraception but inconsistently use birth control.

48. 4. Most teenagers today are open about discussing contraception and sexuality, but may get caught up in the heat of sexuality and forget about birth control measures. A good deal of the information adolescents have related to reproduction and sexuality may have come from their peers and may not be very reliable.
NP: Planning; CN: Physiological integrity; CNS: Reduction of risk potential; CL: Evaluation

49. A sexually active teenager seeks counseling from the school nurse about prevention of sexually transmitted diseases (STDs). Which of the following contraceptive measures should the nurse recommend?

1. Rhythm method
2. Withdrawal method
3. Prophylactic antibiotic use
4. Condom and spermicide use

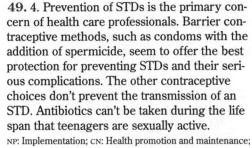

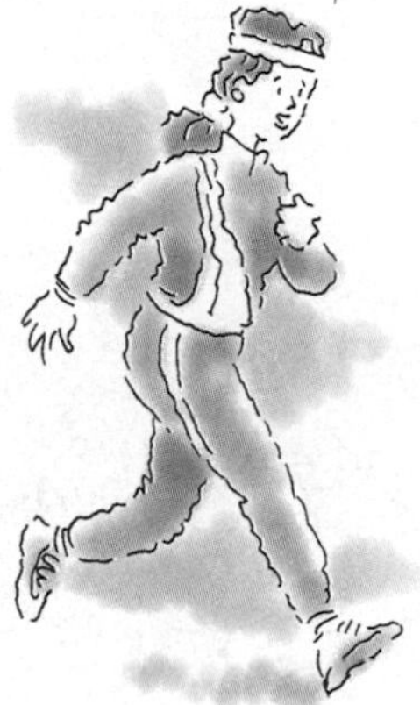

Nice work! You've finished nearly 50 questions already!

49. 4. Prevention of STDs is the primary concern of health care professionals. Barrier contraceptive methods, such as condoms with the addition of spermicide, seem to offer the best protection for preventing STDs and their serious complications. The other contraceptive choices don't prevent the transmission of an STD. Antibiotics can't be taken during the life span that teenagers are sexually active.

NP: Implementation; CN: Health promotion and maintenance; CNS: Prevention and early detection of disease; CL: Application

50. The nurse understands that which of the following developmental rationales explains risk-taking behavior in adolescents?

1. Adolescents are concrete thinkers and concentrate only on what is happening at the time.
2. Belief in their own invulnerability persuades adolescents that they can take risks safely.
3. Risk of parents' anger and disappointment usually deters adolescents from risky behavior.
4. Peer pressure usually doesn't play an important part in a adolescent's decision to become sexually active.

50. 2. Understanding the growth and development of an adolescent helps the nurse see that they feel they're invulnerable. Peer pressure plays an important role in risk-taking behaviors; more so than fear of parents' anger or disappointment. Adolescents think about the future and can formally operate in their thought process.

NP: Evaluation; CN: Health promotion and maintenance; CNS: Growth and development through the life span; CL: Analysis

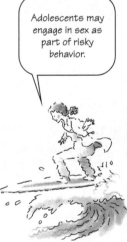

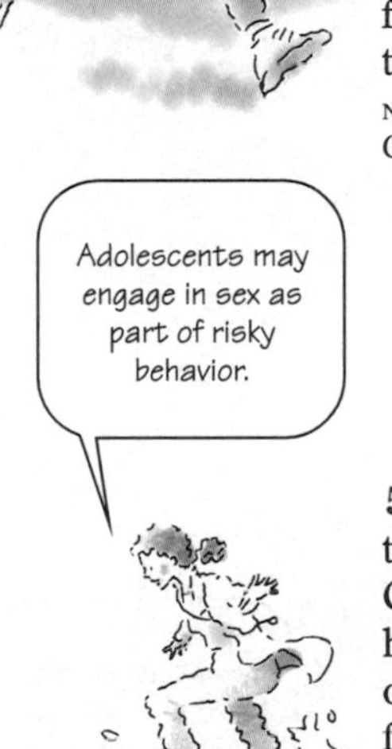

51. Statistics about sexually transmitted diseases (STDs) may not be reliable for which of the following reasons?

1. Most adolescents seek out treatment for their STD.
2. Adolescents are usually honest with their parents about their sexual behavior.
3. All sexually transmitted diseases must be reported to the Centers for Disease Control and Prevention (CDC).
4. Chlamydial infections and human papillomavirus (HPV) infections aren't required to be reported to the CDC.

51. 4. Chlamydial infections and HPV infections aren't required to be reported to the CDC. Most teenagers are afraid to seek out health care for sexual diseases or are unaware of the signs and symptoms of STDs. Teenagers find this a very difficult topic to discuss with their parents and will usually seek out a peer or another adult to obtain information.

NP: Evaluation; CN: Safe, effective care environment; CNS: Safety and infection control; CL: Application

52. It's important for the nurse to include which of the following statements in discharge education for the client who's taking metronidazole (Flagyl) to treat trichomoniasis?

1. Sexual intercourse should stop.
2. Alcohol shouldn't be consumed.
3. Milk products should be avoided.
4. Exposure to sunlight should be limited.

52. 2. While taking metronidazole to treat trichomoniasis, clients shouldn't consume alcohol for at least 48 hours following the last dose. The other choices have no effect on the client while taking this medication.

NP: Implementation; CN: Physiological integrity; CNS: Pharmacological and parenteral therapies; CL: Application

53. Which of the following statements by an adolescent would alert the nurse that more education about sexually transmitted diseases (STDs) is needed?

1. "You always know when you've got gonorrhea."
2. "The most common STD in kids my age is chlamydia infection."
3. "Most of the girls who have *Chlamydia* don't even know it."
4. "If you have symptoms of gonorrhea, they can show up a day or a couple of weeks after you got the infection to begin with."

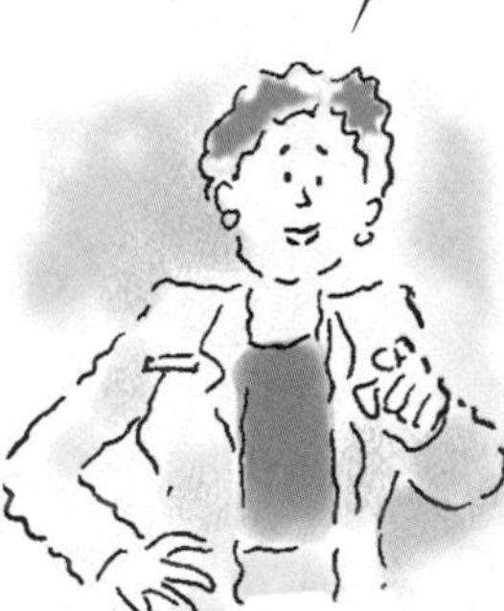

The phrase *more education is needed* indicates that question 53 asks for an incorrect statement.

53. 1. Gonorrhea can occur with or without symptoms. There are four main forms of the disease: asymptomatic, uncomplicated symptomatic, complicated symptomatic, and disseminated disease. All of the other statements are accurate.

NP: Assessment; CN: Health promotion and maintenance; CNS: Prevention and early detection of disease; CL: Application

54. Which of the following assessments describes the method of prevention of sexually transmitted diseases (STDs) by avoiding exposure?

1. The least accepted and most difficult approach
2. The least expensive and most effective approach
3. The most expensive and least effective approach
4. The most difficult and most time-consuming approach

54. 2. Primary prevention of STDs by avoiding exposure is the least expensive and most effective approach. The nurse can play a role in offering this education to young people before they initiate sexual intercourse.

NP: Planning; CN: Safe, effective care environment; CNS: Safety and infection control; CL: Application

55. Which of the following clients would the nurse consider at greater risk for developing acquired immunodeficiency syndrome (AIDS)?

1. Clients who live in crowded housing with poor ventilation
2. A young sexually active client with multiple partners
3. Adolescents who are homeless who live in shelters
4. A young sexually active client with one partner

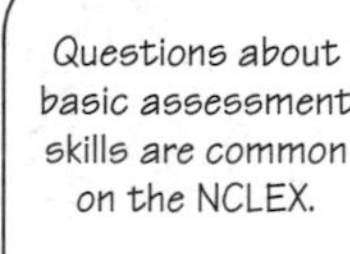

Questions about basic assessment skills are common on the NCLEX.

55. 2. The younger the client when sexual activity begins, the higher the incidence of HIV and AIDS. Also, the more sexual partners, the higher the incidence. Neither crowded living environments nor homeless environments by themselves lead to an increase in the incidence of AIDS.

NP: Assessment; CN: Health promotion and maintenance; CNS: Prevention and early detection of disease; CL: Knowledge

56. When assessing an adolescent for pelvic inflammatory disease (PID), which of the following signs and symptoms should the nurse expect to see?

1. A hard, painless, red defined lesion
2. Small vesicles on genital area with itching
3. Cervical discharge with redness and edema
4. Lower abdominal pain and urinary tract symptoms

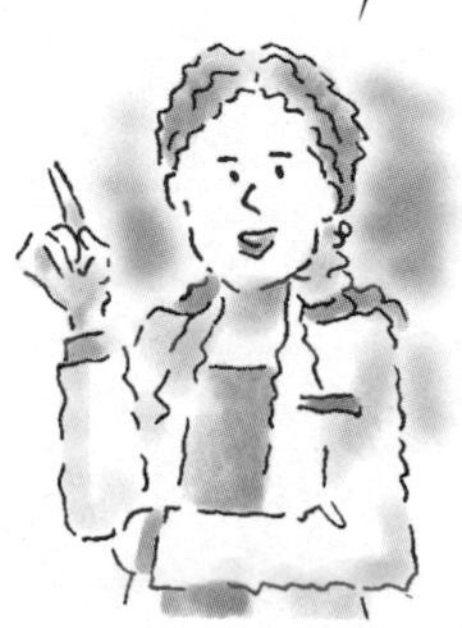

56. 4. PID is an infection of the upper female genital tract most commonly caused by sexually transmitted diseases. Presenting symptoms in the adolescent may be generalized, with fever, abdominal pain, urinary tract symptoms, and vague influenza-like symptoms. Small vesicles on the genital area with itching indicates herpes genitalis. Cervical discharge with redness and edema indicates chlamydia. A hard, painless, red defined lesion indicates syphilis.

NP: Assessment; CN: Health promotion and maintenance; CNS: Prevention and early detection of disease; CL: Application

57. The nurse should include which of the following facts when teaching an adolescent group about the human immunodeficiency virus (HIV)?

1. The incidence of HIV in the adolescent population has declined since 1995.
2. The virus can be spread through many routes, including sexual contact.
3. Knowledge about HIV spread and transmission has led to a decrease in the spread of the virus among adolescents.
4. About 50% of all new HIV infections in the U.S. occurs in people under age 22.

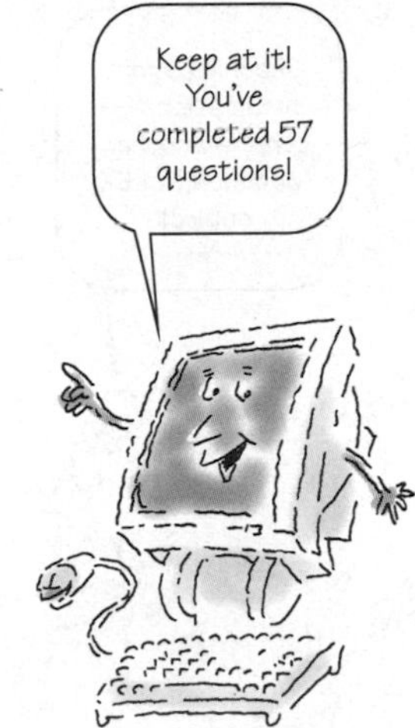
Keep at it!
You've
completed 57
questions!

57. 2. HIV can be spread through many routes, including sexual contact and contact with infected blood or other body fluids. The incidence of HIV in the adolescent population has *increased* since 1995, even though more information about the virus is targeted to reach the adolescent population. Only about 25% of all new HIV infections in the U.S. occurs in people under age 22.

NP: Implementation; CN: Health promotion and maintenance; CNS: Prevention and early detection of disease; CL: Application

58. When planning a program to teach adolescents about acquired immunodeficiency syndrome (AIDS), which of the following actions might lead to better success of the program?

1. Surveying the community to evaluate the level of education
2. Obtaining peer educators to provide information about AIDS
3. Setting up clinics in community centers and having condoms readily available
4. Having primary health care providers host workshops in community centers

58. 2. Peer education programs have noted that teens are more likely to ask questions of peer educators than of adults and that peer education can change personal attitudes and the perception of risk for human immunodeficiency virus infection. The other approaches would be helpful, but not necessarily make the outreach program more successful.

NP: Evaluation; CN: Safe, effective care environment; CNS: Management of care; CL: Analysis

59. Which of the following statements should the nurse include when teaching adolescents about syphilis?

1. Syphilis is rarely transmitted sexually.
2. There is no known cure or treatment for syphilis.
3. The viability of the organism outside the body is long.
4. Affected persons are most infectious during the first year.

59. 4. Affected persons are most infectious during the first year of the disease. Syphilis is treated with penicillin or doxycycline. About 95% of the cases of syphilis are sexually transmitted. Syphilis can be transmitted to a fetus. The viability of the organism outside the body is short.

NP: Implementation; CN: Health promotion and maintenance; CNS: Prevention and early detection of disease; CL: Knowledge

60. In teaching a group of parents about monitoring for urinary tract infection (UTI) in preschoolers, which of the following symptoms would indicate that a child should be evaluated?

1. Voids only twice in any 6-hour period
2. Exhibits incontinence after being toilet trained
3. Has difficulty sitting still for more than a 30-minute period of time
4. Urine smells strongly of ammonia after standing for more than 2 hours

60. 2. A child who exhibits incontinence after being toilet trained should be evaluated for UTI. Most urine smells strongly of ammonia after standing for more than 2 hours, so this doesn't necessarily indicate UTI. The other options aren't reasons for parents to suspect problems with their child's urinary system.

NP: Evaluation; CN: Safe, effective care environment; CNS: Management of care; CL: Application

61. Which of the following instructions should the nurse include in the teaching plan for a client receiving co-trimoxazole (Septra) for a repeated urinary tract infection with *Escherichia coli?*

1. "For the drug to be effective, keep your urine acidic by drinking at least a quart of cranberry juice a day."
2. "Take the medication for 10 days even if your symptoms improve in a few days."
3. "Return to the clinic in 3 days for another urine culture."
4. "Take two of the pills a day now, but keep the rest of the pills to take if the symptoms reappear within 2 weeks."

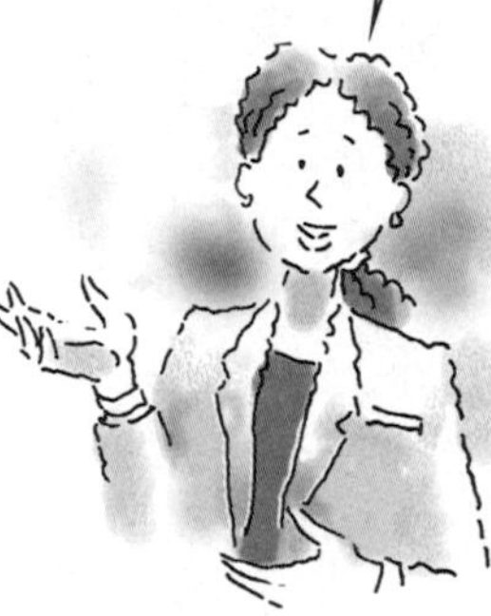

Teaching about medications — that's another common NCLEX subject.

61. 2. Discharge instructions for clients receiving an anti-infective medication should include taking all of the prescribed medication for the prescribed time. The child won't need to have a culture repeated until the medication is completed. Drinking highly acidic juices such as cranberry juice may help maintain urinary health, but won't get rid of an already present infection.

NP: Planning; CN: Physiological integrity; CNS: Pharmacological and parenteral therapies; CL: Application

62. The nurse should include which of the following facts when teaching parents about handling a child with recurrent urinary infection?

1. Antibiotics should be discontinued 48 hours after symptoms subside.
2. Recurrent symptoms should be treated by renewing the antibiotic prescription.
3. Complicated urinary tract infections are related to poor perineal hygiene practice.
4. Follow-up urine cultures are necessary to detect recurrent infections and antibiotic effectiveness.

62. 4. A routine follow-up urine specimen is usually obtained 2 or 3 days after the completion of the antibiotic treatment. All of the antibiotic should be taken as ordered and not stopped when symptoms disappear. If recurrent symptoms appear, a urine culture should be obtained to see if the infection is resistant to antibiotics. Simple, not complicated, urinary tract infections are generally caused by poor perineal hygiene.

NP: Implementation; CN: Health promotion and maintenance; CNS: Prevention and early detection of disease; CL: Application

63. When reviewing the results of a clean-voided urine specimen, which of the following results would indicate to the nurse that the child may have a urinary tract infection (UTI)?

1. A specific gravity of 1.020
2. Cloudy color without odor
3. A large amount of casts present
4. 100,000 bacterial colonies per milliliter

63. 4. The diagnosis of UTI is determined by the detection of bacteria in the urine. Infected urine usually contains more than 100,000 colonies/ml, usually of a single organism. The urine is usually cloudy, hazy, and may have strands of mucus. It also has a foul, fishy odor even when fresh. Casts and increased specific gravity aren't specific to UTI.

NP: Evaluation; CN: Health promotion and maintenance; CNS: Prevention and early detection of disease; CL: Knowledge

64. Which of the following factors should the nurse recognize as predisposing the urinary tract to infections in males or females?

1. Increased fluid intake
2. Short urethra in young females
3. Ingestion of highly acidic juices
4. Frequent emptying of the bladder

64. 2. The urethra is much shorter in females than in males (2 cm in young females, 4 cm in mature women, 20 cm in the adult male). Increased fluid intake would help flush the urinary tract system and frequent emptying of the bladder would decrease the risk of urinary tract infection. Drinking highly acidic juices such as cranberry juice may help maintain urinary health.

NP: Assessment; CN: Health promotion and maintenance; CNS: Prevention and early detection of disease; CL: Comprehension

65. When assessing a child with vesicoureteral reflux, the nurse should understand that this client is at risk for developing which of the following complications?

1. Glomerulonephritis
2. Hemolytic uremia syndrome
3. Nephrotic syndrome
4. Renal infection

65. 4. Reflux of urine into the ureters and then back into the bladder after voiding sets up the client for a urinary tract infection. This can lead to renal damage due to scarring of the parenchyma. Glomerulonephritis is an autoimmune reaction to a beta-hemolytic strep infection. Eighty percent of nephrotic syndrome cases are idiopathic. Hemolytic uremia syndrome may be the result of genetic factors. Bladder infection can lead to renal infections when infected urine refluxes from the bladder into the kidney.

NP: Assessment; CN: Health promotion and maintenance; CNS: Prevention and early detection of disease; CL: Knowledge

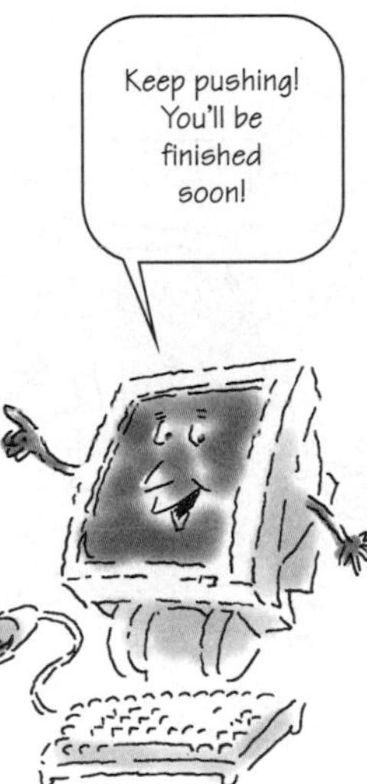
Keep pushing! You'll be finished soon!

66. Nurses should understand that which of the following factors contributes to the increased incidence of urinary tract infections (UTIs) in girls?

1. Vaginal secretions are too acidic.
2. Girls aren't protected by circumcision.
3. The urethra is in close proximity to the anus.
4. Girls touch their genitalia more often than boys do.

66. 3. Girls are especially at risk for bacterial invasion of the urinary tract because of basic anatomical differences; the urethra is short and there is close proximity to the anus. Vaginal secretions are normally acidic and this decreases the risk of infection. There is no documented research that supports that girls touch their genitalia more often than boys do. Circumcision doesn't protect girls *or* boys from UTIs.

NP: Evaluation; CN: Health promotion and maintenance; CNS: Growth and development through the life span; CL: Knowledge

67. A child has been sent to the school nurse for wetting her pants three times in the past 2 days. The nurse should recommend that this child be evaluated for which of the following complications?

1. School phobia
2. Emotional trauma
3. Urinary tract infection
4. Structural defect of the urinary tract

67. 3. Frequent urinary incontinence should be evaluated by the primary health care provider, with the first action being checking the urine for infection. Children exhibit signs of school phobia by complaining of an ailment before school starts and getting better after they're allowed to miss school. After infection, structural defect, and diabetes mellitus have been ruled out, emotional trauma should be investigated.

NP: Implementation; CN: Health promotion and maintenance; CNS: Growth and development through the life span; CL: Application

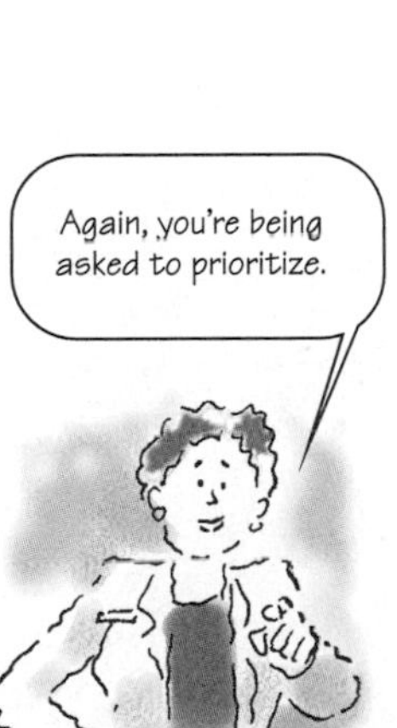
Again, you're being asked to prioritize.

68. When the nurse is teaching parents of children about recurrent urinary tract infections (UTIs), which of the following goals should be included as the most important?

1. Detection
2. Education
3. Prevention
4. Treatment

68. 3. Prevention is the most important goal in primary and recurrent UTIs; most preventive measures are simple, ordinary hygienic habits that should be a routine part of daily care. Treatment, detection, and education are all important, but not the most important goal.

NP: Implementation; CN: Physiological integrity; CNS: Reduction of risk potential; CL: Analysis

69. Which of the following interventions should a nurse recommend to parents of young girls to help prevent urinary tract infections (UTIs)?

1. Limit bathing as much as possible.
2. Increase fluids and decrease salt intake.
3. Have the child wear cotton underpants.
4. Have the child clean her perineum from back to front.

69. 3. Cotton is a more breathable fabric and allows for dampness to be absorbed from the perineum. Increasing fluids would be helpful, but decreasing salt isn't necessary. Bathing shouldn't be limited; however, the use of bubble bath or whirlpool baths should. However, if the child has frequent UTIs, taking a bath should be discouraged and taking a shower encouraged. The perineum should always be cleaned from front to back.

NP: Implementation; CN: Health promotion and maintenance; CNS: Prevention and early detection of disease; CL: Knowledge

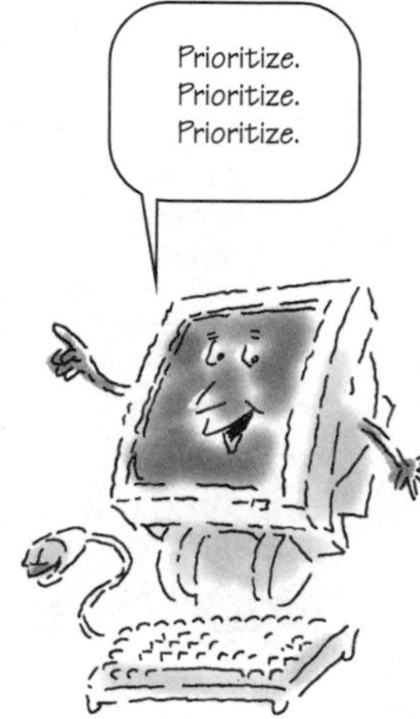
Prioritize.
Prioritize.
Prioritize.

70. The nurse understands that which of the following characteristics is the single most important factor influencing the occurrence of urinary tract infections (UTIs)?

1. Urinary stasis
2. Frequency of baths
3. Uncircumcised males
4. Amount of fluid intake

70. 1. Ordinarily, urine is sterile. However, at 98.6° F, it provides an excellent culture medium. Under normal conditions, the act of completely and repeatedly emptying the bladder flushes away any organisms before they have an opportunity to multiply and invade surrounding tissue. There is an increased incidence of UTI in uncircumcised infants under one year but not after that age. Baths and fluid intake are factors in the development of UTIs, but aren't the most important.

NP: Assessment; CN: Physiological integrity; CNS: Reduction of risk potential; CL: Application

71. When evaluating infants and young toddlers for signs of urinary tract infections (UTIs), the nurse should demonstrate knowledge that which of the following symptoms would be most common?

1. Abdominal pain
2. Feeding problems
3. Frequency
4. Urgency

71. 2. In infants and children less than 2 years old, the signs are characteristically nonspecific, and feeding problems are usually the first indication. Symptoms more nearly resemble GI tract disorders. Abdominal pain, urgency, and frequency are signs that would be observed in the older child with a UTI.

NP: Evaluation; CN: Physiological integrity; CNS: Physiological adaptation; CL: Knowledge

72. When obtaining a urine specimen for culture and sensitivity, the nurse should understand that which of the following methods of collection is best?

1. Bagged urine specimen
2. Clean-catch urine specimen
3. First-voided urine specimen
4. Catheterized urine specimen

72. 4. The most accurate tests of bacterial content are suprapubic aspiration (for children less than 2 years old) and properly performed bladder catheterization. The other methods of obtaining a specimen have a high incidence of contamination not related to infection.

NP: Implementation; CN: Physiological integrity; CNS: Basic care and comfort; CL: Application

73. After collecting a urine specimen, which of the following actions by the nurse is the most appropriate?

1. Take the specimen to the laboratory immediately
2. Send the specimen to the laboratory on the scheduled run
3. Take the specimen to the laboratory on the nurse's next break
4. Keep the specimen in the refrigerator until it can be taken to the laboratory

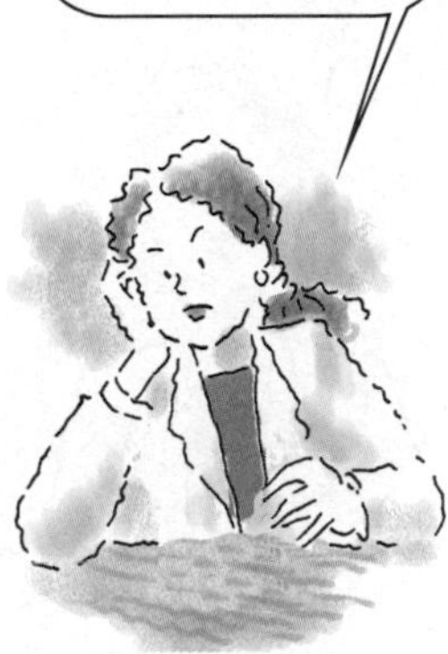

More than one answer for question 73 may seem correct. Choose the best answer.

73. 1. Care of urine specimens obtained for culture is an important nursing aspect related to diagnosis. Specimens should be taken to the laboratory for culture immediately. If the culture is delayed, the specimen can be placed in the refrigerator, but storage can result in a loss of formed elements, such as blood cells and casts.

NP: Implementation; CN: Physiological integrity; CNS: Basic care and comfort; CL: Application

74. When teaching parents of a child with a urinary tract infection (UTI) about fluid intake, which of the following statements by a parent would indicate the need for further teaching?

1. "I should encourage my child to drink about 50 ml per pound of body weight daily."
2. "Clear liquids should be the primary liquids that my child should drink."
3. "I should offer my child carbonated beverages about every 2 hours."
4. "My child should avoid drinking caffeinated beverages."

74. 3. Caffeinated or carbonated beverages are avoided because of their potentially irritating effect on the bladder mucosa. Adequate fluid intake is always indicated during an acute UTI. It is recommended that a person drink approximately 50 ml/lb of body weight daily. The client should primarily drink clear liquids.

NP: Evaluation; CN: Physiological integrity; CNS: Basic care and comfort; CL: Analysis

75. Which of the following treatments should the nurse anticipate in a child who has a history of recurrent urinary tract infections (UTIs)?

1. Frequent catheterizations
2. Prophylactic antibiotics
3. Limited activities
4. Surgical intervention

75. 2. Children who experience recurrent UTIs may require antibiotic therapy for months or years. Recurrent UTIs would be investigated for anatomic abnormalities and surgical intervention may be indicated, but the client would also be placed on antibiotics before the tests. The child's activities aren't limited, and frequent catheterization predisposes a child to infection.

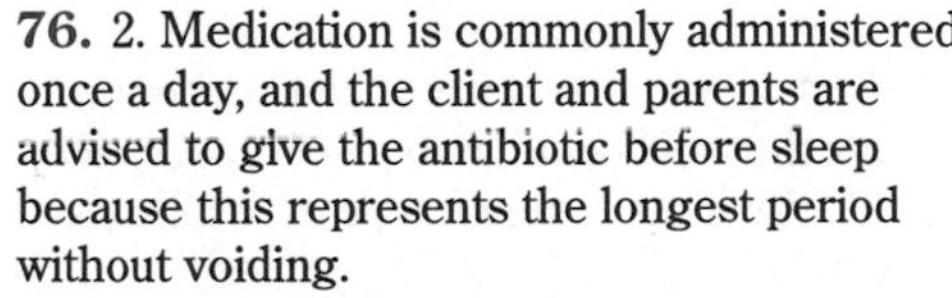

NP: Planning; CN: Physiological integrity; CNS: Pharmacological and parenteral therapies; CL: Application

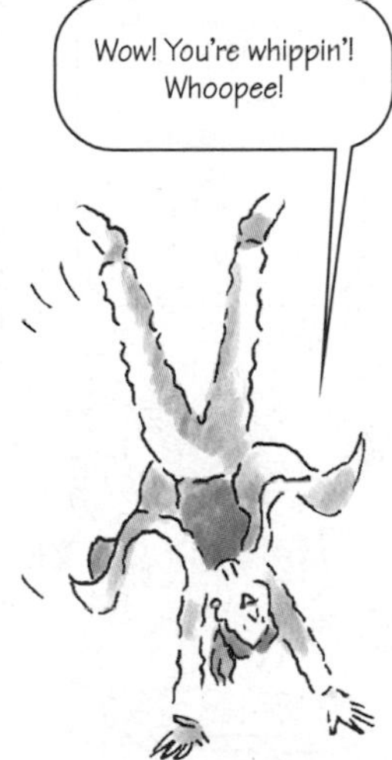

Wow! You're whippin'! Whoopee!

76. When teaching parents about giving medications to children for recurrent urinary tract infections (UTIs), which of the following instructions should be included?

1. The medication should be given first thing in the morning.
2. The medication should be given right before bedtime.
3. The medication is generally given four times a day.
4. It doesn't matter when the medication is given.

76. 2. Medication is commonly administered once a day, and the client and parents are advised to give the antibiotic before sleep because this represents the longest period without voiding.

NP: Implementation; CN: Physiological integrity; CNS: Pharmacological and parenteral therapies; CL: Application

77. The nurse understands that the potential for progressive renal injury is greatest when urinary tract infections (UTIs) occur in which of the following age groups or situations?

1. A school-age child who must get permission to go to the bathroom
2. An adolescent female who has started menstruation
3. Children who compete in competitive sports
4. Young infants and toddlers

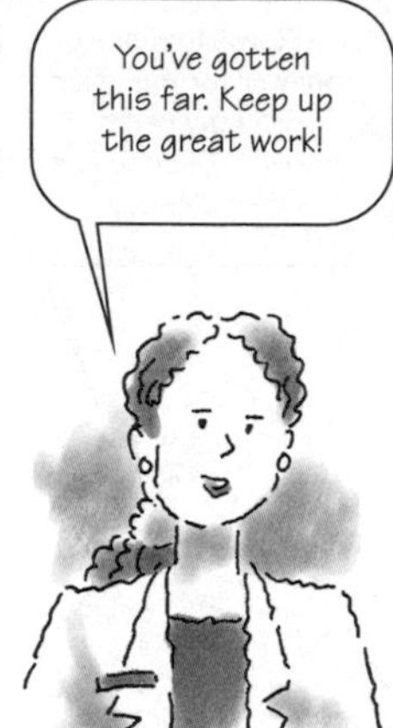

You've gotten this far. Keep up the great work!

77. 4. The hazard of progressive renal injury is greatest when infection occurs in young children, especially those under 2 years old. The first two options might lead to a simple UTI that would need to be treated. Competitive sports have no bearing on a UTI.

NP: Evaluation; CN: Safe, effective care environment; CNS: Safety and infection control; CL: Comprehension

78. Which of the following statements should the nurse make to help parents understand the recovery period after a child has had surgery to remove a Wilms' tumor?

1. "Children will easily lie in bed and restrict their activities."
2. "Recovery is usually fast in spite of the abdominal incision."
3. "Recovery usually takes a great deal of time due to the large incision."
4. "Parents need to perform activities of daily living for about 2 weeks after surgery."

78. 2. Children generally recover very quickly from surgery to remove a Wilms' tumor, even though they may have a large abdominal incision. Children like to get back into the normalcy of being a child, which is through play. Parents need to encourage their children to do as much for themselves as possible, although some regression is expected.

NP: Implementation; CN: Psychosocial integrity; CNS: Coping and adaptation; CL: Analysis

79. When teaching parents about administering co-trimoxazole (Septra) to a child for treatment of a urinary tract infection (UTI), the nurse should include which of the following instructions?

1. Give the medication with food.
2. Give the medication with water.
3. Give the medication with a cola beverage.
4. Give the medication 2 hours after a meal.

79. 2. When giving Septra, the medication should be administered with a full glass of water on an empty stomach. If nausea and vomiting occur, giving the drug with food may decrease gastric distress. Carbonated beverages should be avoided because they irritate the bladder.

NP: Implementation; CN: Physiological integrity; CNS: Pharmacological and parenteral therapies; CL: Application

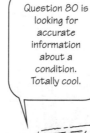

80. The nurse understands that which of the following characteristics is true of the incidence of Wilms' tumor?

1. Peak incidence occurs at 10 years of age.
2. It's the least common type of renal cancer.
3. It's the most common type of renal cancer.
4. It has a decreased incidence among siblings.

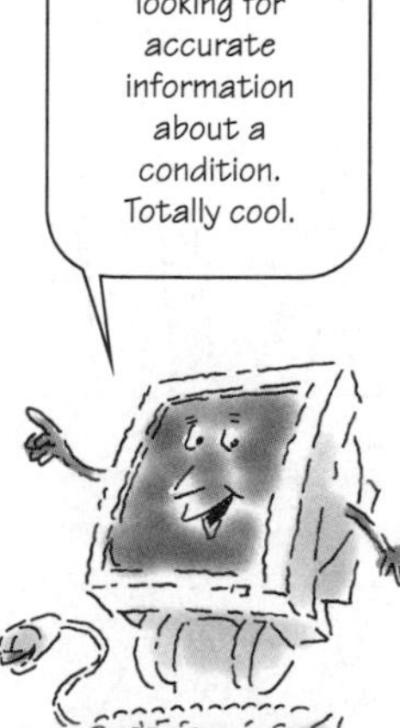

Question 80 is looking for accurate information about a condition. Totally cool.

80. 3. Wilms' tumor is the most frequent intra-abdominal tumor of childhood and the most common type of renal cancer. The peak incidence is 3 years, and there is an increased incidence among siblings and identical twins.

NP: Assessment; CN: Health promotion and maintenance; CNS: Prevention and early detection of disease; CL: Knowledge

81. Which of the following presenting signs is most common with Wilms' tumor?

1. Pain in the abdomen
2. Fever greater than 104° F (40° C)
3. Decreased blood pressure
4. Swelling within the abdomen

81. 4. The most common presenting sign is a swelling or mass within the abdomen. The mass is characteristically firm, nontender, confined to one side, and deep within the flank. A high fever isn't a presenting sign for Wilms' tumor. Blood pressure is characteristically increased, not decreased.

NP: Assessment; CN: Health promotion and maintenance; CNS: Prevention and early detection of disease; CL: Application

82. When the nurse is explaining the diagnosis of Wilms' tumor to parents, which of the following statements by a parent would indicate the need for further teaching?

1. "Wilms' tumor usually involves both kidneys."
2. "Wilms' tumor occurs slightly more often in the left kidney."
3. "Wilms' tumor is staged during surgery for treatment planning."
4. "Wilms' tumor stays encapsulated for an extended period of time."

82. 1. Wilms' tumor usually involves only one kidney and is usually staged during surgery so an effective course of treatment can be established. Wilms' tumor has a slightly higher occurrence in the left kidney and it stays encapsulated for an extended period of time.

NP: Implementation; CN: Health promotion and maintenance; CNS: Prevention and early detection of disease; CL: Knowledge

83. A parent asks the nurse about the prognosis of her child diagnosed with Wilms' tumor. The nurse should base her response on which of the following factors?

1. Usually children with Wilms' tumor only need surgical intervention.
2. Survival rates for Wilms' tumor are the lowest among childhood cancers.
3. Survival rates for Wilms' tumor are the highest among childhood cancers.
4. Children with localized tumor have only a 30% chance of cure with multimodal therapy.

83. 3. Survival rates for Wilms' tumor are the highest among childhood cancers. Usually children with Wilms' tumor who have stage I or II localized tumor have a 90% chance of cure with multimodal therapy.

NP: Implementation; CN: Health promotion and maintenance; CNS: Prevention and early detection of disease; CL: Application

84. If both kidneys are involved with Wilms' tumor, the nurse should understand that treatment prior to surgery might include which of the following methods?

1. Peritoneal dialysis
2. Abdominal gavage
3. Radiation and chemotherapy
4. Antibiotics and I.V. fluid therapy

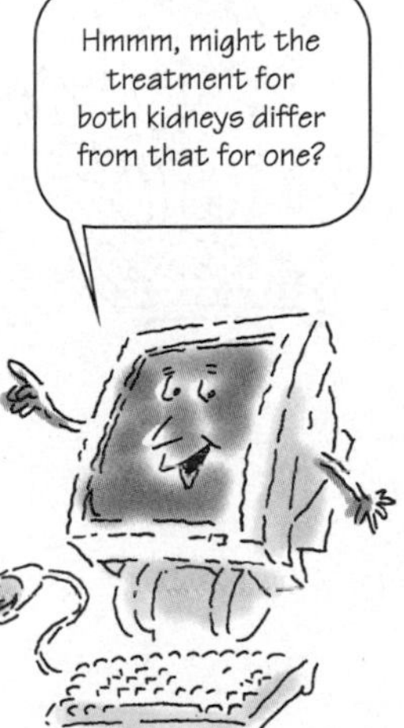
Hmmm, might the treatment for both kidneys differ from that for one?

84. 3. If both kidneys are involved, the child may be treated with radiation therapy or chemotherapy preoperatively to shrink the tumor, allowing more conservative therapy. Antibiotics aren't needed because Wilms' tumor isn't an infection. Peritoneal dialysis would only be needed if the kidneys aren't functioning. Abdominal gavage wouldn't be indicated.

NP: Implementation; CN: Safe, effective care environment; CNS: Management of care; CL: Application

85. When caring for the child with Wilms' tumor preoperatively, which of the following nursing interventions would be most important?

1. Avoid abdominal palpation.
2. Closely monitor arterial blood gases (ABGs).
3. Prepare child and family for long-term dialysis.
4. Prepare child and family for renal transplantation.

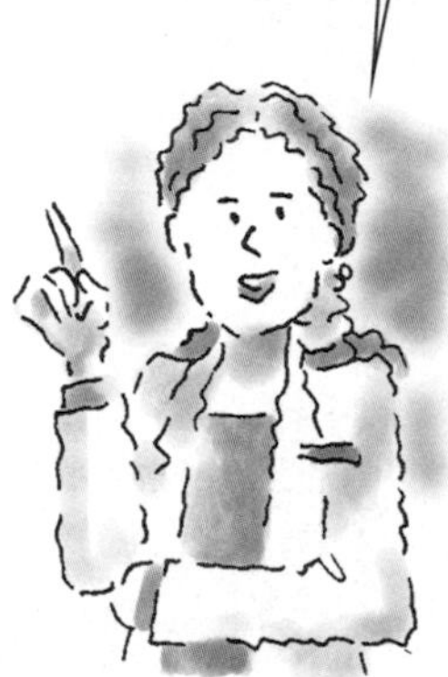
Note the word
preoperatively
in question 85.

85. 1. After the diagnosis of Wilms' tumor is made, the abdomen shouldn't be palpated. Palpation of the tumor might lead to rupture, which will cause the cancerous cells to spread throughout the abdomen. ABGs shouldn't be affected. If surgery is successful, there won't be a need for long-term dialysis or renal transplantation.

NP: Implementation; CN: Physiological integrity; CNS: Reduction of risk potential; CL: Application

86. A child is scheduled for surgery to remove a Wilms' tumor from one kidney. The parents ask the nurse what treatment, if any, they should expect after their child recovers from surgery. Which of the following responses would be most accurate?

1. "Chemotherapy may be necessary."
2. "Kidney transplant is indicated eventually."
3. "No additional treatments are usually necessary."
4. "Chemotherapy with or without radiation therapy is indicated."

86. 4. Because radiation therapy and chemotherapy are usually begun immediately after surgery, parents need an explanation of what to expect, such as major benefits and adverse effects. Kidney transplant isn't usually necessary.

NP: Implementation; CN: Safe, effective care environment; CNS: Management of care; CL: Application

87. When assessing the abdomen of a child with a potential diagnosis of Wilms' tumor, which of the following factors might lead to a different diagnosis?

1. The mass is on one side of the abdomen.
2. There is a mass on both sides of the abdomen.
3. The mass crosses the midline of the abdomen.
4. There is no pain associated with palpation of the mass.

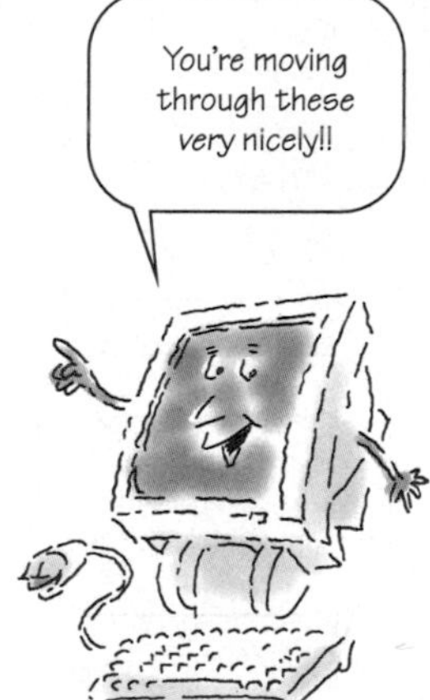
You're moving
through these
very nicely!!

87. 3. When an abdominal mass crosses the midline, a neuroblastoma should be suspected; not a Wilms' tumor. A Wilms' tumor arises off the kidneys and can be on one side or both sides but doesn't cross the mid-line. Pain isn't usually associated with Wilms' tumor.

NP: Assessment; CN: Health promotion and maintenance; CNS: Prevention and early detection of disease; CL: Analysis

88. The parent of a child with Wilms' tumor asks the nurse about surgery. Which of the following statements best explains the need for surgery for Wilms' tumor?

1. Surgery isn't indicated in children with Wilms' tumor.
2. Surgery is usually performed within 24 to 48 hours of admission.
3. Surgery is the least favorable therapy for the treatment of Wilms' tumor.
4. Surgery will be delayed until the client's overall health status improves.

88. 2. Surgery is the preferred treatment and is scheduled as soon as possible after confirmation of a renal mass, usually within 24 to 48 hours of admission, to be sure the encapsulated tumor remains intact.

NP: Implementation; CN: Safe, effective care environment; CNS: Management of care; CL: Comprehension

89. A 3-year-old client has had surgery to remove a Wilms' tumor. Which of the following actions should the nurse take first when the mother asks for pain medication for the child?

1. Get the pain medication ready for administration.
2. Assess the client's pain using a pain scale of 1 to 10.
3. Assess the client's pain using a smiley face pain scale.
4. Check for the last time pain medication was administered.

89. 3. The first action of the nurse should be to assess the client for pain. A 3-year-old child is too young to use a pain scale from 1 to 10 but can easily use the smiley face pain scale. After assessing the pain, the nurse should then investigate the time the pain medication was last given and administer the medication accordingly.

NP: Assessment; CN: Physiological integrity; CNS: Pharmacological and parenteral therapies; CL: Application

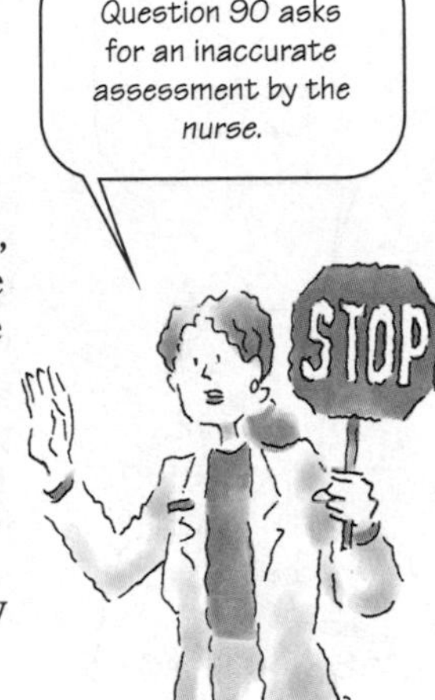

Question 90 asks for an inaccurate assessment by the nurse.
STOP

90. A child has been diagnosed with a Wilms' tumor. Because of the parents' religious beliefs, they choose not to treat the child. Which of the following statements by the nurse indicates the need for further discussion?

1. "I know this is a lot of information in a short period of time."
2. "I don't think parents have the legal right to make these kinds of decisions."
3. "These parents just don't understand how easily treated a Wilms' tumor is."
4. "I think the parents are in shock."

90. 2. Parents *do* have the legal right to make decisions regarding the health issues for their child. Religion plays an important role in many peoples lives and decisions about surgery and treatment for cancer are sometimes made that scientifically don't make sense to the health care provider. The parents are probably in a state of shock because a lot of information has been given and this is a cancer that requires decisions to be made quickly, especially surgical intervention.

NP: Evaluation; CN: Psychosocial integrity; CNS: Coping and adaptation; CL: Analysis

91. A child with a Wilms' tumor has had surgery to remove a kidney and has received chemotherapy. The nurse should include which of the following instructions at discharge?

1. Avoid contact sports
2. Decrease fluid intake
3. Decrease sodium intake
4. Avoid contact with other children

91. 1. Because the child is left with only one kidney, certain precautions such as avoiding contact sports are recommended to prevent injury to the remaining kidney. Decreasing fluid intake wouldn't be indicated; fluid intake is essential for renal function. Avoiding other children is unnecessary and will make the child feel self-conscious and may lead to regressive behavior. The child's sodium intake shouldn't be reduced.

NP: Implementation; CN: Health promotion and maintenance; CNS: Prevention and early detection of disease; CL: Application

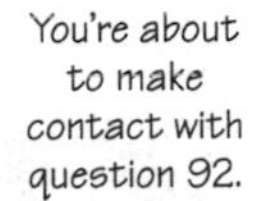

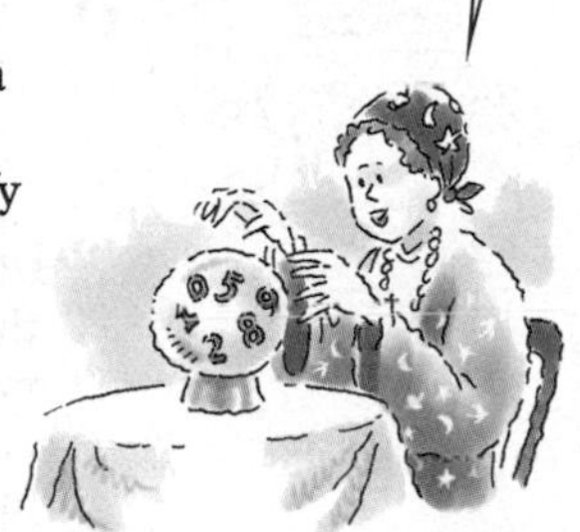

You're about to make contact with question 92.

92. When caring for a child after removal of a Wilms' tumor, which of the following assessment findings would indicate the need to notify the primary care provider?

1. Fever of 101° F (38.3° C)
2. Absence of bowel sounds
3. Slight congestion in the lungs
4. Complaints of pain when moving

92. 2. This child is at risk for intestinal obstruction. GI abnormalities require notification of the primary health care provider. A slight fever following surgery isn't uncommon, nor are slight congestion in the lungs and complaints of pain.

NP: Assessment; CN: Physiological integrity; CNS: Reduction of risk potential; CL: Application

93. Because surgery is performed for a Wilms' tumor within 24 to 48 hours of admission, the nurse must prepare the family and child quickly for procedures. Which of the following statements should guide the nurse in her preparation of the family?

1. Because the parents are in a state of shock, they don't need explanations.
2. Explanations should be kept simple and should be repeated often.
3. Scientific terminology should be used with drawings and models.
4. The play therapist is the best person to prepare this family.

93. 2. Decisions are made rapidly after the diagnosis of Wilms' tumor is made. Parents are typically in shock at this time. Explanations should be kept simple and repeated often. The play therapist might become involved with this family, especially postoperatively. There generally is no time to prepare the play therapist for the role of educator in this situation.

NP: Implementation; CN: Health promotion and maintenance; CNS: Prevention and early detection of disease; CL: Application

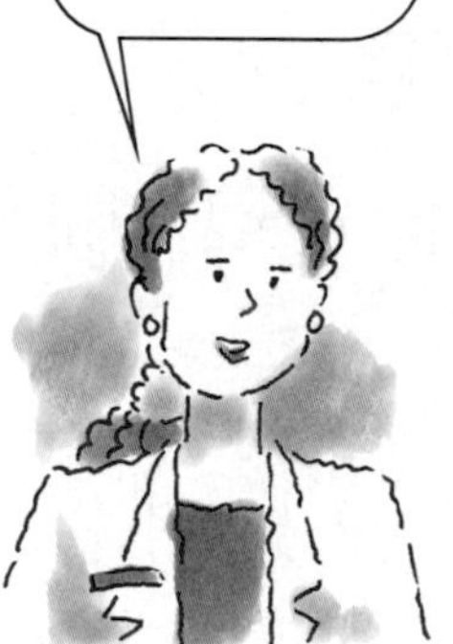

Be sensitive to the needs of a client's family when delivering bad news.

94. Which statement made by the primary care provider to the parents of a child who has had a Wilms' tumor removed would be the most difficult for the parents to hear and might require nursing intervention?

1. "We will start chemotherapy within the next 24 to 48 hours."
2. "The tumor was a stage IV, which indicates other organ involvement."
3. "We were able to remove all of the tumor, but we had to take the kidney as well."
4. "The incision is long, and the dressing will need to be changed daily."

94. 2. Surgery is an anxiety-producing to parents. It also marks the confirmation of the stage of the tumor. A stage IV tumor has a poor prognosis because other organs are involved. This statement, above all others, would be the most difficult for the parents to hear.

NP: Evaluation; CN: Psychosocial integrity; CNS: Coping and adaptation; CL: Analysis

95. In providing psychosocial care to a 6-year-old client who has had abdominal surgery for Wilms' tumor, which activity would be the most appropriate?

1. Allowing the child to watch a 2-hour movie without interruptions
2. Giving the child a puzzle with 5 pieces to encourage him to move while in bed
3. Telling the child that you can give him enough medication so that he feels no pain
4. Providing the child with puppets and supplies and asking him to draw how he feels

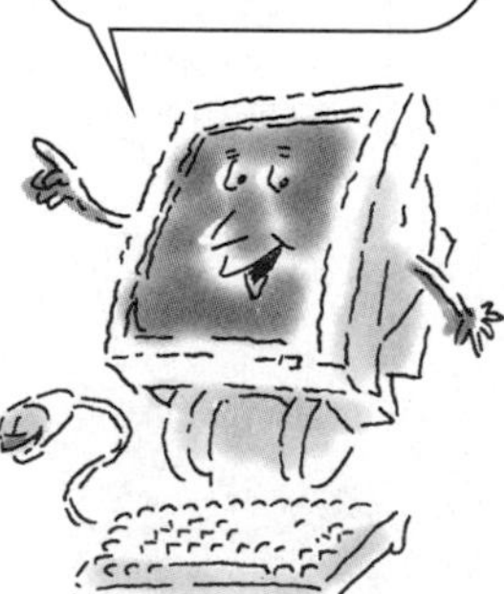

This question is looking for the *most appropriate* answer. In other words, prioritize.

95. 4. A movie is a good diversion, but giving puppets and encouraging the child to draw his feelings is a better outlet. Many procedures have been performed on this client since admission. You probably can't give enough pain medication so that a person who has had surgery will feel no pain. A puzzle with only 5 pieces is too basic for a 6-year-old child and wouldn't hold his interest.

NP: Evaluation; CN: Psychosocial integrity; CNS: Coping and adaptation; CL: Application

96. A nurse should understand that staging of a Wilms' tumor helps to determine which of the following parameters?

1. Size of tumor
2. Level of treatment
3. Length of incision
4. Amount of anesthesia

96. 2. Staging of the tumor helps to determine the level of treatment because it provides information about the level of involvement. The other choices are insignificant in staging of the tumor.

NP: Planning; CN: Health promotion and maintenance; CNS: Prevention and early detection of disease; CL: Knowledge

NP: Nursing process CN: Client needs category CNS: Client needs subcategory CL: Cognitive level

97. The nurse is educating parents about Wilms' tumor. Which of the following statements made by a parent would indicate the need for further teaching?
1. "My child could have inherited this disease."
2. "Wilms' tumor can be associated with other congenital anomalies."
3. "This disease could have been a result of trauma to the baby in utero."
4. "There is no method of identification of gene carriers of Wilms' tumor."

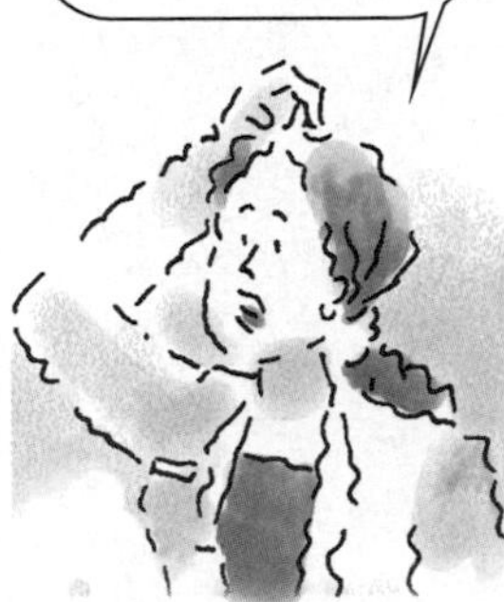

Further teaching is so important that you'll see similar questions more than once.

97. 3. Wilms' tumor isn't a result of trauma to the fetus in utero. Wilms' tumor can be genetically inherited and is associated with other congenital anomalies. There is, however, no method of identification of gene carriers of Wilms' tumor at this time.

NP: Implementation; CN: Psychosocial integrity; CNS: Psychosocial adaptation; CL: Application

98. Which of the following assessment findings will aid in the differentiation of a Wilms' tumor from the liver when doing an abdominal assessment?
1. The liver moves with respiration.
2. The liver is a more encapsulated organ.
3. A Wilms' tumor isn't as deep as the liver.
4. A Wilms' tumor usually isn't well defined.

98. 1. It's difficult to distinguish a Wilms' tumor from the liver if the tumor is on the right side of the body. One difference is that the liver will move with respirations and a Wilms' tumor won't. A Wilms' tumor is deep in the abdomen and is usually well-defined and encapsulated.

NP: Assessment; CN: Health promotion and maintenance; CNS: Prevention and early detection of disease; CL: Application

99. Which of the following actions by the nurse would be appropriate to take in a child diagnosed with a Wilms' tumor?
1. Take blood pressure in the right arm only.
2. Only offer clear liquids at room temperature.
3. Post a sign over the bed that reads, "Don't palpate abdomen."
4. Allow the child to participate in group activities in the playroom.

99. 3. To reinforce the need for caution, it may be necessary to post a sign over the bed that reads, "Don't palpate abdomen." Careful bathing and handling are also important in preventing trauma to the tumor site; thus, group activities should be discouraged. The blood pressure could be taken in any extremity and, prior to surgery, there are usually no dietary restrictions.

NP: Assessment; CN: Health promotion and maintenance; CNS: Prevention and early detection of disease; CL: Application

100. A 6-year-old girl has a history of repeated urinary tract infections (UTIs). She has been diagnosed with vesicoureteral reflux. Which of the following nursing responses would be most accurate to the mother who asks what the major complications are?
1. Damage to the ovaries that could lead to fertility problems
2. Minimal change nephrosis, which results in kidney damage and hypertension
3. Development of pyelonephritis and possible renal damage from the reflux of urine
4. Hemolytic syndrome that results in damage to the kidneys and abnormal spilling of protein

100. 3. Vesicoureteral reflux is the abnormal reflux of urine from the bladder back up the ureters and possibly into the kidneys. Residual urine that isn't voided promotes growth of bacteria and results in a high incidence of UTIs. This infected urine could reflux into the kidneys, resulting in pyelonephritis. Vesicoureteral reflux isn't associated with hemolytic syndrome, minimal change nephrosis, or damage to the ovaries.

NP: Implementation; CN: Physiological integrity; CNS: Physiological adaptation; CL: Knowledge

101. Which of the following treatments is administered for the correction of minimal change nephrosis?

1. Diuretics are given until the urine is free from protein.
2. Steroids are administered until the urine is free from protein.
3. Antihypertensives are given until hypertension is resolved.
4. Ibuprofen is administered for the anti-inflammatory effect until the hematuria resolves.

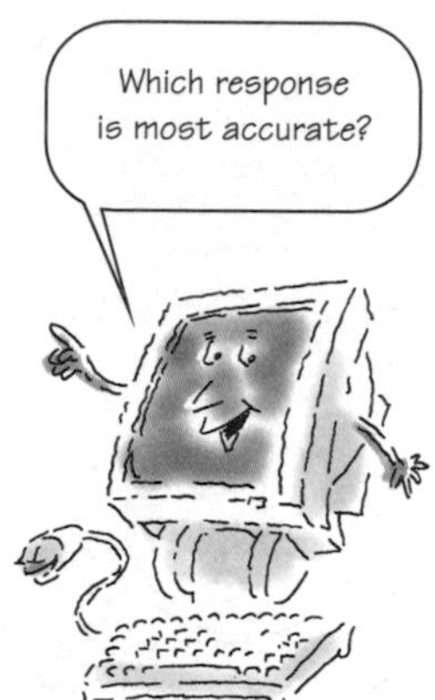
Which response
is most accurate?

101. 2. Nephrotic syndrome is characteristic of glomerular damage that results in increased permeability to protein. Steroids are given until the urine is protein-free for several weeks. Ibuprofen doesn't treat hematuria. Diuretics don't treat glomerular permeability to protein. Antihypertensives are given as needed, but the evaluation criterion is protein in the urine.
NP: Analysis; CN: Physiological integrity; CNS: Physiological adaptation; CL: Knowledge

102. Which of the following play activities would be appropriate for a 2-year-old child waiting for surgery for the removal of a Wilms' tumor?

1. Playing a group game in the playroom
2. Riding the toy scooter in the playroom
3. Playing in the playroom on the jungle gym
4. Playing with clay and cookie cutters in his room

102. 4. A child with a diagnosis of a Wilms' tumor must be treated with extreme caution to prevent injury to the encapsulated tumor. Even palpation of the abdomen could result in spreading of the tumor. Therefore, the least active choice is playing with clay. The other choices are more physical activities that would carry a high risk of injury or falling.
NP: Planning; CN: Physiological integrity; CNS: Reduction of risk potential; CL: Application

103. A 6-year-old child with nephritic syndrome has been hospitalized. She presents with a distended abdomen, periorbital edema, proteinuria, anorexia, and fatigue. Which nursing measure would be **most** appropriate?

1. Daily measurement of weight and abdominal girth
2. A high-calorie diet
3. Daily walks and play therapy
4. Promotion of adequate fluid intake

103. 1. Careful monitoring of weight, abdominal girth, and intake and output are essential. A diet high in protein, not calories, will help restore the body's plasma oncotic pressure. A child with severe edema is on bed rest, instead of walks, to promote diuresis. Play therapy is important but should be done at bedside. Fluids are restricted based on the child's symptoms.
NP: Implementation; CN: Physiological integrity; CNS: Physiological adaptation; CL: Comprehension

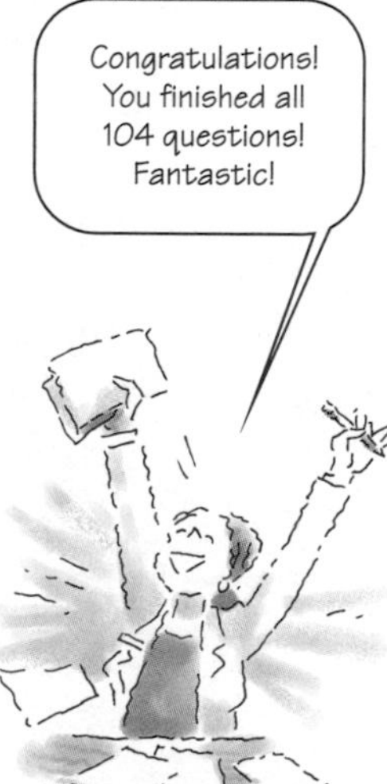
Congratulations!
You finished all
104 questions!
Fantastic!

104. A 13-year-old child with end-stage renal disease (ESRD) is admitted to the pediatric unit. When discussing the care plan with the client's mother, the nurse shares which information about the **purpose** of weighing the child?

1. To measure adequacy of nutritional management
2. To check the accuracy of the fluid intake record
3. To impress on the child the importance of eating well
4. To determine changes in the amount of edema

104. 4. Measuring daily weight is the most accurate way to assess edema and fluid shifts. Weight is a factor in determining nutritional management but isn't the primary reason for daily weighing. Weight doesn't accurately reflect fluid intake, only a strict intake record does. Weighing a child won't encourage a child to eat more. A child in ESRD doesn't have much appetite and his weight won't reflect his disinterest in eating.
NP: Planning; CN: Physiological integrity; CNS: Basic care and comfort; CL: Comprehension

NP: Nursing process CN: Client needs category CNS: Client needs subcategory CL: Cognitive level

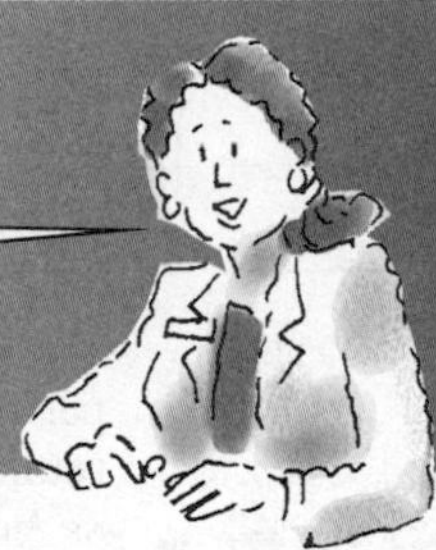

Chapter 35 Integumentary disorders

1. A 3-year-old child gets a burn at the angle of the mouth from chewing on an electrical cord. Which of the following findings should the nurse expect 10 days after the injury?

1. Normal granular tissue
2. Contracture of the injury site
3. Ulceration with serous drainage
4. Profuse bleeding from the injury site

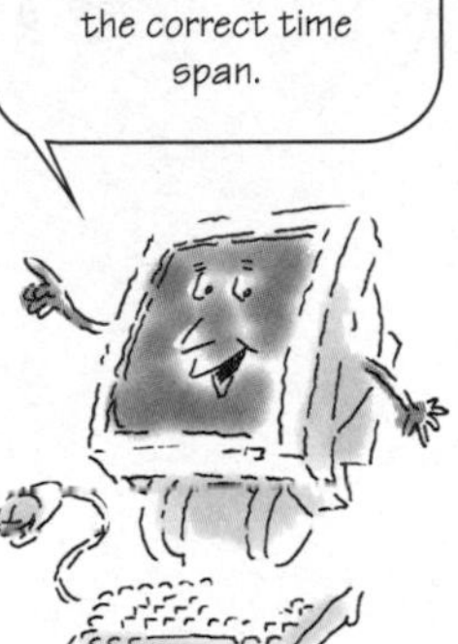

Limit your answer to the correct time span.

1. 4. Ten days after oral burns from electrical cords, the eschar falls off, exposing arteries and veins. Burns to the oral cavity heal rapidly, but with contractures and scarring. Although contractures are likely, they're not seen 10 days postinjury.

NP: Assessment; CN: Physiological integrity; CNS: Physiological adaptation; CL: Knowledge

2. Providing adequate nutrition is essential for a burn client. Which of the following statements best describes the nutritional needs of a burn client?

1. A child needs 100 cal/kg during hospitalization.
2. The hypermetabolic state after a burn injury leads to poor healing.
3. Caloric needs can be lowered by controlling environmental temperature.
4. Maintaining a hypermetabolic rate will lower the child's risk for infection.

2. 2. A burn injury causes a hypermetabolic state leading to protein and lipid catabolism, which affects wound healing. Caloric intake should be 1½ to 2 times the basal metabolic rate, with a minimum of 1.5 to 2 g/kg of body weight of protein daily. High metabolic rates increase the risk for infection. Keeping the temperature within a normal range lets the body function efficiently and use calories for healing and normal physiological processes. If the temperature is too warm or cold, energy must be used for warming or cooling, taking energy away from tissue repair.

NP: Analysis; CN: Physiological integrity; CNS: Basic care and comfort; CL: Knowledge

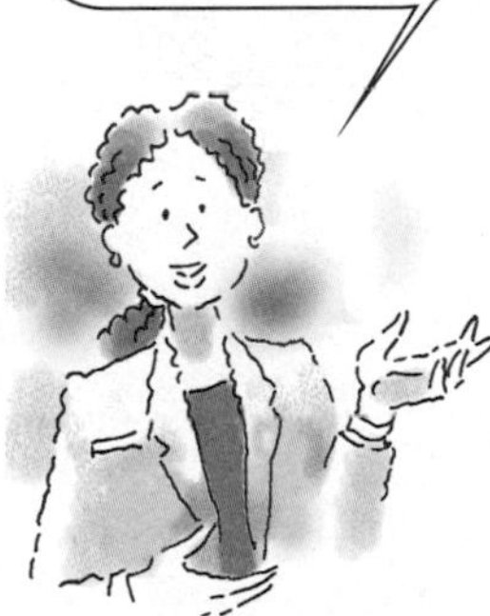

Measuring burns in children is different than measuring burns in adults.

3. A 1-year-old child is treated in the clinic for a burn to the left leg. Which of the following ways to measure burn size would be accurate for this child?

1. The rule of nines
2. Percentage based on the child's weight
3. The child's palm equals 1% of the child's body surface area
4. Percentage can't be determined without knowing the type of burn

3. 3. The palm of a child is equal to 1% of that child's body surface. The rule of nines is used for children ages 14 years and older. Burn type doesn't determine the percentage of body surface involved. The child's weight is important to calculate fluid replacement for extensive burns, not to estimate total body surface area.

NP: Analysis; CN: Physiological integrity; CNS: Physiological adaptation; CL: Knowledge

NP: Nursing process CN: Client needs category CNS: Client needs subcategory CL: Cognitive level

4. An 18-month-old child is admitted to the hospital for full-thickness burns to the anterior chest. The mother asks how the burn will heal. Which of the following statements is accurate about healing for full-thickness burns?

1. Surgical closure and grafting are usually needed.
2. Healing takes 10 to 12 days, with little or no scarring.
3. Pigment in a black client will return to the injured area.
4. Healing can take up to 6 weeks, with a high incidence of scarring.

You don't need a crystal ball to answer question 4.

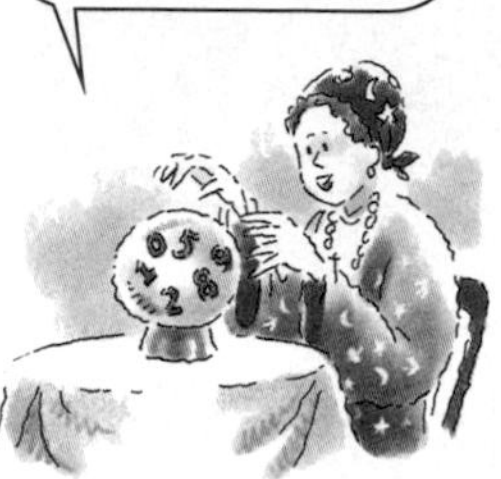

4. 1. Full thickness burns usually need surgical closure and grafting for complete healing. Deep partial-thickness burns heal in 6 weeks, with scarring. Healing in 10 to 12 weeks with little or no scarring is associated with superficial partial-thickness burns. With superficial partial-thickness burns, pigment is expected to return to the injured area after healing.

NP: Analysis; CN: Physiological integrity; CNS: Physiological adaptation; CL: Knowledge

5. A 9-year-old child is admitted to the hospital with deep partial-thickness burns to 25% of his body. Which of the following assessment findings is consistent with a deep partial-thickness burn?

1. Erythema and pain
2. Minimal damage to the epidermis
3. Necrosis through all layers of skin
4. Tissue necrosis through most of the dermis

5. 4. A client with a deep partial-thickness burn will have tissue necrosis to the epidermis and dermis layers. Necrosis through all skin layers is seen with full-thickness injuries. Erythema and pain are characteristic of superficial injury. With deep burns, the nerve fibers are destroyed and the client won't feel pain in the affected area. Superficial burns are characteristic of slight epidermal damage.

NP: Analysis; CN: Physiological integrity; CNS: Physiological adaptation; CL: Knowledge

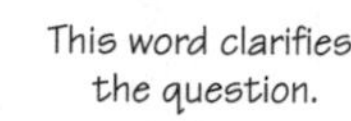
This word clarifies the question.

6. A 4-year-old child is admitted to the burn unit with a circumferential burn to the left forearm. Which of the following findings should be reported to the physician?

1. Numbness of fingers
2. +2 radial and ulnar pulses
3. Full range of motion and no pain
4. Bilateral capillary refill less then 2 seconds

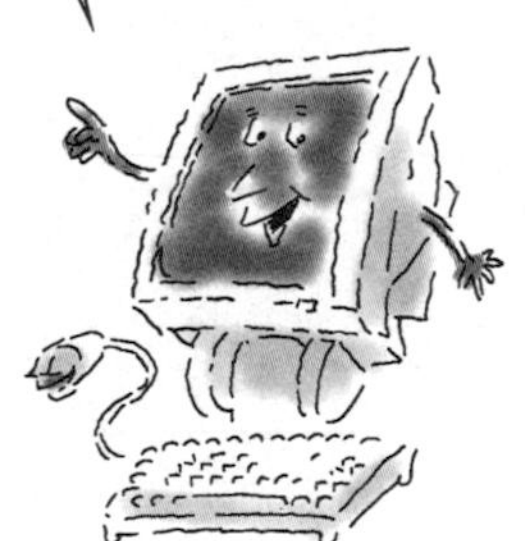

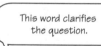

6. 1. Circumferential burns can compromise blood flow to an extremity, causing numbness. Capillary refill less then 2 seconds indicates a normal vascular blood flow. Absence of pain and full range of motion implies good tissue oxygenation from intact circulation. +2 Pulses indicate normal circulation.

NP: Assessment; CN: Physiological integrity; CNS: Physiological adaptation; CL: Knowledge

7. Which of the following facts should be given to the parents of a child with fifth disease?

1. There is a possible reappearance of the rash for up to 1 week.
2. Isolation of high-risk contacts should be avoided for 4 to 10 days.
3. Pregnant client are at risk for fetal death if infected with fifth disease.
4. Children with fifth disease are contagious only while the rash is present.

7. 3. There is a 3% to 5% risk for fetal death from hydrops fetalis if a pregnant client is exposed during the first trimester. The cutaneous eruption of fifth disease can reappear for up to 4 months. A child with fifth disease is contagious during the first stage, when symptoms of headache, body aches, fever, and chills are present, not after the rash. The child should be isolated from pregnant women, immunocompromised clients, and clients with chronic anemia for up to 2 weeks.

NP: Analysis; CN: Safe, effective care environment; CNS: Safety and infection control; CL: Knowledge

NP: Nursing process CN: Client needs category CNS: Client needs subcategory CL: Cognitive level

8. A mother is concerned that her 3-year-old daughter has been exposed to erythema infectiosum (fifth disease). Which of the following symptoms are characteristic of this viral infection?

1. A fine, erythematous rash with a sandpaper-like texture
2. Intense redness of both checks that may spread to the extremities
3. Low-grade fever, followed by vesicular lesions of the trunk, face, and scalp
4. Three- to five-day history of sustained fever, followed by a diffuse erythematous maculopapular rash

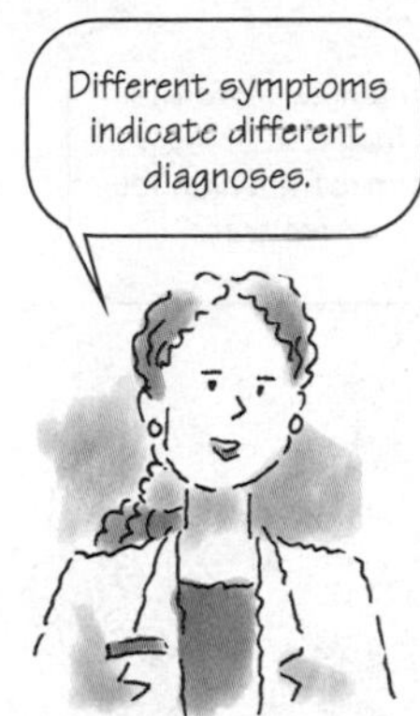
Different symptoms indicate different diagnoses.

8. 2. The classic symptoms of erythema infectiosum begin with intense redness of both checks. An erythematous rash after a fever is characteristic of roseola. Children with varicella typically have vesicular lesions of the trunk, face, and scalp after a low-grade fever. An erythematous rash with a sandpaper-like texture is associated with scarlet fever, which is a bacterial infection.

NP: Analysis; CN: Physiological integrity; CNS: Physiological adaptation; CL: Knowledge

9. A family that recently went camping brings their child to the clinic with a complaint of a rash after a tick bite. Lyme disease is suspected. Which of the following assessment findings would be seen with Lyme disease?

1. Erythematous rash surrounding a necrotic lesion
2. Bright rash with red outer border circling the bite site
3. Onset of a diffuse rash over the entire body 2 months after exposure
4. A linear rash of papules and vesicles that occur 1 to 3 days after exposure

9. 2. A bull's eye rash is a classic symptom of Lyme disease. Necrotic, painful rashes are associated with the bite of a brown recluse spider. In Lyme disease, the rash is located primarily at the site of the bite. A linear, papular, vesicular rash indicates exposure to the leaves of poison ivy.

NP: Assessment; CN: Physiological integrity; CNS: Physiological adaptation; CL: Knowledge

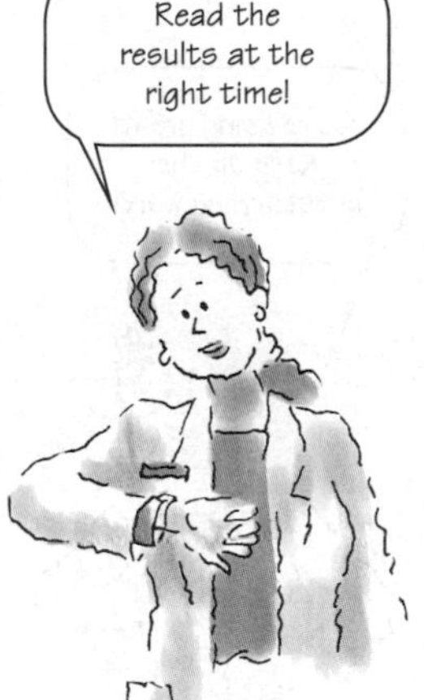
Read the results at the right time!

10. A Mantoux test is ordered for a 6-year-old child. Which of the following directions about this test is accurate?

1. Read results within 24 hours
2. Read results 48 to 72 hours later
3. Use the large muscle of the upper leg
4. Massage the site to increase absorption

10. 2. The test should be read 48 to 72 hours after placement by measuring the diameter of the induration that develops at the site. The purified protein derivative is injected intradermally on the volar surface of the forearm. Massaging the site could cause leakage from the injection site.

NP: Analysis; CN: Physiological integrity; CNS: Reduction of risk potential; CL: Knowledge

11. Which of the following statements about Kawasaki syndrome is true?

1. It's highly contagious.
2. It's an afebrile condition with cardiac involvement.
3. It usually occurs in children older than 5 years.
4. Prolonged fever, with peeling of the fingers and toes, are the initial symptoms.

11. 4. To be diagnosed with Kawasaki syndrome, the child must have a fever for 5 days or more, plus four of the following five symptoms: bilateral conjunctivitis, changes in the oral mucosa and peripheral extremities, rash, and lymphadenopathy. Kawasaki syndrome is more likely to occur in children aged younger than 5 years. The syndrome isn't contagious.

NP: Analysis; CN: Physiological integrity; CNS: Physiological adaptation; CL: Knowledge

12. A 22-pound child is diagnosed with Kawasaki syndrome and started on gamma globulin therapy. The physician orders an I.V. infusion of gamma globulin, 2 g/kg, to run over 12 hours. Which of the following doses is correct?

1. 11 g
2. 20 g
3. 22 g
4. 44 g

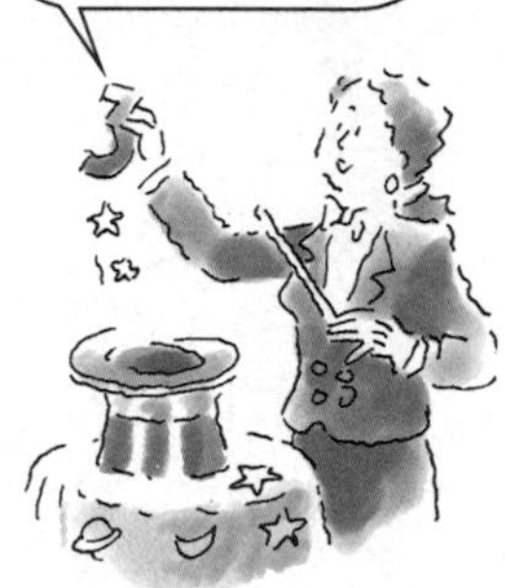

You need more than
magic to find the
correct dosage. You
need math.

12. 2. One kilogram equals 2.2 pounds, so a 22-pound child weighs 10 kg. 2 g × 10 kg = 20 g. Convert the weight to kilograms, 22 (lb) ÷2.2 = 10 (kg). Calculate the dose: 2 g × 10 = 20 g.

NP: Implementation; CN: Physiological integrity; CNS: Pharmacological and parenteral therapies; CL: Application

13. A mother is concerned because her child was exposed to varicella in day care. Which of the following statements is true about varicella?

1. The rash is nonvesicular.
2. The treatment of choice is aspirin.
3. Varicella has an incubation period of 5 to 10 days.
4. A child is no longer contagious once the rash has crusted over.

13. 4. Once every varicella lesion is crusted over, the child is no longer considered contagious. The incubation period is 10 to 20 days. Use of aspirin has been associated with Reye's syndrome and is contraindicated in varicella. The rash is typically a maculopapular vesicular rash.

NP: Analysis; CN: Physiological integrity; CNS: Physiological adaptation; CL: Knowledge

14. Which of the following statements is correct about the rash associated with varicella?

1. It's diagnostic in the presence of Koplik's spots in the oral mucosa.
2. It's a macular papular rash starting on the scalp and hairline and spreading downward.
3. It's a vesicular macular papular rash that appears abruptly on the trunk, face, and scalp.
4. It appears as yellow ulcers surrounded by red halos on the surface of the hands and feet.

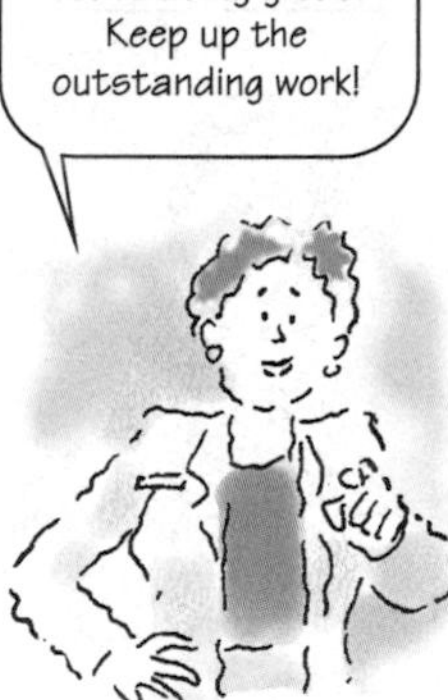

You're doing great!
Keep up the
outstanding work!

14. 3. Teardrop vesicles on an erythematous base generally begin on the trunk, face, and scalp, with minimal involvement of the extremities. A descending macular papular rash is characteristic of rubeola. Koplik's spots are diagnostic of rubeola. Yellow ulcers of the hands and feet are associated with hand-foot-and-mouth caused by the coxsackievirus.

NP: Analysis; CN: Physiological integrity; CNS: Physiological adaptation; CL: Knowledge

15. A child is brought to the emergency department after an extended period of sledding. Frostbite of the hands is suspected. Which of the following statements is true about frostbite?

1. The skin is white.
2. The skin looks deeply flushed and red.
3. Frostbite is helped by rubbing to increase circulation.
4. Slow gradual rewarming of the extremities with hot water is needed.

15. 1. Signs and symptoms of frostbite include tingling, numbness, burning sensation, and white skin. Gradual rewarming by exposure to hot water can lead to more tissue damage. Treatment includes very gentle handling of the affected area. Rubbing is contraindicated as it can damage fragile tissue.

NP: Analysis; CN: Physiological integrity; CNS: Physiological adaptation; CL: Knowledge

16. A mother brings her child to the physician's office because the child complains of pain, redness, and tenderness of the left index finger. The child is diagnosed with a paronychia. Which of the following organisms is the most likely cause of this superficial abscess of the cuticle?

1. *Borrelia burgdorferi*
2. *Escherichia coli*
3. *Pseudomonas* species
4. *Staphylococcus* species

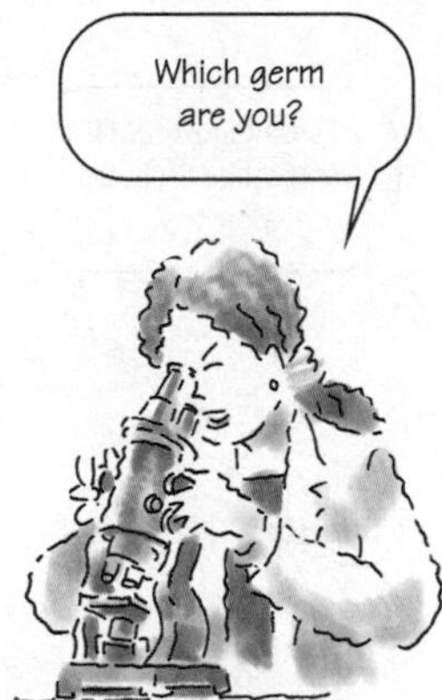
Which germ
are you?

16. 4. A paronychia is a localized infection of the nail bed caused by either staphylococci or streptococci. *Pseudomonas* species are associated with ecthyma. *Escherichia coli* is associated with urinary tract infections. *Borrelia burgdorferi* is responsible for Lyme disease.

NP: Assessment; CN: Physiological integrity; CNS: Physiological adaptation; CL: Knowledge

17. Which of the following treatments for paronychia would be the most appropriate?

1. Give warm soaks.
2. Splint and put ice on the affected finger.
3. Allow the infection to resolve without treatment.
4. Admit the child to the hospital for I.V. antibiotic therapy.

17. 1. Giving warm soaks is the treatment of choice for paronychia. Untreated, the local abscess can spread beneath the nail bed, called secondary lymphangitis. I.V. antibiotic therapy isn't needed if the abscess is kept from spreading. Splinting and icing aren't indicated.

NP: Planning; CN: Physiological integrity; CNS: Physiological adaptation; CL: Knowledge

18. A mother is concerned that her 9-month-old infant has scabies. Which of the following assessment findings is associated with this infestation?

1. Diffuse pruritic wheals
2. Oval white dots stuck to the hair shafts
3. Pain, erythema, and edema with an embedded stinger
4. Pruritic papules, pustules, and linear burrows of the finger and toe webs

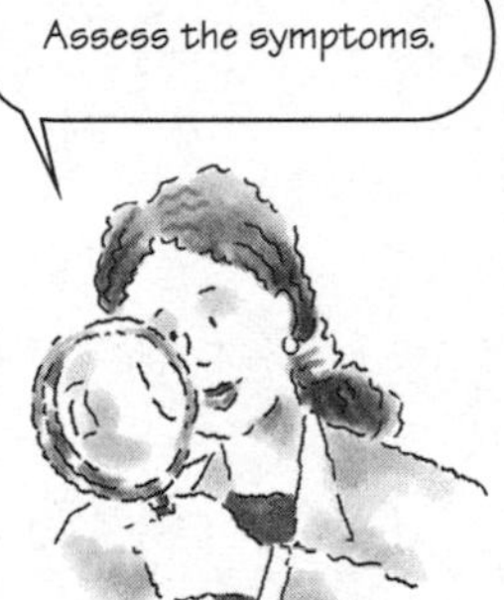
Assess the symptoms.

18. 4. Pruritic papules, vesicles, and linear burrows are diagnostic for scabies. Nits, seen as white oval dots, are characteristic of head lice. Urticaria is associated with an allergic reaction. Bites from honeybees are associated with a stinger, pain, and erythema.

NP: Assessment; CN: Physiological integrity; CNS: Physiological adaptation; CL: Knowledge

19. After treatment with permethrin (Elimite) for scabies, the mother of a 16-month-old child is concerned the cream didn't work because the child is still scratching. Which of the following explanations or instructions would be correct?

1. Continue the application daily until the rash disappears.
2. Pruritus caused by secondary reactions of the mites can be present for weeks.
3. Stop treatment because the cream is unsafe for children younger than 2 years of age.
4. Pruritus caused by permethrin is usually present in children younger than 5 years of age.

19. 2. Sensitization of the host is the cause of the intense itching and can last for weeks. Permethrin is the recommended treatment for scabies in infants as young as 2 months. It can safely be repeated after 2 weeks.

NP: Analysis; CN: Physiological integrity; CNS: Pharmacological and parenteral therapies; CL: Knowledge

20. The mother of a 5-month-old infant is planning a trip to the beach and asks for advice about sunscreen. Which of the following instructions should the nurse give the mother?

1. The sunscreen protection factor (SPF) of the sunscreen should be at least 10.
2. Apply sunscreen to the exposed areas of the skin.
3. Sunscreen shouldn't be applied to infants younger than 6 months of age.
4. Sunscreen needs to be applied heavily only once one half hour before going out in the sun.

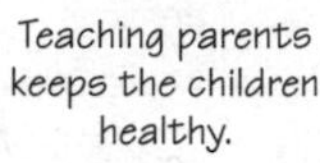

Teaching parents keeps the children healthy.

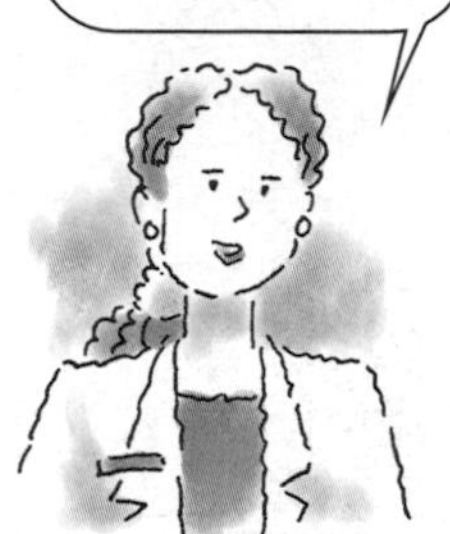

20. 3. Sunscreen isn't recommended for use in infants younger than 6 months of age. These children should be dressed in cool light clothes and kept in the shade. Sunscreen should be applied evenly throughout the day and each time the child is in the water. The SPF for children should be 15 or greater. Sunscreen should be applied to all areas of the skin.

NP: Analysis; CN: Health promotion and maintenance; CNS: Prevention and early detection of disease; CL: Knowledge

21. An infant is being treated with antibiotic therapy for otitis media and develops an erythematous, fine, raised rash in the groin and suprapubic area. Which of the following instructions or explanations will most likely be given to the mother?

1. The infant has candidiasis.
2. Change the brand of diapers.
3. Use an over-the-counter diaper remedy.
4. Stop the antibiotic therapy immediately.

21. 1. Candidiasis, caused by yeast-like fungi, can occur with the use of antibiotics. Changing the brand of diapers or suggesting that the parent use an over-the-counter remedy would be appropriate for treating diaper rash, not candidiasis. Antibiotic therapy shouldn't be stopped. The treatment for candidiasis is topical nystatin ointment.

NP: Assessment; CN: Physiological integrity; CNS: Physiological adaptation; CL: Knowledge

22. The skin in the diaper area of a 6-month-old infant is excoriated and red. Which of the following instructions would the nurse give to the mother?

1. Change the diaper more often.
2. Apply talcum powder with diaper changes.
3. Wash the area vigorously with each diaper change.
4. Decrease the infant's fluid intake to decrease saturating diapers.

22. 1. Simply decreasing the amount of time the skin comes in contact with wet soiled diapers will help heal the irritation. Gentle cleaning of the irritated skin should be encouraged. Infants shouldn't have fluid intake restrictions. Talc is contraindicated in children because of the risks of inhaling the fine powder.

NP: Assessment; CN: Safe, effective care environment; CNS: Safety and infection control; CL: Application

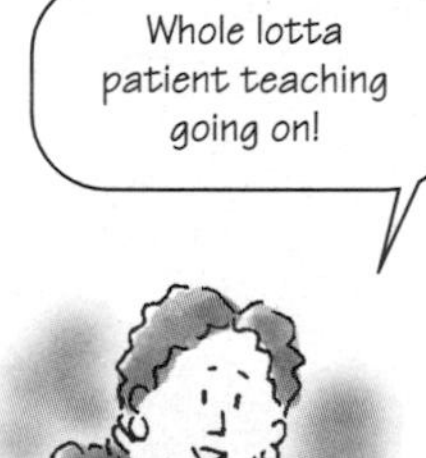

Whole lotta patient teaching going on!

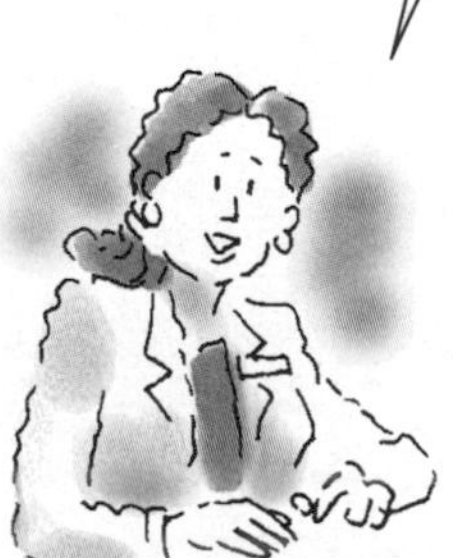

23. A 9-year-old child is being discharged from the hospital after severe urticaria caused by allergy to nuts. Which of the following instructions would be included in discharge teaching for the child's parents?

1. Use emollient lotions and baths.
2. Apply topical steroids to the lesions as needed.
3. Apply over-the-counter products such as diphenhydramine hydrochloride (Benadryl).
4. Use an epinephrine administration kit and follow up with an allergist.

23. 4. Children who have urticaria in response to nuts, seafood, or bee stings should be warned about the possibility of anaphylactic reactions to future exposure. The use of epinephrine pens should be taught to the parents and older children. Other treatment choices, such as Benadryl, topical steroids, and emollients, are for the treatment of mild urticaria.

NP: Analysis; CN: Health promotion and maintenance; CNS: Prevention and early detection of disease; CL: Application

24. When examining a nursery school-age child, the nurse finds multiple contusions over the body. Child abuse is suspected. Which of the following statements indicate which findings should be documented?

1. Contusions confined to one body area are typically suspicious.
2. All lesions, including location, shape, and color, should be documented.
3. Natural injuries usually have straight linear lines, while injuries from abuse have multiple curved lines.
4. The depth, location, and amount of bleeding that initially occurs is constant, but the sequence of color change is variable.

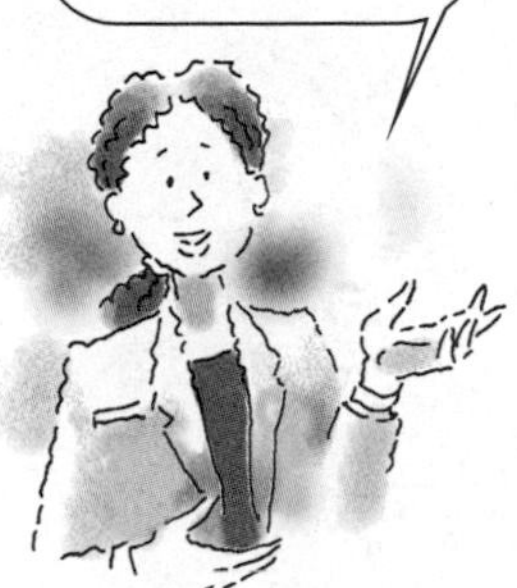

Be aware of the signs of child abuse. It's the nurse's responsibility to report it.

25. A 7-year-old child is diagnosed with head lice. The mother asks how to get the nits out of the hair. The nits represent which of the following parts of the life cycle of the louse?

1. Adult
2. Empty egg shells
3. Newly laid eggs
4. Nymph

26. For which of the following reasons is lindane (G-well) shampoo used only as a second-line treatment for lice?

1. Lindane causes alopecia.
2. Lindane causes hypertension.
3. Lindane is associated with seizures.
4. Lindane increases liver function test (LFT) results.

What do we need to know about lice treatment?

27. Which of the following instructions should be given to the parents about the treatment of hair lice?

1. The treatment should be repeated in 7 to 12 days.
2. Treatment should be repeated every day for 1 week.
3. If treated with a shampoo, combing to remove eggs isn't necessary.
4. All contacts with the infested child should be treated even without evidence of infestation.

24. 2. An accurate precise examination must be properly documented as a legal document. Injuries from normal falls are usually not linear in nature. The bleeding can cause variations, but the color change is consistent. Contusions that result from falls are typically confined to a single body area and are considered a reasonable finding of a child still learning to walk.

NP: Assessment; CN: Health promotion and maintenance; CNS: Prevention and early detection of disease; CL: Application

25. 2. The mother is finding empty eggshells in the child's hair. Adults are the last stage of development, living about 30 days. Nymphs are the newly hatched lice and become adults in 8 to 9 days. Newly laid eggs are small, translucent, and difficult to see.

NP: Analysis; CN: Physiological integrity; CNS: Physiological adaptation; CL: Knowledge

26. 3. Lindane is associated with seizures after absorption with topical use. Alopecia, increased LFT results, and hypertension aren't associated with the use of lindane.

NP: Analysis; CN: Physiological integrity; CNS: Pharmacological and parenteral therapies; CL: Knowledge

27. 1. Treatment should be repeated in 7 to 12 days to ensure that all eggs are killed. Combing the hair thoroughly is necessary to remove the lice eggs. People exposed to head lice should be examined to assess the presence of infestation before treatment.

NP: Analysis; CN: Physiological integrity; CNS: Physiological adaptation; CL: Knowledge

28. A mother reports that her 4-year-old child has been scratching at his rectum recently. Which of the following infestations or conditions would the nurse suspect?

1. Anal fissure
2. Lice
3. Pinworms
4. Scabies

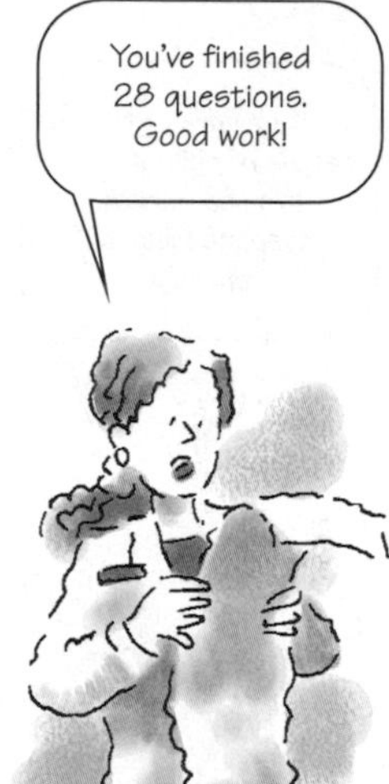

28. 3. The clinical sign of pinworms is perianal itching that increases at night. Scabies are associated with a pruritic rash characterized as linear burrows of the webs of the fingers and toes. Lice are infestations of the hair. Anal fissures are associated with rectal bleeding and pain with bowel movements.
NP: Analysis; CN: Physiological integrity; CNS: Physiological adaptation; CL: Knowledge

29. Diagnosing pinworms by the clear cellophane tape test is preferred. How many tests are necessary to detect infestations at virtually 100% accuracy?

1. One
2. Three
3. Five
4. Ten

29. 3. Detection is virtually 100% accurate with five tests. Three tests should detect infestations at about 90% accuracy. One test is only 50% accurate.
NP: Analysis; CN: Health promotion and maintenance; CNS: Prevention and early detection of disease; CL: Application

30. Each member of the family of a child diagnosed with pinworms is prescribed a single dose of pyrantel pamoate (Antiminth). Which of the following statements is correct about pyrantel pamoate?

1. The drug may stain the feces red.
2. The dose may be repeated in 2 weeks.
3. Fever and rash are common adverse effects.
4. The medicine will kill the eggs in about 48 hours.

30. 2. Pyrantel is effective against the adult worms only, so treatment can be repeated to eradicate any emerging parasites in 2 weeks. Common adverse effects are headaches and abdominal complaints. Staining the feces is associated with pyrvinium pamoate.
NP: Analysis; CN: Physiological integrity; CNS: Pharmacological and parenteral therapies; CL: Knowledge

31. A child received a bite to the hand from a large dog. Which of the following types of injury is associated with bites from large dogs?

1. Abrasion
2. Crush injury
3. Fracture
4. Puncture wound

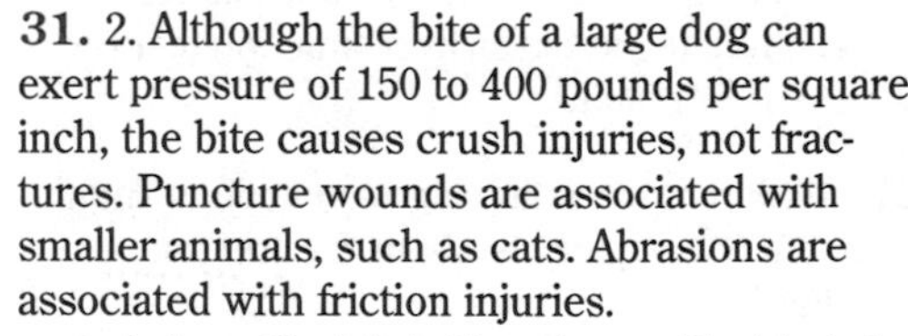

31. 2. Although the bite of a large dog can exert pressure of 150 to 400 pounds per square inch, the bite causes crush injuries, not fractures. Puncture wounds are associated with smaller animals, such as cats. Abrasions are associated with friction injuries.
NP: Analysis; CN: Physiological integrity; CNS: Physiological adaptation; CL: Knowledge

32. The nurse knows that bites from dogs are at risk for infection. Which of the following interventions should be done to help prevent infection?

1. Give the rabies vaccine.
2. Give antibiotics immediately.
3. Clean and irrigate the wounds.
4. Nothing; bites from dogs have a low incidence of infection.

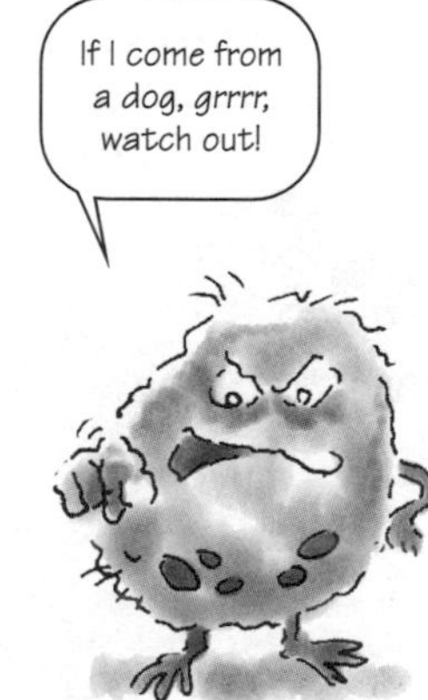

If I come from
a dog, grrrr,
watch out!

32. 3. Not every dog bite requires antibiotic therapy, but cleaning the wound is necessary for all injuries involving a break in the skin. Rabies vaccine is used if there is a suspicion the dog has rabies. The infection rate for dog bites has been reported to be as high as 50%.
NP: Implementation; CN: Physiological integrity; CNS: Reduction of risk potential; CL: Application

NP: Nursing process CN: Client needs category CNS: Client needs subcategory CL: Cognitive level

33. Which of the following organisms is believed responsible for up to 50% of the infections resulting from dog bites?

1. *Escherichia coli*
2. *Francisella tularensis*
3. *Pasteurella multocida*
4. *Rochalimaea henselae*

33. 3. *Pasteurella multocida* is associated with infection in up to 50% of the bites from dogs. *E. coli* is more likely to cause infections of the urinary tract. *Rochalimaea henselae*, a gram-negative rickettsial bacterium, is associated with cat-scratch disease. *Francisella tularensis* is found in such animals as rabbits, hares, and muskrats.

NP: Analysis; CN: Physiological integrity; CNS: Physiological adaptation; CL: Knowledge

34. A child is brought to the physician's office for multiple scratches and bites from a kitten. Which of the following symptoms is primarily found on assessment with cat-scratch disease?

1. Abdominal pain
2. Adenitis
3. Fever
4. Pruritus

34. 2. Adenitis is the primary feature of cat-scratch disease. Although low-grade fever has been associated with cat-scratch disease, it's only present 25% of the time. Pruritus and abdominal pain aren't symptoms of cat-scratch disease.

NP: Analysis; CN: Physiological integrity; CNS: Physiological adaptation; CL: Knowledge

35. In which of the following populations is giardiasis the most common parasitic intestinal infection in the United States?

1. Children riding a school bus
2. Children playing on a playground
3. Children attending a sporting event
4. Children attending group day care or nursery school

35. 4. The most common intestinal parasitic infection in the United States is giardiasis, prevalent among children attending group day care or nursery school. Playgrounds, sporting events, and school buses don't present unusual risk of giardiasis.

NP: Analysis; CN: Physiological integrity; CNS: Physiological adaptation; CL: Knowledge

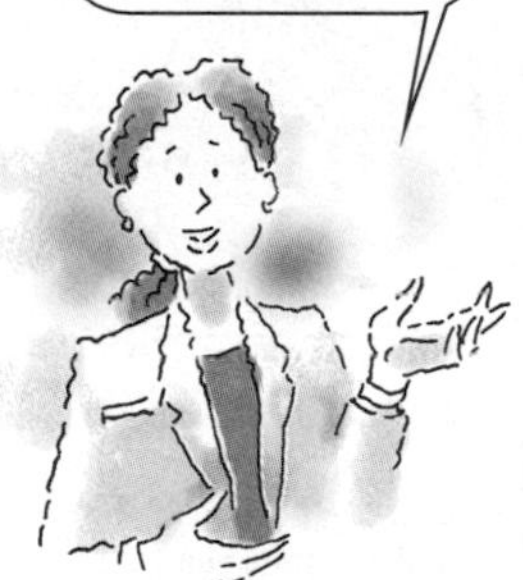

You need to know the correct terms to share information with clients and other health care providers.

36. Which of the following characteristics would apply to lesions such as papules, nodules, and tumors?

1. Palpable elevated masses
2. Loss of the epidermis layer
3. Fluid-filled elevations of the skin
4. Nonpalpable flat changes in skin color

36. 1. Papules are elevated up to 0.5 cm. Nodules and tumors are elevated more than 0.5 cm. Macules and patches are described as nonpalpable flat changes in skin color. Fluid-filled lesions are vesicles and pustules. Erosions are characterized as loss of the epidermis layer.

NP: Analysis; CN: Health promotion and maintenance; CNS: Prevention and early detection of disease; CL: Knowledge

37. A child is diagnosed with impetigo. Pustules are the primary lesions found on this child. Which of the following descriptions is correct for pustules?

1. Lesion filled with pus
2. Superficial area of localized edema
3. Serous-filled lesion less than 0.5 cm
4. Serous-filled lesion greater than 0.5 cm

37. 1. Pustules are pus-filled lesions, such as acne and impetigo. Bullae are serous-filled lesions greater than 0.5 cm in diameter. A wheal is a superficial area of localized edema. Vesicles are serous-filled lesions up to 0.5 cm in diameter.

NP: Analysis; CN: Physiological integrity; CNS: Physiological adaptation; CL: Knowledge

38. A 3-month-old infant is noted to have café-au-lait spots on examination. The presence of 6 or more of these lesions with a diameter greater then 1.5 cm is suggestive of which of the following disorders?
1. Meningococcemia
2. Neurofibromatosis
3. Tinea versicolor
4. Vitiligo

38. 2. Six or more uniformly pigmented patches with irregular borders, known as café-au-lait spots, with diameters greater then 1.5 cm are associated with neurofibromatosis. Tinea versicolor is a superficial fungus infection. Meningococcemia has petechiae, not café-au-lait spots. Depigmented areas are signs of vitiligo.
NP: Assessment; CN: Health promotion and maintenance; CNS: Prevention and early detection of disease; CL: Knowledge

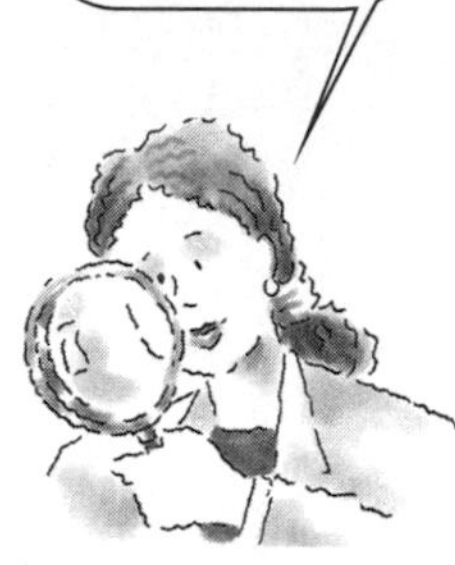

Assessment is an enormously important skill.

39. A child is brought to the physician's office for treatment of a rash. Many petechiae are seen over his entire body. Multiple petechiae would be consistent with which of the following conditions or symptoms?
1. Bleeding disorder
2. Scabies
3. Varicella
4. Vomiting

39. 1. Petechiae are caused by blood outside a vessel, associated with low platelet counts and bleeding disorders. Petechiae aren't found with varicella disease or scabies. Petechiae can be associated with vomiting, but they'd be present on the face, not the entire body.
NP: Assessment; CN: Physiological integrity; CNS: Physiological adaptation; CL: Knowledge

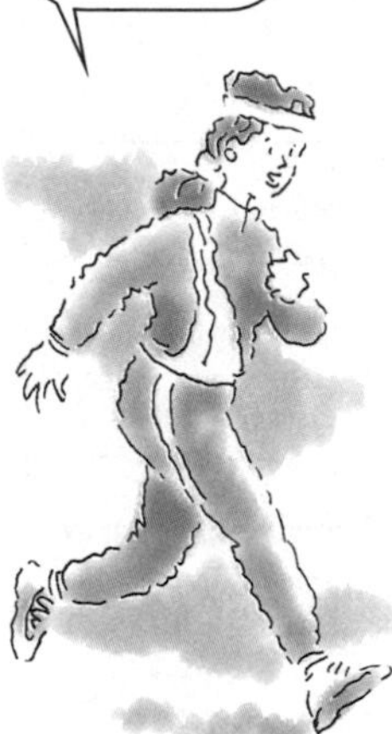

Don't fall down now! Keep at it!

40. A child fell at camp and sustained a bruise to his thigh. Which of the following descriptions would accurately describe the bruise after 1 week?
1. Resolved
2. Reddish blue
3. Greenish yellow
4. Dark blue to bluish brown

40. 3. After 7 to 10 days, the bruise becomes greenish yellow. Resolution can take up to 2 weeks. Initially after the fall, there's a reddish blue discoloration, followed by dark blue to bluish brown at days 1 to 3.
NP: Analysis; CN: Physiological integrity; CNS: Physiological adaptation; CL: Application

41. Which of the following factors about contusions are suggestive of child abuse?
1. Multiple contusions of the shins
2. Contusions of the back and buttocks
3. Contusions at the same stages of healing
4. Large contusion and hematoma of the forehead

41. 2. Contusions of the back and buttocks are highly suspicious of abuse related to punishment. Contusions at various stages of healing are red flags to potential abuse. Contusions of the shins and forehead are usually related to an active toddler falling and bumping into objects.
NP: Assessment; CN: Health promotion and maintenance; CNS: Prevention and early detection of disease; CL: Knowledge

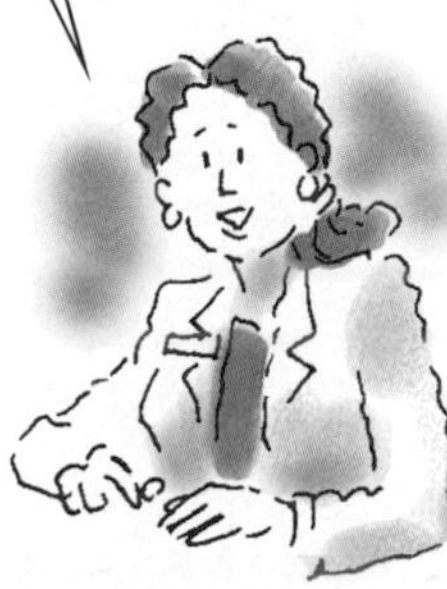

Know what to tell a family when an infant is born with salmon patches.

42. Which of the following statements about salmon patches (stork bites) is correct?
1. They're benign and usually fade in adult life.
2. They're commonly associated with syndromes of the newborn.
3. They can cause mild hypertrophy of the muscle associated with the lesion.
4. They're treatable with laser pulse surgery in late adolescence and adulthood.

42. 1. Salmon patches occur over the back of the neck in 40% of infants and are harmless, needing no intervention. Port wine stains are associated with syndromes of neonates such as Sturge-Weber syndrome. Port wine stains found on the face or extremities may be associated with soft tissue and bone hypertrophy. Laser pulse surgery isn't recommended for salmon patches because they typically fade on their own in adulthood.
NP: Analysis; CN: Health promotion and maintenance; CNS: Growth and development through the life span; CL: Knowledge

43. A neonate is born with a blue-black macular lesion over the lower lumbar sacral region. Which of the following terms applies to this lesion?

1. Café-au-lait spots
2. Mongolian spots
3. Nevis of Ota spot
4. Stork bites

43. 2. Mongolian spots are large blue-black macular lesions generally located over the lumbosacral areas, buttocks, and limbs. Café-au-lait spots occur between the ages of 2 and 16 years, not in infancy. Nevis of Ota is found surrounding the eyes. Stork bites or salmon patches occur at the neck and hairline area.

NP: Assessment; CN: Health promotion and maintenance; CNS: Growth and development through the life span; CL: Knowledge

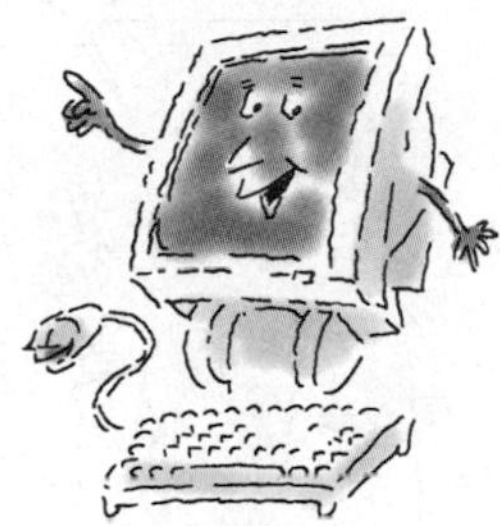

The word *severe* is a clue to the correct answer.

44. Which of the following findings indicate severe dehydration in a child?

1. Gray skin and decreased tears
2. Capillary refill less than 2 seconds
3. Mottled skin and tenting of the skin
4. Pale skin with dry mucous membranes

44. 3. Severe dehydration is associated with mottling and tenting of the skin. Pale skin with dry mucous membranes is a sign of mild dehydration. Malnutrition is characterized by gray skin and tenting of the skin. Capillary refill less then 2 seconds is normal.

NP: Analysis; CN: Health promotion and maintenance; CNS: Prevention and early detection of disease; CL: Knowledge

45. Isotretinoin (Accutane) is associated with which of the following adverse effects?

1. GI upset
2. Gram-negative folliculitis
3. Teratogenicity
4. Vaginal candidiasis

45. 3. The use of even small amounts of isotretinoin has been associated with severe birth defects. Most female clients are prescribed oral contraceptives. Cleocin T, another medicine used in the treatment of acne, is associated with both diarrhea and gram-negative folliculitis. Tetracycline is associated with yeast infections.

NP: Analysis; CN: Health promotion and maintenance; CNS: Growth and development through the life span; CL: Knowledge

46. Which of the following characteristics is often responsible for the failure of treatment for acne in teenagers?

1. Topical treatment
2. Systemic treatment
3. A dominant parent who wants treatment and a passive teenager who doesn't
4. A dominant teenager who wants treatment and a passive uninterested parent

46. 3. The active participation of a teenager is needed for the successful treatment of acne. Systemic and topical therapy are needed in most acne treatment.

NP: Analysis; CN: Health promotion and maintenance; CNS: Growth and development through the life span; CL: Knowledge

47. Which of the following information should be given to a teenager about acne?

1. Acne is caused by diet.
2. Acne is related to gender.
3. Acne is caused by poor hygiene.
4. Acne is caused by hormonal changes.

47. 4. Acne is caused by hormonal changes in sebaceous gland anatomy and the biochemistry of the glands. These changes lead to a blockage in the follicular canal and cause an inflammatory response. Diet, hygiene, and the client's gender don't cause acne.

NP: Analysis; CN: Health promotion and maintenance; CNS: Growth and development through the life span; CL: Knowledge

48. When teaching a client about tetracycline for severe inflammatory acne, which of the following instructions must be given?

1. Take the drug with or without meals.
2. Take the drug with milk and milk products.
3. Take the drug on an empty stomach with small amounts of water.
4. Take the drug 1 hour before or 2 hours after meals with large amounts of water.

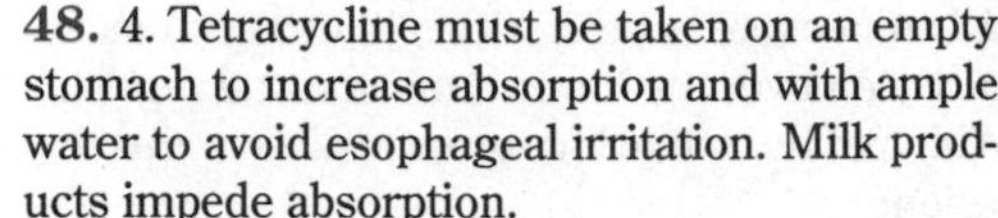

48. 4. Tetracycline must be taken on an empty stomach to increase absorption and with ample water to avoid esophageal irritation. Milk products impede absorption.

NP: Implementation; CN: Physiological integrity; CNS: Pharmacological and parenteral therapies; CL: Application

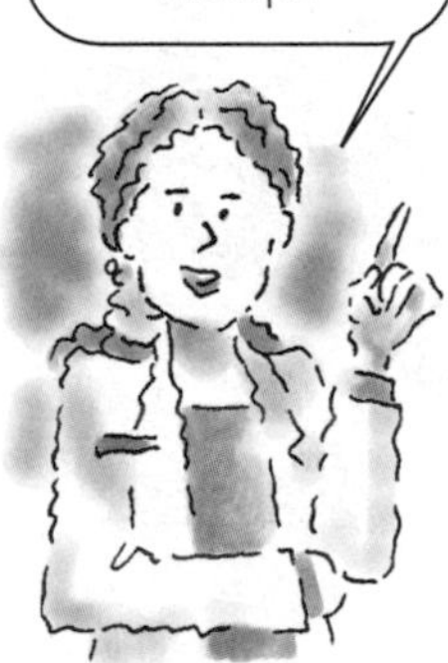
Parent teaching prevents future mishaps.

49. When advising parents about the prevention of burns from tap water, which of the following instructions should be given?

1. Set the water-heater temperature at 130° F or less.
2. Run the hot water first, then adjust the temperature with cold water.
3. Before you put your infant in the tub, first test the water with your hand.
4. Supervise an infant in the bathroom, only leaving him for a few seconds, if needed.

49. 3. Instruct the parents to fill the tub with water first and then test all of the water in the tub with their hand for hot spots. Water heaters should be set at 120° F. Never leave an infant alone in the bathroom, even for a second. The cold water should be run first and then adjusted with hot water.

NP: Analysis; CN: Health promotion and maintenance; CNS: Prevention and early detection of disease; CL: Knowledge

50. While caring for a 2-day-old neonate, the nurse notices the left side of the neonate becomes reddened for 2 to 3 minutes. Which of the following factors or conditions would cause this?

1. Contact dermatitis
2. Environmental conditions
3. Harlequin color change
4. Tet spells

Hip! Hip! Hurray for you! You've reached question 50.

50. 3. Harlequin color change is a benign disorder related to the immaturity of hypothalamic centers that control the tone of peripheral blood vessels. Tet spells are associated with tetralogy of Fallot and cause cyanotic changes. Changes in environmental conditions can cause diffuse bilateral mottling of the skin. Contact dermatitis isn't short-lived.

NP: Assessment; CN: Health promotion and maintenance; CNS: Growth and development through the life span; CL: Knowledge

51. A 15-month-old child is diagnosed with pediculosis of the eyebrows. Which of the following interventions are included in the treatment?

1. Use lindane.
2. Use petroleum jelly.
3. Shave the eyebrows.
4. No treatment is needed.

51. 2. Petroleum jelly should be applied twice daily for 8 days, followed by manual removal of nits. The eyebrow should never be shaved because of the uncertainty of hair return. Lindane is contraindicated because of the risk for seizures.

NP: Analysis; CN: Physiological integrity; CNS: Physiological adaptation; CL: Knowledge

52. A 5-year-old child appears with hair loss and a 6-cm boggy honey-colored mass on the scalp. With which of the following conditions is this mass associated?

1. Alopecia areata
2. Bullous impetigo
3. Cradle cap
4. Kerion

52. 4. A kerion is a boggy inflammatory mass over the tinea. It's associated with the inflammatory reaction of the fungal infection. Bullous impetigo and cradle cap aren't associated with hair loss. Alopecia areata is hair loss without inflammation or associated rash.

NP: Assessment; CN: Physiological integrity; CNS: Physiological adaptation; CL: Knowledge

53. Which of the following changes in the mouth is consistent with Kawasaki syndrome?
1. Koplik's spots
2. Tonsillar exudate
3. Vesicular lesions
4. Dry cracked lips, strawberry tongue

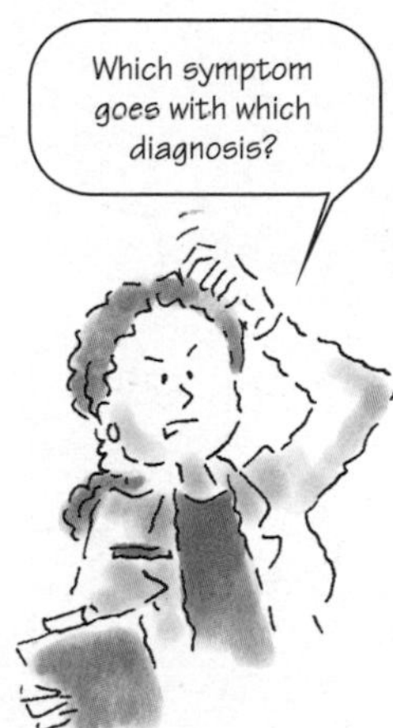

Which symptom goes with which diagnosis?

53. 4. Oral changes associated with Kawasaki syndrome include an injected pharynx, injected lips, dry fissured lips, and strawberry tongue. Koplik's spots are consistent with measles. Vesicular lesions are associated with coxsackievirus. Tonsillar exudate is consistent with pharyngitis caused by group A beta hemolytic streptococci.

NP: Analysis; CN: Physiological integrity; CNS: Physiological adaptation; CL: Knowledge

54. A 3-year-old child has palpable purpura of the buttocks and lower extremities. These findings are a classic symptom of which of the following disorders?
1. Child abuse
2. Henoch-Schönlein purpura (HSP)
3. Idiopathic thrombocytopenic purpura (ITP)
4. Rocky Mountain spotted fever

54. 2. The rash associated with HSP is believed to occur in every client and allows for a definitive diagnosis. It begins as petechiae and progresses to purpuric lesions of the buttocks and lower extremities. The lesions of child abuse are painful and nonraised. Petechiae or purpura associated with ITP are distributed over the entire body. The rash in Rocky Mountain spotted fever is a nonraised macular papular rash spread over the body.

NP: Assessment; CN: Physiological integrity; CNS: Physiological adaptation; CL: Knowledge

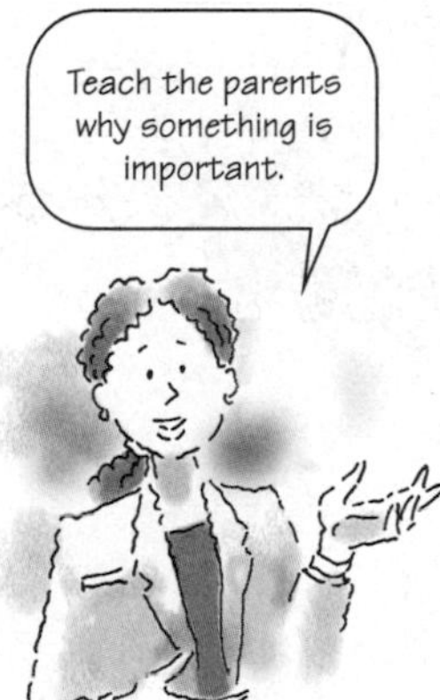

Teach the parents why something is important.

55. Topical treatment with 2.5% hydrocortisone is prescribed for a 6-month-old infant with eczema. The mother is instructed to use the cream for not more than 1 week. Why is this time limit appropriate?
1. The drug loses its efficacy after prolonged use
2. To reduce adverse effects, such as skin atrophy and fragility
3. If no improvement is seen, a stronger concentration will be prescribed
4. If no improvement is seen after 1 week, an antibiotic will be prescribed

55. 2. Hydrocortisone cream should be used for brief periods to decrease adverse effects, such as atrophy of the skin. The drug doesn't lose efficacy after prolonged use, a stronger concentration may not be prescribed if no improvement is seen, and an antibiotic would be inappropriate in this instance.

NP: Analysis; CN: Physiological integrity; CNS: Pharmacological and parenteral therapies; CL: Knowledge

56. A 9-year-old child is examined because her mother noticed lesions on her tongue. Painless, slightly depressed, red lesions bordered with white bands are seen on examination. The mother reports the patterns were different yesterday. Which of the following conditions is suspected?
1. Geographic tongue
2. Koplik's spots
3. Scald burns
4. Stomatitis

56. 1. This benign disorder is caused by loss of filiform papules. The configuration is known to change from day to day. Scald burns are painful lesions from hot liquids. Koplik's spots and stomatitis lesions don't change patterns.

NP: Assessment; CN: Physiological integrity; CNS: Physiological adaptation; CL: Knowledge

57. A 4-year-old child had a subungual hemorrhage of the toe after a jar fell on his foot. Electrocautery is performed. For which of the following reasons is electrocautery done?

1. Prevent loss of nail growth
2. Prevent spread of the infection
3. Relieve pain and reduce the risk for infection
4. Prevent permanent discoloration of the nail bed

57. 3. The hematoma is treated with electrocautery to relieve pain and reduce risk for infection. The discoloration seen with subungual hemorrhage is from the collection of blood under the nail bed. It's not permanent and doesn't affect nail growth. Infections of the nail beds are called paronychia.

NP: Analysis; CN: Physiological integrity; CNS: Physiological adaptation; CL: Knowledge

58. A 9-month-old infant is brought to the physician's office. He has painful, hot, tense, bright-red lesions on his cheeks. Which of the following infections does this symptom indicate?

1. Erysipelas
2. Fifth disease
3. Impetigo
4. Lupus

58. 1. Erysipelas is a superficial cellulitis of the skin characterized by painful, hot, tense, bright red lesions. The infection tends to occur on the face and scalp but can appear on any surface. The rashes of fifth disease and lupus don't have the signs of infection, such as pain, heat, and tension. Impetigo appears as pustules.

NP: Assessment; CN: Physiological integrity; CNS: Physiological adaptation; CL: Knowledge

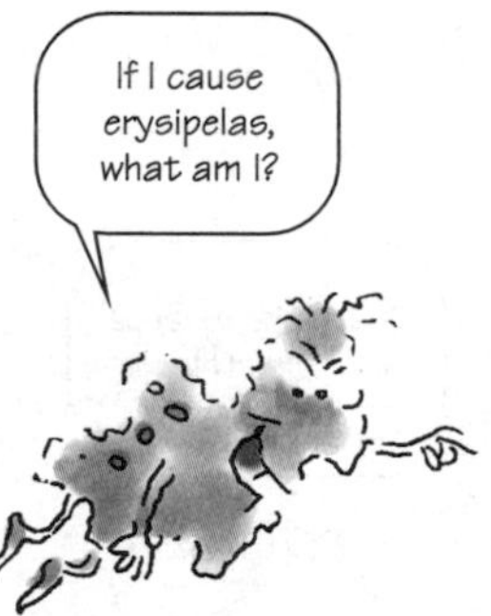
If I cause erysipelas, what am I?

59. A 16-month-old child is diagnosed with erysipelas. Which of the following organisms causes this superficial cellulitis?

1. *Haemophilus influenzae*
2. *Staphylococcus aureus*
3. Group B streptococcus
4. Group A beta streptococcus

59. 4. Erysipelas is caused by group A beta streptococci. *H. influenza*, *S. aureus*, and *Streptococcus pneumoniae* don't cause this superficial cellulitis of the skin.

NP: Analysis; CN: Physiological integrity; CNS: Physiological adaptation; CL: Knowledge

60. A mother of a 4-month-old infant asks about the strawberry hemangioma on his cheek. Which statement is correct?

1. The lesion will continue to grow for 3 years, then need surgical removal.
2. If the lesion continues to enlarge, referral to a pediatric oncologist is warranted.
3. Surgery is indicated before age 12 months if the diameter of the lesion is greater then 3 cm.
4. The lesion will continue to grow until age 12 months, then begin to resolve by age 2 to 3 years.

60. 4. These rapidly growing vascular lesions reach maximum growth by age 1 year. The growth period is then followed by an involution period of 6 to 12 months. Lesions show complete involution by age 2 or 3 years. These benign lesions don't need surgical or oncologic referrals.

NP: Assessment; CN: Health promotion and maintenance; CNS: Growth and development through the life span; CL: Knowledge

61. A 3-year-old child is being discharged from the emergency department after receiving three sutures for a scalp laceration. In how many days would the nurse tell the family to return for suture removal?

1. 1 to 3 days
2. 5 to 7 days
3. 8 to 10 days
4. 10 to 14 days

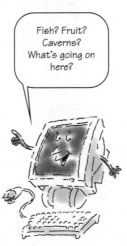

61. 2. The recommended healing time for this type of laceration is 5 to 7 days. Sutures need longer than 1 to 3 days to form an effective bond. Eight to 10 days is needed for sutures of the fingertips and feet, and 10 to 14 days is the recommended time for extensor surfaces of the knees and elbows.

NP: Analysis; CN: Physiological integrity; CNS: Physiological adaptation; CL: Knowledge

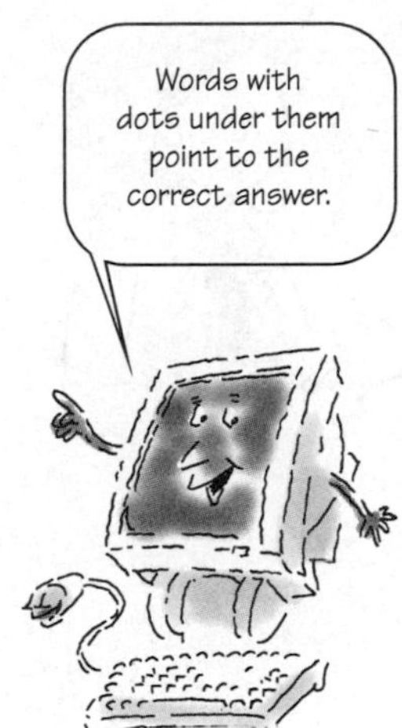

Words with dots under them point to the correct answer.

62. Which of the following symptoms are early signs of infection of a laceration?

1. Fever
2. Copious drainage
3. Excessive discomfort
4. Local nodal enlargement

62. 3. The first sign of infection is usually excessive discomfort. Nodal enlargement, fever, and copious drainage are advanced signs of infection.

NP: Analysis; CN: Health promotion and maintenance; CNS: Prevention and early detection of disease; CL: Knowledge

63. A mother calls the physician to report an erythematous macular, papular rash on the trunk of her 2-day-old neonate. Which of the following conditions is indicated?

1. Erythema toxicum neonatorum
2. Cutis marmorata
3. Milia
4. Miliaria rubra

63. 1. Erythema toxicum neonatorum is an asymptomatic benign self-limiting cutaneous eruption most frequently seen on days 3 and 4 after birth. Miliaria rubra has erythematous papules, vesicles caused by obstruction of sweat ducts. Milia are 1- to 2-mm white papules on the face. Cutis marmorata is mottled skin.

NP: Analysis; CN: Physiological integrity; CNS: Physiological adaptation; CL: Knowledge

64. When being examined, a 6-year-old child was noted to have a papulovesicular eruption on the left anterior lateral chest, with complaints of pain and tenderness of the lesion. Which of the following disorders would these findings indicate?

1. Contusion
2. Herpes zoster
3. Scabies
4. Varicella

64. 2. Herpes zoster is caused by the varicella zoster virus. It has papulovesicular lesions that erupt along a dermatome, usually with hyperesthesia, pain, and tenderness. Scabies appear as linear burrows of the fingers and toes caused by a mite. Contusions aren't found with papulovesicular lesions. The papulovesicular lesions of varicella are distributed over the entire trunk, face, and scalp and don't follow a dermatome.

NP: Assessment; CN: Physiological integrity; CNS: Physiological adaptation; CL: Knowledge

Fish? Fruit? Caverns? What's going on here?

65. During an examination of a 5-month-old infant, a flat, dull pink, macular lesion is noted on the infant's forehead. Which of the following conditions does this lesion indicate?

1. Cavernous hemangioma
2. Nevus flammeus
3. Salmon patch
4. Strawberry hemangioma

65. 3. Salmon patches are common vascular lesions in infants. They appear as flat, dull pink, macular lesions in various regions of the face and head. When they appear on the nape of the neck, they're commonly called "stork bites." These lesions fade by the first year of life. Nevus flammeus, or port wine stains, are reddish-purple lesions that don't fade. Both strawberry and cavernous hemangiomas are raised lesions.

NP: Assessment; CN: Physiological integrity; CNS: Physiological adaptation; CL: Knowledge

66. A child's parents ask for advice on the use of an insect repellent that contains deet. Which of the following statements would be correct?

1. Spray the child's clothing instead of the skin.
2. The repellent works better as the temperature increases.
3. The repellent isn't effective against the ticks responsible for Lyme disease.
4. Apply insect repellent as you would sunscreen, with frequent applications.

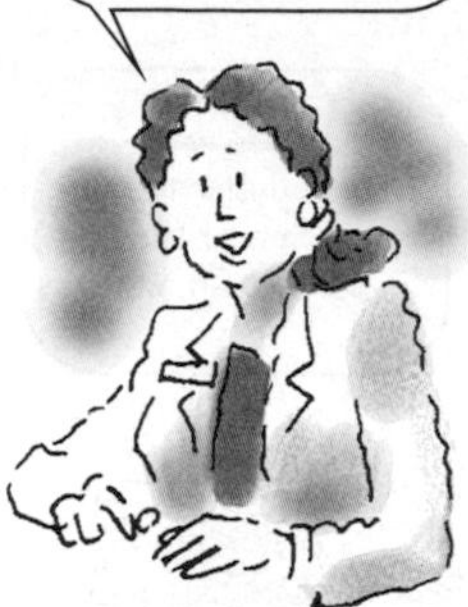

You're almost at question 70. That was quick!

66. 1. Deet spray has been approved for use on children. It should be used sparingly on all skin surfaces. By concentrating the spray on clothing and camping equipment, the adverse effects and potential toxic buildup is significantly reduced. Repellent is lost to evaporation, wind, heat, and perspiration. With each 10° F increase in temperature, it leads to as much as a 50% reduction in protection time. Deet is very effective as a tick repellent.

NP: Analysis; CN: Physiological integrity; CNS: Reduction of risk potential; CL: Knowledge

67. Deet-containing products such as insect repellent should be used in which of the following concentrations on a child's skin for optimal results?

1. 10%
2. 15%
3. 20%
4. 30%

67. 1. The highest concentration approved by the Food and Drug Administration for children is 10%. Because of thinner skin and greater surface area to mass ratio in children, parents should use deet products sparingly.

NP: Analysis; CN: Physiological integrity; CNS: Reduction of risk potential; CL: Knowledge

68. Which of the following statements about warts is correct?

1. Cutting the wart is the preferred treatment for children.
2. There is no treatment that specifically kills the wart virus.
3. Warts are caused by a virus affecting the inner layer of skin.
4. Warts are harmless and usually last 2 to 4 years if untreated.

68. 2. The goal of treatment is to kill the skin that contains the wart virus. Warts are harmless and last 1 to 2 years if untreated. Cutting the wart is likely to spread the virus. The virus that causes warts affects the outer layer of the skin.

NP: Analysis; CN: Physiological integrity; CNS: Physiological adaptation; CL: Knowledge

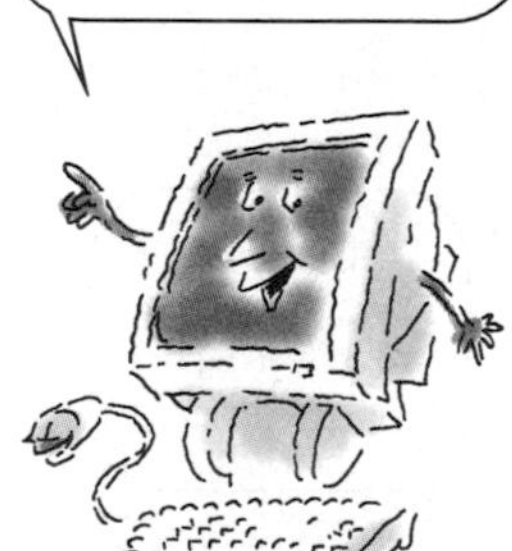

69. Which of the following factors cause tooth decay and gum disease when allowed to remain on the teeth for prolonged periods?

1. Breast milk
2. Pacifiers
3. Thumb or other fingers
4. Water

69. 1. Tooth decay and gum disease result when the carbohydrates in breast milk, formula, cow's milk, and fruit juices remain on the teeth for a prolonged period. Water is harmless and pacifiers and fingers don't cause tooth decay and gum disease, but may contribute to malocclusion.

NP: Assessment; CN: Health promotion and maintenance; CNS: Prevention and early detection of disease; CL: Knowledge

70. What are the classic signs of cellulitis in a child?

1. Pale, irritated, cold to touch
2. Vesicular blisters at the site of the injury
3. Fever, edema, tenderness, warmth at the site
4. Swelling, redness, with well-defined borders

70. 3. Cellulitis is a deep, locally diffuse infection of the skin. It's associated with redness, fever, edema, tenderness, and warmth at the site of the injury. Vesicular blisters suggest impetigo. Cellulitis has no well-defined borders.

NP: Assessment; CN: Physiological integrity; CNS: Physiological adaptation; CL: Knowledge

71. A 2-year-old child has cellulitis of the finger. Which of the following organisms or conditions is the most likely cause of the infection?
1. Parainfluenza virus
2. Respiratory syncytial virus
3. *Escherichia coli*
4. *Streptococcus*

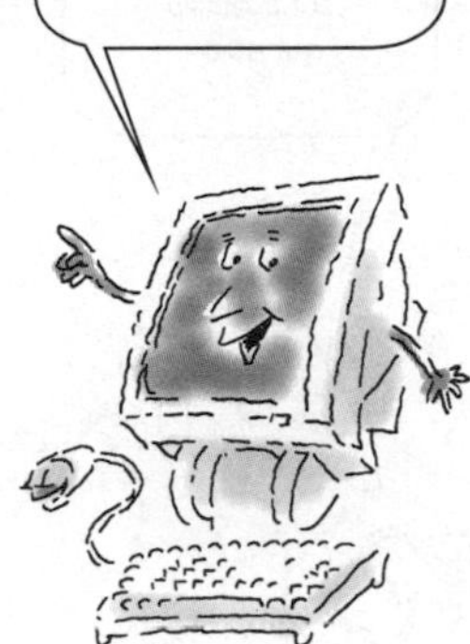

Note that this question asks about most likely causes, not the only ones.

71. 4. *Streptococcus* cause most cases of cellulitis. Parainfluenza and respiratory syncytial virus cause infections of the respiratory tract. *E. coli* is a cause of bladder infections.

NP: Assessment; CN: Physiological integrity; CNS: Physiological adaptation; CL: Knowledge

72. A child has a desquamation rash of the hands and feet. Which of the following symptoms best describes desquamation rash?
1. Peeling skin
2. Thin, flaking layers of epidermis
3. Thick skin with deep visible burrows
4. Thinning skin that may appear translucent

72. 1. Desquamation is characteristic in diseases such as Stevens-Johnson syndrome. Thickening of the skin with burrows is defined as lichenification. Scaling is thin, flaking layers of epidermis. Thinning skin is best described as atrophy of the skin.

NP: Assessment; CN: Physiological integrity; CNS: Physiological adaptation; CL: Knowledge

73. Which of the following instructions about the administration of nystatin oral solution is correct?
1. Give the solution immediately after feedings.
2. Give the solution immediately before feedings.
3. Mix the solution with small amounts of the feeding.
4. Give half the solution before and half the solution after the feeding.

73. 1. Nystatin oral solution should be swabbed onto the mouth after feedings to allow for optimal contact with mucous membranes. Before meals and with meals doesn't give the best contact with the mucous membranes.

NP: Implementation; CN: Physiological integrity; CNS: Pharmacological and parenteral therapies; CL: Application

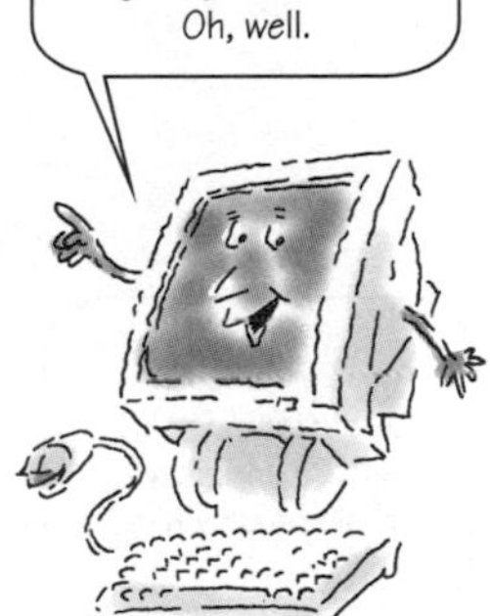

Petechiae. Even the word sounds small, doesn't it? Oops, I gave you a hint. Oh, well.

74. An infant is examined and found to have a petechial rash. Which of the following descriptions is correct for petechia?
1. Purple macular lesion larger than 1 cm in diameter
2. A purple to brown bruise, macular or papular, various sizes
3. Collection of blood from ruptured blood vessels larger than 1 cm in diameter
4. A pinpoint, pink to purple, nonblanching macular lesion 1 to 3 mm in diameter

74. 4. Petechiae are small 1- to 3-mm macular lesions. A bruise is defined as ecchymosis. Purple macular lesions greater than 1 cm are defined as purpura. A hematoma is a collection of blood.

NP: Assessment; CN: Physiological integrity; CNS: Physiological adaptation; CL: Knowledge

75. A child has a red rash in a circular shape on his legs. The lesions aren't connected. Which of the following classifications is the most appropriate for this rash?
1. A linear rash
2. A diffuse rash
3. An annular rash
4. A confluent rash

75. 3. An annular rash is ring-shaped. Linear rashes are lesions arranged in a line. A diffuse rash usually has scattered, widely distributed lesions. Confluent lesions are touching or adjacent to each other.

NP: Assessment; CN: Physiological integrity; CNS: Physiological adaptation; CL: Knowledge

76. A mother noticed her teenager is losing hair in small round areas on the scalp. This symptom is characteristic of which of the following conditions?

1. Alopecia
2. Amblyopia
3. Exotropia
4. Seborrhea dermatitis

76. 1. Alopecia is the correct term for thinning hair loss. Seborrhea dermatitis is cradle cap and occurs in infants. Exotropia and amblyopia are eye disorders.

NP: Analysis; CN: Physiological integrity; CNS: Physiological adaptation; CL: Knowledge

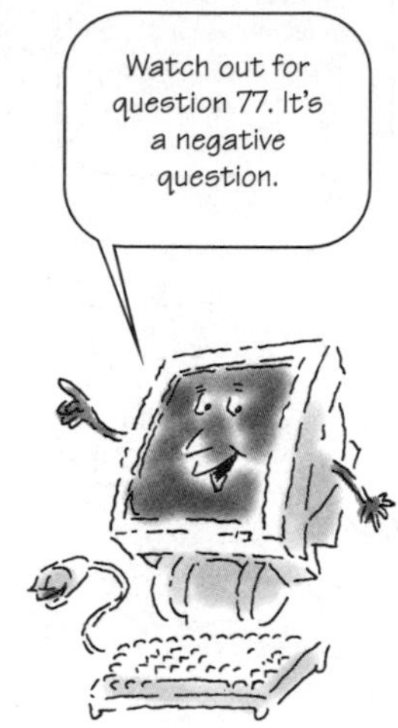

Watch out for question 77. It's a negative question.

77. Which of the following rashes doesn't show dermatological changes of the palms?

1. Coxsackievirus
2. Measles
3. Rocky Mountain spotted fever
4. Syphilis

77. 2. Rocky Mountain spotted fever, syphilis, and coxsackievirus show changes on the palms and soles of the feet. The rash in measles occurs on the face, trunk, and extremities.

NP: Analysis; CN: Physiological integrity; CNS: Physiological adaptation; CL: Knowledge

78. Atopic dermatitis can be characterized as which of the following types of disorder?

1. Fungal infection
2. Hereditary disorder
3. Sex-linked disorder
4. Viral infection

78. 2. Atopic dermatitis is a hereditary disorder associated with a family history of asthma, allergic rhinitis, or atopic dermatitis. Viral and fungal infections don't cause atopic dermatitis.

NP: Analysis; CN: Physiological integrity; CNS: Physiological adaptation; CL: Knowledge

79. The mother of a 6-month-old infant with atopic dermatitis asks for advice on bathing the child. Which instruction should be given?

1. Bathe the infant twice daily.
2. Bathe the infant every other day.
3. Use bubble baths to decrease itching.
4. The frequency of the infant's baths isn't important in atopic dermatitis.

79. 2. Bathing removes lipoprotein complexes that hold water in the stratum corneum and increase water loss. Decreasing bathing to every other day can help prevent the removal of lipoprotein complexes. Soap and bubble bath should be used sparingly while bathing the child.

NP: Analysis; CN: Physiological integrity; CNS: Basic care and comfort; CL: Application

80. Discharge instructions for a child with atopic dermatitis include keeping the fingernails cut short. Which of the following statements would explain the reason for this intervention?

1. Prevent infection of the nail bed
2. Prevent the spread of the disorder
3. Prevent the child from causing a corneal abrasion
4. Reduce breaks in skin from scratching that may lead to secondary bacterial infections

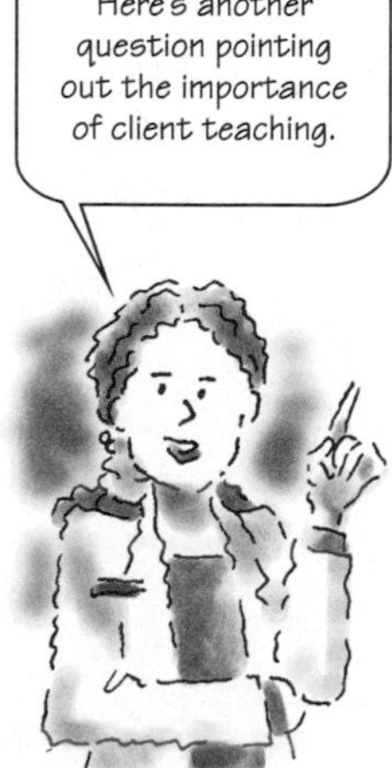

Here's another question pointing out the importance of client teaching.

80. 4. Keeping fingernails cut short will prevent breaks in the skin when a child scratches. Atopic dermatitis can be found in various areas of the skin, but isn't spread from one area to another. Cutting fingernails too short or cutting the skin around the nail can increase the risk of infection. Keeping fingernails short is a good way to reduce corneal abrasions, but doesn't apply to atopic dermatitis.

NP: Analysis; CN: Physiological integrity; CNS: Physiological adaptation; CL: Knowledge

NP: Nursing process CN: Client needs category CNS: Client needs subcategory CL: Cognitive level

81. A 10-year-old child is being treated for common warts. Which of the following viruses causes this condition?

1. Coxsackievirus
2. Human herpesvirus (HHV)
3. Human immunodeficiency virus (HIV)
4. Human papillomavirus (HPV)

81. 4. HPV is responsible for various forms of warts. HIV infections aren't associated with epithelial tumors known as warts. coxsackievirus is associated with hand-foot-mouth disease. HHV is associated with varicella and herpes zoster.

NP: Analysis; CN: Physiological integrity; CNS: Physiological adaptation; CL: Knowledge

82. A 6-year-old child has a spiny projection from the skin suspended from a narrow stalk on the forehead. Which of the following types of wart is this skin projection?

1. Filiform wart
2. Flat wart
3. Plantar wart
4. Venereal warts

82. 1. Filiform warts are long spiny projections from the skin surface. Plantar warts are rough papules, commonly found on the soles of the feet. Flat warts are flat-topped smooth-surfaced lesions. Venereal warts appear on the genital mucosa and are confluent papules with rough surfaces.

NP: Assessment; CN: Physiological integrity; CNS: Physiological adaptation; CL: Knowledge

83. An adolescent says his feet itch, sweat a lot, and have a foul odor. Which of the following terms applies to this condition?

1. Candidiasis
2. Tinea corporis
3. Tinea pedis
4. Molluscum contagiosum

83. 3. Tinea pedis is a superficial fungal infection on the feet, commonly called athletes' foot. Candidiasis is a fungal infection of the skin or mucous membranes commonly found in the oral, vaginal, and intestinal mucosal tissue. Molluscum contagiosum is a viral skin infection with lesions that are small red papules. Tinea corporis, or ringworm, is a flat scaling papular lesion with raised borders.

NP: Analysis; CN: Physiological integrity; CNS: Physiological adaptation; CL: Knowledge

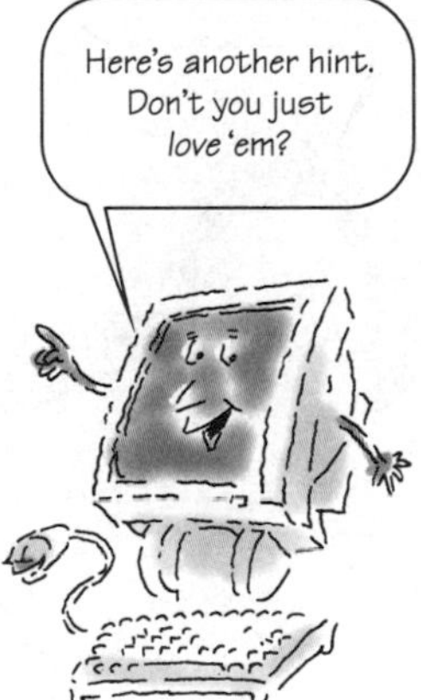

Here's another hint. Don't you just love 'em?

84. Which of the following treatments would best control hypertrophic scarring?

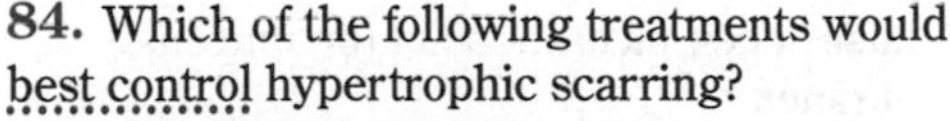

1. Compression garments
2. Moisturizing creams
3. Physiotherapy
4. Splints

84. 1. Compression garments are worn for up to 1 year to control hypertrophic scarring. Physiotherapy and splints help keep joints and limbs supple. Moisturizing creams help decrease hyperpigmentation.

NP: Analysis; CN: Physiological integrity; CNS: Physiological adaptation; CL: Knowledge

85. During a physical examination, a child is noted to have nails with "ice-pick" pits and ridges. The nails are thick and discolored and have splintered hemorrhages easily separated from the nail bed. Which of the following conditions would cause this condition?

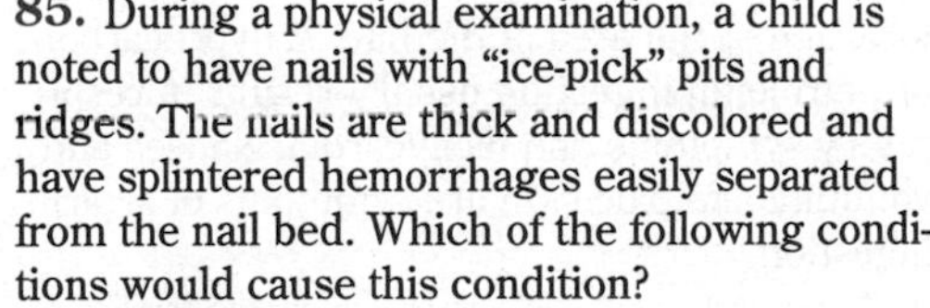

1. Paronychia
2. Psoriasis
3. Scabies
4. Seborrhea

85. 2. Psoriasis is a chronic skin disorder with an unknown cause that shows these characteristic skin changes. Scabies are mites that burrow under the skin, usually between the webbing of the fingers and toes. A paronychia is a bacterial infection of the nail bed. Seborrhea is a chronic inflammatory dermatitis or cradle cap.

NP: Assessment; CN: Physiological integrity; CNS: Physiological adaptation; CL: Knowledge

86. A neonate is examined and noted to have bruising on the scalp, along with diffuse swelling of the soft tissue that crosses over the suture line. Which of the following assessments is most accurate?

1. Caput succedaneum
2. Cephalhematoma
3. Craniotabes
4. Hydrocephalus

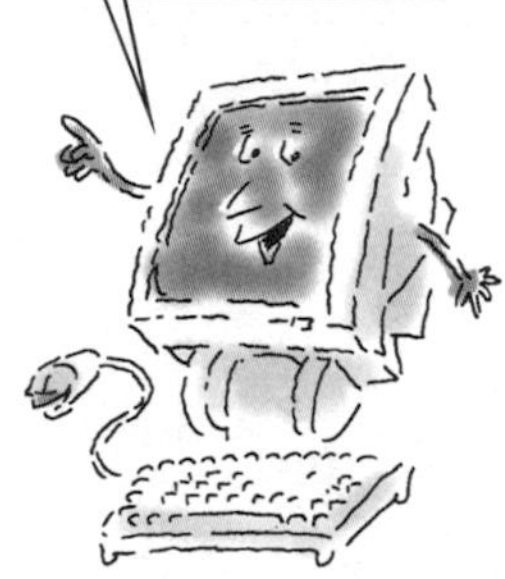

The words most accurate give you a bit of a clue to this question.

86. 1. Caput succedaneum originates from trauma to the neonate while descending through the birth canal. It's usually a benign injury that spontaneously resolves over time. Cephalhematoma is a collection of blood in the periosteum of the scalp that doesn't cross over the suture line. Hydrocephalus is an increased volume of cerebrospinal fluid (CSF) or the obstruction of the flow of the CSF and isn't related to soft tissue swelling. Craniotabes is the thinning of the bone of the scalp.

NP: Assessment; CN: Physiological integrity; CNS: Physiological adaptation; CL: Knowledge

87. A child has a healed wound from a traumatic injury. A lesion formed over the wound is pink, thickened, smooth, and rubbery in nature. Which of the following conditions best describes this wound?

1. Erosion
2. Fissure
3. Keloids
4. Striae

87. 3. Keloids are an exaggerated connective tissue response to skin injury. Striae are linear depressions of the skin. An erosion is a depressed vesicular lesion. A fissure is a cleavage in the surface of skin.

NP: Assessment; CN: Physiological integrity; CNS: Physiological adaptation; CL: Knowledge

88. The mother of an infant gives a history of poor feeding for a few days. A complete physical examination shows white plaques in the mouth with an erythematous base. The plaques stick to the mucous membranes tightly and bleed when scraped. Which of the following conditions best describes the plaques?

1. Chickenpox
2. Herpes lesions
3. Measles
4. Oral candidiasis

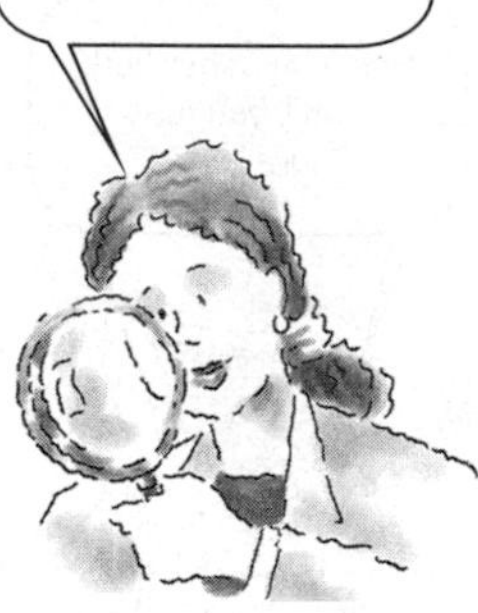

88. 4. Oral candidiasis, or thrush, is a painful inflammation that can affect the tongue, soft and hard palates, and buccal mucosa. Herpes lesions are usually vesicular ulcerations of the oral mucosa around the lips. Measles that form Koplik's spots can be identified as pinpoint white elevated lesions. Chickenpox, or varicella, causes open ulcerations of the mucous membranes.

NP: Assessment; CN: Physiological integrity; CNS: Physiological adaptation; CL: Knowledge

89. A child was found unconscious at home and brought to the emergency department by the fire and rescue unit. Physical examination showed cherry-red mucous membranes, nail beds, and skin. Which of the following causes is the most likely explanation for the child's condition?

1. Aspirin ingestion
2. Carbon monoxide poisoning
3. Hydrocarbon ingestion
4. Spider bite

89. 2. Cherry-red skin changes are seen when a child has been exposed to high levels of carbon monoxide. Spider-bite reactions are usually localized to the area of the bite. A hydrocarbon or petroleum ingestion usually results in respiratory symptoms and tachycardia. Nausea and vomiting and pale skin are symptoms of aspirin ingestion.

NP: Assessment; CN: Physiological integrity; CNS: Physiological adaptation; CL: Knowledge

90. A teenager asks advice about getting a tattoo. Which of the following statements about tattoos is a common misperception?

1. Human immunodeficiency syndrome (HIV) is a possible risk factor.
2. Hepatitis B is a possible risk factor.
3. Tattoos are easily removed with laser surgery.
4. Allergic response to pigments is a possible risk factor.

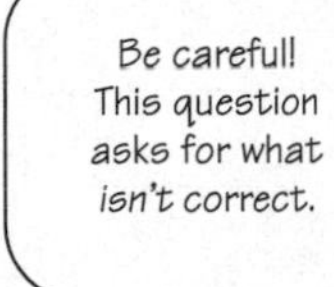
Be careful!
This question
asks for what
isn't correct.

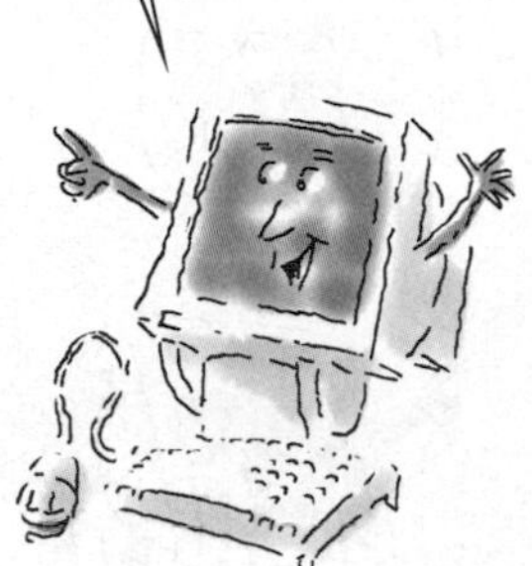

90. 3. The removal of tattoos isn't easily done, and most people are left with a significant scar. The cost is expensive and not covered by insurance. Because of the moderate amount of bleeding with a tattoo, both hepatitis B and HIV are potential risks if proper techniques aren't followed. Allergic reactions have been seen when establishments don't use Food and Drug Administration–approved pigments for tattoo coloring. Reactions can also occur in clients who are hypersensitive to the pigments or tools used.

NP: Assessment; CN: Health promotion and maintenance; CNS: Safety and infection control; CL: Knowledge

91. Which of the following terms describes a fungal infection found on the upper arm?

1. Tinea capitis
2. Tinea corporis
3. Tinea cruris
4. Tinea pedis

91. 2. Tinea corporis describes fungal infections of the body. Tinea capitis describes fungal infections of the scalp. Tinea pedis is the term for fungal infections of the foot. Tinea cruris is used to describe fungal infections of the inner thigh and inguinal creases.

NP: Analysis; CN: Physiological integrity; CNS: Physiological adaptation; CL: Application

92. A 15-kg infant is started on amoxicillin/clavulanate potassium (Augmentin) therapy, 200 mg/5 ml, for cellulitis. The dose is 40 mg/kg over 24 hours given three times daily. How many milliliters would be given for each dose?

1. 2.5 ml
2. 5 ml
3. 15 ml
4. 20 ml

92. 2. The dose is first calculated by multiplying the weight times the milligrams. It's then divided by three even doses. The milligrams are then used to determine the milliliters based on the concentration of the medicine. 40 mg × 15 kg = 600/3 doses = 200 mg/dose. The concentration is 200 mg in every 5 ml.

NP: Analysis; CN: Physiological integrity; CNS: Pharmacological and parenteral therapies; CL: Knowledge

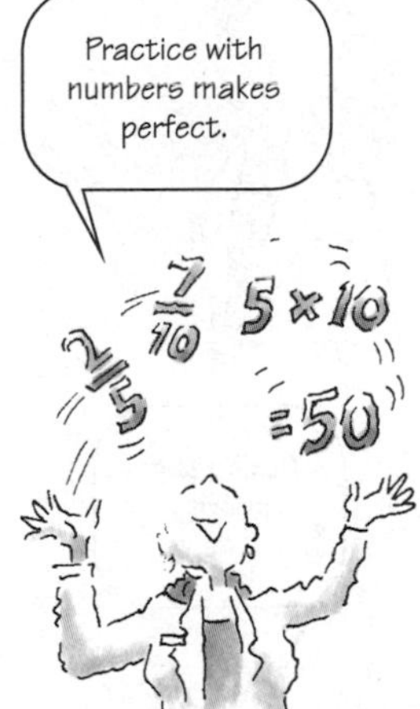
Practice with
numbers makes
perfect.
5 × 10
= 50

93. At what stage of acquired syphilis are chancres found?

1. Tertiary syphilis
2. Primary acquired syphilis
3. Secondary acquired syphilis
4. Chancres aren't found in syphilis

93. 2. A chancre is a painless shallow ulcer that develops in primary syphilis and appears 3 weeks after exposure. In secondary syphilis, nodular, pustular, and annular lesions are seen. Tertiary stages are rare in children.

NP: Analysis; CN: Physiological integrity; CNS: Physiological adaptation; CL: Knowledge

94. A 4-year-old child has a tick embedded in the scalp. Which of the following methods is the preferred way of removing the tick?

1. Burning the tick at the skin surface
2. Surgically removing the tick
3. Grasping the tick with tweezers and applying slow, outward pressure
4. Grasping the tick with tweezers and quickly pulling the tick out

94. 3. Applying gentle outward pressure prevents injury to the skin, and the retention of tick parts occurs. Surgical removal is indicated for retention of tick parts. Burning the tick and quickly pulling the tick out may cause injury to the skin and should be avoided.

NP: Assessment; CN: Physiological integrity; CNS: Physiological adaptation; CL: Knowledge

95. A child with hives is prescribed diphenhydramine (Benadryl) 5 mg/kg over 24 hours in divided doses every 6 hours. The child weighs 8 kg. How many milligrams should be given with each dose?

1. 4.5 mg
2. 10 mg
3. 22 mg
4. 40 mg

95. 2. Multiplying 5 mg by the weight (8 kg) gives the amount of milligrams for 24 hours (40 mg). Divided this by the number of doses per day (4), giving 10 mg/dose. 5 mg × 8 kg = 40 mg/4 doses = 10 mg/dose.

NP: Implementation; CN: Physiological integrity; CNS: Pharmacological and parenteral therapies; CL: Application

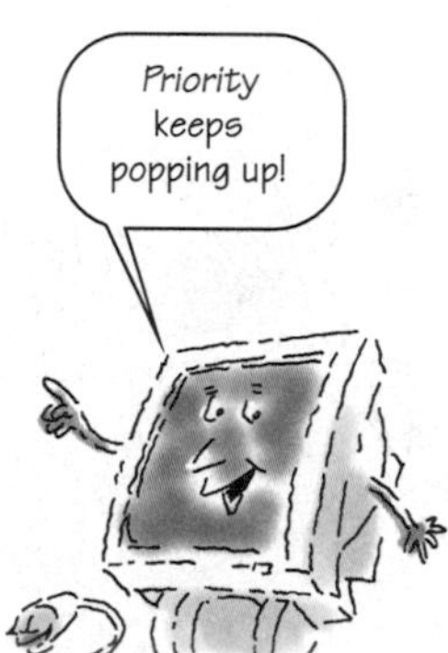

Priority keeps popping up!

96. An 8-year-old child arrives at the emergency department with chemical burns to both legs. Which of the following treatments has priority for this child?

1. Dilute the burns
2. Apply sterile dressings
3. Apply topical antibiotics
4. Debride and graft the burns

96. 1. Diluting the chemical is the first treatment. It will help remove the chemical and stop the burning process. The remaining treatments are initiated after dilution.

NP: Assessment; CN: Physiological integrity; CNS: Physiological adaptation; CL: Knowledge

97. A 12-year-old child with full-thickness, circumferential burns to the chest has difficulty breathing. Which of the following procedures will most likely be performed?

1. Chest tube insertion
2. Escharotomy
3. Intubation
4. Needle thoracocentesis

97. 2. Escharotomy is a surgical incision used to relieve pressure from edema. It's needed with circumferential burns that prevent chest expansion or cause circulatory compromise. Intubation is performed to maintain a patent airway. Insertion of a chest tube and needle thoracocentesis are performed to relieve a pneumothorax.

NP: Assessment; CN: Physiological integrity; CNS: Physiological adaptation; CL: Knowledge

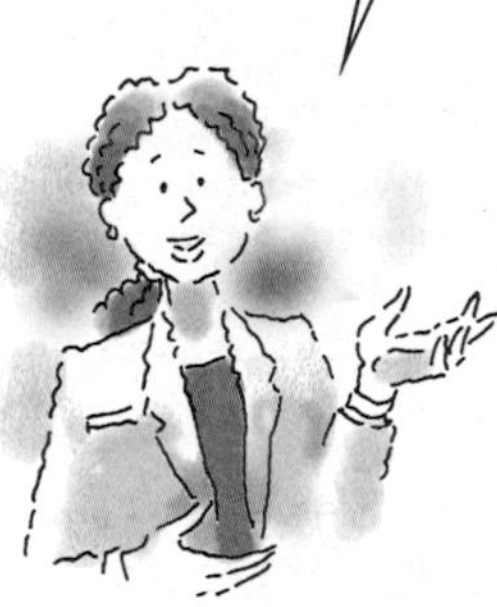

Knowing why something happens allows you to teach more effectively.

98. A 6-year-old child is evaluated after sustaining burns to his left shoulder. The parents are instructed to use moisturizing cream and protect the burn from sunlight. What is the purpose of this treatment?

1. To avoid keloids
2. To avoid scarring
3. To avoid hypopigmentation
4. To avoid hyperpigmentation

98. 4. Healed or grafted burns would require creams and protection from the sun to decrease hyperpigmentation. Scarring, hypopigmentation, and keloids aren't treated with moisturizing creams and avoidance of sunlight.

NP: Analysis; CN: Physiological integrity; CNS: Physiological adaptation; CL: Knowledge

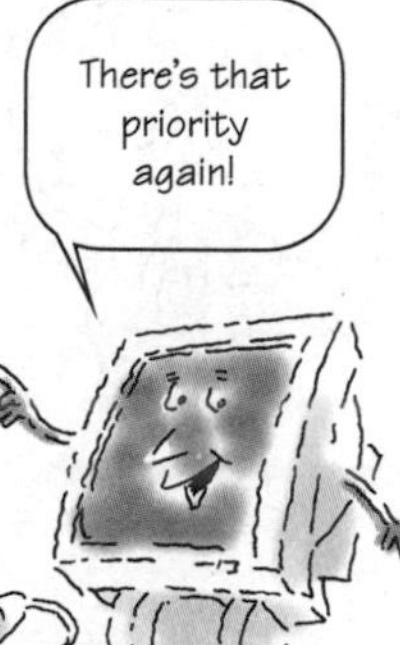

There's that priority again!

99. A child arrives in the emergency department 20 minutes after sustaining a major burn injury to 40% of his body. After initiating an I.V. line, which intervention would the nurse perform next?

1. Insert an indwelling catheter.
2. Apply Silvadene cream to the burn.
3. Shave the hair around the burn wound.
4. Obtain cultures from the deepest burn area.

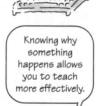

99. 1. I.V. fluids must be started immediately on all children who sustain a major burn injury to prevent the child from going into hypovolemic shock. The fluids are titrated based on urine output. To monitor this output exactly, an indwelling urinary catheter must be inserted. The other interventions will be performed, but not immediately.

NP: Implementation; CN: Physiological integrity; CNS: Reduction of risk potential; CL: Application

NP: Nursing process CN: Client needs category CNS: Client needs subcategory CL: Cognitive level

100. A 12-year-old child sustains a moderate burn injury. The mother reports that the child last received a tetanus injection when he was 5 years old. An appropriate nursing intervention would be to administer which of the following immunizations?

1. 0.5 ml of tetanus toxoid I.M.
2. 0.5 ml of tetanus toxoid I.V.
3. 250 U of Hyper-Tet I.M.
4. 250 U of Hyper-Tet I.V.

100. 1. Tetanus prophylaxis is given to all clients with moderate to severe burn injuries if it's longer than 5 years since the last immunization or if there is no history of immunization. The correct dosage is 0.5 ml I.M. one time if the child was immunized within 10 years. If it's more than 10 years or the child hasn't received tetanus immunization, the dosage is 250 U of Hyper-Tet one time. There is no I.V. form of tetanus available.

NP: Implementation; CN: Physiological integrity; CNS: Pharmacological and parenteral therapies; CL: Analysis

101. A child arrives in the emergency department after sustaining a major burn injury. For which of the following metabolic alterations must the nurse assess during the first 8 hours?

1. Hyponatremia and hypokalemia
2. Hyponatremia and hyperkalemia
3. Hypernatremia and hypokalemia
4. Hypernatremia and hyperkalemia

101. 2. Capillary permeability increases during the first 48 hours postburn, allowing fluids to shift from the plasma to the interstitial spaces. This fluid is high in sodium, causing the client's serum sodium level to decrease. Potassium also leaks from the cells into the plasma, causing hyperkalemia.

NP: Assessment; CN: Physiological integrity; CNS: Physiological adaptation; CL: Analysis

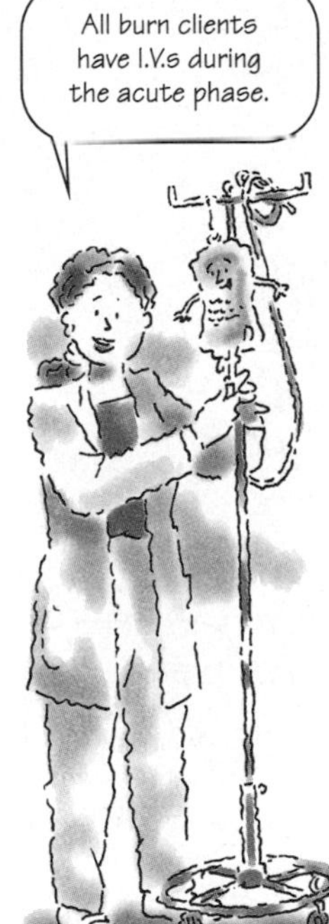

All burn clients have I.V.s during the acute phase.

102. A child weighing 10 kg has a deep partial-thickness burn to 40% of his body surface area. The nurse will titrate this child's I.V. fluids to achieve which of the following hourly urinary outputs?

1. 5 ml
2. 10 ml
3. 30 ml
4. 50 ml

102. 2. Fluid resuscitation should be started on all clients with burns over more than 20% of their body surface area. In children, an hourly urine output of 1 to 2 ml/kg of body weight shows adequate kidney perfusion and fluid resuscitation. Adults should have an hourly urine output of 30 to 50 ml.

NP: Implementation; CN: Physiological integrity; CNS: Physiological adaptation; CL: Knowledge

103. A team of nurses is preparing a trauma room for the arrival of a client with partial-thickness burns to both lower extremities and portions of the trunk. Which of the following fluids should be ready for immediate use?

1. Albumin
2. Dextrose 5% and ½ normal saline
3. Lactated Ringer's solution
4. Normal saline with 2 mEq KCl/100 ml

103. 3. Lactated Ringer's solution is recommended because it replaces the lost sodium and corrects the metabolic acidosis. The use of albumin is controversial. If albumin is given, it's as adjunct therapy and not for primary fluid replacement. The stress from a burn injury affects the glucose metabolism. Dextrose shouldn't be given during the first 24 hours as it can put the client into pseudodiabetes. The client is hyperkalemic from the potassium shift from the intracellular spaces to the plasma, and additional potassium would be detrimental.

NP: Implementation; CN: Physiological integrity; CNS: Pharmacological and parenteral therapies; CL: Application

104. A client states that she recently received information that hand-foot-and-mouth disease has been diagnosed in a few of her child's preschool classmates. This viral infection has which characteristics?

1. Low-grade fever, followed by vesicular lesions on the trunk, face and scalp
2. Mild, self-limited eruption of vesicles on the buccal mucosa, tongue, soft palate, hands and feet
3. Purpuric, maculopapular lesions with GI symptoms and joint pain
4. Bright red rash with a red outer border circling a bite mark

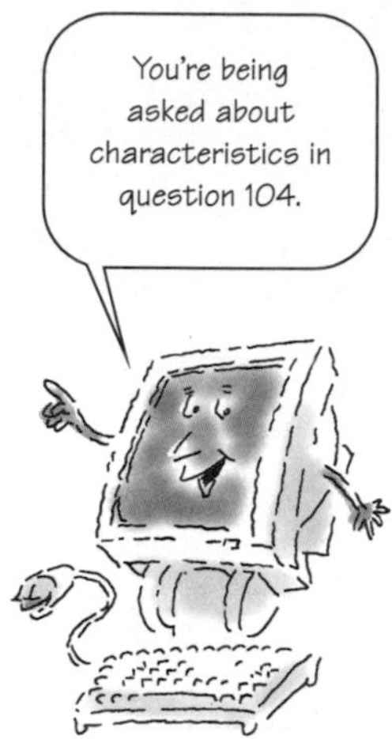

You're being asked about characteristics in question 104.

104. 2. Hand-foot-and-mouth disease is caused by coxsackievirus and usually occurs in preschool children. Vesicular lesions accompanied by a low-grade fever are typically signs of varicella. Purpura, GI symptoms, and joint pain are symptoms of Henoch-Schoenlein purpura. A bright-red bull's eye rash is a classic symptom of Lyme disease.

NP: Analysis; CN: Physiological integrity; CNS: Physiological adaptation; CL: Knowledge

105. A 27½-lb child is receiving antibiotics for cellulitis. The order reads Pen-Vee K 40 mg/kg/day divided every 6 hours. Which dosage of antibiotics should this child receive with each dose?

1. 225 mg
2. 500 mg
3. 125 mg
4. 12.5 mg

105. 3. One kilogram equals 2.2 pounds so a 27½-lb child weighs 12.5 kg. 40 mg/kg/day equals a total of 500 mg given every 6 hours or 4 times in a 24 hour time period. 500 mg divided by 4 equals 125 mg.

NP: Implementation; CN: Physiological integrity; CNS: Pharmacological and parenteral therapies; CL: Application

106. A neonate presents with jaundice. The nurse should give the parents which information about jaundice?

1. An excess of bilirubin causes jaundice requiring additional feedings and phototherapy to help resolve the condition.
2. Jaundice is a form of birthmark that will resolve over time.
3. Jaundice is a sign of infection, and the infant will need to be hospitalized for treatment.
4. Jaundice is a normal physiological process that every neonate goes through.

106. 1. Jaundice is a physiological response to higher levels of circulating bilirubin. Not every neonate requires intervention but high levels of bilirubin may produce kernicterus with subsequent brain damage. High levels of bilirubin may also be a sign of infection. Jaundice isn't a birthmark nor is it a sign of infection. Although jaundice is a physiologic response, it isn't a normal response unless the neonate has a higher level of bilirubin than normal.

NP: Analysis; CN: Physiological integrity; CNS: Physiological adaptation; CL: Knowledge

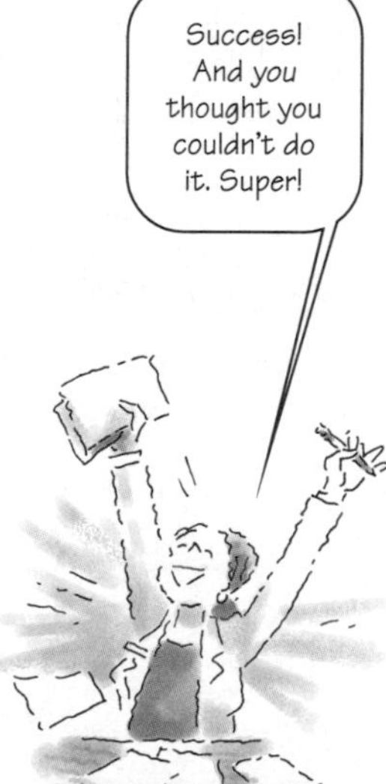

Success! And you thought you couldn't do it. Super!

107. A child has been diagnosed with urticaria. Which statement best describes the wheals that commonly accompany urticaria?

1. An elevated, firm, circumscribed lesion 1 to 2 cm in diameter
2. A flat, nonpalpable irregularly shaped lesion more than 1 cm in diameter
3. An elevated, irregular shaped area of cutaneous edema, solid, transient, and of variable diameter
4. An elevated, circumscribed lesion in the dermis or subcutaneous layer, filled with liquid or semisolid material

107. 3. A wheal is an elevated, irregular shaped area of cutaneous edema that's solid and transient; the diameter varies. An elevated firm lesion in the dermis 1 to 2 cm in size is consistent with a nodule. Flat lesions greater than 1 cm describe a patch. Cysts are the same description as nodules but are filled with a liquid or semisolid material.

NP: Analysis; CN: Physiological integrity; CNS: Physiological adaptation; CL: Knowledge

Part VI Issues in nursing

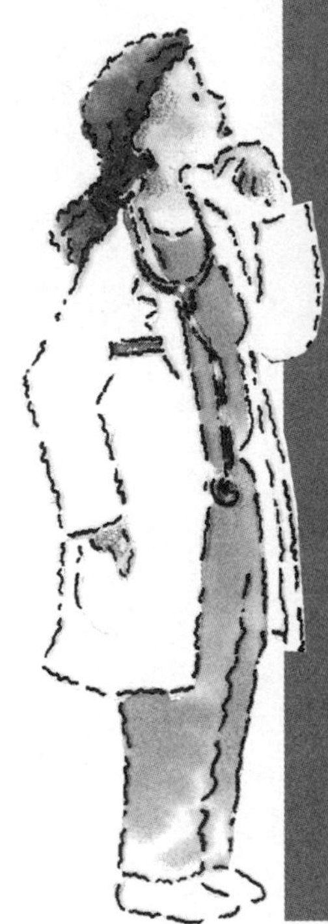

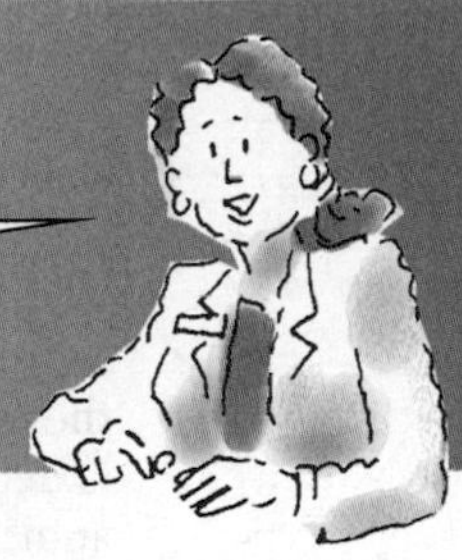

Chapter 36
Management & leadership

1. The nurse-manager of a 20-bed coronary care unit isn't on duty when a staff nurse makes a serious medication error. The client, who received an overdose of medication, nearly dies. Which statement accurately reflects the accountability of the nurse-manager?

1. The nursing supervisor on duty will call the nurse-manager at home and apprise her of the problem.
2. Because the nurse-manager is off duty, she isn't accountable for incidents that occur in her absence. Therefore, the nurse-manager won't be notified.
3. The nurse-manager will be informed of the incident when returning to work on Monday because the nurse-manager was officially off duty when the incident took place.
4. Although the nurse-manager is off duty, the nursing supervisor decides to call the nurse-manager if time permits; the supervisor believes that the manager has no responsibility for what happened during the manager's absence.

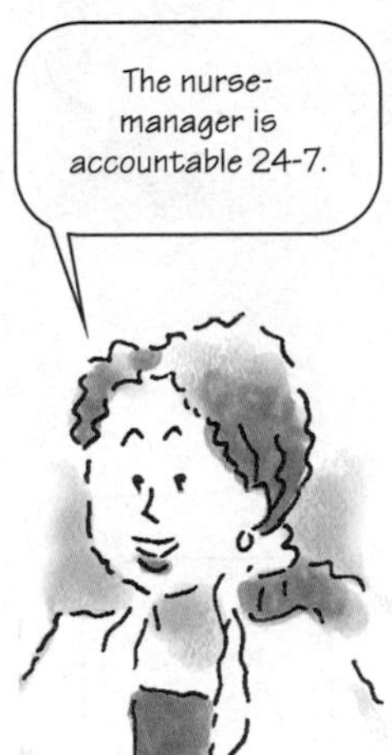

1. 1. The nurse-manager is accountable for what happens on the unit 24 hours per day, 7 days per week. If a serious problem occurs, the nurse-manager should be notified as soon as possible. The other choices don't accurately reflect the accountability of the nurse-manager's position.

NP: Analysis; CN: Safe, effective care environment; CNS: Safety and infection control; CL: Analysis

2. A community health nurse is working with disaster relief following a flood. Finding safe housing for survivors, providing support for families, organizing counseling, and securing physical care are examples of which type of prevention?

1. Aggregate care prevention
2. Primary prevention
3. Secondary prevention
4. Tertiary prevention

2. 4. Tertiary prevention involves reducing the degree and quantity of injury, disability, and damage following a disaster or crisis. Aggregate prevention isn't a level of care prevention. Primary prevention focuses on keeping the crisis or disaster from happening. The goal of secondary prevention is to reduce the duration and intensity of the disaster or crisis.

NP: Analysis; CN: Safe, effective care environment; CNS: Management of care; CL: Application

3. A staff nurse on a busy pediatric unit is an excellent role model for her colleagues. She encourages them to participate in the unit's decision-making process and helps them improve their clinical skills. This nurse is functioning effectively in which role?

1. Manager
2. Autocrat
3. Leader
4. Authority

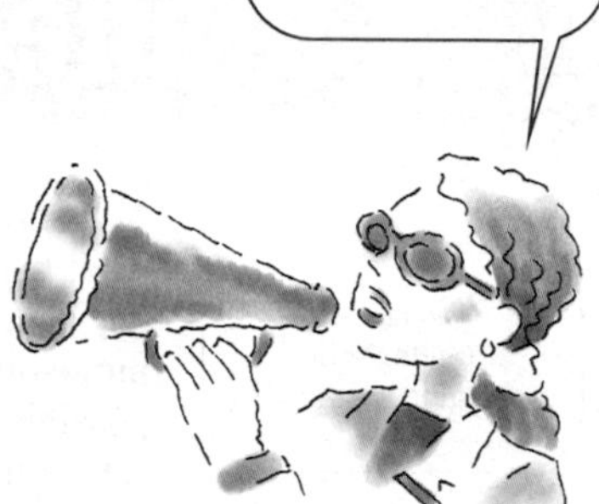
As a staff
nurse, you play an
excellent role!

3. 3. A leader doesn't have formal power and authority but influences the success of a unit by being an excellent role model and by guiding, encouraging, and facilitating professional growth and development. A manager has formal power and authority from the status within the organization and such power and authority is detailed in the manager's job description. An autocrat isn't interested in guiding or encouraging staff or in being an effective role model. Authority, a characteristic of a managerial position, is given by virtue of position within an organization.

NP: Analysis; CN: Safe, effective care environment; CNS: Management of care; CL: Application

4. The managers of the physical and occupational therapy neurologic departments have expressed concern to the nurse-manager of an adult neurologic rehabilitation unit that clients have been arriving late for therapy. In response, the nursing staff of the rehabilitation unit has complained that therapy schedules don't allow sufficient time for performing nursing interventions. Which action by the nurse-manager is the best solution to this problem?

1. Meet with the managers of physical and occupational therapy and determine how to reschedule clients. The nurse-manager will inform the staff of the changes.
2. Tell the nursing staff that they need to determine how to transport clients to therapy according to the schedules developed by the therapists.
3. Meet with the managers of physical and occupational therapy and identify several possible ways to solve the problem. Ask the adult neurologic rehabilitation staff for input and then make the final decision in conjunction with the therapy managers.
4. Ask several of the nursing leaders in the adult neurologic rehabilitation unit to work with the therapy staff to identify the best way to solve this problem. Ask the rehabilitation staff to solicit input from their colleagues and to keep the nurse-manager informed as they work on this project. Let the rehabilitation staff know that the nurse-manager is available as a resource.

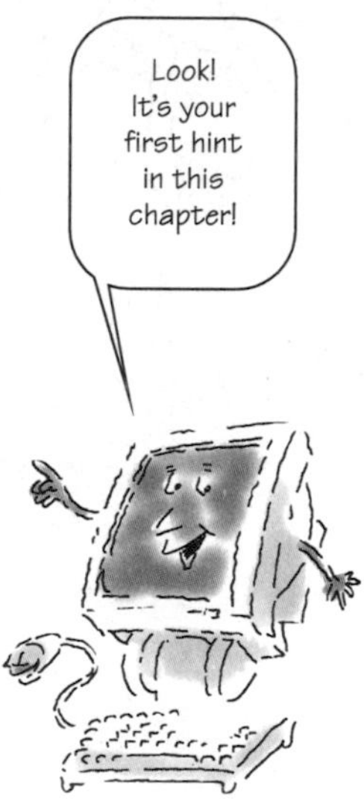
Look!
It's your
first hint
in this
chapter!

4. 4. In this situation, functioning as a democratic leader is best. The nursing and therapy staffs who deal with the day-to-day problems of direct client care have the best grasp of the situation and should have autonomy to solve problems. The manager, however, should be available to help. Option 1 reflects an autocratic manager. Without staff input, the nurse-manager won't have the necessary information to identify the best solution. By simply telling the nursing staff to follow the therapists' schedules, the nurse-manager has abdicated responsibility for problem solving (laissez-faire manager), yet the problem still exists. Determining problem-solving options without staff input is indicative of a participative manager. A participative manager asks staff members for opinions, but they don't have input into actual problem solving. This lack of input may lead to resentment and frustration.

NP: Analysis; CN: Safe, effective care environment; CNS: Management of care; CL: Analysis

5. The staff of an outpatient clinic has formed a task force to develop new procedures for swift, safe evacuation of the unit. The new procedures haven't been reviewed, approved, or shared with all personnel. When the nurse-manager receives word of a bomb threat, the task force members push for evacuating the unit using the new procedures. Which action should the nurse-manager take?

1. Determine that the procedures currently in place must be followed and direct staff to follow them without question.
2. Tell staff members to use whatever procedures they feel are best.
3. Ask staff members to quickly meet among themselves and decide what procedures to follow.
4. Tell staff members to assemble in the staff lounge; there the nurse-manager will quickly gather opinions about evacuation procedures before deciding what to do.

5. 1. In an emergency, such as a bomb scare, the nurse-manager must determine, without hesitation, the best action for the safety and welfare of clients and staff. Allowing staff members to do whatever they think best will cause confusion and inefficient client evacuation because no one will know how to function effectively as a team during the crisis. Taking time to have staff meet is wasting valuable time.

NP: Analysis; CN: Safe, effective care environment; CNS: Safety and infection control; CL: Analysis

6. The selection of a nursing care delivery system (NCDS) is critical to the success of a nursing area. Which factor is essential to the evaluation of a NCDS?

1. Determining how planned absences, such as vacation time, will be scheduled so that all staff are treated fairly
2. Identifying who will be responsible for making client care decisions
3. Deciding what type of dress code will be implemented
4. Identifying salary ranges for various types of staff

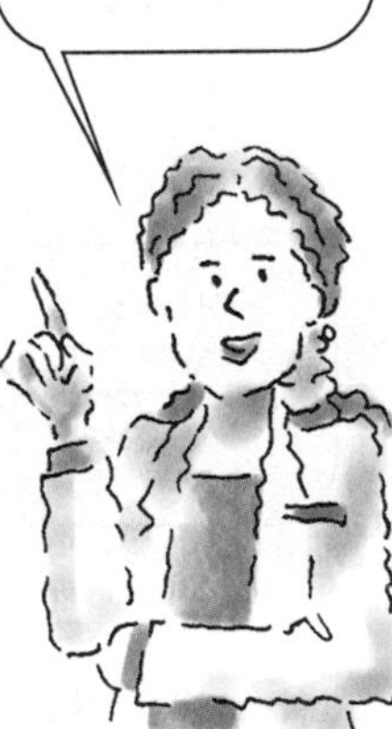

In question 6, it's essential that you read into this hint.

6. 2. Determining who has responsibility for making decisions regarding client care is an essential element of all client care delivery systems. Dress code, salary, and scheduling planned staff absences are important to any organization but aren't actually determined by the NCDS.

NP: Analysis; CN: Safe, effective care environment; CNS: Management of care; CL: Application

7. A nurse-manager on an oncology unit has been informed that she must determine which nursing care delivery system (NCDS) is best for efficient client care, client satisfaction, and cost reduction. Knowing that 2 or 3 registered nurses, 4 licensed practical nurses, and 5 nursing assistants are generally on duty on each shift and that the clients can be grouped fairly easily by geographic location and client care needs, the nurse-manager and her staff appropriately decide to implement which NCDS?

1. Functional nursing
2. Case management
3. Team nursing
4. Primary nursing

7. 3. Team nursing is efficient and costs less to implement than primary or case management systems. Because the staff members know each other well, they can function effectively as a team. Although functional nursing is the most cost effective, care is commonly fragmented and client satisfaction decreased. Case management and primary nursing require more registered nurses than are available.

NP: Analysis; CN: Safe, effective care environment; CNS: Management of care; CL: Analysis

8. A winter storm has prevented most of the staff members from getting to work on a busy medical-surgical unit. One registered nurse, 2 licensed practical nurses, and 3 nursing assistants have been able to get to work. The nurse-manager must decide which nursing care delivery system should be implemented for the best possible client care during this staffing crisis. The nurse-manager directs the staff to implement which delivery system?

1. Team nursing
2. Primary nursing
3. Functional nursing
4. Case management

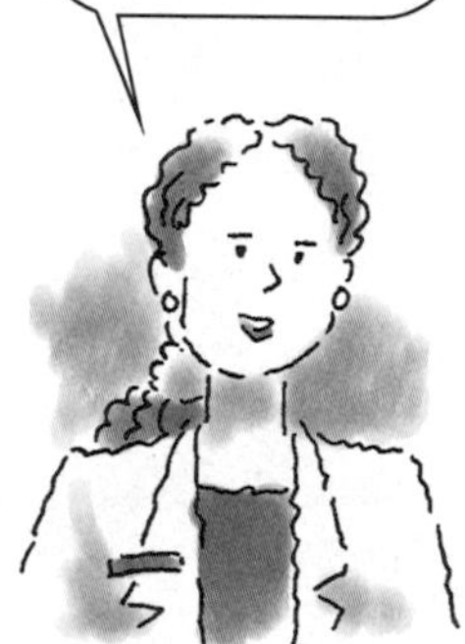

During a crisis, which delivery system functions the best? That's a hint!

8. 3. Functional nursing best uses the skills of all staff in a timely manner during this crisis. This delivery system requires the least staff and delegates tasks to those who can best perform them. Team nursing doesn't allow for the best use of a limited number of staff who must care for a large number of clients. Primary nursing and case management require more registered nurses than are currently available.
NP: Analysis; CN: Safe, effective care environment; CNS: Management of care; CL: Analysis

9. The nurse-manager in the office of a group of surgeons has received complaints from discharged clients about inadequate instructions for performing home care. Knowing the importance of good, timely client education, the nurse should take which steps?

1. Contact the nurses who work in the facility and tell them that client education should be implemented as soon as the clients are admitted to either the hospital or the outpatient surgical center.
2. Review and revise the way client education is conducted in the surgeons' office.
3. Because no serious damage was done to any of the clients, the nurse-manager can safely ignore their complaints.
4. Work with the surgeons' and nursing staff in the hospital and outpatient surgical center to evaluate current client education practices and revise as needed.

9. 4. Client education is the responsibility of all nurses providing care to the client, and the nurses must work together to establish the best methods. The most appropriate response is to contact the nurse manager, not the nursing staff, at the facility. Evaluating client education in one setting only doesn't consider the entire process and the staff providing it. No complaint should be ignored; patient education is an important nursing responsibility.
NP: Analysis; CN: Safe, effective care environment; CNS: Safety and infection control; CL: Application

10. A nurse-manager of an intensive care unit (ICU) can't be held legally responsible in a court of law for which action performed by the unit's staff?

1. A nursing assistant administers medications to a client in ICU.
2. A staff nurse refuses to follow a physician's order to administer medication because administering the dosage ordered could seriously harm the client.
3. A nursing assistant attempts to initiate I.V. therapy.
4. A staff nurse fills a client prescription at the hospital pharmacy because the pharmacist on duty is busy.

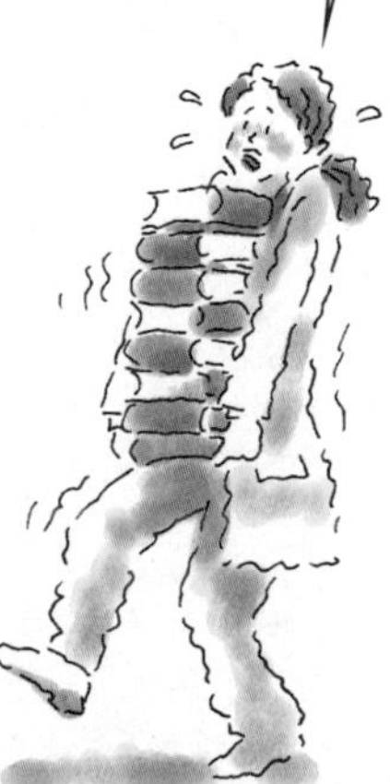

I'd like to delegate this work. Maybe it's too much?

10. 2. The nurse-manager is legally responsible for actions that fall within the scope of practice of the staff members who perform them. A nurse may not knowingly administer or perform tasks that will harm a client. It's within a nurse's scope of practice to refuse to carry out such orders. Administering medications and initiating I.V. therapy aren't within the scope of practice for nursing assistants. A staff nurse isn't licensed to fill prescriptions.
NP: Analysis; CN: Safe, effective care environment; CNS: Management of care; CL: Analysis

NP: Nursing process CN: Client needs category CNS: Client needs subcategory CL: Cognitive level

11. A primary nurse in the unit tells the nurse-manager that a newly hired registered nurse needs an additional week of orientation to function effectively on the staff. Which action is most appropriate for the nurse-manager?

1. Tell the primary nurse that the new nurse must finish orientation in 6 weeks because of a staffing shortage.
2. Meet with the new nurse and the primary nurse and help set up an additional week of orientation.
3. Fire the new nurse because the unit is short-staffed and nurses who can complete the orientation process in the normal length of time are needed.
4. Schedule a staff meeting to find out if there are problems with the orientation process.

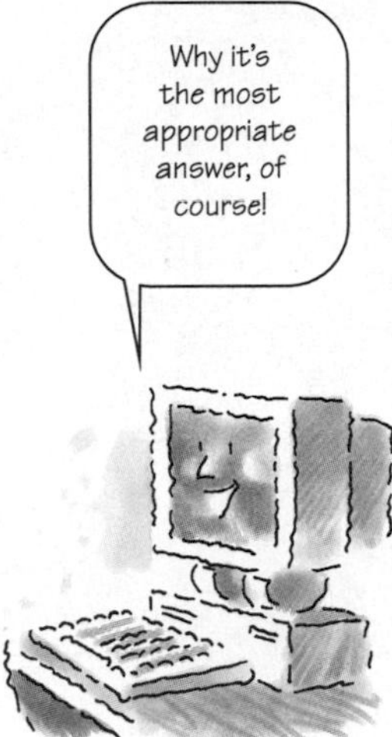

Why it's the most appropriate answer, of course!

11. 2. The nurse-manager is responsible for adequate orientation of new staff. Needing additional orientation doesn't mean that a nurse isn't competent. However, the new nurse should know what's expected of her and the time frame in which she must accomplish the expectations. Firing the new nurse isn't the answer because she's apparently close to completing orientation and the primary nurse says the nurse has good skills. Periodically reviewing and revising the orientation process is a good idea. However, in this case, the most appropriate course of action is to help the new nurse complete her orientation as efficiently as possible.

NP: Analysis; CN: Safe, effective care environment; CNS: Management of care; CL: Analysis

12. Delegation is the process of transferring work to subordinates. A nurse-manager can appropriately delegate which task?

1. Scheduling staff assignments for the next month
2. Terminating a nursing assistant for insubordination
3. Deciding on salary increases for licensed practical nurses after they complete orientation
4. Telling a staff nurse to initiate disciplinary action against one of her peers

12. 1. Scheduling may be safely and appropriately delegated. Termination, disciplinary action, and salary increases shouldn't be delegated to staff, who don't have the power and authority to take such actions.

NP: Analysis; CN: Safe, effective care environment; CNS: Management of care; CL: Analysis

13. A nurse-manager appropriately behaves as an autocrat in which situation?

1. Planning vacation time for staff
2. Directing staff activities if a client has a cardiac arrest
3. Evaluating a new medication administration process
4. Identifying the strengths and weaknesses of a client education video

13. 2. In a crisis situation, the nurse-manager should take command for the benefit of the client. Planning vacation time and evaluating procedures and client resources require staff input characteristic of a democratic or participative manager.

NP: Analysis; CN: Safe, effective care environment; CNS: Management of care; CL: Application

14. The nurse-manager of a home health facility includes which item in the capital budget?

1. Salaries and benefits for her staff
2. A $1,200 computer upgrade
3. Office supplies
4. Client education materials costing $300

14. 2. Capital budgets generally include items valued at more than $500. Salaries and benefits are part of the personnel budget. Office supplies and client education materials are part of the operating budget.

NP: Analysis; CN: Safe, effective care environment; CNS: Management of care; CL: Application

15. A nurse-manager delegates responsibility for the review and revision of the surgical unit's client education materials. Which statement illustrates the **best** method of delegation?

1. Tell the nursing staff they're responsible for the review and revision and that their recommendations for improving the materials are welcome.
2. Ask two of the best staff nurses to form a task force to review and revise client education materials. Explain that they should solicit input from clients and staff members, complete this task within 6 weeks, and submit recommendations in writing.
3. Tell the nursing staff that the education materials aren't satisfactory. Explain that the staff should select people to review them and make recommendations for change. Tell them that the nurse-manager will make the final decisions about changes.
4. Ask the assistant manager to develop a plan for the review and revision of client education materials.

15. 2. Delegation must be done clearly and precisely. The nurse-manager must assign responsibility, identify the task to be accomplished, explain what outcomes are needed, and the time frame for completing the work. The remaining options don't give clear explanations of work to be done, don't clearly assign responsibility or the specific outcomes desired, or establish a time frame for completion of the task.

NP: Analysis; CN: Safe, effective care environment; CNS: Management of care; CL: Application

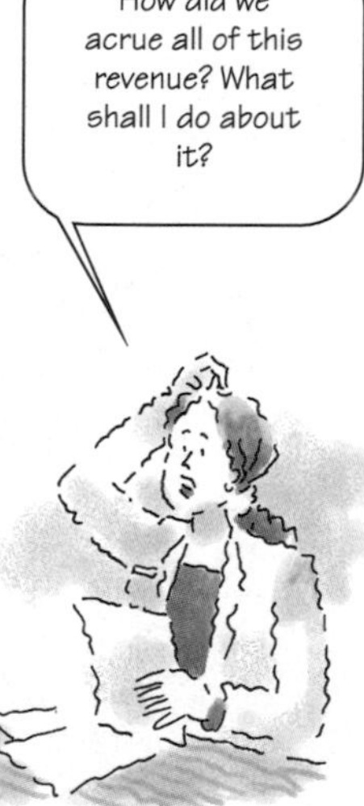

How did we acrue all of this revenue? What shall I do about it?

16. A nurse-manager works for a nonprofit health care corporation in which there has been significant revenue over expenses for the year. The nurse-manager has been told to anticipate which action?

1. Receipt a portion of the revenue to improve client services on the unit.
2. Revenue will be identified as profit.
3. Revenue will be divided among stockholders as dividends.
4. Reduction of operating expenses to help the organization pay taxes on the revenue.

16. 1. Revenue over expenses in a nonprofit organization is tax-exempt and is usually reinvested in the organization and used to improve services. A for-profit organization calls its revenue over expenses a profit and the revenue can be divided as a dividend among stockholders or reinvested in the organization.

NP: Analysis; CN: Safe, effective care environment; CNS: Management of care; CL: Application

17. A nurse-manager must include which items as part of the personnel budget?

1. Anticipated overtime payments for staff
2. Computers for staff use
3. Office supplies for secretarial use
4. Videos for staff education

17. 1. Personnel budgets include salaries, benefits, anticipated overtime costs, and potential salary increases. Office supplies and videos are part of the day-to-day operating budget. Any expense or single item of equipment costing more than $500 is part of the capital budget

NP: Analysis; CN: Safe, effective care environment; CNS: Management of care; CL: Application

18. The nurse-manager of an outpatient physical medicine and rehabilitation facility isn't satisfied with the policies and procedures of discharge planning. The manager knows other managers at similar facilities that are regarded as the "best" in the country. As part of a quality-improvement process she decides to take which steps?

1. Contact the nurse-managers at the best facilities and compare their discharge planning policies and procedures with those of her facility. After making the comparison, the nurse-manager will share the information with her staff and together they'll make recommendations.
2. Ask her staff nurses to investigate discharge policies and procedures at other outpatient rehabilitation facilities and provide recommendations for changes. The nurse-manager will present staff findings to administration.
3. Contact the nurse-managers at the best facilities and ask them for copies of their discharge planning policies and procedures. Then the nurse-manager can change her policies and procedures to match those at the best facilities.
4. Ask the staff nurses to form a task force for reviewing and revising the current discharge policies and procedures.

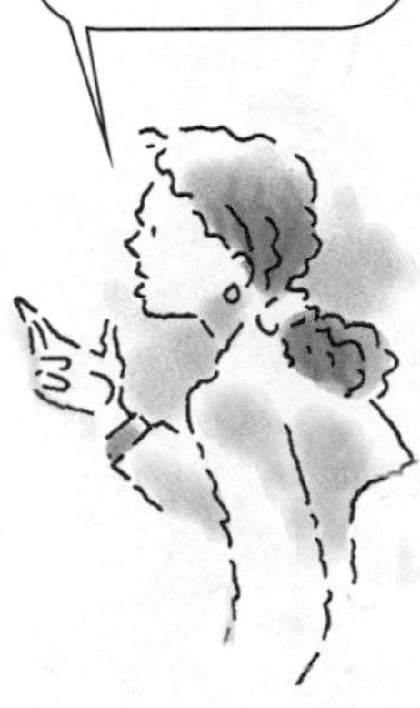

It's time for a change around here. Which steps should be taken to achieve the best results?

18. 1. Benchmarking is a good approach for the nurse-manager to take. ***Benchmarking*** is the process of comparing the delivery of client care practices in one organization to those in the best health care organizations. Because the nurse-manager already has contacts at the best facilities, she's the most appropriate person to obtain the necessary information. The nurse-manager, however, shouldn't automatically change her policies and procedures to match those of the best facilities. Instead, she should evaluate the policies to determine which ones might be implemented at her facility, then make recommendations for change in conjunction with her staff. Asking her staff to form a task force is a good idea, but benchmarking is a practice that saves time and effort and allows information to be obtained from excellent resources.

NP: Analysis; CN: Safe, effective care environment; CNS: Management of care; CL: Application

19. As the nurse-manager of a medical-surgical unit reviews this month's risk management data, she notices that a number of incident reports have been completed because 6 p.m. medications were administered late. Dinner is served between 5:30 p.m. and 6 p.m. Staff take their dinner breaks between 5 p.m. and 6:30 p.m. Based on this information, which is the most appropriate action from the nurse-manager?

1. Terminate the nurses responsible for failing to administer medications on time.
2. Decide that the staff must not take dinner breaks until at least 7 p.m.
3. Decide that the kitchen staff must change the time they deliver supper trays.
4. Review the process of administering medication including the time medications are administered, staff and client dinner times, the number of medications to be administered at 6 p.m., and the number of staff available between 5 and 6 p.m.

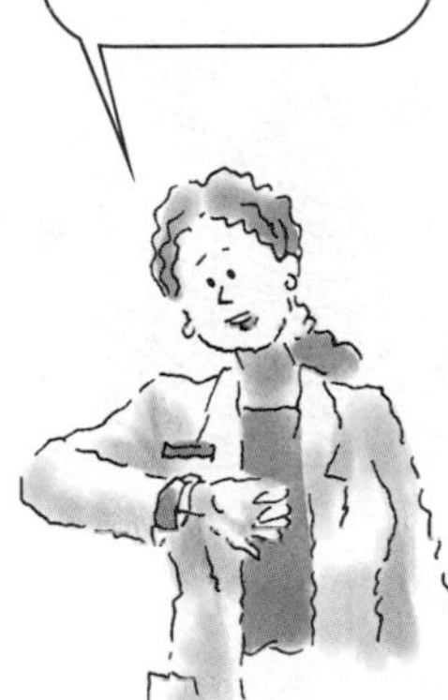

Be sensitive to time when evaluating risk management findings.

19. 4. An effective nurse-manager knows that to evaluate risk management findings accurately she must look at the entire process and circumstances surrounding each incident. Terminating staff without such evaluation doesn't resolve all of the factors contributing to the problem. She can't change dinner breaks or kitchen delivery times unless she has evaluated how these factors influence medication administration.

NP: Analysis; CN: Safe, effective care environment; CNS: Management of care; CL: Analysis

20. Performance improvement is an important component of continuous quality improvement. Which action should an effective nurse-manager take when conducting performance evaluations?

1. Conduct performance evaluations in a group setting so input from peers and subordinates is considered when evaluating a staff member's effectiveness.
2. Provide feedback on strengths as well as areas for improvement and clarify what the staff member is expected to accomplish before the next performance evaluation.
3. Document areas for improvement in writing. Areas of strength don't need to be documented because these areas are complementary and don't describe actions the staff member must take to improve.
4. Delegate responsibility for conducting performance evaluations to primary nurses whenever possible to help them grow professionally.

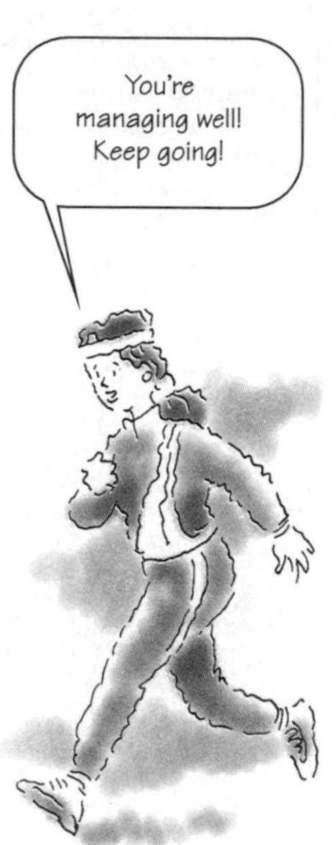

You're managing well! Keep going!

20. 2. An effective performance evaluation provides recognition of strengths, identifies areas for improvement, and clarifies performance expectations. Performance evaluations should be done in private, not in front of others. All components of a performance evaluation should be documented in writing. Although input from staff members can be useful in preparing performance evaluations, delegating all responsibility to others is inappropriate. The nurse-manager is responsible for the performance of the staff.

NP: Analysis; CN: Safe, effective care environment; CNS: Management of care; CL: Application

21. The manager of an outpatient clinic is explaining the various health care delivery systems to a client who's interested in joining a system with a reasonable fixed capitation rate. Which organization is the client primarily interested in joining?

1. A preferred provider organization (PPO)
2. A managed-care organization
3. A health-maintenance organization (HMO)
4. A privately funded insurance company

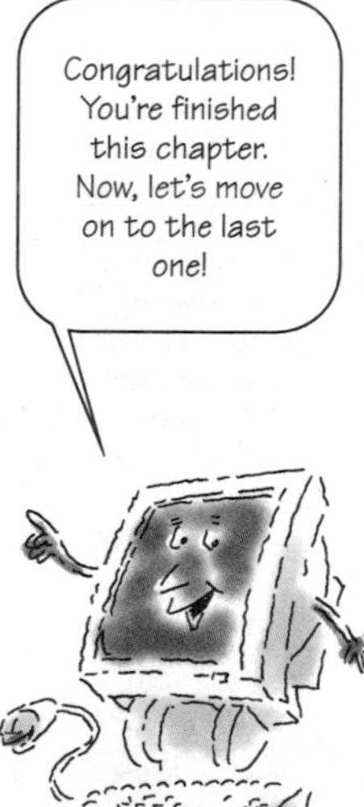

Congratulations! You're finished this chapter. Now, let's move on to the last one!

21. 3. An HMO provides comprehensive health services for a fixed rate of payment or capitation. A PPO pays health care expenses for members if they use a provider who's under contract to that PPO. Managed care provides beneficiaries with a variety of services for an established, agreed upon payment. A privately funded insurance company won't offer services for a fixed rate.

NP: Analysis; CN: Safe, effective care environment; CNS: Management of care; CL: Application

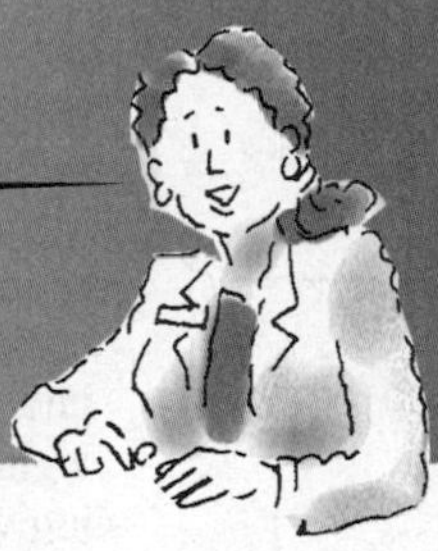

We saved the best, and
most challenging, topic for
last! Don't stress — you've
done an excellent job!

Chapter 37 Ethical & legal issues

1. An elderly client has been admitted to the medical-surgical unit from the postanesthesia care unit. While the nurse is off the floor, the client falls out of bed and fractures his right leg and right wrist. The nurse finding him states that the "side rails were down and the bed was in the high position." Legal charges are filed against the nurse and the hospital. Which charge is the most appropriate for her actions?

1. Collective liability
2. Comparative negligence
3. Battery
4. Negligence

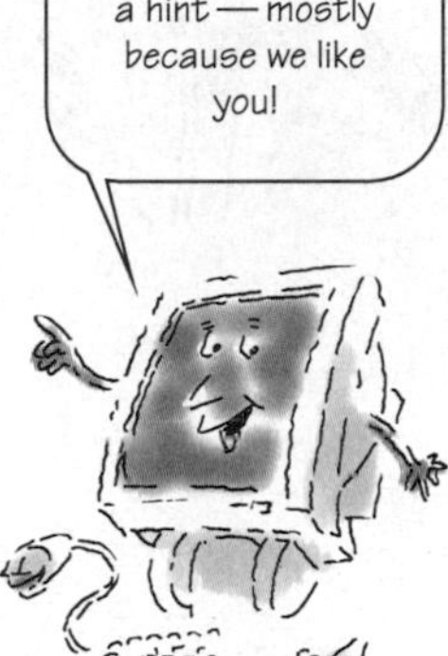

We've given you
a hint — mostly
because we like

1. 4. *Negligence* is a general term that denotes conduct lacking in due care. Carelessness is interpreted as a deviation from the standard of care that a reasonable person would use in a particular set of circumstances. Battery involves harmful or unwarranted contact with the client. Comparative negligence holds the injured parties accountable for their fault in the injury. Collective liability stems from cooperation by several manufacturers in a wrongful activity that by its nature requires group participation.

NP: Evaluation; CN: Safe, effective care environment; CNS: Safety and infection control; CL: Analysis

2. A client's attorney can file a lawsuit within which time frame?

1. Discovery rule
2. Statute of limitations
3. Grace period
4. Alternative dispute resolution

2. 2. Statute of limitations is the time period during which a case must be filed or the injured party is barred from bringing the lawsuit. Discovery rule is the actual term for the client's discovery of the injury. The statute of limitations typically gives clients 2 years from the time of discovery to file a lawsuit; however, the time may vary from state to state. Grace period refers to any period specified in a contract during which payment is permitted, without penalty, beyond the due date of the debt. Alternative dispute resolution refers to any means of settling disputes outside the courtroom setting.

NP: Analysis; CN: Safe, effective care environment; CNS: Safety and infection control; CL: Comprehension

3. A client's attorney must prove which elements for a professional negligence action?

1. Duty, breach of duty, damages, and causation
2. Duty, damages, and causation
3. Duty, breach of duty, and damages
4. Breach of duty, damages, and causation

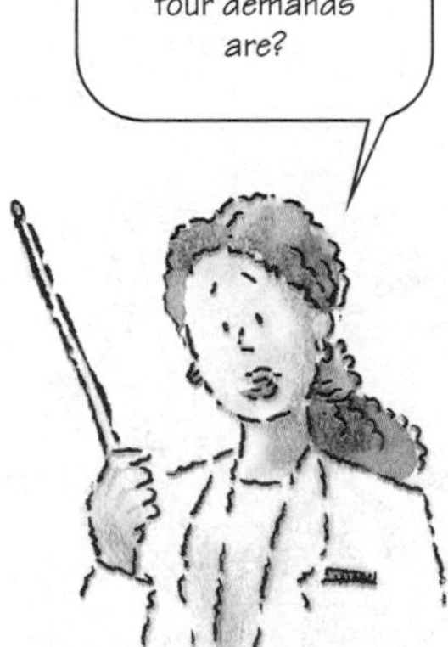

Let's go over
that again. The
four demands
are?

3. 1. Any professional negligence action must meet four demands — commonly known as the four D's — to be considered negligence and result in legal action: a **d**uty for the health care professional to provide care to the person making the claim, a **d**ereliction (breach) of that duty, the breach of duty resulted in **d**amages, and the damages were caused by a **d**irect result of the negligence (causation).

NP: Evaluation; CN: Safe, effective care environment; CNS: Management of care; CL: Application

NP: Nursing process CN: Client needs category CNS: Client needs subcategory CL: Cognitive level

4. Which guidelines define and regulate the scope of the nursing professional practice (that is, set rules on what the nurse can and can't do as a professional)?

1. State legislature
2. Facilities policies and procedures
3. Standards of Care
4. Nurse Practice Act

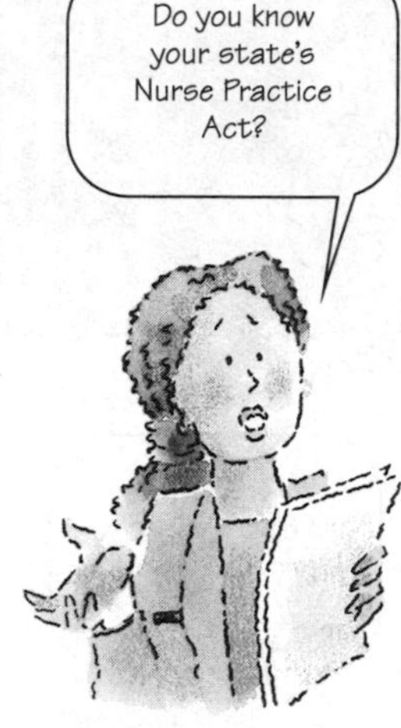
Do you know your state's Nurse Practice Act?

4. 4. The Nurse Practice Act is a series of statutes, enacted by each state legislature, that outline the legal scope of nursing practice within a particular state. The act sets educational requirements for the nurse, distinguishes between nursing practice and medical practice, and defines the scope of nursing practice. State legislatures set acts that create boards of nursing within each state but they don't regulate the scope of nursing. Facility policies govern the practice in that particular facility. Standards of Care, which are criteria that serve as a basis for comparison when evaluating the quality of nursing practice, are established by federal, accreditation, state, and professional organizations.

NP: Evaluation; CN: Safe, effective care environment; CNS: Management of care; CL: Application

5. A client who's a member of the Jehovah's Witnesses refuses a blood transfusion based on his religious beliefs and practices. His decision must be followed based on which ethical principle?

1. The right to die
2. Advance directive
3. The right to refuse treatment
4. Substituted judgment

5. 3. The right to refuse treatment is an ethical principle of respect for the autonomy of the individual. The client can refuse treatment if he's competent and aware of the risks and complications associated with that refusal. The right to die involves whether to initiate or withhold life-sustaining treatment for a client who is irreversibly comatose, vegetative, or suffering with end-stage terminal illness. An advance directive is a document used as a guideline for starting or continuing life-sustaining medical care; the client commonly has a terminal disease or disability and can't indicate his own wishes. Substituted judgment is an ethical principle used when a decision is made for an incapacitated client.

NP: Implementation; CN: Safe, effective care environment; CNS: Management of care; CL: Application

6. A nurse gives a client the wrong medication. After assessing the client, the nurse completes an incident report. Which statement describes what will occur next?

1. The incident will be reported to the state board of nursing for disciplinary action.
2. The incident will be documented in the nurse's personnel file.
3. The medication error will result in the nurse being suspended and, possibly, terminated from employment at the facility.
4. The incident report is a method of promoting quality care and risk management.

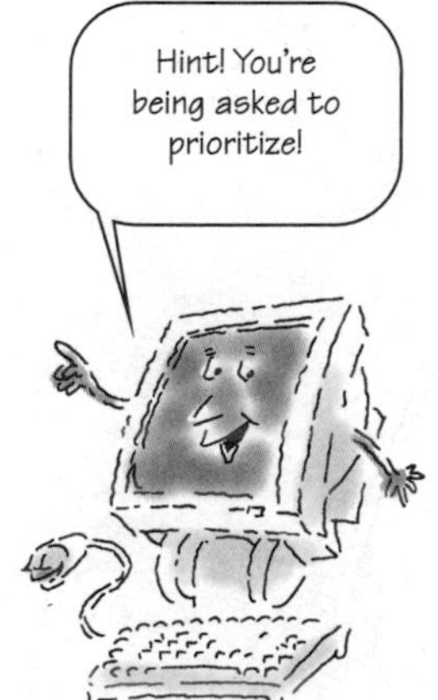
Hint! You're being asked to prioritize!

6. 4. Unusual occurrences and deviations from care are documented on incident reports. Incident reports are internal to the facility and are used to evaluate care, determine potential risks, or system problems that could have contributed to the error. This type of error won't result in a report to the state board of nursing or in suspension of the nurse. Some facilities do track the number of errors by a nurse or on particular units; the purpose of tracking errors is to provide appropriate education and to improve the nursing process.

NP: Evaluation; CN: Safe, effective care environment; CNS: Management of care; CL: Analysis

NP: Nursing process CN: Client needs category CNS: Client needs subcategory CL: Cognitive level

7. A client has suffered an extensive brain injury and can't make his own treatment choices. Which written document is recognized by state law and provides directions for provision of care at a time when the client can't make his own choices?

1. Advance directive
2. Living will
3. Durable power of attorney
4. Patient self-determination

7. 1. An advance directive is a document written or completed by the client and used by a facility to provide care at a time when the client can't make his own choices. The living will and durable power of attorney are both examples of advance directives. A living will is a document that's prepared by a competent adult and provides direction regarding medical care if the client becomes incapacitated. Durable power of attorney is an authorization enabling any competent individual to name someone else to exercise decision-making authority on the individual's behalf under specific circumstances. The Patient Self-Determination Act of 1990 allows clients to write instructions for their care and treatment for a time when they become unable to make their own decisions.

NP: Assessment; CN: Safe, effective care environment; CNS: Management of care; CL: Knowledge

8. In which way do nurses play a key role in error prevention?

1. Identifying incorrect dosages or potential interactions of prescribed medications
2. Never questioning the order of a physician because he's ultimately responsible for the client outcome
3. Notifying the Occupational Safety and Health Association (OSHA) of violations in the workplace
4. Informing the client of his bill of rights as a client

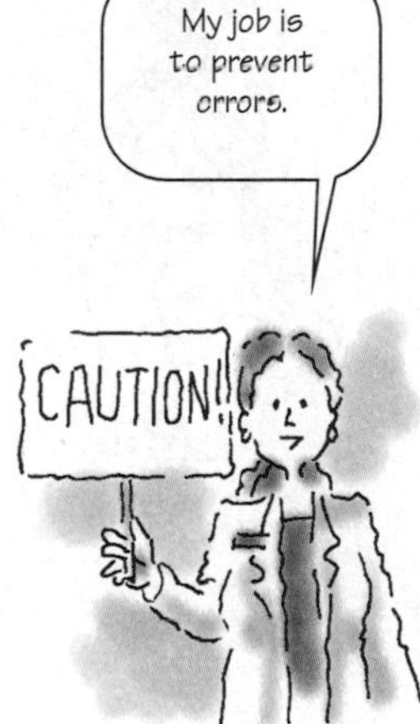
My job is to prevent errors.
CAUTION!

8. 1. Nurses must be knowledgeable about drug dosages and possible interactions when administering medications; they must follow appropriate policies to correct dosage errors or potential interactions. The nurse is responsible for questioning unclear or ambiguous physician orders and should never carry out an order for which she's uncomfortable. Notifying OSHA doesn't solve medication errors. OSHA establishes comprehensive safety and health standards, inspects workplaces, and requires employers to eliminate safety hazards. The client should be aware of his rights as a client, but that awareness doesn't play a key role in error prevention.

NP: Evaluation; CN: Safe, effective care environment; CNS: Safety and infection control; CL: Application

9. Which statement is true concerning informed consent?

1. Minors are permitted to give informed consent.
2. The professional nurse and physician may both obtain informed consent.
3. The client must be fully informed regarding treatment, tests, surgery, and the risks and benefits prior to giving informed consent.
4. Mentally competent and incompetent clients can legally give informed consent.

9. 3. When the professional nurse is involved in the informed consent process, the nurse is only witnessing the consent process and doesn't actually obtain the consent. Only a minor who is married or emancipated can give informed consent. Obtaining consent is the responsibility of the physician. Legally, the client must be mentally competent to give consent for procedures.

NP: Planning; CN: Safe, effective care environment; CNS: Management of care; CL: Comprehension

10. Which statement is correct regarding the Omnibus Reconciliation Act of 1986?

1. All families of clients who are nearing death, or have died, must be approached with the option of organ and tissue donation.
2. The medical examiner should be notified of all potential organ donors.
3. A request must be made to the family regarding release of the donor's name.
4. Hospitals aren't responsible for establishing designated requesters for donation.

10. 1. The federal Omnibus Reconciliation Act of 1986 mandates that all hospitals establish written protocols for the identification of potential organ and tissue donors. The act sets standards for organ procurement agencies. The medical examiner should be notified if the client is a potential organ or tissue donor only if the medical examiner is involved in the case. Requesters for donation are health care professionals who have received special training on properly approaching family members regarding organ or tissue donation.

NP: Implementation; CN: Safe, effective care environment; CNS: Management of care; CL: Comprehension

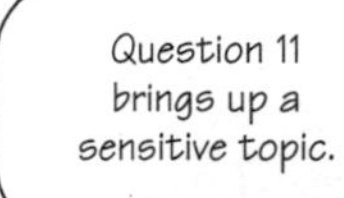
Question 11
brings up a
sensitive topic.

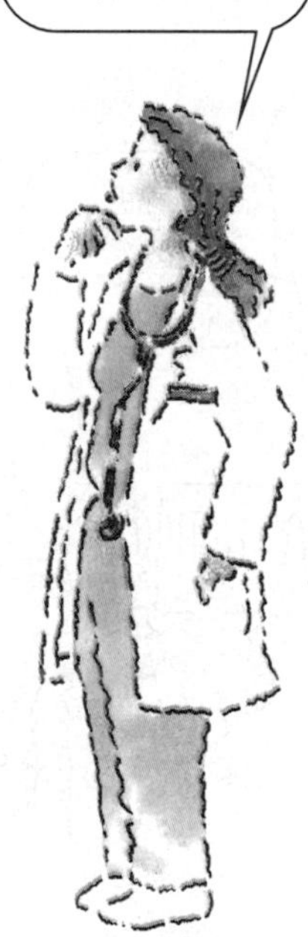

11. When approaching a family for organ or tissue donation, the nurse should keep in mind which guideline?

1. Approaching a family is done only with a physician's approval and written order.
2. The requester doesn't have to believe in the benefits of organ donation but should support the process with a positive attitude.
3. The requester is knowledgeable about the basics of organ and tissue donation and is capable of educating the family members about brain death early in the organ donation process.
4. The family is offered an opportunity to speak with an organ procurement coordinator.

11. 4. The family should be offered an opportunity to speak with an organ procurement coordinator. An organ procurement coordinator is knowledgeable about the organ donation process and should have exceptional interpersonal skills for dealing with grieving family members. Physician support in the process is desirable but consent or written orders aren't necessary for a referral to the organ procurement organization. The requestor must believe in the benefits of organ donation and support the process with a positive attitude. The family should be approached about speaking to an organ procurement coordinator only after the family has been made aware of the client's condition and prognosis. Approaching a family member who believes there's still hope for recovery will likely result in a negative outcome.

NP: Evaluation; CN: Safe, effective care environment; CNS: Management of care; CL: Analysis

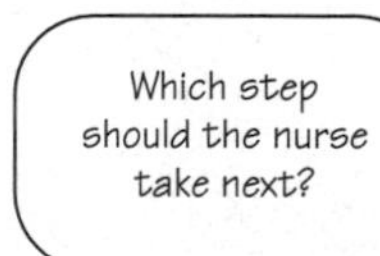
Which step
should the nurse
take next?

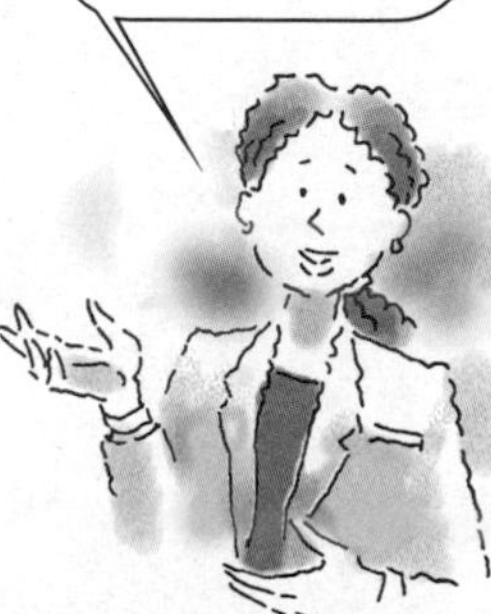

12. Which are the stages of grief that a client or family member goes through?

1. Acceptance, depression, anger, bargaining, and denial
2. Denial, anger, decreased interaction, depression, and mourning
3. Acceptance, anger, denial, and bargaining
4. Denial, anger, bargaining, depression, and acceptance

12. 4. Denial is the avoidance of death's inevitability and is the first step of the grieving process. Anger, the most intense grief reaction, arises when people realize that death and loss will actually occur or has occurred for a family member. Bargaining happens when family members attempt to stall or manipulate the outcome or death. Depression is a response to loss that's expressed as profound sadness or deep suffering. Acceptance is the final stage, and it's the ability to overcome the grief and accept what has happened.

NP: Assessment; CN: Psychosocial integrity; CNS: Coping and adaptation; CL: Comprehension

13. While performing an assessment of a 75-year-old female in the emergency department, the nurse notes many bruises in various stages of healing on the client's body. After documenting the locations of the bruises in the medical record, which step should the nurse take next?

1. Notify the nursing supervisor immediately.
2. Notify the physician.
3. Try to obtain more information from the client as to when and how these bruises occurred.
4. Follow the facility's policy and procedures for reporting elder abuse.

13. 3. The nurse should try to obtain more information from the client to complete the assessment. Without the information, she shouldn't assume that the bruises are from abuse, and she shouldn't notify her nursing supervisor until she has obtained additional facts. She should, however, inform the physician so he can examine the client. She should follow the facility's policy and procedure for reporting abuse. However, reporting should be done after the assessment if the nurse has a strong suspicion that abuse is the cause.

NP: Assessment; CN: Psychosocial integrity; CNS: Psychosocial adaptation; CL: Application

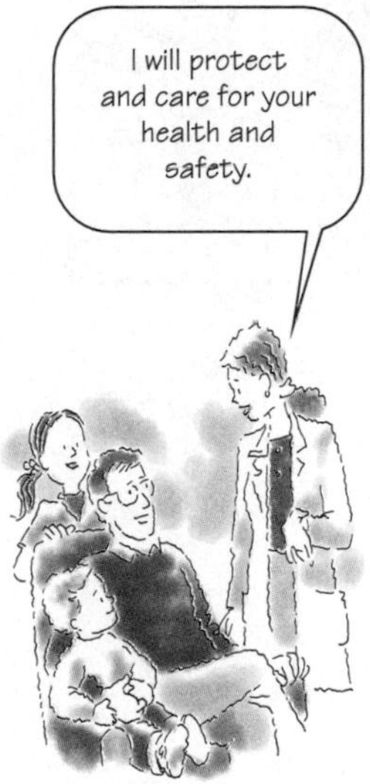

14. Which concept refers to the role of the professional nurse in client advocacy?

1. The nurse makes decisions for clients who can't make decisions for themselves
2. The nurse follows the basic standards of care and hospital policies and procedures for providing care for clients.
3. The nurse promotes and protects the client's interests and rights.
4. The nurse adapts a paternalistic approach to the care of clients.

I will protect and care for your health and safety.

14. 3. The nurse who understands the advocacy role promotes, protects, and, thereby, advocates a client's interests and rights in an effort to make the client well. The nurse doesn't make decisions for clients but provides care for the acutely ill client with the consent of his significant other, a power of attorney, or his living will. Standards of care are the basis for providing safe competent nursing care and set minimum criteria for proficiency on the job, enabling the nurse and others to judge the quality of care provided. Paternalism violates self-determination and advocacy by acting for another.

NP: Analysis; CN: Safe, effective care environment; CNS: Management of care; CL: Application

15. A client with a history of heart disease is scheduled for cataract surgery when he tells the nurse that he's experiencing chest discomfort and shortness of breath. The nurse administers a nitroglycerin tablet sublingually as ordered by the admitting physician but fails to notify the physician, surgeon, or anesthesiologist. If the client suffers a massive heart attack during surgery, the nurse could be held liable for which malpractice charge?

1. Failure to act as a client advocate
2. Failure to communicate with the client
3. Failure to assess, monitor, and communicate
4. Failure to protect from harm

15. 3. The nurse has a responsibility to assess, monitor, and communicate a client's status under her care. In this case, the change in the client's status could influence care during surgery and the potential outcomes. Failure to act as a client advocate has been recognized by the courts when the nurse fails to develop and implement nursing diagnoses, and fails to exercise good judgment on the client's behalf. Failure to communicate with the client refers to not adequately educating him about care, procedures, or discharge instructions. Failure to protect from harm occurs when health care providers must protect a client because of the client's vulnerable state and inability to distinguish potentially harmful situations.

NP: Assessment; CN: Safe, effective care environment; CNS: Management of care; CL: Application

16. In which circumstance may the nurse legally and ethically disclose confidential information about a client?

1. The human immunodeficiency virus (HIV)–status of a single male client to his family members.
2. The diagnosis of pancreatic cancer to the client's significant other.
3. The diagnosis of an uncontrolled seizure disorder of a taxi driver to a state agency.
4. The client is 32 weeks pregnant with twins and is legally separated.

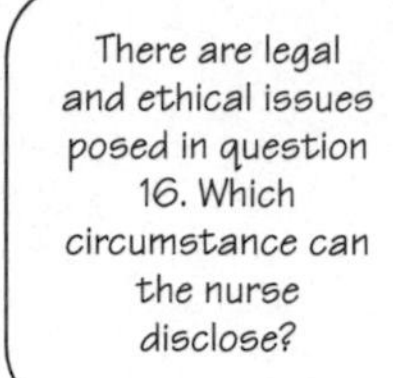

There are legal and ethical issues posed in question 16. Which circumstance can the nurse disclose?

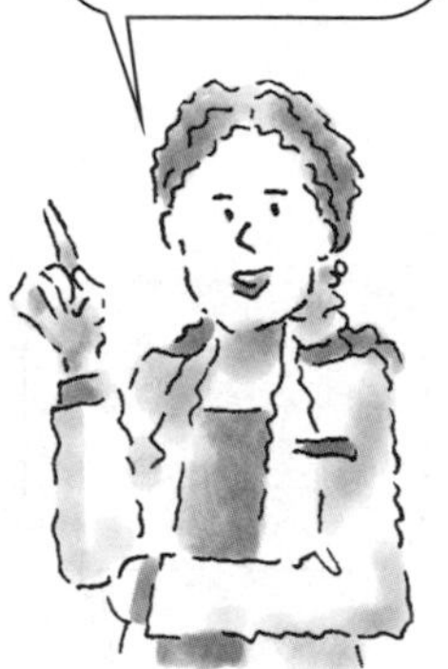

16. 3. The nurse may lawfully disclose confidential information about a client when the welfare of a person is at stake. The physician is required to inform the Department of Motor Vehicles that the taxi driver has an uncontrolled seizure disorder because it's in the best interest of the public's and client's safety. Options 2 and 4 don't affect the welfare of a group of people. Confidentiality of HIV testing is required, but the client should be encouraged to share the information with others. A positive HIV test can mean the loss of a job, medical insurance, financial security, and even housing because family, friends, and the public may fear the HIV positive person.

NP: Evaluation; CN: Safe, effective care environment; CNS: Management of care; CL: Application

17. A client in a long-term care facility refuses to take his oral medications. The nurse threatens the client and tells him that, if the medication isn't taken, restraints will be applied and the medication will be given by injection. The nurse's statement constitutes which legal tort?

1. Assault
2. Battery
3. Negligence
4. Right to refuse care

17. 1. Assault occurs when a person puts another person in fear of harmful or threatening contact. Battery is the actual contact with one's body. If the nurse actually carried out the threat, battery would also apply. Negligence involves actions below the standard of care. The client has the legal right to refuse care. In this situation, the correct action is to try to calm the client, allow him time to talk, and then determine if he will take the medications. If the client still won't take the medications, the nurse should document his refusal, note the medications, and notify the physician and nursing supervisor.

NP: Evaluation; CN: Safe, effective care environment; CNS: Management of care; CL: Comprehension

18. Entering the client's room to get the neonate for an examination by the physician, the nurse on the maternity unit sees the client holding the crying neonate and slapping his face. Which action is most appropriate?

1. Take the neonate to the nursery, tell the physician so he can examine the neonate for injuries, and notify social services.
2. Leave the room without the neonate and notify the nursing supervisor.
3. Confront the client by asking her what she's doing and why.
4. Take the neonate to the nursery and tell coworkers to observe the client for further incidents.

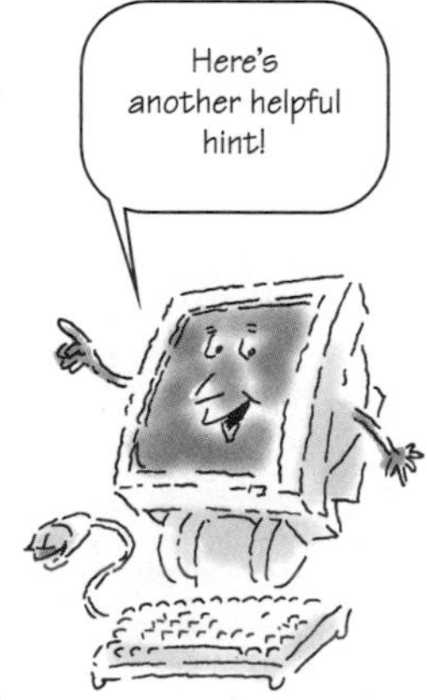

Here's another helpful hint!

18. 1. The neonate's safety and protection is the first priority. The nurse should immediately take neonate to the nursery and inform the physician of the abuse. By being the neonate's advocate, the nurse allows the physician to examine him for injuries resulting from the incident. Social services should be notified. Follow the facility's policy and procedure for reporting suspected and actual child abuse. Although the incident may be part of the revised care plan, it requires immediate intervention, not simple notification of coworkers.

NP: Implementation; CN: Psychosocial integrity; CNS: Psychosocial adaptation; CL: Analysis

NP: Nursing process CN: Client needs category CNS: Client needs subcategory CL: Cognitive level

19. The care plan is revised for a client who has difficulty dealing with a crying neonate. Which strategy should the new care plan include **early** in the client's hospital stay?

1. Anger management therapy
2. Proper care of a crying infant
3. Proper methods for dealing with stressful situations such as crying infants
4. Assessment of the client's strengths and weaknesses in coping mechanisms and the presence of support systems

19. 4. Assessment of the client's strengths and weaknesses in her coping mechanisms and the presence of support systems is important in the implementation process. Assessment will also help identify situations that the client perceives as stressors. Providing education about alternatives to expressing feelings and about crisis hotlines and community support systems should also be part of the care plan. It hasn't been established that the client is angry, so anger management therapy isn't necessary. Proper care of a crying infant is necessary, but assessing the client's coping will help provide the basis for teaching.

NP: Evaluation; CN: Psychosocial integrity; CNS: Coping and adaptation; CL: Analysis

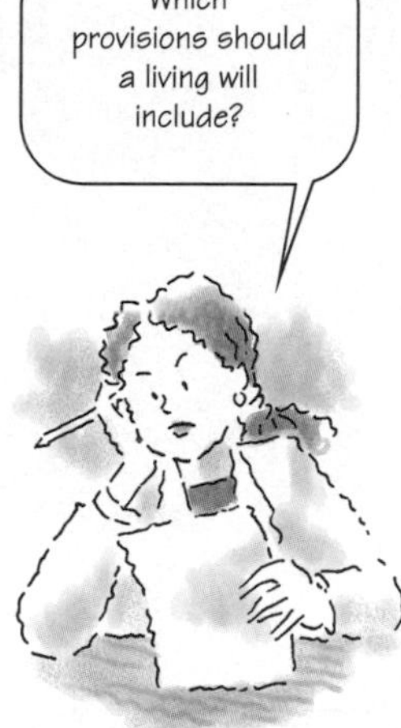
Which provisions should a living will include?

20. Although living will laws vary from state to state, they generally include which provisions?

1. Instructions on when and how the living will should be executed
2. Who may uphold a living will declaration
3. How long the living will is in effect
4. What will happen to the client's valuables after death

20. 1. Living wills include instructions on when and how it should be executed, the witness and testator requirements, immunity from liability for following a living will directive, documentation requirements, and under what circumstances it will take effect. A living will doesn't state who may uphold the declaration or how long it's in effect. A living will doesn't dictate what will happen to the client's valuables.

NP: Analysis; CN: Safe, effective care environment; CNS: Management of care; CL: Knowledge

21. Which is the role of the nurse in a domestic abuse situation?

1. Document the situation and provide support for the victim.
2. Protect the client' privacy by not documenting the abuse.
3. Provide counseling to the person committing the abuse.
4. Provide counseling for the victim.

21. 1. The nurse must carefully and adequately document the assessment of the abused victim. The documentation must include statements from the victim, physical and psychological assessment findings, and observations relative to the abuse situation. The victim should be provided with local community resources, social agencies, and legal services as necessary to prevent recurrence of physical abuse. The professional nurse isn't qualified to counsel the abuser or the victim. The abuser and victim should be referred for therapy.

NP: Analysis; CN: Psychosocial integrity; CNS: Psychosocial adaptation; CL: Analysis

22. A day shift nurse gives a client a medication injection for pain and forgets to document it on the medication administration record (MAR). The day shift nurse reports to the evening shift nurse that she gave the client 4 mg of morphine at 2 p.m. for postoperative pain but didn't document it. The evening shift nurse puts the day shift nurse's initials, date, and time the dose was administered in the MAR. The action by the evening shift nurse is considered to be which type of documentation error?

1. Omission
2. Late entry
3. Improper correction
4. Unauthorized entry

22. 4. This action is an unauthorized entry. A nurse shouldn't document for another nurse, except for an authorized entry in an emergency. Omission is a documentation error in which information is missing from the medical record. A late entry refers to an entry entered at a time later than it should have been. If a late entry is necessary, identify it as a "late entry" and document the reference date and time. An improper correction is an entry corrected in an incorrect manner, such as erasing, using "white out," or obliterating the error with a marking pen.

NP: Analysis; CN: Safe, effective care environment; CNS: Management of care; CL: Analysis

23. A pediatric nurse is asked to work temporarily (float) in the intensive care unit (ICU) The nurse has never worked in the ICU and has no critical care experience. Which action is most appropriate for this nurse?

1. Refuse to float to ICU.
2. Notify the nursing supervisor that she feels unqualified and untrained for the assignment.
3. Go to ICU and take a total client assignment; ask the critical care nurses for assistance when necessary.
4. Go to ICU, tell the ICU nurses she has never worked in the ICU, and let the nurses decide what tasks she can perform.

23. 2. The pediatric nurse should notify the nursing supervisor about feeling unqualified and untrained. The nursing supervisor can guide the pediatric nurse as to the tasks the pediatric nurse is qualified to perform in the ICU without jeopardizing her license. When the census on a unit is low, many facilities use staff to float to another unit as a cost-effective and reasonable manner for managing resources. A nurse should never take responsibility for a total client care assignment if the nurse doesn't have the skills to plan and deliver that care. Option 4 puts the decision and responsibility for performance on ICU nurses. However, the nursing supervisor should make those decisions because she knows the overall needs of the facility and can allocate nursing resources.

NP: Analysis; CN: Safe, effective care environment; CNS: Management of care; CL: Application

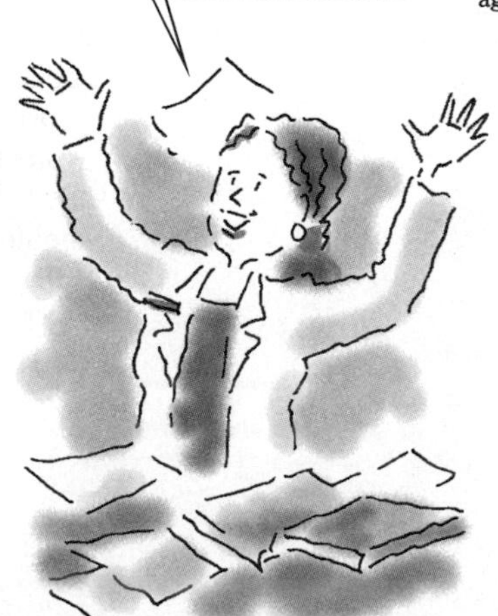

You did it! You finished the final chapter! Now, for more fun, try the six comprehensive tests that follow!

Appendices

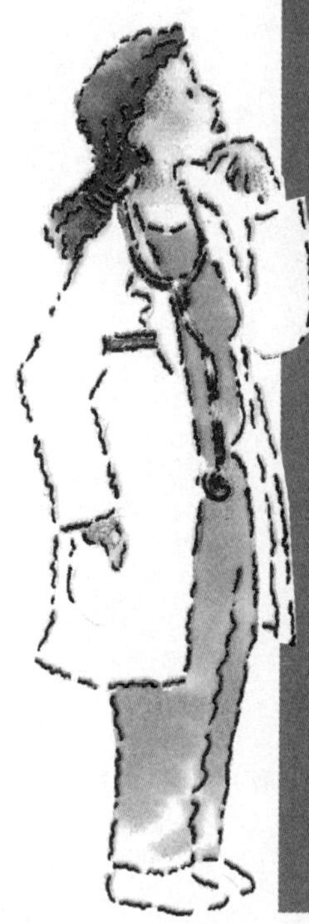

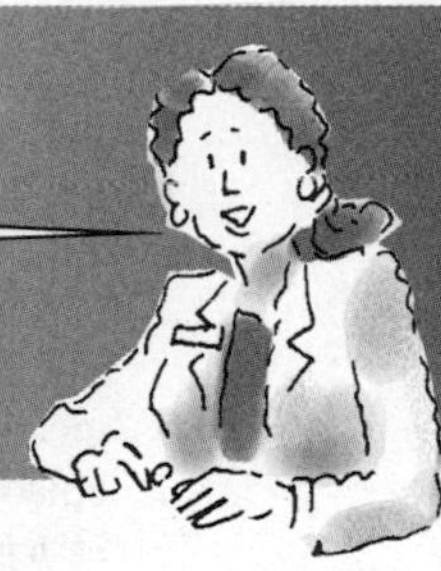
This comprehensive test,
the first of six,
is just like a real NCLEX
test. It's a great way to
practice!

COMPREHENSIVE Test 1

1. A 43-year-old client with blunt chest trauma from a motor vehicle accident has sinus tachycardia, is hypotensive, and has developed muffled heart sounds. There are no obvious signs of bleeding. Which of the following conditions is suspected?

1. Heart failure
2. Pneumothorax
3. Cardiac tamponade
4. Myocardial infarction (MI)

1. 3. Cardiac tamponade results in signs of obvious shock and muffled heart sounds. In an MI, the client may complain of chest pain. An electrocardiogram could confirm changes consistent with an MI. Heart failure would result in inspiratory crackles, pulmonary edema, and jugular vein distention. Pneumothorax would result in diminished breath sounds in the affected lung, respiratory distress, and tracheal displacement.

NP: Assessment; CN: Physiological integrity; CNS: Physiological adaptation; CL: Analysis

2. Which of the following types of shock is associated with tamponade?

1. Anaphylactic
2. Cardiogenic
3. Hypovolemic
4. Septic

2. 2. Fluid accumulates in the pericardial sac, hindering motion of the heart muscle and causing it to pump inefficiently, resulting in signs of cardiogenic shock. Hypovolemic shock involves the actual loss of fluid. Anaphylactic and septic are types of distributive shock in which fluid is displaced from the capillaries and leaks into surrounding tissues.

NP: Assessment; CN: Physiological integrity; CNS: Physiological adaptation; CL: Knowledge

3. Which of the following diagnostic tests is used to detect cardiac tamponade?

1. Chest X-ray
2. Echocardiography
3. Electrocardiogram (ECG)
4. Pulmonary artery pressure monitoring

3. 1. Chest X-rays show a slightly widened mediastinum and enlarged cardiac silhouette. Echocardiography records pericardial effusion with signs of right ventricular and atrial compression. An ECG can rule out other cardiac disorders. Pulmonary artery monitoring shows increased right atrial or central venous pressure and right ventricular diastolic pressure.

NP: Assessment; CN: Physiological integrity; CNS: Reduction of risk potential; CL: Knowledge

NP: Nursing process CN: Client needs category CNS: Client needs subcategory CL: Cognitive level

4. Which of the following interventions or medications is the emergency treatment for cardiac tamponade?
1. Surgery
2. Dopamine
3. Blood transfusion
4. Pericardiocentesis

4. 4. Pericardiocentesis, or needle aspiration of the pericardial cavity, is done to relieve tamponade. Dopamine is used to restore blood pressure in normovolemic individuals. Blood transfusions may be given if the client is hypovolemic from blood loss. An opening is created surgically if the client continues to have recurrent episodes of tamponade.
NP: Implementation; CN: Physiological integrity; CNS: Physiological adaptation; CL: Knowledge

5. A nurse is teaching a 50-year-old client how to decrease risk factors for coronary artery disease. He's an executive who smokes, has a type A personality, and is hypertensive. Which of the following risk factors can't be changed?
1. Age
2. Hypertension
3. Personality
4. Smoking

5. 1. Age is a risk factor that can't be changed. Type A personality, hypertension, and smoking factors can be controlled.
NP: Assessment; CN: Health promotion and maintenance; CNS: Prevention and early detection of disease; CL: Comprehension

6. A client says he's stressed by his job but enjoys the challenge. Which of the following suggestions is best to help the client?
1. Switch job positions.
2. Take stress management classes.
3. Spend more time with his family.
4. Don't take his work home with him.

6. 2. Stress management classes will teach the client how to better manage the stress in his life, after identifying the factors that contribute to it. Alternatives may be found to leaving his job, which he enjoys. Not spending enough time with his family and not taking his job home with him haven't yet been identified as contributing factors.
NP: Implementation; CN: Physiological integrity; CNS: Reduction of risk potential; CL: Application

7. Which of the following nursing diagnoses is correctly worded?
1. Anger related to terminal illness
2. Pain related to alteration in comfort
3. Red sacrum related to improper positioning
4. Social isolation related to inability to speak because of laryngectomy

7. 4. This is a correctly worded nursing diagnosis. The first option identifies anger as an unhealthy response when it may be an appropriate and socially acceptable response. The second option is incorrect because both parts of this diagnosis relate to pain and say the same thing. The third option is improperly written; it's a legally inadvisable statement.
NP: Analysis; CN: Safe, effective care environment; CNS: Management of care; CL: Application

8. A 28-year-old client with human immunodeficiency virus (HIV) is admitted to the hospital with flulike symptoms. He has dyspnea and a cough. He's placed on a 100% nonrebreather mask and arterial blood gases are drawn. Which of the following results indicates the client needs intubation?

1. Pao_2, 90 mm Hg; $Paco_2$, 40 mm Hg
2. Pao_2, 85 mm Hg; $Paco_2$, 45 mm Hg
3. Pao_2, 80 mm Hg; $Paco_2$, 45 mm Hg
4. Pao_2, 70 mm Hg; $Paco_2$, 55 mm Hg

8. 4. An increasing $Paco_2$ and decreasing Pao_2 indicate poor oxygen perfusion. Normal Pao_2 levels are 80 to 100 mm Hg and normal $Paco_2$ levels are 35 to 45 mm Hg.

NP: Assessment; CN: Physiological integrity; CNS: Physiological adaptation; CL: Analysis

9. Which of the following substances most commonly transmits the human immunodeficiency virus (HIV)?

1. Blood
2. Feces
3. Saliva
4. Urine

9. 1. HIV is transmitted by contact with infected blood. It exists in all body fluids but transmission through saliva, urine, and feces is much less likely to occur than through blood.

NP: Assessment; CN: Safe, effective care environment; CNS: Safety and infection control; CL: Knowledge

10. Which of the following opportunistic diseases is caused by protozoa in clients with acquired immunodeficiency syndrome?

1. Tuberculosis (TB)
2. Histoplasmosis
3. Kaposi's sarcoma
4. *Pneumocystis carinii* infection

10. 4. *P. carinii* infection is caused by protozoa. TB is caused by bacteria. Histoplasmosis is a fungal infection. Kaposi's sarcoma is a neoplasm.

NP: Assessment; CN: Physiological integrity; CNS: Physiological adaptation; CL: Knowledge

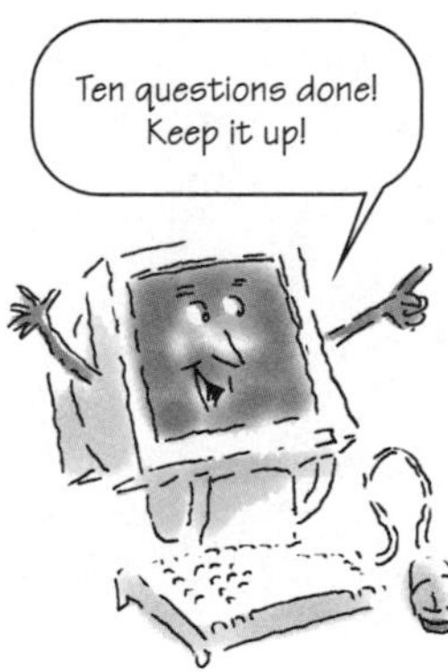
Ten questions done!
Keep it up!

11. A client with acquired immunodeficiency syndrome is intubated, leaving him prone to skin breakdown from the endotracheal tube. Which of the following interventions is best to prevent this?

1. Use lubricant on the lips.
2. Provide oral care every 2 hours.
3. Suction the oral cavity every 2 hours.
4. Reposition the endotracheal tube every 24 hours.

11. 4. Pressure causes skin breakdown. However, repositioning the endotracheal tube from one side of the mouth to the other or to the center of the mouth can relieve pressure in one area for a time. Extreme care must be taken to move the tube only laterally; it must not be pushed in or pulled out. The tape securing the tube must be changed daily. Two nurses should perform this procedure. Oral care, suctioning, and lubricant help keep skin clean and intact and reduce the risk of further infection.

NP: Implementation; CN: Physiological integrity; CNS: Basic care and comfort; CL: Application

12. Which of the following medications is given with pentamidine isethionate to clients with acquired immunodeficiency syndrome for *Pneumocystis carinii* pneumonia?

1. Amphotericin B
2. Co-trimoxazole
3. Fluconazole
4. Sulfadiazine

12. 2. Co-trimoxazole is given orally or I.V. for *P. carinii* pneumonia. Sulfadiazine is used to treat toxoplasmosis. Fluconazole and amphotericin B are used for coccidioidomycosis.

NP: Implementation; CN: Physiological integrity; CNS: Pharmacological and parenteral therapies; CL: Knowledge

13. A client receiving pentamidine isethionate should have which of the following parameters monitored frequently?

1. Heart rate
2. Electrolyte levels
3. Blood sugar levels
4. Complete blood count (CBC)

13. 3. Pentamidine isethionate can cause permanent diabetes mellitus and requires monitoring of blood sugar levels. The client's CBC, heart rate, and electrolyte levels can be monitored less frequently.

NP: Implementation; CN: Physiological integrity; CNS: Pharmacological and parenteral therapies; CL: Comprehension

14. A nurse caring for a client with acquired immunodeficiency syndrome is working with a nursing student. She notes the student doesn't attempt to suction or assist with care of the client. Which of the following actions is appropriate?

1. Talk to the student.
2. Talk to the charge nurse.
3. Address a coworker with the concerns.
4. Seek advice from the student's instructor.

14. 1. The nurse should approach the student to determine her feelings and experience in caring for this client. The charge nurse and coworkers aren't familiar with the student's abilities, but the instructor may be approached if the nurse can't communicate with the student.

NP: Implementation; CN: Safe, effective care environment; CNS: Management of care; CL: Analysis

15. A client's significant other is tearful over the client's condition and lack of improvement. He says he feels very powerless and unable to help his friend. Which of the following responses by the nurse is the best?

1. Agree with the person.
2. Tell him there's nothing he can do.
3. State she understands how he must feel.
4. Ask if he would like to help with some comfort measures.

15. 4. The significant other expresses a need to help and the nurse can encourage him to do whatever he feels comfortable with, such as putting lubricant on lips, moist cloth on forehead, or lotion on skin. The nurse may not understand his situation, and agreeing with a person doesn't diminish powerlessness. There are many ways the significant other can help if he wants to.

NP: Implementation; CN: Psychosocial integrity; CNS: Coping and adaptation; CL: Analysis

16. A 31-year-old client is admitted to the hospital with respiratory failure. He's intubated in the emergency department, placed on 100% FIO_2, and is coughing up copious secretions. Which of the following interventions has priority?

1. Get an X-ray.
2. Suction the client.
3. Restrain the client.
4. Obtain an arterial blood gas (ABG) analysis.

16. 2. Secretions can cut off the oxygen supply to the client and result in hypoxia so suctioning the client is your first priority. After the client has acclimated to his ventilator settings, ABGs can be drawn. X-rays are a priority to check placement of the endotracheal tube. Restraints are warranted if the client is a threat to his safety.

NP: Implementation; CN: Physiological integrity; CNS: Reduction of risk potential; CL: Analysis

17. A client with an endotracheal tube has copious, brown-tinged secretions. Which of the following interventions is a priority?

1. Use a trap to obtain a specimen.
2. Instill saline to break up secretions.
3. Culture the specimen with a culturette swab.
4. Obtain an order for a liquefying agent for the sputum.

17. 1. Suspicious secretions should be sent for culture and sensitivity using a sterile technique such as a trap. Swab culturettes are useful for wound cultures — not endotracheal cultures. Saline would dilute the specimen. Various agents are available to help break up secretions, and respiratory therapists can usually help recommend the right agent, but this isn't a priority.

NP: Implementation; CN: Safe, effective care environment; CNS: Safety and infection control; CL: Analysis

18. An X-ray shows an endotracheal (ET) tube is 2 cm above the carina, and there are nodular lesions and patchy infiltrates in the upper lobe. Which of the following interpretations of the X-ray is accurate?

1. The X-ray is inconclusive.
2. The client has a disease process going on.
3. The ET tube needs to be advanced.
4. The ET tube needs to be pulled back.

18. 2. The X-ray is suggestive of tuberculosis. At 2 cm, the ET tube is at an adequate level in the trachea and doesn't have to be advanced or pulled back.

NP: Evaluation; CN: Health promotion and maintenance; CNS: Prevention and early detection of disease; CL: Analysis

19. A client has copious secretions. X-ray results indicate tuberculosis (TB). Which of the following interventions should be performed first?

1. Repeat X-ray
2. Tracheostomy
3. Bronchoscopy
4. Arterial blood gas (ABG) analysis

19. 3. Bronchoscopy can help diagnose TB and obtain specimens while clearing the bronchial tree of secretions. Tracheostomy may be done if the client remains on the ventilator for a prolonged period. A change in condition or treatment may require an ABG analysis. X-rays may be repeated periodically to determine lung and endotracheal tube status.

NP: Planning; CN: Physiological integrity; CNS: Reduction of risk potential; CL: Comprehension

20. A nurse is aware that family members of a client diagnosed with tuberculosis, as well as staff members, may have been exposed to the disease. A tuberculin skin test may show which of the following conditions?

1. Active disease
2. Recent infection
3. Extent of the infection
4. Infection at some point

20. 4. A tuberculin skin test shows the presence of infection at some point; a positive skin test doesn't guarantee that an infection is *currently* present, however. Some people have false-positive results. Active disease may be viewed on a chest X-ray. Computed tomography or magnetic resonance imaging can evaluate the extent of lung damage.

NP: Assessment; CN: Safe, effective care environment; CNS: Safety and infection control; CL: Knowledge

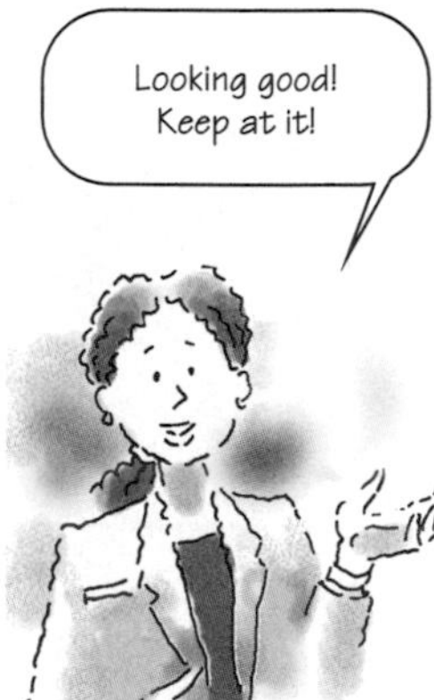

21. A client is diagnosed with tuberculosis (TB). In addition to recommending skin testing of the family members, TB should be reported to which of the following individuals or agencies?

1. Centers for Disease Control and Prevention (CDC)
2. Local health department
3. Infection-control nurse
4. Client's physician

21. 2. The local health department must be informed of an outbreak of TB because it's a reportable disease. They, in turn, inform the CDC. The infection-control nurse or employee health department may request that staff be tested if exposed. Generally, the client's family can inform his physician.

NP: Planning; CN: Safe, effective care environment; CNS: Safety and infection control; CL: Application

22. The usual treatment for tuberculosis (TB) includes the use of isoniazid (INH) and which of the following therapies?

1. Theophylline inhaler
2. I.M. penicillin
3. Three other antibacterial agents
4. Aerosol treatments with pentamidine

22. 3. Because TB has become resistant to many antibacterial agents, the initial treatment includes the use of multiple antituberculotic or antibacterial drugs. These may include rifampin, ethambutol hydrochloride, pyrazinamide, cycloserine, clofazimine, and streptomycin. Pentamidine is used in the treatment of *Pneumocystis carinii* pneumonia. Theophylline is a bronchodilator used to treat asthma and chronic obstructive pulmonary disease. Penicillins are used to treat *Staphylococcus aureus* — not TB.

NP: Implementation; CN: Physiological integrity; CNS: Pharmacological and parenteral therapies; CL: Knowledge

23. How long do most clients receive treatment for tuberculosis (TB)?

1. 2 to 4 months
2. 9 to 12 months
3. 18 to 24 months
4. More than 2 years

23. 2. Treatment for TB is usually continued for at least 9 to 12 months.

NP: Implementation; CN: Physiological integrity; CNS: Pharmacological and parenteral therapies; CL: Knowledge

24. For what length of time is a client considered infectious after treatment for tuberculosis is started?

1. 72 hours
2. 1 week
3. 2 weeks
4. 4 weeks

24. 4. After 4 weeks, the disease is no longer infectious but the client must continue to take the medication.

NP: Implementation; CN: Safe, effective care environment; CNS: Safety and infection control; CL: Knowledge

25. A client tells his nurse that his tuberculosis medications are so expensive that he can't afford to take them. Which of the following interventions by the nurse is best?

1. Refer the client to social services.
2. Tell the client to apply for Medicaid.
3. Refer the client to the local or county health department.
4. Tell the client to follow his insurance rules and regulations.

25. 3. The local and county health departments provide treatment and follow-up free of charge for all residents to ensure proper care. Insurance can be an alternative source to help pay for treatment, but the client may not be insured or the policy may not cover prescriptions. Medicaid or medical assistance is another avenue for the client, *if* he qualifies. Social services can help seek alternative methods of payment and reimbursement but would probably first refer the client to the local and county health departments.

NP: Implementation; CN: Safe, effective care environment; CNS: Management of care; CL: Knowledge

26. A 62-year-old client is admitted to the hospital with pneumonia. He has a history of Parkinson's disease, which his family says is progressively worsening. Which of the following assessments is expected?

1. Impaired speech
2. Muscle flaccidity
3. Pleasant and smiling demeanor
4. Tremors in the fingers that increase with purposeful movement

26. 1. In Parkinson's disease, dysarthria, or impaired speech, is due to a disturbance in muscle control. Muscle rigidity results in resistance to passive muscle stretching. The client may have a masklike appearance. Tremors should decrease with purposeful movement and sleep.

NP: Assessment; CN: Physiological integrity; CNS: Physiological adaptation; CL: Application

27. Which of the following terms describes a clinical judgment that an individual, family, or community is more vulnerable to develop a certain problem than others in the same or similar situation?

1. Risk nursing diagnosis
2. Actual nursing diagnosis
3. Possible nursing diagnosis
4. Wellness nursing diagnosis

27. 1. Risk nursing diagnosis refers to the vulnerability of a client, family, or community to health problems. An actual nursing diagnosis describes a human response to a health problem being manifested. Possible nursing diagnoses are made when there isn't enough evidence to support the presence of the problem, but the nurse believes the problem is highly probable and wants to collect more data. A wellness nursing diagnosis is a diagnostic statement describing the human response to levels of wellness in an individual, family, or community that have a potential for enhancement to a higher state.

NP: Analysis; CN: Safe, effective care environment; CNS: Management of care; CL: Knowledge

28. Which of the following interventions is best to decrease a client's risk for skin breakdown?

1. Use a specialty mattress.
2. Position the client in alignment.
3. Reposition the client every 4 hours.
4. Massage bony prominences every shift.

28. 1. Specialty beds, such as fluid, air, and egg crate mattresses, can protect pressure areas on the client. Pressure areas on the client should be padded to prevent skin breakdown. The client should be turned every 2 hours. Massaging bony prominences causes friction and may irritate tissues.

NP: Implementation; CN: Physiological integrity; CNS: Reduction of risk potential; CL: Application

29. An 82-year-old male client with Parkinson's disease is frequently incontinent of urine. Which of the following interventions is appropriate?

1. Diaper the client.
2. Apply a condom catheter.
3. Insert an indwelling urinary catheter.
4. Provide skin care every 4 hours.

29. 2. A condom catheter uses a condom-type device to drain urine away from the client. Diapering the client may keep urine away from the body but may also be demeaning if the client is alert or the family objects. Because the client with Parkinson's disease is already prone to urinary tract infections, an indwelling urinary catheter should be avoided because it may promote this. Skin care must be provided as soon as the client is incontinent to prevent skin maceration and breakdown.

NP: Implementation; CN: Physiological integrity; CNS: Basic care and comfort; CL: Analysis

30. Family members report exhaustion and difficulty taking care of a dependent family member. Which of the following approaches is in the best interest of the client?

1. Ask the client what he wishes.
2. Have the family members discuss it among themselves.
3. Tell the family the client should go to a nursing care facility.
4. Call a family conference and ask social services for assistance.

30. 4. A family conference with social services can enlighten the family to all prospects of care available to them. The family may not be aware of alternative care measures for the client so a discussion among themselves may not be helpful. The client should supply input if he's able but this may not help solve the problems of exhaustion and care difficulties. The client may not qualify for a nursing care facility because of stringent criteria.

NP: Planning; CN: Safe, effective care environment; CNS: Management of care; CL: Analysis

31. A 30-year-old primagravida in her second trimester tells a nurse her fingers feel tight and sometimes she feels as though her heart skips a beat. She has a history of rheumatic fever. Which of the following indicates the client may be experiencing cardiovascular disease?

1. Clear lungs
2. Sinus tachycardia
3. Increased dyspnea on exertion
4. Runs of paroxysmal atrial tachycardia

31. 3. Increasing dyspnea on exertion should alert the nurse to cardiovascular compromise. Cardiac arrhythmias (other than sinus tachycardia or paroxysmal atrial tachycardia) and persistent crackles at the bases are also symptoms of cardiovascular disease.

NP: Assessment; CN: Health promotion and maintenance; CNS: Growth and development through the life span; CL: Analysis

32. Which of the following diagnostic tests determines the extent of cardiovascular disease during pregnancy?
1. Stress test
2. Chest X-ray
3. Echocardiography
4. Cardiac catheterization

32. 3. Echocardiography is less invasive than X-rays and other methods and provides the information needed to determine cardiovascular disease, especially valvular disorders. Cardiac catheterization and stress tests may be postponed until after delivery.
NP: Planning; CN: Physiological integrity; CNS: Physiological adaptation; CL: Knowledge

33. Which of the following factors is assessed to determine the effect of a client's heart condition on the fetus?
1. Urinalysis
2. Fetal heart tones
3. Laboratory test results of the mother
4. Other signs and symptoms of the client

33. 2. Fetal heart tones show how the fetus is responding to the environment. Assessing other signs and symptoms of the mother, including laboratory test results and urinalysis, can only determine the effect on the mother.
NP: Assessment; CN: Health promotion and maintenance; CNS: Growth and development through the life span; CL: Comprehension

34. Which of the following factors is an example of subjective data in a nursing assessment?
1. Laboratory study results
2. Physical assessment data
3. Report of a diagnostic procedure
4. Client's feelings and statements about health problems

34. 4. Subjective data, also known as symptoms or covert cues, include the client's own verbatim statements about the health problems. Physical assessment data, laboratory study results, and diagnostic procedure reports are observable, perceptible, and measurable and can be verified and validated by others.
NP: Assessment; CN: Safe, effective care environment; CNS: Management of care; CL: Comprehension

35. Which of the following classifications of medication may be used safely for a pregnant client with cardiovascular disease?
1. Antibiotics
2. Warfarin (Coumadin)
3. Cardiac glycosides
4. Diuretics

You're cruisin'! Keep up the good work!

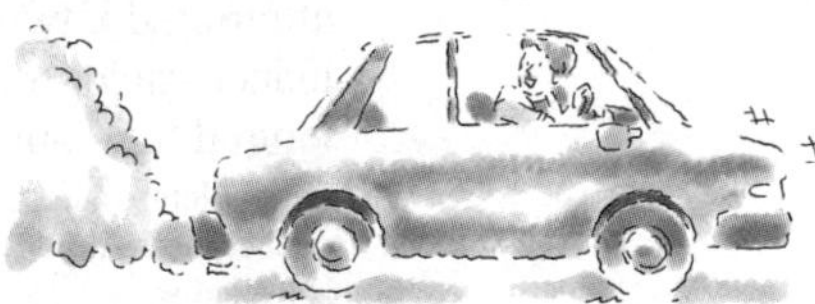

35. 3. Cardiac glycosides and common antiarrhythmics, such as procainamide and quinidine, may be used. Diuretics should be used with extreme caution, if at all, because of the potential for causing uterine contractions. If anticoagulants are needed, heparin is the drug of choice — not warfarin. Prophylactic antibiotics are reserved for clients susceptible to endocarditis.
NP: Planning; CN: Physiological integrity; CNS: Pharmacological and parenteral therapies; CL: Comprehension

36. A client arrives at the emergency department in her third trimester with painless vaginal bleeding. Which of the following conditions is suspected?
1. Placenta previa
2. Premature labor
3. Abruptio placentae
4. A sexually transmitted disease

36. 1. Placenta previa presents with painless vaginal bleeding. Abruptio placentae usually includes vague abdominal discomfort and tenderness. Sexually transmitted diseases and premature labor usually don't cause bleeding.
NP: Assessment; CN: Health promotion and maintenance; CNS: Prevention and early detection of disease; CL: Knowledge

37. After assessing vital signs and applying an external monitor, which of the following interventions is a priority for a client with suspected placenta previa?

1. Insert an indwelling urinary catheter.
2. Plan for an immediate cesarean delivery.
3. Place the client in Trendelenburg position.
4. Obtain blood work and start I.V. catheters.

37. 4. Blood for hemoglobin, hematocrit, type, and crossmatch should be collected and I.V. catheters inserted. The nurse shouldn't attempt Trendelenburg positioning or urinary catheterization. The client may be placed on her left side. Depending on the degree of bleeding and fetal maturity, a cesarean delivery may be required.

NP: Implementation; CN: Physiological integrity; CNS: Reduction of risk potential; CL: Application

38. A pregnant client with vaginal bleeding asks a nurse how the fetus is doing. Which of the following responses is best?

1. "I don't know for sure."
2. "I can't answer that question."
3. "It's too early to tell anything."
4. Tell the client what the monitors show.

38. 4. The client deserves a truthful answer and the nurse should be objective without giving opinions. Vague answers may be misleading and aren't therapeutic.

NP: Implementation; CN: Psychosocial integrity; CNS: Coping and adaptation; CL: Analysis

39. A client with placenta previa is hospitalized, and a cesarean delivery is planned. In addition to the routine neonatal assessment, the neonate should be assessed for which of the following conditions?

1. Prematurity
2. Congenital anomalies
3. Respiratory distress
4. Aspiration pneumonia

39. 3. Hypoxia, resulting in respiratory distress, is a potential risk due to decreased blood volume and prematurity. Congenital anomalies aren't necessarily associated with placenta previa. Aspiration pneumonia isn't considered a threat unless the amniotic fluid is meconium-stained. The age of maturity can be determined through established maternal dates.

NP: Assessment; CN: Physiological integrity; CNS: Reduction of risk potential; CL: Application

40. A neonate requires blood transfusions after birth. Which of the following cannulation sites is most preferred?

1. Scalp veins
2. Intraosseous
3. Umbilical cord
4. Subclavian cutdown

40. 3. The umbilical cord may be easily cannulated and is the preferred site. Scalp veins may also be used. Intraosseous cannulation is attempted if two attempts at other sites prove inaccessible. A subclavian cutdown takes a prolonged time and is the least desired.

NP: Implementation; CN: Health promotion and maintenance; CNS: Growth and development through the life span; CL: Knowledge

41. A nurse working in the triage area of an emergency department sees that several pediatric clients arrive simultaneously. Which of the following clients is treated first?

1. A crying 4-year-old child with a laceration on his scalp
2. A 3-year-old child with a barking cough and flushed appearance
3. A 3-year-old child with Down syndrome who's pale and asleep in his mother's arms
4. A 2-year-old infant with stridorous breath sounds, sitting up in his mother's arms and drooling

41. 4. The infant with the airway emergency should be treated first, because of the risk of epiglottiditis. The 3-year-old with the barking cough and fever should be suspected of having croup and should be seen promptly, as should the child with the laceration. The nurse would need to gather information about the child with Down syndrome to determine the priority of care.

NP: Assessment; CN: Safe, effective care environment; CNS: Management of care; CL: Analysis

42. A 2-year-old child is being examined in the emergency department for epiglottiditis. Which of the following assessment findings supports this diagnosis?

1. Mild fever
2. Clear speech
3. Tripod position
4. Gradual onset of symptoms

42. 3. The tripod position (sitting up and leaning forward) facilitates breathing. Epiglottiditis presents with a sudden onset of symptoms, high fever, and muffled speech. Additional symptoms are inspiratory stridor and drooling.

NP: Assessment; CN: Physiological integrity; CNS: Physiological adaptation; CL: Application

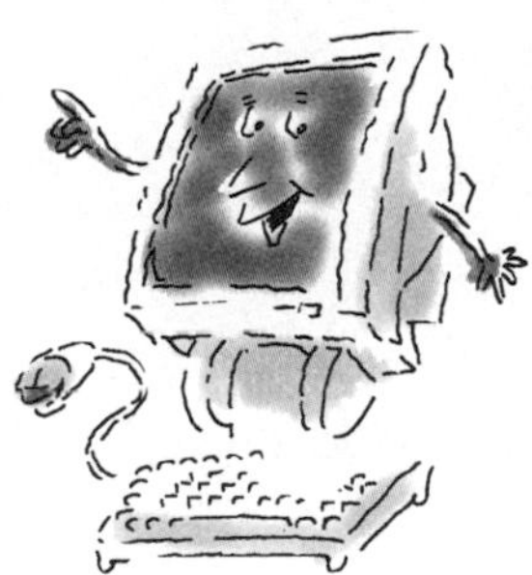

Way to go! You're more than halfway finished!

43. Which of the following methods is best when approaching a 2-year-old child to listen to breath sounds?

1. Tell the child it's time to listen to his lungs now.
2. Tell the child to lie down while the nurse listens to his lungs.
3. Ask the caregiver to wait outside while the nurse listens to his lungs.
4. Ask if he would like the nurse to listen to the front or the back of his chest first.

43. 4. The 2-year-old child needs to feel in control, and this approach best supports the child's independence. Giving the child no choice may make him uncooperative. The caregiver should be allowed to remain with the child because fear of separation is common in 2-year-olds. The child should be allowed to remain in the tripod position to facilitate breathing.

NP: Implementation; CN: Health promotion and maintenance; CNS: Growth and development through the life span; CL: Application

44. A mother says a 2-year-old child is up to date with his vaccines. Which of the following immunizations should be included?

1. Diptheria-pertussis-tetanus (DPT), inactivated polio (IPV), measles-mumps-rubella (MMR)
2. DPT, IPV, MMR, Hemophilus influenza type B (Hib), varicella, pneumococcal, hepatitis B
3. DPT, hepatitis B, IPV
4. MMR, IPV, hepatitis B

44. 2. By the age of 2, the DPT, IPV, MMR, Hib, varicella, pneumococcal, and hepatitis B vaccines should have been received. The nurse should clarify this with the mother or caregiver.

NP: Assessment; CN: Safe, effective care environment; CNS: Safety and infection control; CL: Knowledge

45. A child with epiglottiditis is at risk for which of the following conditions?

1. Airway obstruction
2. Dehydration
3. Malnutrition
4. Seizures

45. 1. The biggest threat to the child is airway obstruction because of the inflammation and swelling of the epiglottis and surrounding tissue. Dehydration can be prevented with I.V. therapy and seizures averted by decreasing the fever. Malnutrition is least likely to occur because epiglottiditis is a short-lived situation.
NP: Planning; CN: Physiological integrity; CNS: Reduction of risk potential; CL: Comprehension

46. Which of the following methods is used to diagnose epiglottiditis?

1. Lateral neck X-ray
2. Direct visualization
3. History of sudden onset
4. Presenting signs and symptoms

46. 4. The presenting symptoms are diagnostic of epiglottiditis. Only an anesthesiologist or physician skilled in intubation should do direct visualization. Lateral neck X-rays aren't necessary. History of sudden onset helps support the assessment, but a history alone wouldn't be sufficient to make a diagnosis.
NP: Assessment; CN: Health promotion and maintenance; CNS: Prevention and early detection of disease; CL: Knowledge

47. A student nurse working with a registered nurse is assessing a child with epiglottiditis. The student tells the client she needs to look at his throat. Which of the following interventions by the registered nurse is best?

1. Hand her a flashlight and tongue blade.
2. Give her a sterile tongue blade and culturette swab.
3. Tell the student that the registered nurse will visualize the child's throat.
4. Tell the student visualization will be done by the anesthesiologist.

47. 4. Direct visualization of the epiglottis can trigger a complete airway obstruction and should only be done in a controlled environment by an anesthesiologist or a physician skilled in pediatric intubation.
NP: Implementation; CN: Safe, effective care environment; CNS: Management of care; CL: Application

48. The mother of a 2-year-old child with epiglottiditis says she needs to pick up her older child from school. The 2-year-old child begins to cry and appears more stridorous. Which of the following interventions by the nurse is best?

1. Ask the mother how long she may be gone.
2. Tell the 2-year-old everything will be all right.
3. Tell the 2-year-old the nurse will stay with him.
4. Ask the mother if there's anyone else who can meet the older child.

48. 4. Increased anxiety and agitation should be avoided in the child to prevent airway obstruction. A 2-year-old child fears separation from parents, so the mother should be encouraged to stay. Other means of picking up the older child need to be found. Telling the child that everything will be all right may not decrease his agitation. The mother is the primary caregiver and important to the child for emotional and security reasons.
NP: Implementation; CN: Health promotion and maintenance; CNS: Growth and development through the life span; CL: Analysis

49. A father arrives in a busy emergency department and is upset with his wife for bringing their 2-year-old child with epiglottiditis in for treatment. Which of the following interventions by the nurse is best?

1. Leave the room.
2. Call for security.
3. Recognize the father's behavior as his attempt to cope with the situation.
4. Tell both parents to leave because they're upsetting the child.

49. 3. Lack of control over his son's situation results in irrational behavior. The nurse should try to calm both parents and let them know they did the right thing due to the seriousness of their child's situation. Calling for security, sending the parents out, or leaving the room won't help the child nor will it reduce frustration or inappropriate behavior.

NP: Implementation; CN: Psychosocial integrity; CNS: Coping and adaptation; CL: Analysis

50. A 40-year-old client is being treated for GI bleeding. On his fifth day of hospitalization, he begins to have tremors, is agitated, and is experiencing hallucinations. These signs suggest which of the following conditions?

1. Alcohol withdrawal
2. Allergic response
3. Alzheimer's disease
4. Hypoxia

50. 1. These are signs of alcohol withdrawal syndrome, which can begin 5 to 7 days after the last drink. An allergic reaction would cause difficulty breathing, skin rash, or edema as primary symptoms. Alzheimer's disease occurs in older individuals and has other psychosocial signs, such as a masklike face and altered mentation. Hypoxia would cause symptoms of respiratory distress.

NP: Assessment; CN: Psychosocial integrity; CNS: Psychosocial adaptation; CL: Analysis

51. If a nurse suspects a client is experiencing alcohol withdrawal syndrome, which of the following actions is appropriate?

1. Verify it with family.
2. Inform social services.
3. Ask the client about his drinking.
4. Tell the client everything will be all right.

51. 3. Confirming suspicions with the client is the most beneficial to help in diagnosis and treatment. If the client isn't cooperative, verification can be sought with the family. Social services aren't required at this time but may be helpful in discharge planning. Giving false reassurance isn't therapeutic for the client.

NP: Assessment; CN: Psychosocial integrity; CNS: Psychosocial adaptation; CL: Application

52. A client experiencing alcohol withdrawal syndrome says he sees cockroaches on the ceiling. Which of the following responses is appropriate?

1. Ask the client where he sees them.
2. Ask the client if the cockroaches are still there.
3. Tell the client there are no cockroaches on the ceiling.
4. Tell the client it's dim in the room and turn on the overhead lights.

52. 4. Try to reorient the client to reality and minimize distortions. Don't support the client's hallucinations or place the client on the defensive but try to present reality gently without agitating the client.

NP: Implementation; CN: Psychosocial integrity; CNS: Psychosocial adaptation; CL: Application

53. A client experiencing alcohol withdrawal syndrome says he's itching everywhere from the bugs on his bed. Which of the following responses is appropriate?

1. Examine the client's skin.
2. Ask what kind of bugs he thinks they are.
3. Tell the client there are no bugs on his bed.
4. Tell the client he's having tactile hallucinations.

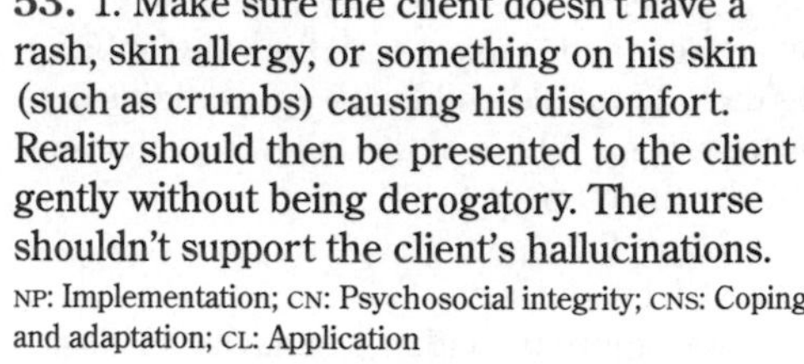

53. 1. Make sure the client doesn't have a rash, skin allergy, or something on his skin (such as crumbs) causing his discomfort. Reality should then be presented to the client gently without being derogatory. The nurse shouldn't support the client's hallucinations.
NP: Implementation; CN: Psychosocial integrity; CNS: Coping and adaptation; CL: Application

54. A client with alcohol withdrawal syndrome is pulling at his central venous catheter saying he's swatting the spiders crawling over him. Which of the following interventions is most appropriate?

1. Encourage the client to rest.
2. Protect the client from harm.
3. Tell the client there are no spiders.
4. Tell the client he's pulling the I.V. tubing.

54. 2. During periods of alcohol withdrawal syndrome, the client needs to be protected from harm. If the client dislodges the central venous catheter, he may incur an air embolus, which can be life threatening. Although reality should be presented to the client, telling him that there are no spiders and that he's pulling the I.V. tubing may not make him stop; therefore, his safety is still at risk. The client may need to be restrained if continued observation during this time isn't available. The client should also be encouraged to rest; however, this intervention doesn't take priority over safety.
NP: Implementation; CN: Psychosocial integrity; CNS: Psychosocial adaptation; CL: Analysis

55. A client who experienced alcohol withdrawal syndrome is no longer having hallucinations or tremors and says he would like to enter a rehabilitation facility to stop drinking. Which of the following interventions is appropriate?

1. Ask about his insurance.
2. Tell him he should talk with his family.
3. Refer him to Alcoholics Anonymous (AA).
4. Promote participation in a treatment program.

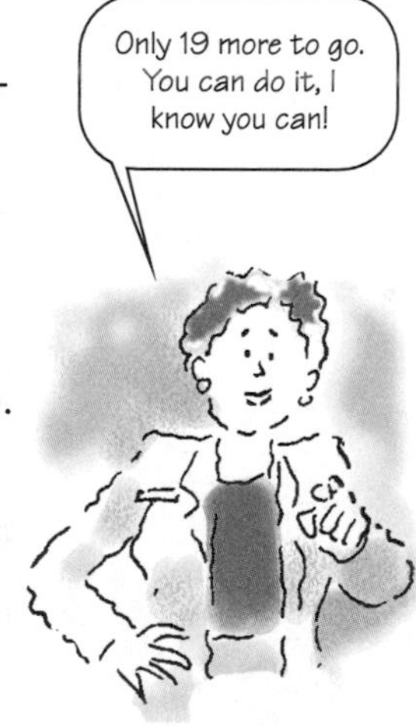

Only 19 more to go. You can do it, I know you can!

55. 4. The client should be encouraged to enter a facility if that's in his best interest. Arrangements can be made and discussed with the social service coordinator and his physician. The client can inform his family, and support should be encouraged. Referral to AA should be considered after rehabilitation takes place.
NP: Planning; CN: Psychosocial integrity; CNS: Psychosocial adaptation; CL: Application

56. A 72-year-old man with cirrhosis is admitted to the hospital in a hepatic coma. Which of the following nursing interventions has priority?

1. Perform a neurologic check.
2. Complete the client admission.
3. Orient the client to his environment.
4. Check airway, breathing, and circulation.

56. 4. Priorities include airway, breathing, and circulation. Once these are ensured, a neurologic check is needed to determine status. Depending on the client's alertness, orientation to the environment may need to be kept simple (where he is, date, time). General orientation and completing the admission may require the help and affirmation of family members.
NP: Assessment; CN: Physiological integrity; CNS: Reduction of risk potential; CL: Comprehension

57. A client with cirrhosis is restless and at times tries to climb out of bed. Which of the following interventions is best to promote safety?

1. Use leather restraints.
2. Use soft wrist restraints.
3. Use a vest restraint device.
4. Use a sheet tied across the client's chest.

57. 3. The client may require gentle reminders not to get out of bed to prevent a fall. The vest restraint would help in this endeavor. Soft wrist restraints may not stop the client from sitting up or trying to swing his legs over the bed rails. Leather restraints are only warranted for extremely combative and unsafe clients. A sheet tied across the client's chest can hamper breathing or may asphyxiate the client if he slides down in the bed.

NP: Implementation; CN: Safe, effective care environment; CNS: Management of care; CL: Analysis

58. Which of the following assessment findings in a client with cirrhosis indicates late-stage symptoms?

1. Constipation
2. Diarrhea
3. Hypoxia
4. Vomiting

58. 3. Fluid in the lungs and weak chest expansion can lead to hypoxia. Diarrhea, vomiting, and constipation are early signs and symptoms of cirrhosis.

NP: Assessment; CN: Physiological integrity; CNS: Physiological adaptation; CL: Knowledge

59. A client with cirrhosis is jaundiced and edematous. He's experiencing severe itching and dryness. Which of the following interventions is best to help the client?

1. Put mitts on his hands.
2. Use alcohol-free body lotion.
3. Lubricate the skin with baby oil.
4. Wash the skin with soap and water.

59. 2. Alcohol-free body lotion applied to the skin can help relieve dryness and is absorbed without oiliness. Mitts may help keep the client from scratching his skin open. Soap dries out the skin. Baby oil doesn't allow excretions through the skin and may block pores.

NP: Implementation; CN: Physiological integrity; CNS: Basic care and comfort; CL: Knowledge

60. A 20-year-old client with a spinal cord injury sustained in a previous motorcycle accident is hospitalized for renal calculi, or kidney stones. To reduce the client's risk for developing recurrent kidney stones, which of the following instructions is correct?

1. Eat yogurt daily.
2. Drink cranberry juice.
3. Eat more fresh fruits and vegetables.
4. Increase the intake of dairy products.

60. 2. Acid urine decreases the potential for kidney stones. The majority of renal calculi form in alkaline urine. Cranberries, prunes, and plums promote acidic urine. Yogurt helps restore pH balance to secretions in yeast infections. Fruits and vegetables increase fiber in the diet and promote alkaline urine. Dairy products may contribute to the formation of kidney stones.

NP: Implementation; CN: Physiological integrity; CNS: Reduction of risk potential; CL: Application

61. A client with a spinal cord injury says he has difficulty recognizing the symptoms of urinary tract infection (UTI) before it's too late. Which of the following symptoms is an early sign of UTI?

1. Lower back pain
2. Burning on urination
3. Frequency of urination
4. Fever and change in the clarity of urine

61. 4. The client with a spinal cord injury should recognize fever and change in the clarity of urine as early signs of UTI. Lower back pain is a late sign. The client with a spinal cord injury may not have burning or frequency of urination.

NP: Implementation; CN: Physiological integrity; CNS: Reduction of risk potential; CL: Application

62. A client tells a nurse he boils his urinary catheters to keep them sterile. Which of the following questions should the nurse ask?

1. "What technique is used for catheterization?"
2. "What temperature are the catheters boiled at?"
3. "Why aren't prepackaged sterile catheters used?"
4. "Are the catheters dried and stored in a clean, dry place?"

62. 1. The client should describe his procedure to make sure aseptic technique is used. Water boils at 212° F (100° C), but the nurse should make sure the client is boiling the catheters for an appropriate amount of time. Catheters should be boiled just before use and allowed to cool before using. Prepackaged sterile catheters aren't necessary if the proper sterilization techniques are used.

NP: Evaluation; CN: Physiological integrity; CNS: Reduction of risk potential; CL: Analysis

63. A 60-year-old client had a colostomy 4 days ago due to rectal cancer and is having trouble adjusting to it. Which of the following conditions is most common?

1. Anxiety
2. Low self-esteem
3. Alteration in comfort
4. Alteration in body image

63. 4. Alteration in body image is most common with a new colostomy and dealing with its care. Low self-esteem may also be a concern for the client. The client should be having less discomfort postoperatively. The client shouldn't have signs of anxiety but he may not be comfortable caring for the colostomy.

NP: Assessment; CN: Psychosocial integrity; CNS: Coping and adaptation; CL: Comprehension

64. A nurse approaches a client with a recent colostomy for a routine assessment and finds him tearful. Which of the following actions is appropriate?

1. State she'll come back another time.
2. Ask the client if he's having pain or discomfort.
3. Tell the client she needs to perform an assessment.
4. Sit down with the client and ask if he'd like to talk about anything.

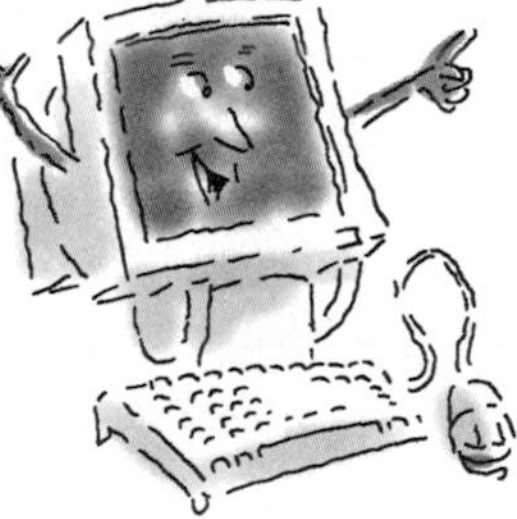
You're almost finished. Keep pluggin' away!

64. 4. Asking open-ended questions and appearing interested in what the client has to say will encourage verbalization of feelings. Leaving the client may make him feel unaccepted. Asking closed-ended questions won't encourage verbalization of feelings. Ignoring the client's present state isn't therapeutic for the client.

NP: Implementation; CN: Psychosocial integrity; CNS: Coping and adaptation; CL: Application

65. After a review of colostomy care, a client says she doesn't know if she'll be able to care for herself at home without help. Which of the following nursing interventions is most appropriate to ensure continuity of care?

1. Review care with the client again.
2. Provide written instructions for the client.
3. Ask the client if there's anyone who can help.
4. Arrange for home health care to visit the client.

65. 4. Although all of these interventions may benefit the patient, arranging for home health care will best ensure continuity of care.

NP: Assessment; CN: Safe, effective care environment; CNS: Management of care; CL: Application

66. A client is experiencing mild diarrhea through his colostomy. Which of the following instructions is correct?

1. Eat prunes.
2. Drink apple juice.
3. Increase lettuce intake.
4. Increase intake of bananas.

66. 4. Bananas help make formed stool and aren't irritating to the bowel. Apple juice and prunes can increase the frequency of diarrhea. Lettuce acts as a fiber and can increase the looseness of stools.

NP: Implementation; CN: Physiological integrity; CNS: Basic care and comfort; CL: Application

67. A client reports a lot of gas in her colostomy bag. Which of the following instructions is best?

1. Burp the bag.
2. Eat less beans.
3. Replace the bag.
4. Put a tiny hole in the top of the bag.

67. 1. Letting air out of the bag by opening it and burping it is the best solution. Replacing the bag is costly. Putting a hole in the bag will also cause fluids to leak out. The client can be encouraged to note which foods are causing gas and to eat less gas-forming foods.

NP: Implementation; CN: Physiological integrity; CNS: Basic care and comfort; CL: Knowledge

68. A client at a routine blood glucose screening for diabetes mellitus tells a nurse she has excessive urination and excessive thirst. The nurse should ask about which of the following symptoms first?

1. Weakness
2. Weight loss
3. Vision changes
4. Excessive hunger

68. 4. Polyuria, polydipsia, and polyphagia are the three hallmark signs of diabetes mellitus. Weight loss, weakness, and vision changes also occur with diabetes mellitus.

NP: Assessment; CN: Health promotion and maintenance; CNS: Prevention and early detection of disease; CL: Knowledge

69. Which of the following factors places a client at greatest risk for developing diabetes mellitus?

1. Obesity
2. Japanese descent
3. A great-grandparent with diabetes mellitus
4. Delivery of a neonate weighing more than 10 pounds

69. 1. Obesity is a risk factor associated with diabetes mellitus. Delivery of a neonate weighing more than 9 lb, a family history of diabetes mellitus (mother, father, or sibling), and those of Native American, Black, Asian, or Hispanic descent are at high risk for developing diabetes mellitus, but obesity puts the client at greatest risk.

NP: Assessment; CN: Health promotion and maintenance; CNS: Prevention and early detection of disease; CL: Knowledge

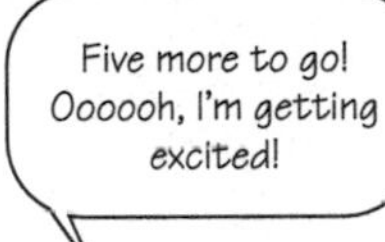

Five more to go!
Oooooh, I'm getting excited!

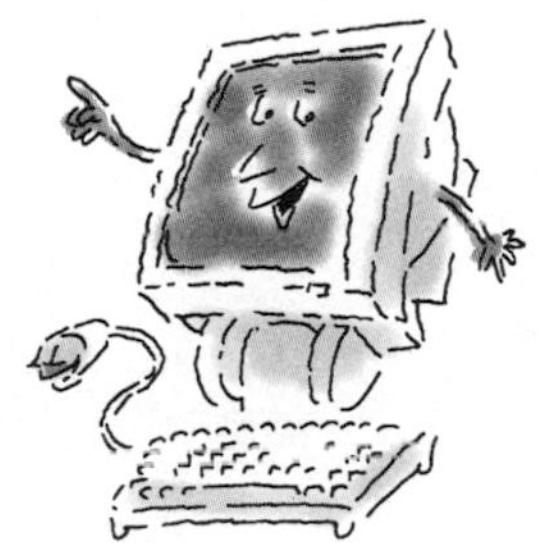

70. Which of the following blood glucose levels is considered within normal limits?

1. 70 to 125 mg/dl
2. 130 to 135 mg/dl
3. 135 to 140 mg/dl
4. 140 to 145 mg/dl

70. 1. A blood glucose level more than 126 mg/dl should prompt the nurse to refer the client to the physician for follow-up due to the risk of diabetes mellitus.

NP: Assessment; CN: Health promotion and maintenance; CNS: Prevention and early detection of disease; CL: Knowledge

71. A client asks what diabetes mellitus does to the body over time. Which of the following conditions is a common chronic complication of diabetes mellitus?

1. Multiple sclerosis
2. Diabetic ketoacidosis
3. Cardiovascular disease
4. Hyperosmolar hyperglycemic nonketotic syndrome (HHNS)

71. 3. Cardiovascular disease is a common chronic complication of diabetes mellitus. Diabetic ketoacidosis and HHNS are acute complications that can occur. There's no known relationship between multiple sclerosis and diabetes mellitus.

NP: Assessment; CN: Health promotion and maintenance; CNS: Prevention and early detection of disease; CL: Knowledge

72. A client asks how she may decrease the risk of developing diabetes mellitus, which runs in her family. Which of the following responses is appropriate?

1. "Eat only poultry and fish."
2. "Omit carbohydrates from your diet."
3. "Start a moderate exercise program."
4. "Check blood glucose levels every month."

72. 3. Exercise and weight control are the goals in preventing and treating diabetes mellitus. Red meat can be eaten but should be limited because it contributes to cardiovascular disease. Complex carbohydrates account for a large portion of the diabetic diet and shouldn't be omitted. Checking blood glucose levels will help monitor the development of diabetes mellitus but won't prevent or decrease the chance of it occurring.

NP: Implementation; CN: Physiological integrity; CNS: Reduction of risk potential; CL: Knowledge

73. An 83-year-old client fractured a hip after a fall in her home. Because of her extensive cardiac history and chronic obstructive pulmonary disease, surgery isn't an option. The client tells a nurse she doesn't know how she's going to get better. Which of the following responses is best?

1. "You're doing fine."
2. "What's your biggest concern right now?"
3. "Just give it some time and you'll be okay."
4. "You don't believe you're doing well?"

73. 2. Open-ended questions allow the client to have control over what she wants to discuss and help the nurse determine care needs. Telling the client she's doing fine or that she just needs more time doesn't encourage her to verbalize concerns. A reiteration of the client's concerns may not be helpful in encouraging the client to verbalize feelings.

NP: Implementation; CN: Health promotion and maintenance; CNS: Growth and development through the life span; CL: Comprehension

74. A client says she slipped on a throw rug while going to the bathroom at night. Which of the following factors needs assessment?

1. If the home is safe
2. If the client is confused
3. If the client hit her head
4. If the client has a urinary tract infection (UTI)

74. 1. A safety assessment of the home can determine if changes need to be made to ensure the client doesn't fall again. Going to the bathroom at night isn't necessarily a sign of UTI. The nurse may determine if the client has experienced a head injury or confusion by asking how the accident occurred.

NP: Assessment; CN: Health promotion and maintenance; CNS: Safety and infection control; CL: Application

75. A client in her third trimester of pregnancy is having contractions 5 minutes apart that began suddenly. The nurse identifies that it's the client's seventh month. She's admitted directly to the obstetric department. Which of the following interventions has priority?

1. Call the obstetrician.
2. Time the contractions.
3. Check fetal heart tones.
4. Call the client's husband.

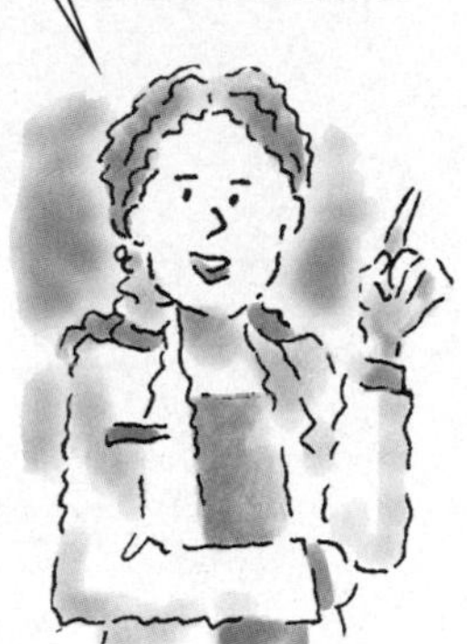

I knew you could do it!
For your first
comprehensive test,
that was outstanding.
Congratulations!

75. 3. The nurse should check fetal heart tones and assess the client's vital signs. The client should be placed on a monitor to check contractions and for continuous fetal monitoring. The obstetrician and husband should be notified as soon as possible.

NP: Implementation; CN: Health promotion and maintenance; CNS: Growth and development through the life span; CL: Application

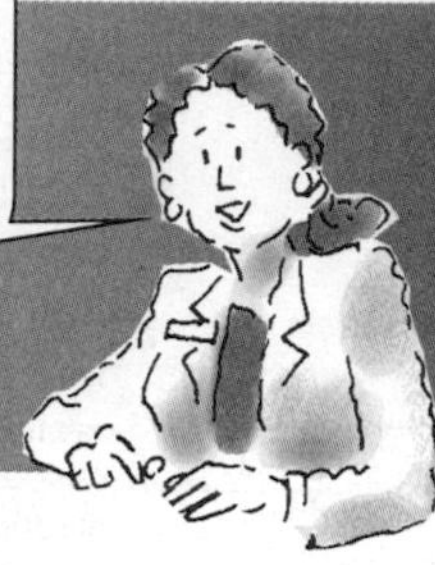
Here's another
comprehensive test to
help you get ready to take
the NCLEX test.
Good luck!

COMPREHENSIVE Test 2

1. A young client with anorexia nervosa is being treated using family therapy. Which of the following descriptions applies to anorexia nervosa, according to the social theory of causation?

1. A repressed issue
2. A learned maladaptive behavior
3. A reaction related to poor school achievements
4. A sign of pain within the whole family system

1. 4. The social theory of causation recognizes that difficulties within families are generally expressed by one member showing symptoms. Behavioral theory considers anorexia nervosa a learned maladaptive behavior, and psychoanalytic theory considers it a sign of repression. Anorexia nervosa is associated with a high level of achievement in school.

NP: Assessment; CN: Psychosocial integrity; CNS: Psychosocial adaptation; CL: Comprehension

2. Which of the following diagnostic tests is performed first to detect transposition of the great vessels (TGV)?

1. Blood cultures
2. Cardiac catheterization
3. Chest X-ray
4. Echocardiogram

2. 3. Chest X-ray would be done first to visualize congenital heart diseases such as TGV. Cardiac catheterization and an echocardiogram would be done after TGV is seen on the chest X-ray. Blood cultures won't diagnose TGV.

NP: Planning; CN: Health promotion and maintenance; CNS: Prevention and early detection of disease; CL: Application

3. Four 6-month-old children arrive at the clinic for diphtheria-pertussis-tetanus (DPT) immunization. Which of the following children can safely receive the immunization at this time?

1. The child with a temperature of 103° F (39.4° C)
2. The child with a runny nose and cough
3. The child taking prednisone for the treatment of leukemia
4. The child with difficulty breathing after the last immunization

3. 2. Children with cold symptoms can safely receive DPT immunization. Children with a temperature more than 102° F, serious reactions to previous immunizations, or immunosuppressive therapy shouldn't receive DPT immunization.

NP: Analysis; CN: Health promotion and maintenance; CNS: Prevention and early detection of disease; CL: Analysis

4. A nurse is giving discharge instructions to parents of a child who had a tonsillectomy. Which of the following instructions is the most important?

1. The child should drink extra milk.
2. The child shouldn't drink from straws.
3. Orange juice should be given to provide pain control.
4. The child's mouth should be rinsed with salt water to provide pain relief.

4. 2. Straws and other sharp objects inserted into the mouth could disrupt the clot at the operative site. Extra milk wouldn't promote healing and may encourage mucus production. Drinking orange juice and rinsing with salt water will irritate the tissue at the operative site.

NP: Implementation; CN: Physiological adaptation; CNS: Basic care and comfort; CL: Application

5. A 2-year-old child is diagnosed with bronchiolitis caused by respiratory syncytial virus (RSV). The family also includes an 8-year-old child. Which of the following statements is correct?

1. RSV isn't highly communicable in infants.
2. RSV isn't communicable to older children and adults.
3. The 2-year-old client must be admitted to the hospital for isolation.
4. The children should be separated to prevent the spread of the infection.

5. 4. Toddlers easily transmit and contract RSV and so they should be separated from other children. RSV is also communicable to older children and adults, but these clients may exhibit only mild symptoms of the disorder. Hospitalization is indicated only for children who need oxygen and I.V. therapy.

NP: Planning; CN: Safe, effective care environment; CNS: Safety and infection control; CL: Analysis

6. A child with asthma uses a peak expiratory flowmeter in school. The results indicate his peak flow is in the yellow zone. Which of the following interventions by the school nurse is appropriate?

1. Follow the child's routine asthma treatment plan.
2. Monitor the child for signs and symptoms of an acute attack.
3. Call 911 and prepare for transport to the nearest emergency department.
4. Call the child's mother to take the child to the family physician immediately.

6. 2. The child should be monitored to determine if an asthma attack is imminent. The routine treatment plan may be insufficient when the peak flow is in the yellow zone (50% to 80% of personal best). There's no immediate need to see the physician if the child is asymptomatic. This isn't an emergency situation.

NP: Implementation; CN: Physiological integrity; CNS: Reduction of risk potential; CL: Application

7. Parents of a child with asthma are trying to identify possible allergens in their household. Which of the following inhaled allergens is the most common?

1. Perfume
2. Dust mites
3. Passive smoke
4. Dog or cat dander

7. 2. The household dust mite is the most commonly inhaled allergen that can cause an asthma attack. Animal dander, passive smoke, and perfume are sometimes allergens causing asthma attacks but aren't as common as dust mites.

NP: Implementation; CN: Physiological integrity; CNS: Reduction of risk potential; CL: Application

8. A nurse is verifying orders from a physician. Which of the following diets is correct for a child newly diagnosed with celiac disease?

1. Low-fat diet
2. No-gluten diet
3. High-protein diet
4. No-phenylalanine diet

8. 2. The intestinal cells of individuals with celiac disease become inflamed when the child eats products containing gluten, such as wheat, rye, barley, or oats. The child with celiac disease needs normal amounts of fat and protein in the diet for growth and development. Omitting phenylalanine products would be appropriate for the client with phenylketonuria.

NP: Planning; CN: Safe, effective care environment; CNS: Safety and infection control; CL: Application

9. A client is undergoing a thoracentesis at the bedside. A nurse assists the client to an upright position with a table and pillow in front of him to support his arms. Which of the following rationales for this intervention is correct?

1. Fluid will accumulate at the base.
2. There's less chance to injure lung tissue.
3. It allows for better expansion of the lung.
4. It's less painful for the client in this position.

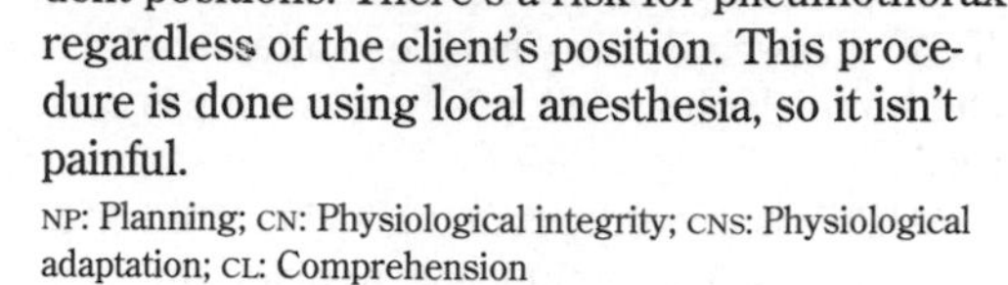

9. 1. Fluids will drain and collect in the dependent positions. There's a risk for pneumothorax regardless of the client's position. This procedure is done using local anesthesia, so it isn't painful.

NP: Planning; CN: Physiological integrity; CNS: Physiological adaptation; CL: Comprehension

10. Which of the following leisure activities is recommended for a school-age child with hemophilia?

1. Baseball
2. Cross-country running
3. Football
4. Swimming

10. 4. Swimming is a noncontact sport with low risk for traumatic injury. Baseball, cross-country running, and football all involve a risk for trauma from falling, sliding, or contact.

NP: Implementation; CN: Physiological integrity; CNS: Physiological adaptation; CL: Application

11. Which of the following assessments is important for an infant in sickle cell crisis?

1. The infant has no bruises.
2. The infant has normal skin turgor.
3. The infant participates in exercise.
4. The infant maintains bladder control.

11. 2. Normal skin turgor indicates the infant isn't severely dehydrated. Dehydration may cause sickle cell crisis or worsen a crisis. Bruising isn't associated with sickle cell crisis. Bed rest is preferable during a sickle cell crisis. Bladder control may be lost when oral or I.V. fluid intake is increased during a sickle cell crisis.

NP: Planning; CN: Physiological integrity; CNS: Physiological adaptation; CL: Analysis

12. A client has arterial blood gases drawn. The results are as follows: pH, 7.52; Pa_{O_2}, 50 mm Hg; Pa_{CO_2}, 28 mm Hg; HCO_3^-, 24 mEq/L. Which of the following conditions is indicated?

1. Metabolic acidosis
2. Metabolic alkalosis
3. Respiratory acidosis
4. Respiratory alkalosis

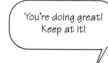

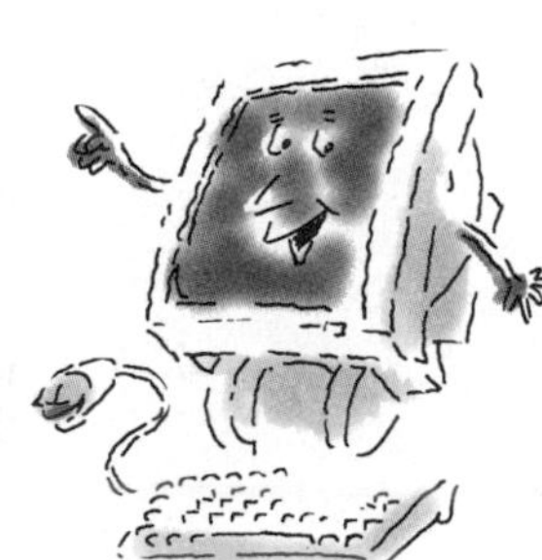
You're doing great! Keep at it!

12. 4. A pH greater than 7.45 and a Pa_{CO_2} less than 35 mm Hg indicate respiratory alkalosis. A pH less than 7.35 and an HCO_3^- less than 22 mEq/L indicate metabolic acidosis. A pH greater than 7.45 and an HCO_3^- greater than 24 mEq/L indicate metabolic alkalosis. A pH less than 7.35 and a Pa_{CO_2} greater than 45 mm Hg indicate respiratory acidosis.

NP: Analysis; CN: Physiological integrity; CNS: Physiological adaptation; CL: Knowledge

13. A client with chronic alcohol abuse is admitted to the hospital for detoxification. Later that day, his blood pressure increases and he's given an as-needed medication to prevent which of the following complications?

1. Stroke
2. Seizure
3. Fainting
4. Anxiety reaction

13. 2. During detoxification from alcohol, changes in the client's physiologic status, especially an increase in blood pressure, may indicate a possible seizure. Clients are treated with benzodiazepines such as chlordiazepoxide (Librium) to prevent this. Stroke, fainting, and anxiety aren't the primary concerns when withdrawing from alcohol.

NP: Implementation; CN: Physiological integrity; CNS: Physiological adaptation; CL: Application

14. An adolescent client ingests a large number of acetaminophen tablets in an attempt to commit suicide. Which of the following laboratory results is associated with acetaminophen overdose?

1. Metabolic acidosis
2. Elevated liver enzyme levels
3. Increased serum creatinine level
4. Increased white blood cell (WBC) count

14. 2. Elevated liver enzyme levels, which could indicate liver damage, are associated with acetaminophen overdose. Metabolic acidosis isn't associated with acetaminophen overdose. An increased WBC count indicates infection. An increased serum creatinine level may indicate renal damage.

NP: Assessment; CN: Physiological integrity; CNS: Pharmacological and parenteral therapies; CL: Comprehension

15. A nurse is caring for a client recently diagnosed with acute pancreatitis. Which of the following statements indicates that a short-term goal of nursing care has been met?

1. The client denies abdominal pain.
2. The client doesn't complain of thirst.
3. The client denies pain at McBurney's point.
4. The client swallows liquids without coughing.

15. 1. Pancreatitis is accompanied by acute pain from autodigestion by pancreatic enzymes. When the client denies abdominal pain, the short-term goal of pain control is met. Pain at McBurney's point accompanies appendicitis. Clients with acute pancreatitis receive I.V. fluids and may not have a sensation of thirst. Clients with acute pancreatitis receive nothing by mouth during initial therapy.

NP: Evaluation; CN: Physiological integrity; CNS: Physiological adaptation; CL: Application

16. A client is to take 8 ounces of magnesium sulfate solution. The calibrations on the measuring device are in milliliters. How many milliliters should the nurse give?

1. 8 ml
2. 80 ml
3. 240 ml
4. 480 ml

16. 3. One ounce = 30 ml. Eight times 30 = 240 ml.

NP: Planning; CN: Physiological integrity; CNS: Pharmacological and parenteral therapies; CL: Application

17. A man stepped on a piece of sharp glass while walking barefoot. He comes to the emergency department with a deep laceration on the bottom of his foot. Which of the following questions is the most important for the nurse to ask?

1. "Was the glass dirty?"
2. "Are you immune to tetanus?"
3. "When did you have your last tetanus shot?"
4. "How many diphtheria-pertussis-tetanus (DPT) shots did you receive as a child?"

17. 3. Questioning the client about the date of his last tetanus immunization is important because the booster immunization should be received every 10 years in adulthood or at the time of the injury if the last booster immunization was given more than 5 years before the injury. A client wouldn't know his tetanus immunity status. DPT immunizations in childhood don't give lifelong immunization to tetanus. Whether the client noticed dirt on the glass is immaterial because all deep lacerations require a tetanus immunization or booster.

NP: Assessment; CN: Safe, effective care environment; CNS: Safety and infection control; CL: Application

18. A postmenopausal client asks a nurse how to prevent osteoporosis. Which of the following responses is best?
1. "Take a multivitamin daily."
2. "After menopause, there's no way to prevent osteoporosis."
3. "Drink two glasses of milk each day and swim three times a week."
4. "Take hormones as directed by the physician and do weight-bearing exercise regularly."

18. 4. Hormone replacement therapy and weight-bearing exercise are recommended for the prevention of osteoporosis. Two glasses of milk per day don't provide the daily requirements for adult women, and swimming isn't a weight-bearing exercise. A multivitamin doesn't provide adequate calcium for a postmenopausal woman, and calcium alone won't prevent osteoporosis.

NP: Implementation; CN: Health promotion and maintenance; CNS: Prevention and early detection of disease; CL: Application

19. A client diagnosed with cardiomyopathy saw a posting on the Internet describing research about a new herbal treatment for the disorder. When the client asks about this research, which of the following responses is most appropriate?
1. "Herbs are often used to treat cardiomyopathy."
2. "Cardiomyopathy can be treated only by heart surgery."
3. "The Internet is a reliable source of research, so try this treatment."
4. "Research found on the Internet should be verified with a physician."

19. 4. Although the Internet contains some valid medical research, there's no control over the validity of information posted on it. The research should be discussed with a physician, who has access to medical research and can verify the accuracy of the information. Cardiomyopathy is treatable with drugs or surgery. Herbs aren't standard treatment for cardiomyopathy.

NP: Implementation; CN: Safe, effective care environment; CNS: Management of care; CL: Application

20. A young adult client received her first chemotherapy treatment for breast cancer. Which of the following statements by the client requires further exploration by the nurse?
1. "I'm thinking about joining a dance club."
2. "I don't think I'm going to work tomorrow."
3. "I don't care about the side effects of drugs."
4. "I want to return to school for a college degree."

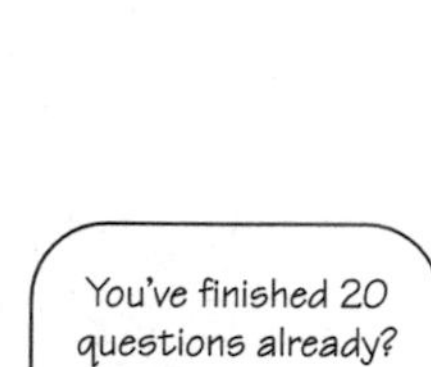

You've finished 20 questions already? Wow, super!

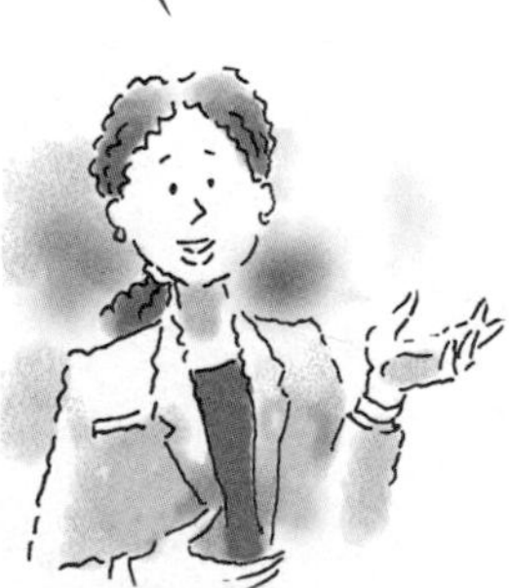

20. 3. Adverse effects of chemotherapy may occur after treatment and should be discussed with the client because some can be treated, controlled, or prevented. The nurse needs to explore what the client means by this statement. The client may feel poorly after chemotherapy and may want to take time off from work until feeling better. Joining social clubs is typical behavior for a young adult. Returning to school is also typical of a young adult.

NP: Assessment; CN: Health promotion and maintenance; CNS: Growth and development through the life span; CL: Analysis

21. A male client has been diagnosed with panhypopituitarism. Which of the following hormones will be given to the client orally?
1. Estrogen
2. Levothyroxine
3. Serotonin
4. Testosterone

21. 2. Thyroid hormone release depends on the release of thyroid-stimulating hormone (TSH) by the anterior pituitary. TSH is absent from the pituitary when panhypopituitarism exists, so levothyroxine should be given orally. Serotonin release isn't controlled by the pituitary gland. Testosterone is given by injection or topically by patch. Estrogen isn't indicated for a male client.

NP: Implementation; CN: Physiological integrity; CNS: Pharmacological and parenteral therapies; CL: Application

NP: Nursing process CN: Client needs category CNS: Client needs subcategory CL: Cognitive level

22. Which of the following nursing interventions is appropriate for an adult client with chronic renal failure?

1. Weigh the client daily before breakfast.
2. Offer foods high in calcium and phosphorous.
3. Serve the client large meals and a bedtime snack.
4. Encourage the client to drink large amounts of fluids.

22. 1. Daily weights are obtained to monitor fluid retention. Fluids should be restricted for the client with chronic renal failure. To improve food intake, meals and snacks should be given in small portions. Calcium intake is encouraged, but clients with chronic renal failure have difficulty excreting phosphorous. Therefore, phosphorous must be restricted.

NP: Implementation; CN: Physiological integrity; CNS: Physiological adaptation; CL: Application

23. During an admission interview, the nurse gathers data from a male client. Which of the following findings is a risk factor for testicular cancer?

1. Obesity
2. Cryptorchidism
3. History of alcoholism
4. History of cigarette smoking

23. 2. Cryptorchidism, or an undescended testicle, is a risk factor for testicular cancer. Cigarette smoking, obesity, and alcoholism aren't risk factors for developing testicular cancer.

NP: Assessment; CN: Health promotion; CNS: Prevention and detection of disease; CL: Comprehension

24. Which of the following assessment findings indicates an increased risk for skin cancer?

1. A deep sunburn
2. A dark mole on the client's back
3. An irregular scar on the client's abdomen
4. White irregular patches on the client's arm

24. 1. A deep sunburn is a risk factor for skin cancer. A dark mole or an irregular scar are benign findings. White irregular patches are abnormal but aren't a risk factor for skin cancer.

NP: Assessment; CN: Health promotion; CNS: Prevention and detection of disease; CL: Application

25. Which of the following behaviors is consistent with the diagnosis of conduct disorder in a child?

1. Enuresis
2. Suicidal ideation
3. Cruelty to animals
4. Fear of going to school

25. 3. Cruelty to animals is a symptom of conduct disorder. Fear of going to school is school phobia. Enuresis and suicidal ideation aren't usually associated with conduct disorder.

NP: Assessment; CN: Psychosocial integrity; CNS: Psychosocial adaptation; CL: Application

26. Which of the following symptoms is associated with a genital chlamydia infection?

1. Genital warts
2. No symptoms
3. Purulent discharge
4. Fluid-filled blisters

26. 3. Purulent discharge from the cervix, urethra, or Bartholin's gland is associated with several sexually transmitted diseases, including chlamydia. Fluid-filled blisters are a sign of herpes infection. Genital warts are a sign of human papillomavirus. Although some women with genital chlamydia infection are asymptomatic, this isn't the usual course of this condition.

NP: Planning; CN: Health promotion and maintenance; CNS: Prevention and early detection of disease; CL: Comprehension

27. Which of the following outcomes is appropriate for a client with a diagnosis of depression and attempted suicide?

1. The client will never feel suicidal again.
2. The client will find a group home to live in.
3. The client will remain hospitalized for at least 6 months.
4. The client will verbalize an absence of suicidal ideation, plan, and intent.

27. 4. An appropriate outcome is that the client will verbalize that he no longer feels suicidal. It's unrealistic to ask that he never feels suicidal. There's no reason for a group home or 6 months of hospitalization.

NP: Analysis; CN: Physiological integrity; CNS: Coping and adaptation; CL: Application

28. An adult client has a hip spica cast applied for treatment of a fractured femur. Which of the following precautions is included in the client's plan of care?

1. Use the bar to aid in turning the client.
2. Provide skin care around the cast edges.
3. Sedate the client while the cast is drying.
4. Encourage the client to turn frequently while the cast is drying.

28. 2. Skin care prevents pressure ulcers at the edges of the cast. Using the bar as a turning aid potentially can break the connection in the cast. The client in a hip spica cast won't be able to turn alone. Sedation will depress respiratory effort.

NP: Planning; CN: Physiological integrity; CNS: Reduction of risk potential; CL: Application

29. A registered nurse (RN) is supervising the care of a licensed practical nurse (LPN). The LPN is caring for a client diagnosed with a terminal illness. Which of the following statements by the LPN should be corrected by the RN?

1. "Some clients write a living will indicating their end-of-life preferences."
2. "The law says you have to write a new living will each time you go to the hospital."
3. "You could designate another person to make end-of-life decisions when you can't make them yourself."
4. "Some people choose to tell their physician they don't want to have cardiopulmonary resuscitation."

29. 2. One living will is sufficient for all hospitalizations unless the client wishes to make changes. The "No Code" or "Do Not Resuscitate" status is discussed with the physician, who then enters this in the client's chart. A living will explains a person's end-of-life preferences. A durable power of attorney for health care can be written to designate who will make health care decisions for the client in the event the client can't make decisions for himself.

NP: Evaluation; CN: Safe, effective care environment; CNS: Management of care; CL: Analysis

30. An elderly client's husband tells the nurse he's concerned because his wife insists on talking about events that happened to her years in the past. The nurse assesses the client and finds her alert, oriented, and answering questions appropriately. Which of the following statements made to the husband is correct?

1. "Your wife is reviewing her life."
2. "A spiritual advisor should be notified."
3. "Your wife should be discouraged from talking about the past."
4. "Your wife is regressing to a more comfortable time in the past."

30. 1. Life review or reminiscing is characteristic of elderly people and the dying. A spiritual advisor might comfort the client but isn't necessary for a life review. Discouraging the client from talking would block communication. Regression occurs when a client returns to behaviors typical of another developmental stage.

NP: Implementation; CN: Health promotion and maintenance; CNS: Growth and development through the life span; CL: Application

31. A client with a new colostomy asks a nurse how to avoid leakage from the ostomy bag. Which of the following instructions is correct?

1. Limit fluid intake.
2. Eat more fruits and vegetables.
3. Empty the bag when it's about half full.
4. Tape the end of the bag to the surrounding skin.

31. 3. Emptying the bag when partially full will prevent the bag from becoming heavy and detaching from the skin or skin barrier. Limiting fluids may cause constipation but won't prevent leakage. Increasing fruits and vegetables in the diet will help prevent constipation, not leakage. Taping the bag to the skin will secure the bag to the skin but won't prevent leakage.

NP: Implementation; CN: Physiological integrity; CNS: Basic care and comfort; CL: Application

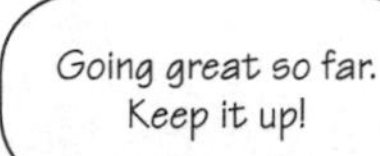
Going great so far.
Keep it up!

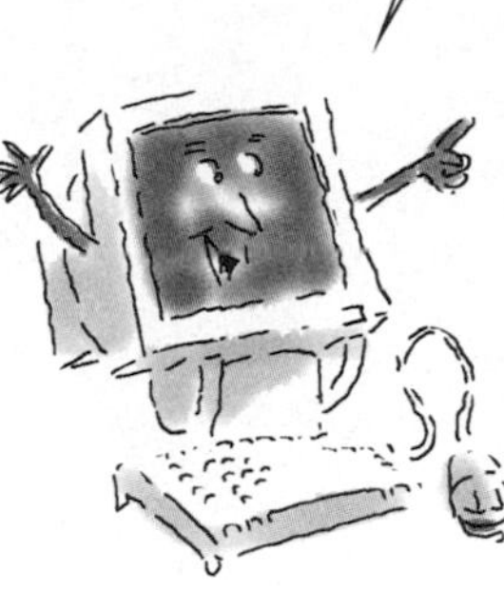

32. A nurse must obtain the blood pressure of a client in airborne isolation. Which of the following methods is best to prevent transmission of infection to other clients by the equipment?

1. Dispose of the equipment after each use.
2. Wear gloves while handling the equipment.
3. Use the equipment only with other clients in airborne isolation.
4. Leave the equipment in the room for use only with that client.

32. 4. Leaving equipment in the room is appropriate to avoid organism transmission by inanimate objects. Disposing of equipment after each use prevents the transmission of organisms but isn't cost-effective. Wearing gloves protects the nurse, not other clients. Using equipment for other clients spreads infectious organisms among clients.

NP: Implementation; CN: Safe, effective care environment; CNS: Safety and infection control; CL: Application

33. To prevent circulatory impairment in an arm when applying an elastic bandage, which of the following methods is best?

1. Wrap the bandage around the arm loosely.
2. Apply the bandage while stretching it slightly.
3. Apply heavy pressure with each turn of the bandage.
4. Start applying the bandage at the upper arm and work toward the lower arm.

33. 2. Stretching the bandage slightly maintains uniform tension on the bandage. Wrapping the bandage loosely wouldn't secure the bandage on the arm. Using heavy pressure would cause circulatory impairment. Beginning the wrapping at the upper arm would cause uneven application of the bandage. For example, elastic stockings are applied distal to proximal to promote venous return.

NP: Implementation; CN: Physiological integrity; CNS: Reduction of risk potential; CL: Application

34. A client needs to use an incentive spirometer after abdominal surgery. Which of the following statements about incentive spirometry is correct?

1. It's a substitute for early postoperative ambulation.
2. It's better than deep breathing to prevent atelectasis.
3. It causes less discomfort for the client than deep breathing.
4. It helps the client visualize deep breathing to prevent atelectasis.

34. 4. Incentive spirometry helps the client see inspiratory effort using floating balls, lights, or bellows. Early ambulation is still indicated for this postoperative client. Incentive spirometry is no more effective than deep breathing without equipment. Deep breathing and incentive spirometry cause equal discomfort during inspiration.

NP: Implementation; CN: Physiological integrity; CNS: Reduction of risk potential; CL: Comprehension

35. A client complains of an inability to sleep while on the medical unit. Which intervention to promote sleep has priority?

1. Offer a sedative routinely at bedtime.
2. Give the client a backrub before bedtime.
3. Question the client about sleeping habits.
4. Move the client to a bed farthest from the nurses' station.

35. 3. Interviewing the client about sleeping habits may give more information about the causes of the inability to sleep. A backrub may promote sleep but may not address this client's problem. Sedatives should be given as a last option. Moving the client may not address the client's specific problem.

NP: Implementation; CN: Physiological integrity; CNS: Basic care and comfort; CL: Application

36. To assess the function of the optic nerve, which of the following equipment is used?

1. Finger, to test the cardinal fields
2. Flashlight, to test corneal reflexes
3. Snellen's chart, to test visual acuity
4. Piece of cotton, to test corneal sensitivity

36. 3. The Snellen's chart is used to test the function of the optic nerve. Testing the cardinal fields assesses the oculomotor, trochlear, and abducens nerves. Corneal light reflex reflects the function of the oculomotor nerve. Corneal sensitivity is controlled by the trigeminal and facial nerves.

NP: Assessment; CN: Physiological integrity; CNS: Basic care and comfort; CL: Comprehension

37. Which of the following descriptions is correct for the prone position?

1. Sitting upright
2. Lying on the side
3. Lying on the back
4. Lying on the abdomen

37. 4. Prone position is lying on the abdomen. Sitting upright is known as Fowler's or high-Fowler's position. Side lying is also known as the lateral position. Lying on the back is the supine position.

NP: Implementation; CN: Safe, effective care environment; CNS: Management of care; CL: Comprehension

38. Which of the following interventions is best to prevent bladder infections for a client with an indwelling urinary catheter?

1. Limit fluid intake.
2. Encourage showers rather than tub baths.
3. Open the drainage system to obtain a urine specimen.
4. Irrigate the catheter twice daily with sterile saline solution.

38. 2. A shower would prevent bacteria in the bath water from sustaining contact with the urinary meatus and the catheter, while a tub bath may allow easier transit of bacteria into the urinary tract. Catheter irrigation is performed only with an order from the physician to keep the catheter patent. Opening the drainage system would provide a pathway for the entry of bacteria. Increased — not limited — fluid intake is recommended for a client with an indwelling urinary catheter.

NP: Planning; CN: Physiological integrity; CNS: Reduction of risk potential; CL: Comprehension

39. A nurse wants to use a waist restraint for a client who wanders at night. Which of the following factors or interventions should be considered before applying the restraint?

1. The nurse's convenience
2. The client's reason for getting out of bed
3. A sleeping medication ordered as needed at bedtime
4. The lack of nursing assistants on the night shift

39. 2. The nurse should question the client's reason for getting out of bed because the client may be looking for a bathroom. Lack of adequate staffing and convenience aren't reasons for applying restraints. Sleeping medications are chemical restraints that should be used only if the client is unable to go to sleep and stay asleep.

NP: Evaluation; CN: Safe, effective care environment; CNS: Safety and infection control; CL: Application

NP: Nursing process CN: Client needs category CNS: Client needs subcategory CL: Cognitive level

40. Six months after the death of her infant son, a client is diagnosed with dysfunctional grieving. Which of the following behaviors is expected?
1. She goes to the infant's grave weekly.
2. She cries when talking about the loss.
3. She's overactive without a sense of loss.
4. She states the infant will always be part of the family.

40. 3. One of the signs of dysfunctional grieving is overactivity without a sense of loss. Including the infant as a part of the family, going to the grave, and crying are all normal responses.

NP: Assessment; CN: Psychosocial integrity; CNS: Coping and adaptation; CL: Comprehension

41. A nurse notices a client has been crying. Which of the following responses is the most therapeutic?
1. None; this is a private matter.
2. "You seem sad, would you like to talk?"
3. "Why are you crying and upsetting yourself?"
4. "It's hard being in the hospital, but you must keep your chin up."

41. 2. Therapeutic communication is a primary tool of nursing. The nurse must recognize the client's nonverbal behaviors indicate a need to talk. Asking "why" is often interpreted as an accusation. Ignoring the client's nonverbal cues or giving opinions and advice are barriers to communication.

NP: Implementation; CN: Psychosocial integrity; CNS: Psychosocial adaptation; CL: Application

42. A nurse gives the wrong medication to a client. Another nurse employed by the hospital as a risk manager will expect to receive which of the following communications?
1. Incident report
2. Oral report from the nurse
3. Copy of the medication Kardex
4. Order change signed by the physician

42. 1. Incident reports are tools used by risk managers when a client might be harmed. They're used to determine how future problems can be avoided. An oral report won't serve as legal documentation. A copy of the medication Kardex wouldn't be sent with the incident report to the risk manager. A physician won't change an order to cover the nurse's mistake.

NP: Implementation; CN: Safe, effective care environment; CNS: Management of care; CL: Application

43. Performing a procedure on a client in the absence of informed consent can lead to which of the following charges?
1. Fraud
2. Harassment
3. Assault and battery
4. Breach of confidentiality

43. 3. Performing a procedure on a client without informed consent can be grounds for charges of assault and battery. Breach of confidentiality refers to conveying information about the client, harassment means to annoy or disturb, and fraud is to cheat.

NP: Implementation; CN: Safe, effective care environment; CNS: Management of care; CL: Comprehension

44. A surgical client newly diagnosed with cancer tells a nurse she knows the laboratory made a mistake about her diagnosis. Which of the following terms describes this reaction?
1. Denial
2. Intellectualization
3. Regression
4. Repression

44. 1. Cancer clients often deny this diagnosis when first made. Such a response may benefit the client in that it allows energy for surgical healing. Repression describes not remembering being diagnosed, regression describes childlike behavior, and intellectualization describes speaking of the disease as if reading a textbook.

NP: Assessment; CN: Psychosocial integrity; CNS: Coping and adaptation; CL: Comprehension

45. A single client delivers a premature neonate. Which of the following interventions is included in her treatment plan?

1. An early postpartum physician visit
2. Referral to the health department
3. Request for a social service visit in the hospital
4. Request for a home health visit the day after discharge

45. 3. Due to the client's marital status and premature condition of the neonate, a social service visit is appropriate. The social service visit will determine if there's a need for a referral to the health department. The mother has no physical indications for an early postpartum visit or need for an early home visit.

NP: Planning; CN: Safe, effective care environment; CNS: Management of care; CL: Analysis

46. Which of the following statements made by a client about her neonate indicates the need for further teaching?

1. "I'll trim the baby's nails when he's sleeping."
2. "I'll remember to place the baby on his back when he sleeps."
3. "Our infant car seat must be placed in the back seat of the car."
4. "The first thing I'm going to do when we get home is give the baby a tub bath."

46. 4. Neonates shouldn't be placed in a tub bath until after the cord is off and completely healed to prevent infection. It's correct to place a neonate on his back, cut his nails while he sleeps, and place the car seat in the back.

NP: Evaluation; CN: Safe, effective care environment; CNS: Safety and infection control; CL: Analysis

47. A client in labor is receiving oxytocin (Pitocin) to augment her labor. A nurse notes a change in her contraction pattern. The fetal heart monitor indicates that her contractions are lasting 2 minutes, with a notable rise in the baseline. Based on this finding, which of the following actions has priority?

1. Notify the physician.
2. Give oxygen through a mask.
3. Turn off the oxytocin (Pitocin).
4. Turn the client on her left side.

47. 3. The first action must be to stop the oxytocin, to prevent fetal hypoxia or possible rupture of the uterus. The client would then be placed on her left side, given oxygen to prevent fetal hypoxia, and the physician would be notified.

NP: Implementation; CN: Health promotion and maintenance; CNS: Growth and development through the life span; CL: Analysis

48. A client who just delivered is concerned about her neonate's Apgar scores of 7 and 8. She says she's been told scores lower than 9 are associated with learning difficulties in later life. Which of the following responses is best?

1. "You shouldn't worry so much, your infant is perfectly fine."
2. "You should ask about placing the infant in a follow-up diagnostic program."
3. "You're right in being concerned, but there are good special education programs available."
4. "Apgar scores are used to indicate a need for resuscitation at birth. Scores of 7 and above indicate no problem."

48. 4. Apgar scores don't indicate future learning difficulties; they're for rapid assessment of the need for resuscitation. An Apgar score of 7 and 8 is normal and doesn't indicate a need for intervention. It's inappropriate to just tell a client not to worry.

NP: Implementation; CN: Health promotion and maintenance; CNS: Growth and development through the life span; CL: Application

49. After delivering a neonate with a cleft palate and cleft lip, a client has minimal contact with her neonate. She asks the nurse to do most of the neonate's care. Which of the following nursing diagnoses is appropriate?

1. Anxiety related to fear of harming the neonate
2. Knowledge deficit related to neonate's potential
3. Risk for altered parenting related to birth defect
4. Ineffective individual coping related to birth defect

49. 3. Neonates born with birth defects are at risk for altered parenting. The parents must work through issues of not producing the perfect dream child and guilt associated with this. There's nothing in the question that indicates the client felt anxious about caring for the neonate or had ineffective individual coping problems or knowledge deficit.

NP: Analysis; CN: Health promotion and maintenance; CNS: Growth and development through the life span; CL: Application

50. A breast-feeding client asks how she can do breast self-examination (BSE) while nursing. Which of the following responses is best?

1. "You should do BSE after the infant has emptied the breast."
2. "You don't have to do BSE until after you stop breast-feeding."
3. "You should continue to do BSE the way you did before becoming pregnant."
4. "Your physician will examine your breasts until after you stop breast-feeding."

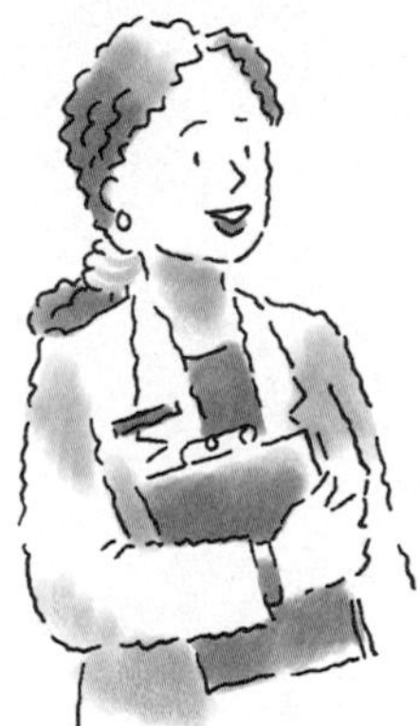

You've now completed 50 questions and are two-thirds finished. Groovy!

50. 1. During breast-feeding, the client should examine each breast after the neonate has emptied the breast. Women must continue to examine their breasts, even if they're lactating. Contrary to how it's performed before pregnancy, BSE should be done on the same day of the month until the menstrual cycle returns. Breast examination shouldn't be done solely by the physician.

NP: Implementation; CN: Health promotion and maintenance; CNS: Prevention and early detection of disease; CL: Comprehension

51. A prenatal client says she can't believe she has such mixed feelings about being pregnant. She tried for 10 years to become pregnant and now she feels guilty for her conflicting reactions. Which of the following responses is best?

1. "You need to talk to your midwife about these feelings."
2. "You're experiencing the normal ambivalence pregnant mothers feel."
3. "These feelings are expected only in women who have had difficulty becoming pregnant."
4. "Let's make an appointment with a counselor."

51. 2. Conflicting, ambivalent feelings regarding pregnancy are normal for all pregnant women. These feelings don't call for counseling or other professional interventions. Ambivalence is felt by most pregnant women, not only mothers who had difficulty becoming pregnant.

NP: Implementation; CN: Psychosocial integrity; CNS: Coping and adaptation; CL: Application

52. A maternity client says her husband is behaving in strange ways since she became pregnant. He's having morning sickness, has put on weight, complains of intestinal pains, and is acting like he's pregnant. Which of the following terms describes this reaction?

1. Extreme anxiety
2. Normal couvade
3. Signs of reaction formation
4. Abnormal, needing counseling

52. 2. The father's adjustment may include behaviors referred to as couvade. Historically, there have been different cultural couvades. Today, the term is associated with the father developing pregnancy-like symptoms. Because the behavior is normal and isn't reaction formation or anxiety, there's no need for counseling.

NP: Evaluation; CN: Psychosocial integrity; CNS: Psychosocial adaptation; CL: Analysis

53. Three days after discharge, a client bottle-feeding her neonate calls the postpartum floor, asking what she can do for breast engorgement. Which of the following instructions is correct?

1. Put a tight binder around her breasts.
2. Get under a warm shower and let the water flow on her breasts.
3. Stop drinking milk because it contributes to breast engorgement.
4. Contact her physician; she shouldn't be engorged at this late date.

53. 1. A tight binder is recommended for the client bottle-feeding her neonate to reduce engorgement. A warm shower will stimulate milk production. It's normal to become engorged during the first few days after delivery; drinking milk isn't the cause.
NP: Implementation; CN: Physiological integrity; CNS: Basic care and comfort; CL: Application

54. A pregnant client complains of leg cramps that wake her from sleep. Which of the following instructions is correct?

1. Dorsiflex the foot.
2. Elevate the legs at night.
3. Point the toes until the cramp releases.
4. Drink more than 1 quart of milk a day.

54. 1. Dorsiflexion of the foot is the recommended intervention to relieve a leg cramp during pregnancy. Drinking more than 1 quart of milk and pointing the toes are associated with causing leg cramps. Elevating the legs isn't a usual treatment.
NP: Implementation; CN: Physiological integrity; CNS: Basic care and comfort; CL: Application

55. A client is being treated for premature labor with ritodrine (Yutopar). After receiving this medication for 12 hours, her blood pressure is slightly elevated, her chest is clear, and her pulse is 120 beats/minute. She complains of a little nausea, and the fetal heart rate is 145 beats/minute. Which of the following interventions is correct?

1. Continue routine monitoring.
2. Contact the physician immediately.
3. Turn the client on her left side and give oxygen.
4. Increase the flow rate of the I.V. and give oxygen.

55. 1. These findings are normal adverse effects to the medication and don't call for interventions at this time except to continue close monitoring. Contacting the physician, placing the client on her left side, changing the I.V. flow rate, and giving oxygen are all interventions for abnormal assessment findings.
NP: Evaluation; CN: Physiological integrity; CNS: Pharmacological and parental therapies; CL: Analysis

56. At 6 cm of dilation, the client in labor receives a lumbar epidural for pain control. Which of the following nursing diagnoses is possible?

1. Risk for injury related to rapid delivery
2. Acute pain related to wearing off of anesthesia
3. Hyperthermia related to effects of anesthesia
4. Altered tissue perfusion related to effects of anesthesia

56. 4. A disadvantage of a lumbar epidural is the risk for hypotension, which can lead to altered tissue perfusion. Epidurals are associated with a longer labor and hypothermia. There's no pain involved with the anesthesia wearing off.
NP: Analysis; CN: Physiological integrity; CNS: Pharmacological and parenteral therapies; CL: Application

57. When assessing a client who just delivered, a nurse finds the following: blood pressure, 110/70 mm Hg; pulse, 60 beats/minute; respirations, 16 breaths/minute; lochia, moderate rubra; fundus, above the umbilicus to the right; and negative Homans' sign. Which of the following interventions is correct?

1. Nothing, all findings are normal.
2. Have the client void and recheck the fundus.
3. Turn the client on her left side to decrease the blood pressure.
4. Rub the fundus to decrease lochia flow and prevent hemorrhage.

57. 2. A fundus up and to the right indicates a full bladder. The client should empty her bladder and be reassessed. Lochia flow and blood pressure are normal. Placement of the uterus at the umbilicus and to the right isn't a normal finding.

NP: Implementation; CN: Physiological integrity; CNS: Reduction of risk potential; CL: Analysis

58. A client with diabetes delivers a 9-pound, 6-ounce neonate. The neonate is assessed for which of the following conditions?

1. Hyperglycemia
2. Hypoglycemia
3. Hyperthermia
4. Hypothermia

58. 2. Neonates of mothers with diabetes and large neonates are at risk for hypoglycemia related to increased production of insulin by the neonate in utero. Hypothermia, hyperthermia, and hyperglycemia aren't primary concerns.

NP: Assessment; CN: Physiological integrity; CNS: Reduction of risk potential; CL: Application

59. A prenatal client, age 13, asks about getting fat while she's pregnant. A nurse tells her she needs to gain enough weight to be in the upper portions of her recommended weight due to her age to prevent which of the following conditions?

1. A premature neonate
2. A difficult delivery
3. A low birth-weight neonate
4. Pregnancy-induced hypertension (PIH)

59. 3. Adolescent girls, especially those age younger than 15 years, are at higher risk for delivering low birth-weight neonates unless they gain adequate weight during pregnancy. Gaining weight isn't associated with having an easier delivery, risk for PIH, or a premature neonate.

NP: Implementation; CN: Physiological integrity; CNS: Reduction of risk potential; CL: Application

60. A neonate receiving phototherapy develops loose stools. Which of the following statements is correct about loose stools during phototherapy?

1. They're abnormal and may indicate an infection.
2. They're associated with an adverse reaction to formula.
3. They're common when receiving phototherapy treatments.
4. They're abnormal and phototherapy should be discontinued.

60. 3. While receiving phototherapy, a breakdown of bilirubin often results in loose stools. The neonate must be monitored for diarrhea and dehydration when under the lights. The loose stools wouldn't be considered related to infection or formula at this time.

NP: Assessment; CN: Physiological integrity; CNS: Physiological adaptation; CL: Comprehension

61. A client who's 36 weeks pregnant chokes on her food while eating at a restaurant. Which of the following statements is correct about performing the Heimlich maneuver on a pregnant client?

1. Chest thrusts are used when the client is pregnant.
2. Only back thrusts are used when the client is pregnant.
3. The Heimlich maneuver is performed the same as when not pregnant.
4. The Heimlich maneuver can't be performed on a pregnant client.

61. 1. During pregnancy, chest thrusts are used instead of abdominal thrusts. Abdominal thrusts compress the abdomen, which would harm the fetus. Because of this, the Heimlich is adjusted for the pregnant woman. A fist is made with one hand, placing thumb side against the center of the breastbone. The fist is grabbed with the other hand and thrust inward. Avoid the lower tip of the breastbone. Back thrusts aren't done as they may result in dislodgment of the obstruction, further obstructing the airway.

NP: Implementation; CN: Physiological integrity; CNS: Reduction of risk potential; CL: Application

62. A nurse works in a mental health facility that uses a therapeutic community (milieu) approach to client care. Which of the following statements describes the nurse's role in this facility?

1. Primary caregiver
2. Member of the milieu
3. Supervision more than counseling
4. Distinctly separate from the psychiatrist

62. 2. In a therapeutic community, everything focuses on the client's treatment. Staff and clients work together as a team or member of the milieu. The nurse wouldn't be a primary caregiver, but would work with the psychiatrist. The nurse's role could be that of supervision as well as counseling.

NP: Implementation; CN: Safe, effective care environment; CNS: Management of care; CL: Comprehension

63. A client with a substance abuse problem is being discharged from the state mental hospital. His discharge plans should include which of the following interventions?

1. Referral to Al-Anon
2. Weekly urine testing for drug use
3. Day hospital treatment for 6 months
4. Participation in a support group like Alcoholics Anonymous (AA)

63. 4. AA is a major support group for alcoholics after treatment. Membership in AA is associated with relapse prevention. Al-Anon is a support group for the family of the abuser of alcohol. Weekly urine testing or day hospital treatment isn't usual.

NP: Planning; CN: Safe, effective care environment; CNS: Management of care; CL: Application

64. A community mental health nurse visits a client diagnosed with paranoid schizophrenia. When she arrives at his house, he calls her Satan, shouts at her, and tells her to back away. Which of the following interventions has priority?

1. Use his phone and call the police.
2. Remain safe by leaving the house.
3. Talk to him in a calm voice to reduce his agitation.
4. Remind him who she is and that he has nothing to fear.

64. 2. Safety is the first priority during any home visit, so the nurse should leave. Attempting to talk with the client, reminding him who she is, or using the phone places the nurse at risk for harm. After the nurse has ensured her safety, arrangements should be made to provide help for the client.

NP: Implementation; CN: Safe, effective care environment; CNS: Safety and infection control; CL: Analysis

NP: Nursing process CN: Client needs category CNS: Client needs subcategory CL: Cognitive level

65. A client is scheduled to retire in the next month. He phones his nurse therapist and says he can't cope; his whole world is falling apart. The therapist recognizes this reaction as which of the following conditions?

1. Panic reaction
2. Situational crisis
3. Normal separation anxiety
4. Maturational crisis

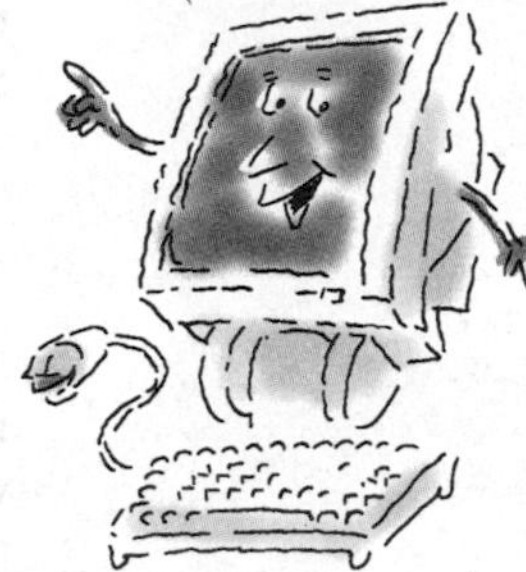

Only 10 more to go!
Oh, my, I just can't wait!

65. 4. A maturational (developmental) crisis is one that occurs at a predictable milestone during a life span; birth, marriage, and retirement are examples. Separation anxiety is a childhood disorder; a situational crisis is caused by events such as an earthquake. A panic reaction would also involve physical symptoms.

NP: Evaluation; CN: Health promotion and maintenance; CNS: Growth and development through the life span; CL: Analysis

66. A client with a phobic condition is being treated with behavior modification therapy. Which of the following treatments is expected?

1. Dream analysis
2. Free association
3. Systematic desensitization
4. Electroconvulsive therapy (ECT)

66. 3. Systematic desensitization is a behavior therapy used in the treatment of phobias. ECT is used with depression. Dream analysis and free association are techniques used in psychoanalytic therapy.

NP: Planning; CN: Psychosocial integrity; CNS: Psychosocial adaptation; CL: Comprehension

67. A severely depressed client rarely leaves her chair. To prevent physiologic complications associated with psychomotor retardation, which of the following goals is appropriate?

1. Restrict coffee intake.
2. Increase calcium intake.
3. Rest in bed three times per day.
4. Empty the bladder on a schedule.

67. 4. To prevent bladder infections associated with stasis of urine, the client should be encouraged to routinely empty her bladder. Resting in bed is another form of psychomotor retardation. Neither calcium nor coffee intake are directly related to the psychological effects associated with this condition.

NP: Planning; CN: Health promotion and maintenance; CNS: Prevention and early detection of disease; CL: Application

68. During the termination phase of a therapeutic nurse-client relationship, which of the following interventions is avoided?

1. Refer the client to support groups.
2. Address new issues with the client.
3. Review what has been accomplished during this relationship.
4. Have the client express sadness that the relationship is ending.

68. 2. During the termination phase, new issues shouldn't be explored. A normal response is sadness. It's appropriate to refer the client to support groups. To review what has been accomplished is a goal of this phase.

NP: Implementation; CN: Psychosocial integrity; CNS: Coping and adaptation; CL: Application

69. The behavior of a client with borderline personality disorder causes a nurse to feel angry toward the client. Which of the following responses by the nurse is the most therapeutic?

1. Ignore the client's irritating behavior.
2. Restrict the client to her room until supper.
3. Report her feelings to the client's physician.
4. Tell the client how her behavior makes the nurse feel.

69. 4. A nursing intervention used with personality disorders is to help the client recognize how her behavior affects others. Restricting the client to her room, ignoring the client, and reporting feelings to the physician aren't appropriate interventions at this time.

NP: Implementation; CN: Psychosocial integrity; CNS: Psychosocial adaptation; CL: Application

70. During a manic state, a client paced around the dayroom for 3 days. He talked to the furniture, proclaimed he was a king, and refused to partake in unit activities. Which of the following nursing diagnoses has priority?

1. Hypertension related to hyperactivity
2. Risk for violence related to manic state
3. Altered nutrition related to hyperactivity
4. Ineffective individual coping related to manic state

70. 3. During a manic state, clients are at risk for malnutrition due to not taking in enough calories for the energy they're expending. This client isn't showing violent behavior. Individual coping issues aren't the primary concern at this time. Hypertension isn't an approved nursing diagnosis.

NP: Analysis; CN: Physiological integrity; CNS: Basic care and comfort; CL: Application

71. A client with a panic disorder is having difficulty falling asleep. Which of the following nursing interventions should be performed first?

1. Call the client's psychotherapist.
2. Teach the client progressive relaxation.
3. Allow the client to stay up and watch television.
4. Obtain an order for a sleeping medication as needed.

71. 2. Relaxation techniques work very well with a client showing anxiety. If this doesn't work, then pharmacological interventions, diversionary activities, and contacting the psychotherapist would be in order.

NP: Implementation; CN: Psychological integrity; CNS: Coping and adaptation; CL: Application

72. A 65-year-old client with major depression hasn't responded to antidepressants. Which of the following interventions used to treat major depression might be added to the treatment plan?

1. Electroconvulsive therapy (ECT)
2. Electroencephalography (EEG)
3. Electromyography (EMG)
4. Tranquilizers

72. 1. ECT is commonly used for treatment of major depression for clients who haven't responded to antidepressants or who have medical problems that contraindicate the use of antidepressants. EEG is a technique used to treat clients with anxiety, general tension, stuttering, insomnia, and chronic pain. EMG is used in biofeedback. Major tranquilizers are used to treat schizophrenia or anxiety disorders.

NP: Implementation; CN: Physiological integrity; CNS: Physiological adaptation; CL: Comprehension

73. A client diagnosed with bipolar disease is receiving a maintenance dosage of lithium carbonate. His wife calls the community mental health nurse to report that her husband is hyperactive and hyperverbal. Which of the following interventions is appropriate?

1. Mental status examination
2. Measurement of lithium blood levels
3. Evaluation at the local emergency room
4. Admission to the hospital for observation

73. 2. Increased activity might indicate a need for an increased dose of lithium or that the client isn't taking his medications; blood levels will determine this. He doesn't need to go to the emergency room, have a mental status examination, or be admitted to the hospital at this time.

NP: Implementation; CN: Physiological integrity; CNS: Pharmacological and parenteral therapies; CL: Analysis

74. After electroconvulsive therapy (ECT), which of the following nursing interventions is correct?

1. Assess the client's vital signs.
2. Let the client sleep undisturbed.
3. Allow the family to visit immediately.
4. Restrain the client until completely awake.

74. 1. Vital signs are monitored carefully for approximately 1 hour after ECT or until stable. The client shouldn't be restrained or left alone. Visitors should be allowed when the client is awake and ready.

NP: Implementation; CN: Physiological integrity; CNS: Reduction of risk potential; CL: Application

75. A client with schizophrenia has been taking an antipsychotic medication for 2 years. She develops muscle rigidity, a temperature of 105° F (40.6° C), fluctuating blood pressure, tachycardia, and tachypnea. These symptoms indicate which of the following conditions?

1. Agranulocytosis
2. Tardive dyskinesia (TD)
3. Neuroleptic malignant syndrome (NMS)
4. Normal adverse effects to antipsychotics

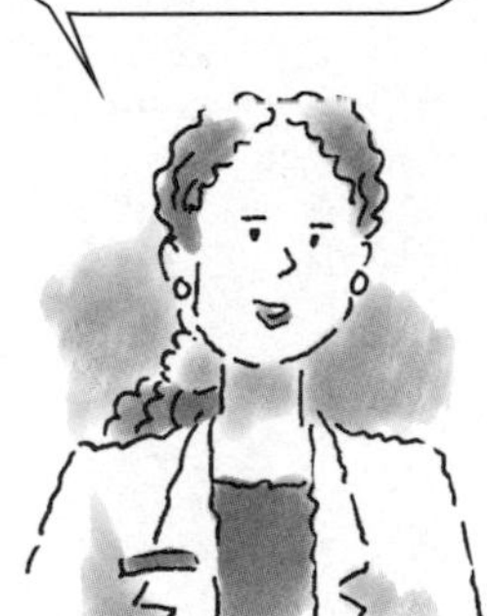

I knew you could do it! Super job! You're well on your way to total confidence for the NCLEX.

75. 3. Muscle rigidity, high temperature, fluctuating blood pressure, tachycardia, and tachypnea are all signs of NMS. Agranulocytosis is a decrease in the production of leukocytes. These symptoms aren't normal adverse effects of antipsychotics. TD is involuntary oral, buccal, or lingual chewing movements.

NP: Analysis; CN: Physiological integrity; CNS: Reduction of risk potential; CL: Analysis

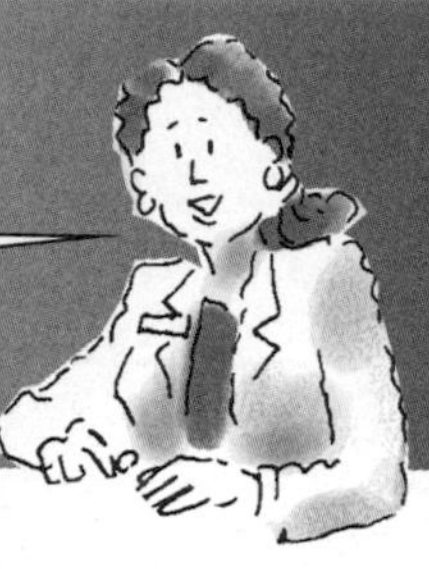
Here's another challenging comprehensive test with a variety of questions like a real NCLEX test. Have a go at it!

COMPREHENSIVE Test 3

1. A client in the postoperative phase of abdominal surgery is to advance his diet as tolerated. The client has tolerated ice chips and a clear liquid diet. Which of the following diets is given next?

1. Fluid restricted
2. Full liquids
3. General
4. Soft

1. 2. Clear liquid diets are nutritionally inadequate but minimally irritating to the stomach. Clients are advanced to the full liquid diet next, adding bland and protein foods. A soft diet comes next, which omits foods that are hard to chew or digest. A regular or general diet has no limitations. A fluid restriction is ordered in addition to the diet order for clients in renal failure or congestive heart failure.

NP: Implementation; CN: Physiological integrity; CNS: Basic care and comfort; CL: Comprehension

2. The following information is recorded on an intake and output record: milk, 180 ml; orange juice, 60 ml; 1 serving scrambled eggs; 1 slice toast; 1 can Ensure oral nutritional supplement, 240 ml; I.V. dextrose 5% in water at 100 ml/hour; 50 ml water after twice daily medications. Medications are given at 9:00 a.m. and 9:00 p.m. What is the client's total intake for the 7:00 a.m. to 3:00 p.m. shift?

1. 1,000 ml
2. 1,250 ml
3. 1,330 ml
4. 1,380 ml

2. 3. 180 + 60 + 240 + 800 + 50 = 1,330.

NP: Evaluation; CN: Physiological integrity; CNS: Basic care and comfort; CL: Analysis

3. A pediatrician writes an order for digoxin (Lanoxin), 2.5 mg, for a neonate. The nurse questions the order with the pharmacist and physician taking the call. Which of the following legal standards is most relevant?

1. American Medical Association
2. American Nurses Association (ANA)
3. American Pharmaceutical Association
4. Nurse Practice Act

3. 4. Each state has a Nurse Practice Act that dictates a nurse's scope of practice. Each nurse must practice competent standards based on her state's Nurse Practice Act. The ANA is an organization of nurses that offers credentialing and nursing education. It doesn't set standards of nursing practice. Physicians and pharmacists must practice competency based on the standards established by their professional organizations.

NP: Implementation; CN: Safe, effective care environment; CNS: Management of care; CL: Application

4. In checking a client's chart, the nurse notes that there's no record of a narcotic being given to the client even though the previous nurse signed for one. The client denies receiving anything for pain since the previous night. Which of the following actions should be taken next?

1. Notify the physician that a narcotic is missing.
2. Notify the supervisor that the client didn't receive the prescribed pain medication.
3. Notify the pharmacist that the client didn't receive the prescribed pain medication.
4. Approach the nurse who signed out the narcotic to seek clarification about the missing drug.

4. 4. The nurse needs to seek clarification in a nonthreatening manner. If the nurse who signed out the narcotic can't give a plausible explanation, the nurse who discovered the error must then notify the supervisor. The nurse who signed out the narcotic may have a drug problem. The appropriate line of communication is to the hospital supervisor. The physician needs to be notified if the client didn't receive the prescribed medication. The pharmacist needs to be notified of discrepancies in the narcotic count.

NP: Implementation; CN: Safe, effective care environment; CNS: Management of care; CL: Application

5. A client is seen in the emergency department with bruises on her face and back. She has the signs of a battered wife. Which of the following community resources could provide assistance to the client?

1. Alcoholics Anonymous (AA)
2. Crime Task Force
3. Lifeline Emergency Aid
4. Women's shelter

5. 4. A women's shelter can house women and children who need protection from an abusive partner or parent. AA is a support group for alcoholics and their families. The Crime Task Force and Lifeline Emergency Aid don't provide housing for women or children who want to leave an abusive relationship.

NP: Planning; CN: Safe, effective care environment; CNS: Management of care; CL: Application

6. Multidisciplinary team meetings are used frequently as a method of communication among health care disciplines. Which of the following units uses this method of communication?

1. Hemodialysis
2. Home health care services
3. Labor and delivery units
4. Outpatient surgical units

6. 2. Home health care services and restorative care services (such as rehabilitation units) that use different disciplines are required by the Joint Commission on Accreditation of Healthcare Organizations or Medicare to hold multidisciplinary team meetings. This serves as a means of communicating the client's diagnosis, plan of care, and discharge needs, using all disciplines for input. Hemodialysis units, outpatient surgical units, and labor and delivery units use between-shift reporting as a method of communicating.

NP: Implementation; CN: Safe, effective care environment; CNS: Management of care; CL: Application

7. A nurse finds a client crying after she was told hemodialysis is needed due to the development of acute renal failure. Which of the following interventions is best?

1. Sit quietly with the client.
2. Refer the client to the hemodialysis team.
3. Remind the client this is a temporary situation.
4. Discuss with the client the other abilities she has.

7. 1. Sitting with the client shows compassion and concern, and may help the nurse establish therapeutic communication. Making a referral doesn't allow the client to explore feelings with the nurse. The nurse can't guarantee the acute renal failure is temporary. Discussing the client's other abilities is diverting the emphasis away from the primary issue for this client.

NP: Implementation; CN: Psychosocial integrity; CNS: Coping and adaptation; CL: Knowledge

8. A client was admitted to a mental health ward for hyperexcitability, increasing agitation, and distractibility. Which of the following nursing interventions has priority?

1. Involve the client in a group activity.
2. Be direct, firm, and set rules for the client.
3. Use a quiet room for the client away from others.
4. Channel the client's energy toward a planned activity.

8. 3. Being in a quiet environment away from stimuli facilitates helping the client regain a sense of control. If the nurse attempts to be firm and set rules for this client, it will most likely heighten the agitation. The client is too excited to focus at this time; group activities or other activities may worsen the client's situation.

NP: Implementation.; CN: Psychosocial integrity; CNS: Psychosocial adaptation; CL: Knowledge

9. Which of the following controllable risk factors identified on a client history may contribute to heart disease?

1. Race
2. Prostate cancer
3. Diabetes mellitus
4. Previous myocardial infarction (MI)

9. 3. Diabetes mellitus, if uncontrolled, can lead to heart disease. Race is a factor that can't be controlled. Previous MI and history of prostate cancer aren't risk factors.

NP: Assessment; CN: Health promotion and maintenance; CNS: Prevention and early detection of disease; CL: Knowledge

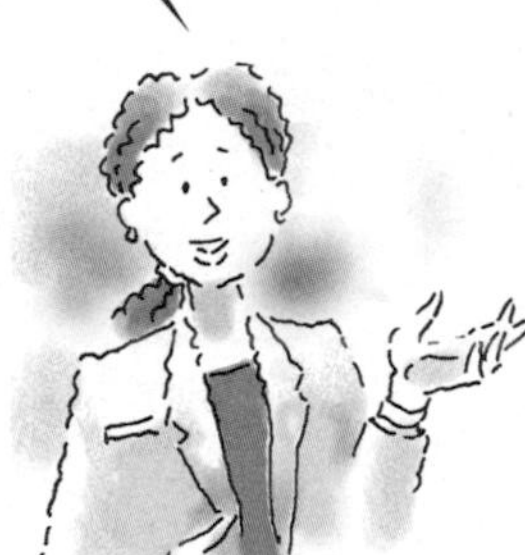
You've finished 10 questions already! Good job!

10. A public health nurse visiting a new postpartum client notices that the client has two children under age 4. The nurse notices one infant playing in the cabinet under the sink. Which of the following instructions should the public health nurse give the client?

1. Cover the infant's hands with gloves.
2. Make sure all liquid cleaners are labeled.
3. Tighten all cap tops on the bottles under the sink.
4. Remove all liquid cleaners that could be ingested orally.

10. 4. All liquid cleaners must be removed to reduce the risk for poisoning. Safety locks should be placed on cabinets to prevent young children from opening the cabinets or the bottles. Infants can't read danger labels.

NP: Implementation; CN: Safe, effective care environment; CNS: Safety and infection control; CL: Application

11. A nurse arrives at a motor vehicle accident involving a school bus and a large truck. The school bus is lying on its side. Several people had been thrown from the windows of the school bus. Which of the following victims needs priority care?

1. A girl crying hysterically
2. A boy who's unconscious
3. A boy with a laceration of the scalp
4. A girl with an obvious open fracture

11. 2. The unconscious child should be assessed for breathing and circulation status. An unconscious or unresponsive client always needs assistance first. Once help arrives, the girl's fracture can be stabilized, pressure can be applied to the laceration of the scalp to stop the bleeding, and emotional support can be given to the girl crying hysterically.

NP: Assessment; CN: Safe, effective care environment; CNS: Safety and infection control; CL: Application

12. Which of the following statements from a newly diagnosed client with diabetes indicates more instruction is needed?

1. "I need to check my feet daily for sores."
2. "I need to store my insulin in the refrigerator."
3. "I can use my plastic insulin syringe more than once."
4. "I need to see my physician for follow-up examinations."

12. 2. Insulin only needs to be stored in the refrigerator if it won't be used within 6 weeks after being opened; it should be at room temperature when given to decrease pain and prevent lipodystrophy. According to a poll by the Juvenile Diabetes Foundation, a very high percentage of diabetics reuse their insulin syringes. However, it's recommended they be carefully recapped and placed in the refrigerator to prevent bacterial growth. The remaining statements show that the client understands his condition and the importance of preventing complications.

NP: Evaluation; CN: Safe, effective care environment; CNS: Safety and infection control; CL: Analysis

13. A client with terminal cancer is receiving large doses of narcotics for pain control. He becomes agitated and continues trying to get out of bed but can't stand without a two-person assistance. To reduce the risk of falling, which of the following types of restraint is the most beneficial?

1. Leg restraints
2. Chemical restraints
3. Mechanical restraints
4. Tying him in bed with a sheet

13. 2. Antianxiety medication can be used to calm the client. Chemical restraints are effective, especially with highly agitated clients receiving large doses of narcotics. Other forms of restraint will only increase the client's agitation and hostility, thus increasing the safety risk.

NP: Implementation; CN: Safe, effective care environment; CNS: Safety and infection control; CL: Application

14. A client who had a heart transplant is in reverse isolation postoperatively. Which of the following explanations for this is correct?

1. To protect the client from his own bacteria
2. To protect the hospital staff from the client
3. To protect the other clients on the nursing unit
4. To protect the client from outside infections from others

14. 4. Immunosuppressed clients need to be protected from infections from others. Infections can occur if strict handwashing techniques aren't observed, especially with hospital staff going from one room to the next. Protective isolation is used to protect the hospital staff and other clients from an infected client.

NP: Planning; CN: Safe, effective care environment; CNS: Safety and infection control; CL: Application

15. A physician ordered a sterile dressing tray set up in a client's room to insert a subclavian central venous catheter. Which of the following steps is done first to set up the sterile field?

1. Open the tray toward the nurse.
2. Use correct handwashing technique.
3. Put on sterile gloves before opening the tray.
4. Place the sterile dressing tray on an overbed table.

15. 2. Use appropriate handwashing technique before participating in a sterile procedure. Clean the area with an appropriate antiseptic, place the tray in the center of the clean area, and open it away from the nurse. After the dressing tray is opened, put on sterile gloves to assist the physician.

NP: Implementation; CN: Safe, effective care environment; CNS: Safety and infection control; CL: Application

16. The nurse is instructing a homebound client on safety precautions for chemotherapy. Which color plastic bag is universally used for handling chemotherapy supplies?

1. Blue
2. Purple
3. Red
4. White

16. 3. Biohazardous waste products are placed in red biohazard bags. White bags are used for normal trash products and blue bags are used for recycling plastics. Purple bags aren't used for biohazardous waste products.

NP: Planning; CN: Safe, effective care environment; CNS: Safety and infection control; CL: Knowledge

17. A public health nurse is interviewing a young Pakistani client in her home. The nurse notices the client and the infant wear long skirts and coverings over their heads. The home isn't air-conditioned and the room is very warm. The dress code is recognized as part of which of the following characteristics?

1. Culture
2. Economic status
3. Race
4. Socialization

17. 1. Many cultures have specific dress codes. The client's dress, as described, doesn't indicate economic status. Race refers to a group of people with similar physical characteristics such as skin color. Socialization is the process by which individuals learn the ways of a given society to function within that group.

NP: Analysis; CN: Health promotion and maintenance; CNS: Growth and development through the life span; CL: Application

18. Which of the following actions is included in the assessment step of the nursing process?

1. Identify actual or potential health problems specific to the individual client.
2. Judge the effectiveness of nursing interventions that have been implemented.
3. Identify goals and interventions specific to the individualized needs of the client.
4. Systematically collect subjective and objective data with the goal of making a clinical nursing judgment.

18. 4. Assessment involves data collection, organization, and validation. Evaluation involves judging the effectiveness of nursing interventions and whether the goals of the plan of care have been achieved. The nurse and client work together to identify goals, outcomes, and intervention strategies that will reduce identified client problems in the planning step. The diagnosis step of the nursing process involves the identification of actual or potential health problems.

NP: Assessment; CN: Safe, effective care environment; CNS: Management of care; CL: Knowledge

19. During an interdepartmental team meeting at a hospice, a nurse who practices Catholicism verbalizes concern for the spiritual needs of a terminally ill infant and her non-Catholic family. She suggests the infant be baptized before death. Which of the following recommendations of the multidisciplinary team is most likely?

1. Insist the infant obtain baptism before death occurs.
2. Bathe the infant with special oil to prepare for death.
3. Schedule an appointment with a Catholic priest to see the family.
4. Recognize that not all religions practice infant baptism.

19. 4. Many religious organizations (for example, Baptist, Adventist, Buddhist, Quaker) don't practice baptism or only baptize an individual when he or she is an adult. Hospice organizations use the family's religious leader as a choice for spiritual directions. Seventh Day Adventists believe in divine healing and anointing with oil. Deciding whether to baptize the infant isn't the nurse's responsibility. It's important to honor all customs and religious beliefs of families.

NP: Assessment; CN: Psychosocial integrity; CNS: Coping and adaptation; CL: Comprehension

20. A home health client asks a nurse for information on sources of financial support. The client has an elderly parent who's blind living with her. Which of the following programs is the client referred to?

1. Medicare
2. Meals on Wheels
3. Supplemental Security Income
4. Aid to Families with Dependent Children

20. 3. Supplemental Security Income is a governmental subsidy assisting the poor and medically disabled. Aid to Families with Dependent Children is a state subsidy given to poor families with dependent children. Meals on Wheels is a nonprofit organization that delivers food to the poor. Medicare is available to elderly individuals age 65 years and older and individuals younger than 65 years with long-term disabilities or end-stage renal disease.

NP: Implementation; CN: Health promotion and maintenance; CNS: Growth and development through the life span; CL: Application

21. Giving hearing and vision screening to elementary school children is an example of which of the following types of prevention strategy?

1. Primary
2. Secondary
3. Tertiary
4. None of the above

21. 2. Screening is a major secondary prevention strategy. Secondary prevention is aimed at early detection and treatment of illness. Primary prevention strategies are aimed at preventing the disease from the beginning by avoiding or modifying risk factors. Tertiary prevention strategies focus on rehabilitation and prevention of complications arising from advanced disease.

NP: Assessment; CN: Health promotion and maintenance; CNS: Growth and development through the life span; CL: Application

22. Which of the following nursing actions is most appropriate in relieving pain related to cancer?

1. Use heat or cold on painful areas.
2. Keep a hard bedroll behind the client's back.
3. Allow the client to stay in one position to prevent pain.
4. Keep bright lights on in the room so the nurse can assess the client more quickly.

22. 1. Using either heat or cold can reduce inflammatory responses, which will reduce pain. Avoid pressure (such as bedrolls) on painful areas. Change the client's position frequently. Coordinate activity with pain medication. Reduce bright lights and noise to prevent anxiety, which can increase pain.

NP: Implementation; CN: Physiological integrity; CNS: Physiological adaptation; CL: Application

Stay focused, now. You're nearly one-third finished!

23. Which of the following definitions is correct for "validation of nursing assessment data"?

1. The process of confirming the accuracy of assessment data collected
2. A method for guiding the nursing interview and physical examination
3. A recording method for assessment data that becomes a permanent part of the medical record
4. The use of insight, instinct, and clinical experience to make clinical judgments about clients

23. 1. In validation, the nurse verifies that the cues and inferences are correct. The second option refers to a format for performing or recording an interview and health assessment. The third option refers to a framework or outline for recording data and facilitating its use by other nurses caring for the client. The fourth option refers to the use of intuition, a legitimate aspect of nursing practice, to problem solve and make clinical decisions when assessment data are incomplete or ambiguous.

NP: Assessment; CN: Safe, effective care environment; CNS: Management of care; CL: Comprehension

24. A local community health nurse is asked to speak to a group of adolescent girls on the topic of preventing pregnancy. Which of the following statements indicates the adolescents need more information on this topic?

1. "I can get pregnant even on the first time we have sex."
2. "I can get pregnant even though I don't have sex regularly."
3. "I can't get pregnant because my menstrual cycle isn't regular yet."
4. "I can get pregnant even if my boyfriend withdraws before he comes."

24. 3. Many adolescents have misunderstandings related to risk periods and timing, including periods of susceptibility during the menstrual cycle, age-related susceptibility, and timing of male ejaculation.

NP: Evaluation; CN: Health promotion and maintenance; CNS: Growth and development through the life span; CL: Comprehension

25. Which of the following nursing actions is most appropriate in stimulating the appetite of a child with cancer?

1. Use food as a reward system.
2. Serve large meals frequently.
3. Prepare foods appropriate to the age of the child.
4. Place the child on a rigid time schedule for eating.

25. 3. It's important to prepare foods appropriate to children in certain age groups. Involve the child in food preparation and selection. Encourage parents to relax pressures placed on eating by stressing the legitimate nature of loss of appetite. Let the child eat all food that can be tolerated. Assess the family's beliefs about food habits. Take advantage of a hungry period and serve small snacks.

NP: Implementation; CN: Physiological integrity; CNS: Physiological adaptation; CL: Application

26. A nurse working in a public health clinic is planning tuberculosis (TB) screening. Screening is indicated for which of the following groups?

1. All clients coming into the clinic
2. People living in a homeless shelter
3. Clients who haven't received the TB vaccine
4. Clients suspected of having human immunodeficiency virus (HIV)

26. 4. Clients with HIV infection or suspected of having HIV are at greater risk of developing TB. A screening test should be done and, if positive, treatment with isoniazid (Nydrazid) given. Clients coming to the clinic don't need to be tested unless they're at high risk—for example, living with someone infected with TB, abusing I.V. drugs, or suffering from chronic health conditions, such as diabetes mellitus and end-stage renal disease. Clients living in a homeless shelter aren't necessarily at greater risk unless other residents in the shelter have TB. The TB vaccine isn't widely used in the United States.

NP: Assessment; CN: Health promotion and maintenance; CNS: Prevention and early detection of disease; CL: Application

27. A professional nurse should report positive tuberculosis (TB) smears or cultures to the health department within which of the following time periods?

1. 12 hours
2. 48 hours
3. 1 week
4. 10 to 14 days

27. 2. A client is considered contagious if he has a positive TB smear or culture, so the results must be reported within 24 to 48 hours. One week or 10 to 14 days is too long to wait. The smear or culture may not have grown an organism in 12 hours.

NP: Implementation; CN: Health promotion and maintenance; CNS: Prevention and early detection of disease; CL: Application

28. Which of the following methods is used for the Mantoux test, tuberculin skin testing used to identify clients infected with *Mycobacterium tuberculosis*?

1. Intradermal injection
2. Multiple puncture test
3. I.V. infusion
4. I.M. injection

28. 1. A Mantoux test is given intradermally, not I.M., I.V., or by multiple puncture test.
NP: Implementation; CN: Health promotion and maintenance; CNS: Prevention and early detection of disease; CL: Knowledge

29. A home health nurse must have expertise in many roles. In which of the following nurse-client interactions is the home health nurse showing a secondary intervention as an advocate?

1. Contacting the local church to borrow a walker for the client to use
2. Listening to a client express feelings of frustration over the limitations imposed by his condition
3. Giving I.V. antibiotic therapy every 12 hours with attention to sterile technique and prevention of complications
4. Teaching a client with chronic obstructive pulmonary disease the effect of abdominal distention on breathing and ways to help bowel function

29. 1. Referral to community agencies is an advocacy role for home health nurses. The role of the advocate implies the home care nurse is able to advise clients how to find alternative sources of care. Instructing clients about disease processes, giving emotional support, and giving therapies to clients are direct care activities.
NP: Implementation; CN: Safe, effective care environment; CNS: Management of care; CL: Application

30. A home health nurse's role includes direct and indirect care functions. Which of the following actions is an example of indirect care function?

1. Supervising a home health aide
2. Participating in a team conference about a client
3. Showing the home health aide body positioning for the client
4. Teaching the care provider how to read a food label for sodium content

30. 2. Participating in a team conference is an example of indirect care. Direct care is defined as the actual nursing care given to clients in their homes. Direct care may involve assessment of physical or psychosocial status, performance of skilled interventions, supervision of other disciplines, and teaching.
NP: Implementation; CN: Safe, effective care environment; CNS: Management of care; CL: Application

31. A young pregnant client attending prenatal classes is concerned about her alcohol intake. Which of the following statements indicates the client's child is at high risk of fetal alcohol syndrome (FAS)?

1. "I just snort once or twice a day."
2. "I had one glass of wine with dinner last week."
3. "I drink a six pack of beer daily to settle my nerves."
4. "I smoke marijuana with my boyfriend and his friends."

31. 3. Ingestion of alcohol on a daily basis increases the risk of FAS. Other forms of addictive behavior, such as the ingestion of cocaine and smoking marijuana, increase the risk of fetal abuse — not fetal alcohol syndrome.
NP: Evaluation; CN: Health promotion and maintenance; CNS: Prevention and early detection of disease; CL: Comprehension

32. According to the Centers for Disease Control and Prevention, which of the following groups doesn't need preventive therapy for tuberculosis (TB)?

1. Clients with human immunodeficiency virus (HIV) infection
2. Recent tuberculin skin test converters
3. Persons with no contact with infectious TB cases
4. Previously untreated or inadequately treated clients with abnormal chest X-rays

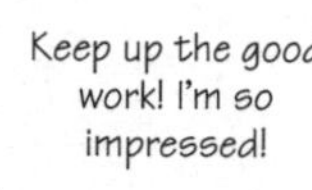

Keep up the good work! I'm so impressed!

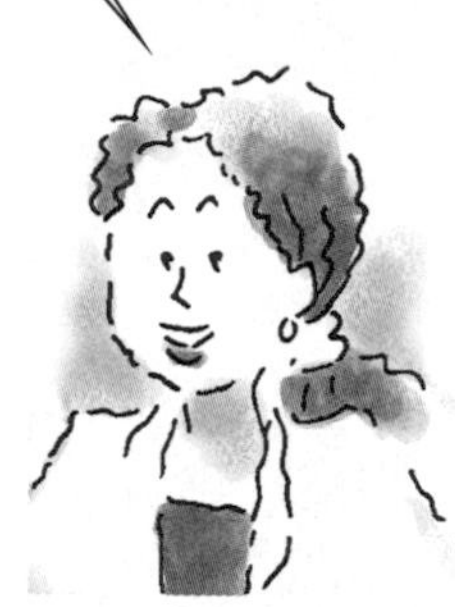

32. 3. Clients with no contact with infectious TB cases aren't at high risk of developing TB. Preventive therapy should be initiated for recent tuberculin skin test converters, previously untreated or inadequately treated clients with abnormal chest X-rays, and clients infected with HIV.

NP: Implementation; CN: Health promotion and maintenance; CNS: Prevention and early detection of disease; CL: Application

33. Which of the following psychosocial approaches should the emergency department nurse use when dealing with suspected family violence?

1. Punitive
2. Supportive treatment
3. Disgust and avoidance
4. Get the facts at all costs

33. 2. Emotional support is a nonthreatening approach when dealing with suspected family violence. Aggressive, punitive, and disdainful approaches can increase the anxiety of the perpetrator, increasing the risk of more violence.

NP: Implementation; CN: Psychosocial integrity; CNS: Coping and adaptation; CL: Application

34. A concerned client called the school asking that the nurse assess her 13-year-old son for signs of depression. Which of the following symptoms would the nurse expect to see?

1. Becomes angry at peers easily
2. Seeks out support from peers
3. Eats several small meals daily
4. Feels he can control everything in his life

34. 1. Adolescents experiencing depression may experience and express anger at peers. Adolescents feel a lack of control over their current situation, so they isolate themselves from their peers. The adolescent often has an intake of nutrients insufficient to meet metabolic needs.

NP: Assessment; CN: Psychosocial integrity; CNS: Coping and adaptation; CL: Analysis

35. A 56-year-old client recently lost his 82-year-old father to lung cancer. In counseling the client, the bereavement nurse expects which of the following signs of grief?

1. Decreased libido
2. Absence of anger and hostility
3. Difficulty crying or controlling crying
4. Clear dreams and imagery of the deceased

35. 4. A grieving client usually has vivid, clear dreams and fantasies. He also has a good capacity for imagery, particularly involving the loss. Difficulty crying or controlling crying, absence of anger and hostility, and decreased libido are signs of depression.

NP: Assessment; CN: Psychosocial integrity; CNS: Coping and adaptation; CL: Analysis

36. A 72-year-old client experienced the death of her husband 1 year ago. She now needs home health services due to severe osteoarthritis. Which of the following statements indicates the client will need further bereavement counseling?

1. "I'm lucky my children live so close."
2. "I really don't have anything to live for."
3. "My health isn't very good, but I can live with it."
4. "I've always had trouble remembering where I placed things."

36. 2. Wishing for death is a sign of depression. Usually after a year, most individuals accept the death of their loved ones and begin restoring their lives. Being grateful for good health and close family ties is a sign of acceptance of a new life that one experiences after the loss of a loved one. Memory loss can be a sign of dementia or depression.

NP: Analysis; CN: Psychosocial integrity; CNS: Coping and adaptation; CL: Analysis

37. Which of the following drugs and routes of administration is best to treat secondary syphilis?
1. Penicillin G orally
2. Penicillin G rectally
3. Cephalexin (Keflex) I.V.
4. Penicillin G I.M.

37. 4. Penicillin is the drug of choice to treat syphilis. Because of the long-term consequences of inadequate treatment, penicillin is usually given either I.M. or I.V., especially for syphilis of the nervous system or secondary syphilis. Keflex isn't the drug of choice for syphilis.
NP: Implementation; CN: Physiological integrity; CNS: Pharmacological and parenteral therapies; CL: Knowledge

38. Which of the following nursing actions is most appropriate for handling chemotherapeutic agents?
1. Wear disposable gloves and protective clothing.
2. Break needles after the infusion is discontinued.
3. Disconnect I.V. tubing with gloved hands.
4. Throw I.V. tubing in the trash after the infusion is discontinued.

38. 1. A nurse must wear disposable gloves and protective clothing to protect skin contact with the chemotherapeutic agent. Don't recap or break needles. Contaminated needles, syringes, I.V. tubes, and other contaminated equipment must be disposed of in a leak-proof, puncture-resistant container. Use a sterile gauze pad when priming I.V. tubing, connecting and disconnecting tubing, inserting syringes into vials, breaking glass ampules, or other procedures in which chemotherapeutic agents are being handled.
NP: Implementation; CN: Physiological integrity; CNS: Physiological adaptation; CL: Application

39. A client developed oral ulcerations secondary to chemotherapy agents. Which of the following nursing actions is most appropriate for reducing pain and irritation in the mouth?
1. Serve a high-fiber diet.
2. Use a toothbrush to clean teeth.
3. Avoid taking oral temperatures.
4. Rinse the mouth with hydrogen peroxide and water.

39. 3. If oral ulcers are present, taking oral temperatures will be painful. Use the axillary region, rectum, or ear as sites for temperature readings. Use a soft-sponge toothbrush, cotton-tipped applicator, or gauze-wrapped finger to clean teeth. Give normal saline solution mouthwashes and rinses to reduce pain and inflammation. Hydrogen peroxide mixed with water is too irritating if oral ulcers are present.
NP: Implementation; CN: Physiological integrity; CNS: Physiological adaptation; CL: Application

40. A client is admitted to the emergency department after being sexually assaulted. A policewoman accompanies her. The nurse realizes that several important tasks should be done in a sexual assault case. Which of the following nursing interventions receives priority?
1. Assisting with medical treatment
2. Collecting and preparing evidence for the police
3. Attempting to reduce the client's anxiety from a panic to a moderate level
4. Providing anticipatory guidance to the client about normal responses to sexual assault

40. 3. Reducing anxiety will help the client participate in medical, forensic, and legal follow-up activities. Medical treatment should begin as soon as the client's anxiety decreases below the panic level. Collecting and preparing evidence and providing anticipatory guidance aren't high-priority interventions.
NP: Implementation; CN: Psychosocial integrity; CNS: Coping and adaptation; CL: Comprehension

41. A school nurse is giving an educational forum on attention deficit hyperactivity disorder (ADHD) to the local school board. Which of the following behaviors is most common in children with ADHD?

1. Lethargy
2. Long attention span
3. Short attention span
4. Preoccupation with body parts

41. 3. Short attention span is a common characteristic of ADHD due to difficulty concentrating. Children with this disorder are distracted by environmental stimuli, so they won't be concentrating on their body parts. These children show hyperexcitability, not lethargy.

NP: Assessment; CN: Psychosocial integrity; CNS: Psychosocial adaptation; CL: Comprehension

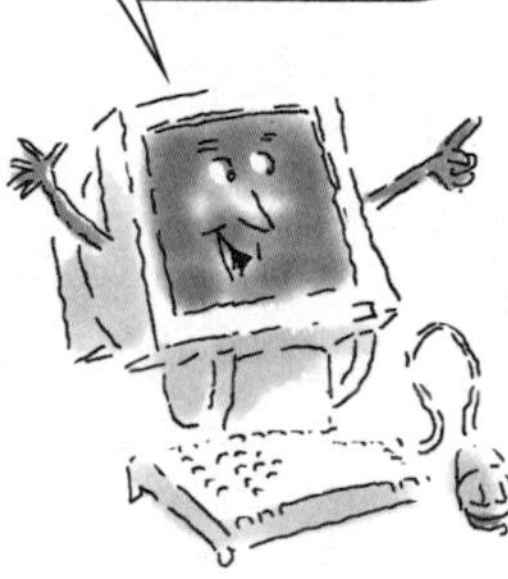

Excellent! You're more than halfway to the end. You should feel proud — and motivated!

42. A client with burns on 50% of his body is receiving total parenteral nutrition (TPN). Which of the following symptoms indicates the client is having a complication of TPN?

1. Pain
2. Absent bowel sounds
3. Abdominal cramping
4. Increased urine glucose

42. 4. Glycosuria, increased urine glucose, is associated with high blood glucose levels, a complication of TPN. Absent bowel sounds are an indication to begin TPN. Pain from major burns is expected. Abdominal cramping is associated with diarrhea or constipation.

NP: Evaluation; CN: Physiological integrity; CNS: Basic care and comfort; CL: Application

43. A 35-year-old woman is admitted to an inpatient substance abuse unit with a diagnosis of alcohol dependence. Which of the following comments by the client supports this diagnosis?

1. "I don't drink more than two beers when I'm out."
2. "I always remember what happens the next day."
3. "I always ask a friend to drive me home when I'm drinking."
4. "I've had four tickets for driving while intoxicated last month."

43. 4. Driving while intoxicated can be seen as a symptom of alcohol dependence. Designating drivers and limiting alcohol consumption are self-responsible actions, but don't address the underlying problem. By asking someone to drive them home, clients with alcohol dependence rationalize that it's okay to drink if they're responsible. The amount one drinks doesn't matter. An alcoholic experiences blackouts, which are periods of amnesia about experiences while intoxicated.

NP: Assessment; CN: Psychosocial integrity; CNS: Psychosocial adaptation; CL: Analysis

44. A nurse is working with a client with alcoholism in an acute care mental health unit. The client has been referred to Alcoholics Anonymous (AA). Which of the following statements by the client indicates that the client is ready to begin the AA program?

1. "I know I'm powerless over alcohol and need help."
2. "I think it will be interesting and helpful to join AA."
3. "I'd like to sponsor another alcoholic with this same problem."
4. "My family is very supportive and will attend meetings with me."

44. 1. In step 1 of AA, a person admits his powerlessness over alcohol and is ready to accept help. This should occur before he begins AA. A supportive family and a desire to help others with the same problem are good for the client, but they don't necessarily indicate readiness to participate in the program.

NP: Implementation; CN: Psychosocial integrity; CNS: Psychosocial adaptation; CL: Application

45. In planning care for a client diagnosed with paranoid schizophrenia, which of the following actions is correct for the psychiatric home health nurse?
1. Confront the client about her hallucinations.
2. Ask the minister to provide spiritual direction.
3. Instruct family members to discourage delusions.
4. Affirm when client's perceptions and thinking are in touch with reality.

45. 4. The nursing plan of care focuses on reinforcing perceptions and thinking that are in touch with reality. Confronting a client about her hallucinations and delusions isn't effective or therapeutic. Using family members could create distrust between the client and the family. Spiritual direction is important, but a client with paranoid schizophrenia may have issues surrounding her religious or spiritual orientation. Therefore, asking a minister to provide spiritual direction may not be effective or therapeutic.

NP: Planning; CN: Psychosocial integrity; CNS: Psychosocial adaptation; CL: Application

46. A psychiatric home health nurse finds a client with bipolar disorder sitting on the porch. The client is wearing a red polka dot dress, large yellow hat, and heavy makeup with large gold jewelry. Which of the following phases of the illness is the client most likely in?
1. Delusional
2. Depressive
3. Manic
4. Suspicious

46. 3. Extreme labile moods are characteristic of clients in the manic phase of bipolar disorder. Hyperactivity, verbosity, and drawing attention to oneself through dress are typical of the manic phase. In the depressive phase, clients are withdrawn, cry, and may not eat. Delusions and suspiciousness may be seen in bipolar disorder, but are more commonly seen in schizophrenia. Visual or auditory hallucinations, delusional thoughts, and extreme suspiciousness are behaviors seen in clients diagnosed with paranoid schizophrenia.

NP: Assessment; CN: Psychosocial integrity; CNS: Psychosocial adaptation; CL: Analysis

47. A nurse is assessing a 4-week-old neonate for signs of acute pain. Which of the following symptoms is expected?
1. Whimpering
2. Eyes opened wide
3. Limp body posture
4. Wanting to breast-feed frequently

47. 1. Crying, whimpering, and groaning are vocal expressions of acute pain in the neonate. Eyes tightly closed, changes in feeding behavior, and fist clenching with rigidity also are signs of acute pain in the neonate.

NP: Assessment; CN: Health promotion and maintenance; CNS: Growth and development through the life span; CL: Application

48. A home health nurse is instructing a client about positioning her child, who's diagnosed with juvenile rheumatoid arthritis (JRA). Which of the following positions or equipment is needed to maintain posture for a child with JRA?
1. Soft mattress
2. Prone position
3. Large fluffy pillows
4. Semi-Fowler's position

48. 2. Lying in the prone position is encouraged to straighten hips and knees. Semi-Fowler's position increases pressure on the hip joints and should be avoided. A firm mattress is needed to maintain good alignment of spine, hips, and knees, and no pillow or a very thin pillow should be used.

NP: Implementation; CN: Physiological integrity; CNS: Basic care and comfort; CL: Application

49. Which of the following comfort measures is best to reduce pain and stiffness for a child with juvenile rheumatoid arthritis (JRA)?
1. Hot packs
2. Cool baths
3. Cold compresses
4. Immersion in lukewarm water for 10 minutes

49. 1. Heat is beneficial to children with arthritis. Moist heat is best for relieving pain and stiffness. The most efficient and practical method is in the bathtub. Cold, cool, or lukewarm treatment isn't beneficial in relieving pain or stiffness in children with JRA.
NP: Implementation; CN: Physiological integrity; CNS: Basic care and comfort; CL: Application

50. While putting an elderly client with an indwelling urinary catheter in bed, a nurse notices the tubing hanging below the bed. She places the tubing in a loop on the bed with the client and makes sure the client won't lie on the tubing. Which of the following rationales explains the nurse's action?
1. To inhibit drainage
2. To allow drainage to occur
3. To allow the urine to collect in the tubing
4. To have the client check the tubing for urine

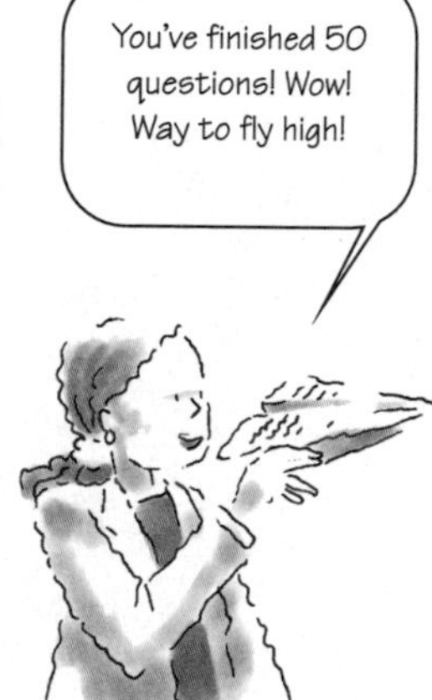

You've finished 50 questions! Wow! Way to fly high!

50. 2. Catheter tubing shouldn't be allowed to develop dependent loops or kinks because this inhibits proper drainage by requiring the urine to travel against gravity to empty into the bag. Permitting the urine to collect in the tubing increases the risk of infection. Observing the catheter and tubing is the responsibility of the nurse.
NP: Implementation; CN: Physiological integrity; CNS: Reduction of risk potential; CL: Application

51. A client complains of severe burning on urination. Which of the following instructions is best to give the client?
1. Wear only nylon panties.
2. Drink coffee to increase urination.
3. Soak in warm water with bubble bath.
4. Drink 2,500 to 3,000 ml of water per day.

51. 4. Drinking large amounts of water will help flush bacteria from the urinary tract. Avoid nylon underwear; wear only cotton undergarments to decrease the warm, moist environment. Avoid using bubble baths, perfumed soaps, or bath powders in the perineal area. The scent in toiletries can be irritating to the urinary meatus. Avoid tea, coffee, carbonated drinks, and alcoholic beverages because of bladder irritation.
NP: Implementation; CN: Physiological integrity; CNS: Basic care and comfort; CL: Application

52. Which of the following instructions is given to a client with a hearing aid?
1. Clean the hearing aid with baby oil.
2. Wear the hearing aid while sleeping.
3. Keep the hearing aid out of direct sunlight.
4. Leave the hearing aid in place while showering.

52. 3. The hearing aid should be kept out of direct sunlight and away from high temperatures. Solvents or lubricants shouldn't be used on the aid. If there is a detachable ear mold, it can be washed in warm, soapy water and dried with a soft cloth. The hearing aid should be left in place while the client is awake, except when showering.
NP: Implementation; CN: Physiological integrity; CNS: Basic care and comfort; CL: Application

53. A 72-year-old client is being discharged from same-day surgery after having a cataract removed from her right eye. Which of the following discharge instructions does the nurse give the client?

1. Sleep on the operative side.
2. Resume all activities as before.
3. Don't rub or place pressure on the eyes.
4. Wear an eye shield all day and remove it at night.

53. 3. Rubbing or placing pressure on the eyes increases the risk of accidental injury to ocular structures. The nurse should also caution against lifting objects, straining, strenuous exercise, and sexual activity because such activities can increase intraocular pressure. Glasses or shaded lenses should be worn to protect the eye during waking hours after the eye dressing is removed. An eye shield should be worn at night. Caution against sleeping on the operative side to reduce the risk of accidental injury to ocular structures.

NP: Implementation; CN: Physiological integrity; CNS: Reduction of risk potential; CL: Application

54. Which of the following benzodiazepines can be given parenterally?

1. Alprazolam (Xanax)
2. Buspirone (BuSpar)
3. Chlordiazepoxide (Librium)
4. Oxazepam (Serax)

54. 3. Chlordiazepoxide (Librium) can be given parenterally (I.M. or I.V.). Alprazolam (Xanax), buspirone (BuSpar), and oxazepam (Serax) must be given orally.

NP: Implementation; CN: Physiological integrity; CNS: Pharmacological and parenteral therapies; CL: Knowledge

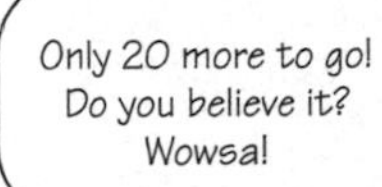

Only 20 more to go!
Do you believe it?
Wowsa!

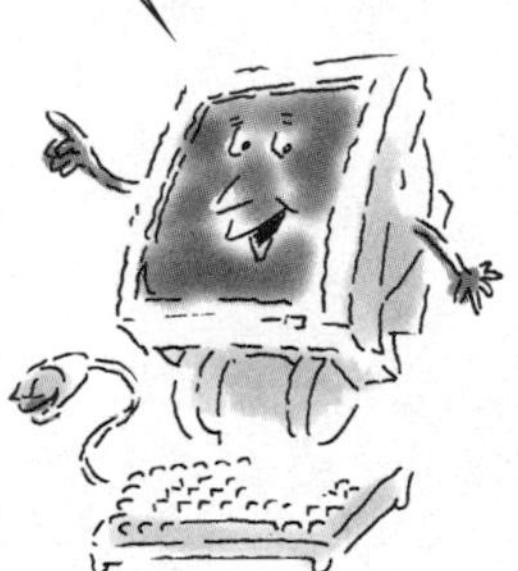

55. Which of the following instructions is correct for a client taking nortriptyline (Pamelor) for depression?

1. Be aware that this drug can cause a slow heart rate.
2. This drug will work immediately to treat depression.
3. Take this drug in the morning because it causes drowsiness.
4. Wear protective clothing and sunscreen when out in the sun.

55. 4. A common adverse effect of this drug is sensitivity to the sun. Protective clothing and sunscreen are worn in the sun. This drug can cause an irregular heart rate. It doesn't work immediately, but takes 2 to 3 weeks to achieve the desired effect. Take this drug at bedtime if it causes drowsiness.

NP: Implementation; CN: Physiological integrity; CNS: Pharmacological and parenteral therapies; CL: Application

56. Which of the following instructions is correct for a client receiving lithium for bipolar disorder?

1. Avoid drugs containing ibuprofen.
2. Drink at least two cups of coffee daily.
3. Be aware that you may experience increased alertness.
4. It isn't necessary to monitor the blood level of this drug.

56. 1. Avoid drugs that alter the effect of lithium, such as ibuprofen (Advil, Motrin, Nuprin) and sodium bicarbonate or other antacids containing sodium. Lithium can decrease alertness and coordination. Avoid beverages with caffeine because they increase urination, which may alter the effect of lithium. Lithium levels may need to be monitored every 2 weeks, especially if adverse effects occur. The dose may need to be regulated.

NP: Implementation; CN: Physiological integrity; CNS: Pharmacological and parenteral therapies; CL: Application

57. A physician ordered nitroprusside I.V. for a client in cardiogenic shock. Which of the following nursing interventions is needed to give this drug safely?

1. Give only with other drugs.
2. Mix the drug in an alkaline solution.
3. Mix the drug only in normal saline solution.
4. Cover the drug-containing I.V. solution with an opaque wrapper.

57. 4. The nurse should cover the drug-containing I.V. solution with an opaque wrapper because the drug is light-sensitive. Only dilute the drug in dextrose 5% in water; no other fluid should be used. Nitroprusside can't be mixed in alkaline solutions, and shouldn't be given with other drugs.

NP: Implementation; CN: Physiological integrity; CNS: Pharmacological and parenteral therapies; CL: Application

58. Which of the following nursing interventions is correct for a client receiving total parenteral nutrition (TPN)?

1. Discard TPN solutions after 24 hours.
2. Discard lipid emulsions after 20 hours.
3. Inspect the TPN solution for clearness and visibility.
4. Teach the client to blow out during expiration when the tubing is disconnected.

58. 1. TPN solutions are good media for fungi, so they should be discarded after 24 hours. The nurse should teach the client to perform Valsalva's maneuver, taking a deep breath and holding it, when the tubing is disconnected. Valsalva's maneuver increases intrathoracic pressure, which prevents air entry. Inspect TPN solutions for cloudiness, cracks, or leaks before hanging. Lipid emulsions are also good media for fungi and should be discarded after 12 hours.

NP: Implementation; CN: Physiological integrity; CNS: Pharmacological and parenteral therapies; CL: Application

59. Which of the following narcotic analgesics may be given parenterally to an older client to be more useful?

1. Hydromorphone (Dilaudid)
2. Meperidine (Demerol)
3. Morphine
4. Oxycodone (Percocet)

59. 1. Dilaudid is a fast-acting drug and is a useful alternative to morphine or Demerol. Morphine and Demerol can increase the risk of confusion in the elderly. Oxycodone is given only orally or rectally.

NP: Implementation; CN: Physiological integrity; CNS: Pharmacological and parenteral therapies; CL: Application

60. Which of the following diagnostic tests is used to diagnose bacterial endocarditis?

1. Electrolytes
2. Blood cultures
3. Prothrombin time (PT)
4. Venereal Disease Research Laboratory (VDRL)

60. 2. Blood cultures are crucial in diagnosing bacterial endocarditis. Electrolyte levels indicate abnormalities that occur with drug therapy as well as with complications associated with heart failure. A positive VDRL may be evidence of syphilitic heart disease. PT values are useful in monitoring anticoagulant therapy.

NP: Evaluation; CN: Physiological integrity; CNS: Reduction of risk potential; CL: Application

61. In preparing a client for cardiac catheterization, which of the following statements or questions is most appropriate?

1. "Are you allergic to contrast dyes or shellfish?"
2. "Have you ever had this kind of procedure before?"
3. "You'll need to fast 24 hours before the procedure."
4. "You'll be given medication to help you sleep during the procedure."

61. 1. The nurse must assess the client for allergies to iodine before the procedure because the dye used during catheterization contains iodine. The client needs to stay awake during the procedure to follow directions, such as taking a deep breath and holding it during injection of the dye, and to report chest, neck, or jaw discomfort. The client is instructed to fast for 6 hours before the procedure. The client will be asked to empty his bladder before the procedure. Knowing the client's history and prior experience with this procedure would be helpful, but knowing the client's allergies is more important.

NP: Implementation; CN: Physiological integrity; CNS: Reduction of risk potential; CL: Application

62. Which of the following techniques is considered a noninvasive diagnostic method to evaluate cardiac changes?

1. Cardiac biopsy
2. Cardiac catheterization
3. Magnetic resonance imaging (MRI)
4. Pericardiocentesis

62. 3. MRI is a noninvasive procedure that aids in the diagnosis and detection of thoracic aortic aneurysm and evaluation of coronary artery disease, pericardial disease, and cardiac masses. Cardiac biopsy, cardiac catheterization, and pericardiocentesis are invasive techniques used to evaluate cardiac changes.

NP: Analysis; CN: Health promotion and maintenance; CNS: Prevention and early detection of disease; CL: Knowledge

63. In evaluating an electrocardiogram (ECG) strip in a telemetry unit, a nurse notices a client is having premature ventricular contractions (PVCs). Which of the following criteria is used to evaluate the presence of PVCs on the ECG strip?

1. There's no PR interval.
2. The R-R interval is irregular.
3. Ventricular rate is slower than atrial rate.
4. The QRS complex is followed by a compensatory pause.

63. 4. The QRS complex is followed by a compensatory pause that ends when the underlying rhythm resumes. This is one of the ECG criteria used to evaluate PVCs. The remaining responses are ECG criteria used to evaluate atrial flutter.

NP: Evaluation; CN: Physiological integrity; CNS: Reduction of risk potential; CL: Analysis

64. In evaluating an electrocardiogram (ECG) strip for the presence of a pacemaker, which of the following criteria indicates a malfunction?

1. Short T waves
2. Normal sinus rhythm
3. Pacing spikes appearing at different times during a cardiac cycle
4. Pacing spike followed by a wide QRS complex

64. 3. When pacing spikes appear at different times during a cardiac cycle, it indicates a failure to capture. Failure to capture may result in inappropriate pacing; the ECG would show a pacing spike delivered on time but not followed by a wide QRS complex. Tall T waves or an irregular heart rate indicate a failure-to-sense malfunction.

NP: Evaluation; CN: Physiological integrity; CNS: Reduction of risk potential; CL: Analysis

65. In caring for a client with arterial insufficiency, which of the following instructions is most appropriate for home health teaching?
1. "You may leave your feet open to the air."
2. "It's best to sit and rest for several hours a day."
3. "Avoid crossing your legs at the knees or ankles."
4. "It's best to wear tight socks instead of no socks."

65. 3. Leg crossing should be avoided because it compresses the vessels in the legs. Feet and extremities must be protected to reduce the risk of trauma. Avoid constrictive clothing, such as tight elastic on socks, to prevent compression of vessels in the legs. Injury to the extremity will require more blood to heal than to keep the tissue intact; an extremity with compromised circulation may not be able to provide the extra blood required.
NP: Implementation; CN: Physiological integrity; CNS: Reduction of risk potential; CL: Application

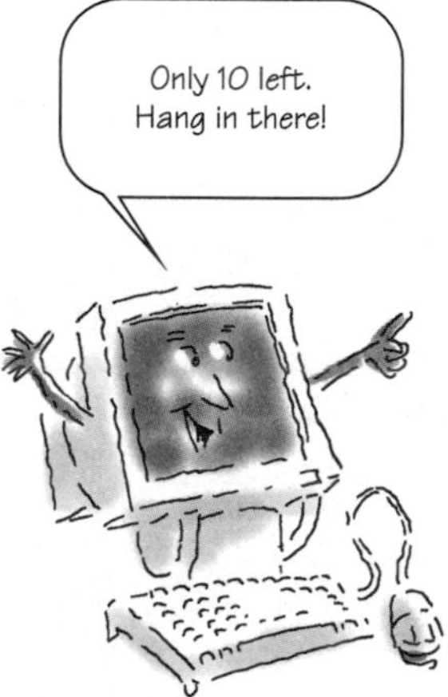
Only 10 left.
Hang in there!

66. Which of the following instructions is correct for home health teaching for a client taking oral anticoagulants?
1. "You may shave with a standard razor."
2. "You may take ibuprofen or aspirin for pain."
3. "Take the anticoagulant at the same time each day."
4. "It's important to eat a large quantity of green leafy vegetables."

66. 3. It's important to take the anticoagulant at the same time each day to maintain an adequate blood level. Avoid taking aspirin or ibuprofen because these drugs decrease clotting time. Eating a large amount of green leafy vegetables, which contain vitamin K, increases the clotting time, thus requiring more anticoagulants. An electric razor reduces the risk of cutting the skin. Avoid the use of standard razors.
NP: Implementation; CN: Physiological integrity; CNS: Reduction of risk potential; CL: Application

67. Which of the following actions is most appropriate to reduce sensory deprivation for a visually impaired elderly client in the hospital?
1. Keep the lights dimmed.
2. Close the curtains or blinds on windows to reduce glare.
3. Open the hospital door so bright light can shine in the room.
4. Open the curtains during the day so the sun can shine brightly.

67. 2. Closing curtains or blinds on windows can reduce glare and improve vision for the older client. Controlled lighting can help the older client see better in the hospital. Adequate background lighting helps the older client decrease visual accommodation when moving from brightly lit to dimly lit rooms and hallways.
NP: Implementation; CN: Physiological integrity; CNS: Reduction of risk potential; CL: Application

68. Which of the following actions is most appropriate to reduce sensory overload for a hearing-impaired elderly client in the coronary care unit?
1. Keep the overhead light on continuously.
2. Discuss the client's condition at the bedside.
3. Allow all family members to stay with the client.
4. Limit bedside conversation to that directed to the client.

68. 4. Limiting bedside conversation to that directed to the client creates fewer disturbances, thus reducing sensory overload. Turning off or dimming the overhead lights further reduces visual stimulation and facilitates day and night light fluctuations. Although fostering family interaction with the client is necessary, only one or two family members should be allowed to visit with the client at one time. Crowding of people in the client's room may precipitate a loss of privacy and control for the client.
NP: Implementation; CN: Physiological integrity; CNS: Reduction of risk potential; CL: Application

69. Which of the following instructions is most appropriate in home health teaching for a client with osteoarthritis of the left knee?

1. Use cold on joints.
2. Keep the knee extended.
3. Develop a weight-reduction plan.
4. Have someone help the client in activities of daily living.

69. 3. Reducing weight decreases joint stress. Local moist heat provides pain relief and will decrease stiffness. The client should perform muscle-strengthening exercises, which help prevent joint stiffness. The nurse should allow the client to perform activities of daily living with less assistance.

NP: Implementation; CN: Physiological integrity; CNS: Reduction of risk potential; CL: Application

70. A home care aide notified the agency that she found the client lying on the floor. When the home health nurse arrives, the newly diagnosed diabetic client is semicomatose, with a fast heart rate and low blood pressure. The client's skin is warm and dry. Which of the following conditions is indicated?

1. Hypoglycemia
2. Cardiogenic shock
3. Diabetic ketoacidosis (DKA)
4. Hyperosmolar hypoglycemic nonketotic syndrome (HHNS)

70. 3. DKA develops as a result of severe insulin deficiency. The incidence of DKA generally results from undiagnosed diabetes and inadequacy of prescribed medication and dietary therapies. HHNS is a deadly complication of diabetes distinguished by severe hyperglycemia, dehydration, and changed mental status. Hypoglycemia involves episodes of low blood glucose levels caused by erratic or altered absorption of insulin. In cardiogenic shock, the client has pale, cool, and moist skin.

NP: Implementation; CN: Physiological integrity; CNS: Physiological adaptation; CL: Application

71. A nurse is standing next to a person eating fried shrimp at a parade. Suddenly, the man clutches at his throat and is unable to speak, cough, or breathe. The nurse asks the man if he's choking and he nods yes. Which of the following responses is most appropriate?

1. Attempt rescue breathing.
2. Perform the Heimlich maneuver.
3. Deliver external chest compressions.
4. Use the head tilt-chin lift maneuver to establish the airway.

71. 2. If a conscious victim acknowledges that he's choking, the best response is to perform the Heimlich maneuver to relieve the airway obstruction. The other options are used for an unresponsive victim with absent heart rate and breathing.

NP: Implementation; CN: Physiological integrity; CNS: Physiological adaptation; CL: Application

72. Preparation is the key to successful resuscitation. Which of the following responses is most appropriate to prepare for a cardiopulmonary emergency?

1. Have nasal oxygen ready when needed.
2. Place an oropharyngeal airway at the bedside.
3. Keep the medication cart locked up for safety.
4. Don't start an I.V. line unless necessary.

72. 2. A nurse should learn to anticipate clinical deterioration before overt signs and symptoms are apparent. If a client is having breathing difficulties, the nurse should place an oropharyngeal airway at the bedside while the client is monitored for deterioration. The emergency cart should be placed outside the client's room for easy access. If breathing stops, the client will need to be intubated and placed on a respirator, if necessary. The client should have a stable I.V. line for administration of emergency drugs.

NP: Implementation; CN: Physiological integrity; CNS: Physiological adaptation; CL: Analysis

73. In preparing for cardioversion, which of the following actions is most appropriate?

1. Keep the client awake and alert.
2. Keep the side rails up for client safety.
3. Set the machine on SYNC and charge at 200 watts.
4. Set the machine on DEFIB and charge at 400 watts.

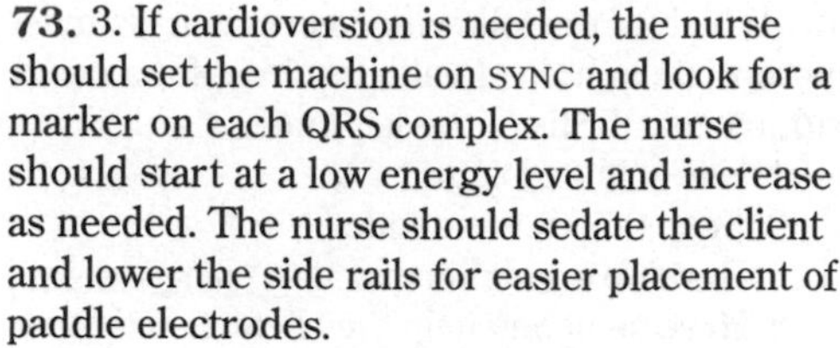

73. 3. If cardioversion is needed, the nurse should set the machine on SYNC and look for a marker on each QRS complex. The nurse should start at a low energy level and increase as needed. The nurse should sedate the client and lower the side rails for easier placement of paddle electrodes.

NP: Implementation; CN: Physiological integrity; CNS: Physiological adaptation; CL: Application

74. A young client is admitted to the emergency department unconscious from an overdose of salicylates. The physician orders dialysis. Which of the following dialysis methods is most appropriate?

1. Hemodialysis
2. Peritoneal dialysis
3. Continuous hemofiltration
4. Continuous ambulatory peritoneal dialysis

74. 1. Hemodialysis is a rapid method to correct fluid and electrolyte problems. It's also a fast way to treat accidental or intentional poisonings as a means of clearing drugs or toxins from the body. Peritoneal dialysis, continuous ambulatory peritoneal dialysis, and continuous hemofiltration are slow methods of removing toxins.

NP: Implementation; CN: Physiological integrity; CNS: Physiological adaptation; CL: Application

75. Which of the following nursing actions is most appropriate for a low birth-weight neonate?

1. Keep the temperature cool.
2. Gavage feed the neonate if he has a weak sucking reflex.
3. Keep the neonate uncovered in the humidified incubator.
4. Keep the I.V. infusion at a keep-vein-open rate.

75. 2. To maintain adequate nutrition, a low birth-weight neonate may need to be gavage fed. The neonate should be kept warm. The nurse should avoid situations that might predispose the neonate to chilling, such as exposure to cool air. Maintain adequate parenteral fluids to prevent dehydration.

NP: Implementation; CN: Physiological integrity; CNS: Physiological adaptation; CL: Application

Congratulations! You did a great job, and I'm totally proud of you! Yaaaaaaaay!

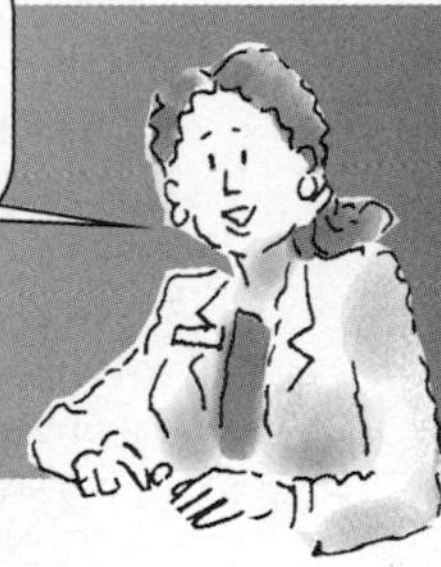
Here's another
comprehensive test to
practice for the NCLEX.
Check it out!

COMPREHENSIVE Test 4

1. A nurse-manager has identified several personal problems with a staff member. Which of the following approaches is best for the nurse-manager to take?

1. Map out a plan of action for each problem and discuss it.
2. Begin to solve the first problem and work through the list.
3. Ask the staff member to select the problem she would like to resolve.
4. Prioritize the problems with the staff member and begin to work on them together.

1. 4. It's important for the nurse-manager and staff member to agree on which problem is a priority and work on its resolution together. Mapping out the problem without input from the staff member leaves the possibility that the staff member might not be committed to work on its resolution.

NP: Planning; CN: Safe, effective care environment; CNS: Management of care; CL: Application

2. A team leader notes increasing unrest among the staff members. Which of the following actions is best for the team leader to take?

1. Discuss the problem with a coworker.
2. Report the problem to the nurse-manager.
3. Bring the group together and discuss the team leader's perception.
4. Ignore the problem and hope the attitude won't interfere with the functioning of the floor.

2. 3. The leader should comment to the group on the observed behavior. This is a firm approach but one that shows concern. Ignoring problems or discussing them with someone else doesn't confront the issue at hand.

NP: Implementation; CN: Safe, effective care environment; CNS: Management of care; CL: Application

3. A physician ordered a urine specimen for culture and sensitivity stat. Which of the following approaches is best for the nurse to use in delegating this task?

1. "We need a stat urine culture on the client in room 101."
2. "Please get the urine for culture for the client in room 101."
3. "A stat urine was ordered for the client in room 101. Would you get it?"
4. "We need a urine for culture stat on the client in room 101. Tell me when you send it to the lab."

3. 4. This option not only delegates the task, but also provides a checkpoint. To effectively delegate, you need to follow up on what someone else is doing. The other options don't provide for feedback, which is essential for communication and delegation.

NP: Implementation; CN: Safe, effective care environment; CNS: Management of care; CL: Application

4. A 67-year-old widow is visiting a physician for an annual check up. The client asks the nurse, "Do you think it's wrong to masturbate?" Which of the following responses by the nurse is best?

1. "How do you feel about that?"
2. "Do you really want to do that?"
3. "I think you're a little too old for that."
4. "Why don't you ask your physician?"

4. 1. It's essential in communication to find out how the client thinks and feels. The second and third options are biased in their reply and put the client down. The last option tells the client the nurse isn't interested. The client might be too uncomfortable to discuss this topic with the physician.

NP: Implementation; CN: Psychosocial integrity; CNS: Coping and adaptation; CL: Comprehension

5. A client on a clear liquid diet is writing his menu. Which choice indicates that he needs further teaching?

1. Gelatin dessert
2. Milkshake
3. Popsicle or similar frozen dessert
4. Tea

5. 2. Full-liquid diets contain milk, cereal, gruel, clear liquids, and plain frozen desserts. The clear-liquid diet contains only foods that are clear and liquid at room or body temperature, such as gelatin, fat-free broth, bouillon, popsicles or similar frozen desserts, tea, and regular or decaffeinated coffee.

NP: Planning; CN: Safe, effective care environment; CNS: Management of care; CL: Knowledge

6. Which of the following medications should a nurse withhold from a client 6 hours before a series of pulmonary function tests (PFTs)?

1. Antibiotics
2. Antitussives
3. Bronchodilators
4. Corticosteroids

6. 3. PFTs measure the volume and capacity of air. If a bronchodilator is given, it will improve the bronchial airflow and alter the test results. The other drugs would have no effect on the bronchial tree with regard to PFT results.

NP: Assessment; CN: Physiological integrity; CNS: Pharmacological and parenteral therapies; CL: Comprehension

7. A client returns to a nursing unit after a bronchoscopy and is expectorating pink-tinged mucus. Which of the following actions by the nurse is most appropriate?

1. Notify the physician as soon as possible.
2. Take the client's vital signs, then call the physician.
3. Auscultate the client's lung fields for possible pulmonary edema.
4. Tell the client this is expected after the procedure, but continue to monitor the client.

7. 4. Pink-tinged mucus is an expected outcome after a bronchoscopy due to irritation of the bronchial tree. The client should be told this is common, but that he'll be monitored. The physician doesn't need to be called with this finding. This symptom isn't related to pulmonary edema.

NP: Assessment; CN: Health promotion and maintenance; CNS: Prevention and early detection of disease; CL: Comprehension

8. The assessment of a client on the first day after thoracotomy shows a temperature of 100°F (37.8° C); heart rate, 96 beats/minute; blood pressure, 136/86 mm Hg; and shallow respirations at 24 breaths/minute, with rhonchi at the bases. The client complains of incisional pain. Which of the following nursing actions has priority?

1. Medicate the client for pain.
2. Help the client get out of bed.
3. Give ibuprofen (Motrin) as ordered to reduce the fever.
4. Encourage the client to cough and deep-breathe.

8. 1. Although all the interventions are incorporated in this client's care plan, the priority is to relieve pain and make the client comfortable. This would give the client the energy and stamina to achieve the other objectives.

NP: Assessment; CN: Physiological integrity; CNS: Basic care and comfort; CL: Application

9. Which of the following interventions is most important to include in a care plan for a client with atelectasis?

1. Give oxygen continuously at 3 L/minute.
2. Cough and deep-breathe every 4 hours.
3. Use the incentive spirometer every hour.
4. Get the client out of bed to a chair every day.

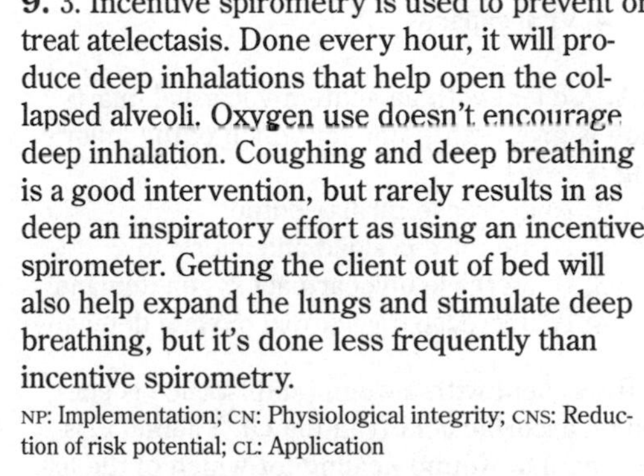

9. 3. Incentive spirometry is used to prevent or treat atelectasis. Done every hour, it will produce deep inhalations that help open the collapsed alveoli. Oxygen use doesn't encourage deep inhalation. Coughing and deep breathing is a good intervention, but rarely results in as deep an inspiratory effort as using an incentive spirometer. Getting the client out of bed will also help expand the lungs and stimulate deep breathing, but it's done less frequently than incentive spirometry.

NP: Implementation; CN: Physiological integrity; CNS: Reduction of risk potential; CL: Application

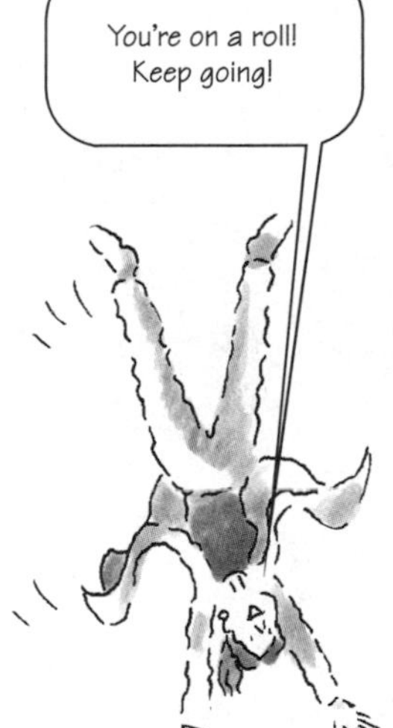
You're on a roll!
Keep going!

10. Two hours after submucous resection, the client's nostrils are packed and a drip pad is anchored under the nose. Which of the following assessments alerts the nurse that the surgical site is bleeding?

1. Frequent swallowing
2. Dry mucous membranes
3. Decrease in urine output
4. Temperature elevation

10. 1. Frequent swallowing is a sign of hemorrhage in this surgery. Decreased urine output and dry mucous membranes, as well as temperature elevation, are usually signs of dehydration.

NP: Analysis; CN: Physiological integrity; CNS: Reduction of risk potential; CL: Analysis

11. A bedridden client develops disuse osteoporosis. Which of the following interventions is most important for this client?

1. Turn, cough, and deep breathe.
2. Increase fluids to 3,000 ml daily.
3. Promote venous return by elevating the legs.
4. Provide active and passive range-of-motion exercise.

11. 4. All the interventions listed are good for a bedridden client. However, active and passive range-of-motion exercises provide the mechanical stresses of weight bearing that are absent and lead to disuse osteoporosis.

NP: Implementation; CN: Health promotion and maintenance; CNS: Prevention and early detection of disease; CL: Application

12. An elderly client on bed rest for a week after a bout of pneumonia is in a negative nitrogen balance. Which of the following complications has highest priority?
1. Constipation
2. Renal calculi
3. Muscle wasting
4. Vitamin B_6 deficiency

12. 3. Negative nitrogen balance leads to muscle wasting. The body breaks down muscle tissue to use as energy. Renal calculi can be a complication of bed rest and demineralization of the bone but treating a negative nitrogen balance takes priority. Constipation and vitamin B_6 deficiency also need to be corrected but aren't of the highest priority.

NP: Implementation; CN: Physiological integrity; CNS: Physiological adaptation; CL: Comprehension

13. The Pao_2 of a client with asthma gives information on which of the following factors?
1. Respiratory excursion
2. Tidal volume
3. Efficiency of gas exchange
4. Vital capacity

13. 3. The Pao_2 reflects the gas exchange ventilation and perfusion. It doesn't measure the respiratory excursion, tidal volume, or vital capacity.

NP: Assessment; CN: Health promotion and maintenance; CNS: Prevention and early detection of disease; CL: Knowledge

14. A client with an acute myocardial infarction is given morphine for which of the following reasons?
1. To decrease cardiac output
2. To increase preload and afterload
3. To increase myocardial oxygen demand
4. To decrease myocardial oxygen demand

14. 4. Morphine sulfate will calm and relax the client and decrease respiratory rate, anxiety, and stress, thus decreasing myocardial oxygen demand.

NP: Implementation; CN: Physiological integrity; CNS: Pharmacological and parenteral therapies; CL: Comprehension

15. A client with a wound dehiscence is started on ascorbic acid (vitamin C). Vitamin C is essential to wound healing for which of the following reasons?
1. Vitamin C reduces edema.
2. Vitamin C enhances oxygen transport.
3. Vitamin C enhances protein synthesis.
4. Vitamin C restores the inflammatory process.

15. 3. Vitamin C enhances the synthesis of protein and is essential for the maturation and repair of tissue. It doesn't affect the inflammatory process or oxygen transport or reduce edema.

NP: Implementation; CN: Physiological integrity; CNS: Pharmacological and parenteral therapies; CL: Comprehension

16. A client with which of the following conditions is expected to have an increase of tactile fremitus?
1. Atelectasis
2. Emphysema
3. Pneumonia
4. Pneumothorax

16. 3. Pneumonia produces a consolidation of mucus and debris. Mucus causes the lung field to have an increase in tactile fremitus. The other diseases involve air, which would decrease tactile fremitus.

NP: Assessment; CN: Health promotion and maintenance; CNS: Prevention and early detection of disease; CL: Comprehension

17. Which of the following injuries is least likely to become infected?

1. Contusion of the ankle in an 18-year-old client
2. Laceration from glass in a 6-year-old client
3. Stab wound in the leg of a 37-year-old client
4. Cat bite to the left hand of an elderly client

18. A client is hospitalized for 5 days with mononucleosis. Which of the following assessment findings indicates a possibly serious consequence?

1. Vomiting
2. Dark brown urine
3. Temperature of 101° F (38.3° C)
4. Cervical lymphadenopathy

19. A nurse is teaching a client about lifestyle changes that need to be made after a myocardial infarction (MI). The diagnosis of ineffective individual coping is supported when the client is observed in which of the following actions?

1. Reading a book about meal planning
2. Pacing the floor of his room on occasion
3. Sitting quietly in his room for a short time
4. Telling his family he didn't have an MI

20. A client with a history of myasthenia gravis is admitted to the emergency department with complaints of respiratory distress. The client's condition worsens and arterial blood gases are drawn. Which of the following conditions is expected?

1. Metabolic acidosis
2. Metabolic alkalosis
3. Respiratory acidosis
4. Respiratory alkalosis

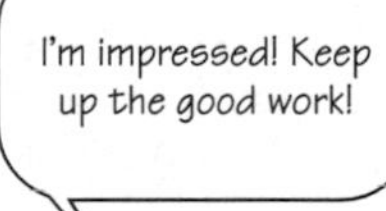

I'm impressed! Keep up the good work!

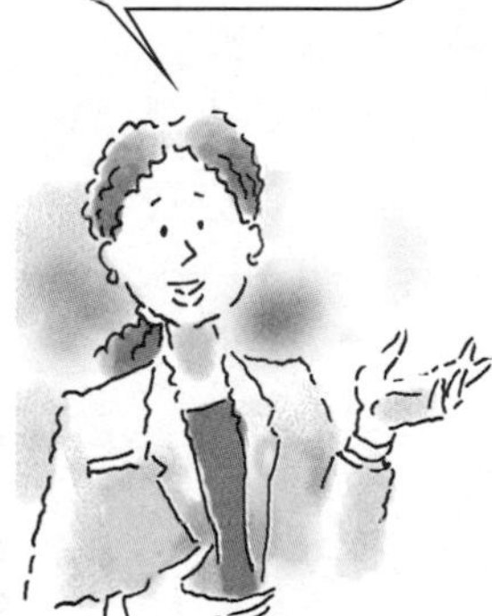

17. 1. A contusion doesn't involve a break in the skin. The other options all involve a break in the skin that could lead to infection.

NP: Assessment; CN: Physiological integrity; CNS: Reduction of risk potential; CL: Comprehension

18. 2. Dark brown urine could indicate the presence of bilirubin and implicate liver involvement. The other answers are typical findings for a client with this diagnosis.

NP: Assessment; CN: Physiological integrity; CNS: Physiological adaptation; CL: Analysis

19. 4. The client is showing the defense mechanism of denial. Reading a book on meal planning is a positive intervention. Sitting quietly is a normal behavior. The client needs time to come to terms with his diagnosis. Pacing the floor on occasion is a form of anxiety that's normal for the client to experience.

NP: Evaluation; CN: Psychosocial integrity; CNS: Coping and adaptation; CL: Analysis

20. 3. The client has a restrictive lung problem because of myasthenia gravis. This is aggravated by respiratory distress. Because of the restrictive problem, the client won't be able to exhale efficiently and carbon dioxide will build up, causing respiratory acidosis. Metabolic acidosis is a metabolic condition that occurs with either accumulation of acids or excessive loss of bases in the body, such as in diarrhea or renal failure. Metabolic alkalosis occurs due to excessive acid loss or base retention, such as from vomiting. Respiratory alkalosis results from a decreased carbon dioxide level, which could occur if the patient were hyperventilating.

NP: Analysis; CN: Physiological integrity; CNS: Physiological adaptation; CL: Analysis

21. A client who had a thoracotomy is using oxygen and having an arterial blood gas (ABG) analysis. Which of the following is correct to tell the client?

1. "The nurse will shave the puncture site before the test."
2. "You need to keep the oxygen mask on for the entire test."
3. "You'll be suctioned immediately before the blood is drawn."
4. "You won't be allowed to drink anything for 2 hours before the blood is drawn."

21. 2. To determine the effectiveness of oxygen therapy, ABGs are drawn with the oxygen in use. This also needs to be written on the test form. Suctioning decreases available oxygen. No special preparations for the test with regard to skin preparation or diet are needed.

NP: Implementation; CN: Physiological integrity; CNS: Basic care and comfort; CL: Application

22. Which of the following conditions causes heart failure after a myocardial infarction (MI)?

1. Increased workload of the heart
2. Increased oxygen demands of the heart
3. Inability of the heart chambers to adequately fill
4. Impairment of contractile function of the damaged myocardium

22. 4. After an MI, the injured myocardium is replaced by scar tissue. This scar tissue causes the ventricle to pump less efficiently. After an MI has resolved, oxygen and workload demands should normalize and the heart's chambers should fill adequately.

NP: Assessment; CN: Physiological integrity; CNS: Physiological adaptation; CL: Comprehension

23. A client is admitted to the emergency department with severe epistaxis. The physician inserts posterior packing. Later, the client is anxious and says he doesn't feel he's breathing right. Which of the following nursing actions is appropriate?

1. Cut the packing strings and remove the packing.
2. Reassure the client what he's experiencing is normal.
3. Ask the client to fully explain what he means by "right."
4. Use a flashlight and inspect the posterior oral cavity of the client.

23. 4. The nurse must assess the patency of the airway. The packing might have become dislodged. The client is too anxious to explain what he means. The nurse shouldn't remove the packing or give the client false reassurance.

NP: Implementation; CN: Physiological integrity; CNS: Reduction of risk potential; CL: Analysis

24. A registered nurse is teaching another nurse how to measure pulmonary artery pressures. She explains the wedge pressure is a reflection of which of the following pressures?

1. Systemic vascular resistance
2. Right ventricular end pressure
3. Right atrial presystolic pressure
4. Left ventricular end-diastolic pressure

24. 4. The pulmonary capillary wedge pressure is the reflection of the pressure in the left ventricle at rest, which is end diastole. Wedge pressure doesn't reflect pressures in the right side of the heart or systemic vascular resistance.

NP: Assessment; CN: Physiological integrity; CNS: Physiological adaptation; CL: Knowledge

25. Which of the following actions correctly explains the purpose of diaphragmatic breathing exercises for a client with chronic obstructive pulmonary disease (COPD)?
1. Dilate the bronchioles.
2. Decrease vital capacity.
3. Increase residual volume.
4. Decrease alveolar ventilation.

25. 1. In COPD, the bronchioles constrict during exhalation due to pressure changes in the lungs. Diaphragmatic breathing exercises keep the bronchioles open during exhalation. These exercises aren't performed for the other reasons stated.

NP: Assessment; CN: Physiological integrity; CNS: Reduction of risk potential; CL: Comprehension

26. A client with chronic obstructive pulmonary disease (COPD) is being discharged from the hospital. The nurse provided teaching on medications, diet, and exercise. Which of the following statements by the client indicates more teaching is needed?
1. "I'll eat six small meals a day."
2. "I'll get a flu shot every winter."
3. "I'll walk every morning before breakfast."
4. "I'll call my physician if I get cold symptoms."

26. 3. The worst time of the day for a client with COPD is morning. Exercise is important, but should be done later in the day. All other choices are appropriate for the client with COPD.

NP: Evaluation; CN: Physiological integrity; CNS: Basic care and comfort; CL: Comprehension

27. A client is showing symptoms of bronchial obstruction. Which of the following assessment findings is expected?
1. Hacking cough
2. Diminished breath sounds
3. Production of rust-colored sputum
4. Decreased use of accessory muscles

27. 2. Bronchial obstruction means no passage of air through the bronchi, so diminished or no breath sounds would be heard. There would be increased use of accessory muscles. A hacking cough is often associated with upper respiratory tract infection and dryness in the upper airways. Rust-colored sputum is a sign of pneumococcal pneumonia.

NP: Assessment; CN: Physiological integrity; CNS: Physiological adaptation; CL: Knowledge

28. A client has just started treatment for tuberculosis. Rifampin is the drug ordered by the physician. Which of the following statements indicates the client has a good understanding of his medication?
1. "I won't go to family gatherings for 6 months."
2. "My urine will look orange because of the medication."
3. "Now I don't need to cover my mouth or nose when I sneeze or cough."
4. "I told my wife to throw away all the spoons and forks before I come home."

28. 2. Rifampin discolors body fluids, such as urine and tears. The client can go to family functions and eat with normal utensils. The client should cover his mouth and nose when coughing and sneezing until he has been on the medication at least 2 weeks.

NP: Implementation; CN: Physiological integrity; CNS: Pharmacological and parenteral therapies; CL: Application

29. Which of the following actions should be initiated before feeding a client with Parkinson's disease?

1. Sit the client upright.
2. Have suction available.
3. Order a clear liquid diet.
4. Have a speech therapist evaluate the client.

29. 4. A speech therapist can evaluate the client's swallowing and make recommendations before the client is fed. Aspiration due to involuntary movement is common. Sitting the client upright and having suction available are helpful when feeding the client, but evaluation of the client's swallowing ability should come first. Clear liquids may be too difficult for the client; semisoft foods may be easier to swallow.

NP: Implementation; CN: Physiological integrity; CNS: Reduction of risk potential; CL: Knowledge

30. Management of a pregnant client with cardiovascular disease focuses on which of the following treatments?

1. Rest
2. Hospitalization
3. Therapeutic abortion
4. Continuous cardiac monitoring

30. 1. The goal of antepartum management is to prevent complications and minimize the strain on the client. This is done with rest. Hospitalization may be required in older women or those with previous decompensation. Therapeutic abortion is considered in severe dysfunction, especially in the first trimester. Continuous cardiac monitoring isn't necessary.

NP: Implementation; CN: Physiological integrity; CNS: Reduction of risk potential; CL: Knowledge

31. Which of the following assessment findings most likely indicates a urinary tract infection (UTI) in a 5-year-old child?

1. Incontinence
2. Lack of thirst
3. Concentrated urine
4. Subnormal temperature

31. 1. Incontinence in a toilet-trained child is associated with UTI. Subnormal temperature isn't a sign of UTI. Concentrated urine is a sign of dehydration. Lack of thirst wouldn't be expected in a child with UTI.

NP: Assessment; CN: Health promotion and maintenance; CNS: Prevention and early detection of disease; CL: Application

32. During a home health visit, a nurse assesses a client's medication and notes the client has two prescriptions for fluid retention. One prescription reads "Lasix, 40 mg, one tablet daily." The next prescription reads "Furosemide, 40 mg, one tablet daily." Which of the following instructions is given to the client?

1. Take both medications as ordered.
2. Lasix and furosemide are the same drug.
3. Use Lasix one day and furosemide the next day.
4. Throw away one of the drugs to avoid confusing the client.

32. 2. Using generic names for medications is common, especially for home health clients. It's the responsibility of the nurse to teach the client both brand and generic names of drugs. Setting up medications in a medication tray, using only one pharmacy to dispense medications, and using all medications until the bottle is emptied will reduce medication errors.

NP: Implementation; CN: Physiological integrity; CNS: Pharmacological and parenteral therapies; CL: Analysis

33. A school nurse is called to assess a preadolescent Vietnamese girl attending a new school in an affluent district. A teacher tells the nurse the student sits in the back of the class and won't speak when spoken to, although her parents confirmed the student speaks English. Which of the following assessment findings is most likely?

1. The student is experiencing cultural shock.
2. The student is developing a peer support system.
3. The student is going through a socialization period.
4. The student is becoming acculturated to the new school.

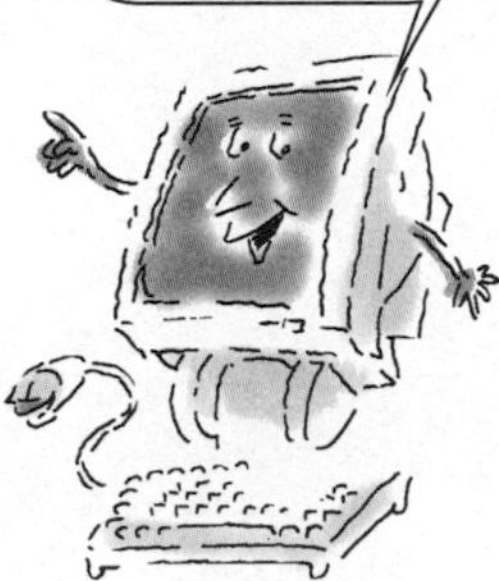
You're doing
sensationally! I
mean, I should do
so well, eh?
My, my, my.

33. 1. Cultural shock is a feeling of helplessness, discomfort, and a state of disorientation when an outsider attempts to comprehend or adapt to a new cultural situation. Acculturation occurs when there's a blending of cultural or ethnic backgrounds. This process takes time to develop. Peer groups usually develop based on the background, interests, and capabilities of its members. Developing peer cultures is part of the socialization process.

NP: Analysis; CN: Health promotion and maintenance; CNS: Growth and development through the life span; CL: Application

34. A school nurse is screening for hearing and vision at a local middle school. Which of the following techniques is used to communicate effectively with this age group?

1. Give undivided attention to each student.
2. Have the parents present during the screening.
3. Have several adolescents listen to each other's health histories.
4. Use puppets or dolls to show how the screening is going to take place.

34. 1. Give undivided attention to communicate effectively with adolescents. Respect their privacy. The presence of parents and use of puppets or dolls can be used to effectively communicate with younger children.

NP: Assessment; CN: Health promotion and maintenance; CNS: Growth and development through the life span; CL: Application

35. A nurse practitioner at a local rural health clinic is screening an 18-month-old infant for developmental problems. Which of the following developmental screening tests is used?

1. Goodenough-Harris Draw-a-Person Test
2. Denver Developmental Screening Test (DDST)
3. McCarthy Scales of Children's Abilities (MSCA)
4. Preschool readiness screening scales

35. 2. The DDST is applicable for children from birth through age 6. Preschool readiness screening scales are designed for screening 5-year-old children for readiness for school. The Goodenough-Harris Draw-a-Person test is used to assess intellectual ability in children ages 3 to 10. The MSCA is a developmental tool for children ages 2½ to 8½.

NP: Assessment; CN: Health promotion and maintenance; CNS: Growth and development through the life span; CL: Application

36. In preparing educational intervention for college students, the nurse understands that drinking alcoholic beverages may be a behavior commonly associated with the relief of which of the following problems?

1. Fatigue
2. Anxiety
3. Headache
4. Stomach pain

36. 2. Drinking alcoholic beverages is commonly thought to alleviate anxiety. These beverages aren't commonly used to relieve fatigue, headache, or stomach pain.

NP: Assessment; CN: Psychosocial integrity; CNS: Coping and adaptation; CL: Application

37. An educational forum about relaxation techniques is provided for college students preparing for their final exams. Which of the following relaxation techniques is used to counteract anxiety?
1. Meditation
2. Music therapy
3. Dance therapy
4. Reality orientation

37. 1. Meditation is a relaxation therapy used to counteract anxiety related to stress-inducing internal and external stimuli. Music therapy, dance therapy, and reality orientation are used as adjuncts to psychiatric care.
NP: Analysis; CN: Psychosocial integrity; CNS: Coping and adaptation; CL: Application

38. During the interview of a parent of a 12-year-old child, a teacher discovers the child has a history of conduct disorder. Which of the following behaviors is characteristic of this disorder?
1. Plays well with peers
2. No aggressive behavior
3. Obsessed with making fires
4. Becomes competitive in sports

38. 3. Adolescents with conduct disorder commonly become obsessed with making fires. They also have difficulty establishing relationships. These children aren't just competitive, but physically aggressive in sports, violating the rights of others.
NP: Assessment; CN: Psychosocial integrity; CNS: Psychosocial adaptation; CL: Comprehension

39. A 40-year-old client is admitted to the local women's shelter after being raped by her estranged husband. The client describes the traumatic event. Which of the following responses by the nurse is best?
1. Change the subject to prevent the client from crying.
2. Listen attentively while the client describes the event.
3. Arrange for the client to tell her story in group therapy.
4. Medicate the client with a tranquilizer to prevent hysteria.

39. 2. Retelling the event is part of the healing process. Giving medication and changing the subject don't allow the client to integrate the experience into her life. Group therapy may be helpful, but the best nursing response is to listen and convey empathy.
NP: Implementation; CN: Psychosocial integrity; CNS: Psychosocial adaptation; CL: Application

40. A nurse is assessing a client with manic-depressive disorder. The client tells the nurse her family physician prescribed lithium. Which of the following symptoms indicates the client is developing lithium toxicity?
1. Lethargy
2. Hypertension
3. Hyperexcitability
4. Low urine output

40. 1. Nausea, vomiting, diarrhea, thirst, polyuria, lethargy, slurred speech, hypotension, muscle weakness, and fine hand tremors are signs of lithium toxicity.
NP: Assessment; CN: Physiological integrity; CNS: Pharmacological and parenteral therapies; CL: Application

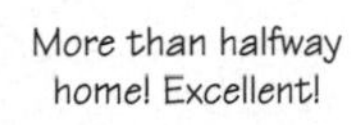
More than halfway
home! Excellent!

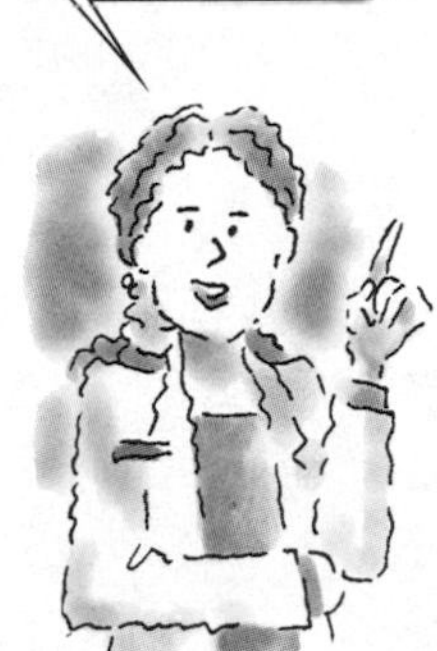

41. Which of the following interventions is used during assessment of a pediatric client?

1. Ask the parents to leave the room during health assessment.
2. Position the client on an examination table or bed at all times.
3. Organize the health assessment in the same way for every infant or child.
4. Identify the source (child, parent, caregiver, guardian) and indicate the reliability of the information obtained.

41. 4. Document the source of information obtained for the nursing assessment of a child. Depending on the child's age, parents may help position and hold the child, facilitating assessment. Separation from the parent may cause anxiety and increase the child's fear and distrust. Organization of the assessment is changed to accommodate the individual child's age and development.

NP: Assessment; CN: Health promotion and maintenance; CNS: Growth and development through the life span; CL: Comprehension

42. Which of the following interventions is used during assessment of an elderly client?

1. Ask the client to change positions quickly.
2. Keep the room temperature cool during health assessment.
3. Speak loudly and quickly to facilitate understanding of directions.
4. Change the height of the examination table or modify the client's position.

42. 4. You may need to change the height of the examination table or use a different position when assessing an elderly client. Physiologically, an older client is prone to falls and dizziness due to decreased ability to respond to sudden movements and position changes. The room temperature should be warm because older clients become hypothermic easily. Speak in a slow, normal tone of voice to facilitate communication.

NP: Assessment; CN: Health promotion and maintenance; CNS: Growth and development through the life span; CL: Comprehension

43. Which of the following nursing diagnoses is appropriate for a client with chronic obstructive pulmonary disease who is anxious, dyspneic, and hypoxic?

1. Ineffective breathing pattern related to anxiety
2. Risk for aspiration related to absence of protective mechanisms
3. Impaired gas exchange related to altered oxygen-carrying capacity of the blood
4. Ineffective airway clearance related to presence of tracheobronchial obstruction or secretions

43. 3. The correct nursing diagnosis for this client is based on the impaired oxygenation at the cellular level. The first option applies to a client whose inhalation or exhalation pattern doesn't enable adequate pulmonary inflation or emptying. The second option applies if the client is at risk for aspirating gastric or pharyngeal secretions, food, or fluids into the tracheobronchial passages. The last option is appropriate for a client who's unable to clear secretions or obstructions from the respiratory tract.

NP: Planning; CN: Physiological integrity; CNS: Reduction of risk potential; CL: Application

44. Which of the following statements is a wellness nursing diagnosis?

1. Potential for enhanced spiritual well-being
2. Risk for activity intolerance related to prolonged bed rest
3. Possible self-care deficits: grooming related to fatigue and muscular weakness
4. Constipation related to decreased activity and fluid intake as manifested by hard, formed stool every 3 days

44. 1. Wellness diagnoses are one-part statements containing the label only and begin with "Potential for enhanced," followed by the higher level of wellness desired for the individual or group. The second option is a "risk for" nursing diagnosis. The third option describes a suspected problem for which additional data are needed for confirmation. The last option describes a manifested health problem validated by identifiable major defining characteristics.

NP: Analysis; CN: Psychosocial integrity; CNS: Psychosocial adaptation; CL: Application

45. Which of the following definitions is correct for collaborative problems?

1. Unusual or unexpected human responses to pharmacological agents
2. Pathophysiological responses of body organs or systems for which physicians have ultimate responsibility
3. Human responses for which registered nurses are capable of intervening legally and independently of physicians
4. Certain physiological responses or complications of body organs or systems for which nurses intervene in association with physicians and other disciplines

45. 4. This option describes a collaborative problem that requires physician and nurse prescribed actions. The first option describes an adverse reaction to a pharmacological agent. The second option describes the focus of a medical diagnosis. The third option describes a nursing diagnosis; interventions for nursing diagnoses fall within the scope of practice of registered nurses.

NP: Analysis; CN: Safe, effective care environment; CNS: Management of care; CL: Comprehension

46. An intake nurse at a local mental health facility is admitting a client with psychosis. Which of the following assessment techniques is most valuable to use when planning this client's care?

1. Rorschach test
2. Interview with the client
3. Mental Status Examination (MSE)
4. Review old records of the client

46. 3. The MSE is a basis for planning care with a mental health client, especially one who's psychotic. An interview with a client with psychosis would be unreliable. The Rorschach test is used for depression. Review of old records won't assess the current state on which interventions are planned.

NP: Assessment; CN: Psychosocial integrity; CNS: Psychosocial adaptation; CL: Comprehension

47. Which of the following actions best describes the planning step of the nursing process?

1. Collect client health data.
2. Implement the interventions identified in the plan of care.
3. Evaluate the client's progress toward attainment of the outcomes.
4. Identify the expected goals or outcomes individualized for the client and family.

47. 4. Client goals or outcomes are identified in the planning step of the nursing process. Health data are collected in the assessment step of the nursing process. Planned interventions are done in the implementation step of the nursing process. A client's achievement of outcomes or goals is determined in the evaluation step of the nursing process.

NP: Planning; CN: Safe, effective care environment; CNS: Management of care; CL: Knowledge

48. Which of the following patient outcomes or goals is correct for a client with the nursing diagnosis "risk for disuse syndrome"?

1. The client will be free of musculoskeletal complications.
2. The client will experience shorter periods of immobility and inactivity.
3. The nurse will stress the importance of maintaining adequate fluid intake.
4. The nurse will provide holistic care by collaborating with the health care team.

48. 2. This is an appropriate outcome for a client with this nursing diagnosis. Disuse syndrome, a result of prolonged or unavoidable immobility or inactivity, can be prevented. Musculoskeletal complications indicate actual disuse or complications of immobility. The last two options describe a nursing goal, not a patient outcome.

NP: Planning; CN: Physiological integrity; CNS: Reduction of risk potential; CL: Application

49. A 42-year-old client who underwent a right modified mastectomy with insertion of a Hemovac drain will be hospitalized overnight because of minor complications. Which of the following goal statements is correct?

1. Teach proper care of the incision site and drain by October 12.
2. The client will know how to care for the incision site and drain by October 12.
3. The client will show the proper care of the incision site and drain by October 12.
4. The client will care for the incision site and contend with psychological loss by October 12.

49. 3. This statement contains a specific measurable verb, clearly identifies the client behavior, and includes a date. Option 1 is a nursing goal as written, not a client-centered goal. The client goal of option 2 isn't measurable as stated. Option 4 includes two goals that need to be addressed separately under the appropriate nursing diagnosis and it contains nonmeasurable verbs.

NP: Planning; CN: Physiological integrity; CNS: Basic care and comfort; CL: Application

50. Which of the following expected outcomes or goals is correct for a client with the nursing diagnosis "risk for injury related to lack of awareness of environmental hazards"?

1. Encourage the client to discuss safety rules with children.
2. Help the client learn safety precautions to take in the home.
3. The client will eliminate safety hazards in their surroundings.
4. Refer the client to community resources for more information.

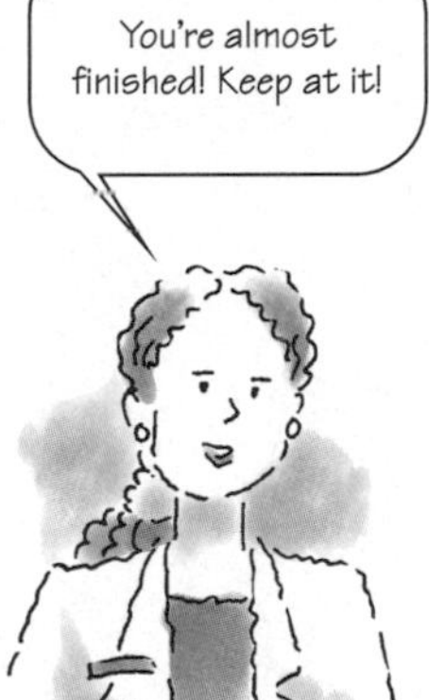
You're almost
finished! Keep at it!

50. 3. This goal is appropriate and measurable as written and focuses on the client. The other options are nursing interventions as written.

NP: Planning; CN: Health promotion and maintenance; CNS: Prevention and early detection of disease; CL: Application

51. Which of the following activities is performed in the planning step of the nursing process?

1. Collect, validate, and organize data.
2. Establish priorities, client goals, and outcome identification.
3. Set priorities, perform nursing interventions, and record actions.
4. Identify problems and synthesize the data gathered during the assessment.

51. 2. Establishing priorities, client goals, and outcome identification are activities of the planning step of the nursing process. Options 1 and 4 describe activities of the assessment step of the nursing process. Option 3 describes activities of the implementation step of the nursing process.

NP: Planning; CN: Safe, effective care environment; CNS: Management of care; CL: Comprehension

52. A client with heart failure is given furosemide (Lasix) 40 mg I.V. daily. The morning serum potassium level is 2.8 mEq/L. Which of the following actions is the most appropriate?
1. Question the physician about the dosage.
2. Give 20 mg of the ordered dose and recheck the laboratory test results.
3. Notify the physician, repeat the potassium as ordered, then give the furosemide.
4. Give the furosemide and get an order for sodium polystyrene sulfonate.

52. 3. Furosemide is a diuretic. As water is lost, so is potassium. Diuresis is a treatment for heart failure. Notifying the physician of the low potassium level and getting an order for potassium chloride is the appropriate action before giving the furosemide. Furosemide, 40 mg, is an appropriate dose for the treatment of heart failure. The nurse shouldn't give half the dose without an order. Giving furosemide and sodium polystyrene sulfonate together would further lower the potassium level.
NP: Analysis; CN: Physiological integrity; CNS: Pharmacological and parenteral therapies; CL: Application

53. Which of the following clients is at greatest risk for developing respiratory alkalosis?
1. A client in labor
2. A client with diabetes
3. A client with renal failure
4. An immediate postoperative client

53. 1. A client's respirations at certain stages of labor increase in volume, causing the $Paco_2$ to decrease, increasing the pH. Diabetes often causes a metabolic imbalance, resulting in metabolic acidosis. The respirations of a postoperative client are usually shallow after anesthesia and, because of pain, often cause respiratory acidosis. In renal failure, the inability of the kidneys to eliminate wastes increases the risk of developing metabolic acidosis.
NP: Analysis; CN: Physiological integrity; CNS: Physiological adaptation; CL: Application

54. Which of the following conditions indicates that a sterile field has been contaminated?
1. Sterile objects are held above the waist of the nurse.
2. Sterile packages are opened with the first edge away from the nurse.
3. The outer inch of the sterile towel hangs over the side of the table.
4. Wetness on the sterile cloth on top of the nonsterile table has been noted.

54. 4. Moisture outside the sterile package and field contaminates it because fluid can be wicked into the sterile field. The outer inch of the drape is considered contaminated but doesn't indicate that the sterile field itself has been contaminated. Bacteria tend to settle, so there's less contamination above waist level and away from the nurse.
NP: Assessment; CN: Safe, effective care environment; CNS: Safety and infection control; CL: Knowledge

55. Which of the following interventions is helpful for a client to retain carbon dioxide?
1. Have the client breathe into a paper bag.
2. Give one ampule of bicarbonate as ordered.
3. Give oxygen at 3 L/minute through a nasal cannula.
4. Reposition the client in a high Fowler's position.

55. 1. By breathing into a paper bag, the client will rebreathe some of his own exhaled carbon dioxide and increase the carbon dioxide in his blood, which will correct his respiratory alkalosis. Giving oxygen won't increase the carbon dioxide to correct the imbalance. Giving one ampule of bicarbonate will worsen the alkalosis. Repositioning the client won't help him retain carbon dioxide.
NP: Implementation; CN: Physiological integrity; CNS: Physiological adaptation; CL: Comprehension

56. A nurse is checking the results of urine studies done on a client with dehydration. Which of the following results reflects an alteration in fluid balance?

1. Protein levels
2. Ketones levels
3. Specific gravity levels
4. Culture and sensitivity levels

56. 3. Specific gravity measures the concentration of urine. A dehydrated client will concentrate urine and decrease urine output to prevent further dehydration. Culture results indicate the presence or absence of an infection and aren't affected by fluid status. Protein may or may not be present in the urine and doesn't fluctuate with changes in fluid status. Ketones aren't present in the urine, and these levels don't fluctuate with fluid status.

NP: Assessment; CN: Physiological integrity; CN: Physiological adaptation; CL: Knowledge

57. A client admitted with hypoparathyroidism is being monitored for hypocalcemia. Which of the following signs is used to check for hypocalcemia?

1. Battle's sign
2. Brudzinski's sign
3. Chvostek's sign
4. Homans' sign

57. 3. Hypocalcemia can cause Chvostek's sign, abnormal facial muscle and nerve spasms elicited when the facial nerve is tapped. A positive Homans' sign indicates deep vein thrombosis. Brudzinski's sign is the flexion of the hips and knees in response to flexion of the head and neck toward the chest, indicating meningeal irritation. Battle's sign is bruising over the temporal bone in the presence of a basilar skull fracture.

NP: Analysis; CN: Physiological integrity; CNS: Reduction of risk potential; CL: Application

58. A client is complaining of pain 1 day after a colostomy. The nurse gives meperidine (Demerol) I.M. and, 30 minutes later, finds the respiratory rate at 8 breaths/minute, with the nasal cannula on the floor. Arterial blood gas (ABG) results are pH, 7.23; Pao_2, 58 mm Hg; $Paco_2$, 61 mm Hg; HCO_3^-, 24 mEq/L. Which of the following groups of factors contributes most to this client's ABG results?

1. Colostomy, pain, and Demerol
2. Meperidine, the nasal cannula on the floor, and the colostomy
3. Meperidine, respiratory rate of 8 breaths/minute, and the nasal cannula on the floor
4. Pain, respiratory rate of 8 breaths/minute, and the nasal cannula on the floor

58. 3. This client has respiratory acidosis. Narcotics can suppress respirations, causing retention of carbon dioxide. A Pao_2 of 58 mm Hg indicates hypoxemia, which is caused by the removal of the client's supplementary oxygen and the decreased respiratory rate. Pain increases — not decreases — the respiratory rate, which causes a decrease in $Paco_2$. Colostomy drainage doesn't start until 2 to 3 days postoperatively, and this drainage would contribute to metabolic alkalosis.

NP: Assessment; CN: Physiological integrity; CNS: Physiological adaptation; CL: Analysis

59. Which of the following arterial blood gas (ABG) results is typical for a client with emphysema?

1. pH, 7.52; $Paco_2$, 18 mm Hg; HCO_3^-, 22 mEq/L
2. pH, 7.50; $Paco_2$, 38 mm Hg; HCO_3^-, 38 mEq/L
3. pH, 7.30; $Paco_2$, 52 mm Hg; HCO_3^-, 30 mEq/L
4. pH, 7.30; $Paco_2$, 40 mm Hg; HCO_3^-, 18 mEq/L

59. 3. Clients with emphysema retain carbon dioxide due to air trapping, causing an elevated $Paco_2$ and respiratory acidosis. Because emphysema is a chronic disease, the kidneys compensate over time for the increased $Paco_2$ by retaining HCO_3^-, thus attempting to normalize the pH. The other ABG results aren't consistent with results found in a client with emphysema.

NP: Assessment; CN: Physiological integrity; CNS: Physiological adaptation; CL: Comprehension

60. Which of the following factors is a major cause of metabolic alkalosis in a client who had a colon resection?

1. Hyperventilation
2. Pain management
3. Nasogastric suction
4. I.V. therapy

60. 3. Removing acidic gastric secretions from the stomach is a metabolic cause of alkalinization of the blood pH. Pain management may further decrease the respiratory rate. Most I.V. fluids don't influence pH. Hyperventilation decreases carbon dioxide and increases the pH, causing respiratory alkalosis.

NP: Analysis; CN: Physiological integrity; CNS: Physiological adaptation; CL: Analysis

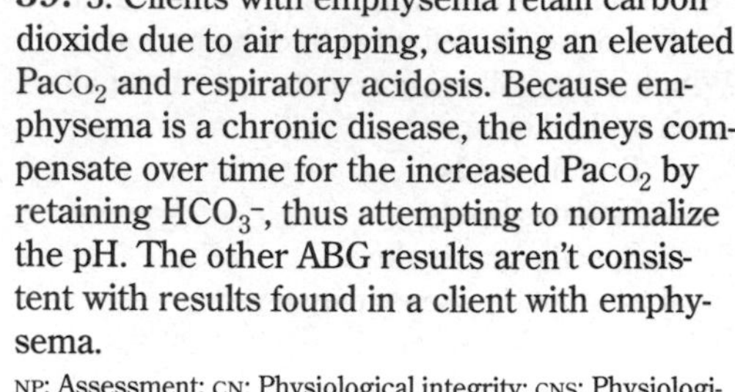

61. Which of the following reasons is correct for using a paper towel to turn off the faucet after hand washing?

1. To clean the faucet after use
2. To maintain sterility of the washed hands
3. To prevent contamination of the faucet handle
4. To prevent transmission of microorganisms from the faucet handle to the hands

61. 4. The faucet has microorganisms on it put there by all the "dirty" hands that touched it when turning it on. Although a paper towel isn't sterile, it's clean and protects the hands from becoming contaminated from the faucet after washing. Hand washing doesn't make the hands sterile. Wiping the faucet after use may make it look cleaner but isn't the reason for using a paper towel to turn off the faucet.

NP: Implementation; CN: Safe, effective care environment; CNS: Safety and infection control; CL: Comprehension

62. After making the bed of a 69-year-old client with dementia, which of the following actions has priority?

1. Put the bed in the lowest position.
2. Put the call button within the client's reach.
3. Put the top side rails in the upright position.
4. Put soiled linen in a hamper or biohazard bag.

62. 1. To reduce the risk of injury due to falls, the bed should be placed in the lowest position. The call button should be in reach of the client, but the immediate safety of the client comes first. All four side rails should be up to prevent accidental falls and to remind clients to stay in bed. Soiled linens should be placed in a hamper or biohazard bag, but client safety is a priority.

NP: Implementation; CN: Safe, effective care environment; CNS: Management of care; CL: Comprehension

63. After emptying urine from the bedpan of a client whose urinary output is being monitored, which of the following steps is done next?

1. Wash hands thoroughly.
2. Apply a clean pair of gloves.
3. Report the amount of urine to the nurse in charge right away.
4. Document the amount and characteristics of urine in the chart.

63. 1. After any procedure is completed, the nurse must wash her hands to prevent transmission of microorganisms. The application of gloves is only necessary if the nurse must attend to another item of personal care before documenting urinary output; even so, hands should be washed first. Crucial information is reported to the charge nurse, not routine intake and output.

NP: Implementation; CN: Safe, effective care environment; CNS: Safety and infection control; CL: Knowledge

64. Which of the following clients should be placed in an orthopneic position?

1. A client with edema of the lower legs and ankles
2. A client with a decubitus ulcer on the coccyx and buttocks
3. An immobilized client with calf tenderness due to a thrombus
4. An elderly client with difficulty breathing unless in a sitting position

64. 4. The orthopneic position, which is appropriate for a client with breathing difficulty, is a sitting position with the arms leaning on a bedside table. Sitting with the legs elevated to decrease edema is appropriate for clients with ankle and lower leg swelling. A client with a decubitus ulcer will need to be positioned on his side and turned every 2 hours. Fowler's or semi-Fowler's positions are most appropriate for a client on complete bed rest.

NP: Planning; CN: Physiological integrity; CNS: Physiological adaptation; CL: Application

65. A client preparing to transfer from the bed to a wheelchair complains of feeling light-headed and dizzy as he rises from a supine to a sitting position. Which of the following actions should the nurse take next?

1. Lift the client quickly into the wheelchair.
2. Return the client to the supine position and apply a safety vest.
3. Ask the client to dangle his legs at the bedside while leaving the room for a few seconds to get assistance.
4. Have the client sit at the side of the bed for a few minutes while supporting his back and shoulders.

65. 4. A quick change in position will decrease the blood pressure, causing momentary lightheadedness and dizziness. An additional change in position may further reduce the client's blood pressure to a level that may require emergency assistance. This can be avoided by waiting with the client in the sitting position until the blood pressure stabilizes. Leaving the room may put the client in danger if the blood pressure decreases further and the client needs emergency assistance. If the client continues to complain of dizziness and lightheadedness, then return the client to bed. A safety vest isn't necessary.

NP: Implementation; CN: Safe, effective care environment; CNS: Management of care; CL: Application

66. Which of the following actions is the most effective infection control measure for preventing the transmission of microorganisms?
1. Change a client's bed linen daily.
2. Wash hands before and after client contact.
3. Wear sterile gloves when touching a client's skin.
4. Wear a mask when in direct contact with infected clients.

66. 2. Most often, the transmission of microorganisms occurs when health care personnel don't wash their hands before and after touching a client or contaminated objects. A daily linen change isn't the most effective method of controlling infection. Sterile gloves and a mask aren't needed during routine client care.
NP: Implementation; CN: Safe, effective care environment; CNS: Safety and infection control; CL: Comprehension

67. Which of the following actions represents a correct implementation of blood-borne pathogen precautions?
1. Wear eye goggles while giving a complete bed bath.
2. Recap a needle used for an injection before disposal.
3. Dispose of blood-contaminated materials in a biohazard container.
4. Use alcohol to decontaminate blood-contaminated steel instruments.

67. 3. Blood-contaminated materials are disposed of in a biohazard container. Recapping needles puts the health care provider at risk for sticking himself. Blood precautions needn't be observed during a bath because of the low risk for exposure to blood. Blood-contaminated steel instruments are decontaminated in an autoclave.
NP: Implementation; CN: Safe, effective care environment; CNS: Safety and infection control; CL: Comprehension

68. A nurse should wear a mask and protective eyewear or a face shield in which of the following situations?
1. When strong odors are emitted from an infected wound
2. When the client has an oral temperature greater than 101° F (38.3° C)
3. If needles or other sharp instruments are to be used in the procedure
4. During a procedure where splashing of blood or body fluid is anticipated

68. 4. Wearing eye goggles or face shields prevents blood or body-fluid splashes into the eyes. Odors don't transmit microorganisms. The use of needles or other sharp instruments doesn't mandate eye protection. A client with a fever won't transmit microorganisms into the eyes any more frequently than a client without a fever.
NP: Implementation; CN: Safe, effective environment; CNS: Management of care; CL: Comprehension

69. A nurse is caring for a client on neutropenic precautions. At which of the following times should the nurse remove the barrier protection when leaving the room?
1. Within the client's room, just inside the doorway
2. Out of the client's room, just outside the doorway
3. In the hallway, a significant distance from the client's room
4. At the bedside, immediately after completing work with the client

69. 2. Disposing of gowns and gloves just outside the doorway provides sufficient distance from the client for all but airborne microorganisms. The client is protected from infection by airborne pathogens by keeping the door shut as much as possible to decrease the chance of exposure. Disposal of barriers at the bedside or inside the door negates the effectiveness of wearing barriers in the first place. It's unnecessary to wear the barriers away from the doorway as the door should remain closed.
NP: Planning; CN: Safe, effective care environment; CNS: Safety and infection control; CL: Knowledge

70. Which of the following time frames is most appropriate for completing client teaching for a client undergoing an open cholecystectomy?

1. The day of discharge
2. A few weeks before the surgery
3. The first 12 hours after surgery
4. Before discharge, 1 to 2 days after the surgery

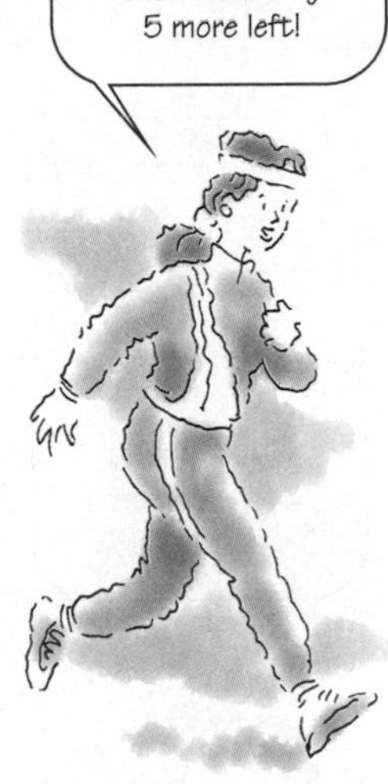

You're nearing the finish! Only 5 more left!

70. 4. Pain levels should have sufficiently subsided 1 to 2 days after the surgical procedure, allowing the client to concentrate on the information. A few weeks before surgery is generally too early to retain information, and teaching within the first 12 hours after surgery isn't likely to produce retention of information, either. The day of discharge is too late, because it doesn't give the client time to ask questions or practice procedures (such as syringe preparation) that may be necessary. Also, the individual may be anxious about returning home, which may interfere with learning.

NP: Planning; CN: Physiological integrity; CNS: Basic care and comfort; CL: Application

71. For which of the following individuals is the use of an oral thermometer contraindicated?

1. A school-age child
2. An unconscious client
3. An alert, oriented client
4. An elderly client in no acute distress

71. 2. Oral thermometers can be broken by an unconscious client. Only a client who can follow directions to hold the thermometer in his mouth should be allowed to do so. The clients in the other three options should have no difficulty.

NP: Assessment; CN: Safe, effective care environment; CNS: Safety and infection control; CL: Knowledge

72. Which of the following techniques is correct for tracheostomy care of a client at home?

1. Septic
2. Antiseptic
3. Medically aseptic
4. Surgically aseptic

72. 3. At home, the procedure of tracheostomy care is clean or medically aseptic because of the cost and difficulty of performing a completely sterile procedure. Septic means infected or dirty. An antiseptic is a solution used to prevent infection. Surgical asepsis can only realistically be practiced in the hospital.

NP: Implementation; CN: Safe, effective care environment; CNS: Safety and infection control; CL: Comprehension

73. A 46-year-old single mother was concerned about her 15-year-old son's behavior. He suddenly decided his mother shouldn't date or have men in the house. He told his mother he was the "man of the house." Which of the following disturbances was occurring in the internal dynamics of the family?

1. Age-appropriate behavior is occurring.
2. The son is powerful in the family system.
3. The son is trying to establish a role reversal.
4. It's culturally acceptable to be the man of the house at age 15.

73. 3. Role reversal occurs when the patterns of expected behavior aren't appropriate to age and ability. Males ages 13 to 17 are developing their identities, and separation from parents becomes necessary for individuation to occur. Males have a better understanding of their roles in relationships and families if they're raised around strong male role models. In healthy families, power is shared appropriate to age until the children are independent.

NP: Analysis; CN: Psychosocial integrity; CNS: Coping and adaptation; CL: Analysis

74. Which of the following behaviors in a preschooler is a cause for concern?
1. Has nightmares
2. Cries and holds tightly to parents
3. Takes toys away from other children
4. Sits quietly and doesn't participate in play activities

74. 4. This could be a sign of despair or hopelessness if observed in a preschooler. During times of stress, it's typical for the preschooler to be frightened at night. It's normal for a child at this stage to show separation anxiety and play typical of preschoolers.

NP: Assessment; CN: Psychosocial integrity; CNS: Psychosocial adaptation; CL: Knowledge

75. Which of the following techniques is appropriate for promoting proper breathing in a client experiencing pain or anxiety?
1. Rapid, light respirations
2. Rapid, deep respirations
3. In through the mouth and out through the nose
4. In through the nose and out through the mouth

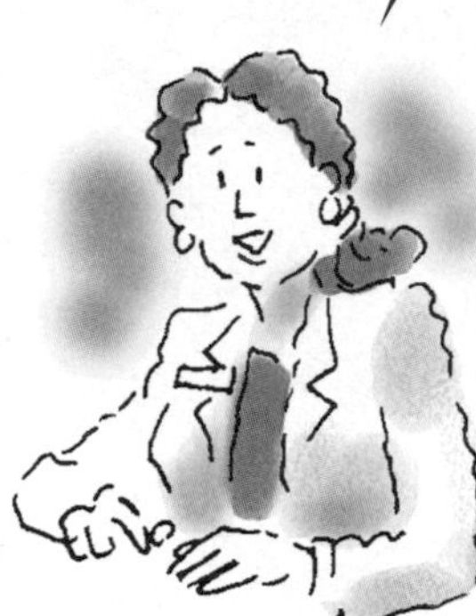

You did a wonderful job! Only two more tests left!

75. 4. Air inhaled through the nose is warmed, humidified, and filtered for large particles with the nasal hairs, conditioning the air for delivery to the lungs. Exhaling through the mouth after inhaling through the nose requires some concentration and provides a focus to distract a client experiencing pain and anxiety. This method is used to control respiratory rates when clients are anxious or in pain and optimizes air exchange. Rapid, light, or deep respirations cause the client to lose oxygen exchange time while continuing to blow off carbon dioxide. This leads to hypoxemia and respiratory alkalosis.

NP: Implementation; CN: Physiological integrity; CNS: Physiological adaptation; CL: Application

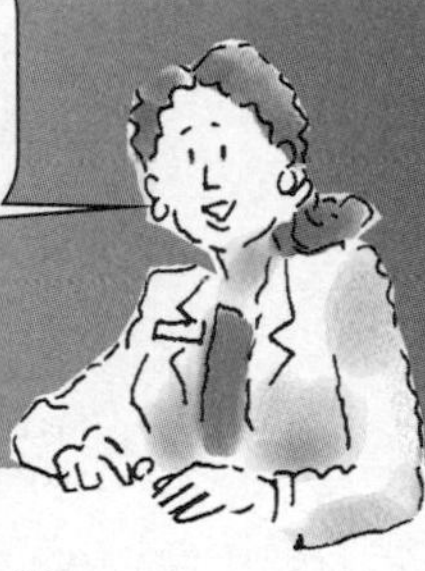
This is the next to
last comprehensive
test. Go for it, and
good luck!

COMPREHENSIVE Test 5

1. Which information about vital signs should be reported to the physician?

1. Blood pressure of 120/72 mm Hg in a healthy man
2. Pulse of 110 beats/minute on awakening in the morning
3. Blood pressure of 110/68 mm Hg in a healthy woman
4. Pulse of 120 beats/minute after 30 minutes of aerobic exercise

1. 2. The normal range for a pulse is 60 to 100 beats/minute and, in the morning, the rate is at its lowest. Blood pressures of 120/72 mm Hg for a healthy man and 110/68 mm Hg for a healthy woman are normal. Aerobic exercise increases the heart rate over the normal range of 60 to 100 beats/minute. The formula for maximum aerobic heart rate is: 210 – age × 80%. A person shouldn't go over the maximum heart rate during aerobic exercise.

NP: Analysis; CN: Physiological integrity; CNS: Physiological adaptation; CL: Comprehension

2. Which of the following actions shows the primary value of the dorsalis pedis and posterior tibial pulses during assessment?

1. Assessing heart rate
2. Evaluating pulse rate
3. Assessing circulation to the lower extremities
4. Identifying the presence of tachycardia in the client

2. 3. These pulses represent peripheral circulation and are rated by their quality from 0 (absent) to 4 (bounding). Heart rate and pulse rate are used interchangeably and assessed through the radial or apical pulses. Tachycardia is a fast pulse rate best assessed at the apical or radial locations.

NP: Assessment; CN: Physiological integrity; CNS: Physiological adaptation; CL: Knowledge

3. A nurse is preparing to bathe a client who's hospitalized for emphysema. Which of the following nursing interventions is correct?

1. Remove the oxygen and proceed with the bath.
2. Increase the flow of oxygen to 6 L/minute by nasal cannula.
3. Keep the head of the bed slightly elevated during the procedure.
4. Lower the head of the bed and roll the client to his left side to increase oxygenation.

3. 3. The elasticity of the lungs is lost for clients with emphysema, who can't tolerate lying flat because the abdominal organs compress the lungs. The best position is one with the head slightly elevated. The rate of oxygen delivery shouldn't be increased or decreased without an order from the physician. Increasing oxygen flow on a client with emphysema may also suppress the hypoxic drive to breathe. Positioning the client on his left side with the head of the bed flat would decrease oxygenation.

NP: Analysis; CN: Physiological integrity; CNS: Physiological adaptation; CL: Application

NP: Nursing process CN: Client needs category CNS: Client needs subcategory CL: Cognitive level

4. A 40-year-old client is scheduled to have elective facial surgery later in the morning. The nurse notes the pulse rate is 130 beats/minute. Which of the following reasons best explains the tachycardia?

1. Age
2. Anxiety
3. Exercise
4. Pain

4. 2. Anxiety tends to increase heart rate, temperature, and respirations. Exercise will increase the heart rate but most likely won't occur preoperatively. The normal heart rate for a client this age is 60 to 100 beats/minute. The client shouldn't be in any pain preoperatively.

NP: Assessment; CN: Physiological integrity; CNS: Physiological adaptation; CL: Comprehension

5. A thin client is sitting up in bed talking on the phone and has a blood pressure of 90/50 mm Hg. Which of the following nursing actions is correct?

1. Increase fluids.
2. Call the physician.
3. Consider this a normal variation.
4. Suspect orthostatic hypotension.

5. 3. A thin client can have a blood pressure as low as 88/46 mm Hg and remain asymptomatic. Calling the physician with this information is inappropriate, as is increasing fluids. Orthostatic hypotension is a decrease in blood pressure and increase in heart rate that occur with a sudden change in position from lying to sitting. It might indicate some dehydration, but this client had been sitting up without symptoms for a while.

NP: Assessment; CN: Health promotion and maintenance; CNS: Prevention and early detection of disease; CL: Application

6. A nurse is checking a rectal temperature with a mercury (glass) thermometer. Which of the following actions by the nurse is incorrect?

1. Insert the thermometer through the anal sphincter.
2. Read the thermometer with the mercury at eye level.
3. Apply water-soluble lubricant to the thermometer before insertion.
4. Leave the thermometer in place for 5 to 10 minutes before reading.

6. 4. To obtain a rectal reading, 2 to 3 minutes are adequate; 5 to 10 minutes are needed for axillary temperatures. The rest of the answers are correct for rectal temperature readings.

NP: Implementation; CN: Safe, effective care environment; CNS: Management of care; CL: Knowledge

7. The vital signs of a 56-year-old client are: temperature, 98.6° F (37° C) orally; pulse, 80 beats/minute, and respirations, 30 breaths/minute. Which of the following interpretations of these values is correct?

1. Pulse is above normal range.
2. Temperature is above normal range.
3. Respirations are above normal range.
4. Respirations and pulse are above normal range.

7. 3. Normal vital signs for an adult client are: temperature, 96.6° to 99° F (36° to 37° C); pulse, 60 to 100 beats/minute; respirations, 16 to 20 breaths/minute.

NP: Assessment; CN: Health promotion and maintenance; CNS: Growth and development through the life span; CL: Knowledge

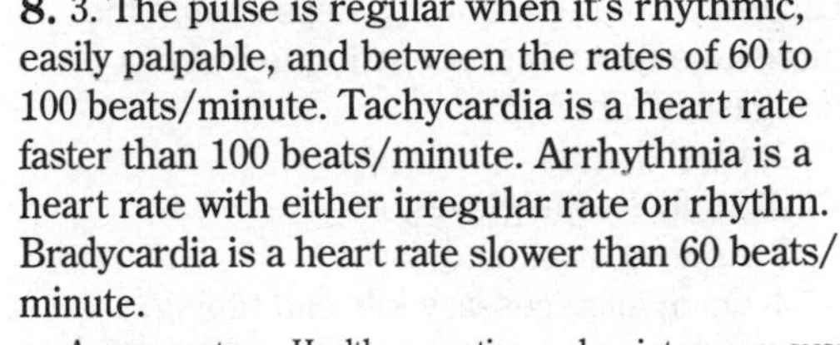

8. A nurse notes a client's pulse is regular and readily palpable at a rate of 84 beats/minute. Which of the following terms best describes this pulse?
1. Arrhythmia
2. Bradycardia
3. Regular
4. Tachycardia

8. 3. The pulse is regular when it's rhythmic, easily palpable, and between the rates of 60 to 100 beats/minute. Tachycardia is a heart rate faster than 100 beats/minute. Arrhythmia is a heart rate with either irregular rate or rhythm. Bradycardia is a heart rate slower than 60 beats/minute.

NP: Assessment; CN: Health promotion and maintenance; CNS: Growth and development through the life span; CL: Knowledge

9. Which of the following actions is correct for performing tracheal suctioning?
1. Apply suction during insertion of the catheter.
2. Limit suctioning to 10 to 15 seconds' duration.
3. Resterilize the suction catheter in alcohol after use.
4. Repeat suctioning intervals every 15 minutes until clear.

9. 2. The length of time a client should be able to tolerate the suction procedure is 10 to 15 seconds. Any longer may cause hypoxia. Suctioning during insertion can cause trauma to the mucosa and removes oxygen from the respiratory tract. Suctioning intervals with supplemental oxygen between suctions is performed after at least 1-minute intervals to allow the client to rest. Suction catheters are disposed of after each use and are cleansed in normal saline solution after each pass.

NP: Implementation; CN: Physiological integrity; CNS: Physiological adaptation; CL: Application

10. While performing nasopharyngeal suction, a nurse hears a client's pulse oximeter alarm. The pulse oximeter indicates the client's oxygen saturation reading is 86%. Which of the following actions should the nurse take?
1. Stop suctioning and give oxygen to the client.
2. Withdraw the suction catheter and tell the client to cough several times.
3. Continue suctioning for 10 to 15 more seconds and then withdraw the suction catheter.
4. Keep the suction catheter inserted and wait a few seconds before beginning suctioning.

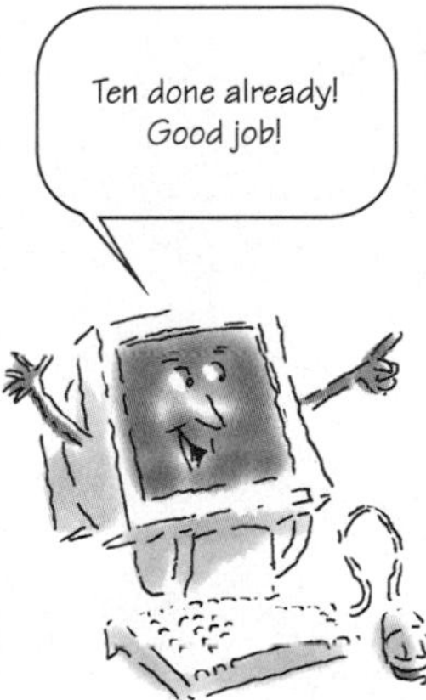
Ten done already! Good job!

10. 1. The pulse oximeter reading indicates the client isn't oxygenating well, so the nurse must stop suctioning and give oxygen to increase the saturation. The normal range for oxygen saturation is 90% to 100%. Suctioning draws air as well as secretions from the lungs, reducing oxygen saturation in the blood. Withdrawing the suction catheter will stop the removal of oxygen, but coughing will delay an increase in saturation. The suction catheter occupies space in the airway, making it harder for the client to breathe when it's left in place. Further suctioning will reduce the oxygen level even further.

NP: Evaluation; CN: Physiological integrity; CNS: Physiological adaptation; CL: Application

11. Which of the following positions is optimal for a client having a nasogastric tube inserted?
1. Fowler's
2. Prone
3. Side-lying
4. Supine

11. 1. The upright, or Fowler's, position is more natural for swallowing and protects against aspiration. Positioning the client on his back, stomach, or side places him at risk for aspiration if he should gag. It's also difficult to swallow in these positions.

NP: Implementation; CN: Physiological integrity; CNS: Basic care and comfort; CL: Comprehension

12. Which of the following steps should the nurse take first when preparing to insert a nasogastric tube?
1. Wash hands.
2. Apply sterile gloves.
3. Apply a mask and gown.
4. Open all necessary kits and tubing.

12. 1. The first intervention before a procedure is hand washing. Clean gloves are used because the mouth and nasopharynx aren't considered sterile. Opening all the equipment is the next step before inserting the nasogastric tube. A mask and gown aren't required.
NP: Implementation; CN: Safe, effective care environment; CNS: Safety and infection control; CL: Comprehension

13. As a nurse is inserting a nasogastric tube, the client begins to gag. Which action should the nurse take?
1. Remove the inserted tube and notify the physician of the client's status.
2. Stop the insertion, allow the client to rest, then continue inserting the tube.
3. Encourage the client to take deep breaths through the mouth while the tube is being inserted.
4. Pause until the gagging stops, tell the client to take a few sips of water and swallow as the tube is inserted.

13. 4. Swallowing helps advance the tube by causing the epiglottis to cover the opening of the trachea, thus helping to eliminate gagging and coughing. Removing the tube or stopping the insertion is unnecessary as gagging is an expected response to this procedure. Deep breathing opens the trachea, allowing the tube to possibly advance into the lungs.
NP: Evaluation; CN: Safe, effective care environment; CNS: Safety and infection control; CL: Application

14. Which of the following steps, if taken by the nurse after insertion of a nasogastric tube, could harm the client?
1. Affix the nasogastric tube to the nose with tape.
2. Check tube placement by aspirating stomach contents using a piston syringe.
3. Check tube placement by instilling 100 ml of water into the tube to check for stomach filling.
4. Document in the chart the insertion, method used to check tube placement, and client's response to the procedure.

14. 3. Should the tube be located in the lungs, instilling water would flood the lungs, precipitating choking, coughing, hypoxemia and, possibly, pneumonia. Withdrawing stomach contents from the nasogastric tube double-checks the correct placement. Anchoring the tube after placement to the nose with tape or a manufactured device prevents the tube from becoming dislodged. Documentation is required for any procedure.
NP: Evaluation; CN: Safe, effective care environment; CNS: Management of care; CL: Comprehension

15. A new graduate is assigned to a nursing unit. A nurse manager assesses that the graduate's skills are deficient. Which action is most appropriate for the nurse manager to take?
1. Talk with the supervisor about terminating the new graduate.
2. Discuss with the graduate that a transfer to another unit is necessary.
3. Work with the graduate and develop a plan to improve the graduate's deficiencies.
4. Counsel the graduate that, if performance doesn't improve, the graduate will be terminated.

15. 3. A principle of leadership involves mastery over ignorance by working with people. The leader needs to work with the new graduate and provide opportunities for the graduate to grow and develop. The other responses wouldn't give the new graduate the opportunity and support needed for improvement.
NP: Implementation; CN: Safe, effective care environment; CNS: Management of care; CL: Application

16. A client recently placed on a cardiac monitor has a heart rate of 170 beats/minute, with frequent premature contractions. Which of the following nursing actions is best?

1. Call the client's physician immediately.
2. See the client and make a full assessment.
3. Delegate one of the nurses' aides to take the client's vital signs.
4. Notify the supervisor about the change in the client's condition.

16. 2. Because a change has occurred in the client's status, the nurse must assess the client first. This shouldn't be delegated to unlicensed personnel. Before the physician or supervisor is notified, a full assessment must be made.
NP: Implementation; CN: Safe, effective care environment; CNS: Management of care; CL: Application

17. A client is hospitalized with an acute sinus infection. Which of the following assessments made by the nurse indicates serious complications?

1. Orbital edema
2. Nuchal rigidity
3. Fever of 102° F (39° C)
4. Frontal headache

17. 2. Nuchal rigidity indicates neurologic involvement, possibly meningitis. The other symptoms are typical of a sinus infection.
NP: Analysis; CN: Physiological integrity; CNS: Physiological adaptation; CL: Comprehension

18. Which of the following statements by a client who had nasal surgery indicates the client needs further teaching about postoperative care?

1. "I'll do frequent mouth care."
2. "I'll eat two oranges a day."
3. "I'll eat two bananas a day."
4. "I'll drink at least 8 glasses of fluid a day."

18. 3. After nasal surgery, the client shouldn't strain or bear down as this will increase the risk for bleeding. Bananas can cause severe constipation, which could lead to straining. The other interventions would be appropriate postoperative care for this client.
NP: Evaluation; CN: Physiological integrity; CNS: Reduction of risk potential; CL: Comprehension

19. Which of the following actions is correct when collecting a urine specimen from a client's indwelling urinary catheter?

1. Collect urine from the drainage collection bag.
2. Disconnect the catheter from the drainage tubing to collect urine.
3. Remove the indwelling catheter and insert a sterile straight catheter to collect urine.
4. Insert a sterile needle with syringe through a tubing drainage port cleaned with alcohol to collect the specimen.

19. 4. Wearing clean gloves, cleaning the port with alcohol, and then obtaining the specimen with a sterile needle ensures the specimen and the closed urinary drainage system won't be contaminated. A urine sample must be new urine, and the urine in the bag could be several hours old and growing bacteria. The urinary drainage system must be kept closed to prevent microorganisms from entering. A straight catheter is used to relieve urinary retention, obtain sterile urine specimens, measure the amount of postvoid residual urine, and empty the bladder for certain procedures. It isn't necessary to remove an indwelling catheter to obtain a sterile urine specimen unless the physician requests the whole system be changed.
NP: Implementation; CN: Safe, effective care environment; CNS: Safety and infection control; CL: Comprehension

20. A client recovering from surgery tells a nurse, "I feel like I have to urinate more often than usual, and it burns when I urinate." The nurse should plan to obtain a urinary specimen for which of the following factors?

1. Culture
2. Glucose
3. Ketones
4. Specific gravity

20. 1. The signs and symptoms of this client are those of a urinary tract infection, and a culture will probably show a bacterial infection. Ketones and glucose in the urine don't cause the client to complain of burning and frequency. Specific gravity is a measure of the concentration of the urine. A high or low specific gravity won't cause these symptoms.

NP: Implementation; CN: Physiological integrity; CNS: Reduction of risk potential; CL: Comprehension

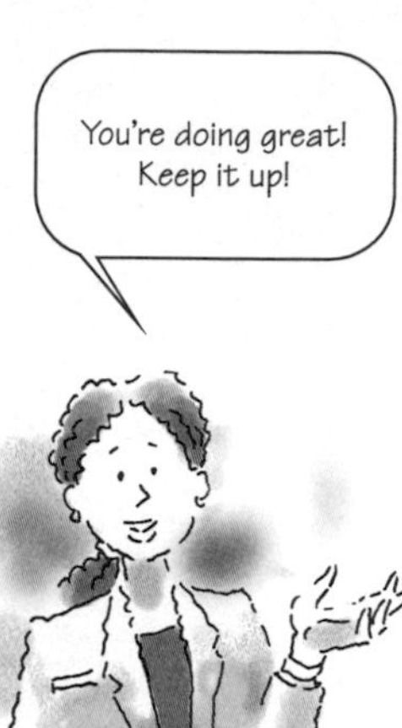
You're doing great!
Keep it up!

21. A client recovering from a knee replacement has normal saline solution ordered to run at 125 ml/hour I.V. The I.V. bag was hung at 8:00 a.m. It's now 3:00 p.m., and 300 ml have been infused. A nurse has just come on her shift at 3:00 p.m. Which of the following actions is correct?

1. Discontinue the I.V. infusion when the bag is complete.
2. Instruct the client to increase his fluid intake.
3. Speed up the rate of the I.V. fluids.
4. Notify the physician of the client's status.

21. 4. At 125 ml/hour over 7 hours, 875 ml should have been infused. The I.V. fluid is 575 ml behind. The physician will determine how the I.V. fluids will be adjusted and will want to know why the client didn't get the prescribed fluids. Legally, the nurse can't change the rate of I.V. fluids. The order is for I.V. fluids — not oral fluids — and the route change can only be authorized by a physician.

NP: Evaluation; CN: Safe, effective care environment; CNS: Management of care; CL: Application

22. A nurse is removing an indwelling urinary catheter. Which of the following actions is appropriate?

1. Wear sterile gloves.
2. Cut the lumen of the balloon.
3. Document the time of removal.
4. Position the client on the left side.

22. 3. The client should void within 8 hours of the removal of an indwelling urinary catheter. Documenting the time of removal allows the nurse and physician to verify the duration of elapsed time since removal, thus contributing to continuity of care. Clean, disposable gloves are required because it isn't a sterile procedure. The client should be positioned comfortably on his back, and privacy should be provided. The catheter may retrograde into the bladder, requiring surgical removal, if the balloon is cut from the lumen and the catheter isn't secured.

NP: Implementation; CN: Safe, effective care environment; CNS: Safety and infection control; CL: Comprehension

23. Which of the following foods can alter results when stool is checked for occult blood?

1. Red meat
2. Dairy products, canned fruit, and pretzels
3. Horseradish, raw fruits, and vegetables
4. Potatoes, orange juice, and decaffeinated coffee

23. 1. Consumption of red meat has caused false-positive readings. Avoid foods that are high in iron. The other foods don't cause false-positive readings.

NP: Evaluation; CN: Physiological integrity; CNS: Basic care and comfort; CL: Comprehension

24. A client complains of excessive flatulence. Which food, if consumed regularly, may be responsible for this?

1. Cauliflower
2. Ice cream
3. Meat
4. Potatoes

24. 1. Cauliflower is the only food listed that often results in flatulence.

NP: Evaluation; CN: Physiological integrity; CNS: Basic care and comfort; CL: Comprehension

25. Which of the following techniques is correct for postoperative coughing and deep breathing exercises?

1. Splint the incision and cough.
2. Splint the incision, take a deep breath, and then cough.
3. Lie prone, splint the incision, take a deep breath, and then cough.
4. Lie supine, splint the incision, take a deep breath, and then cough.

25. 2. Splinting the incision with a pillow will protect the incision while the client coughs. Taking a deep breath will help open the alveoli, which promotes oxygen exchange and prevents atelectasis. Coughing and deep breathing exercises are best accomplished in a sitting or semisitting position. Expectoration of secretions will be facilitated in a sitting position, as will splinting and taking deep breaths.

NP: Planning; CN: Physiological integrity; CNS: Reduction of risk potential; CL: Application

26. Which of the following characteristics of the client goal in the care plan is correct?

1. Nurse-focused, flexible, measurable, and realistic
2. Client-focused, flexible, realistic, and measurable
3. Nurse-focused, time-limited, realistic, and measurable
4. Client-focused, time-limited, realistic, and measurable

26. 4. All goals should be client focused, allowing the client to understand what needs to be accomplished. Specify a time limit for when this task should be achieved. Be realistic, so the client may be successful in reaching the goal. The goal must be measurable so all staff can evaluate the client's progress. Nurse flexibility is an important attribute and necessary for reassessing needs and approaches for the client's optimal recovery. However, in the actual goal, specific criteria must be identified to allow all staff to work from the same data for achieving client goals.

NP: Planning; CN: Health promotion and maintenance; CNS: Prevention and early detection of disease; CL: Knowledge

27. A nurse is performing an admission assessment on a client with exacerbation of asthma. Which of the following times is ideal to begin discharge planning?

1. At the time of admission
2. The day before discharge
3. After the acute episode is resolved
4. When the discharge order is written

27. 1. Discharge planning should begin as soon as the client is admitted. Client stays are increasingly shorter, giving the interdisciplinary team less time to accomplish care goals. Beginning discharge planning as early as possible will give staff the greatest amount of time and make appropriate resources available. Waiting until the acute episode is resolved will greatly diminish the time available for discharge planning. Also, waiting for a discharge order or deferring planning until the end of the client's stay doesn't allow sufficient time.

NP: Planning; CN: Safe, effective care environment; CNS: Management of care; CL: Comprehension

28. Which of the following actions is an example of developmentally based care?

1. Provide books to a 9-year-old client.
2. Walk a 10-year-old client according to written orders.
3. Provide a pureed diet to a postoperative 13-year-old client.
4. Change a surgical dressing on a 15-year-old client every 4 hours as ordered.

28. 1. Providing books to a 9-year-old client facilitates her reading skills and helps her grow developmentally. Changing a surgical dressing, walking a client, and providing a pureed diet are routine care tasks, which don't necessarily promote further development of the individual.
NP: Analysis; CN: Health promotion and maintenance; CNS: Growth and development through the life span; CL: Comprehension

29. A nurse is witnessing consent from a client before a cardiac catheterization. Which of the following factors is a component of informed consent?

1. Freedom from coercion
2. Durable power of attorney
3. Private insurance coverage
4. Disclosure of previous answers given by the client

29. 1. The client must give consent voluntarily without any type of outside influences from persons involved with the procedure or research. The client must also be of sound mind and not under the influence of types of medications that may interfere with reasoning. Private insurance coverage shouldn't be a factor in informed consent. All clients (or another appointed individual) have the right to make their own decisions regardless of type of insurance. A durable power of attorney may be indicated if a client is unable to make decisions for himself. Previous answers given by the individual shouldn't be an influencing factor in the informed consent process.
NP: Analysis; CN: Safe, effective care environment; CNS: Management of care; CL: Knowledge

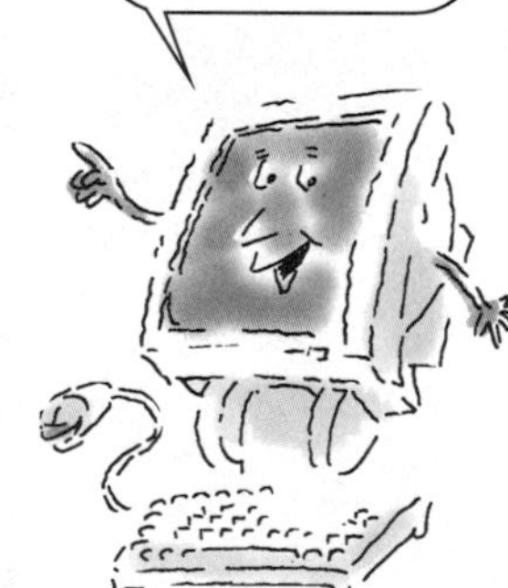

Way to go! You've finished 30 questions already! I'll bet even you don't believe it!

30. A client on complete bed rest complains of excessive flatulence. Which of the following positions would be helpful to the client?

1. Fowler's
2. Knee-chest
3. Semi-Fowler's
4. Trendelenburg's

30. 2. Because gas rises, the knee-chest position facilitates the passage of flatus. In Trendelenburg's position the client lies flat with his head lower than his feet. Semi-Fowler's and Fowler's positions inhibit gas passage.
NP: Implementation; CN: Physiological integrity; CNS: Basic care and comfort; CL: Knowledge

31. A client had a laxative prescribed that acts by causing stool to absorb water and swell. Which of the following terms describes this type of laxative?

1. Bulk forming
2. Emollient
3. Lubricant
4. Stimulant

31. 1. Bulk-forming laxatives cause stool to absorb water and swell. Emollients lubricate the stool; lubricants soften the stool, making it easier to pass; and stimulants promote peristalsis by irritating the intestinal mucosa or stimulating nerve endings in the intestinal wall.
NP: Analysis; CN: Physiological integrity; CNS: Basic care and comfort; CL: Knowledge

32. A nurse encourages a client to avoid foods that have a laxative effect, including which of the following?

1. Alcohol
2. Cheese
3. Eggs
4. Pasta

32. 1. All the foods listed except alcohol have a constipating effect.

NP: Implementation; CN: Physiological integrity; CNS: Basic care and comfort; CL: Comprehension

33. A client is complaining of moderate pain. Which of the following assessment findings indicates a physiological response to pain?

1. Restlessness
2. Decreased pulse rate
3. Increased blood pressure
4. Protection of the painful area

33. 3. Increased blood pressure is a physiological, or involuntary, response to moderate pain. Restlessness and protection of the painful area are behavioral responses. Decreased pulse rate occurs when pain is severe and deep.

NP: Assessment; CN: Physiological integrity; CNS: Physiological adaptation; CL: Comprehension

34. A client with long-standing rheumatoid arthritis has frequent complaints of joint pain. The nurse's plan of treatment is based on the understanding that chronic pain is most effectively relieved when analgesics are administered in which of the following ways?

1. Conservatively
2. I.M.
3. On an as-needed basis
4. At regularly scheduled intervals

34. 4. To control chronic pain and prevent cycled pain, regularly scheduled intervals are most effective. As-needed and conservative methods aren't effective means to manage chronic pain because the pain isn't relieved regularly. I.M. administration isn't practical on a long-term basis.

NP: Analysis; CN: Physiological integrity; CNS: Pharmacological and parenteral therapies; CL: Application

35. A nurse notes crackles in the lung bases and pedal edema during client assessment. Which of the following is a common cause of fluid volume excess?

1. Prolonged fever
2. Hyperventilation
3. Excessive I.V. infusion
4. Fluid volume shifts secondary to vomiting

35. 3. Fluid volume excess can result from excess I.V. fluids, especially in a compromised client. Vomiting, fever, and hyperventilation will result in loss of body fluids, leading to a fluid volume deficit.

NP: Assessment; CN: Physiological integrity; CNS: Basic care and comfort; CL: Application

36. Which of the following nursing interventions is correct for clients receiving I.V. therapy?

1. Change the tubing every 8 hours.
2. Monitor the flow rate at least every hour.
3. Change the I.V. catheter and entry site daily.
4. Increase the rate to catch up if the correct amount hasn't been infused at the end of the shift.

36. 2. Closely observing the rate of infusion prevents underhydration and overhydration. The I.V. catheter and entry site should be changed every 48 to 72 hours in most situations. Tubing is changed according to agency policy but not at the frequency of every 8 hours. Increasing the rate may lead to fluid overload.

NP: Implementation; CN: Physiological integrity; CNS: Pharmacological and parenteral therapies; CL: Comprehension

37. A client is given instructions for a low-sodium diet. Which of the following statements best shows the client understands the diet instruction?

1. "Meat, fish, and chicken are high in sodium."
2. "I'll miss eating fruits."
3. "I'll enjoy eating at restaurants more often now."
4. "I'll avoid dairy products, potato chips, and carrots."

37. 4. Dairy products, potato chips, carrots, and restaurant food are all high in sodium. Meat, fish, chicken, and fruits aren't.

NP: Evaluation; CN: Physiological integrity; CNS: Basic care and comfort; CL: Knowledge

38. A nursing student asks a nurse what tetany indicates. Which of the following responses is correct?

1. Hypokalemia
2. Hypocalcemia
3. Decrease in sodium level
4. Muscle cramps and tingling of the fingers

38. 2. Tetany, muscle cramps, and tingling of the fingers are signs and symptoms of hypocalcemia. Hypokalemia is manifested by muscle weakness, cardiac arrhythmias, lethargy, anorexia, nausea, and vomiting. Low sodium levels may cause seizures.

NP: Implementation; CN: Physiological integrity; CNS: Physiological adaptation; CL: Comprehension

39. A client must choose a meal that follows his diet orders of a high-calorie, high-protein, decreased-sodium, and low-potassium diet. Which of the following choices indicates the client understands the dietary guidelines?

1. Halibut, salad, rice, and instant coffee
2. Crab, beets, spinach, and baked potato
3. Salmon, rice, green beans, sourdough bread, coffee, and ice cream
4. Sirloin steak, salad, baked potato with butter, and chocolate ice cream

39. 3. The best choice of these meals is salmon with rice and green beans, which is high in protein, and the sourdough bread and ice cream add calories. Halibut, instant coffee, and potatoes are high in potassium, and beets are high in sodium.

NP: Evaluation; CN: Health promotion and maintenance; CNS: Prevention and early detection of disease; CL: Comprehension

40. A client with terminal cancer tells a nurse, "I've given up. I have no hope left. I'm ready to die." Which of the following responses is most therapeutic?

1. "You've given up hope?"
2. "We should talk about dying to a social worker."
3. "You should talk to your physician about your fears of dying so soon."
4. "Now, you shouldn't give up hope. There are cures for cancer found every day."

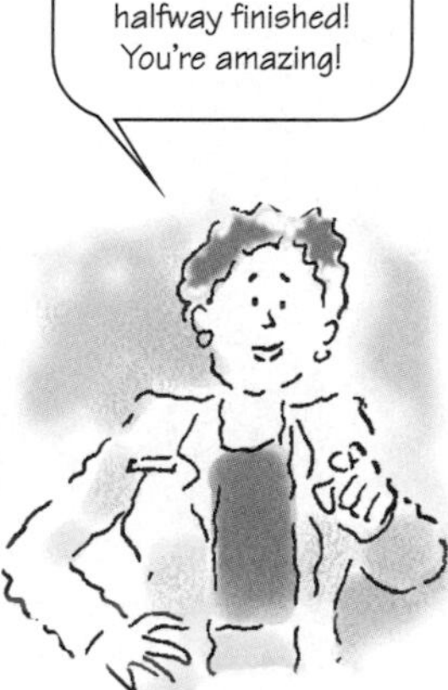

You're more than halfway finished! You're amazing!

40. 1. The use of reflection invites the client to talk more about his concerns. Deferring the conversation to a social worker or physician closes the conversation. Telling the client the cure for cancer is right around the corner gives false hope.

NP: Implementation; CN: Psychosocial integrity; CNS: Coping and adaptation; CL: Comprehension

41. A client's laboratory values are the following: calcium, 18 mg/dl; potassium, 3 mEq/L; and magnesium, 4 mEq/L. These values put this client most at risk for which of the following complications?

1. Bleeding
2. Renal failure
3. Cardiac arrhythmia
4. Respiratory distress

41. 3. Low potassium, magnesium, and calcium levels cause the heart muscle to become irritable, resulting in arrhythmias. Renal failure isn't caused by low electrolyte levels. Respiratory weakness may occur with a low potassium level. Bleeding is seen with a low calcium level.

NP: Evaluation; CN: Health promotion and maintenance; CNS: Prevention and early detection of disease; CL: Comprehension

42. Which of the following laboratory values for a newly diagnosed client with diabetes requires intervention?

1. pH, 7.45
2. Sodium, 118 mEq/L
3. Glucose, 120 mg/dl
4. Potassium, 3.9 mEq/L

42. 2. The normal range for sodium is 135 to 145 mEq/L. The rest of the results are within normal limits.

NP: Assessment; CN: Health promotion and maintenance; CNS: Prevention and early detection of disease; CL: Comprehension

43. A client is 2 days postoperative from a femoral popliteal bypass. The nurse's assessment finds the client's left leg cold and pale. Which of the following actions has priority?

1. Check distal pulses.
2. Notify the physician.
3. Elevate the foot of the bed.
4. Wrap the leg in a warm blanket.

43. 1. The client has arterial disease and had vascular surgery. The nurse must assess the client for complications. A potential problem would be a clot at the surgical site, so the nurse must assess circulation by checking for distal pulses. Before the physician is notified, the nurse should determine if distal pulses are present. Elevating the foot of the bed would promote venous return but decrease arterial blood flow and shouldn't be done. The leg can be covered lightly after circulation is assessed.

NP: Implementation; CN: Physiological integrity; CNS: Physiological adaptation; CL: Application

44. Which of the following drug forms can be administered through a nasogastric tube?

1. Enteric coated
2. Oral
3. Parenteral
4. Sublingual

44. 2. Most oral medications can be given through a nasogastric tube because they're intended for passage into the stomach. Some oral drugs have special coatings intended to keep the pill intact until it passes into the small intestine; these enteric-coated pills shouldn't be crushed and put through a nasogastric tube. Sublingual means under the tongue and parenteral means I.V., I.M., and subcutaneous. Some parenteral medications, such as insulin, may be destroyed by gastric juices.

NP: Implementation; CN: Physiological integrity; CNS: Pharmacological and parenteral therapies; CL: Comprehension

45. A client requiring the highest possible concentration of oxygen will need which of the following delivery systems?

1. Face tent
2. Venturi mask
3. Nasal cannula
4. Mask with reservoir bag

45. 4. A mask with a reservoir bag administers 70% to 100% oxygen at flow rates of 8 to 10 L/minute. The nasal cannula maximum rate is 44% at 6 L/minute, the Venturi mask maximum rate is 24% to 55%, and a face tent maximum delivery is 22% to 34%.

NP: Analysis; CN: Physiological integrity; CNS: Pharmacological and parenteral therapies; CL: Comprehension

46. To ensure the safe administration of medications, which of the following actions is correct?

1. Make sure the client is in the right room.
2. Check the name band of the client.
3. Have the client repeat his name.
4. Note the physician's name.

46. 2. The five rights for proper administration of medications and therapies are the right client, right dose, right time, right route, and right medication. Checking the name band is the most reliable way to verify client identification.

NP: Implementation; CN: Physiological integrity; CNS: Pharmacological and parenteral therapies; CL: Knowledge

47. A client with difficulty breathing has a respiratory rate of 34 breaths/minute and seems very anxious. She's refusing all her medications, claiming they're making her worse. Which of the following nursing actions is best?

1. Notify the physician of the status of this client.
2. Hold the medication until the next scheduled dose.
3. Encourage the client to take some of her medications.
4. Put the medicine in applesauce to give it without the client's knowledge.

47. 1. Notifying the physician of the client's condition and her refusal to take her medications allows the physician to decide what alternatives should be instituted. Holding a medication requires the physician to be notified. Giving medications in applesauce destroys trust between the nurse and client. Even if the client takes some of the medications, the physician will still need to be notified. It needs to be explored why the client believes the medications are making her worse.

NP: Implementation; CN: Physiological integrity; CNS: Pharmacological and parenteral therapies; CL: Application

48. Which of the following statements is an example of a key element in the nursing plan of care?

1. Advance diet to regular as tolerated.
2. Ambulate 30′ with walker by discharge.
3. Give furosemide (Lasix) 40 mg I.V. now.
4. Discontinue I.V. fluids when tolerating oral fluids.

48. 2. Ambulating 30′ with a walker by discharge is a measurable expected outcome or goal, a key element of a nursing care plan. Other key elements include nursing diagnoses and interventions. The other options are physician's orders, not key elements of care plans.

NP: Planning; CN: Safe, effective care environment; CNS: Management of care; CL: Application

49. A client hasn't had a bowel movement for 3 days. Which of the following medications may contribute to the constipation?

1. Folic acid
2. Iron
3. Potassium
4. Vitamin E

49. 2. Iron may cause constipation when supplements are taken at 100% of the RDA. Vitamin E, folic acid, and potassium don't increase the likelihood of constipation.

NP: Planning; CN: Physiological integrity; CNS: Pharmacological and parenteral therapies; CL: Knowledge

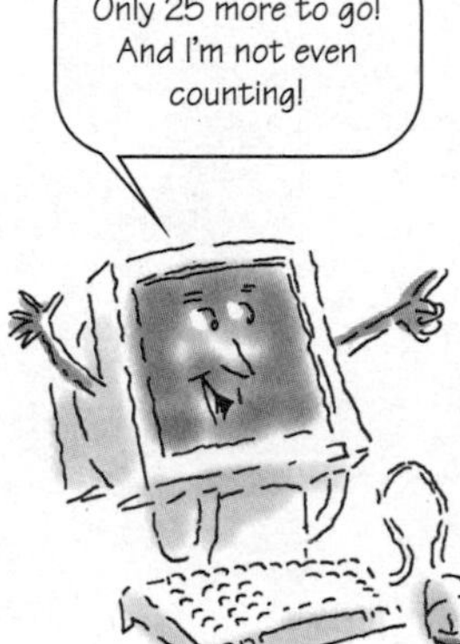

Only 25 more to go! And I'm not even counting!

50. A client had an appendectomy 24 hours ago. Which of the following goals is appropriate for this client?

1. The client will be able to walk in the hallway.
2. The client will be able to attend physical therapy.
3. The client will be able to accomplish all activities of daily living.
4. The client will be able to state the rationale for all postoperative medications.

50. 1. A 24-hour postoperative client is expected to be able to walk in the hallway. It's too early to expect a client to state the rationale for all postoperative medications, especially if the client is elderly. A client who just had an appendectomy shouldn't need physical therapy unless deconditioning was evident. At 24 hours, a client should begin to assume responsibility for activities of daily living, but shouldn't necessarily be responsible for all activities.

NP: Planning; CN: Physiological integrity; CNS: Basic care and comfort; CL: Application

51. Which of the following actions is included in the principles of asepsis?

1. Maintain a sterile environment.
2. Keep the environment as clean as possible.
3. Test for microorganisms in the environment.
4. Clean an environment until it's free from germs.

51. 2. Asepsis is the process of avoiding contamination from outside sources by keeping the environment clean. A clean environment has a reduced number of microorganisms, but isn't necessarily sterile (the absence of all microorganisms). Testing for microorganisms or culturing isn't indicated in the promotion of asepsis.

NP: Analysis; CN: Safe, effective care environment; CNS: Safety and infection control; CL: Comprehension

52. A nurse is helping another nurse transfer a client from the bed to a stretcher. Which of the following principles of body mechanics is correct?

1. Bend from the waist.
2. Pull rather than push.
3. Stretch to reach an object.
4. Use large muscles in the legs for leverage.

52. 4. Keeping one's back straight and using the large muscles in the legs will help avoid back injury, as the muscles in one's back are relatively small compared with the larger muscles of the thighs. Pulling isn't the best option and may cause straining. When feasible, one should push an object rather than pull it. Stretching to reach an object increases the risk for injury. Bending from the waist can cause stress on the back muscles causing a potential injury.

NP: Planning; CN: Safe, effective care environment; CNS: Safety and infection control; CL: Comprehension

53. A registered nurse (RN) is supervising an unlicensed care provider. The role of the RN includes which of the following principles?

1. The RN must directly supervise all delegated tasks.
2. After a task is delegated, it's no longer the RN's responsibility.
3. The RN is responsible for delegating tasks to adjunct personnel.
4. Follow-up with a delegated task is necessary only if the assistive personnel are untrustworthy.

53. 3. The RN must delegate tasks that are within the scope of practice of the unlicensed personnel. Even when the task is delegated, the RN retains responsibility for the successful completion of the task. The RN need not directly supervise all delegated tasks as that would negate the benefits of delegation. The RN must always follow up with the assistive personnel to ensure the task was completed appropriately, not only in instances of mistrust.

NP: Planning; CN: Safe, effective care environment; CNS: Management of care; CL: Comprehension

54. An elderly client had recent surgery and is on bed rest. When planning care for the client, which of the following nursing interventions is included?

1. Daily assessment of the wound site
2. Foot and ankle range-of-motion (ROM) exercises
3. Wound cleansing with hydrogen peroxide
4. Coughing and deep breathing in the prone position

54. 2. Foot and ankle ROM exercises are standard protocol for clients who remain in bed for an extended period of time. ROM exercises promote blood flow to the area, prevent atrophy, and lessen the potential for edema. Coughing and deep breathing aren't generally recommended in the prone position. Wound cleaning with hydrogen peroxide isn't generally recommended. The wound site should be assessed every shift.

NP: Planning; CN: Physiological integrity; CNS: Reduction of risk potential; CL: Application

55. A client receiving phenothiazine has become restless and fidgety and has been pacing the hallway continuously for the past hour. This behavior suggests that the client may be experiencing which of the following adverse reactions to phenothiazine?

1. Dystonia
2. Akathisia
3. Parkinsonian effects
4. Tardive dyskinesia

55. 2. The client's behavior suggests akathisia — an adverse effect of phenothiazines. Dystonia appears as excessive salivation, difficulty speaking, and involuntary movements of the face, neck, arms and legs. Parkinsonian effects include a shuffling gait, hand tremors, drooling, rigidity, and loose arm movements. Tardive dyskinesia is characterized by odd facial and tongue movements.

NP: Analysis; CN: Physiological integrity; CNS: Reduction of risk potential; CL: Comprehension

56. A client who had her gallbladder removed two days ago now complains of pain in the right calf. Which of the following responses has priority?

1. Assess the client for Homans' sign.
2. Instruct the client to flex her knee and hip.
3. Apply a warm compress and call the physician.
4. Gently massage the calf and notify the physician.

56. 1. Pain in the calf is a symptom of possible deep vein thrombosis. The nurse must assess further. Assessing the client for Homans' sign would be the next intervention. Never massage the calf muscle as the clot could be dislodged. Making the client flex her knee and hip won't help assess for the presence of a clot. Warm compresses may be ordered after a diagnosis of deep vein thrombosis is made.

NP: Implementation; CN: Physiological integrity; CNS: Reduction of risk potential; CL: Analysis

57. A nurse deflates the balloon on a pulmonary artery catheter after obtaining a wedge pressure reading. Which of the following rationales for this is most accurate?

1. Prevent cardiac arrhythmias.
2. Prevent pulmonary tissue infarction.
3. Obtain cardiac output measurements.
4. Obtain accurate left ventricular pressure readings.

57. 2. If the balloon on the pulmonary artery catheter is left inflated, it would stay in a wedged position and occlude the area distal to it. This would result in infarction of tissue. The functions of a pulmonary artery catheter include obtaining left ventricular pressure readings and cardiac output measurements, but this isn't why the balloon is deflated. Preventing cardiac arrhythmias is secondary.

NP: Implementation; CN: Physiological integrity; CNS: Reduction of risk potential; CL: Comprehension

58. Which of the following statements by a client with chronic arterial disease indicates further teaching is needed?

1. "I'm going to stop smoking."
2. "I'm going to have the podiatrist check my feet."
3. "I'm going to keep the heat in my house at 80° F."
4. "I'm going to walk short distances every morning."

58. 3. Clients with peripheral vascular disease need to be at a comfortable temperature because of impaired circulation. Having the heat at 80° F is too warm. The other choices are all appropriate interventions for a client with peripheral vascular disease.

NP: Evaluation; CN: Physiological integrity; CNS: Reduction of risk potential; CL: Application

59. A registered nurse is in charge of eight clients. The nurse has a licensed practical nurse (LPN) and a client care assistant working under her. Which of the following activities would the nurse assign to herself rather than delegate to the staff?

1. Consoling a grieving visitor.
2. Assessing a newly admitted client.
3. Irrigating a Salem sump to continuous drainage.
4. Giving a tap water enema to a preoperative client.

59. 2. Assessment of a new admission can't be delegated to an LPN. Consoling a visitor and giving a tap water enema are within the scope of practice of an LPN and client care assistant. Irrigation of a Salem sump is under the scope of practice of an LPN.

NP: Planning; CN: Safe, effective care environment; CNS: Management of care; CL: Application

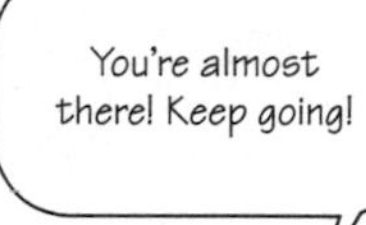
You're almost there! Keep going!

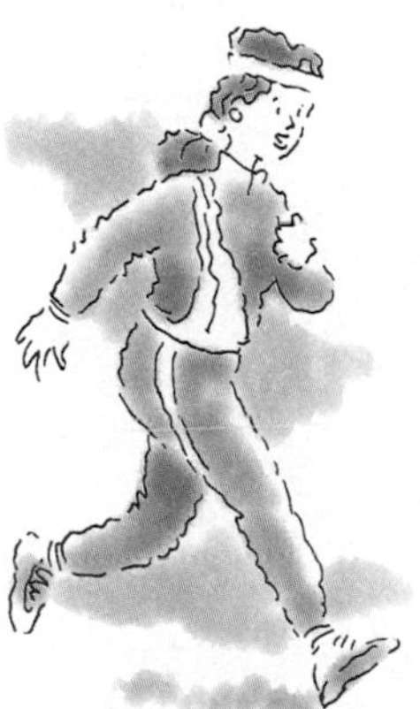

60. A 6-year-old child needs diabetic teaching. Which of the following factors is considered when the nurse plans the teaching?

1. Another child with diabetes can teach the client.
2. The child can teach his parents after the nurse teaches him.
3. The child and parents should be recipients of teaching.
4. Teaching should be directed to the parents, who then can teach the child.

60. 3. The parents and child should participate in the nurse's teaching to ensure accuracy of teaching and that the child has educated adult caregivers. Another school-aged child couldn't be entrusted to teach this child, although their input would be valuable. Parents should be included in the teaching plan but shouldn't be responsible for the teaching. The school-aged child shouldn't be the sole provider of teaching to the parents.

NP: Planning; CN: Health promotion and maintenance; CNS: Growth and development through the life span; CL: Application

61. Parents of a toddler are having problems putting the him to bed at night. Which of the following interventions is most appropriate?

1. Stop the afternoon naps.
2. Allow the toddler to have a tantrum for ½ hour.
3. Encourage the parents to develop nighttime rituals.
4. Allow the toddler to have some control over bedtime.

61. 3. Rituals are extremely important for toddlers to feel secure and relaxed. Allowing a toddler to make small decisions, such as choosing the order of the ritual and color of pajamas, will give him the feeling of some control. The toddler must clearly understand that tantrums won't get him what he wants. Stopping the naps may be helpful, depending on the toddler's needs.

NP: Implementation; CN: Psychosocial integrity; CNS: Coping and adaptation; CL: Knowledge

62. After abdominal surgery for repair of an aortic aneurysm, a client may show maladaptive coping behavior in response to body changes related to the surgery. Which of the following nursing interventions is best?

1. Let the client express his feelings.
2. Explain that a psychological referral would be beneficial.
3. Instruct the client on how to use positive coping strategies.
4. Encourage the client to participate in diversionary activities.

62. 1. Allowing verbalization of feelings is the most therapeutic nursing intervention. Providing diversionary activities doesn't foster effective coping. Making a referral may help, but initially the client should be allowed to express feelings. Giving advice may stop therapeutic communication.

NP: Implementation; CN: Psychosocial integrity; CNS: Coping and adaptation.; CL: Analysis

63. A new nurse graduate has started at the medical center and is assigned to a preceptor. The preceptor and other staff report that the nurse is uncooperative and unwilling to take direction. Which of the following actions by the preceptor is appropriate?

1. Explain the behavior won't be tolerated.
2. Ask the nurse why she wants to work here.
3. Reestablish goals with the nurse.
4. Begin the disciplinary process with this nurse.

63. 3. This is a new graduate in orientation and the preceptor should help this nurse learn the responsibilities and routines and reestablish goals. If the behavior continues, the nurse may need career counseling. This person isn't experienced and therefore shouldn't be reprimanded. Asking the nurse "why" in relation to working is inappropriate; it's the behavior that's creating the problem. This nurse shouldn't be disciplined as an initial step.

NP: Analysis; CN: Psychosocial integrity; CNS: Psychosocial adaptation; CL: Application

64. A client with a history of bipolar disorder rushes into the mental health clinic waiting room scantily dressed and makes loud, obscene remarks to other clients. Which of the following responses by the nurse has priority?

1. Encourage the other clients to ignore the behavior.
2. Confront the behavior and make the client take a seat.
3. Tell the client to sit down and stop upsetting the others.
4. Quietly escort the client to a private area and help put on a gown.

64. 4. The client with bipolar disorder is highly excitable. The nurse needs to be firm yet distracting, and this is best done in a private area, which also preserves the client's dignity. Telling the client to sit down may cause the client to be more resistive and even heighten the behavior. Confronting the behavior isn't desired as this client lacks judgment and insight. Having the others ignore the client won't alter the problem.

NP: Implementation; CN: Psychosocial integrity; CNS: Psychosocial adaptation; CL: Analysis

65. A nurse is reviewing treatment of hypercyanotic spells (tet spells) with the parents of a 4-month-old client being discharged from the hospital. Which of the following discharge instructions is correct?

1. "Calm the baby down by holding her and placing her knees up to her chest."
2. "Call 911 immediately and begin cardiopulmonary resuscitation (CPR) on the baby."
3. "You'll need to administer four back blows to the baby if she begins having a tet spell."
4. "You don't need to worry about these spells yet because the baby is too young. You'll need to watch for them when she becomes more mobile."

65. 1. Tet spells are acute episodes of cyanosis and hypoxia that occur when the infant's oxygen demand exceeds the available supply. They may occur when the infant is crying or eating. Tet spells are emergency situations that require immediate intervention. Begin by calming the infant down and placing the infant in the knee-chest position, which increases systemic vascular resistance by limiting venous return. This decreases the right to left shunting and improves oxygenation. Back blows are given to infants who have something lodged in their trachea. CPR won't calm the infant down or improve oxygenation.

NP: Implementation; CN: Physiological integrity; CNS: Reduction of risk potential; CL: Application

66. Which of the following nursing interventions is used to treat gout?

1. Antibiotics, high fluid intake, narcotics
2. Antihyperuricemic drugs, low-purine diet, narcotics
3. High fluid intake, low-purine diet, antihyperuricemic drugs
4. High-purine diet, nonsteroidal anti-inflammatory drugs, prednisone

66. 3. A low-purine diet decreases uric acid formation, and the high fluid intake increases urinary output to flush out the uric acid. Drugs such as antihyperuricemics are used to reduce serum urate concentrations. Anti-inflammatory medications are used during acute phases, but because this is a long-term condition, narcotics aren't generally given.

NP: Implementation; CN: Physiological integrity; CNS: Reduction of risk potential; CL: Application

67. Which of the following symptoms is a late sign of compartment syndrome?

1. Sudden decrease in pain
2. Swelling of toes or fingers
3. Inability to move fingers or toes
4. Change in skin color and diminished distal pulses

67. 4. Compartment syndrome is a complication of a cast that places pressure on the blood vessels and nerves to the extremity. Symptoms include pain not relieved by analgesics and swelling of the extremity. A late symptom is a change in skin color with diminished distal pulses. After a fracture, some swelling and pain result, but pulses need to be monitored, as well as color, sensation, and movement.

NP: Evaluation; CN: Physiological integrity; CNS: Reduction of risk potential; CL: Analysis

68. A client with an arm cast complains of severe pain in the affected extremity and decreased sensation and motion are noted. Swelling in the fingers is also increased. Which of the following interventions has priority?

1. Elevate the arm.
2. Remove the cast.
3. Give an analgesic.
4. Call the physician.

68. 4. The cast may be too tight and may need to be split or removed by the physician. The arm should already be elevated. Notify the physician when circulation, sensation, or motion is impaired. Giving analgesics wouldn't be the first step as they may mask the signs of a serious problem.

NP: Implementation; CN: Physiological integrity; CNS: Reduction of risk potential; CL: Application

69. Which of the following characteristics is correct for preoperative teaching of a 4-year-old child scheduled for a cardiac catheterization?

1. Basic and performed close to the implementation of the procedure
2. Done several days before the procedure so the child will have time to prepare
3. Detailed in regard to the actual procedure so the child will know exactly what to expect
4. Directed at the child's parents because the child is too young to understand the procedure

69. 1. Four-year-old children are in Piaget's cognitive stage of preoperational thought. Their thinking is concrete and tangible, and they're unable to make deductions or generalizations and are egocentric. They need simple explanations of procedures in relationship to how the procedure will affect them. They don't have a concept for the future so explanations need to be done close to the time of the procedure, not days in advance.

NP: Planning; CN: Health promotion and maintenance; CNS: Growth and development through the life span; CL: Comprehension

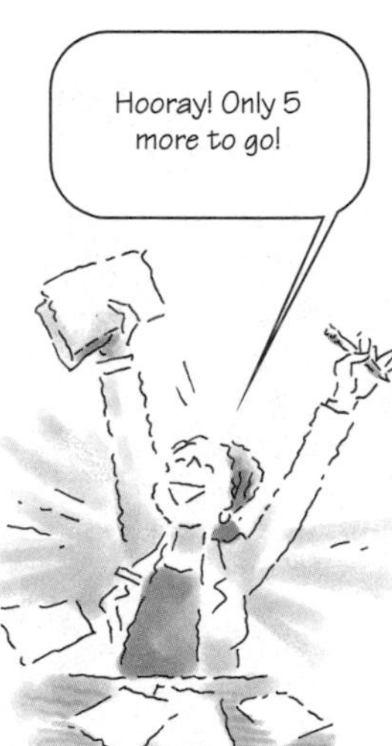

70. The registered nurse is directing unlicensed personnel to draw the morning blood work for a 4-year-old child in the hospital. The nurse emphasizes the procedure is to be done in the treatment room. Which of the following rationales is correct?

1. The procedure will be faster.
2. The child won't fear painful procedures done while he's in his bed.
3. The child can only be restrained on the examination table.
4. The parents won't observe the procedure and upset the child.

70. 2. This implementation is based on the concept of "atraumatic care" and growth and development principles. Small children need to have a safe zone in their beds to relax and rest in their rooms. The treatment room is used instead. Parental support is important and needs to be encouraged during stressful and painful procedures. It won't be faster to draw blood in the treatment room; it would take the same amount of time regardless of where it's done. The child could be restrained in his room, but it isn't appropriate.

NP: Implementation; CN: Psychosocial integrity; CNS: Coping and adaptation; CL: Comprehension

71. A client tells a nurse, "My medical illness is the result of something bad I did to someone in the past." Which of the following responses by the nurse is the most appropriate?

1. "What did you do wrong?"
2. "Let's talk about your concerns."
3. "That's silly! Don't believe that!"
4. "You're suffering from a psychiatric delusion. Relax, it will end soon."

71. 2. The nurse must be aware of cultural variations that relate to illness so she can appropriately address the client's needs. Calling the client silly or asking the client what he did wrong would likely escalate the client's concerns. Telling the client it will end soon gives false reassurance.

NP: Assessment; CN: Psychosocial integrity; CNS: Psychosocial adaptation; CL: Application

72. A client on a psychiatric unit asks a nurse about the medications another client takes. Which of the following responses is best?

1. "How close are the two of you?"
2. "I can't give you that information, I must protect her privacy."
3. "Let me ask her if it's OK for me to tell you about her condition and medications."
4. "The client is taking insulin for her diabetes and digitalis for her heart condition."

72. 2. Revealing one client's medication to another client is violating procedures of client confidentiality. Seeking the client's permission to release confidential information is an inappropriate action. Asking the client the nature of his relationship to the other client won't help the client understand the purpose of protecting confidentiality. Assuring the client that the hospital has an obligation to protect not only his confidentiality but that of others will provide the client with a sense of comfort.

NP: Implementation; CN: Psychosocial integrity; CNS: Psychosocial adaptation; CL: Application

NP: Nursing process CN: Client needs category CNS: Client needs subcategory CL: Cognitive level

73. A client's goal is to interact verbally at least once in each group therapy session by a certain date. The client attended the group session, maintained eye contact with the group members, followed the conversation nonverbally as indicated by head nodding, and spoke once to the group leader by giving a one-word answer. Which of the following judgments by the nurse about goal attainment is correct?

1. The goal was partially met.
2. The goal was completely met.
3. The goal was completely unmet.
4. New problems or nursing diagnoses have developed.

73. 1. This goal was partially met because the client must verbally participate more in the group. For a goal to be completely met, the client must show the subjective and objective data indicating the goal has been clearly attained. A completely unmet goal indicates the client's complete lack of behavior change and absence of subjective and objective data to indicate the achievement of the goal. In this case, no new problems or new nursing diagnoses were evident.

NP: Evaluation; CN: Psychosocial integrity; CNS: Coping and adaptation; CL: Analysis

74. Two days after admission to a psychiatric unit, a client with bipolar disorder becomes verbally aggressive during a group therapy session. Which nursing response is best?

1. "You're behaving in an unacceptable manner, and you need to control yourself."
2. "You're scaring everyone in the group. You can't participate until you know how to act."
3. "This is why you have relationship troubles; you don't know how to talk to people."
4. "You're disturbing the other clients. Let's go to the exercise room to help you release some of your energy."

74. 4. This response shows the nurse finds the client's behavior unacceptable, yet still regards the client as worthy of help. The third option is judgmental and not therapeutic. The other options give the false impression that the client is in control of the behavior; the client hasn't been in treatment long enough to control the behavior.

NP: Implementation; CN: Psychosocial integrity; CNS: Coping and adaptation; CL: Evaluation

75. A client visits a physician's office to seek treatment for depression, feelings of hopelessness, poor appetite, insomnia, low self-esteem, and difficulty making decisions. The client says that these symptoms began at least 2 years ago. Which of the following disorders is suspected?

1. Major depression
2. Dysthymic disorder
3. Cyclothymic disorder
4. Atypical affective disorder

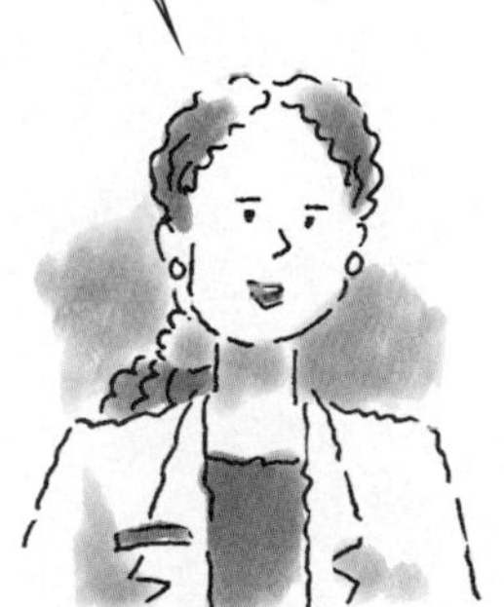

You're terrific! I knew you could do it! Only one more test to take. Go for it!

75. 2. Dysthymic disorder is marked by feelings of depression lasting at least 2 years, accompanied by at least two of the following symptoms: sleep disturbance, appetite disturbance, low energy or fatigue, low self-esteem, poor concentration, difficulty making decisions, and hopelessness. Cyclothymic disorder is a chronic mood disturbance of at least 2 years' duration marked by numerous periods of depression and hypomania. Major depression is a recurring, persistent sadness or loss of interest or pleasure in almost all activities, with signs and symptoms recurring for at least 2 weeks. Manic signs and symptoms characterize atypical affective disorder.

NP: Assessment; CN: Psychosocial integrity; CNS: Psychosocial adaptation; CL: Knowledge

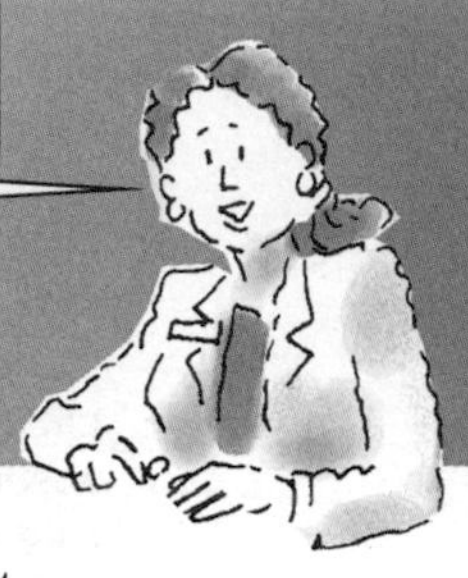
This is the LAST
comprehensive test.
Good luck! I know
you're ready for it.

COMPREHENSIVE Test 6

1. A nurse is teaching clients about hypertension. When she's explaining the importance of modifying risk factors, which factor would not be included?

1. High sodium intake
2. Sedentary lifestyle
3. Tobacco use
4. Family history

1. 4. Family history is a risk factor for hypertension that can't be modified. Risk factors that can be modified include high-sodium intake, sedentary lifestyle, and tobacco use.

NP: Implementation; CN: Health promotion and maintenance; CNS: Prevention and early detection of disease; CL: Application

2. A client experienced an acute inferior myocardial infarction at a local community hospital. After antithrombolytic therapy fails, the physician wants to transfer the client to a neighboring hospital for emergency cardiac catheterization. Which member of the health care team must accompany the client?

1. Physician
2. Paramedic
3. Registered nurse (RN)
4. Licensed practical nurse (LPN)

2. 3. During transfer, the client must receive the same level of care that he received in the hospital; therefore, an RN must accompany him. It isn't necessary for a physician to accompany the client. A paramedic, although not required, will most likely accompany the nurse. An LPN is below the standard of care for this situation.

NP: Implementation; CN: Safe, effective care environment; CNS: Management of care; CL: Application

3. A 56-year-old client with heart failure is allergic to sulfa-based medications. Which type of diuretic should he avoid?

1. Osmotic diuretics
2. Thiazide and thiazide-like diuretics
3. Potassium-sparing diuretics
4. Loop diuretics

3. 2. Thiazide and thiazide-like diuretics are sulfonamide derivatives, so their use should be avoided in clients allergic to sulfa-based medications. Osmotic, potassium-sparing, and loop diuretics can be safely administered to these clients. Loop diuretics, however, are most commonly administered for treatment of heart failure.

NP: Planning; CN: Physiological integrity; CNS: Pharmacological and parenteral therapies; CL: Application

4. A client with heart failure says he sleeps with two pillows because he experiences difficulty breathing when lying flat. The nurse documents which type of breathing?

1. Bradypnea
2. Dyspnea on exertion
3. Paroxysmal nocturnal dyspnea
4. Orthopnea

4. 4. A client with orthopnea has shortness of breath when lying flat, so he prefers sleeping with the upper body elevated. Bradypnea is decreased but regular breathing. Dyspnea on exertion occurs when the client has difficulty breathing with activity. Paroxysmal nocturnal dyspnea occurs when the client awakens at night and feels short of breath.

NP: Assessment; CN: Health promotion and maintenance; CNS: Prevention and early detection of disease; CL: Application

5. During an initial assessment of a neonate, the nurse notes a respiratory rate of 62 breaths/minute. How should the nurse intervene?

1. Notify the physician immediately.
2. Do nothing; this is a normal respiratory rate for a neonate.
3. Position the isolette so the neonate's head is elevated.
4. Prepare for emergency endotracheal intubation.

5. 2. A normal respiratory rate for a neonate is 30 to 80 breaths/minute, so notifying the physician or elevating the neonate's head isn't necessary. The nurse should prepare for endotracheal intubation if the neonate has signs of imminent respiratory distress such as an expiratory grunt.

NP: Implementation; CN: Health promotion and maintenance; CNS: Growth and development through the life span; CL: Analysis

6. During a neonate's 1-month checkup, the pediatrician flexes the neonate's legs to right angles at the hips and knees, and abducts both hips until the knees touch the table. Which statement describes the purpose of this test?

1. To check the neonate's flexibility
2. To assess leg strength
3. To check for congenital hip dislocation
4. To examine the neonate for a hydrocele

6. 3. This test assesses for congenital hip dislocation. If dislocation is present, the physician can see, feel, and sometimes hear a click. Although a neonate's flexibility and leg strength may be assessed at age 1 month, the examination techniques differ from those described here. To identify a hydrocele, the physician palpates the neonate's testes.

NP: Assessment; CN: Physiological integrity; CNS: Physiological adaptation; CL: Analysis

7. At which age should initial screening for idiopathic juvenile scoliosis take place?

1. 7 years
2. 10 years
3. 13 years
4. 16 years

7. 2. Children should have initial screening at age 10—immediately before the adolescent growth spurt—when promontory signs of scoliosis may become apparent. By age 13, a child may have significantly developed scoliosis that requires surgery.

NP: Assessment; CN: Health promotion and maintenance; CNS: Growth and development through the life span; CL: Application

8. Which position is correct for scoliosis screening of a 10-year-old male?

1. Facing away from the examiner, standing upright with his arms held out straight in front of his body
2. Facing away from the examiner, bending forward in 50% flexion with his arms and head dangling
3. Facing the examiner, standing upright with his arms held straight at his sides
4. Sitting in a chair with feet flat on the floor and his back at a 90-degree angle

8. 2. Assessing a client's back for asymmetry, or a "razorback" hump, is best done with the client bending at the waist in 50% flexion with the arms and head dangling. This assessment can also be done with the arms hanging dependently at the sides so the examiner can check for asymmetry at the shoulders, waist folds, and space between the arms and waist.

NP: Assessment; CN: Health promotion and maintenance; CNS: Prevention and early detection of disease; CL: Application

9. Parents bring their infant to the clinic for a checkup after she was hospitalized with a new onset of type 1 diabetes mellitus. Which statement would indicate an understanding of their child's current situation?

1. "The physician was wrong about the diagnosis because all of my child's fingersticks have been normal."
2. "My child has experienced a honeymoon period, which could last a month to a year, and hasn't required any insulin injections."
3. "Nobody in our family has diabetes, so how can my child have it?"
4. "If our child lives a careful, sedentary lifestyle, she won't need as much insulin."

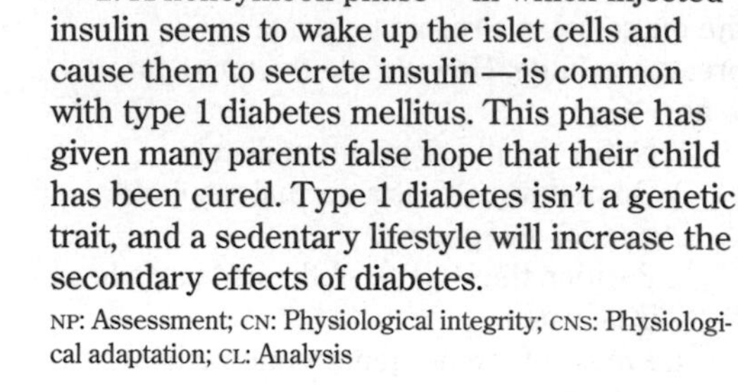

9. 2. A honeymoon phase—in which injected insulin seems to wake up the islet cells and cause them to secrete insulin—is common with type 1 diabetes mellitus. This phase has given many parents false hope that their child has been cured. Type 1 diabetes isn't a genetic trait, and a sedentary lifestyle will increase the secondary effects of diabetes.

NP: Assessment; CN: Physiological integrity; CNS: Physiological adaptation; CL: Analysis

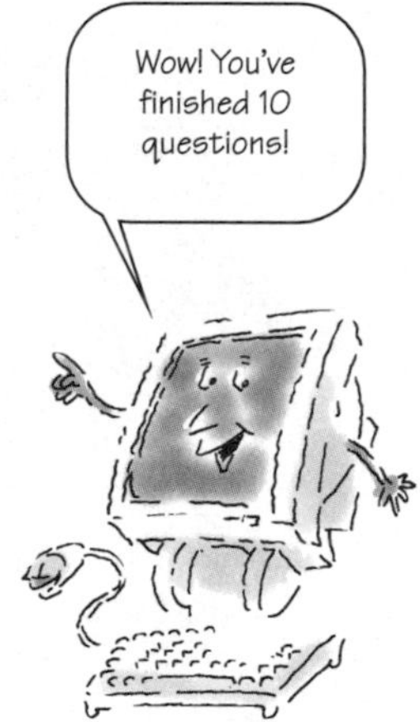
Wow! You've finished 10 questions!

10. A client with dyspnea, diaphoresis, stridor, hypotension, and cyanosis comes to the emergency department. His wife states that 2 days ago he complained of fever, malaise, cough, and mild chest discomfort; however, he seemed to be better then he developed his present symptoms. Based on his presentation, which diagnosis is most likely?

1. Smallpox
2. Inhalation anthrax
3. Botulism
4. Pneumonic plague

10. 2. This client's clinical presentation is consistent with inhalation anthrax. Signs and symptoms include fever, malaise, cough, mild chest discomfort, and a short recovery phase. The recovery phase is followed by the onset of dyspnea, diaphoresis, stridor, cyanosis, and shock. Death typically occurs 24 to 36 hours after the onset of severe symptoms. Smallpox causes fever, back pain, vomiting, malaise, headache, and rigors. Papules form 2 to 3 days later; the papules are initially abundant on the face and extremities and progress to pustular vesicles. The initial signs and symptoms of botulism are ptosis, blurred vision, diplopia, generalized weakness, dizziness, dysarthria (difficulty speaking), dysphonia (hoarseness), and dysphagia (difficulty swallowing). These signs and symptoms are followed by symmetrical descending flaccid paralysis and respiratory failure. The client with pneumonic plague presents with high fever, chills, headache, hemoptysis, and toxemia. A rapid progression to dyspnea, stridor, and cyanosis occurs. Without treatment, the client with pneumonic plague will die from respiratory failure, shock, and bleeding in 12 to 24 hours

NP: Assessment; CN: Physiological integrity; CNS: Physiological adaptation; CL: Analysis

NP: Nursing process CN: Client needs category CNS: Client needs subcategory CL: Cognitive level

11. A 2-year-old male child is admitted for surgical removal of a Wilms' tumor. Wilms' tumor is an adenosarcoma located in which organ?

1. Liver
2. Kidney
3. Pancreas
4. Duodenum

11. 2. Wilms' tumor is found in the kidney and kidney area. It isn't found in the liver, pancreas, or any part of the small intestine.

NP: Assessment; CN: Health promotion and maintenance; CNS: Prevention and early detection of disease; CL: Knowledge

12. Two days after undergoing a left thoracotomy, a client's temperature reaches 102° F (38.9° C). The nurse notifies the physician who orders two sets of blood cultures. How much blood is necessary for the cultures?

1. 2 ml
2. 5 ml
3. 10 ml
4. 20 ml

12. 3. When an adult client requires blood cultures, the nurse should draw 10 ml of blood; 5 ml should be injected into an anaerobic (without oxygen) bottle and 5 ml injected into an aerobic (with oxygen) bottle.

NP: Implementation; CN: Physiological integrity; CNS: Reduction of risk potential; CL: Knowledge

13. The charge nurse is developing the client-care assignments for her shift. Which client is most appropriately assigned to a licensed practical nurse (LPN)?

1. a newly admitted client with a cerebrovascular accident and do-not-resuscitate (DNR) status
2. a client who underwent cerebral arteriography 1 hour ago
3. a client who underwent carotid endarterectomy 4 hours ago
4. a client who underwent craniotomy 3 days ago and has just been transferred from the critical care unit

13. 1. The most appropriate client to assign to the LPN is the newly admitted client with DNR status; typically, a newly admitted client is assigned to a registered nurse (RN) because the client requires frequent assessments. The client who recently underwent cerebral arteriography and the client who recently underwent carotid endarterectomy require frequent assessments by an RN. The client just transferred from the critical care unit has the potential for becoming unstable; therefore, an RN should care for this client.

NP: Assessment; CN: Safe, effective care environment; CNS: Management of care; CL: Analysis

14. A physician prescribes carbamazepine (Tegretol) 1,200 mg P.O. b.i.d. for a client with trigeminal neuralgia. Which action should the nurse take first?

1. Administer the medication with meals.
2. Encourage the client to promptly report unusual bleeding, bruising, fever, or chills.
3. Question the order because the dose exceeds the recommended daily dose.
4. Store the drug in a cool, dry place.

14. 3. The first intervention by the nurse should be to question the order because it exceeds the recommended daily dose. Clients with trigeminal neuralgia should receive no more than 1,200 mg/day. After the nurse obtains an appropriate order, she should encourage the client to take the drug at equally spaced intervals with food to avoid GI distress. The nurse should also encourage the client to promptly report unusual bleeding, bruising, jaundice, dark urine, pale stools, abdominal pain, impotence, fever, chills, sore throat, mouth ulcers, edema, or disturbances in mood, alertness, or coordination. The drug should be stored in a cool, dry place.

NP: Implementation; CN: Physiological integrity; CNS: Pharmacological and parenteral therapies; CL: Analysis

15. Emergency medical system (EMS) personnel have used the Cincinnati prehospital stroke scale to assess a client and have alerted the hospital that they're transporting a client with a possible stroke. The treatment goal is to administer fibrinolytics within which time period?

1. 4 hours of the onset of symptoms
2. 60 minutes of arrival in the emergency department (ED)
3. 2 hours of arrival in the ED
4. 25 minutes of arrival in the ED

15. 2. The goal for initiating fibrinolytic therapy is within 60 minutes of arrival in the ED. Fibrinolytics must be administered within 3 hours of the onset of symptoms.

NP: Implementation; CN: Physiological integrity; CNS: Pharmacological and parenteral therapies; CL: Application

16. A client with an above-the-knee amputation visits the orthopedic surgeon for a followup. Which comment would indicate the client is properly caring for the stump and prosthetic leg?

1. "I inspect the stump weekly to look for signs of redness, blistering, or abrasions."
2. "I put my prosthesis on before I get out of bed."
3. "I wash the stump every day with an antiseptic soap."
4. "I wipe out the socket of my prosthesis with a damp, soapy cloth weekly."

16. 2. The prosthesis should be applied upon rising in the morning. The stump and prosthesis should be inspected daily and cleaned daily with a mild soap. The prosthesis should be kept clean to prevent irritation or pressure areas from dirt or bacteria.

NP: Evaluation; CN: Health promotion and maintenance; CNS: Prevention and early detection of disease; CL: Analysis

17. The nurse is caring for a client after a total knee replacement. The extremity was placed in a continuous passive motion (CPM) machine in the postanesthesia care unit, and the physician has provided orders for degree of flexion and hours per day (cycle) of CPM use. Which action is one of the nurse's responsibilities?

1. Check the cycle and range-of-motion settings every morning.
2. Increase the degrees of flexion daily guided by client level of tolerance.
3. Instruct the family on how and when the CPM should be cycled.
4. Turn the machine off when the client is eating a meal.

17. 4. The CPM machine can be turned off during meals to improve client comfort. The cycle and degrees of flexion should be checked every shift, and either the physician or physical therapist determine how and when the degrees of flexion can be increased. To prevent injury to the client, only health care professionals should manipulate the CPM.

NP: Implementation; CN: Physiological integrity; CNS: Basic care and comfort; CL: Application

18. A client has multiple myeloma. Which action is a sign that he may not be coping well with his prognosis?

1. He becomes tearful when discussing his condition.
2. He asks questions about his prognosis.
3. He shows concerns about his family.
4. He avoids any conversation concerning his health.

18. 4. A client who avoids conversation about his health may be denying his condition and not coping well with his prognosis. Crying is a normal response to his disease. Asking questions about his prognosis and showing concern for his family are normal coping responses.

NP: Assessment; CN: Psychological integrity; CNS: Psychosocial adaptation; CL: Analysis

19. A client presents with intermittent lower back pain and limited motion of the lumbar spine. He asks the nurse if he might have ankylosing spondylitis. Which client is at greatest risk for developing ankylosing spondylitis?

1. White female age 4
2. Black male age 20
3. Asian male age 70
4. White female age 25

19. 4. Ankylosing spondylitis usually begins between ages 15 to 30 and the prevalence is highest in Whites.

NP: Assessment; CN: Health promotion and maintenance; CNS: Prevention and early detection of disease; CL: Knowledge

20. A client with pernicious anemia undergoes gastrectomy. Which route should the nurse use to administer cyanocobalamin (vitamin B_{12}) after the surgery?

1. Buccal route
2. Transdermal route
3. Oral route
4. Parenteral route

20. 4. A client who has undergone gastrectomy is no longer able to produce the intrinsic factor necessary for vitamin B_{12} absorption through the GI tract; therefore, the parenteral route (intramuscular or deep subcutaneous injections) is required. This medication isn't available for buccal or transdermal routes.

NP: Planning; CN: Physiological integrity; CNS: Pharmacological and parenteral therapies; CL: Application

21. After the nurse teaches a client with diverticular disease about proper diet, he fills out his lunch menu. Which selection by the client demonstrates the need for further teaching?

1. Tossed salad with tomatoes, sunflower seeds, and tuna
2. Egg salad on whole wheat bread and an apple
3. Cottage cheese with apple, pear, and plum slices
4. Ham salad served with whole wheat crackers and a banana

21. 1. Clients with diverticular disease should avoid high-roughage foods, such as nuts, seeds, popcorn, and raw celery. They should, however, consume high-fiber foods, such as fresh fruit with skins (apples, pears, and plums), bananas, dried fruits, whole wheat bread and crackers, and raw vegetables (lettuce, carrots, and cauliflower).

NP: Evaluation; CN: Physiological integrity; CNS: Basic care and comfort; CL: Application

22. A nurse is teaching nursing students about maintaining a healthy liver. Which measure should the nurse include in her teaching?

1. Take over-the-counter medication as needed.
2. Take prescribed medications according to instructions.
3. Add a nutritional supplement to the diet to ensure adequate nutrition.
4. Consume a low-protein diet that contains moderate carbohydrate and fat.

22. 2. Taking these measures will help maintain a healthy liver: take prescribed medications according to instructions; avoid taking unnecessary over-the-counter medications; eat a balanced diet that's moderate to high in protein, moderate in carbohydrate and fat, and adequate in vitamins; and take a nutritional supplement only if advised to do so by a physician.

NP: Implementation; CN: Health promotion and maintenance; CNS: Prevention and early detection of disease; CL: Application

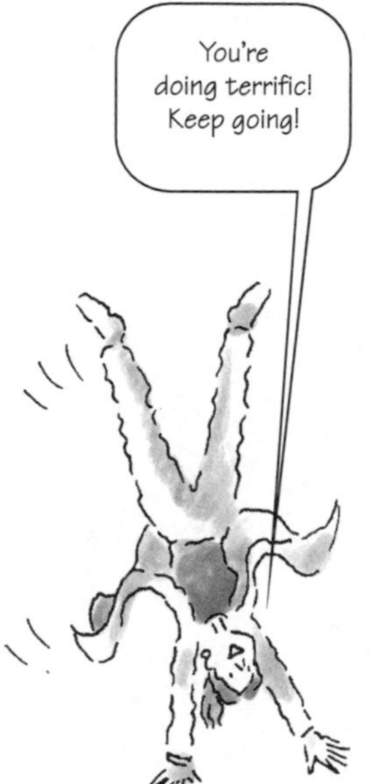
You're doing terrific! Keep going!

23. A 28-year-old female complaining of a racing heart and nervousness is admitted to the telemetry floor. Her telemetry shows a heart rate of 130 beats/minute in sinus tachycardia. Her skin is very warm, dry, and her eyes appear to be bulging. Which nursing action is the most important upon admission?

1. Inserting a urinary catheter and assessing appearance of urine
2. Observing the client's gait
3. Reaching out and feeling the client's neck
4. Standing behind the client and gently palpating the cricothyroid area

23. 4. The client shows signs of hyperthyroidism, and standing behind her and palpating the cricothyroid area is the correct way to assess for an enlarged thyroid gland. Inserting a catheter isn't necessary; assessing the client's urine, which would be concentrated because of dehydration, can be done after she voids. Observing the client's gait isn't necessary at this time.

NP: Assessment; CN: Physiological integrity; CNS: Physiological adaptation; CL: Analysis

24. A client is unemployed, has no health insurance, hasn't filled her levothyroxine (Synthroid) prescription for some time, and has been getting "sicker by the day." Which problem is probably related to her not taking her medication?

1 Diarrhea and vomiting
2. Rapid heart rate
3. Warm, dry, flushed skin
4. Rectal temperature of 94° F (34.4° C)

24. 4. Hypothyroidism leads to a hypodynamic state, so a low body temperature is expected after the levothyroxine has been metabolized. Each of the other symptoms is indicative of a hypermetabolic state and, although the client may exhibit these problems, they're probably related to infection and dehydration.

NP: Evaluation; CN: Physiological integrity; CNS: Physiological adaptation; CL: Application

25. A child with chronic renal failure is scheduled for hemodialysis with an external shunt three times per week. As part of the discharge planning, the nurse should tell the family to perform which step?

1. Assess the site daily for symptoms of redness.
2. Wash the serum at the shunt site with normal saline.
3. Assess the child's blood pressure on the same side as the shunt.
4. Keep a clean dressing in place over the shunt site.

25. 1. The child and parents should assess the shunt site for redness daily because a color change may indicate infection. Serum at the shunt site should be washed away with half strength hydrogen peroxide and an antibiotic ointment applied. Blood pressure shouldn't be taken in the arm with the shunt. A sterile dressing should be placed over the shunt site.

NP: Planning; CN: Safe, effective care environment; CNS: Safety and infection control; CL: Application

26. A 17-year-old client tells the nurse that she has vulvar itching and a thick, cream-cheese–like vaginal discharge. This condition is usually treated with which medication?

1. Metronidazole (Flagyl)
2. Erythromycin (Ery-Tab)
3. Miconazole (Monistat)
4. Amoxicillin (Amoxil)

26. 3. The client most likely has *candidiasis*, which produces a thick cream-cheese–like vaginal discharge and is treated with miconazole or nystatin (Mycostatin). Metronidazole is used to treat *Trichomonas vaginalis*. Erythromycin, amoxicillin, or other antibiotic therapy can contribute to *candidiasis* infections and isn't used to treat this infection.

NP: Implementation; CN: Physiological integrity; CNS: Pharmacological and parenteral therapies; CL: Application

27. When assessing a 5-hour-old neonate, which finding is a concern?

1. Color is dusky, axillary temperature is 96.8° F (37° C), and the baby is spitting up mucus.
2. Hands and feet are cyanotic, abdomen is rounded, and the infant hasn't voided or passed meconium.
3. Anterior fontanel is ¾" (2 cm) wide, head is molded, and sutures are overriding.
4. Irregular abdominal respirations and intermittent tremors in the extremities.

27. 1. Skin color should be pink tinged or ruddy and saliva should be scant. The normal axillary temperature ranges from 97.7° to 98.6° F (36.5° to 37° C). Acrocyanosis may be present for 2 to 6 hours. Overriding sutures and molding, when present, may persist for a few days. The neonate should pass meconium and void within 24 hours. Neonatal tremors are normal in the neonate; however, they must be evaluated to differentiate them from seizures.

NP: Assessment; CN: Health promotion and maintenance; CNS: Growth and development through the life span; CL: Application

28. A mother calls the pediatrician because there's an outbreak of scabies at her child's school. The nurse should tell the mother to check for which finding?

1. Pain, erythema, and edema at the site of the bite
2. Oval white dots that adhere to hair shafts
3. Diffuse pruritic wheals
4. Pruritic papules, vesicles, and linear burrows on the finger and toe webs

28. 4. The mother should check her child for pruritic papules, vesicles, and linear burrows on the finger and toe webs. Oval white dots that adhere to the hair shaft can indicate head lice.

NP: Analysis; CN: Health promotion and maintenance; CNS: Prevention and early detection of disease; CL: Knowledge

29. A young child with a rash that's raised and has circumscribed areas filled with fluid comes to the school health room. Which type of rash should the nurse document?

1. Vesicular rash
2. Papular rash
3. Macular rash
4. Petechial rash

29. 1. A vesicular rash contains small raised, circumscribed lesions filled with clear fluid. A papular rash contains raised solid lesions with color changes in circumscribed areas. A macular rash is flat with color changes in circumscribed areas. Petechiae are pinpoint purple or red spots on the skin caused by multiple hemorrhages.

NP: Assessment; CN: Physiological integrity; CNS: Reduction of risk potential; CL: Comprehension

30. A 20-month-old toddler has been treated with Nix for scabies. Because he continues to scratch, his mother wonders whether the drug is working. Which response by the nurse is most appropriate?

1. "Stop treatment because the drug isn't safe for children under age 2."
2. "Pruritus can be present for weeks after treatment."
3. "Apply the drug every day until the rash and itching disappears."
4. "Pruritus is common in children under age 5 treated with Nix."

30. 2. Pruritus may be present for weeks in a child treated with Nix for scabies. The drug is safe for use in infants as young as age 2 months. Treatment with Nix can be safely repeated in 2 weeks. Pruritus is caused by secondary reactions of the mites.

NP: Analysis; CN: Health promotion and maintenance; CNS: Prevention and early detection of disease; CL: Application

31. An 8-year-old child was sent home after the school reported the presence of head lice. Which information is most helpful to the parents?

1. The child should remain isolated for 1 week after treatment.
2. Lindane (Kwell) is the treatment of choice for head lice.
3. Treatment with a pediculicide followed by combing the hair with a fine-tooth comb will usually kill all lice and remove the nits. Retreatment in 7 to 10 days may be necessary to kill newly hatched lice.
4. The only way to get rid of head lice is to cut the hair.

31. 3. Treatment with a pediculicide followed by combing the hair with a fine-tooth comb will usually kill all lice and remove the nits. Retreatment in 7 to 10 days may be necessary to kill newly hatched lice. After the infestation has been appropriately treated, there's no reason to isolate the child. Lindane isn't the drug of choice because of its potential for neurotoxicity. The hair should be cut in severe cases only.

NP: Implementation; CN: Physiological integrity; CNS: Reduction of risk potential; CL: Application

32. A client needs an increased amount of a psychoactive substance to achieve the desired effects. Which term is the name for this need?

1. Withdrawal
2. Abuse
3. Dependence
4. Tolerance

32. 4. Tolerance is the need for increasing amounts of a substance to achieve the desired effects. Withdrawal is a characteristic syndrome that occurs after substance use is abruptly discontinued or dosage is dramatically reduced. Abuse is the continuing use of a substance even when it interferes with occupational and social functioning. The client abusing a substance can stop using it without experiencing symptoms of withdrawal. Dependence is a maladaptive pattern of substance use that leads to clinically significant impairment or distress.

NP: Assessment; CN: Psychosocial integrity; CNS: Coping and adaptation; CL: Comprehension

33. Which word best describes the type of schizophrenia identified by marked negativism, rigidity, excitement, stupor, or posturing?

1. Catatonic
2. Undifferentiated
3. Disorganized
4. Paranoid

33. 1. Catatonic schizophrenia is a state of psychologically induced immobilization, which is, at times, interrupted by episodes of extreme agitation, such as negativism, rigidity, excitement, stupor, or posturing. Undifferentiated schizophrenia occurs when no single clinical presentation dominates (paranoid, disorganized, or catatonic). Disorganized schizophrenia is characterized by disorganized speech, disorganized behavior, and inappropriate affect. The dominant theme in paranoid schizophrenia is one of delusions and hallucinations.

NP: Assessment; CN: Psychosocial integrity; CNS: Psychosocial adaptation; CL: Comprehension

34. A client is diagnosed with a somatoform disorder. This diagnosis has which primary gain?

1. Illness allows reprieve from responsibilities.
2. Sick role allows for dependency needs to be met.
3. The symptoms may serve to control others or to stabilize relationships.
4. The client becomes increasingly socialized.

34. 1. The primary gain in somatoform disorders is that the illness allows reprieve from responsibilities. The secondary gain is that the sick role allows for dependency needs to be met. In somatoform disorders, the client's symptoms may serve to control others, but this has nothing to do with primary gain. As the illness progresses, the client becomes increasingly socially isolated.

NP: Assessment; CN: Psychosocial integrity; CNS: Psychosocial adaptation; CL: Knowledge

35. A client complains of chronic lower back pain and fatigue and has seen multiple care providers without relief of symptoms. The client insists that something is "terribly wrong." Which action should the nurse take first?

1. Refer the client for a psychiatric evaluation.
2. Initiate group therapy for behavior modification.
3. Obtain a thorough health assessment to rule out physical illnesses.
4. Refer the client to physical therapy.

35. 3. The first action by the nurse should be to take a thorough health assessment including laboratory studies to rule out physical illnesses. The other actions aren't appropriate until a diagnosis is made.

NP: Analysis; CN: Psychosocial integrity; CNS: Psychosocial adaptation; CL: Comprehension

36. The nurse is discussing diet and nutrition with a client who's taking lithium and tells him that he should include adequate amounts of which nutrient in his diet?

1. Sugar
2. Salt
3. Protein
4. Fiber

36. 2. As lithium concentration increases, sodium concentration decreases. Thus, an adequate intake of salt (sodium) is necessary to avoid lithium toxicity. Lithium doesn't affect sugar, protein, or fiber intake.

NP: Implementation; CN: Physiological integrity; CNS: Pharmacological and parenteral therapies; CL: Knowledge

37. A client with bipolar disorder is taking lithium and tells the nurse, "I can stop taking the medicine when I feel better." Which response by the nurse is best?

1. "That's correct. When you feel better, you can stop taking the medication."
2. "Take the medication for 1 week after you feel better to be sure there's enough medication in your system."
3. "Bipolar clients may take lithium indefinitely to prevent relapses."
4. "This medication is given as needed. That means that you can take it when you feel that you need it."

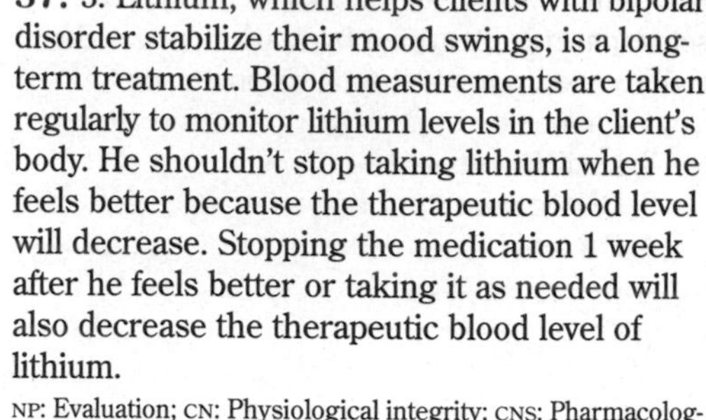

37. 3. Lithium, which helps clients with bipolar disorder stabilize their mood swings, is a long-term treatment. Blood measurements are taken regularly to monitor lithium levels in the client's body. He shouldn't stop taking lithium when he feels better because the therapeutic blood level will decrease. Stopping the medication 1 week after he feels better or taking it as needed will also decrease the therapeutic blood level of lithium.

NP: Evaluation; CN: Physiological integrity; CNS: Pharmacological and parenteral therapies; CL: Analysis

You're making great progress!

38. A client's condition is becoming stabilized after an episode of substance-induced delirium. During the initial recovery period, the nurse should assess the client for which psychosocial health problem?

1. Flashbacks
2. Depression
3. Nightmares
4. Dissociation

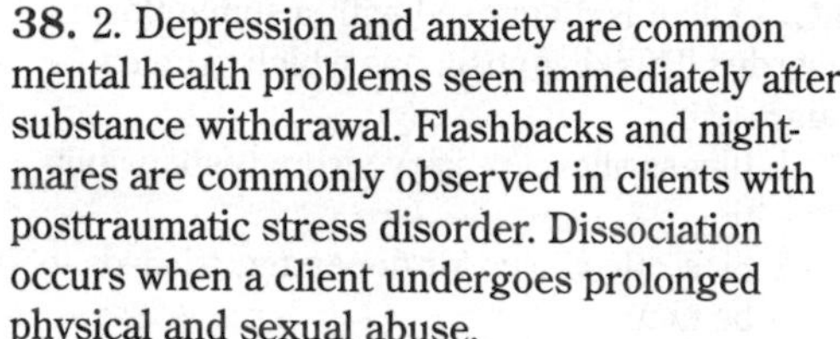

38. 2. Depression and anxiety are common mental health problems seen immediately after substance withdrawal. Flashbacks and nightmares are commonly observed in clients with posttraumatic stress disorder. Dissociation occurs when a client undergoes prolonged physical and sexual abuse.

NP: Assessment; CN: Psychosocial integrity; CNS: Coping and adaptation; CL: Analysis

39. A client with a history of depression demonstrates some inconsistent symptoms of cognitive impairment. The nurse should expect which situation when the depression is treated?

1. Delusional thinking ceases
2. Recognition of objects improves
3. Memory problems resolve
4. Suicidal ideation is no longer a problem

39. 3. In a condition called *pseudodementia,* a client treated for depression will have a dramatic improvement in memory. Delusional thinking and object-recognition problems aren't characteristic of pseudodementia. The nurse must assess all clients with depression for suicidal ideation because they're at some degree of risk for suicide.

NP: Assessment; CN: Psychosocial integrity; CNS: Coping and adaptation; CL: Application

40. A client with borderline personality disorder has extreme views of herself and her situation. Which behavior indicates that the client is a candidate for medication?

1. Disorientation
2. Hyperactivity
3. Regression
4. Mood swings

40. 4. Medications aren't typically given to clients with personality disorders. However, clients with mood swings, hallucinations, or psychotic behaviors are appropriate candidates for medications. Disorientation, hyperactivity and regression aren't necessarily seen in clients with borderline personality disorders.

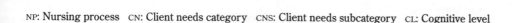

NP: Evaluation; CN: Psychosocial integrity; CNS: Psychosocial adaptation; CL: Application

41. A client has traits of an avoidant personality disorder. Which family intervention should be given priority in the care plan?

1. Explaining that the family should teach the client social skills.
2. Recommending that the family recognize the client's high sensitivity to criticism.
3. Exploring ways for the family to help the client express true feelings.
4. Asking the family to keep a daily log of the client's adjustment difficulties.

41. 2. A client with traits of an avoidant personality disorder is very sensitive to criticism and disapproval but doesn't typically have learning or social skills problems. Such a client may have difficulty expressing feelings and may have few friends or only family members for interaction. Having the family keep a log of the client's adjustment difficulties isn't an appropriate intervention; the list may be interpreted as a statement of rejection.

NP: Planning; CN: Psychosocial integrity; CNS: Coping and adaptation; CL: Analysis

42. A client with a substance abuse disorder says the problem doesn't really exist. Which intervention should be the nurse's initial one?

1. Educating about the principles of mental health
2. Examining the use of defense mechanisms
3. Recognizing and discussing feelings of resentment
4. Discussing the need for a caretaker while in recovery

42. 2. Defense mechanisms contribute to the client's denial. Education won't be well received unless the client recognizes the problem and determines that the nurse's teaching would be useful. The client can't recognize and discuss feelings of resentment when denying that a problem exists. The client needs to become responsible for his own behavior and take care of himself.

NP: Implementation; CN: Psychosocial integrity; CNS: Coping and adaptation; CL: Application

43. The nurse is evaluating drug therapy effectiveness in a client undergoing alcohol detoxification. Which finding indicates that drug therapy isn't successful?

1. There are signs of toxicity from the drug.
2. The drug prevents the occurrence of further problems.
3. During the course of treatment, the dosage has increased.
4. The drug facilitates the client's interactions with staff.

43. 1. Signs of toxicity from drug therapy may occur during the detoxification period. The medication is working if it prevents further problems. Sometimes the dosage must be adjusted to obtain the maximum benefit. If the drug enables the client to have therapeutic interactions with the staff, the client is benefiting from the therapy.

NP: Evaluation; CN: Physiological integrity; CNS: Pharmacological and parenteral therapies; CL: Application

44. The nurse explains the unit's rules to a client with bulimia nervosa. Which action by the client indicates that learning has occurred?

1. The client asks to be accompanied to the bathroom after lunch.
2. The client writes down every food item eaten in the past 24 hours.
3. The client decides to help the dietitian plan the unit's meals.
4. The client discusses current problems with the nurse before mealtime.

44. 1. When the client asks to be accompanied to the bathroom after a meal, the client is following protocol for restoring healthy eating and promoting adequate nutrition. This action indicates the client's commitment to not purging after a meal. Recording the food eaten in a 24-hour period would be appropriate for a client with anorexia nervosa, not a client with bulimia nervosa. It's inappropriate for a client to plan meals for the unit's clients. The client can discuss problems any time, not just before mealtimes.

NP: Evaluation; CN: Psychosocial integrity; CNS: Coping and adaptation; CL: Analysis

45. The nurse is teaching a client with an eating disorder about cues that trigger unhealthy eating behaviors. Which example explains social cues?

1. Diet advertisements
2. Troublesome memories
3. Interpersonal conflict
4. Frustration fatigue

45. 3. Social cues that trigger maladaptive behavior include feelings of isolation and conflict with family or friends. Diet advertisements are considered situational cues. Troublesome memories are psychological cues. Frustration fatigue is an example of a physiological cue.
NP: Implementation; CN: Psychosocial integrity; CNS: Coping and adaptation; CL: Application

46. A schizophrenic client states, "The voices keep talking to me. They're telling me that I have to leave here and that I shouldn't talk to you. Don't you hear what they're saying?" Which response is best?

1. "You didn't take your medicine this morning, did you?"
2. "The voices aren't real. You're sick and they're part of your illness."
3. "Are you hearing voices again?"
4. " I don't hear the voices, but I see that you are upset."

46. 4. The nurse should be honest and tell the client that she doesn't hear the voices while acknowledging the client's feelings. Asking if the client took his medication or explaining his illness doesn't allow the client to feel valued by the nurse. Asking him if he hears voices makes him feel that the nurse wasn't listening.
NP: Implementation; CN: Psychosocial integrity; CNS: Psychosocial adaptation; CL: Application

47. A nurse is teaching caregivers about the signs and symptoms of schizophrenia relapse. The caregivers should report which signs and symptoms to a mental health professional?

1. Changes in appetite resulting in weight loss or gain
2. Loss of interest in sexual activities
3. Increased socialization
4. Feelings of tenseness and difficulty sleeping

47. 4. Signs and symptoms of schizophrenia relapse include difficulty concentrating and sleeping, feelings of tenseness, and increased bizarre thinking and withdrawal. The other choices aren't signs and symptoms of schizophrenia.
NP: Assessment; CN: Psychosocial integrity; CNS: Psychosocial adaptation; CL: Knowledge

48. A client with schizophrenia has been prescribed risperidone (Risperdal). The client's symptoms include hallucinations, delusions, and withdrawal. The medication will help improve which symptoms?

1. Negative symptoms
2. Positive symptoms
3. Negative and positive symptoms
4. Paranoid symptoms

48. 3. Risperidone (Risperdal) targets both negative and positive symptoms. Positive symptoms include delusions, hallucinations, and bizarre behaviors. Negative symptoms indicate a loss or lack of normal functioning such as lack of motivation and social withdrawal.
NP: Assessment; CN: Physiological integrity; CNS: Pharmacological and parenteral therapies; CL: Application

49. A newly graduated nurse is caring for a client recently diagnosed with dissociative identity disorder. The nurse asks the preceptor about discussing a client's traumatic childhood with the client. Which advice from the preceptor is best?

1. "Ask pointed questions and demand specific answers."
2. "If the client begins talking about it, just listen and be supportive."
3. "Tell the client that you suspect that much of his memory is exaggerated."
4. "Tell the client that those issues can be discussed with a physician only."

49. 2. If the subject is painful, the client will discuss it when he feels comfortable and ready. Forcing him to talk about the subject will cause severe anxiety and result in distrust. The other choices don't facilitate a trusting relationship between the nurse and the client.

NP: Analysis. CN: Psychosocial integrity, CNS: Psychosocial adaptation, CL: Application

50. A client with dissociative identity disorder frequently switches from one personality to another. The nurse can identify the switch by which finding?

1. Episodes of orthostatic hypotension
2. Blinking or rolling the eyes frequently
3. Dystonic reactions
4. Episodes of tachycardia

50. 2 Switching from one personality to another is manifested in a number of ways including blinking, facial movements, and changes in voice. Changes in blood pressure or pulse or dystonic reactions aren't indicative of switching from one personality to another.

NP: Assessment; CN: Psychosocial integrity; CNS: Psychosocial adaptation; CL: Application

51. A 38-year-old female is scheduled to have a hysterectomy and is concerned about no longer being a "whole woman." Which intervention by the nurse is best?

1. Tell her to talk to her husband about the permanent changes that will be taking place with her body.
2. Refer her to group therapy.
3. Encourage her to discuss her concerns and feelings.
4. Give her information to read and leave the room.

51. 3. The nurse should encourage the client to express her feelings. Telling her to talk to her husband will cause the client added concern and anxiety. Referring her to group therapy isn't an appropriate intervention at this time. Giving her information and leaving the room doesn't allow her to ask questions and express concerns.

NP: Analysis; C: Psychosocial integrity; CNS: Psychosocial adaptation; CL: Analysis

52. A 23-year-old woman is seen in the emergency department for rape. The woman is very calm and appears emotionally unaffected by the event. Which assessment of the client's behavior is appropriate?

1. The client probably isn't telling the truth but is trying to get the perpetrator in trouble.
2. The client was a willing partner.
3. The client's initially deceptive calm may be masking distress, denial, or emotional shock.
4. The client is pregnant and is trying to blame the pregnancy on a rape.

52. 3. One of the immediate consequences of rape is deceptive calmness. This behavior usually masks emotional shock, denial, or distress. The other responses are judgmental opinions. Nurses are to remain nonjudgmental in providing care.

NP: Assessment; CN: Psychosocial integrity; CNS: Psychosocial adaptation; CL: Analysis

53. A full-term neonate was just admitted to the transitional nursery. He has a large meningomyelocele covered by an intact sac. The nurse knows immediately to place this baby on his stomach with hips slightly elevated. Which statement describes the rationale for this position?

1. To prevent the sac covering the defect from rupturing
2. To preserve urine and bowel control
3. To assess neurological functioning more easily
4. To prevent further neurological damage

53. 1. The sac covering the defect is the only barrier preventing bacteria from directly entering the neonate's central nervous system and causing meningitis and encephalitis. A large defect will result in loss of urine and bowel control. The nurse can assess neurological functioning when the child is on his back or stomach. The damage to the neurological system happened in utero, and the nurse should prevent further damage by placing the infant on his stomach until after surgery; but preventing neurological damage isn't the priority.

NP: Implementation; CN: Physiological integrity; CNS: Reduction of risk potential; CL: Analysis

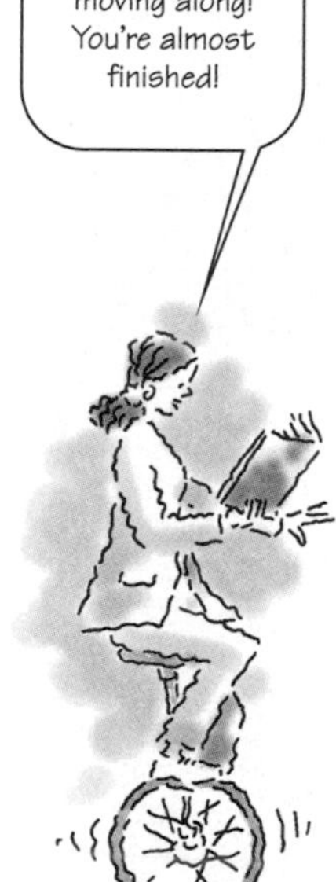
Keep moving along! You're almost finished!

54. The nurse is teaching the mother of a neonate with a cleft palate how to feed him. Which instruction should she give the mother?

1. Feed the neonate in a semi-reclining position with his head resting on the mother's curved elbow.
2. Feed the neonate in an upright position.
3. Feed the neonate lying on his stomach with his head turned toward his mother.
4. Feed the neonate in any position that the mother and child are comfortable.

54. 2. Feed the neonate with a cleft palate in an upright position. Incorrect feeding can allow formula to slip through the palate opening, enter the upper respiratory tract and lungs, and cause aspiration pneumonia. Any of the other positions is placing the neonate at risk for aspiration pneumonia.

NP: Implementation; CN: Physiological integrity; CNS: Reduction of risk potential; CL: Analysis

55. A nurse observes school-age children playing. Which activity is typical of this age-group?

1. Barbie dolls
2. Monopoly
3. Sony Play Station video games
4. Hot Wheels cars

55. 2. School-age children engage in competitive play with established rules and goals. Monopoly is an excellent example of play that pulls these elements together. Playing with Barbie dolls is an example of associative play, which preschoolers engage in. Solitary play of video games is seen in adolescents. Playing with Hot Wheels cars is more indicative of toddlers' parallel play.

NP: Assessment; CN: Health promotion and maintenance; CNS: Growth and development through the life span; CL: Application

56. A nurse is assessing an infant's growth and development. Which action by the nurse indicates the best understanding of a 4-month-old's stage of growth and development?

1. Eliciting a social smile
2. Allowing the infant to hold his own bottle
3. Playing peek-a-boo with the infant
4. Letting the infant sit without support

56. 1. A social smile should be seen in a 4-month-old. An infant can't hold his own bottle until age 6 to 7 months, and he'll engage in peek-a-boo activity at age 10 to 12 months. He can sit without support at about 8 months of age.

NP: Planning; CN: Health promotion and maintenance; CNS: Growth and development through the life span; CL: Application

57. Serial ultrasonography can help a physician follow the progress of a pregnancy. Which process isn't generally followed by ultrasound examinations?

1. Fetal growth
2. Amniotic fluid volume
3. Placental location
4. Umbilical cord length

57. 4. Umbilical cord length isn't followed by ultrasound examinations. Fetal growth and amniotic fluid volume can be followed with sequential ultrasonography to evaluate progressive changes. Placental location can also be followed, especially when placenta previa is present.

NP: Assessment; CN: Physiological integrity; CNS: Physiological adaptation; CL: Knowledge

58. At the pelvic inlet, the fetus must present the narrowest diameter of the fetal skull. Which diameter is the narrowest?

1. Occipitomental diameter
2. Occipitofrontal diameter
3. Anteroposterior diameter
4. Biparietal diameter

58. 4. The biparietal diameter is the narrowest portion of the fetal skull. The occipitomental diameter is usually the widest. The occipitofrontal diameter is usually 12 cm and not the narrowest diameter. The anteroposterior diameter is wider than the biparietal diameter.

NP: Assessment; CN: Physiological integrity; CNS: Physiological adaptation; CL: Knowledge

59. A client is in active labor. Which observation indicates fetal distress?

1. Fetal heart rate of 144 beats/minute
2. Accelerations of the fetal heart rate with contractions
3. Fetal scalp pH of 7.14
4. Presence of long-term variability

59. 3. A scalp pH below 7.25 indicates acidosis and fetal hypoxia. A fetal heart rate of 144 beats/minute, acceleration of the fetal heartbeat with contractions, and the presence of long-term variability with contractions are normal responses of a healthy fetus to labor.

NP: Assessment; CN: Health promotion and maintenance; CNS: Prevention and early detection of disease; CL: Knowledge

60. During a routine examination, the mother of a 3-month-old child asks the nurse, "How soon will she have her first tooth?" The first tooth usually erupts at which age?

1. 4 months
2. 5 months
3. 6 months
4. 7 months

60. 3. The first tooth typically erupts at age 6 months, though some infants do get their first tooth when a little younger or older.

NP: Assessment; CN: Health promotion and maintenance; CNS: Growth and development through the life span; CL: Knowledge

61. A nurse assesses an 18-month-old toddler and determines that the child is exhibiting normal growth and development patterns. Which activity does the nurse observe?

1. Running and jumping in place
2. Jumping down from a chair
3. Naming a specific color
4. Saying his full name

61. 1. An 18-month-old child should be able to run and jump in place. Typically, a child of 30 months is able to jump down from a chair, can name one color, and knows his full name.

NP: Assessment; CN: Health promotion and maintenance; CNS: Growth and development through the life span; CL: Knowledge

62. A mother was diagnosed with polyhydramnios during her pregnancy and just delivered a preterm male neonate. In which manner should the nurse assess a neonate for tracheoesophageal fistula?

1. Observing the neonate during the first formula feeding
2. Determining if cyanosis is present at birth
3. Inserting a catheter through the esophagus to the stomach
4. Assessing lung sounds to determine if possible pneumonia is present

62. 3. Tracheoesophageal fistula is present if a catheter can't be passed through the neonate's esophagus to the stomach. A barium swallow or a bronchial endoscopy examination will reveal the blind-end esophagus. The condition should be diagnosed before the infant is fed; otherwise, the infant will cough and may become cyanotic during feeding. Immediately after birth, pneumonia shouldn't be present with a tracheoesophageal fistula. Emergency surgery is essential to prevent pneumonia caused by the stomach's contents leaking into the lungs.

NP: Assessment; CN: Health promotion and maintenance; CNS: Prevention and early detection of disease; CL: Analysis

63. Which statement about hypertrophic cardiomyopathy is correct?

1. It's characterized by decreased contractility and ventricular dilation.
2. A family history is rarely positive for the disease.
3. Beta-adrenergic blockers are the treatment of choice.
4. Physical activity isn't restricted.

63. 3. Beta-adrenergic blockers (propranolol and atenolol) are the treatment of choice because they reduce the degree of outflow tract obstruction and have antiarrhythmic effects. Hypertrophic cardiomyopathy is characterized by enhanced contractility and impaired ventricular filling; dilated cardiomyopathy is characterized by decreased contractility and ventricular dilatation. There's a strong family history for the disease in 30% to 60% of clients. Moderate exercise limitations are placed on clients with hypertrophic cardiomyopathy.

NP: Assessment; CN: Physiological integrity; CNS: Physiological adaptation; CL: Knowledge

64. Which cause of myocarditis is the most common?

1. Bacteria
2. Parasite
3. Fungus
4. Virus

64. 4. Myocarditis (inflammation of the myocardium) is usually caused by a virus. Of all the viruses, coxsackieviruses and echoviruses are the most common agents. Bacteria, parasites, and fungi may cause myocarditis, but they aren't the most common causes.

NP: Evaluation: CN: Physiological integrity; CNS: Physiological adaptation; CL: Analysis

65. Measures to prevent hemorrhagic cystitis in a school-age child receiving the antineoplastic drug cyclophosphamide (Cytoxan) include administering the detoxifying agent mesna (Mesnex) and taking which action?

1 Transfusing platelets before administering the drug
2. Giving the child cranberry juice to drink
3. Encouraging the child to void frequently
4. Limiting the child's fluid intake

65. 3. Hemorrhagic cystitis can result when the by-products of Cytoxan metabolism remain in the bladder; therefore, emptying the bladder at least every 2 hours when the child is awake can help prevent this painful condition. The child should be encouraged to void as soon as the urge is felt. Bacteria or low platelets don't cause the condition, so transfusing platelets and giving cranberry juice aren't correct. Limiting fluid is contraindicated. Instead, the child will be given fluids liberally, usually by I.V. infusion, and encouraged to drink; a high intake of fluids will increase elimination of the drug's toxic by-products.

NP: Implementation; CN: Physiological integrity; CNS: Pharmacological and parenteral therapies; CL: Application

66. When protective isolation isn't indicated, which activity is recommended for the child receiving chemotherapy?

1. Bed rest
2. Activity as tolerated
3. Walk to bathroom only
4. Out of bed for brief periods

66. 2. Children should be able to engage in activities of interest and maintain as much independence and autonomy as possible; they'll limit their activity when they feel tired or ill. Limiting their activities to bed rest, walking to bathroom only, or only out of bed for brief periods isn't necessary and restricts activity unnecessarily. Whenever possible, include children in planning their care. These children should avoid adults and other children with infections.

NP: Implementation; CN: Health promotion and maintenance; CNS: Growth and development through the life span; CL: Application

67. A child is intubated and placed on a ventilator after a near drowning. The physician's order is to suction every 3 to 4 hours. Which phrase describes the purpose of suctioning?

1. To keep the client free of infection
2. To keep the client from experiencing cardiac arrhythmias
3. To keep the client's airway patent
4. To maintain fluid and electrolyte balance

67. 3. Because of the increased secretions from drowning, the airway is more prone to obstruction, and suctioning is essential for maintaining patency. Suctioning won't prevent infection and may even cause it. Suctioning can cause bradycardia; therefore, preoxygenation is essential to prevent arrhythmias. Suctioning doesn't affect fluid and electrolyte balance.

NP: Implementation; CN: Physiological integrity; CNS: Reduction of risk potential; CL: Comprehension

68. A child with cystic fibrosis has a bronchodilator, steroids ordered by metered-dose inhaler, and chest physiotherapy. In which order should these medications and treatments be administered?

1. Perform chest physiotherapy first.
2. Administer the bronchodilator first.
3. Administer the steroid first.
4. Let the client eat lunch first and then perform chest physiotherapy.

68. 2. Administer the bronchodilator to dilate the bronchi. The steroid can then reach further down the respiratory tract. After each medication is given, perform chest physiotherapy to expectorate secretions in the lower airways. Administer the medications and chest physiotherapy before meals to prevent aspiration.

NP: Implementation; CN: Physiological integrity; CNS: Pharmacological and parental therapies; CL: Application

69. The nurse is teaching nutrition to neurologic nurses. Which condition is a ketogenic diet sometimes used to treat?

1. Anorexia nervosa
2. Nephrotic syndrome
3. Epilepsy
4. Ulcerative colitis

69. 3. A ketogenic diet is typically suggested as a method of treatment for epilepsy. Anorexia nervosa is treated with counseling and slowly reintroducing food. Children with nephrotic syndrome are usually on a low-sodium diet. Ulcerative colitis is treated with a low-residue diet.

NP: Implementation; CN: Physiological integrity; CNS: Reduction of risk potential; CL: Application

70. A child is unable to walk without assistance because of decreased oxygen at birth. Which disorder is characterized by a malfunction of the brain's motor center from hypoxia?

1. Down syndrome
2. Cerebral palsy
3. Sickle cell anemia
4. Osteogenesis imperfecta

70. 2. Cerebral palsy affects the motor center of the brain and is usually caused by brain trauma. Down syndrome is a chromosomal abnormality. Sickle cell anemia is a genetic disorder of red blood cells. Osteogenesis imperfecta is a congenital anomaly involving decreased calcium in the bones and leads to multiple fractures at birth.

NP: Assessment; CN: Physiological integrity; CNS: Physiological adaptation; CL: Application

71. A 17-year-old client who injured her right knee during a basketball game is scheduled for an arthroscopy. This procedure involves which step?

1. An X-ray using a contrast media
2. Visualization of the joint with a small instrument
3. Inserting a needle and withdrawing fluid for biopsy
4. Aspirating synovial fluid from the bursa

71. 2. After a small incision is made in the knee, a small tube-shaped instrument is inserted for viewing the knee and surrounding cartilage, tendon, and ligaments. Contrast media is typically used for X-rays of joints. Biopsies are taken if cancer is a concern. Synovial fluid is collected for culture if an infection or inflammation is a concern.

NP: Planning; CN: Physiological integrity; CNS: Physiological adaptation; CL: Comprehension

72. The nurse is assessing a 13-year-old child 12 hours after surgery for a compound-fracture repair of the right arm. Which finding requires immediate attention?

1. Bruising of the fingers
2. Capillary refill of 3 seconds
3. Pallor of the nail beds
4. Edema of the extremity

72. 3. Pallor suggests a decrease in circulation to the extremity, and the surgeon should be notified. Bruising can be expected with a compound fracture. The fingers should be observed for further discoloration indicating decreased circulation. Capillary refill of 3 seconds is normal. Edema is expected but should be watched; increased edema might impair circulation.

NP: Assessment; CNS: Physiological integrity; CNS: Reduction of risk potential; CL: Application

73. A 3-year-old child has diarrhea, and the pediatrician has recommended a BRAT diet for the next 24 hours. BRAT stands for which foods?

1. Bran, rice crispies, apple juice, and tomato juice
2. Beans, red meat, apples, and tomatoes
3. Bananas, rice, applesauce, and toast
4. Broccoli, red ice pops, apple butter, and tacos

73. 3. BRAT stands for bananas, rice, applesauce, and toast. This diet is commonly used for children with diarrhea because these foods add some form to the stool without further irritating the bowel. The other diet choices can cause gas, irritation, and inflammation in the already inflamed bowel.

NP: Implementation; CN: Physiological integrity; CNS: Basic care and comfort; CL: Knowledge

74. A mother brings her 4-month-old son into the emergency department (ED) because he's been crying for several hours as if in pain. The nurse notes that he's crying uncontrollably and his knees are pulled to his chest. She learns from the mother that the child has been vomiting almost all feedings and he had a strange-looking stool just before coming to the ED. The nurse suspects intussusception and asks the mother to describe the stool. Which description does the nurse expect?

1. Pale colored, almost white
2. Very frothy, foul smelling
3. Bright green, loose
4. Dark red with little seeds similar to currants

74. 4. Intussusception is a telescoping of one part of the bowel into the other and it causes bloody stools that look like currant jelly. Pale-colored stools indicate a liver problem. A frothy, foul-smelling stool indicates a problem with lipid metabolism. Bright green, loose stools suggest a viral or bacterial infection.

NP: Assessment; CN: Physiological integrity; CNS: Physiological adaptation; CL: Analysis

75. A mother asks why her child has congenital hypothyroidism. Which explanation is best?

1. It's the result of poor prenatal care.
2. It's the result of failure of embryonic development of the thyroid.
3. It's the result of tobacco use during pregnancy.
4. It's genetic in origin and all children born to you will have congenital hypothyroidism.

75. 2. Congenital hypothyroidism is commonly idiopathic. Prenatal care, tobacco use, and dominant genetic traits haven't been linked to this disorder.

NP: Implementation; CN: Psychosocial integrity; CNS: Coping and adaptation; CL: Knowledge

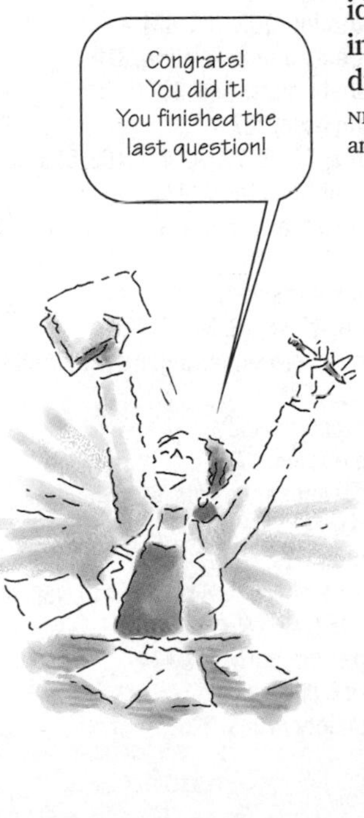

Index

B

C

D

E

F

I